EMBALMING

HISTORY, THEORY, AND PRACTICE

EMBALMING

HISTORY, THEORY, AND PRACTICE

Fifth Edition

Robert G. Mayer, CFSP, FBIE

Licensed Embalmer and Funeral Director
Pittsburgh, Pennsylvania

Adjunct Professor
Pittsburgh Institute of Mortuary Science
Pittsburgh, Pennsylvania

With a Foreword by

John D. Reed, Sr., CFSP, CPC

Funeral Director – Embalmer
Dodd and Reed Funeral Home
Webster Springs, West Virginia

Past President – National Funeral Directors Association
Brookfield, Wisconsin

New York Chicago San Francisco Lisbon London Madrid Mexico City Milan
New Delhi San Juan Seoul Singapore Sydney Toronto

Embalming: History, Theory, and Practice, Fifth Edition

Copyright © 2012 by The McGraw-Hill Companies, Inc. All rights reserved. Printed in the United States of America. Except as permitted under the United States Copyright Act of 1976, no part of this publication may be reproduced or distributed in any form or by any means, or stored in a data base or retrieval system, without the prior written permission of the publisher.

Previous editions copyright © 2006, 2000 by The McGraw-Hill Companies, Inc., copyright © 1996, 1990 by Appleton & Lange.

2 3 4 5 6 7 8 9 0   QVR/LEH   16 15 14 13 12

ISBN 978-0-07-174139-2
MHID 0-07-174139-9

This book was set in Times Roman by Aptara, Inc.
The editors were Joe Morita and Regina Y. Brown.
The production supervisor was Catherine H. Saggese.
Project management was provided by Samir Roy, Aptara, Inc.
The cover designer was Anthony Landi.
Quad/Graphics was printer and binder.

This book is printed on acid-free paper.

Library of Congress Cataloging-in-Publication Data

Mayer, Robert G.
    Embalming: history, theory, and practice/Robert G. Mayer. – 5th ed.
       p. ; cm.
    Includes bibliographical references and index.
    ISBN 978-0-07-174139-2 (hardcover : alk. paper)
    ISBN 0-07-174139-9 (hardcover : alk. paper)
    I. Title.
    [DNLM: 1. Embalming. WA 844]
  614′.6—dc23
                                   2011053519

McGraw-Hill books are available at special quantity discounts to use as premiums and sales promotions, or for use in corporate trainning programs. To contact a representative please e-mail us at bulksales@mcgraw-hill.com.

This edition is dedicated to the staff and personnel of the
Air Force Mortuary Affairs Operations at the Charles C. Carson
Center for Mortuary Affairs, Dover Air Force Base Port Mortuary.
Their commitment continues to ensure dignity, honor,
and respect in the care and preparation of those fallen
in the service of their country, the United States of America.

And to those special persons who have educated, mentored,
challenged, and supported my career in funeral service:

Alfred H. Davis, Paul H. Velker and John T. Rebol,
William J. Neff, William J. Musmanno,
J. Sheridan and Dorothy D. Mayer,
Edward C. and Gail R. Johnson, Melissa Johnson,
Dr. Emory S. James, Lester Wakeham,
Robert J. Inman, Peter J. Ball, C. Richard Sanders,
David G. Hicks, William Zwicharowski,
William A. Smith, and David G. Williams

CONTENTS

David G. Hicks
Chair of Embalming Sciences
Cincinnati College of Mortuary Science
Cincinnati, Ohio

Patty S. Hutcheson
President
American Board of Funeral Service Education
President
Gupton-Jones College of Funeral Service
Decatur, Georgia

Melissa Johnson
Funeral Director/Embalmer
Executive Director
American Society of Embalmers
Forest Park, Illinois

Eugene C. Ogrodnik
President and CEO
Pittsburgh Institute of Mortuary Science
Pittsburgh, Pennsylvania

Alta Williams
Curriculum Chair
American Board of Funeral Service Education
Associate Professor
City Colleges of Chicago
Malcolm X and Richard J. Daley Campuses
Chicago, Illinois

CONTRIBUTORS

These persons have made contributions to the development of this textbook throughout its four editions 1990–2006. They are listed with their titles at the time of their initial contribution to the text.

John Alsobrookd, MS
Associate Professor, Funeral Service
  Program
Vincennes University Junior College
Vincennes, Indiana

R. Stanley Barnes
Funeral Director
Canton, Ohio

Daniel Buchanan, MA
President
Gupton-Jones College of Funeral Service
Decatur, Georgia

Jeff Chancellor
The Dodge Company
Fresno, California

Paul Cimiluca, BS, MA
Adjunct Professor of Chemistry
Cincinnati College of Mortuary Science
Cincinnati, Ohio

William Counce, PhD
Funeral Service Education Department
Jefferson State College
Birmingham, Alabama

Emmet Crahan
Dodge Chemical Company
Jay, New York

Kenneth Curl, PhD
Chairman
Funeral Service Education Department
University of Central Oklahoma
Edmond, Oklahoma

James M. Dorn, MS
Chairman, Embalming Sciences
Cincinnati College of Mortuary Science
Cincinnati, Ohio

Donald E. Douthit, MS
Supervisor of Clinical Services
Cincinnati College of Mortuary Science
Cincinnati, Ohio

Dan Flory, PhD
President
Cincinnati College of Mortuary Science
Cincinnati, Ohio

Vernie R. Fountain
Founder/Instructor
Fountain National Academy of Professional
  Embalming Skills
Springfield, Missouri

Jerome F. Fredrick, PhD
Director of Chemical Research
Dodge Chemical Company
Bronx, New York

Arthur Grabowski
Mortuary Science Department
State University of New York College of
  Technology
Canton, New York

Marvin E. Grant, Med
Mortuary Science Department
East Mississippi Community College
Scooba, Mississippi

David G. Hicks, MSEd
Chair of Embalming Sciences
Cincinnati College of Mortuary Science
Cincinnati, Ohio

Barbara M. Hopkins, PhD
Associate Professor and Chair
Chemistry Department
Xavier University
Cincinnati, Ohio

Edward C. Johnson
Funeral Director—Instructor of Embalming,
  Restorative Art
Chicago, Illinois

Gail R. Johnson
Funeral Director—Instructor of
  Clinical Embalming
Chicago, Illinois

Melissa Johnson, CFSP
Funeral Director/Embalmer
Chicago, Illinois
Executive Director, Co-Founder
American Society of Embalmers
Forest Park, Illinois

Ralph Klicker, MSEd
Director
Thanos Institute
Buffalo, New York

John M. Kroshus, PhD
Assistant Professor and Director
Program of Mortuary Science
University of Minnesota
Minneapolis, Minnesota

Michael Kubasak
Funeral Director/Embalmer
Kubasak Associates
Mesquite, Nevada

Michael Landon
Chairman
Department of Funeral
  Service Education
Fayetteville Technical Community
  College
Fayetteville, North Carolina

Daniel Lawlor
Funeral Director/Embalmer
Providence, Rhode Island

Terry McEnany, MA
Dean Simmons Institute
Syracuse, New York

Michael C. Mathews, MA
Assistant Professor
Program of Mortuary Science
University of Minnesota
Minneapolis, Minnesota

Robert G. Mayer, CFSP, FBIE
Embalmer and Funeral Director
Pittsburgh, Pennsylvania
Faculty
Pittsburgh Institute of Mortuary Science
Pittsburgh, Pennsylvania

Nathan Minnich
Funeral Director/Embalmer
Elizabeth, Pennsylvania

Louis Misantone
President,
  Funeral Institute of the North East
Westwood, Massachusetts

Stuart E. Moen, MA
Dean
Commonwealth Institute of Funeral Service
Houston, Texas

Frank P. Nagy, PhD
Associate Professor
Department of Anatomy
Wright State University Medical School
Dayton, Ohio

Shun Newbern
Funeral Director/Embalmer
Rose Hills Memorial Park
Whittier, California

Robert W. Ninker
Executive Director
Illinois Funeral Directors Association
Springfield, Illinois

John B. Pludeman
Instructor
Milwaukee Area Technical College
Milwaukee, Wisconsin

George H. Poston, PhD
President
Commonwealth Institute of Funeral Service
Houston, Texas

Leandro Rendon, MS
Director of Research and Educational Programs
The Champion Company
Williamsburg, Virginia

N. Thomas Rogness, MA
Instructor
Institute of Funeral Service
Houston, Texas

Gordon Rose, PhD
Former Professor and Chairman
Mortuary Science Department
Wayne State University
Detroit, Michigan

Curtis D. Rostad
Funeral Director/Embalmer
Executive Director
Wyoming Funeral Directors Association
Highlands Ranch, Colorado

Shelly J. Roy
Funeral Director
York, Alabama

C. Richard Sanders
The Dodge Company
Largo, Florida

Donald W. Sawyer
Director of Embalming Education
Dodge Chemical Company
Castro Valley, California

Dale E. Stroud
Former Associate Professor
Mortuary Science Department
University of Minnesota
Minneapolis, Minnesota

Brenda L. Tersine, MA
Former Instructor
Mortuary Science Department
Hudson Valley Community College
Troy, New York

John R. Trout
Funeral Service Education Department
Northampton Area Community College
Bethlehem, Pennsylvania

Todd W. VanBeck, MA
Director
New England Institute of Funeral Service Education
Mount Ida College
Newton Centre, Massachusetts

Michael Weakland
Funeral Director
Winter Funeral Home, P.C.
Pittsburgh, Pennsylvania

Karl Wenzel
McEachnie Funeral Home
Ajax, Ontario

Larry Whitaker
The Dodge Company
Beaverton, Oregon

Kenneth R. Whittaker
Dean of Students
Dallas Institute of Funeral Service
Dallas, Texas

This text written initially and edited for four subsequent printings by its primary author, Robert G. Mayer, former instructor at Pittsburgh Institute of Mortuary Science, has proven to be the most comprehensive text, relevant and up to date on the subject of embalming deceased human beings. Following the curriculum guidelines of the American Board of Funeral Service Education, versions of this text are being used in all mortuary schools in America as well as Canada, Japan, Australia, Great Britain, Korea, Ireland, South America and many other international countries supports that.

The thirst for embalming knowledge and skill is overwhelming in international markets. Educators, Tutors and Practitioners in those international markets have demonstrated a profound desire to advance their knowledge and technical skills to the level of American Funeral Directors and Embalmers. The universal use of this text will enhance the technical skills in those markets allowing it to become a reference manual for the Professional Embalmer and the lay reader.

Embalming, as one would expect, is not a subject discussed outside of funeral service circles, However, I personally feel that Embalming should not be taken lightly by the Professional Embalmer. We as practicing Embalmers do Embalm bodies daily. A family experiences a death occasionally and when a family chooses embalming with viewing it should be performed to the best of our ability and *should lessen the ravages of illness and trauma*. The memory picture left with that family following a funeral service will be in their minds forever.

It may influence whether a service with embalming and viewing would be selected in the event of another death in the family.

Being both humbled and honored to serve as a volunteer embalmer at the Port Mortuary, Dover Air Force Base, Dover DE for a week in July 2008. I spent several hours at the bulletin board reading letters and cards from families of fallen soldiers expressing their gratitude and heartfelt appreciation to the staff under the direction of William Zwicharowski and Matt Genereaux. It was the most heart wrenching time I have ever spent. Throughout that week, more so then ever before, it became crystal clear to me how vitally important it is for families to be able to view their loved ones body. Men and women who studied from and were inspired by this text or others rendered excellent Professional Technical Skills for those families.

Throughout time many Funeral Service Practitioners have given expressions that have been seamlessly integrated into our profession like the Gladstone statement and others. One I particularly like is "You must express grief at the death of a loved one, and then you must go on. The eyes of the deceased must be gently closed and the eyes of the living must be gently opened" (Jan Brugler 1973). That sense of academic awareness present in this text will continue to inspire Funeral Professionals for expressions and the excellent performance of our Technical Skills for years to come.

John D. Reed, Sr. CFSP-CPC
NFDA President 2008/2009

This book covers embalming as no other book ever has. It is useful as a teaching text and, in that regard, follows the American Board of Funeral Service education curriculum guide on this subject. It is also useful as a historical or technical reference for the funeral service practitioner or the lay reader.

Gordon S. Bigelow, PhD
Executive Director
American Board of Funeral Service Education
March 1996

This book is a most impressive work. It covers the subject broadly, thoroughly, and with the highest degree of professionalism. It is outstanding in every respect.

Eugene C. Ogrodnik
President and CEO
Pittsburgh Institute of Mortuary Science
January 2011

You must express your grief at the death of a loved one, and then you must go on. The eyes of the dead must be gently closed and the eyes of the living must be gently opened.

Jan Brugler, 1973

Since its inception in 1987 this textbook project has allowed me the unique opportunity to integrate onto the printed page three segments of my professional life. First, since 1968 I have served funeral homes in the greater Pittsburgh area through my trade embalming service. Second, from 1967 to 1982 I was a full-time faculty member with the Pittsburgh Institute of Mortuary Science and remain there in an adjunct position. Third, for the past 40 years I have participated, both as a presenter and as an attendee, in continuing education programs throughout the United States, England, and Ireland. Thus, I have been able to combine theory with current ideas from many individuals along with my hands-on experiences in the preparation room. . . . It all makes for a very unique mixture.

Nothing is more certain than change. This fifth edition is updated with new techniques, and information relative to the history, theory, and practice of embalming, inclusive of the subjects of restorative art and mortuary cosmetology. Special attention has been given to the creation of a safe working environment – from the standpoint of ergonomics, personal hygiene and safe use of embalming chemicals. Expanded technical areas of the text will assist the embalmer in the preparation of tissue and organ donors and the preparation of the body for viewing without using standard embalming chemicals.

Ron Hast, editor of *Mortuary* Management, has stated, "Embalming is the best known method of presenting a deceased person well throughout the memorial event." It is incumbent on us not to overstate the purpose and results of embalming as longer terms of preservation. Artistic value coupled with preservation is primary. In time, nature consumes all who die back unto itself. Embalming was once considered a method for the prevention of the spread of virulent diseases amongst the general public. Better understanding of the causative agents, virulence and transmission of disease have demonstrated caution for those who have direct contact with the dead human body, however, only in rare instances and with warning from agencies such as the Centers for Disease Control would the presence of the unembalmed body be considered a health hazard to the general public.

Embalming is a choice. Those we are privileged to serve need to know the values of this process to make intelligent decisions. Consistent, masterful presentation

of each decedent entrusted to our care builds positive reputations.

Like many of our long held community traditions – because of cultural, social, political, religious and economic factors – the presence of the embalmed deceased is no longer the central focus of the twenty-first century funeral ceremony, as it had once been in America in the twentieth century. Hence the memorial service, with the absence of the body, has now become as familiar as the funeral service with the body present. Temporary means of preservation are now being requested using refrigeration and wet and dry ice to satisfy the wishes of environmental groups and those with interest in Green and Natural burial. Within funeral service itself, safer chemicals are gradually replacing chemicals long known to be toxic and may very well in time be proven to be carcinogenic to the practitioner.

Embalming: History, Theory, & Practice, is designed as a basic textbook for the mortuary science student and as a reference source for the practitioner. Incorporated throughout this work is the American Board of Funeral Service Education: *Embalming Basic Course Content Curriculum and Glossary (2008)* and portions of the *Restorative Art Basic Course Content Curriculum and Glossary (2006).* The three interdisciplinary mortuary arts and sciences of embalming, restorative art, and mortuary cosmetology are presented in this single volume. Restoration of the body as well as cosmetic treatments are interdependent with the embalming of the remains. In the words of the noted Chicago embalmer and educator Edward C. Johnson, "restorative art and mortuary cosmetology are simply a continuation of embalming . . . each is dependent upon good embalming – they are extensions of the process"

It has been stated that the **art** of embalming is the raising of a vessel for injection but the **science** of embalming is knowing which vessel to raise! It has been the foundation of this text from its inception that the dead human body needs to "tell" the practitioner what embalming protocols need to be employed for successful preparation of the remains. The embalming case analysis at the very beginning, during, and following the preparation is the important factor. The embalmer needs to learn to observe, analyze the observation, develop a plan of implementation, and finally observe the obtained results. In the preparation of each body it becomes the responsibility of the embalmer to determine the thoroughness, effectiveness, and quality of the work.

Some things have not changed! Simon Mendelsohn, writing in 1944 on *Embalming Fluids* for Ciba Pharmaceuticals, stated that embalming serves four purposes—it provides time for friends and family to gather with the body present and viewable for ceremonies; it permits the body to be shipped back to a hometown or home country for disposition and viewing if desired; it is a means of sanitizing the deceased; and it can improve the appearance of the deceased following trauma or the effects of disease. These reasons for embalming remain. The very definition of embalming established by the American Board of Funeral Service Education establishes the goals: temporary preservation, sanitation, and restoration of the deceased to an acceptable appearance.

Arterial embalming served the early anatomists – such as Dr. John Hunter (1728–1793). Preservation allowed Hunter and his students to dissect thousands of bodies. His discoveries included collateral circulation, lymphatic system and numerous successful surgical techniques. His embalming and preservative techniques still allow students of the 21st century to study Hunter's anatomical specimens – housed at the Hunterian Museum in the Royal College of Surgeons, London. An interesting aside is that formaldehyde would not be discovered for almost 75 years after Hunter's death! Embalming today still allows for anatomical study of the human body.

In America the infancy of arterial embalming was at the time of the Civil War. It allowed the fallen soldier to be transported in a preserved state to home for burial. Arterial embalming today allows the fallen military hero to be transported from a distant foreign field or waters to the hometown often with the possibility of the viewing of the remains. The work done at the Charles C. Carson Center for Mortuary Affairs located at Dover Air Force Base in Dover, Delaware, houses the largest and only Port Mortuary under the United States Department of Defense within the continental United States. There a team of experienced embalmers and mortuary personal perform what could very often be called the miraculous through the use of embalming. Presently William Zwicharowski, a former student of mine, holds the position of Branch Chief of Mortuary Operations.

The writer, poet, funeral director, and embalmer Thomas Lynch says in his book, *Bodies In Motion and At Rest*, ". . . 'But remembering him the way he was,' I say, slowly, deliberately as if the listener were breakable, 'begins by dealing with the way he *is*.' I'm an apostle of the present tense. After years and years of directing funerals, I've come to the conclusion that seeing is the hardest and most helpful part. The truth, even when it hurts, has a healing in it, better than fiction or fantasy. When someone dies, it is not them we fear seeing, it is them ***dead***. It is the death. We fear that seeing will be believing." The science and art that the embalmer employs affords friends and family the opportunity to gather and the opportunity to see the reality by one last comforting look on the face of a loved one at their ceremony of farewell. This confrontation with the deceased, for many, begins the process of closure that leads to healing.

Robert G. Mayer
Pittsburgh, Pennsylvania
December 2011

Embalming: History, Theory and Practice is a product of the American Board of Funeral Service Education–presently located in St. Joseph, Missouri. This organization is the accrediting agency for the colleges of mortuary science in the United States–currently there are 57 institutions. Working committees of the ABFSE develop and keep current the basic core curricula. ABFSE Executive Directors Dr. Gordon Bigelow, Dr. George Connick and Dr. Michael Smith have all overseen the development and production of this text. Dr. Gretchen L. Warner, present ABFSE Executive Director, has seen this edition through the final year of preparation and publication.

During the past 50 years a number of individuals have contributed and encouraged my professional career. The dedication of this book lists some of the most influential. During the preparation of this edition of *Embalming: History, Theory, and Practice* some of those who have encouraged me and in their own way made additions to these printed pages include: Peter J. Ball of High Bentham in the U.K., and David G. Hicks of the Cincinnati College of Mortuary Science and Eugene C. Ogrodnik of the Pittsburgh Institute of Mortuary Science. In particular I am grateful for the preparation skills of David G. Williams, Melissa Johnson, and William Smith, embalmers extraordinaire.

Several organizations have made generous contributions to this text through their continuing education programs–The Dodge Sunshine Seminars (over 50 years in existence); Ohio Embalmers Association (80 years of programming); British Institute of Embalmers and the American Society of Embalmers. Their speakers have kept the embalmer up-to-date on all aspects of embalming topics and developments. They have been most valuable to this author.

This project began with the present primary author/editor in 1987, after being approached by Glenn G. McMillen, a former mortuary school classmate (1962) and past president of the National Funeral Directors Association. The first edition was published in 1990 by Appleton & Lange. Seed moneys and underwriting for the first edition was made possible by The Heritage Club of the National Funeral Directors Association. The National Funeral Directors Association has continued to support this project during the past 22 years.

I am most proud of the Selected Readings portion of this text. In this edition There are 20 in depth articles on a number of subjects relative to embalming and restorative art. Four recent articles are printed in this text for the first time.

The third edition of this text, published in 2000 by McGraw-Hill, combined for the first time in any textbook the subjects of embalming, restorative art, and mortuary cosmetology. These three divisions of the mortuary preparation sciences and arts are also contained in this fifth edition. Contributions on the topic of restorative art has been enhanced by the work of Vernie Fountain and C. Richard Sanders. Fifty-one persons have contributed to this text, in whole or in part. New contributors include, Paul Cimiluca, David G. Hicks, Shun Newbern and Karl Wenzel.

Three readers from the American Board of Funeral Service Education have reviewed the changes made in this edition–Patty S. Hutchison, Alta Williams and Eugene C. Ogrodnik.

Original artwork by Jeffrey C. Pierce of Pittsburgh and Jude Waples of Oakville, Ontario remains in this edition. Transcription work complete by Brockton A. Shaffer, of Clearfield, Pennsylvania. Finally a special thanks must be given to David E. Mahlstedt of Pittsburgh, Pennsylvania for his computer and editing skills, without whose help this edition would not have been possible. Ralph Yearick of Yearick-Milea Co. in Pittsburgh provided the necessary technical computer support.

I am grateful for Edward Eckenrode, who has assumed a substantial amount of my business activities making it possible for me to devote time to the preparation of this edition.

A special thanks to Eugene C. Ogrodnik, a former student of mine, now President and CEO of my alma mater the Pittsburgh Institute of Mortuary Science. He willingly read every word of the manuscript, for this fifth edition, making numerous editorial and grammatical adjustments.

Finally, I wish to thank John Reed of Webster Springs, West Virginia for preparing the foreword for this edition. John was a 1971 graduate of the Pittsburgh Institute of Mortuary Science and has served funeral service at the local, state and national levels. He is a past president of the National Funeral Directors Association.

Robert G. Mayer
Pittsburgh, Pennsylvania
December 2011

PART

I

THE THEORY AND PRACTICE
OF EMBALMING

SECTION I

CHAPTER 1

EMBALMING: SOCIAL, PSYCHOLOGICAL, ETHICAL, AND REGULATORY STANDARDS

► EMBALMING

Embalming and funeral historian Edward C. Johnson has written that, "embalming is a means of artificially preserving the dead human body and it is one of humankind's longest practiced arts."*

The following two statements demonstrate the reverence and respect afforded to the dead human body by two civilized societies separated by 5,000 years. The art of embalming was and is practiced to some extent within both of these societies.

An exhibit at the National Archeological Museum in Athens, Greece describes the care of the dead by the society of Ancient Egypt, circa 3000 BCE.

"The ancient Egyptians did not regard death as the end of life, but as an intermediary stage towards a better eternal life. Eternity was achieved by those who had lived a virtuous life and were able to furnish their tombs and receive funerary offerings from their relatives. The poor attained immortality through the mercy of the gods. Released after death, the spiritual elements continued to exist **so long as the body remained in a recognizable state,** hence the development of mummification." Ancient Egyptians: 3000 BCE.

"All the world fears Time, but Time fears the Pyramids", so says an ancient Arab proverb. Resting within those ancient tombs of stone, the embalmed and mummified dead, just as old as the pyramids themselves, await eternal life. The purpose of embalming, as practiced by those ancient Egyptians, was religious.

Dr. Thomas G. Long in 2009 writes, "Rituals of death rest on the basic need, recognized by all societies, to remove the bodies of the dead from among the living. A corpse must be taken fairly quickly from here, the place of death, to somewhere else. But no healthy society has ever treated this as a perfunctory task, a matter of mere disposal. Indeed, from the beginning, humans have used poetry, song, and prayer to describe the journey of the dead from "here" to "there" in symbolic, even sacred, terms. The dead are not simply being carted to the pit, the fire, or the river; they are traveling toward the next world or the Mystery or the Great Beyond or heaven or the communion of the saints.

And we are accompanying them the last mile of the way. Every generation re-imagines these images of what lies beyond this life, but what persists is the conviction that the dead are not refused to be discarded; they are human treasures traveling somewhere and it is our holy responsibility to go with them all the way to the place of farewell."[†]

Embalming is a chemical method of bringing about a temporary preservation of the dead. It has been and is employed by various cultures and for various reasons throughout the world. In America during the second

---

*See, **The Origin and History of Embalming,** Section II, Embalming: History, Theory, and Practice.

[†]Thomas G Long, "Chronicle of a Death We Can't Accept," **New York Times,** 31 Oct. 2009.

half of the nineteenth century and most of the twentieth century, embalming and viewing of the body was a vital part of the American funeral. Since the latter-half of the twentieth century, there has been a gradual movement toward more simplified disposition of the dead often minimizing viewing of the deceased and if viewed, doing so with or without standard embalming practices.

Embalming, as practiced today, is defined by the American Board of Funeral Service Education as: "the chemical treatment of the dead human body to **reduce** the presence and growth of microorganisms, to **temporarily** inhibit organic decomposition, and to restore the dead human body to an **acceptable** physical appearance."*

Embalming suspends in time, the deceased human body, in a temporary state of preservation. This process makes the following possible:

- temporary preservation and sanitation of the deceased body
- renders the body inoffensive by slowing postmortem changes
- seeing the body allows the family and friends to accept the finality of death,
- allows time to organize ceremony and ritual with the body present
- time for friends and relatives to gather for funeral ceremonies and if desired view the deceased remains
- moving the deceased to a distant location for final disposition and if desired, viewing
- restores a favorable body image by removing the adverse effects of disease, trauma, or postmortem changes
- preservation for anatomical study and research by medical institutions
- a slow breakdown of the body over time; desiccation rather than putrefaction

The Author and Editor Ron Hast has stated, "Embalming is the best known method of presenting the decedent well through the memorial event."†‡

We now turn to an examination of the psychosocial, religious, and philosophical reasons a culture continues with the practice of embalming its dead, the role this scientific and artistic treatment of the dead plays in the final ceremonial rites of disposition, and the impact it can have on the adjustment and well-being of the survivors.

---

*American Board of Funeral Service Education, **Embalming Syllabus:** Approved, March 2008.

†American Board of Funeral Service Education, **Embalming Syllabus:** Approved March 2008.

‡Ron Hast, "The Art of Embalming and its Purpose, **Mortuary Management,** September 2006, 6–9.

▶ SOCIAL AND PSYCHOLOGICAL PERFORMANCE STANDARDS— REVERENCE FOR THE DEAD

Here, we describe the ethical, psychosocial, and practical values of embalming to help provide its practitioners the opportunity to define and articulate to the community the great social value of their work, and why it has been and continues to be an important mainstay of the funeral service profession. This material helps the reader to develop a clear, balanced understanding of the social advantages of embalming and basic care for the dead, and the importance of having the body embalmed and present at death rituals.

Reverence for the dead is the basic ethical axiom of the funeral service profession. Preparation of the deceased human remains is humankind's means of ethically fulfilling our ingrained, ancient, emotive instinct to care for the dead. As funeral service practitioners, we are charged with the maintenance of this moral and ethical responsibility, and it is important that students and practitioners actively embrace this concept.

Ethical Model

Every profession has a primary and supreme ethic of paramount importance in the disposition of its duties. Medicine, for example, bases its professional practice on the Hippocratic oath, which articulates the ethic of healing. Law bases its practice on the ethic of justice. The supreme ethic for the funeral service profession has come to be known as reverence for the dead. The ethical question "What should be done with the dead?" can be controversial. Some people believe the dead should be buried; others believe that the dead should be cremated. Still others endorse donating the dead to medical schools, and some people avoid the question altogether.

Human Nature

In Western culture, there is an attitude of denial and defiance toward death and dying. The American culture, in particular, places tremendous value on things that are new, shiny, and healthy while devaluing things that are old, dull, and dead. Consequently, the value of a human corpse is often morally downgraded, because the dead human body symbolizes that which is abhorrent to our materialistically shallow culture—death—precisely what the culture is trying to avoid.

In addition, the dead human body represents a psychological and ethical paradox for people, stemming from the fact that the living are simultaneously attracted, yet sometimes repulsed, when viewing the dead. The dead represents defeat and despair, and because human beings do not deal well with defeat and despair, we have devised an elaborate system of barriers to help us cope with the situation.

Reverence for the dead, however, is deeply ingrained in human nature, no matter how much we profess our ignorance, apathy, or even disgust. What we call the ethical or reverential care of the dead has been discovered to exist as far back in our ancestry as Neanderthal humans. Anthropological study shows that the burial of the human body is the oldest of all religious customs, and was practiced as far back as about 60,000 BC by **Homo sapiens neanderthalensis.** In Shandiar Cave in northern Iraq, researchers discovered corpses adorned with elk antlers and shoulder blades. Also found were pollen fragments from flowers that were probably used as gifts to the dead and to mask unpleasant odors during the burial ritual. Neanderthals exhibited the primal behaviors characteristic of our natural and instinctual drive to treat the dead with great reverence. That genetic and instinctive legacy continues today, tempered by our modern culture and intellect.

Consequences of the Act

When one examines the reasons behind the decline of the governmental and sociological order, historically, the neglect of reverence for the dead and its consequences is clearly a major contributing factor. History shows us that the ultimate destruction of many civilizations was heralded by a rise in the community's apathy about the care of their dead. Ancient Rome, Greece, and Nazi Germany are examples that fit this pattern. In examining the downfall of each of these powerful regimes, the lack of proper care for the dead was commonplace. Time and again, the annals of history show that the rites, rituals, and ceremonies mourning the dead serve as excellent barometers of the accomplishments of past cultures.

The ethical, moral, and sociological consequences of neglecting the importance of proper care for the dead was summed up concisely by the eminent British Prime Minister, William Evart Gladstone (1809–1898) when he wrote:

> "Show me the manner in which a nation or community cares for its dead and I will measure with mathematical exactness the tender sympathies of its people, their respect for the laws of the land, and their loyalty to high ideals."

Because this quote embodies a great ethical truth with power and eloquence, it has been cited many times by funeral service practitioners, and no matter how often these words are uttered, their impact on our profession, our society, and humanity as a whole never wanes.

▶ UNIVERSAL CONVICTIONS

All of the world's cultures attend to the proper care of the dead and each has developed its own rituals to implement this care. Anthropological, archaeological, and religious literatures all describe the importance to a culture of its chosen forms of funeralization ceremonies, and the significance of the presence of the dead body in helping the community overcome the overwhelming experience of the death of one of its members.

Every civilization ever studied has been found to maintain sacred locations where the bodies and the relics of the dead were placed, including cemeteries, mausoleums, and columbaria. All cultures commemorate their dead through the creation of art, music, and literature, including monuments and memorials, requiem masses and funeral hymns, and biographies and elegies. In fact, human customs and rituals concerning basic care for and commemoration of the dead are so diverse and widespread that no one publication could possibly document all of them in complete detail.

This universal ethic of reverence for the dead is ingrained in the human psyche, and though the ways different cultures manifest this reverence may vary widely, it is a basic thread binding together all of humanity.

Morality

The issue of morality in reference to reverential care of the dead is embodied in the conflict between logic and emotion. The logical mind might well dismiss the corpse as nothing more than a mass of dead tissue, but our emotional selves will not allow such easy dismissal of something so inherent to our humanity, and this leads to an internal conflict between our logical and our emotional selves. When we feel this clash of logic and emotion, we should realize that our deepest emotions are crying out for recognition. In other words, this conflict should serve to shock us into listening to our deepest emotions, as the Neanderthal did, to avoid falling into the trap of rationalization and denial.

An illustration of the power of the emotions associated with death was seen in 1963, a year of supreme importance for the funeral service profession. Jessica Mitford published **The American Way of Death,** a savage and relentless attack on the profession, causing a counterattack on Mitford herself by America's funeral directors. Then came November 22, 1963, and the shocking assassination and subsequent funeral of President John F. Kennedy, an act that rocked our entire nation's moral and emotional foundations. The public did not feel comfortable criticizing funeral directors, symbols of death and funerals, when the nation was in the throes of mourning a slain president. To describe President Kennedy's body merely as "dead tissue" and to dispose of it without ceremony would have been morally irresponsible and blasphemous. This same need for public mourning and ritual is still evident following the deaths of other celebrities. These moral feelings representing our instinct to reverently care for the dead also emerge at other times. For example, if a body is missing due to war or a tragic accident, the community can be distraught beyond description. Thousands of taxpayers' dollars are spent on search and recovery efforts, and there is anxiety and remorse if these efforts fail. If we view this from a strictly logical viewpoint, and reduce the issue to one of the costs of such an effort, accepting the notion that the dead body has no value, then these magnanimous recovery efforts make little sense, and may be viewed as a waste of taxpayers' dollars. Without a body, an essential element to the grieving process is missing; an important piece of the bereavement puzzle is missing.

The Neanderthals made memorials with elk antlers and shoulder blades; today we use granite or marble. The ethic is the same; only the materials are different. We have an innate ethical drive to care for the dead; it is simply part of our humanity.

Religion

Religious convictions are important to consider in this discussion, because for centuries the funeral has been an essentially religious ritual, is certainly so within the Judeo-Christian tradition, and is so within all of the world's religions. Specific reference to embalming is made twice in the Old Testament. Genesis 50:2–3 recounts the death of Jacob, who was also known as Israel: "And Joseph commanded his servants the physicians to embalm his father. So the physicians embalmed Israel." Genesis 50:26 also refers to embalming in connection with Joseph's death: "So Joseph died, being one hundred and ten years old and they embalmed him, and he was put in a coffin in Egypt." Of course, we should not confuse the embalming described in the Old Testament with the modern procedure, but the intent to care reverently for the dead is the same, regardless of current technology.

In addition, the New Testament contains references that reflect the Judeo-Christian tradition to care reverently for the dead. John 11:44 describes burial preparations for Lazarus similar to those in use today, including the use of grave straps to bind the arms, feet, and chin, allowing the body to be manipulated into a normal appearance. The description of Jesus' funerary preparations mirror those used today in some cultures: his body was bound and dressed in fine white linens, and anointed with spices, fragrant oils, and myrrh.

So, we see the tradition of treating the dead with great reverence and respect is an age-old custom, as old as humanity itself. Funeral service professionals must always be cognizant of and maintain this high level of dignity and veneration of the dead in all our practices. To put this basic tenet of funeral service succinctly: Reverence for the dead is expressed through the consistent application and practice of showing respect and honor for, as well as maintaining the dignity of, the dead.

Psychosocial Model

Human beings are basically social creatures. We talk, live, work, and play with other people. Our social interactions take on many different dimensions. We can have shallow or very deep interactions; we can act with indifference or with profound sympathy. In the course of a single day, we may exhibit these and a thousand other characteristics. It is through this complex web of daily interactions that we experience life and create attachments to others. The quality of these attachments varies from one relationship to another; some are deep, some shallow, others indifferent, joyful, or painful. Here, we shall explore the role "embalming" plays in the process of helping us separate from these attached relationships.

Within the realm of attachments between people are the so-called "deep links." Here, our attachments are strong and profoundly interwoven psychological bonds that are extremely powerful. In these circumstances, our needs for security and devotion are satisfied, and virtually every part of the human psyche is involved. Through daily visual and interactive reinforcement of these deep attachments, our relationships with significant persons undergo a kind of layering process in our brains. The thoughts and feelings create perceptual patterns of recognition. These patterns of recognition that develop between people become so familiar that there are instances in which the individual involved is frequently unaware of the depth of these attachments until the relationship is terminated through separation by death or physical or emotional distance.

The how and why of attachments are baffling. Attachments are among our most rudimentary attributes, they flourish throughout our lives, and they can be so powerful as to continue even beyond the grave. The magnitude of these attachments is often unrealized by the person, and individuals are often unaware of how deeply their behaviors and attitudes are affected. Attachments arise from countless life experiences; from suckling at the mother's breast, to seeing someone every day, to sleeping with them every night. They are created by the sound of a voice, the color of someone's eyes, the texture of someone's hair, and in their style and manner of dress and movement. It is fortunate indeed that humans have the capacity to develop these attachments, because they often culminate in deeply cherished, singular relationships with others; feelings of **love**. It is from this type of deep relationship that we experience the joy of love, but it is equally true that from these same deep attachments, we also experience the inevitable anguish of separation and loss. As painful as it is at times, a fact of human existence is that attachments cannot exist without grief.

It is through continual life experiences shared with significant others that our attachments become rooted. As the theories of attachment demonstrate, our ability to connect with our fellow humans goes very deep. Through this process, familiarity with the characteristics of the significant other is **imprinted** in our minds. This imprinting is caused by constant exposure to the attached person, and a mental photograph develops in our hearts and minds. In funeral service, this mental photograph is referred to as the **body image**.

The body image that develops is reinforced unconsciously and consciously through our personal interactions with the attached person; we relate and respond to their created sensory image. The sightless are particularly talented at creating a body image using sensory data derived from the senses other than sight, and their verbal descriptions of what they imagine with their mind's eye are remarkably accurate.

We habitually relate to, recognize, and identify our significant others based on the familiar body image to which our perceptions have become attached. Due to this constant exposure to the body image and because our culture promotes death denial, people often form an unrealistic expectation of permanency in the attached relationship.

It becomes simple for individuals who are profoundly attached to one another to feel confident that the relationship will last forever, irrational as this may seem. Although we know subconsciously that such permanence in even the strongest relationship is simply not possible, many prefer to live under the blissful misconception that death will not end the attachment. Human relationships, however, are not limitless; they too must die, either through physical or psychological separation or through death.

It is crucial that the funeral service practitioner appreciates the complex processes behind these human attachments and separations. It is these psychological processes on which the ethic of reverence for the dead is based, and which necessitate the need for funeralization. Without human attachments, there would be little, if any, need for funerals. A funeral is, in its most elementary form, a social function that reflects the reality of our capacity to form deep attachments, and that most human need to grieve and mourn our dead.

Death brings with it a finality that challenges our means to cope psychologically. With death comes the realization that what was once thought to be permanent and everlasting is in truth temporary and finite, and after death comes the long and often painful process of grief and mourning.

During the mourning process, the bereaved are challenged to divest themselves of their close attachments to the dead person and are asked to rechannel that emotional energy into relationships with other people. The process of mourning is vital and necessary for healthy grieving. Grieving begins in the bereaved psyche by sensory (visual and tactile) confrontation with the dead person's retained body image.

It is often said that it is better to remember the dead as they were when they were alive. The comment, "I would rather remember them alive," is a form of death denial. For honest confrontation of the reality of death, it is necessary for the mourners to see the deceased person (or a symbol of the deceased person in cases where it is impossible to view the body) to bring home the reality of death. By seeing or touching the deceased, the mourners have the visual and physical opportunity that is crucial in verifying the stark reality of death. If the body of the deceased is lost forever and there is no chance to establish the reality of death, there is a risk of complicated bereavement, and mourners may feel a lack of resolution.

Viewing the Body

Honest confrontation of the reality of death requires the mourners to see the deceased or a symbol of the deceased. Viewing and touching a dead human body is the **best** way for the bereaved to overcome any death denial feelings. It is common in the study of grief to observe bereaved persons denying the significance of the death of someone to whom they were strongly attached. The process of denial takes many forms.

Denial frequently manifests as an avoidance of contact with the reality of death—namely, the dead person's body. At first glance, this avoidance may appear to reflect the fact that the bereaved is endeavoring to maintain his or her composure. Unfortunately, the bereaved are often rewarded for this type of rationalizing behavior. Bereavement is not a simple enough process to be adequately managed by rational thought alone; grief is an emotional, not a rational, process. It is important that the funeral service practitioner recognizes this attitude for what it truly is—the denial of the significance of death.

The comprehension of human separation can never fully be accomplished through intellectual rationalizations. Often, the people who are most aggrieved by the death, are the ones who most need to accept the reality of death, and are precisely the people who take the path of least resistance, by avoiding visual and tactile confrontation of the dead body image. Establishing the reality of death is always an issue of need more than want.

Dr. Erich Lindemann, a pioneer in the study of grief management, has suggested that there is really no escaping the slow wisdom of grief. Lindemann postulates that avoidance of the dead body is always done at the psychological peril of the aggrieved, and that this avoidance may appear at first to be consoling in the initial phase of acute grief. But in truth, Lindemann says, this consolation is just an illusion. In time, the necessity to view the body becomes a major issue in postbereavement care.

Lindemann says that a common characteristic in persons experiencing complicated bereavement is an inability to recall a clear mental image of the body in death. Establishment of this mental image is an essential ingredient in creating a strong foundation for subsequent steps in the grieving process. An unclear image of the deceased person or no image at all, fosters a lack of full acceptance of the reality of death.

Lindemann believed that the most significant benefit of funeralization and embalming is achieved at that moment when the finality of the death is fully comprehended by the bereaved person. It is this moment of truth, this awareness of the reality of death that serves as the psychological framework for the validation of embalming.

Many believe, as does the Reverend Paul Irion, that the embalmer's task is to make the body "presentable" for viewing. This is similar to other life situations, such as when a person prepares for social activity by bathing and combing their hair before greeting people in public. The ethical concepts of reverence for the dead, decent disposition, and dignity in death, all demand that the dead body be prepared for viewing so it will not be offensive to mourners during the process of funeralization.

The embalmed body image permits an open, realistic acceptance of death. In this type of stark confrontation, there is no denying the finality of death. Embalming the body permits time for family and friends to engage in the valuable process of leave-taking. The embalmed body image challenges the denial of death and promotes an atmosphere of emotional stability. By confronting the frightening, lonely feelings caused by the emotional conflict of death's denial, the embalmed body image acts as a catharsis for the strong emotions of panic, fear, frustration, and guilt. An embalmer's ultimate purpose, then, is to make the body presentable for viewing, and through the technical work of the embalmer, the realization of the finality of death takes place practically and tastefully.

The Author, Poet, and Funeral Director, Thomas Lynch, in his book **Bodies in Motion and at Rest**, says:

"'but remembering him the way he was,' I say, slowly, deliberately, as if the listener were breakable, 'begins by denying with the way he is.' I'm an apostle of the present tense. After years and years of directing funerals, I've come to the conclusion that seeing is the hardest and most helpful part. The truth, even when it hurts, has a healing in it, better than fiction or fantasy. When someone dies, it is not them we fear seeing, it is them **dead**. It is the death. We fear that seeing will be believing."

▶ RITUALS AND CEREMONIES

Nowhere do we see the need to be social in order to live a happy, balanced life more than in the rituals and rites performed by human beings. So entrenched in the makeup of humankind is ritualistic behavior that a breakdown or corruption of these rituals may result in human cataclysm.

Dr. Carl Jung, a pioneer in psychology, saw human psychological life as a universal phenomenon whereby identification with what he termed the "collective unconscious" linked all humanity together. Although we may differ in ethnicity, religion, or social attitudes, some constants exist in our mentality that all of us can identify with and understand. An archetype of our collective unconscious is funeralization and its associated issues.

Practical Model
To fully implement the ethical, psychological, and sociological values of funeralization, **people need time**. People need time to organize funerals, think about them, participate in them, and make decisions about how they should be carried out. Time is also required for the bereaved to assimilate all that has happened, and acknowledge the ramifications in their own lives.

Embalming slows decomposition and thus affords the bereaved the time to make important decisions. It also serves the practical purpose of rendering the body inoffensive and making it presentable for viewing. Embalming serves as an emotional buffer for the bereaved when the reality of traumatic death might be burdensome, because embalming restores the body image, not to mask reality, but to give the bereaved a body image they can more easily accept. The embalmed body affords the aggrieved the opportunity to accept the finality of death, and does so in a discreet and professional manner.

Embalming also serves a practical need when the body must be transported to another location, offering extended time for transport, and the assurance that the body will remain intact while arrangements are made and during final transportation.

Finally, modern embalming reflects the technology of the age. Today, instead of using herbs and spices as was done in antiquity, we use sophisticated chemicals. As licensed funeral directors and embalmers, we assume the primary responsibility for care of the dead, and that responsibility carries with it a valuable and impressive professional heritage.

▶ THE ETHICAL PERFORMANCE STANDARD

Embalmer Ethics

In the United States, where Judeo-Christian tradition has fostered respect for the human dead and considerations of public health require protection of the living against infection or contagion, the preparation of dead human bodies is entrusted to a specialized group called "licensed embalmers."

Ethical Practice. Ethics is the science of rectitude and duty. Its subject is morality and its sphere is virtuous conduct. It is concerned with the various aspects of rights and obligations. In essence, ethics is a set of principles that governs conduct for the purpose of establishing harmony in all human relations. For practical purposes, ethics is fair play.

In the absence of a specific set of rules by which men and women are governed or through which they learn to govern themselves in their relations with others, they are dependent upon traditional customs and practices as rules of conduct. This chapter, therefore, is intended to suggest some desirable uniform rules of conduct by which any embalmer may be guided in the practice of embalming. No code can specify all the duties of the embalmer in every circumstance that confronts him or her. It can serve as a guide in promoting professional attitudes and ensuring ethical conduct in many of the situations where neither custom nor tradition has provided a standard of practice that serves the best interests of the public and the profession.

Judicious Counsel. Experience qualifies embalmers to be of great value to those whom they serve and it is their professional obligation to give judicious counsel. In accordance with the wishes of the family, the embalmer should advise them concerning their expectations for a visitation, with viewing, when circumstances dictate the need for special attention such as restoration, any necessary invasive procedures, or the embalmer's need for available photos of the deceased to aid him or her in the embalming and feature setting, taking into account any of the deceased's cosmetic or hairdressing preferences.

Whenever the service is made challenging, because of the circumstances of death, the embalmer should communicate realistic expectations to the family directly or through the arranging funeral director. Representations concerning embalming and restoration should be full and factual. Misrepresentations are unethical and unprofessional and should be avoided at all times.

Body Donation, Organ Donation, and Autopsy

The embalmer needs to maintain a neutral position and follow the directions of the family wishing to donate organs or tissue of a deceased family member for the benefit of others. Such instances are opportunities for the embalmer to demonstrate his or her professionalism in serving not only the individual family but the public in general. It is not only ethical for an embalmer to take the time for cooperative efforts with organ procurement organizations, but also a professional expression of the embalmer's responsibilities as a licensee. A neutral position should also be taken when the family wishes to donate the whole deceased human body to a medical college for anatomical dissection and study. Some medical institutions permit embalming (with restrictions) for funeral services with viewing prior to delivery to the medical facility. Another option that can be offered is preparation without embalming for a viewing, if desired, by the family and friends.

Respect and consideration must also be given to the family where they have given consent for an autopsy or partial autopsy. It has been said that the autopsy is the "final diagnosis." Genetic disease within a family may be confirmed by autopsy. The autopsy can also confirm a specific pathological cause of the death. Under certain conditions, the coroner or medical examiner may demand an autopsy—sometimes with great resistance from the family. The funeral director here needs to remain neutral. Sudden or traumatic deaths can have legal ramifications and may be very necessary for insurance benefits.

The embalmer shares with all medical and hospital personnel the professional responsibility of cooperating with all groups and in supporting all measures that promote health, safety, and public welfare. Courtesy, tact, and discretion should characterize all of the embalmer's professional actions.

Misrepresentation

Embalmers should never aid or abet an unlicensed person who attempts to represent himself or herself as a licensed embalmer or to engage in practices reserved to the holder of an embalming license, when licensure is required to engage in such activities or to represent oneself as a licensed embalmer.

Confidentiality

The family members must be able to rely on confidentiality among themselves, the funeral director, and the embalmer on all matters relating to cause and manner of death, surrounding circumstances, condition of the body, and any other issues raised. The embalmer may be privy to other matters shared with him or her by the family. All such confidences must be ensured by the embalmer and funeral director.

Defamation of Others

Comments by one embalmer concerning another funeral director or embalmer should always be selected with care. Insinuations, nonfactual statements, or overplay of facts that have the intent or effect of harming another professional should be avoided at all times.

Enticement of Another Embalmer

It is unethical for an embalmer to willfully entice the employees of another firm with the purpose of unduly hampering, injuring, or prejudicing that firm or professional.

Accommodation of the Family

Not every family may wish or be able to pay for a visitation with viewing, but may express an earnest desire to view the remains in the preparation room. To the extent possible, embalmers should attempt to accommodate families in this regard and should present the remains with features set and whatever other helpful preparations are feasible. Such accommodation may be considered the family's right to check the embalmer's performance.

Identification

The embalmer has the responsibility to ascertain that he or she has a properly identified body and must manage the care and internal identification of the remains such that there can be no mistake, especially when viewing is not planned or cremation is the method of final disposition. (see Selected Readings, **Identification: An Essential Part of What We Do,** by Michael Kubasak).

Observing Laws, Rules, and Regulations

The embalmer is duty-bound and legally responsible to ensure that he or she observes all legal and regulatory requirements of federal, state, or local government. The embalmer also has the responsibility of informing the funeral home owner of the resources or capital investments required to meet Occupational Safety and Health Administration (OSHA) standards, any applicable Environmental Protection Agency (EPA) requirements, or other measures needed to be in compliance.

Maintaining Competence

The embalmer has a moral and ethical responsibility to assure that he or she receives whatever continuing education is necessary to maintain skills commensurate with professional practice. State-of-the-art practices and procedures should be known to and practiced by the embalmer at all times.

Health Protection and Sanitation

The embalmer is ethically responsible for protecting the health of any person allowed to enter the preparation room for any reason, and for restricting entry to any person not authorized to be there. That responsibility includes following appropriate sanitation procedures to maintain a safe working area for any individual. The embalmer is responsible for safe sheltering so that no unauthorized person has access to the human remains in his or her care.

Proper Care of the Deceased and Documentation

The embalmer should deliver and document quality care of the deceased body. The embalming procedures used should be documented on an embalming report for possible future reference. An embalming report needs to be completed for each deceased body brought into the preparation room or embalming facility; this includes bodies being sheltered and not embalmed and bodies which have been embalmed at another facility. A record of clothing or other personal articles or valuables received by the firm would be appropriate. In addition, written permission to embalm or a record of the expressed permission must be obtained. When embalming is not desired, permission needs to be obtained for those minimum care treatments necessary for identification of or viewing the body.

Handling the Remains of the Deceased Human Body

Funeral practitioners are charged with the task of removing the body from the place of death and ensuring that in the moving process the body receives the respect and care. The movement of the remains from a hospital, home, hospice or nursing home, or public morgue should be accomplished with the same degree of care as if the person were a patient being transferred. All equipment—cots, sheets, pillows, pouches, and so on—should be clean.

The remains should be protected by a wrap or appropriate covering that maintains the modesty of the deceased person. The remains should be handled as if the body were dead from a communicable disease; universal precautions should always be followed by those making the removal. This needs to be practiced only in the immediate wrapping and handling of the remains. After the body is placed in protective wrappings and cover, street wear is acceptable for those removing the body. Failure to observe universal precautions is unprofessional and violates the principle of acknowledging that the public welfare is affected by the acts of the funeral practitioner or his or her representatives. If the removal is in a home, soiled linen may also be removed for cleaning. In these situations, the bedding should be made up so the room looks orderly.

The practitioner or their representative should be prompt in responding to a home call or a call from a nursing home, hospice, or hospital. In this respect, the practitioner should realize that federal rules require a window of opportunity for organ procurement organizations to invite the family to consider organ or tissue donations where circumstances are appropriate for that request. The 1998 requirement has the worthy purpose of increasing the number of organs for transplant available to Americans and others who are in need of these human resources.

Once the remains are in the embalmer's facility, respect for the deceased human body takes on even more importance. The preparation of the remains should be viewed as a right of the deceased person to be cleansed, sanitized, groomed, restored, and embalmed with dignity. Special care should be taken in the presentation of the remains to the family. These efforts are ethically correct whether or not there will be a formal viewing. The embalmer should take into account information or photos from the family that would allow the embalmer to best present the remains in a natural way. Such efforts will benefit the viewers who knew the individual when he or she was alive.

When an embalmer takes responsibility and custody for the body, he or she has the duty to see that the body is carefully handled and secure in its location. Negligent behavior, such as leaving the preparation room door open or accessible to unlicensed persons, is unprofessional and should be avoided at all times. The protection of the deceased human body is as important as the embalming procedure itself. Photos of the deceased should never be taken without permission or direction of the persons in charge of arrangements. Doing so would be unprofessional and make the licensee and the owner subject to suit or discipline. If photos are taken for identification or conditions prior to and following preparation, these should become a part of the confidential files of the funeral home. The embalmer should insist that the proprietor provides adequate means of security for the remains. Any act that would allow an unlicensed person to have access to the deceased human being, without the presence of an embalmer, must be avoided both by policy and practice.

There are many times when the embalmer knows or should anticipate that the final preparation of the remains may require other special handling. Determining what needs to be done and seeing that it *is* done is a professional obligation of the embalmer. For example,

an obese person should, where possible, be moved with overhead lifts rather than engaging several persons to move the individual's remains. The ergonomics of lifting excessive or awkward weight should dictate appropriate procedures, while still handling the remains with respectful care.

Quality control in the removal, transportation, preparation, care, and security of the remains is the primary obligation of the embalmer for which he or she should take full responsibility. The embalmer should recognize that there is no act, provided by any member of the firm that has a greater impact on consumer satisfaction than properly prepared and presented remains. Accordingly, the embalmer should demand and receive whatever resources are necessary to accommodate this professional responsibility. The owner, operator, or manager of the funeral home also has the obligation to search out what special needs the embalmer may have to allow him or her to maximize professional presentation of the remains for viewing. If the visitation is marred by embalming errors, the funeral itself can hardly be fully successful.

The ethical standing of the embalmer is maintained through a consistent demonstration that he or she understands and has incorporated these goals and obligations. Embalming is not only a science, but s also an art. A successful embalmer must have the occupational leeway to take additional time, whenever it is necessary, to adequately restore and present the professionally prepared remains for visitation, shipment, or burial. Owners, even licensed ones, who fail to authorize purchase of the necessary equipment, accessories, fluids, supplies, instruments, or protective procedures do, in effect, unethically inhibit the embalmer from delivering the optimum remains for funeralization. Such negligence shows disrespect for the deceased, marginalizes the embalmer's effectiveness, and fails the legislative intent test for appropriate care of the deceased.

Any licensee who fails to act in an ethical way should be accused by the observer, chastised by the licensing board and agency, and disciplined as a signal to others that unprofessional behavior is intolerable in funeral service. Embalming failures, for whatever reason, are injurious to the health and welfare of the public, create anguish for families, and unfairly expose the profession as a whole to criticism. Peer review, discipline, and cooperation for excellence are remedies that can ensure public confidence. If the embalmer or his or her funeral organization is unable or unwilling to practice embalming excellence, the profession should remove them from practice so that the public welfare is best served. An embalmer, by each act of service, contributes to family satisfaction, serves the public, and contributes immeasurably to the future success of any firm.

* Security *

American Society of Embalmers

Best Practice Embalming Tenets©

- Treat all deceased human remains with thoughtful care, maintain dignity, and show respect at all times
- Be knowledgeable of and in compliance with, all regulatory authorities, (federal, state, and local) that govern the preparation and disposition of a deceased human remains
- Prioritize the use of excellent communications among all funeral professionals involved with the decedent and family
  - Authorizations for embalming and restorative art procedures must be shared with the embalmer, preferably in writing
  - Confirm the identity of the deceased prior to the commencement of any procedures
  - The Preparation Room should be kept private and all local, state, and federal laws should be observed as to its use
  - Share information regarding the care of the deceased between director and embalmer
    - ◦ Obtain information about the overall condition of the remains
    - ◦ Obtain information about cause or nature of death
    - ◦ Obtain the time of services to optimize best presentation
      - – Ensure that adequate time is given to the embalming process
      - – Address and remedy problem embalming and shipping situations immediately
- All documents, photographs, and personal information about the deceased must be kept in strict confidence and under secure storage
  - Only those persons designated and authorized by the funeral establishment or family may be allowed attendance during the preparation of a remains
  - Photographs of deceased remains must never be placed on social media sites or shown in public places to non-funeral professionals outside the educational setting
- Respect and comply, without comment, with the wishes of the family or the deceased requesting organ/tissue donor, hospital or forensic autopsy, or full body donation to science
- Professional conduct will ensure that embalmers will not knowingly allow non-licensed embalmers (exception students or apprentices, under supervision) to practice embalming and that they will not participate in derogatory public comments about other embalmers

- Pursue ongoing and continuing education opportunities for the embalmer
- Practice thorough and complete preservation of the entire remains
  - Use all available embalming methods necessary: arterial, hypodermic, surface
- Document all remains entering the funeral facility on a Preparation Care Form
  - Include remains for: identification only, storage, embalming, shipped-in or shipped-out
- Be knowledgeable of multiple methods of treating all types of embalming cases, regardless of their condition.
  - Practice custodial care; monitor remains until final disposition and make corrections as needed
  - Be willing to ask for assistance when needed
- Protect yourself from any potential hazard, infectious, chemical, and physical
- The establishment ownership and the embalming practitioner agree to have available all the necessary supplies, chemicals, dry goods, and equipment to prepare every type of embalming case
- The preparation room and adjoining facilities will be maintained in a clean and sanitary condition

The Executive Director and Board of Directors of the American Society of Embalmers compiled these Best Practice Embalming Tenets to elevate the formal practice of embalming throughout the profession. This document is a work in progress. As the embalming "environment" changes, this document will be updated to reflect the current practices. February 2011.

Used with permission of the American Society of Embalmers–Melissa Johnson-Williams, Executive Director

▶ REGULATORY BODIES

Legislative Intent

The law is said to be the minimum ethic of a community. Members of a society place their trust and confidence in certain persons, charging them to fulfill in a competent manner their wishes and desires over certain matters, one of them being the responsibility for disposition of the dead. Certain individuals within a community have been appointed by law, and by the trust of the members of the community, to oversee the disposition of the dead in a legal, ethical, reverent, and respectful manner. Certain standards of performance are not only expected but demanded from embalmers and funeral directors.

When a state issues an embalming license to a qualified practitioner, it is declaring the following:

1. Embalming is a practice affecting the public safety and welfare and is subject to regulation and control in the public interest.
2. The preparation, care, and final disposition of a deceased human body should be attended with appropriate observance and understanding, in addition to having due regard and respect for the reverent care of the human body and for those bereaved and the overall spiritual dignity of humankind.
3. As a matter of public interest, the practice of embalming merits and receives the confidence of the public in that only qualified persons be authorized to embalm in their state of practice.
4. The state codes should be liberally construed to best carry out these subjects and purposes.

These declarations form a foundation for the development of specific professional performance standards.

State Regulation

In the United States, the practice of embalming is regulated primarily by the legislatures of the individual states. Two principal bodies may have control of the care and disposition of dead human remains: The Board of Health (or Bureau of Vital Statistics) and the State Board of Embalmers and Funeral Directors (or similar governing body) that regulate the funeral homes and the licensing of funeral directors and embalmers. These two groups promulgate and enforce statutory law as well as rules and regulations governing the disposition of dead human bodies.

States regulate a coroner or a medical examiner and the organ and tissue procurement agencies to take actual custody of the dead human body. They also have authority over the disposition of indigent bodies, and regulate the procurement of bodies for medical school anatomical study.

▶ CORONER OR MEDICAL EXAMINER

The state, the county, or the municipality establishes laws and regulations that require certain causes and manner of death to be reported to a local coroner or a medical examiner. Additionally, the embalmer is also responsible for reporting any suspicious circumstances surrounding the death to the coroner or the medical examiner. It is important that the funeral personnel in charge of arrangements ascertain who will sign the certificate of death if the nature of the death is such that the coroner

or the medical examiner must be notified to investigate. The following list shows the types of death about which the coroner or the medical examiner must be notified of. **It is important that the embalmer be familiar with the requirements of the state in which the practice is conducted.**

I. **Accidental deaths: all forms including death arising from employment such as:**
   A. Anesthetic accident (death on the operating table or prior to recovery from anesthesia)
   B. Blows or other forms of mechanical violence
   C. Burns and scalds
   D. Crushed beneath falling objects
   E. Cutting or stabbing
   F. Drowning (actual or suspected)
   G. Electric shock
   H. Explosion
   I. Exposure
   J. Firearms
   K. Fractures of bones, not pathological (such cases to be reported even when fracture is not primarily responsible for death)
   L. Falls
   M. Carbon monoxide poisoning (resulting from natural gas, automobile exhaust, or other)
   N. Hanging
   O. Heat exhaustion
   P. Insolation (sunstroke)
   Q. Poisoning (food, occupational, narcotic, sedative, and other)
   R. Strangulation
   S. Suffocation (foreign object in bronchi, by bed clothing or other means)
   T. Vehicular accidents (automobile, street car, bus, railroad, motorcycle, bicycle, or other)
II. **Homicidal deaths: including those involving child abuse**
III. **Suicidal deaths**
IV. **Abortions—criminal or self-induced: When the manner of death falls within the above classifications, such death must be reported to the coroner even though the survival period subsequent to onset is 12 months.**
V. **Sudden deaths: When in apparent good health or in any suspicious or unusual manner including:**
   A. Alcoholism
   B. Sudden death on the street, at home, in a public place, at place of employment
   C. Deaths in unknown circumstances, whenever there is no witness or where little or no information can be elicited concerning the deceased person (deaths of this type include those persons whose dead bodies are found in the open, in places of temporary

shelter, or in their home under conditions that offer no clues as to the cause of death)
D. Deaths that follow injuries sustained at the place of employment, whenever the circumstances surrounding such injury may ultimately be the subject of investigation
   1. Industrial infections (anthrax, septicemia following wounds including gas bacillus infections, tetanus, etc.)
   2. Silicosis
   3. Industrial poisonings (acids, alkalies, aniline, benzene, carbon monoxide, carbon tetrachloride, cyanogen, lead, nitrous fumes, etc.)
   4. Contusions, abrasions, fractures, burns (flame, chemical, or electrical) received during employment, which in the opinion of the attending physician are of sufficient import, either as the cause or contributing factor to the cause of death, to warrant certifying them on the death certificate
E. All stillborn infants where there is suspicion of illegal interference
F. Death of persons, where the attending physician cannot be found or death of persons, who have not been attended by a physician within 2 weeks prior to the date of death
G. All deaths occurring within 24 hours of admission to a hospital, unless the patient has been under continuous care of a physician for a natural disease that is responsible for death

Federal Regulation

In recent years, federal agencies have come to play an important role in the activities of the funeral establishment and the preparation room. These agencies include the Centers for Disease Control and Prevention (CDC), EPA, the Federal Trade Commission (FTC), and OSHA. Four divisions of OSHA affect the funeral home: (1) the General Rule, (2) the Hazard Communication Standard, (3) the Formaldehyde Rule, and (4) the Bloodborne Pathogen Rule. Chapter 3, Personal, Public Health and Regulatory Standards, is devoted almost entirely to the regulations set by OSHA. Most recently, the Transportation Security Administration (TSA) requires the funeral home or the embalming facility to register as an "approved shipper" if they are transporting bodies by common carrier.

Federal Trade Commission

In April 1984, the federal government, through the FTC, promulgated a rule governing the activities of funeral directors and embalmers. The rule, which is commonly referred to as the Funeral Rule, was amended by the FTC in 1994. It is most important that all embalmers be fully aware of the statutes and rules and regulations of the state in which they are practicing. These rules differ from state to state, but the Funeral Rule applies to **all** states. For this reason, the following excerpts are reprinted from the **Federal Register:**

Misrepresentations

EMBALMING PROVISIONS—DECEPTIVE ACTS OR PRACTICES. In selling or offering to sell funeral goods or funeral services to the public, it is a deceptive act or practice for a funeral provider to:

1. Represent that state or local law requires that a deceased person be embalmed, when such is not the case
2. Fail to disclose that embalming is not required by law, except in certain special cases

PREVENTIVE REQUIREMENTS. To prevent these deceptive acts or practices as well as the unfair or deceptive acts or practices defined in §453.4(b)(1) and §453.5(2) [of the Funeral Rule], funeral providers must:

1. Not represent that a deceased person is required to be embalmed for:
   A. Direct cremation;
   B. Immediate burial; or
   C. A closed casket funeral without viewing or visitation when refrigeration is available and when state or local law does not require embalming; and
2. Place the following disclosure on the general price list, required by §453.2(b)(4) in immediate conjunction with the price shown for embalming: "Except in certain special cases, embalming is not required by law. Embalming may be necessary, however, if you select certain funeral arrangements, such as a funeral with viewing. If you do not want embalming, you usually have the right to choose an arrangement that does not require you to pay for it, such as direct cremation or immediate burial." The phrase "except in certain special cases" need not be included in this disclosure if state or local laws in the area(s) where the provider does business, do not require embalming under any circumstances.

Services Provided Without Prior Approval

UNFAIR OR DECEPTIVE ACTS OR PRACTICES. In selling or offering to sell funeral goods or funeral services to the public, it is an unfair or deceptive act or practice for any provider to embalm a deceased body for a fee unless:

1. State or local law or regulation requires embalming in the particular circumstances, regardless of

any funeral choice which the family might make; or

2. Prior approval for embalming (expressly so described) from a family member or other authorized person, or

3. The funeral provider is unable to contact a family member or other authorized person after exercising due diligence, has no reason to believe the family does not want embalming performed, and obtains subsequent approval for embalming already performed (expressly so described). In seeking approval, the funeral provider must disclose that a fee will be charged if the family selects a funeral which requires embalming, such as a funeral with viewing, and that no fee will be charged if the family selects a service which does not require embalming, such as direct cremation or immediate burial.

PREVENTIVE REQUIREMENT. To prevent these unfair or deceptive acts or practices, funeral providers must include on the itemized statement of funeral goods and services selected, required by §453.2(b)(5), the statement: "If you selected a funeral that may require embalming, such as a funeral with viewing, you may have to pay for embalming. You do not have to pay for embalming you did not approve if you selected arrangements such as direct cremation or immediate burial. If we charge for embalming, we will explain why below."

Local Regulations

At the local level, the zoning board, the local board of health, the waste disposal board, and the water management board can have involvement with the funeral home or the embalming facility.

▶ DOCUMENTATION

(Note: All documents used in this textbook are generic and only examples. A funeral home or an embalming facility must consult its legal advisor for the drafting of all documents.)

Form 1–1. **Embalming Authorization (Fig. 1–1),** provides permission for embalming the body and indemnification of the funeral home. Note the following

- It expands who may assist in the embalming—mortuary students and/or mortuary interns.
- It also provides for the employment of a trade embalmer (independent contractor).
- It allows the body to be embalmed at the funeral home or at a separate embalming facility.
- It allows for restorative treatments.
- It protects the funeral home if the body has been misidentified.

Form 1–2. **Authorization for Restorative and Cosmetic Care (Fig. 1–2),** gives necessary permission when extensive or operative restoration work may be necessary in the preparation of the body.

Form 1–3-A. **Authorization for Minimum Care Services (Fig. 1–3A),** authorizes minimum care when embalming is not requested. It gives the funeral facility permission to perform certain tasks to prepare the body for identification, viewing, or immediate cremation.

Form 1–3-B. **Minimum Care Authorization When Embalming is Declined (Fig. 1–3B),** authorizes minimum care of the body. It provides a detailed description of "minimum care" that can be performed.

Form 1–4. **Authorization to Prepare Donation Cases for Viewing (Fig. 1–4),** is used when a funeral facility prepares a body where organs and/or tissues have been donated.

Form 1–5. **Green Funeral Release and Indemnification (Fig. 1–5),** gives direction for disposition of the dead human body when a green burial (natural burial) is requested.

Form 1–6. **Identification of Remains of the Decedent (Fig. 1–6),** verifies the identification of a decedent. Note the following with respect to this form:

- states who is making the identification
- states that the body was viewed and identified
- states that the next of kin refuses to identify the remains but authorizes final disposition without positive identification
- indemnifies the funeral facility if the body is incorrectly identified

Form 1–7. **Viewing When NOT Advised Against by the Funeral Home (Fig. 1–7),** used when the funeral home advises against viewing the body, for example, when the remains have been subject to trauma, fire, or decomposition, but the family DOES want to view them. Note that a description of the body is given—this would need to vary depending on the reason why the recommendation was made by the funeral facility not to have the body viewed.

Form 1–8. **Attention Funeral Director (Fig. 1–8),** a form for bodies being shipped to another funeral facility. It describes the condition of the body at the shipping location and requests notification of any problems encountered by the receiving funeral facility. It is to be accompanied by a copy of the Decedent Care Report.

Form 1–9. **Decedent Care Report (Fig. 1–9),** this form MUST be completed for EACH deceased human body brought into a funeral or an embalming facility. A copy of the report MUST accompany the body being shipped or transported to another funeral facility.

(*text continues on page 29*)

EMBALMING AUTHORIZATION

1.   **PARTIES:**

"FUNERAL HOME":_____
                                    (Name of Funeral Home)

"REPRESENTATIVE":_____
(Use Reverse Side   (Name of Representative)
for Additional Names)

"DECEDENT":_____
                                    (Name of Decedent)

2.   **RELATIONSHIP OF REPRESENTATIVE:** The REPRESENTATIVE warrants and represents to the FUNERAL HOME that the relationship between the REPRESENTATIVE and the DECEDENT is as follows: (Check the appropriate box)

☐   Spouse

☐   Next-of-Kin (Closest Living Relative)

☐   Personal Representative of the Next-of-Kin with written authorization of Next-of-Kin to act on his or her behalf.

☐   Other:_____

3.   **AUTHORITY OF REPRESENTATIVE:** The REPRESENTATIVE warrants and represents to FUNERAL HOME that the REPRESENTATIVE is the person or the appointed agent of the person who by law has the paramount right to arrange and direct the disposition of the remains of the DECEDENT and that no other person(s) has a superior right over the right of the REPRESENTATIVE.

4.   **EMBALMING AUTHORIZATION:** The REPRESENTATIVE authorizes and directs the FUNERAL HOME, its employees, independent contractors, and agents (including apprentices and/or mortuary students under the direct supervision of a licensed embalmer), to care for, embalm, perform restorative measures, and prepare the body of the DECEDENT. The REPRESENTATIVE acknowledges that this authorization encompasses permission to embalm at the FUNERAL HOME facility or at another facility equipped for embalming. In providing this authorization, REPRESENTATIVE acknowledges that embalming is not an exact science and that results are dependent upon a number of factors, including, but not limited to the conditions under which the death occurred, time lapse between death and the onset of the embalming procedure, physical condition at the time of death, medications, especially analgesics administered prior to death, life-saving procedures, cause of death, storage procedures of the releasing institution, natural elements, tissue/organ donations, and post-mortem (autopsy) examinations.

5.   **PHOTOGRAPHS:** Unless the box at the end of this paragraph is checked by the REPRESENTATIVE, the FUNERAL HOME has authorization to take photographs of the remains to document the condition of the remains prior to or during embalming.   These photographs will be maintained in the internal records of the FUNERAL HOME. ☐ Permission is denied.

6.   **INDEMNIFICATION:** The REPRESENTATIVE agrees to indemnify and hold harmless the FUNERAL HOME from any claims or causes of action arising or related in any respect to this embalming authorization or the FUNERAL HOME's reliance thereon.

DATE: **SIGNATURE OF REPRESENTATIVE:**

_____   _____

Figure 1–1. Embalming authorization. (**National Funeral Directors Association, Brookfield, WI, 2007, with permission.**)

SAMPLE ONLY

AUTHORIZATION FOR RESTORATIVE AND COSMETIC CARE

I/we _____, hereby authorize the

_____ Funeral Home to perform cosmetic and

restorative work on the remains of _____,

who is related to me a as _____. I/we

hereby acknowledge full responsibility for results of same and do not hold harmless

_____Funeral Home , its owners, employees and

agents for results herewith performed.

I/we hereby represent that I/we are of same and nearest degree of relationship to the

deceased:

_____ (seal)

_____ (seal)   _____ witness

_____ Date   _____ witness

Figure 1–2. Authorization for restorative and cosmetic care. (**The Dodge Company, Cambridge, MA, 1999, with permission.**)

SAMPLE ONLY
AUTHORIZATION FOR MINIMUM CARE SERVICES

1. PARTIES:

FUNERAL HOME: _____
(Name of Funeral Home)

REPRESENTATIVE: _____
(Name of Representative)

DECEDENT: _____
(Name of Decedent)

2. Relationship of Representative: The representative warrants and represents to FUNERAL HOME that the relationship between the REPRESENTATIVE and the DECEDENT is as follows (check the appropriate item):

☐ Spouse

☐ Next of Kin (Closest Living Relative)

☐ Personal Representative

☐ Other: _____

3. Authority of the Representative: The REPRESENTATIVE warrants and represents to FUNERAL HOME that the REPRESENTSTIVE is the person or the appointed agent of the person who by law has the paramount right to arrange and direct the disposition of the remains of the DECEDENT and that no other person(s) has a superior right over the right of the REPRESENTATIVE.

4. Minimum Care Services: If the REPRESENTATIVE has directed that the remains of the DECEDENT are not to be embalmed or if a decision on embalming has not yet been made, there are services that the REPRESENTATIVE may wish to authorize so that the remains may be privately viewed, identified or reposed in a dignified and respectful manner. Below is a list of Minimum Care Services. Please check the box next to these Minimum Care Services that you authorize the FUNERAL HOME to provide for the DECEDENT'S remains:

☐ Removal of exterior medical devices (hearing aids, dentures, IV tubing, etc.)

☐ Removal of internal medical devices (pacemakers, pumps, defibrillators, etc.)

☐ Shaving the face and/or trimming beard and moustache

☐ Manicuring finger nails

☐ Trimming hair of the head

☐ Closing incisions by sutures

☐ Closing the mouth (may require sutures)

☐ Aspirating internal cavities and injecting preservative cavity fluids

☐ Application of cosmetics

☐ Other:_____

5. Indemnification: The REPRESENTATIVE agrees to indemnify and hold harmless the FUNERAL HOME from any claims or causes of action from or related in any respect to this decision to authorize the MINIMUM CARE SERVICES from the FUNERAL HOME.

_____   _____
DATE   **SIGNATURE OF REPRESENTATIVE**

Figure 1-3. Authorization for minimum care services. (**National Funeral Directors Association, Brookfield, WI, 2010, with permission.**)

Minimum Care Authorization When Embalming is Declined

Name of the deceased: _____ Date of death: _____

The undersigned represents and warrants to be the next of kin to the deceased or the person(s) with the right and authority by law to control the disposition of the above-named decedent.

The undersigned has declined embalming of the above-named decedent and authorizes the funeral home, or its designated agent, to provide shelter to the body and minimum care.

The undersigned understands minimum care may include, but not be limited to sheltering the body in a clean, private environment; type of environment: refrigerated or non-refrigerated ; positioning the body; removing exterior tubes, catheters, or other medical devices deemed necessary; closing of eyes and mouth by accepted mortuary practices; aspiration of excess fluids and gasses from the body; inventory of personal effects from the body; use of surface disinfectants or deodorants; wrapping or covering the body in a suitable material. Minimum care does not include chemically treating the body by arterial injection of chemicals and does not retard organic decomposition . Minimum care will not ensure any time for presentation of the body for viewing or preservation as a replacement for arterial embalming.

The undersigned have been provided with the opportunity to ask any questions pertaining to minimum care.

The undersigned releases and discharges the funeral home, its affiliates, officers, directors, employees and agents from any and all liabilities claim, losses, damages, costs, or causes of action arising from the decision to not embalm the body, or arising out of any other decision indicated by this authorization which may result in mental or physical distress or anguish or harm or financial loss to the undersigned or others.

Signature: _____
Relationship to deceased:_____

Signature: _____
Relationship to deceased:_____

Funeral Home Representative: _____

Date signed: _____._____

adopted from M. Kubasak / Lamers , LMG Publishing, 2007.

Figure 1-3. (*Continued*)

AUTHORIZATION TO PREPARE DONATION CASES FOR VIEWING

1. **PARTIES:**
FUNERAL HOME: _____

REPRESENTATIVE: _____

DECEDENT: _____

PROCUREMENT ORGANIZATION: _____

2. **RELATIONSHIP OF REPRESENTATIVE**: The REPRESENTATIVE warrants and represents to the FUNERAL HOME that the relationship between the REPRESENTATIVE and the DECEDENT is as follows: (Check appropriate box).
   [ ]   Spouse
   [ ]   Next of Kin (Closest Living Relative)
   [ ]   Personal Representative of the Next of Kin with written authorization of Next of Kin to act on his/her behalf.
   [ ]   Other:

3. **DONATION:** The DEDEDENT and/or the REPRESENTATIVE has authorized the PROCUREMENT ORGANIZATION to carry out the donation specified below:
   [ ]   Organs
   [ ]   Organs and Tissues
   [ ]   Organs, Tissues and Bone
   [ ]   All Body Parts

4. **Viewing:** The REPRESENTATIVE instructs the FUNERAL HOME to prepare the remains of the DECEDENT for viewing. The REPRESENTATIVE understands and acknowledges that the appearance of the DECEDENT and the benefits of the embalming and restorative services provided by the FUNERAL HOME can be adversely impacted by donation procedures and resulting delays. The REPRESENTATIVE hereby releases and agrees to hold FUNERAL HOME, its owners, employees and agents harmless from any claims or causes of action arising or relating to the embalming and restoration of DECEDENT'S remains or the viewing thereof.

5. **RESTORATION COSTS:** The REPRESENTATIVE acknowledges and agrees that additional cost of restoration may be incurred due to the donation and that such costs will be:
   [ ]   Paid solely by the PROCUREMENT ORGANIZATION
   [ ]   Paid by those responsible for the funeral bill

6. **RELEASE:** The REPRESENTATIVE acknowledges and agrees that FUNERAL HOME, its owners, employees and agents have no legal relationship with the PROCUREMENT ORGANIZATION and are under no obligation or responsibility to insure that the PROCUREMENT ORGANIZATION has obtained informed consent to the donation, has conducted donation procedures in a lawful and ethical manner, and/or will use the donated body parts as required by law and the donation authorization.

SIGNATURE OF REPRESENTATIVE: _____

DATE: _____

Figure 1–4. Authorization to prepare donation cases for viewing. (from Donation Best Practices Manual doc. 2005, Brookfield, WI, National Funeral Directors Association, 2010, with permission.)

GREEN FUNERAL RELEASE AND INDEMNIFICATION

1.Parties:

Funeral Home _____

Representative of decedent _____

Decedent _____

2.Relationship of Representative: The REPRESENTATIVE warrants and represents to the FUNERAL HOME that the relationship between the REPRESENTATIVE and the DECEDENT is as follows:

☐ Spouse

☐Next of Kin (closest living relative)

☐Personal Representative of Next of Kin with written authorization of Next of Kin at act on his or her behalf

☐Other: _____

3. AUTHORITY OF REPRESENTATIVE: The REPRESENTATIVE warrants and represents to FUNERAL HOME that the REPRESENTATIVE is the person or the appointed agent of the person who by law has the paramount right to arrange and direct the disposition of the remains of the DECEDENT and that no other person(s) has a superior right over that right of the REPRESENTATIVE

4. GREEN FUNERAL: While the details involved in a disposition known as a "Green Funeral" may vary, they usually involve minimal preparation of the DECEDENT'S remains; no embalming or preservation services; use of a wood, cardboard, wicker, bamboo or cloth container to hold, transport and bury the body; no use of a vault or outer burial container to encase the remains in the grave; and burial in a woodland or open field setting with grave marked by rocks, trees or flowers as opposed to a permanent marker or monument.

5. ADVISORY: The Green Funeral choice is usually made for environmental reasons and a desire for a simpler disposition. It is an appropriate and meaningful choice for certain families. However, it does preclude certain options and poses several risks that the REPRESENTATIVE has been advised of and is now acknowledging. The REPRESENTATIVE has been advised by the FUNERAL HOME that with a Green Funeral, the FUNERAL HOME can provide no assurances regarding the appearance or the condition of the DECEDENT'S remains; that there will not be a public visitation or viewing of the DECEDENT; that there are possible health risks posed by handling an unembalmed body; that there can be substantial risks of physical injury to pallbearers from holding, carrying and transporting a body in a container that may not be designed to hold the weight or to be safely lifted and carried; that burial of the body in a grave or plot without an outer burial container may lead to the ground settling and sinking over the grave; that the body may not be able to be disinterred and moved at a later date; and that, in later years, it may be difficult or impossible to locate the grave due to the lack of a permanent marker or monument.

6. DRECTION TO ARRANGE AND CARRY OUT GREEN FUNERAL: The REPRESENTATIVE directs and authorizes the FUNERAL HOME to arrange and carry out the Green Funeral described above. In directing and authorizing the Green Funeral, the REPRESENTATIVE understands and appreciates the risks explained in Paragraph 5 above and other risks that may have been described by the FUNERAL HOME to the REPRESENTATIVE. Despite these risks, the REPRESENTATIVE directs the FUNERAL HOME to carry out the REPRESENTATIVE'S directions with regard to the Green Funeral for the DECEDENT.

7. INDEMNIFICATION: The REPRESENTATIVE hereby releases FUNERAL HOME fully from all claims and agrees to indemnify and hold harmless the FUNERAL HOME from any claims or causes of action arising from or related in any respect to the direction of the REPRESENTATIVE to carry out the Green Funeral.

DATE:_____

SIGNATURE OF REPRESENTATIVE: _____

Figure 1–5. Green funeral release and indemnification. (**National Funeral Directors Association, Brookfield, WI, 2010.**)

IDENTIFICATION OF REMAINS OF THE DECEDENT

1. Parties:
   Funeral Home: _____
   (Name of Funeral Home)

   Representative: _____
   (Name of Representative – Use Reverse side for additional Names)

   Decedent: _____

2. Relationship of Representative: The REPRESENTATIVE warrants and represents to the Funeral Home that the relationship between the REPRESENTATIVE and the DECEDENT is as follows:
   (Check appropriate box)

   [ ]   Spouse
   [ ]   Next of Kin (Closest Living Relative)
   [ ]   Personal Representative of the Next of Kin with written authorization of Next of Kin to act on his/her behalf
   [ ]   Other

3. Authority of the Representative: The REPRESENTATIVE warrants and represents to the FUNERAL HOME that the REPRESENTATIVE is the person or the appointed agent of the Person who by law has the paramount right to arrange and direct the disposition of the remains of the DECEDENT and that no other person(s) has a superior right over the right of the REPRESENTATIVE.

4. IDENTIFICATION: The REPRESENTATIVE certifies to the FUNERAL HOME as follows:

   [ ]   The REPRESENTATIVE has viewed the remains and positively identified them as the body of the DECEDENT.

   [ ]   The REPRESENTATIVE elects NOT TO IDENTIFY the remains and authorizes the final disposition of the body of the DECEDENT by the FUNERAL HOME without positive identification.

5. INDEMNIFICATION: The REPRESENTATIVE assumes ALL LIABILITY for incorrectly identifying or for failing to identify the body of the DECEDENT and does hereby agree to indemnify and hold harmless the FUNERAL HOME from any claims or causes of action arising in any respect to the REPRESENTATIVE'S act of identification or omission to identify the remains of the DECEDENT.

SIGNATURE OF REPRESENTATIVE: _____

FUNERAL HOME REPRESENTATIVE: _____

Date: _____

Figure 1–6. Identification of decedent. (**Courtesy of Pennsylvania Funeral Directors Association, Harrisburg, PA.**)

Sample Only - TRAUMA
Viewing without embalming

RELEASE

I, _____ , hereby release, discharge, and forever

hold harmless the _____ Funeral Home and its owners and employees,

from any and all claims resulting **from my viewing of the body**

of _____. I explicitly release and discharge the

_____ Funeral Home and its owners and employees

from any and all claims for loss or damages, including but not limited to personal

injury, illness, mental distress or disability of any type, or death, whether or not caused

by the _____ Funeral Home, its owners or employees.

Specifically, I have been informed that the body has been damaged by fire. I have

been informed that any and all of the remains may be charred and that the superficial layer

of skin/tissue is nonexistent due to the fire.

I have been informed that the body is autopsied. I have been informed that the

body may give off a pungent odor that may be noticeable as soon as I enter the building.

I have been offered the opportunity to view the body via a photograph and decided

to proceed with actual viewing of the body.

I have read this Release and I understand and agree to all of its provisions. If any

portion of this Release shall be held invalid, those parts that are not invalid shall continue

in full force and effect.

_____

Date: _____

Witness: _____

Figure 1–7. Viewing requested without embalming: Trauma example. (**Courtesy Pennsylvania Funeral Directors Association, Harrisburg, PA.**)

<u>SAMPLE ONLY</u>

ATTENTION FUNERAL DIRECTOR

Name of deceased: _____

Date and time of this document: _____
                                   (DATE)   (TIME)

Our embalmer(s) have reviewed the condition of this body immediately prior to transfer to the delivery agent (airport, railroad, private carrier) and have noted any special circumstances below for your convenience. A copy of the EMBALMING CARE REPORT is enclosed.

Occasionally, between the time of departure and arrival, body conditions may change or the transfer may create situations that require additional remedial steps upon arrival. If this body is not satisfactory when received, ***please contact us immediately*** at _____. We will take all necessary steps to correct any deficiencies.

We appreciate this opportunity to serve one of your client families and trust that everything meets with your satisfaction.

Special Notes : _____

Enclosed Items:
The following items have been enclosed within the casket:

☐ Register Book

☐ Thank-You cards

☐ Memorial Folders/Prayer Cards

☐ Flower cards

☐ Personal effects (clothing, etc.)

☐ Crucifix/Cross

☐ Flag

☐ Death Certificates

☐ Other

Note: Burial/Transit permit located in head tag envelope.

Thank you for your assistance. If you have concerns about remains, casket or its contents contact us immediately at _____.

Remains reviewed by:

_____
(shipping embalmer)

Figure 1–8. Attention funeral director. (**Courtesy of Kates-Boylston Publications, Wall NJ, 2006.**)

DECENT CARE REPORT   **SAMPLE ONLY**

Date: _____   Case Number: _____

HISTORY & DESCRIPTION

Name of Deceased: _____

Place of Death: _____

Date: _____ Time: _____ Age: _____ Sex: _____ Race: _____ Approx. Height: _____

Approx. Weight: _____ **Identification on body:** _____

Received at Funeral Home: Date: _____ Time: _____ **In House:** _____ **Ship-In:** _____ **Ship-Out:** _____

Permission to Embalm received on the _____ day of _____, 20__ from: _____

Description of personal items **on the body:** itemize on personal effects envelope; place effects in envelope.
Pacemaker _____ Yes _____ No: Permission to remove for cremation _____ Yes _____ No

CONDITION OF BODY PRIOR TO: ( ) STORAGE: ( ) EMBALMING: ( ) PREPARATION WITHOUT EMBALMING

___ Abrasions*	___ Decubitus Ulcers	___ Gangrene*	___ Surgical drains*
___ Amputation	___ Dehydration	___ Hematoma*	___ Surgical Incision*
___ Ascites	___ Dentures (Upper/Lower)	___ Infectious Disease	___ Swelling*+ Cause
___ Autopsy	___ Discoloration (Face/Hands)	___ IV Leak*	___ Tattoos*
___ Bruising*	___ Distention*	___ Laceration (s)	___ Tissue Gas*
___ Burns*	___ Dropsical (anasarca)	___ Jaundice*	___ Tracheotomy
___ Catheter, IV	___ Ecchymosis	___ Livor Mortis	___ Trauma*
___ Catheter, Urinary	___ Edema* (local)	___ Purge	___ Tumor*
___ Cast*	___ Emaciation*	___ Refrigerated ___ Frozen	
___ Clean Shaven (men)	___ Facial Hair* (men)	___ Rigor mortis*	**TREATMENTS**
___ Colostomy	___ Feeding Tube	___ Scars*	Topical disinfectant used:
___ Decomposition*	___ Fractures*	___ Sink Slip*	_____

* Note Location and/or Description on back of form or separate sheet   ___ Orifices Packed

ORGAN / TISSUE DONATION: _____ Yes _____ No (If Yes, attach paperwork from recovery team.)

EMBALMING TECHNIQUES

Primary Injection: ___One Point   ___Split Injection   ___Six Point   ___Restricted Cervical

Other arteries injected: _____

Arteries Injected: ___Axillary R – L ___Brachial R – L ___Carotid R – L ___Femoral R – L

    ___Iliac R – L ___Radial R – L ___Subclavian R – L ___Ulnar R – L

Drainage: ___Femoral R – L ___Jugular R – L ___Post (Autopsy)

Drainage Technique: ___Concurrent ___Intermittent ___Alternate

Mouth Closure: ___Mandibular Suture ___Muscular Suture ___Needle Injector ___Dental Tie

    ___Cotton ___Mouth Former ___Dentures (Upper/Lower) ___Natural Teeth

Eye Closure: ___Eye Caps ___Cotton ___Other

Fluid Dilutions:

Pre-injection: _____ oz.	Type: _____	
Humectant: _____ oz.	Type: _____	
Co-injection: _____ oz.	Type: _____	
Dye: _____ oz.	Type: _____	
Arterial: _____ oz.	Type: _____	Index: _____
Arterial: _____ oz.	Type: _____	Index: _____
Arterial: _____ oz.	Type: _____	Index: _____

Total Gallons of Fluid Injected: _____

Figure 1–9. Embalming decedent care report. (**Courtesy of Michael Weakland, Pittsburgh, Pennsylvania, 2010, with permission.**)

Hypodermic Treatment: ____Fingers ____Hands ____Face ____Legs ____Torso____Other:_____

Surface Treatment (Manner & Location)**:** _____

Purge During Injection: ____ Yes ____ No   (Location & Treatment): _____

Cavity Treatments: Cavity Fluid: _____oz.   Type: _____

Aspiration: ____ Delayed ____ Immediate   **Re-aspiration:** ____ Yes ____ No

Autopsy: ___Cranial __ Thoracic __ Abdominal __Neck organs__Tongue **Viscera Returned:** ____ Yes ____ No

Disposition of Viscera: _____

Plastic Garments: ___Coverall __Pants __ Capri Garment __ Sleeves __ Stockings ___ Unionall

PREPARATION TIME: Beginning: _____ AM PM   Ending: _____ AM PM

Condition & Comments of Body after Embalming   also   Describe ALL Restorative and Cosmetic Treatments

_____

_____

_____

_____

_____

_____

_____

_____

_____

_____

_____

_____

_____

_____

_____

_____

Embalmers Signature: _____   Date: _____

Hairdresser: _____

Restoration: _____

Cosmetics: _____

Dressing & Casketing: _____

Figure 1–9. (*Continued*)

▶ CONCEPTS FOR STUDY AND DISCUSSION

1. Discuss the value of embalming the dead human body.
2. Embalming is defined as the "temporary preservation" of the dead human body. Discuss how long **should** an embalmed body remain in a recognizable preserved condition?
3. Discuss some of the reasons why embalming, as part of the American funeral, has declined during the past number of years.
4. Discuss some of the causes of death that must be reported to the coroner or medical examiner in your state or community.
5. Discuss the difference between the "cause of death" and the "manner of death."
6. Discuss the difference between "organ donation" and "tissue donation."
7. Discuss the FTC rule for obtaining permission for embalming a body.
8. Under the FTC rule, give the choices a family may have for disposition when they do not wish to give permission for embalming.
9. Under the statutes and rules and regulations of your state, when **must** a body be embalmed?
10. Under the statutes and the rules and regulations of your state, give a list of reasons that the license of an embalmer can be suspended or revoked.
11. List all of the documents that your funeral home should use for the following situations – be as complete as possible: (a) a local death, embalming requested, viewing the embalmed body present followed by cremation; (b) a local death, request for an immediate cremation of the body; (c) a body shipped to your establishment from another funeral home, your firm sells the casket, and burial in a local cemetery; (d) you are called by an out-of-state funeral firm to remove, embalm, and ship a body to them.

▶ BIBLIOGRAPHY

Duncan L. Funerals are for the living. *Women's Health* March 1986:28.

Federal Trade Commission: Funeral Rule: 16CFR Part 453.

Gladstone WE. *Dictionary of Thoughts.* New York: Standard Books, Inc., 1974:213.

Holy Bible, Revised Standard Version. New York: Thomas Nelson and Sons, 1952.

Irion PE. *The Funeral: Vestige or Value?* Nashville, TN: The Parthenon Press, 1966.

Lindemann E. Psychological aspects of mourning. Cited in: Jackson E. *For the Living.* Des Moines, IA: The Channel Press, 1963.

Lynch T. *Bodies in Motion and at Rest.* New York: W.W. Norton, 2000.

Organ and Tissue Procurement Manual. Pittsburgh, PA: Pittsburgh Transplant Foundation, 1987.

Resource Manual. Brookfield, WI: National Funeral Directors Association, 1979.

Roach M. *Stiff: The Curious Lives of Human Cadavers.* New York: W.W. Norton, 2003.

Solecki RS, Leroi-Gourhan A. Paleoclimatology and archeology in the Near East. *Annals of the New York Academy of Sciences* 1961;Vol. XCV(Art. 1):729–739.

Undertaking Ethics. Springfield, IL: Funeral Ethics Association, 1994.

CHAPTER 2

FUNDAMENTALS OF EMBALMING

CHAPTER OBJECTIVES

▶ Classifications of Embalming
▶ Suggested Embalming Protocols
▶ Preparation for Viewing Without Embalming
▶ Minimum Care of the Body Without Embalming
▶ Decedent - Care Document

▶ TERMINOLOGY

- **Embalming***—process of chemically treating the dead human body to reduce the presence and growth of microorganisms, retard organic decomposition, and restore an acceptable physical appearance
- **Embalm**—(14c)[†] (1): to treat (a dead body) so as to protect from decay; (2): to fill with sweet odors: **perfume**; (3): to protect from decay or oblivion: **preserve**; (4): to fix in a static condition—**embalmer** n—embalmment n
- **Decay**—(15c)[†] (1): to undergo destructive dissolution; (2): implies a slow change from a state of soundness
- **Decay***—decomposition of proteins by enzymes of aerobic bacteria
- **Decompose**—(ca. 1751)[†] (1): to separate into constituent parts or elements or into simpler compounds; (2): to break up into constituent parts or as if by a chemical process: decay—**decomposition** n
- **Decomposition***—separation of compounds into simpler substances by the action of microbial and/or autolytic enzymes
- **Enzyme**—(1881)[†] complex proteins that are produced by cells which act as a biological catalyst

- **Preserve**—(14c)[†] (1): to keep safe from injury, harm, or destruction: **protect**; (2a): to keep intact or free from decay; (2b): **maintain**; (3): to keep or save from decomposition—**preservation** n
- **Preservation***—the science of treating the dead human body chemically so as to temporarily inhibit decomposition
- **Preservative**—(15c)[†] (1): something that preserves or has the power of preserving; (2): an additive used to protect against decay, discoloration, or spoilage
- **Preservative***—chemicals that inactivate saprophytic bacteria, render unsuitable for nutrition the media upon which such bacteria thrive, and that will arrest decomposition by altering enzymes and lysins of the body as well as converting the decomposable tissue to a form less susceptible to decomposition
- **Protein**—(1844)[†] one of a class of complex nitrogenous compounds that are synthesized by all living organisms and yield amino acids when hydrolyzed
- **Putrefaction**—(14c)[†] (1): the decomposition of organic matter; (2): the typically anaerobic splitting of proteins by bacteria and fungi with the formation of foul-smelling incompletely oxidized products

---

*From the American Board of Funeral Service Education, embalming course content syllabus, 2001.

[†]Date of earliest recorded use in English: **Merriam-Webster's Collegiate Dictionary,** 11th ed, 2003.

- **Putrefaction***—decomposition of proteins by the action of enzymes from anaerobic bacteria
- **Sanitation**—(1848)[†] a process to promote and establish conditions that minimize or eliminate biohazards
- **Substrate**—(1807)[†] a substance acted upon (e.g., protein, fat, carbohydrate), as by an enzyme in the living organism, or embalming chemicals in preserving the dead body
- **Stabilize**—To prevent or retard an unwanted alteration of a physical state. Slowing the onset of the changes of decomposition by the use of refrigeration, dry or wet ice, and the injection of non-formaldehyde fluids.

Embalming is an applied chemical process used to bring about the preservation and sanitation of the dead human body. The terms **embalming** and **preservation** indicate an indefinite perpetuity of the body, and there are such documented results. However, embalming, as practiced in funeral service today, provides a temporary preservation of the human dead, allowing time for society to perform secular and religious rites and ceremonies. Embalming permits the presence of the human dead at the funeral or ceremony of farewell. Embalming purchases time.

Preservation of the dead human body can occur without chemical treatment under certain natural conditions, dependent on such elements as temperature, moisture, and the surrounding environment. For more than 5500 years, documentation shows that the art and science of embalming by chemical means has been practiced in one form or another. Today, preservation for anatomic or museum study can maintain the integrity of the body for many years. These bodies do not always maintain the recognizable condition they had in life. (See Section II, **The Origin and History of Embalming**.)

The American Board of Funeral Service Education, in defining the term **embalming**, summarizes the procedure as practiced within our society today as "the process of **chemically** treating the dead human body to **reduce** the presence and growth of microorganisms, to **retard** organic decomposition, and to restore an **acceptable** physical appearance." As practiced in the United States and other developed countries, embalming purports to do more than simply preserve the visage of the deceased. The embalmed body should not be offensive to the senses. The preserved body can, if necessary, be moved long distances.

Decomposition is defined as "the separation of compounds into simpler substances by the action of microbial enzymes and/or autolytic enzymes." It begins at death. Embalming retards decomposition. Indefinite preservation, by using standard embalming procedures, is not possible. The length of time during which the body will remain as a preserved recognizable entity by standard funeral service embalming is dependent upon various factors both within the body (intrinsic) and outside of the body (extrinsic). Intrinsic factors include the pathologic processes inside the body, circulatory conditions, amount of body moisture, distribution of the preservative chemicals, and so on. Extrinsic factors include the type of preservatives used, strength and volume of embalming chemicals, and climate and environment within the burial chamber (casket and vault or casket and crypt), such as amount of moisture, molds, bacteria, insects, and air. Under more ideal conditions, the embalmed body may be preserved for a temporary period of time, and some bodies may be preserved for many years. Conversely, under unfavorable conditions, the preservation may be as brief as several days. Science has no way to determine the degree or length of time that preservation of the embalmed body can be maintained.

▶ PRESERVATION AND SANITATION

Embalming preservatives and germicides interact primarily on body proteins. The colloidal nature of the protein changes by establishing many cross-linkages that were not formerly present between adjacent proteins. The chemicals and the proteins combine to form a latticework of inert firm material—the **embalmed tissue**—that can no longer be easily broken down by bacterial or autolytic body enzymes.

Body proteins have many reactive centers and a great affinity to hold water. Embalming destroys these reactive centers, and the new protein-like substance no longer has the ability to retain water. As a result, these new (embalmed) protein structures are more stable and longer-lasting. Thus, the tissues are temporarily preserved. The inability of the embalmed tissue to hold water results in a dryness to the embalmed tissue.

Enzymes have the ability to react with the body proteins, fats, and carbohydrates and cause the decomposition of these body substrates. Enzymes are proteins and they originate from body cells (autolytic enzymes) or bacteria (bacterial enzymes). Chemicals such as germicides and preservatives in embalming fluids effect and inactivate the body enzymes. These same chemicals also destroy bacteria (pathogenic and nonpathogenic) through reactions with the proteins that are a part of these organisms. Thus, the embalmed body becomes sanitized. The likelihood of the body remaining a source of disease-producing microbes or their products is greatly reduced. Through conversion or inactivation (embalming) of (1) protein of the tissues, (2) protein of enzymes, and (3) protein of microbes, the body is sanitized and temporarily preserved. The degree of preservation depends on the number of contacts made between the preservative chemicals and the proteins of the body and the bacteria.

▶ RESTORATION

Restoration of the deceased to an acceptable appearance is also a goal of embalming. Restoration of the dead human body is not so much to make the deceased look lifelike but rather to try to lessen the evidence of devastation caused by long-term disease and illness, extended use of drug therapies, surgery, tumors, trauma, disfigurements, and postmortem changes, which have affected those areas of the body that will be viewed. Injection of the proper embalming chemicals can (1) restore facial tissues, (2) decrease facial swellings, (3) remove postmortem intravascular discolorations, (4) reduce extravascular blood discolorations, and (5) restore natural facial coloring.

▶ CLASSIFICATIONS OF EMBALMING

There are four embalming treatment classifications: **vascular embalming, cavity embalming, hypodermic embalming,** and **surface embalming.** It is possible that one or all four types of treatments can be used in the embalming of an autopsied or unautopsied body.

Vascular (arterial) embalming is the use of the blood vascular system of the body to accomplish temporary preservation, sanitation, and restoration of the dead human body; this is accomplished through injection of an embalming chemical solution into the arteries and drainage of blood from the veins. This method of embalming can be used to preserve the entire body, large body sections, or localized body areas. **Cavity embalming** is the direct treatment, other than vascular injection, of the contents of the body cavities (thoracic, abdominal, and pelvic) and the lumina of the hollow viscera; it is usually accomplished in two phases (aspiration and injection) using a long, hollow instrument called a "trocar." **Hypodermic embalming** is the injection of embalming chemicals directly into the tissues of the dead human body through the use of a syringe and needle (for small areas) or a trocar (for large body areas). This is generally a supplemental embalming procedure used when tissues in the adult body cannot be treated sufficiently by vascular injection. **Surface embalming** is preservation of the body tissues by direct contact with embalming chemicals. Preservative gels or surface packs of absorbent materials saturated with preservative chemicals can be directly placed in contact with the body tissues. Surface embalming is considered a supplemental treatment to vascular injection and is used when vascular injection is unsuccessful or impossible.

Arterial and Cavity Embalming

Through the use of arterial and cavity embalming treatments, complete preservation of the unautopsied body can be accomplished. Arterial (vascular) embalming makes use of the blood vascular system. During arterial embalming, a preservative chemical solution is injected into a major artery(s), and while this is being done the blood is displaced and simultaneously drained from a vein.

Cavity embalming is performed after arterial embalming. It is the direct treatment of the contents of the body cavities (abdominal, thoracic, and pelvic) and the materials in the lumen of the hollow viscera. This is carried out by first **aspirating** the cavities followed by **injecting** concentrated chemicals into the cavities. Both processes use a trocar.

A working description might state that embalming of the unautopsied body is performed in two stages: Stage one is arterial injection (vascular profusion) and stage two is cavity embalming. Arterial embalming consists of injection of 3 to 4 gallons of preservative solution (made by mixing concentrated embalming fluid and water), under pressure, into the circulatory system of the dead human body through a large artery (e.g., carotid, femoral). Blood and a portion of the injected solution are concurrently removed from a large (e.g., internal jugular, femoral) vein to provide room for the preservatives. The preservative solution flows through the arterial, capillary, and venous routes in basically the same course followed by blood in the living body, a basic difference being that the embalming solution does not pass through the heart. The solution travels to the ascending aorta where it places pressure on the aortic semilunar valves, forcing them to close. After the valves are tightly shut, the ascending aorta, arch of the aorta, and the entire aorta get filled with the preservative solution, which now flows into the branches of the circulatory system.

The capillary is the simplest division of the blood vascular system; it is the structural mediator through which the injected preservative chemicals are delivered to the receptive tissue sites. In this sense, arterial embalming might be referred to as **capillary embalming.** Capillaries are simple tubes, whose walls are a single layer of endothelial cells. The capillaries have an average diameter of 7 to 9 micrometers and they connect the terminal arterioles and the venules. The surface area of the capillary network in the human body approaches 6000 square meters or 64,585 square feet. This vast membrane of more than 1.5 acres is the permeable barrier that controls the delivery of preserving and disinfecting chemicals to deep and superficial body tissues. The circulatory system of humans normally contains 5 to 6 quarts of blood, or 8% of the body weight, 85% of which is contained within the capillaries. Obviously, thorough profusion of the soft tissue sites with appropriate concentrations of injection chemicals involves far more than filling the aorta and its primary branches. A portion of the embalming solution passes through the capillaries and enters the tissue spaces. Finally, it is here that the preservative solution will make contact with the cells of the tissues and the body protein.

Cavity embalming is the treatment of the contents of the abdominal and thoracic cavities. Many of these organs are hollow and their contents are not reached by the preservative solution. The contents of these hollow organs along with any liquids or gases that may have accumulated in the body cavities are suctioned out by a process called **aspiration.** A long, hollow, needlelike instrument called a "trocar" is inserted through the abdominal wall. The trocar is used to pierce all abdominal and thoracic organs and all areas of the cavities. After aspirating the contents such as liquids, gases, and semisolids, the cavity fluid is injected into the abdominal and thoracic cavities using the trocar. Cavity fluid is a very concentrated preservative. Under most conditions, approximately 32 to 48 oz of cavity fluid is introduced into the cavities. In some situations, several hours later, the embalmer will reaspirate and possibly reinject the cavities. This is an insurance against a purge of gas or liquid from the nose or the mouth.

Hypodermic and Surface Embalming

Hypodermic embalming is the subcuticular injection of a suitable preservative chemical directly into the tissues. The chemical may be injected by a syringe and a needle, or a variety of trocars. The area of treatment may be localized, such as a finger or area of the cheek, or may be extensive, such as in the abdominal and chest walls (in the autopsied body), or an entire lower extremity. Hypodermic treatment is employed when preservative chemicals do not reach an area by arterial embalming.

Surface embalming is the application of an embalming chemical directly to the surface of the tissues. Embalming chemicals are applied as a spray in aerosol form, painted on the surface by brush in the form of a liquid or gel, or applied on cotton as a surface compress. The preservative can be applied to the skin surface or under the skin in areas such as the eyelids and the mouth. With autopsied bodies, the preservative can be applied to the inner surfaces of the cavity walls and the undersurface of the cranial scalp.

Summary and Expectations of the Embalming Process

In 1928, Professor Charles O. Dhonau, dean of the Cincinnati College of Embalming, defined the functions of embalming fluid and the process by which the fluid reaches the cells of the body. He further explained how the fluid functions to achieve sanitation, preservation, and restoration of the body's tissues. This definition, as relevant today as it was more than 70 years ago, serves well to explain the entire embalming process. The definition reads as follows:

An embalming fluid is a chemical substance
which when given physical application (or injection)
at the right time
at the right temperature
in the right quantity
of the right quality, strength dilution, concentration
so as to receive a complete distribution in arteries,
    capillaries and veins
will diffuse (spread) from the capillaries
to the lymph spaces and to the intercellular spaces
and to the cellular tissues
to unite with the cellular substances
so as to normalize their water content
restore their colors
and so to fix and preserve them that they will be pre-
    served against organized (bacterial)
and unorganized (enzymatic) decompositions
and will be preserved against other kinds of changes
such as in water content; oxidation; from soil chemi-
    cals
just so long as the after-care provides the necessary
    means to protect
what has been embalmed.
A part which has been embalmed will not discolor
from any cause within several weeks; it will not be-
    come
blood discolored; or show dehydration changes;
or show greenish colors from protein decomposi-
    tions;
or become malodorous from protein decomposi-
    tions;
by proteolytic bacterial enzymes by which spore form-
    ing
anaerobes, seeking (bound) oxygen, break up com-
    pounds
containing it and release odorous gasses such as hy-
    drogen sulfide;
or become gas distended from the gaseous decom-
    position of proteins
or carbohydrates (tissue gas); nor will the tissues
    soften and finally liquefy
through the work of organized or unorganized fer-
    ments;
nor will the tissues of the body pass through the cycle
    of changes
which at the end converts the hundred or more body
    compounds into
water, nitrogen, methane and carbon dioxide, as a
    result of all the
oxidations through which decompositions proceed.
A part which has
not been properly embalmed should be thought of
    by the embalmer

as an unsolved embalming problem, to which he or she has

contributed either by lack of understanding, by carelessness or by both.

Cincinnati College of Mortuary Science, 1928, with permission.

From Dhonau CO. **Defining Embalming Fluid**. File 100. Cincinnati, OH.

► ANATOMICAL EMBALMING

The embalming of bodies used for dissection by medical colleges varies from that used for funeral ceremonies. The medical school remains will be kept for several months, and in many situations, for several years. Preservation and sanitation of the tissues are of primary concern, not the appearance of the body. The procedure varies among the medical schools, some even permit embalming for funeral services, but with certain restrictions such as not allowing for cavity embalming, in which case the school will later reembalm the body.

In general, the body willed to a medical college is prepared for embalmment by application of a sanitizing agent in the topical for washing and disinfecting the body. One artery is used for injection of the preservative chemicals; cavity treatment is not performed. The body may or may not be drained of blood. A solution, ranging in volume from 4 to 9 gallons, depending on the size and condition of the body, is injected using a mixture of alcohol, formalin, phenol, wetting agent, and water.

Often, drainage is restricted which allows the tissues to greatly expand as a large volume of solution is injected. This swelling will recede over time as the solution saturates the cavities and tissues. During dissection, additional chemicals may be sprayed or applied as packs on the exposed tissues. These solutions will aid in preventing dehydration and formation of mold. There are more costly and complex methods used by medical colleges and museums for the preservation of organic material; examples include, freeze-drying, vulcanization, and plastination.

► EMBALMING CARE REPORT

Michael Kubasak writes, "the number one reason for lawsuits deals with claims of negligence in rendering professional care to the body of deceased persons. Documentation is essential, especially when dealing with special requests or trauma-difficult circumstances . . . document, document, document!"*

*Kubasak M. **Traversing the Minefield Best Practice: Reducing the Risk in Funeral-Cremation Service,** Malibu, CA: LMG Publishing, 2007.

An embalming care report is a very important document that should be completed for each body. **The embalming care report should be completed for each decedent that comes into the custody of a funeral home or an embalming facility irrespective of whether or not the body is embalmed.** Applicable portions of the report should be completed if the body is not embalmed, for example, identification of the body and description of the postmortem appearance of the remains. If minimal preparation was performed for identification, the body needs to be identified and postmortem conditions noted and a description of any treatments performed. The full report needs to be completed if the body is embalmed for local disposition or shipped to another funeral facility. The embalming report can be of significant value in situations of trauma if the embalmer's testimony as to the condition of the body is necessary in legal proceedings.

When the body is being prepared for shipment, a copy of the report should accompany the remains. **Embalming care reports should be filled out in detail and kept as a permanent record of the funeral home or the embalming facility.** The report should provide information to accurately describe (1) the condition of the body before preparation, (2) manner and methods of the preparation, (3) any postembalming treatments, and (4) date and time of arrival of the body into the funeral home or the embalming facility, starting and ending times of the preparation, and the name and license number of the embalmer and any who assisted in the preparation. Sample embalming care reports are shown in Figure 2–1 and Figure 1–9.

► EMBALMING SEQUENCE

The following embalming chronologies provide an overview of the embalming of autopsied and unautopsied bodies. First, several basics apply to the preparation of all bodies.

- The use of universal precautions and personal protective equipment by the embalmer and any assistants is necessary for the preparation of all bodies—bodies dead from noncontagious, contagious, and/or infectious disease.
- All bodies need to be identified. Check identification on the body—wristbands and toe tags. The funeral home or the embalming facility should also place its own identification tag or band on the body.

All bodies need to be sanitized using a disinfectant topical droplet spray and bathed with a germicidal soap solution. Even the clothing needs to be sprayed with a

(*text continues on page 40*)

EMBALMING REPORT
(Confidential)

Embalmer _____   Master No.: _____

Assisted by _____

FUNERAL HOME _____ IN-HOUSE _____ SHIP-IN _____ SHIP-OUT _____

DATE _____ TIME _____ PERMISSION TO EMBALM _____

PROTECTIVE ATTIRE WORN _____ COMMUNICABLE DISEASE _____

NAME _____ DATE OF DEATH _____ TIME OF DEATH _____

CAUSE OF DEATH _____ DOCTOR/MEDICAL-EXAMINER _____

PERSONAL EFFECTS ON BODY _____

AGE _____ SEX _____ RACE _____ HEIGHT _____ WEIGHT _____ FACIAL HAIR _____

NATURAL TEETH _____ DENTURES _____ NO DENTURES _____ OTHER _____

DESCRIBE HAIR _____ DISTINGUISHING MARKS _____

CONDITIONS PRIOR TO EMBALMING

GENERAL: CLEAN _____ REFRIGERATED _____ RIGOR MORTIS _____ SURGERY _____

EVIDENCE OF DISEASE _____ EVIDENCE OF TRAUMA _____ TRACHEOTOMY _____ PACEMAKER _____

I.V. PUNCTURE(S) _____ STOMACH FEEDING TUBE _____ COLOSTOMY _____ GAS IN TISSUES _____

SKIN SLIP _____ CATHETER (URINARY) _____ DISCOLORATION(S) _____ PURGE _____

OTHER _____

FACE: NORMAL _____ EMACIATED _____ SWOLLEN _____ TRAUMA _____ EDEMA _____ GAS IN TISSUES _____ LESIONS _____

SKIN-SLIP _____ TUBE MARKS _____ DISCOLORATION(S) _____

OTHER _____

AUTOPSEY: CRANIAL _____ THORACIC _____ ABDOMINAL _____ PELVIC _____ SPINAL _____

NECK ORGANS REMOVED _____ TONGUE REMOVED _____ PARTIAL AUTOPSY _____ EYES DRAINED _____ EYE(S) REMOVED _____

VISCERA RETURNED WITH BODY _____ PLACEMENT OF VISCERA (AFTER EMBALMING) _____

TISSUES SAMPLES TAKEN (IF NO AUTOPSY PERFORMED) _____

ORGAN DONOR: _____ DESCRIBE _____

ENUCLEATION (WHOLE EYE) _____ CORNEA ONLY _____

PREPARATION OF THE BODY

SURFACE DISINFECTION _____ BODY WASHED _____ HAIR WASHED _____ NAILS CLEANED _____

NOSTRILS TRIMMED _____ FACE SHAVED _____ METHOD OF EYE CLOSURE _____

MOUTH SUPPORT IF USED _____ METHOD OF MOUTH CLOSURE _____

ALL ORIFICES DISINFECTED AND PACKED _____

Figure 2–1. Sample embalming care report.

PRESERVATIVE TREATMENTS

I. PRIMARY INJECTION PLAN [ARTERY(S)]:

    a. One-point injection _____

    b. Restricted cervical injection _____

    c. Six-point injection _____

    d. Other (describe) _____

    _____

    _____

    TOTAL VOLUME OF SOLUTION INJECTED _____

    SOLUTION MIXTURES USED _____
    (indicate Solution Gallon #)

    DRAINAGE SITE _____

    DRAINAGE METHOD _____

II. IF THE HEAD IS SEPARATELY EMBALMED (RESTRICTED CERVICAL OR AUTOPSY): _____

    SOLUTION MIXTURE USED _____

    VOLUME INJECTED _____

III. AREA(S) RECEIVING AN INADEQUATE AMOUNT OF ARTERIAL SOLUTION: _____

IV. SUPPLEMENTAL ARTERY(S) INJECTED: _____

    TOTAL VOLUME OF SOLUTION INJECTED _____

    SOLUTION MIXTURES USED _____
    (indicate Solution Gallon #)

V. SUPPLEMENTAL EMBALMING TREATMENTS (HYPODERMIC, COMPRESSES, GELS, ETC.) _____

VI. CAVITY TREATMENT (UNAUTOPSIED): IMMEDIATE ASPIRATION _____ ; DELAYED ASPIRATION _____

    NAME OF FLUID INJECTED _____ VOLUME INJECTED _____

ARTERIAL FLUIDS AND SOLUTIONS

FLUID COMPANY AND NAME:

    A. WATER

    B. PRE-INJECTION _____

    C. ARTERIAL #1 _____

    D. ARTERIAL #2 _____

    E. CO-INJECTION _____

    F. WATER SOFTENER _____

    G. HUMECTANT _____

    H. DYE _____

    I. OTHER _____

ARTERIAL SOLUTIONS (MEASURED IN OUNCES PER GALLON; 1 GALLON = 128 FLUID OUNCES) PLACE THE LETTER OF THE FLUID FROM THE LIST ABOVE IN THE LEFT COLUMN; IN THE RIGHT COLUMN PUT THE NUMBER OF OUNCES USED.

GALLON #1	GALLON #2	GALLON #3	GALLON #4	GALLON #5
A__ ___ (oz)	A__ ___ (oz)	A__ ___ (oz)	A__ ___ (oz)	A__ ___ (oz)
___ ___	___ ___	___ ___	___ ___	___ ___
___ ___	___ ___	___ ___	___ ___	___ ___
___ ___	___ ___	___ ___	___ ___	___ ___
___ ___	___ ___	___ ___	___ ___	___ ___

COMPLETION

AREA(S) OF DISTENSION RESULTING FROM ARTERIAL INJECTION _____

PURGE DURING ARTERIAL INJECTION [DESCRIBE] _____

PURGE TREATMENT _____

EYELIDS GLUED _____ LIPS GLUED _____ INCISION SEAL POWDER _____ INCISIONS GLUED _____

PLASTICS USED: _____ ; EMBALMING POWDER IN PLASTICS _____

Figure 2–1. (*Continued*)

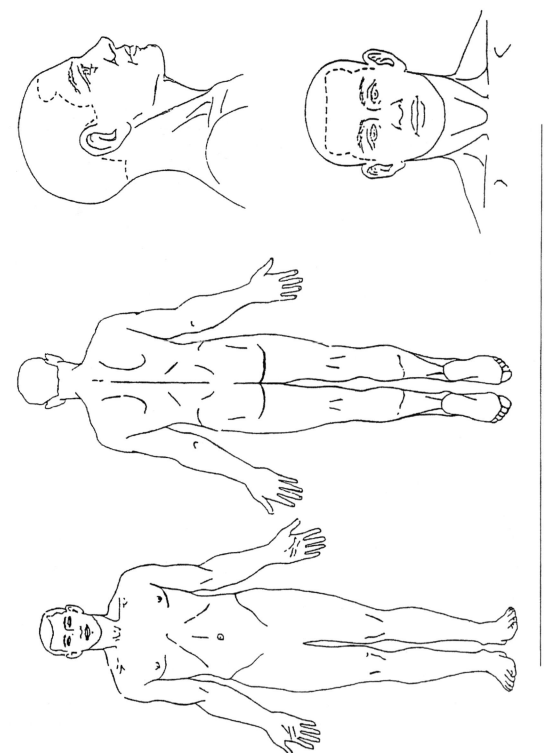

MARK POINTS OF INTEREST &
PLACE COMMENTS ON THE BACK PAGE

Figure 2–1. (*Continued*)

DESCRIPTION OF RESTORATIVE TREATMENTS

DESCRIPTION OF COSMETIC TREATMENTS

SHIP-IN CONDITIONS AND CORRECTIONS

Body received from: _____   City/State _____

Describe problem conditions and their correction:

COMMENTS

Figure 2–1. (*Continued*)

disinfectant prior to removal. Check expiry date of the disinfectants and the duration of contact necessary for them to be the most effective. All contaminated items such as medical waste and body bags need to be disposed of in a biohazard container.

- A decedent care report needs to be completed for each body brought into the funeral home or the embalming facility.
- Embalming analysis is necessary before, during, and after an arterial injection. While in the custody of the funeral facility, the body should continue to be monitored for any postembalming changes.
- The body should be covered at all times, say before and following the embalming process. A modest cloth may be used to cover the genitals during embalming.
- The exhaust ventilation system needs to be in full operation during the embalming process.

Suggested Chronology for Embalming an Unautopsied Adult Body

It should be noted that t he sequence of steps used in embalming does not have to be taken in this recommended order. For example, features of the body (eyes and mouth) can be set before, during, or after arterial embalming. Many embalmers prefer to suture incisions after cavity embalming; aspiration of the organs relieves the pressure on the vascular system and reduces the chance of incision leakage.

After the body has been placed on the embalming table, the following steps are suggested:

1. Remove all clothing from the body. Clothing should be sanitized by application of a disinfectant spray prior to removal. The mouth can be covered with a mask or cotton placed in the oral cavity, so residual air or purge will not escape while undressing
   a. Soiled clothing should either be destroyed or laundered for return to the family.
   b. Contaminated bedding (such as sheets and hospital gowns) should be destroyed or properly laundered.
2. Examine and document any valuables such as watches, rings, rosary beads, and so forth. Valuables should be removed, documented, and stored in a secure place.
3. Disinfect the body using a droplet spray or a disinfectant solution that is sponged onto the body. **Allow time for the disinfectant to work.** Disinfect, clean, and pack all body orifices. A nasal tube aspirator may assist with cleansing of the mouth, throat, and nasal passages.

4. Position the body. Limbs, hands, and facial tissues can be massaged, flexed, bent, rotated, and exercised to relieve the rigor mortis, if present. Elevate the head above the chest and elevate the chest above the abdomen. Slightly tilt the head to the right. The hands can remain at the sides or even down over the table at this point to allow gravitation of blood into the hands, which helps to expand the vessels. Once arterial injection has begun and the hands show signs of fluid distribution, they can be placed in the correct position. Special blocking (using head blocks or towels) may be necessary for arthritic conditions or where limbs have atrophied. Attempt to straighten the arthritic limbs by wrapping them with cloth strips. It is not recommended that any tissue be incised to extend limbs.
5. Wash the body surface using a germicidal, warm-water soapy solution, giving particular attention to face and hands. Shampoo the hair and clean and trim the fingernails. A solvent may be necessary to remove surface stains such as gentian violet or Betadine antiseptic.
6. Shave facial hair. If there is a mustache, goatee, or beard on the deceased, check whether it is to be removed or groomed. If there is any doubt, **do not** remove the facial hair for it can be shaved after embalming once the family has been consulted. (On the first-call information sheet the following question should be asked, for a man, "Are there any instructions regarding facial hair?") Facial hair should also be removed from women and children.
7. Close the mouth, using an appropriate method, such as a needle injector or sutures. If the decedent's dentures are to be used they should be cleaned and disinfected. If dentures or teeth are absent, a mouth former, cotton, or mastic compound can be used as a filler.
   a. If fever blisters are present on the lips or if there is crusted material along the eyelashes, use a soft cloth, gauze, or cotton moistened with warm water to easily remove them. A solvent such as the "dry hair washes" or massage cream can be used to remove scabs, or fever blisters, and to cleanse the skin.
   b. Care should be taken at this point to straighten the nostrils with cotton and to carefully remove visible nostril hairs.
   c. Some embalmers prefer at this time to place a light coating of massage cream over the face, hands, and neck. The cream should not be placed over discolored areas where opaque cosmetics will later be applied.

d. Surface compresses of bleach (phenol or formaldehyde) can be placed on blood or pathologic discolorations at this time. (Some embalmers prefer to do this after the arterial injection.)

8. Clean and close the eyes using cotton or an "eyecap."

9. Select and expose the artery to be used for injection and the vein to be used for drainage.

10. Select the arterial fluids and prepare the embalming solution.

11. Inject the embalming solution. The pressure and rate of flow of the injection are determined by the embalming analysis. Monitor the injection of fluid and look for signs of arterial solution distribution. Where fluid is lacking, change the injection methods (e.g., pressure, rate of flow, drainage) or massage the arteries that supply embalming solution to an area to ensure even distribution of solution throughout the body.

Three questions need to be asked at this stage of embalming:

a. Which body areas **are** and which body areas **are not** receiving arterial solution?

b. Should the strength of the solution be increased?

c. Has the body or body area received sufficient arterial solution?

12. When arterial injection is completed, make a visual and palpable (by touch) analysis of the body to determine whether all areas have received sufficient arterial solution. Areas lacking sufficient fluid may be injected by an artery witch supplies that area. In addition, areas that cannot be reached by arterial injection (e.g., gangrenous limbs) can be embalmed using hypodermic injection and surface preservation techniques at this stage.

13. Remove arterial tubes and drainage instruments. Tie off the vessels used. Dry and tightly suture incisions. Be certain that incision seal powder is placed in the incision to prevent leakage. Sutured incisions may also be covered with glue after the body is washed and dried.

14. Using a trocar, aspirate the body cavities. Some embalmers prefer to delay aspiration for several hours. The condition of the body helps in deciding whether cavity embalming should be done immediately after arterial injection or several hours later.

15. Following aspiration, inject an undiluted cavity fluid into the cavities using the trocar. Size and condition of the body determine the amount of fluid to inject. For an average body, 32 to 48 oz

of cavity fluid is satisfactory. After cavity fluid injection, close the opening(s) in the abdominal wall using a trocar button or suture.

16. Remove any surgical drains, if present, and close the openings by suture or using a multiclosure trocar button. Dispose of the drains in a biohazard container.

a. Remove all intravenous lines or catheters that enter the circulatory system. After removal of these invasive medical devices, seal the point of entry into the body. Dispose of them in a biohazard waste container.

b. If the body is to be cremated, it will be necessary to remove a pacemaker or other medical devices, if present. Permission should be obtained from the family for this procedure.

c. If a colostomy is present, remove the collecting bag and dispose of it in a biohazard waste container. Disinfect the stoma of the colostomy and surrounding area (a concentrated cavity fluid or phenol cautery can be used for this procedure) and close the stoma by sewing a tight purse string suture.

d. If surgical incisions are present and they have not healed completely, remove the surgical sutures, open, drain, disinfect the site, and close by suturing.

e. Pack the anal orifice with cotton saturated with cavity fluid or autopsy gel. Delaying this treatment until this time allows fecal matter to possibly exit.

17. Again, shampoo the hair and wash the body. Dry the body thoroughly, being certain to roll the body to one side so the back shoulders and buttocks can also be dried. After washing and drying, apply surface glue to all sutured areas. Check the mouth to be certain that it is dry and free from any purge material. If there has been purge or blood in the oral cavity, replace any cotton in the mouth and/or throat with clean dry cotton. The mouth and the eyes can now be sealed shut using a lip glue or a superglue.

18. Dress the body in plastic garments (pants, Capri garment, coveralls, stockings, or a unionall). Place embalming powder inside the garment. Dress or cover the body with a clean sheet.

19. Should reaspiration of the cavities be necessary, it is usually performed several hours after completion of the embalming.

20. Flush and clean the embalming machine with clean water. Clean and disinfect all instruments. Dispose of all waste in appropriately covered containers.

21. Cosmetic treatment can follow.

Suggested Chronology for Embalming an Autopsied Adult Body

Note: The statements immediately preceding "Suggested Chronology for Embalming an Unautopsied Adult Body," concerning **universal precautions, identification, embalming care report, embalming analysis, respect for the body, and use of ventilation systems** apply to the preparation of the autopsied body.

Notation needs to be made in the embalming care report as to the type of autopsy performed; organs and tissues removed; and viscera and personal effects that are **returned** with the body.

The autopsied body, as defined in this chronology, is the adult dead human body where the cranial cavity has been opened and the brain removed; thoracic and abdominal cavities have been opened and all visceral organs removed; contents of the pelvic cavity have been removed; and the neck organs and floor of the mouth and tongue have been removed.

1. Place the autopsied body on the center of the preparation table. Spray the remains with a concentrated droplet surface disinfectant. Wash the body with an antiseptic, liquid soap using warm water. Remove any blood on the skin surface. Carefully clean the hands and fingernails. The hair can be rinsed; however, because of the cranial autopsy, the hair will need rewashing after embalming.

2. Open the autopsy temporary sutures and aspirate any liquids that have accumulated within the cavities. Spray the inside walls of the cavities with a droplet disinfectant spray.

3. Examine the extent of the autopsy. If a partial autopsy (one or more organs have been removed or the contents of one body cavity) has been performed, the extent should be evaluated. If the eyes have been removed, the procedure for treatment can begin at this time. Rigor mortis can be relieved by flexing, bending, and massaging the limbs. Position the body.

4. Shave the facial hair (see item #6 in "Suggested Chronology for Embalming the an Unautopsied Adult Body").

5. Clean the oral cavity and replace dentures or, if they are not available, replace missing teeth or dentures with cotton or a "mouth former." The mouth can be held closed by needle injector wires or sutures. Liberally coat the lips with massage cream, inside the buccal cavity, and on the surface of the face.

    a. If the tongue has been removed, the oral cavity can be tightly packed with cotton saturated with cavity fluid, autopsy gel, or a cautery chemical. This cotton is inserted through the neck into the mouth area once the mouth has been closed. Packing this cotton firmly into the oral cavity will assist in preventing the loss of arterial fluid during injection from severed arteries.

6. Clean the areas around the eyes. The eyes can be closed using cotton or an "eyecap."(If the eyes or corneas have been removed, the orbits should be cleaned and a preservative gel or liquid preservative on cotton can be placed into the orbits and the eyelids closed.)

7. Prepare the arterial solution. Strength and quantity depend on conditions of the body. This is established by making an embalming analysis.

8. During arterial injection, fluids that accumulate in the cavities should be aspirated. This will help to protect the embalmer from formaldehyde fumes.

9. Expose the arteries that will be used to inject the legs and their respective veins. Place the arterial tubes into the arteries. Drainage will be done by letting the drainage collect in the body cavities.

10. Inject the legs. Give attention to the distribution of the fluid. Increase pressure or rate of flow to establish a uniform distribution. Areas not reached can be treated by hypodermic injection later. A hemostat can be used to clamp an accompanying vein to control drainage in the hand and help retain the arterial fluid.

11. Expose the arteries that will be used to inject the arms and if possible their accompanying veins—the subclavian arteries or the right and left axillary arteries.

12. Inject the arms. Ascertain good distribution of the fluid is achieved through all the fingers. If distribution is not complete, the radial or ulnar arteries can be raised and injected at this time.

    Drainage can be controlled by the use of a hemostat applied to the accompanying veins. If the subclavian arteries are injected, the respective internal mammary artery and the vertebral artery will need to be clamped to prevent fluid loss.

13. Expose and place arterial tubes into the right and left common carotid arteries. Inject the left side of the head **first and** then inject the right side. Leakage from the internal carotid arteries in the base of the skull can be controlled with hemostats. Leakage from severed branches of the external carotid may also be controlled by hemostats. (If the neck organs and tongue have been removed, cotton saturated with a preservative can be tightly packed into the oral cavity before arterial injection to help control any

leakage from severed vessels during arterial injection.)

14. Prepare a strong preservative solution in the embalming machine. Using a small parietal, infant, or hypo-valve trocar, inject the buttocks, trunk walls, shoulders, and back of the neck (any trunk areas where arterial fluid is absent or insufficient). The trocar can be inserted into the cut skin margins.

15. Aspirate any accumulated fluids and dry the cranial, abdominal, thoracic, and pelvic cavities. A preservative gel or powdered autopsy compound can be applied to the cavity walls.

16. Fill the cavities with an absorbent sheeting. A concentrated preservative such as cavity fluid (or a low-viscosity autopsy gel) can be applied to the surface of the filler—this will allow the filler to act as an internal preservative compress. The neck areas can be filled with cotton or kapok to achieve a natural look; this packing can also be coated with autopsy gel or cavity fluid—the packing will serve as an internal pack to help preserve the neck tissues.

   When the viscera are returned to the thoracic and abdominal cavities, they may be placed in a plastic biohazard bag. The viscera need to be preserved by pouring a concentrated preservative over the organs. Hollow organs can be opened to release any gasses or directly return the organs (without the bag) to the cavities after having first soaked them in a preservative and the excess fluids drained away. If the viscera are returned to the cavities, the neck will have to be packed as mentioned in step #16.*

17. Suture the abdominal and thoracic cavities closed. The baseball suture provides an airtight suture.

18. Fill the cranial cavity with an absorbent material. Anchor the calvarium into position. Suture the scalp closed beginning on the right side of the head and ending on the left. A liberal amount of incision seal powder needs to be placed between the scalp and the calvarium to prevent leakage. A worm suture can be used to close the scalp—it takes up excess skin.

19. Bathe the body and shampoo the hair. The body and hair should be thoroughly dried and the body should be turned and dried underneath.

20. Apply a surface sealer to the autopsy sutures of the thorax and the abdomen.

21. Glue the mouth and the eyes.

22. Dress the body in plastic garments. Place some embalming powder into the garments.

23. The body is now ready for cosmetic application and dressing.

▶ CHRONOLOGY FOR IDENTIFICATION OF THE BODY OR STORAGE IN THE FUNERAL HOME

These guidelines for storage will allow for identification of the body when permission to embalm the body **has not been given.** The guidelines care for the body in such a manner that the body can be stored and once permission **is obtained** the decedent can be embalmed.

Identification of every dead human body received by a funeral establishment is essential. This should be done either by direct confrontation with the body or by identification of a televised image or photograph (digital or Polaroid).

Identification of the deceased by the next of kin or their representative should be documented in writing. Identification is an absolute necessity when disposition is to be by immediate cremation.

The funeral home should note in the embalming or decedent care report the condition of the body. This is especially important when the body is received from a medical institution or a coroner's office. In addition, the funeral home or the embalming establishment **needs to affix its own identification wristband or tag** directly to the decedent.

In instances when permission to embalm is not authorized or such permission is delayed, the deceased human body must be properly cared for. Refrigeration storage of the body is recommended. Proper handling and storage of the body will allow:

- the body to be identified by the next of kin or their designated legal representative
- the body to be viewed, by family or public, if embalming is not desired by the designated legal representative
- the body to be embalmed once authorization is received
- the progress of decomposition to be retarded
- safe, respectful care of the remains

All bodies placed in storage should be positioned with the **head and shoulders elevated** to lessen blood discolorations of the face and the neck. If the body is only to be identified (no arterial embalming) and **permission can be obtained for only cavity treatment** (aspiration and injection), this treatment will lessen gas formation, distension of the abdominal cavity, the possibility of purge, and facial blood discolorations.

If there is a possibility that permission for embalming will be obtained, no cavity treatment should be

---

*There are several types of visceral treatments.

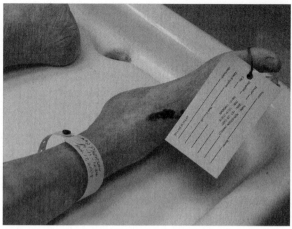

A

B

Figure 2–2. A. Use of Polaroid photo for cremation or burial identification. Digital pictures may also be used. **B.** Identification—medical facility and funeral facility.

performed as it would interfere with arterial embalming of the body.

Shaving of the male face, trimming hair or fingernails, or removing any medical devices (e.g., pacemaker) should not be attempted without first asking for permission. Even closing of the mouth by needle injector or suture should not be done without permission. (See Minimum-care form in Chapter 1.) If the decedent is to be identified by a photograph taken by the funeral home, permission should also be given for this form of identification.

Refrigeration Storage, Identification, or Viewing Without Embalming

1. Disinfect and open the body bag or disinfect and unwrap the decedent. Undress and inspect the remains. Record the physical condition of the remains on an embalming care report. Note medical apparatus (catheters, pacemaker, bandages, etc.).
2. Do **not** remove identification tags or bracelets. Match all tags to ensure all names are correct. Place a **funeral home or embalming facility identification band** on the decedent.
3. Remove and inventory all personal items and store in a secure place in a properly labeled property bag.
4. Disinfect and **pack all orifices**; disinfect the body surface.
5. Remove oropharyngeal tubes, gastric tubes, medical apparatus (see item #7), bandages, and any dressings. If the body is to only be visually identified for cremation or burial and cavity preparation permission **has been given**, cav-

ity aspiration and injection can be done at this time.
6. Do not remove circulatory invasive devices such as IV catheters; these can be taped in place, lessening any exposure to blood or body fluids. If permission is given, after arterial embalming these devices can be removed and properly disposed of in a biohazard container.
7. If a pacemaker is present, it needs to be removed if the body is to be disposed of by cremation. Have the person in charge sign for removal of the pacemaker and give any specific instructions as to its disposition.
8. Bathe the remains; shampoo the hair and clean the nails. (Do not trim nails unless permission is given.)
9. Shave facial hair (if permission has been given) and close the mouth and the eyes.
10. Apply massage cream on the face, neck, and hands. Lips and eyes may be glued at this time.
11. Tape, bandage, superglue, or suture any sites where leakage is present.
12. Place plastic garments on the body. Embalming powder should be placed inside the garment.
13. Place a clean gown on the body.
14. Place a plastic sheet over a cloth sheet (a clean body bag can also be used).
15. Place the body on the plastic and cloth sheets and wrap the remains.
16. Secure the arms and legs of the body with ties around the plastic and sheeting using cloth strips. **Do not tie** around neck. Keep sheets **loose** around the face.

Figure 2–3. A. Identification band remains on the body. **B.** Topical disinfection. **C.** Removal of gastric tube. **D.** Removal of pacemaker, with permission. **E.** Shaving and setting features. **F.** Partial dressing using plastic pants.

G

H

Figure 2–3. (Continued) G. Cotton sheet placed around body enveloped in a body storage bag. **H.** Unembalmed body ready for viewing on dressing table.

17. Attach an ID tag to the wrapped remains and a biohazard tag if the body is not embalmed. Identify the body as "unembalmed" and caution "blood/body infectious material" (Fig. 2–3). If placed in a body pouch, attach an additional identification tag to the exterior of the pouch.
18. Place body in refrigeration unit (Fig. 2–4).

In preparation for viewing or identification of the body where the condition is extreme, some preparation of the body is recommended. With some of these conditions, for example, burns or decomposition, it may be possible to place the body in a unionall and liberally place embalming powder in the garment to assist in con-

trolling offensive odors. The head can be wrapped with gauze bandages, and only if the authorized representative insists can the bandages be removed to expose the damaged tissues.

The family may request that the body be dressed. If this is possible, the body should be first placed in a unionall. If it is not possible to dress the body, this needs to be explained to the family.

(See Selected Readings section of this text for more detailed information in the reprinted article, "Identification: An Essential Part of What We Do," by Michael Kubasak.)

Figure 2–4. Walk-in refrigeration unit.

► KEY TERMS AND CONCEPTS FOR STUDY AND DISCUSSION

1. Define the following terms.
   Arterial embalming
   Cavity embalming
   Embalming
   Hypodermic embalming
   Preservation
   Surface embalming
2. List and define the three primary objectives accomplished by embalming.
3. Outline a basic sequence of steps for embalming an unautopsied body.
4. Outline a basic sequence of steps for embalming an autopsied body.
5. Why is cavity embalming necessary when embalming an unautopsied body? What are the purposes of cavity embalming? Why is reaspiration of the body often recommended?

6. If a family requests viewing but not embalming, (1) what documents should be signed and (2) how would you prepare the deceased?

7. An individual in your town has willed his or her body to the nearest medical college for anatomical study. How do you proceed with such a request?

8. The pathology department at your local hospital requests to meet with your embalming staff: what suggestions might your staff make to the pathology department with respect to procedures that may be done to assist with the embalming of the autopsied body?

9. Explain how you may need to use all the methods of embalming for the preparation of a right arm, which is swollen and black due to a condition of gangrene resulting from diabetes.

10. Historically, when was arterial embalming first employed—with evisceration—for preservation of the dead human body? When was arterial embalming—without evisceration—first used for preservation of the dead human body?

▶ BIBLIOGRAPHY

Bass B. *Death's Acre: Inside the Legendary Forensic Lab, the Body Farm, Where the Dead Do Tell Tales.* New York: Putnams, 2003.

Dhonau CO. *Manual of Case Analysis.* The Embalming Book Company Cincinnati, OH, 1924.

Dorn J, Hopkins B. *Thanatochemistry,* 2nd ed. Upper Saddle River, NJ: Prentice Hall, 1998.

Embalming Course Content Syllabus. Portland, ME: American Board of Funeral Service Education, 2001.

Merriam-Webster's Collegiate Dictionary, 11th ed. Springfield, MA: Merriam Webster, 2003.

Pervier NC. *Textbook of Chemistry for Embalmers.* Minneapolis: University of Minnesota, 1961.

Roach M. *Stiff: The Curious Lives of Human Cadavers.* New York: Norton, 2003.

Spitz WU. *Medicolegal Investigation of Death,* 3rd ed. Springfield, IL: Charles C Thomas, 1993.

Venes D. *Taber's Cyclopedic Medical Dictionary,* 19th ed. Philadelphia: F.A. Davis, 2001.

CHAPTER 3

PERSONAL HEALTH AND REGULATORY STANDARDS

CHAPTER OBJECTIVES

▶ Biological and chemical change to occupational risks.
▶ Workplace health and safety
▶ OSHA: Bloodborne Pathogen Rule
▶ OSHA: Hazard Communication Rule
▶ OSHA: Formaldehyde Standard

Embalming has historically encompassed principles and practices that are part of public health. The embalmer, as a sanitarian, no doubt grew out of two early twentieth century situations—first the pandemic flu of 1919 and second, almost all embalming was first performed in the home. The embalmer cleaned and sanitized the sick room and tended to the dead. The understanding of the manner by which disease was spread and the use of antibiotics did not occur until later in the century. With the understanding of the transmission of diseases today, the risk of the general public contracting a disease by being in the presence of an unembalmed dead human body, with rare exceptions, is very low. The dead human body can be offensive to the senses, but in and by itself, with rare exception, is not dangerous to the health of the observer. (See Selected Readings: The Art of Embalming and Its Purpose by Ron Hast.)

The "at risk" nature for those who have **direct contact** with preparing human remains for disposition has been well documented in medical and public health literatures. The unembalmed dead human body can be a large reservoir of infectious materials that are pathogenic to humans. The process of sanitizing and preserving dead human bodies raises a number of health issues for individuals engaged in the embalming procedure.

The embalmer is professionally responsible for his or her own personal hygiene and health and safety, **because he or she has direct contact with the deceased.**

In certain **rare situations,** when so ordered by the local board of health or the CDC, the embalmer will have the added concern of protecting the family and friends who wish to come into contact with the deceased. A well-embalmed body should not be a health hazard.

Each remains must be thoroughly sanitized and preserved. This can only be accomplished by proper application of chemicals suitable for the task. Use of insufficient quality or quantity of chemicals poses a significant risk to the embalmer. By prudent application of chemicals, maintenance of the work environment that is hygienically clean and safe, and proper disposal of the materials involved in the process, the embalmer protects both public and personal health.

▶ OCCUPATIONAL RISKS

Exposure to Biological Hazards

A 1996 Centers for Disease Control and Prevention (CDC) study reported that there is ample reason for concern about the exposure the embalmers may have to bloodborne and airborne pathogens (McKenna and co-workers, 1996). The CDC analyzed the risk for tuberculosis by determining potential exposure within certain occupational groups, based on historical observation, and the impact that infection within a group could have on public health. The occupational groups were first categorized by their level of risk. The researchers then applied a statistical formula to estimate the number of tuberculosis cases that could be expected within each occupational group. A comparison of the number of cases predicted by statistical formula for an occupational group and the number of actual cases that were reported for each occupational group showed a strong relationship between the occupation and the risk of contracting tuberculosis.

A notable exception to the association between occupational SES (socioeconomic status) and tuberculosis was the occupation of "Funeral director." Even though this occupation was included in the highest SES category of "Executives, administrative, and managerial occupations," 16 cases were allocated to this occupation where only 4.1 were expected (McKenna et al., 1996, p. 590).

The CDC concluded that funeral directors had an elevated risk of contracting tuberculosis as a result of their contact with dead human bodies.

Gershon and colleagues (1998) reported the results in a Johns Hopkins University study which concluded that funeral home employees who worked as embalmers had a greater exposure to tuberculosis than funeral home employees who did not embalm bodies. The study found that 101 out of 864 (11.7%) funeral home employees who volunteered to be tested reacted to the tuberculin skin test. It was determined that the funeral home employees who engaged in embalming were twice as likely to have a positive tuberculin skin test when compared to the funeral home employees who did not embalm bodies.

Beck-Sague and co-workers (1991) also addressed the potential for occupationally acquired infections among embalmers. In particular, this study suggested that embalmers were at potential risk of acquiring infection as a result of their frequent contact with blood (Fig. 3–1). This study reported that 89 of 539 (17%) morticians who responded to a survey reported contracting infectious diseases attributed to their occupation. Among the most frequently reported diseases in the study were hepatitis, staphylococcal and other skin infections, and pulmonary and skin tuberculosis. The most commonly reported exposure was by skin contact with blood (393 out of 539, or 73%). Needle stick injuries were far more common than cuts. Of the 539 morticians who responded to the survey, 212 (39%) reported a needle stick within 12 months prior to the survey, while 61 (11%) morticians reported having been cut.

Turner and colleagues (1989) reported that embalmers in the Boston area were about two times more likely to test positive for hepatitis B (HBV) infection than a blood donor comparison group. The study also reported that the length of time a person had been working as an embalmer elevated the risk of contracting an HBV infection.

Figure 3–1. Secondary infection. Cause of death was listed as leukemia; however, the individual also exhibits the secondary infection of chicken pox.

McDonald (1989) published an editorial which stated that embalmers face much the same risk of exposure to infectious diseases as clinical pathologists. The basis of this finding was the common exposure to blood and body fluids for both pathologists and embalmers. The exposure risk was confirmed when the first documented case of an embalmer being infected with tuberculosis while embalming a dead human body was reported in the **New England Journal of Medicine** on January 27, 2000 by Dr. Timothy Stirling.

Multidrug-resistant pathogens are now commonplace in many regions of the world. The ease of modern global travel and transportation has created a new environment for the spread of these disease-causing organisms and their hosts. Within a period of 24 hours, people, insects and animal vectors, or foodstuffs can be transported from and to anywhere in the world. This rapid movement makes possible the occurrence and transmission of rare and tropical diseases anywhere and at any time. Never before has an embalmer faced such a risk of biological exposure. **Outside Magazine** July 1999 states, "Microbes are still the number three killer in the Western world."

Reported in, **The Forum** December 2009, a publication of the New Jersey Funeral Directors Association: "The incidences of occupationally-contracted infectious, contagious, or communicable disease are low in general and somewhat lower for embalmers than for individuals in other fields, such as healthcare, the Institute of Occupational Medicine, Edinburgh, Scotland reported in 2004. However, when proper protective measures are not used, and given the high probability of percutaneous and mucocutaneous exposures, infectious agent transmission is possible. Therefore, embalmers always should practice universal precautions when handling deceased human bodies, regardless of their known infectious status. "

While each body prepared by the embalmer must be considered a potential danger, several more recently diagnosed diseases need to be mentioned, some of which have reference to the previous discussion of antibiotic resistance:

■ Clostridium difficile produces two toxins and can cause lethal diarrhea often brought on by overuse of antibiotics; found as spores in feces; diapers; and gowns. A new mutation produces 20 times the toxin of the old version

■ Klebsiella pneumoniae, a hospital-borne microbe that can infect the urinary tract, gut, and bloodstream

■ Acinetobacter baumannii, resistant to almost all antibiotics; found in spinal fluid and between the membranes lining the abdominal wall and the urinary tract. Seen in the very seriously ill and trauma injury wounds. Care with urinary catheters and surgical drainage tubes. Soil-borne, infects wounds and can penetrate deep into skin, bone, lungs, and blood

■ Methicillin-resistant **Staphylococcus aureus** (MRSA), a pathologic bacterial staph infection. This premier pathogen causes over 102,000 hospital infections a year. MRSA can be found on the skin, in the nose, in blood and urine, and in exudates or fluid from an infected site. Spread by direct physical contact, or contact with contaminated objects

■ Vancomycin-resistant Enterococci (VRE), a pathologic bacteria, found in open wounds and feces; also associated with invasive devices such as urinary catheters and nasogastric tubes—seen in patients with long-term hospitalization. An especially hardy microbe, it infects blood, urinary tract, and wounds of patients with compromised immune systems

■ Vancomycin-resistant **Staphylococcus aureus** (VRSA), a pathologic bacteria similar to VRE

■ Vancomycin-intermediate Staphylococcus aureus (VISA), a pathologic bacteria, that may be seen in patients with chronic diabetes and kidney disease; found in open wounds

■ Pseudomonas aeruginosa causes deadly lower-respiratory infections in sick patients

■ Creutzfeldt-Jakob disease (CJD), a fatal disease caused by a prion (pathogen smaller than a virus); the causative agent is very difficult, if almost impossible, to destroy. The causative agent appears to be concentrated in cerebrospinal fluid. (See Selected Readings.)

■ Human immunodeficiency virus (HIV), a retrovirus that causes acquired immunodeficiency syndrome (AIDS). HIV was identified in 1984. The disease causes a loss of immune functions and the subsequent development of opportunistic infections. HIV is spread through direct contact with contaminated body fluids.

■ Hepatitis, an inflammation of the liver brought about by several recognized viruses. HAV, hepatitis A; HBV, hepatitis B; HCV, hepatitis C; HDV, hepatitis D: HEV, hepatitis E; HGV, hepatitis G; GBV, hepatitis GBV. Hepatitis A and E are transmitted by the fecal-oral route; hepatitis B, C, D, G, and GBV are bloodborne diseases. Embalmers need to be immunized against hepatitis B.

■ Tuberculosis, caused by **Mycobacterium tuberculosis,** most commonly affects the respiratory system, but it is capable of affecting almost any body system or area. Multidrug-resistant tuberculosis is difficult for physicians to treat. Individuals with lowered immunity can be susceptible to this form of tuberculosis. Worldwide tuberculosis is still a leading cause of death. An embalmer needs to carefully disinfect and dispose of—in a biohazard container—any nasal-oral discharges and sputum when respiratory tuberculosis is present.

The Female Embalmer—Pregnancy

As more and more women enter funeral service, the employer needs to be alert to certain pathogenic microbes and work conditions that may effect a pregnant staff member. The following list of pathogens and diseases has been documented, which can cause potential harm to the fetus.

Cytomegalovirus (CMV), Hepatitis B and C, Herpes viruses, Human Parvovirus B19 (The Fifth Disease), Rubella (German Measles), Syphilis, Toxoplasmosis, and Varicella Zoster virus (Chicken Pox).

The female employee, during pregnancy, should be in consultation with her medical doctor as to what precautions are necessary to protect both the prospective mother and the infant. As of this publication, studies have not demonstrated damage to the fetus by exposure of the pregnant embalmer to formaldehyde. The pregnant employee needs to maintain good personal hygiene standards, wear proper personal protective equipment (PPE), and work in an environment maintained at safe Occupational Safety and Health Administration (OSHA) formaldehyde levels.

Exposure to Chemical Hazards

The objectives of the embalming process are to preserve, sanitize, and restore the dead human body. These objectives are accomplished by the application of chemicals. Many of the chemicals—used in embalming and the related processes—have been categorized or contain components that have been categorized as hazardous substances. Hazards associated with using these substances have been well documented in the health and medical literatures.

A study conducted by Williams and associates (1984) stated that exposure to formaldehyde, particularly, formaldehyde vapor, is probably the most significant of the chemical exposures to which embalmers are subjected. Over the years, a number of other studies have reported on the adverse effects of chronic exposure to formaldehyde (Kerfoot, 1972; Kerfoot and Mooney, 1975; Bender et al., 1983).

Nethercott and Holness (1988) noted that Canadian funeral service workers were more likely to complain about irritations of the nose and eyes than were members of a control group. The study went on to say that those funeral service employees who were in contact with formaldehyde were likely to experience skin and mucous membrane irritation.

Many of the chemicals used in embalming are regulated by the state and the federal OSHA standards. Hazardous substance standards adopted in Minnesota, for example, contain a list of nearly 1100 substances controlled because of the hazards that result from their use (State of Minnesota, 1995). Many of the substances on that list are either used in the embalming process, or are components of products used in the embalming process. Most notable among the health problems that can result from chemicals in the preparation room are contact dermatitis, eye and nose irritations, and upper respiratory irritations.

Since 1987, the United States Environmental Protection Agency has recognized formaldehyde as a potential carcinogen for tumors in the lung, nasopharynx, and nasal passages. In June 2004, the International Agency for Research on Cancer recognized formaldehyde as a human carcinogen. Presently, the European Union, under its Biocides Directive, is examining the health effects of formaldehyde. The National Cancer Institute released in 2009 the findings of an extensive study of workers with a high exposure to formaldehyde—anatomists, pathologists, and funeral personnel. They found these persons to have a statistically increased risk for mortality from lymphohematopoietic malignancies, in particular, myeloid leukemia.

In 2010, the National Academy of Sciences reviewed the EPA findings that linked formaldehyde and leukemia. NAS disagreed with those findings and determined the EPA document needed revision. A separate study published in Toxicological Sciences in 2011 found no connection between formaldehyde and leukemia in animal studies. The United States Department of Health & Human Services in June 2010, added formaldehyde to the National Toxicology Program list of carcinogenic compounds. Research continues, for a positive link between formaldehyde and leukemia has yet to be established.

Exposure to Other Hazards of Embalming

In addition to the hazards associated with biological and chemical agents, embalmers are exposed to hazards including: heat, ionizing radiation, and nonionizing radiation. Although these hazards may not be as prevalent as chemical or biological hazards, they are worth noting, and may necessitate action by a funeral home.

Ventilation and Temperature. Funeral homes must give consideration to the ventilation and temperature in the embalming room. If the temperature of a room is high, an embalmer wearing a full set of PPE may have difficulty ventilating the body heat. This can result in an elevation of core body temperature. Some PPEs can trap body heat within them and that, coupled with any combination of high room temperature, inadequate ventilation, and high humidity can cause some embalmers to feel discomfort, or even lead to fainting.

Ionizing Radiation. There is a possibility that an embalmer might come into contact with a body that has undergone radiation therapy. Hospitals and clinics that administer radiation treatments are supposed to monitor radiation levels. Bodies that have undergone radiation treatment should not be released until such time that they no longer pose a hazard. Communication with the surviving family and health authorities is vital, as the embalmer has no way of telling that a body is hazardous unless it is labeled. If embalmers have questions or concerns about radiation exposure, they should contact the radiation officer at a local hospital or clinic, or contact government agencies that have authority in matters related to radiation exposure.

Nonionizing Radiation. The possibility of adverse exposure to nonionizing radiation is remote. Exposure could result from electromagnetic radiation given off by microwave ovens or computer monitors. Although it is unlikely that either of these sources would cause a major health concern for embalmers, it is still appropriate for funeral homes to consider exposures of this nature.

▶ DEALING WITH EXPOSURE TO EMBALMING HAZARDS—OSHA BLOODBORNE PATHOGEN RULE

Biological Hazards

Health and safety issues associated with embalming are addressed by compliance with **the Bloodborne Pathogen Rule.** The Bloodborne Pathogen Rule is administered by the United States Department of Labor through OSHA. The rule is directly applicable to occupations and professions, including funeral service, where employees are exposed to infectious agents. In addition, many individual states have enacted **EmployeeRight-To-Know** laws that support or expand the scope of federal OSHA regulations. Embalmers must be aware of the duties and responsibilities that are imposed on them by the laws and rules of the various jurisdictions within which they practice. Compliance with the Bloodborne Pathogen Rule, and any state regulations that support or expand it, is required.

Under the Bloodborne Pathogen Rule, employers are required to conduct an evaluation of their workplace(s) to determine if employees have occupational exposure to infectious agents regulated by OSHA. If such exposure exists, a written **Exposure Control Plan** must be developed to control, minimize, or eliminate employee exposure. Exposure control plans, which by law must be accessible to employees, are to be reviewed and updated at least once per year, so that changes in personnel, procedure, and/or work assignments can be documented. The minimum documentation required for an Exposure Control Plan includes exposure determination, methods of compliance, hepatitis B vaccination as well as postexposure evaluation and follow-up, hazard communication, and record keeping.

Exposure Determination. Employers are required to examine workplace(s) to determine (1) if occupational exposure to bloodborne pathogens exists, and (2) what types of duties are being performed when occupational exposure to bloodborne pathogens occurs. If occupational exposure to bloodborne pathogens is identified, employers must then list all job titles or classifications which have exposure. In a funeral home setting, this might include, but not be limited to, embalmers, intern/apprentice embalmers, removal personnel, and any other person having **direct contact** with the unembalmed human remains or with any regulated infectious waste materials. Employers must also identify those employees who have "some" occupational exposure to infectious agents. This might include, but not be limited to, hairdressers, housekeepers, maintenance personnel, funeral directors, drivers, and clerical staff. Employers must identify and list duties that involve exposure to infectious agents. Examples of duties that might appear on such a list include removal of human remains, embalming, hairdressing, cosmetizing, and laundry.

Methods of Compliance. Compliance with the Bloodborne Pathogen Rule is accomplished by the application of (1) universal precautions, (2) engineering controls, and (3) work practice controls. The basic premise of **universal precautions** for the embalmer is to treat all human remains as if they were infected with HIV, HBV, or other pathogens. In other words, **the embalmer should treat all bodies with the same caution that would be applied for extremely hazardous, potentially fatal infections.** By the implementation of this extreme caution, the embalmer attempts "To prevent parenteral, mucous membrane, and nonintact skin exposure" (Code of Federal Regulations, 1992). In other words, the embalmer will avoid needle sticks or cuts that create parenteral exposure by breaking the protective barrier provided by the skin. The embalmer will also avoid other situations that might result in ingestion of contaminated material through the nose or the mouth. The embalmer must take care to avoid allowing infectious agents to invade through the eyes, or be absorbed through or otherwise penetrate the skin. Care must also be taken to prevent infectious agents from invading the host by means of an existing break in the skin, such as cuts, scratches, and so on. To seek protection from possible infection, the embalmer will (1) utilize PPE (2) properly decontaminate infected surfaces, (3) properly handle and dispose of infectious wastes, (4) apply appropriate measures to control leaks, drips, and spills of infectious materials, (5) apply proper work practice skills, and (6) properly handle contaminated laundry.

Engineering controls are those mechanical systems and devices engineered into the architecture of a building. Engineering controls that are used to provide personal and public health protection should be examined and maintained or replaced on a regular schedule. The examination and maintenance should be documented. Doing so will ensure that the systems and devices are offering the most effective means to reduce exposure. The two primary areas of consideration are **adequate ventilation** and **proper plumbing.**

During embalming, there is a possibility that infectious agents can become aerosolized or in some other way become airborne. The purpose of adequate ventilation is to remove contaminated air from the work area and replace it with fresh air. The most important factor in the ventilation system is the location of the exhaust. It should be at the foot of the embalming table and below the level of the tabletop. The air replacement or intake should ideally be high on the opposite wall. Thus, fresh air is being blown toward the embalmer while potentially contaminated air is being drawn down and away from the embalmer's breathing zone (Fig. 3–2).

The number of air exchanges per hour may be determined by (1) the contents of the room, (2) whether more than one embalming will be in progress at the same time, (3) the shape of the room, and (4) other factors, such as hot or cold weather or the preference of the embalmer. As a rough rule of thumb, for a single table room, the number of air changes ranges from 12 to 20 per hour. The Public Health Guidelines have recommended that a ventilation system creates a minimum of six air changes per hour, and preferably more in the preparation room environment. A minimum of 15 air changes per hour is currently recommended for

Figure 3–2. Air exchange system: note that clean air enters at ceiling level, air exhausts from floor and machine levels courtesy of David Hicks, Cincinnati College of Mortuary Science.

the preparation room. (See NFDA Best Formaldehyde Work Practices—2010).

Proper plumbing plays an important role in ensuring that infectious substances and materials commonly associated with embalming do not find their way into the public water supply. Examples of engineering controls that could reduce the possibility of water contamination might include (1) vacuum breakers on the main water line leading into the building, (2) vacuum breakers on hydroaspirators, (3) discharge basins/flush sinks that are in good working order, (4) having a suitable water source for the preparation table, (5) having a proper eyewash station, (6) having a proper drench shower, (7) having a proper hand washing station, and (8) having proper shower room facilities for embalmers to use after the embalming is completed.

Devices such as vacuum breakers on aspiration equipment and on water lines leading into the funeral home help to contain the threat so that any contaminated material could be back-siphoned from the preparation room to other water lines. In many instances, funeral homes may find that the local and the state authorities have extensive plumbing codes that must be satisfied for the protection of public health.

In addition to providing protection for building or public water supplies, plumbing considerations can also assist embalmers in keeping their work areas as clean and hygienic as possible. Adequate water service to preparation room equipment and embalming tables, and suitable sinks or flush basins can offer important aids to sanitation and hygiene.

Work Practice Controls. Work practice controls are common sense steps taken to avoid unnecessary or excessive exposure to infectious agents. Common work practices that contribute to a hygienic environment include

(1) hand washing, (2) proper handling and disposal of contaminated waste and contaminated sharps, (3) avoiding splashing, spraying, or splattering when working with potentially infectious agents, (4) consistent and proper use of PPE, and (5) adequate housekeeping, including a written record of housekeeping provisions. Work practice controls must be spelled out and enforced. Such controls would include immediate hand washing after removal of gloves.

Employees must receive training and instruction on proper hand washing techniques. Sufficient time, water, and antiseptic soap must be used for this process. A general guideline is to wet the hands, apply antiseptic soap, and to sing the song, "Happy Birthday" throughout the lathering procedure. Special attention to scrubbing all hand surfaces with antiseptic soap is required. The hands must be rinsed with warm water. The CDC recommends the following:

1. Using liquid soap and running water at a comfortable temperature, work up a lather and use friction between fingers
2. Rinse using plenty of running water so that no soap remains on the hands. Residual soap can cause skin irritation and chapping
3. Dry well with disposable towels to remove water. This reduced the chapping which may be caused by air drying. Use the towel to turn off the faucet.
4. If chapping or dermatitis occurs, reevaluate your hand washing technique

Employees must receive training and instruction on the use and accessibility of PPE, cleaning and laundering procedures, repair and replacement procedures, procedures to follow when PPE is contaminated or damaged while in use, and procedures for the proper storage of PPE.

Employers are required to provide appropriate PPE suitable in terms of size, use, and application. PPE is considered to be appropriate only if it prevents blood or other potentially infectious substances from passing through, or otherwise reaching, the employee's work clothes, street clothes, undergarments, skin, eyes, mouth, or other mucous membranes under normal conditions of time and use. Further, employers are required to see to it that employees who are performing duties where there is exposure wear the provided PPE. PPE should literally cover the embalmer from head to toe.

Gloves for use during embalming should be of sufficient thickness to provide protection. Latex examination gloves are not suitable for embalming as they are too thin and porous to protect from bloodborne pathogens and embalming chemicals. Heavier (13 mil or greater) latex or nitrile gloves are more protective.

During embalming, the embalmer should wear a surgical cap, hood, or other suitable head covering. All hair should be tucked up underneath the head covering.

Figure 3–3. Attired embalmer.

The mouth, the nose, and the chin should be covered by a tuberculosis (TB) rated surgical mask. The embalmer's forehead, cheeks, and neck should be protected by a face shield. The eyes should be protected by a splash barrier such as safety glasses, goggles, or a combination face-eye shield. The arms, torso, and legs should be protected by a garment or combination of garments that provide suitable coverage. The feet should be covered by a suitable water-resistant, nonslip foot wear or water resistant, nonslip shoe coverings. **A rule of thumb for protective garments is that the embalmer should have no exposed skin.** Employers must make arrangements for cleaning, laundering, or otherwise disposing of contaminated PPE. In addition, employers must make arrangements for damaged PPE to be repaired or replaced (Fig. 3–3).

All PPE must be removed immediately on leaving the work area and placed in a designated area or container for storage, washing, decontamination, or disposal.

Eating, drinking, smoking, application of personal beauty products, and handling of contact lenses are prohibited in work areas. No food or drink should be stored in refrigerators where blood is stored or in other areas of possible contamination.

Employers must ensure that work areas are maintained in a clean and sanitary condition, in accordance with a written schedule for cleaning and disinfection. This could be on completion of embalming or at the end of the work shift.

Used needles and other sharps should not be sheared, bent, broken, recapped, or resheathed by

hand. Sharps are to be disposed in closable, puncture-resistant, disposable containers that are leakproof on the sides and at the bottom and that bear proper warning labels or are color-coded (red).

All procedures involving blood or other potentially infectious body fluids should be performed in such a manner as to minimize splashing, spraying, and aerosolization. Drainage of the body is best achieved by using a drainage tube with a length of plastic or rubber tubing that is sufficient to reach the table drain. Employing this drainage strategy eliminates splashing on the embalming table, thus reducing aerosolization. Use of the newer stainless steel embalming tables along with "body-bridges" allows drainage contents and chemicals to flow onto the table and not down the back of the body. All sinks, basins, or commodes that the embalming table or hydroaspirators and electric aspirators drain into should be covered to eliminate aerosolization of microorganisms as splashing occurs. All instruments, equipment, and environmental and working surfaces must be properly cleaned and disinfected after contact with blood or other potentially infectious materials. All pails, containers, and receptacles intended for reuse and those that have a potential for becoming contaminated with blood or other potentially infectious materials should be inspected, cleaned, and disinfected on a regular basis or as soon as possible on visible contamination.

Hepatitis B Vaccination. Hepatitis B vaccination must be made available to all employees who have occupational exposure. The vaccination program must be (1) offered at no cost to the employee, (2) offered at a reasonable time and place, (3) performed by or under the supervision of a licensed physician, or by or under the supervision of another licensed healthcare professional, and (4) provided according to the recommendations of the U.S. Public Health Service. Employees have the option of accepting or declining the vaccination. If the employee is offered vaccination but declines, a special declination statement should be signed by the employee to document the offer and the choice to decline. If an employee first declines hepatitis B vaccination, but later decides to accept, the declination document is discarded, and the employee must be given the vaccination. It is prudent to have an annual check of immunity levels in the case of HBV. Medical treatments and other factors can reduce the immunity in a person who has undergone HBV vaccinations.

Postexposure Evaluation and Follow-up. In the event that a blood or body fluid exposure incident occurs, employers must immediately implement procedures for post-exposure evaluation and follow-up. The postexposure evaluation and follow-up will include (1) a detailed explanation of the events and circumstances of the exposure, (2) identification and documentation of the source

Figure 3–4. Biohazard symbol.

individual, unless doing so is impossible or prohibited by law, (3) collecting and testing the blood for HBV and HIV, (4) taking steps necessary to assist in the prevention of infection or disease, (5) offering counseling, and (6) conducting an evaluation of any reported illnesses. It is also prudent to review exposure reduction strategies to reduce the potential for future exposure.

Hazard Communication. The following can be used to label or distinguish containers used to store, transport, or ship blood or other potentially infectious agents: (1) fluorescent orange labels, (2) orange and red labels, (3) predominantly orange and red warning labels, (4) labels with lettering and symbols in contrasting colors, or (5) other suitable substitutes for labels, such as red bags or red containers. The labels used to mark infectious hazards must include the legend shown in Fig. 3–4.

In addition to the labeling provisions required by the Bloodborne Pathogen Rule, employers must also provide information and training to those employees who are exposed to infectious hazards in the workplace. Employers will ensure that all employees with occupational exposure receive training related to bloodborne pathogens, and training on methods for dealing with infectious agents. The training must be given at or before the time the employee is assigned a task where exposure exists. Training updates must be repeated at least once per year.

The training program must contain the following components

1. A copy of the regulatory text must be readily available and accessible to employees at all times.
2. A general explanation of the epidemiology and symptoms of bloodborne diseases must be provided.
3. An explanation of the modes of transmission of bloodborne pathogens must be provided. To satisfy the need for information about epidemiology, symptoms, and modes of transmission,

books such as **Control of Communicable Diseases Manual** (Benenson, 1995) have become commonplace in funeral homes as resources that satisfy OSHA compliance standards. This type of reference material provides ready access to information helpful in the identification of infectious agents, as well as information related to the occurrence; reservoir; mode of transmission; incubation period; period of communicability, susceptibility and resistance; and methods of control.

4. An explanation of the employer's exposure control plan and the means by which the employee can obtain a copy of the written plan must be provided.
5. An explanation of the appropriate methods for recognizing tasks and other activities that may involve exposure to blood and other potentially infectious materials must be provided.
6. An explanation of the use and limitations of methods that will prevent or reduce exposure, including appropriate use of engineering controls, work practice controls, and universal precautions must be provided.
7. Information on the types, proper use, location, removal, handling, decontamination, and disposal of PPE.
8. An explanation of the basis for selection of PPE. Not all gloves and masks offer equal protection from microorganisms or chemical exposures.
9. Information on the hepatitis B vaccine, including information on its efficacy, safety, method of administration, the benefits of being vaccinated, and that the vaccine and vaccination will be offered free of charge.
10. Information on the appropriate actions to take and persons to contact in an emergency involving blood or other potentially infectious materials.
11. An explanation of the procedure to follow if an exposure incident occurs, including the method of reporting the incident and the medical follow-up that will be made available.
12. Information on the postexposure evaluation and the follow-up required after an exposure incident.
13. An explanation of the signs, labels, and color coding used to mark biohazardous materials and containers.
14. An opportunity for interactive questions and answers with the person conducting the training session.

Record Keeping. Employers are responsible for establishing and maintaining accurate records for each employee with occupational exposure to bloodborne pathogens. The employee must receive training on the date of hire or date of being responsible for tasks involving exposure; this date may change as a person's duties change. The record must contain (1) the name and the Social Security number of the employee, (2) a copy of the employee's hepatitis B vaccination, (3) results of any examinations, medical testing, and follow-up procedures that occurred as a result of an exposure incident, (4) employer's copy of any healthcare professional's written opinion regarding examinations, medical testing, or follow-up in the aftermath of an exposure incident, and (5) a copy of the healthcare professional's report of any examinations, medical testing, or follow-up in the aftermath of an exposure incident.

Employers must maintain records of each training session. Training records are to be kept for a period of 3 years from the date the training occurred. The record must include (1) the date of each training session, (2) a summary of each training session, (3) the name(s) and qualification(s) of trainer(s), and (4) the names and job titles of all persons attending each training session. Employers are required to make all records available to the employees or their representatives. If either the employment is terminated or the employee transfers to another location or employer, the training records must be made available to the new location or the new employer. If an employer ceases to operate and has no successor, OSHA must be notified so that records can be transferred to an appropriate place and filed for future use.

Embalmers have to make judgments about exposure to potentially infectious agents. Information is vital to the decision making process, and embalmers should have access to as much information as possible.

The assumption in the embalming process is that all bodies contain infectious agents and, therefore, represent reservoirs in which infectious agents can be found. In as much as the embalming procedure is invasive, it is a given that infectious agents will escape from the body during embalming. The embalmer represents a potential host for the escaped infectious agents because the embalmer will be in direct contact with any infectious agents that are released from the body. In spite of the exposure, infectious agents can be prevented from entering the embalmer with the proper application of work practice controls, engineering controls, and universal precautions. In addition to the controls and physical barriers that can be utilized to protect the embalmer, it is important for the embalmer to maintain good personal health to maintain resistance to infection.

Decontamination of instruments, equipment, the work area, and the body are important weapons in the fight against infectious diseases. In preparation room settings where exposure levels are high, decontamination is accomplished by using physical or chemical means (Table 3–1).

Good work practices and universal precautions would dictate that the body, instruments, equipment, counter tops, table tops, walls, floors, light fixtures, sinks, cabinets, and waste receptacles be sanitized and

TABLE 3–1. BREAKING THE CYCLE OF TRANSMISSION OF INFECTIOUS AGENTS IN THE PREPARATION ROOM: PUBLIC HEALTH GUIDELINES FOR THE AT-RISK EMBALMER "HOST"

Portal of "Host" Entry	Infectious Agent
Skin or mucous membrane respiratory tract, alimentary tract, body openings—natural and/or artificial (abrasions, cuts, lacerations, wounds)	Bacteria, fungi (molds and yeasts), viruses, rickettsia, protozoa
Proper "barrier" attire	Personal health practices
Aseptic technique(s)	Personnel health policies
Handwashing, gloves	Environmental sanitation
Disinfection and decontamination	Disinfection and decontamination
Modes of Transmitting the Infectious Agent	Reservoirs of Infectious Agents in the Preparation Room
Direct contact (aerosol or droplet infection) and indirect contact (air, contaminated surfaces) and objects or fomites, body fluids and exudates, insects	Remains, equipment (e.g., hydroaspirators, trocars, razors), instruments, adjacent hard surfaces, air contaminated linens, bandages and dressings, solid and liquid wastes

Proper "barrier" attire
Handwashing, gloves
Proper disposition of wastes
Effective air handling system
Concurrent and terminal disinfection

Note: Proper "barrier" attire may include whole-body covering, head cover, shoe covers, gloves, oral–nasal mask, and eye protection (safety glasses).

TABLE 3–2. ACTIVITY LEVELS OF SELECTED MICROBICIDES

Liquid Microbicide[a]	Use Concentration	Activity Level
Glutaraldehyde, aqueous, e.g., Cidex, Sonacide, Sporicidin	2.0%	High
Formaldehyde + alcohol	8.0% + 70.0%	High
Stabilized hydrogen peroxide	6.0–10.0%	High
Formaldehyde, aqueous	3.0–8.0%	High to intermediate
Iodophors, e.g., Betadine, Wescodyne, HiSine, Losan	75–200 ppm	Intermediate
Iodine + alcohol	0.5% + 70.0%	Intermediate
Chlorine compounds, e.g., sodium hypochlorite as in chlorine bleach	1000–5000 ppm	Intermediate
Phenolic compounds, aqueous, e.g., Amphyl Staphene, O-Syl	0.5–3.0%	Intermediate to low
Quaternary ammonium compounds, e.g., Phemoral, Zepharin Chloride, Diaparine Chloride	0.1–0.2% aqueous	Low
Mercurial compounds, organic and inorganic, e.g., Merthiolate, Mercurochrome, Metaphen	0.1–0.2%	Low

[a]Trade names of certain microbicides are given.
From Block SS: **Disinfection, Sterilization, and Preservation,** 3rd ed. Philadelphia: Lea & Febiger; 1983, with permission.

disinfected. Disinfection and decontamination activity should occur as necessary during an embalming procedure; concurrent disinfection and decontamination, and then terminal disinfection and decontamination must be done thoroughly at the completion of the embalming process.

A quality topical disinfectant should be applied to the deceased human body followed by bathing of the body, during the initial steps of the embalming process. Concurrent cleaning and bathing should occur during the embalming process, followed by a thorough final bathing at the conclusion of the embalming process.

Embalmers could consider steam sterilization or **autoclaving,** for contaminated instruments, **or** immersion of instruments in a suitable cold chemical sterilant. Steam sterilization is seldom used in funeral service, because of two considerations. First, autoclaves are very expensive and second, they are not large enough to hold instruments such as a trocar. Embalmers will find a number of commercially prepared cold chemical sterilants on the market (e.g., Cidex, Sonacide). These cold chemical sterilants have formulations containing acid glutaraldehyde, or alkalinized glutaraldehyde, or formaldehyde in methanol as their active ingredients. Some common microbicides are shown in Table 3–2. (Formaldehyde and methanol (formalin) is only sporicidal (a sterilant) at a concentration of 8% or greater.) Selecting disinfectants that are suited for this application plays an extremely important role. When corrosive disinfectants, such as household bleach are used, the chrome finish on instruments can be damaged. It may nevertheless be advisable to use household bleach when a known CJD case is being embalmed. Anytime instruments appear to be pitted or the chrome finish is worn away, the instruments should be replaced—because when the surface of an instrument is pitted, it becomes difficult to disinfect. The pitted surfaces are ideal hiding places for microorganisms and also permit air bubbles to build up between the disinfecting solution and the surface of the instrument. When one considers the microscopic appearance of these surface pits, it is plain to see that these instruments pose a greater risk for infection during needle sticks or other sharps injuries. For example, a new suture needle will appear quite smooth under the microscope. When a needle stick occurs, there is a squeegee effect when the needle passes through the glove and skin, reducing the number of organisms introduced into the tissues. If the instrument is old or pitted, there is a greatly reduced squeegee effect increasing the quantity of microorganisms transferred into the embalmer or the body being embalmed. To the embalmer, this translates into increased risk of infection. For the body being embalmed, this translates into greater risk of transferring tissue gas bacilli from one body to another.

Following the embalming process, all contaminated surfaces should be decontaminated, cleaned, and disinfected with a suitable disinfectant solution or topical disinfectant (Table 3–3).

The following terms are commonly associated with methods of disinfection and sterilization (Table 3–4).

Asepsis—freedom from infection and from any form of life; sterility

Bactericidal—destructive to bacteria

Bacteriostatic—inhibiting the growth or multiplication of bacteria (no destruction of viability implied)

Cleaning—removal of infectious agents by scrubbing and washing, as with hot water, soap, or a suitable detergent

Concurrent disinfection—the cleaning of the body and instruments at the time of embalming the body

TABLE 3–3. ACCEPTABLE ANTIMICROBIAL PROCEDURES/EXPOSURE INTERVALS

Objects	Vegetative Bacteria and Fungi and Influenza Viruses	Tubercle Bacilli, Enteroviruses Except Hepatitis Viruses, Vegetative Bacteria and Fungi, and Influenza Viruses	Bacterial and Fungal Spores, Hepatitis Viruses, Tubercle Bacilli, Enteroviruses, Vegetative Bacteria and Fungi, and Influenza Viruses
	Disinfection	*Disinfection*	*Sterilization*
Smooth, hard surface objects	A—10 min D—5 min E—10 min F—10 min H—10 min L—5 min M—5 min	B—10 min D—10 min G—10 min H—10 min L—10 min M—10 min	D—18 h J K L—9 h M—10 h
Rubber tubing, rubber catheters	E—10 min F—10 min H—10 min	G—10 min H—10 min	J[a] K
Polyethylene tubing, polyethylene catheters	A—10 min E—10 min F—10 min H—10 min	B—10 min G—10 min H—10 min	D—18 h J[a] K L—9 h M—10 h
Lensed instruments	E—10 min F—10 min H—10 min K M—10 min	K M—10 min	K
Hypodermic needles Thermometers[b]	Sterilization only C—10 min K	Sterilization only C—10 min K	J D—18 h L—9 h M—10 h
Hinged instruments	A—20 min D—10 min E—20 min F—20 min H—20 min L—10 min M—10 min	B—30 min D—20 min G—30 min H—30 min L—20 min M—20 min	J K L—9 h M—10 h
Floors, furniture, other appropriate room surfaces	E—5 min F—5 min H—5 min I—5 min	G—5 min H—5 min	Not necessary or practical

Key
A. Isopropyl alcohol (70–90%) plus 0.2% sodium nitrite to prevent corrosion
B. Ethyl alcohol (70–90%)
C. Isopropyl or ethyl alcohol plus 0.2% iodine
D. Formaldehyde (8%)—alcohol solution plus 0.2% sodium nitrite to prevent corrosion
E. Quaternary ammonium solutions (1:500 aq.) plus 0.2% sodium nitrite to prevent corrosion
F. Iodophor—75 ppm available iodine plus 0.2% sodium nitrite to prevent corrosion
G. Iodophor—450 ppm available iodine plus 0.2% sodium nitrite to prevent corrosion
H. Phenolic solutions (2% aq.) plus 0.5% sodium bicarbonate to prevent corrosion
I. Sodium hypochlorite (1:500 aq.—approximately 100 ppm)[a]
J. Heat sterilization, see manufacturers' recommendations
K. Ethylene oxide gas 6 or technical literature
L. Aqueous formalin (40%)
M. Activated glutaraldehyde (2% aq.)
[a]Investigate thermostability when indicated.
[b]Must be thoroughly wiped, preferably with tincture of soap, before disinfection or sterilization. Alcohol–iodine solution will remove markings on poor-grade thermometers.
Note: 1000 ppm of available chlorine is recommended for inactivation of hepatitis B virus and 5000 ppm for inactivation of HIV (AIDS). Thoroughly rinse all inanimate surfaces of any excess formalin prior to application of the hypochlorite disinfectant. Keene (1973) cautions that when formaldehyde reacts with hydrochloric acid, the compound bis-chloromethyl ether (BCME) may be formed. BCME is a highly toxic, carcinogenic compound.

TABLE 3–4. CHEMICAL AND PHYSICAL METHODS FOR CONTROLLING MICROBIAL CONTAMINATION

Method of Decontamination	Temperature Requirement	Minimum Interval of Exposure (min)									
		0	2	10	12	15	20	90	120	150	180
Sterilization: Complete destruction of all forms of microbial life	285°F (140°C)	—— (instant)									
Saturated steam under pressure (autoclaving)	270°F (132°C)	————									
	250°F (121°C)	——————————— 30 min for hepatitis viruses 2 to 12 h									
Ethylene oxide gas	130°F (54°C)	———————————— 2 h or more									
Hot air, e.g., oven	320°F (160°C)	———————————————————————— 3 to 12 h ——— or more									
Chemical sporicide solution, e.g., 8.0% formaldehyde plus 70% isopropanol, glutaraldehyde[a]	Room temperature										
Disinfection: killing of disease-producing microbial agents, but not resistant spores											
Boiling water or free-flowing steam	212°F (100°C)	———— or more, 30 min for hepatitis viruses									
Chemical germicide solutions, e.g., iodophors, phenylphenols, quarternary ammonium compounds	Room temperature	————— or more									
Sanitization: Chemicals aided by physical methods of soil removal	Maximum of 200°F (93°C)	———————————————									

[a]Recommended for high-level disinfection.
Modified from a chart copyrighted in 1967, Research and Development Section, American Sterilizer Co., Erie, PA.

Decontamination—the use of physical, chemical, or other means to remove, inactivate, or destroy harmful microorganisms or chemicals from a surface

Disinfectant—an agent, usually chemical, applied to inanimate objects/surfaces for the purpose of destroying disease-causing microbial agents, but usually not bacterial spores

Germicide—an agent, usually chemical, applied either to inanimate objects/surfaces or living tissue for the purpose of destroying disease-causing microbial agents, but usually not bacterial spores

Primary disinfection—those disinfection procedures carried out prior to embalming the body. This would include topical disinfection of and washing the deceased human body

Sanitizer—an agent, usually chemical, that possesses disinfecting properties when applied to a precleaned object/surface

Sterilization—a process that renders a substance free from all microorganisms

Terminal disinfection—the cleaning and disinfection of the body, instruments and the embalming room following embalming of the body

Topical Disinfectants in the Preparation Room

Topical disinfectants are used either for the sanitation of the skin and the hair of the dead human body's external orifices or for the sanitation of exposed tissues as a result of trauma, autopsy, organ and/or tissue donation. These chemicals are also used to disinfect body bags, clothing, medical devices, and protective garments (diapers) removed from the body. Instruments, counter tops and embalming tables, and equipment can also be sanitized with a good topical disinfectant.

The disinfectant needs to be broad-spectrum—meaning bactericidal, fungicidal, virucidal, and ideally tuberculocidal. Read the labels carefully. Instructions for use will be explained. These chemicals are also dated and this needs to be noted. There is a period of time in which the chemical needs to be in contact with the object or the surface being disinfected, and this time element should also be listed.

Areas to be treated, ideally need to first be cleaned using a good antiseptic soap. Remove as much contaminated organic matter as possible (blood, sputum, feces, urine, etc.). Apply the chemical as a heavy droplet spray. Give the chemical sufficient time to work. Remove and dry using a disposable towel. Dispose of the towel in a biohazard waste container.

Today, a good topical disinfectant from a mortuary supply company should be effective against tuberculosis,

Staphylococcus aureus, human immunodeficiency virus (HIV), herpes simplex virus, hepatitis B virus (HBV), methicillin-resistant **S. aureus** (MRSA), and vancomycin-resistant **Enterococcus faecalis** (VRE).

QUALITIES OF A GOOD TOPICAL DISINFECTANT

1. It is active, not outdated—should have a long shelf life.
2. Will not corrode or stain instruments.
3. It is effective against a wide range of microbes including viruses and fungi.
4. It destroys microbes and their products quickly.
5. It is a good deodorant for the body.
6. It does not bleach or stain the skin.
7. It is not irritating to the embalmer's skin or respiratory tract.
8. Is not inactivated by the presence of biological debris.

▶ OSHA: HAZARD COMMUNICATION RULE

Chemical Hazards

The federal government has mandated that business and industry, including funeral service, comply with regulations related to the safe handling and use of hazardous substances and materials. The Federal **Hazard Communication Rule** requires that employers communicate to employees the dangers that exist in the workplace as a result of hazardous substances or materials, and directs employers to train employees in the safe use and handling of hazardous substances or materials (Code of Federal Regulations, 1988). Under the Hazard Communication Rule, any chemical or a mixture of chemicals that expose employees to a health or physical risk are considered to be hazardous. Mixtures of chemicals with a composition of 0.1% or more of an ingredient(s) classified as a carcinogen, teratogen, or mutagen are considered to present a physical or a health hazard. Mixtures of chemicals with a composition of 1.0% of an ingredient(s), which although not being classified as a carcinogen, teratogen, or mutagen, but are classified as hazardous substances, are considered to present a physical or a health hazard. Information about the hazards of using certain materials or substances is provided by **Material Safety Data Sheets** (MSDS), labeling, and training.

Material Safety Data Sheets. The Hazard Communication Rule requires manufacturers or suppliers of hazardous materials or substances to include an MSDS with each shipment. The MSDS contains critical information related to the hazards, exposure levels, and symptoms associated with the material or the substance. An MSDS must be kept on file for each hazardous substance or material present in the work area, and must be accessible to employees (Fig. 3–5) (see Appendix 1 page 69).

Labeling. Under the Hazard Communication Rule, all containers that hold hazardous substances or materials must be properly marked with the name of the product as it appears on the MSDS. To be in compliance, any carton of chemicals containing hazmats would be appropriately labeled on the exterior of the box making it clear what the case contained. An MSDS would be found in the carton. Because it is likely that each individual bottle of chemical would be removed from the case and stored separately, each bottle would also need to be clearly labeled.

Training. The Hazard Communication Rule mandates that employers develop a training program that meets the following criteria

1. The employer must identify hazardous substances found in the workplace by their generic, chemical, trade, and/or common names. This information must then be made known to the employees who may potentially have contact with the identified substances.
2. The employer must identify hazardous substances exposure levels that trigger restrictions. There are standards that mandate certain protective procedures and safeguards be put in place when the exposure to hazardous substances approaches, reaches, or exceeds a level that has been determined to be harmful or injurious.
3. The employer must identify the routes of entry, and acute or chronic effects of exposure to hazardous substances. For example, fumes from hazardous substances may be inhaled during normal breathing. Other hazardous substances may be absorbed if they come into direct contact with an employee's skin.
4. The employer must explain the symptoms that accompany exposure. In the case of formaldehyde, the employer might caution the employee to be aware of skin sensitization or irritations of the eyes, nose, and throat.
5. The employer must identify and explain other dangers associated with hazardous substances to which the employee is exposed. Some chemicals, for example, may be flammable or caustic and require special care when being used.
6. The employer must explain emergency treatments that will be employed if there is an exposure incident. If, for example, embalming chemicals get sprayed into the eyes of employees, or onto employees' bodies, training should have already been provided on the proper utilization of an eyewash station or a drench shower.

Material Safety Data Sheet
May be used to comply with
OSHA's Hazard Communication Standard,
29 CFR 1910.1200. Standard must be
Consulted for specific requirements.

U.S. Department of Labor
Occupational Safety and Health Administration
(Non-Mandatory Form)
Form Approved
OMB No. 1218-0072

IDENTITY *(As Used on Label and List)*	*Note: Blank spaces are not permitted. If any item is not applicable, or no information is available, the space must be marked to indicate that.*

Section I

Manufacturer's Name	Emergency Telephone Number
Address *(Number, Street, City, State, and ZIP Code)*	Telephone Number for Information
	Date Prepared
	Signature of Preparer *(optional)*

Section II — Hazardous Ingredients/Identity Information

Hazardous Components (Specific Chemical Identity; Common Name(s))	OSHA PEL	ACGIH TLV	Other Limits Recommended	% *(optional)*

Section III — Physical/Chemical Characteristics

Boiling Point		Specific Gravity (H_2O = 1)	
Vapor Pressure (mm Hg.)		Melting Point	
Vapor Density (AIR = 1)		Evaporation Rate (Butyl Acetate = 1)	

Solubility in Water

Appearance and Odor

Section IV — Fire and Explosion Hazard Data

Flash Point (Method Used)	Flammable Limits	LEL	UEL

Extinguishing Media

Special Fire Fighting Procedures

Unusual Fire and Explosion Hazards

(Reproduce locally)	OSHA 174, Dept. 1985

Figure 3–5. Sample MSDS sheet.

Section V — Reactivity Data

Stability	Unstable		Conditions to Avoid
	Stable		

Incompatibility (*Materials to avoid*)

Hazardous Decomposition or Byproducts

Hazardous Polymerization	May Occur		Conditions to Avoid
	Will Not Occur		

Section VI — Health Hazard Data

Route(s) of Entry: Inhalation?   Skin?   Ingestion?

Health Hazards (*Acute and Chronic*)

Carcinogenicity: NTP?   IARC Monographs?   OSHA Regulated?

Signs and Symptoms of Exposure

Medical Conditions
Generally Aggravated by Exposure

Emergency and First Aid Procedures

Section VII — Precautions for Safe Handling and Use

Steps to Be Taken in Case Material is Released or Spilled

Waste Disposal Method

Precautions to Be Taken in Handling and Storing

Other Precautions

Section VIII — Control Measures

Respiratory Protection (*Specify Type*)

Ventilation	Local Exhaust		Special
	Mechanical (*General*)		Other

Protective Gloves	Eye Protection

Other Protective Clothing or Equipment

Work/Hygienic Practices

* USGPO-1966–491–529/45775

Figure 3–5. (*Continued*)

7. The employer must explain to employees the proper use and handling of hazardous substances. Employees, for example, should be taught methods by which they can protect themselves from the dangers of hazardous substances, such as wearing protective equipment, and avoiding careless or unsafe use of chemicals.

8. The employer must explain cleanup procedures for leaks and spills. An employer, for example, may require that any spill of embalming chemical on the floor of the preparation room be immediately treated by application of a formaldehyde neutralizing spray and wiped up with an absorbent paper towel, which is then placed in a container that is used to handle contaminated materials.

9. The employer must provide information on the name, telephone number, and address of the companies that supply to the workplace those chemicals that are considered hazardous. The employer can easily satisfy this requirement by referring to the manufacturer information section of an MSDS included with chemicals.

10. The employer must inform employees of the existence and location of written materials related to hazardous substances that are found in the workplace. In addition, the employer, upon request, must provide access to copies of training materials for employees, representatives of employees, or regulators.

▶ OSHA: FORMALDEHYDE STANDARD

This standard, which is also part of the federal OSHA requirements, is aimed specifically at addressing hazards associated with exposure to formaldehyde, formaldehyde gas, its solutions, and materials that release formaldehyde. Under the provisions of the Formaldehyde Standard, employers must monitor employees to determine how much exposure exists in the workplace. Studies have shown that exposure to formaldehyde at certain levels will likely cause employees to experience eye, nose, throat, and upper respiratory tract irritation.

Exposure monitoring is accomplished by sampling the air in work spaces where formaldehyde is used. Employers can purchase sampling kits from chemical supply companies and other vendors. Exposure monitoring is intended to determine if the level of exposure to airborne concentrations of formaldehyde in a work area is at or below a specified concentration. The Formaldehyde Standard establishes specific limits on the amount of exposure that is allowed. The specific point at which an 8-hour exposure is unsafe is called the **action level**

(0.5 ppm). If sampling reveals that exposure has reached or exceeded the action level, employers are required to take steps to reduce the exposure. The purpose of requiring exposure reduction at the action level is to insure that exposure does not reach the **permissible exposure limit** (PEL also called the TWA or time-weighted average). The PEL sets the maximum average exposure over 8 hours that is allowed by OSHA or state governments.

There are two types of tests that must occur in every funeral home where any formaldehyde is used: (1) the **time-weighted average** (over a period of 8 hours) (TWA or PEL), and (2) the **short-term exposure level** (over a period of 15 minutes) (STEL). These tests are to be conducted in a "worst case" environment. For example, the TWA testing should be done at a time when there is embalming taking place in the preparation room. When test results document worst-case situations that are within the limits specified by OSHA, it is reasonable to conclude that the air quality of the preparation room at all other times is also acceptable.

Time-weighted Average

Employers are required to take necessary steps to ensure that no employee is exposed to unsafe concentrations of airborne formaldehyde. If the results of the sampling for formaldehyde indicate that the exposure is below 0.5 ppm over an 8-hour period, the action level has not been reached, no additional TWA testing is needed, **except** if (1) the employer receives a report of an employee's symptoms associated with formaldehyde exposure, or (2) there are any changes in procedure, equipment, chemicals, personnel, or other circumstances that affect the work area.

If TWA sampling reveals an exposure that exceeds the STEL or the PEL, the employer is required to implement steps to reduce the exposure. The employer is then required to (1) place formaldehyde warning signs on areas where the concentration of formaldehyde has exceeded these levels, and (2) begin medical surveillance of employees who work in areas where the concentration of formaldehyde has exceeded the STEL or the PEL. These signs must bear the following information

> **Danger**
> **Formaldehyde**
> **Irritant and potential cancer hazard**
> **Authorized personnel only**

Medical surveillance requires that employers take a series of steps aimed at protecting employees. Those steps include having the employees complete a medical questionnaire, which is then reviewed by a physician who can make recommendations based on the employees' responses. The physician can recommend that the employees are having no ill effects and should return to work, or that sufficient cause exists to order that employees be given a medical examination. If the employees are given a medical examination, the physician can recommend that there is no health problem present and employees should return to work, or that a health problem is present and **medical removal** will be ordered.

If medical removal is ordered, the affected employee may not be given preparation duties for up to 6 months. If there is improvement in the physical condition of the employee, the physician may release the employee to return to preparation room duties. If the medical condition of the employee does not improve, (1) the employee may be permanently reassigned to duties other than that in the preparation room, or (2) the employee may be terminated. If employers elect to terminate employees who are medically unable to perform the tasks and duties for which they were hired, there may well be issues related to disability coverage and Worker's Compensation to be addressed.

TIME-WEIGHTED AVERAGE SAMPLING AT OR ABOVE 0.75 PPM. In those cases where TWA sampling reveals airborne concentrations of formaldehyde at or above 0.75 ppm, it shows that the permissible exposure limit has been reached. Employers are then required to (1) post formaldehyde warning signs in and around the work area(s), (2) begin medical surveillance, and (3) provide respirators for employees who are assigned to work in the posted area(s).

RESPIRATORS. There are employers who think that respirators are an easy solution to any problems that arise from formaldehyde concentrations in the preparation area. This is not true! Employers and employees should be aware that OSHA has a respirator standard that must be followed when respirators are put into use in the preparation room. Two of the major provisions of the Respirator Standard are that (1) employees must be fit-tested to see if a respirator is appropriate for them, and (2) a personal respirator must be fitted to each individual employee, and refitted regularly.

THE SHORT-TERM EXPOSURE LEVEL. In addition to the TWA (which is sampled over 8 hours), employers are required to sample for airborne concentrations of formaldehyde over a 15-minute period. If the sampling reveals a concentration of airborne formaldehyde that is **below** 2 ppm, the permissible exposure limit has not been reached and no further short-term exposure limit testing is required, unless (1) the employer receives a report of an employee's symptoms associated with formaldehyde exposure, or (2) there are any changes in procedure, equipment, chemicals, personnel, or other circumstances that affect the work area.

If STEL sampling reveals airborne concentrations of formaldehyde **at or above** 2 ppm the permissible exposure limit has been reached and the employer is required to (1) use formaldehyde warning signs, (2) begin medical surveillance, and (3) require employees assigned to duties in the preparation room to wear respirators.

If the initial testing shows airborne concentrations of formaldehyde above either the action level for the TWA, or the permissible limit for the STEL, employers must begin periodic testing of the employees. Periodic testing means that employers must retest the work area at least every 6 months if exposure is over the action level and every 12 months if exposure is over the STEL. If employers have two consecutive retests, which are conducted at least 7 days apart, that show concentrations below the action level for the TWA, and below the permissible exposure limit for the STEL, the periodic monitoring of employees can be stopped.

See Chapter 7, NFDA Formaldehyde Best Work Practices—2010.

Methods of Compliance with the Formaldehyde Standard

Work Practice Controls. Examples of work practice controls for compliance with the formaldehyde standard include:

1. Wearing appropriate protective equipment when handling chemicals to avoid exposure by contact with the skin.
2. Exercising care when handling and pouring chemicals to avoid spills.
3. Handling and pouring chemicals in a way that prevents vapors from escaping into the room.
4. Keeping instruments and equipment in good working condition to prevent spills and vaporization.
5. Keeping the lid on the embalming machine when embalming solution is in the tank.
6. Recapping fluid bottles.
7. Properly rinsing fluid bottles.
8. Continuously aspirating body cavities during autopsy embalming.
9. Controlling drainage and leakage from the body by utilizing a drainage tube with sufficient length of tubing to reach the bottom of the sink or flush basin reduces chemical splashing.
10. Utilizing a continuous flow of water over the embalming table to rinse and dilute chemicals.
11. Keeping the lid on hazardous waste containers.
12. Maintaining a cover on all sinks and flush basins that the embalming table and aspirator drain into.

Engineering Controls. Examples of engineering controls for compliance with the Formaldehyde Standard are essentially the same as for biological hazards. They can be considered in terms of proper plumbing and adequate ventilation. Plumbing considerations include

1. Providing vacuum breakers on the main water line leading into the building
2. Providing vacuum breakers on hydroaspirators
3. Maintaining discharge basins/flush sinks in good working order
4. Having a suitable water source for the preparation table
5. Having a proper eyewash station
6. Having a proper drench shower
7. Having a proper hand washing station
8. Having proper shower room facilities

Ventilation considerations include having an exhaust for the room located at the foot of the embalming table, **below** the level of the table top. As previously stated, the air replacement vent for the room should ideally be high on the opposite wall. The idea is to introduce fresh air blown toward the embalmer, while the contaminated air is being drawn away from the embalmer. As a rough rule of thumb for a single-table room, the number of air changes ranges from 12 to 20 per hour. The number may vary depending on the contents of the room, the number of bodies that will be embalmed in the room at one time, the shape of the room, weather-related factors, and the preference of the embalmer. Again, the Public Health Guidelines have recommended a ventilation system that creates a minimum of six air changes per hour, and preferably more in a preparation room.

The Formaldehyde Standard also requires employee information and training. Employers must introduce employees, who have occupational exposure, to Material Safety Data Sheets, and identify methods by which employees will have access to the information. Initial training must be provided to employees prior to their being exposed to hazardous substances. In addition, employees must receive additional training if a change in work assignment results in exposure to hazardous substances. Employees must also receive annual updates at intervals of not greater than 1 year. The purpose of the training is to provide employees with information, procedures, and techniques necessary to safely handle substances that contain formaldehyde (see Appendix 1 pages 69–74 for additional hazardous chemicals.)

▶ ENVIRONMENTAL HEALTH AND SAFETY STANDARDS

The National Funeral Directors Association (NFDA) has drafted a set of Environmental Health and Safety Practices. Permission has been given to reproduce those practices. These practices are not intended to fully meet regulatory compliance or legal standards. Individual state statutory and federal regulatory compliance agencies governing funeral service practices need to be consulted.

If observed conscientiously, the following practices will help funeral directors (and embalmers) meet the highest standards of excellence of the funeral service profession.

- **Secure the preparation room.** Do you have procedures in place ensuring that only trained and authorized personnel enter preparation areas? Never enter preparation areas unless you have received proper training, your vaccinations are up-to-date, and you have selected appropriate PPE, including shoe covers. Do not smoke, eat, drink, apply personal makeup, or handle your contact lenses in preparation areas.
- **Evaluate exposure risks.** Are there special risks or diseases associated with the procedure you are performing? Universal precautions must always be observed, but they may or may not be sufficient to keep you safe.
- **Know the products you are using.** Are you familiar with the labels and the Material Safety Data Sheets (MSDSs) for the products you use? Always retain the current MSDS your supplier ships in each new box of chemicals. MSDSs for all products you use must be present and readily accessible on the work site. Make sure all containers are labeled properly. Labels and MSDSs tell you about the chemicals that the products contain—how to handle and dispose of them, and what to do in the case of an emergency.
- **Prepare for emergencies.** When was the last time your emergency equipment was tested? Know where to find and how to operate drench showers, eyewash stations, fire extinguishers, spill cleanup, and all other emergency equipment. Know exactly where your MSDSs are located. Post emergency telephone numbers by all phones.
- **Limit toxicity and waste.** How much of each product are you using and why? Use only the amount of product needed to assure the procedure you are performing is carried out properly. Try to avoid the use of products containing phenol and cresol. Ask your supplier about substitute products that are environmentally friendly. Keep covers on embalming machines. Make sure ventilation systems are clean and running properly. Conduct formaldehyde exposure testing annually. Remember that changes in ventilation, the design of your preparation room, or even volume

of work can change exposure levels. Testing should be performed immediately following such changes.

■ **Avoid solvents and chlorinated compounds.** Are you certain that solvents and chlorinated compounds—such as trichloroethylene (TCE) and perchloroethylene (Perc)—are not going down the drain? Found in some cosmetics, adhesives, tissue builders, and cleaning products, these compounds should only be used topically—if used at all. Make sure solvents and chlorinated compounds are never introduced, even in trace amounts, into drains, sinks, embalming tanks, or groundwater. Gauze or cotton containing these compounds and residue in empty containers should never be tossed into a dumpster or commingled with other wastes. Check MSDSs to determine whether special handling or disposal is required for products containing these compounds.

■ **Know how to manage you wastewater.** Do you know the composition of your wastewater and the proper disposal practices? Permits and reports may be required. Your disposal system should be sized properly, operated correctly, and maintained regularly. Think of the drain as the beginning—not the end—of your sanitary and embalming waste stream. Even the smallest disposal system problems should be investigated and corrected immediately, by using the services of a trained licensed professional. Remember that funeral home expansion may require wastewater disposal system expansion. Septic tanks must be pumped regularly, no less often than every 3 years.

■ **Handle sharps carefully.** Are sharps clean, disinfected, and stored safely? Always use appropriate engineering and safety devices for sharps. Syringe caps and scalpel blade removal/disposal devices that do not require manual handling of the blade are a must. Sharps must be discarded in properly designed and labeled containers for contaminated sharps.

■ **Think before you flip the switch.** Are you being as careful as you should with power-assisted devices? Always follow manufacturer instructions when using power-assisted equipment.

■ **Do not just toss it in the trash.** Do you know where to discard recycled materials, biomedical waste, hazardous waste, contaminated PPE, and potentially contaminated laundry? Be sure to differentiate among the waste you produce, as different rules apply to different wastes. Appropriate, clearly labeled waste containers must be present in the work area. Use licensed and reputable disposal firms. Know where wastes are being taken for disposal and ask about the compliance status of the disposal facility. Keep copies of all waste disposal receipts. Manifests must be maintained and ready for inspection.

■ **Recycle.** Do you have a recycling program? Talk to your supplier about recycling the products you are purchasing and find out about community recycling programs. Do not throw away materials that should be recycled.

■ **Keep it clean.** Are you keeping the work area clean and disinfected? Decontaminate work surfaces immediately if they are overtly contaminated, after any spill and after completing preparation procedures. Wash your hands after every procedure and before you leave the area.

■ **Document your work.** Do you always complete embalming reports and file them in the business office? Report any and all incidents and/or accidents to your supervisor immediately to initiate appropriate follow-up action.

▶ CONCLUSION

The dictates of logic, reason, and research all demand that the dead human body be considered a source of pathogenic microorganisms. Embalmers are charged by the same dictates and by law with the responsibility to implement protective and thorough procedures to ensure that the potential for contagion through exposure to the body is minimized.

$$\text{RISK} = \text{Toxicity} \times \text{Exposure}$$

Proper utilization of the PPE and good disinfectants reduces both toxicity and exposure, thus creating a managed risk.

See Selected Readings section of this text, for detailed studies dealing with topics of hazards of infection, treatment of CJD cases, and ventilation and disinfectant studies.

▶ KEY TERMS AND CONCEPTS FOR STUDY AND DISCUSSION

1. Define the following terms
   Action level
   Airborne pathogen
   Aerosolization
   Asepsis
   Bactericidal
   Bacteriostatic
   Biological hazard
   Bloodborne pathogen
   Bloodborne Pathogen Rule

Cold chemical sterilant
Concurrent disinfection/decontamination
Decontamination
Disinfect
Employee Right-To-Know laws
Engineering controls
Exposure control plan
Formaldehyde Standard
Germicide
Hazard Communication Rule
MSDS
OSHA
PEL
Respirator Standard
Sanitizer
Squeegee effect
STEL
Sterilization
Terminal disinfection/decontamination
TWA
Universal precautions
Work practice controls

2. Describe the research findings documenting the occupational risk faced by embalmers as a result of their exposure to biological hazards.

3. Describe the research findings documenting the occupational risks faced by embalmers as a result of their exposure to chemical hazards.

4. In addition to biological and chemical hazards, what other occupational hazards do embalmers face?

5. What is the minimum documentation required for a Bloodborne Pathogen Exposure Control Plan?

6. Describe the basic premise of universal precautions.

7. What are the two primary areas of consideration for engineering controls?

8. Name five common work practice controls that would contribute to a hygienic environment in the embalming room.

9. List the six areas of training and instruction required for Personal Protective Equipment.

10. Describe the provisions of hepatitis B vaccination and postexposure evaluation and follow-up.

11. List the four types of labeling provisions that can be used to communicate the hazards of potentially infectious agents.

12. With regard to hazardous chemicals, what are the two main requirements of the Hazard Communication Rule?

13. At what concentration does formaldehyde vapor in a room constitute a potential health hazard to the embalmer?

14. Describe the provisions that make up the medical surveillance of employees who are exposed to formaldehyde vapor in the embalming room?

15. Describe the three categories of training required under the Formaldehyde Standard.

▶ BIBLIOGRAPHY

An Embalmer's Odds of Contracting Diseases. *The Forum,* December 2009.

Beck-Sague C, Jarvis W, Fruehling J, et al. Universal precautions and mortuary practitioners: Influence on practices and risk of occupationally acquired infection. *J Occup Med* 1991;33:874-878.

Bender JR, Mullin LS, Grapel GJ, et al. Eye irritation response in humans to formaldehyde. *Am Ind Hygiene Assoc J* 1983;44:463-465.

Benenson AS, ed. *Control of Communicable Diseases Manual,* 16th ed. American Public Health Association, 1995.

The Bloodborne Pathogen Rule. Code of Federal Regulations. Title 29 CFR Part 1910, Occupational Safety and Health Administration, Department of Labor, Toxic and Hazardous Substances. The Bloodborne Pathogen Rule 1910.1030, 1992.

Burke P, Sheffner A. The anti-microbial effects of embalming chemicals and topical disinfectants on the microbial Flora of human remains. *Health Laboratory Sciences* October 1976.

Code of Federal Regulations. Title 29: Subtitle B—Regulations Relating to Labor: Chapter XVII—Occupational Safety and Health Administration, Department of Labor; Part 1910, Hazard Communication 1910.1200, 1988.

Collison K, Adams J. The CDC advises us not to panic about CJD. *Dodge Mag* September 1999.

Collison K. Hepatitis A to G. *Dodge Mag* January 1999.

Environmental Health and Safety Practices. Brookville, WI: National Funeral Directors Association, 2004.

Gershon R, Vlahov D, Escamilla-Cejudo J, et al. Tuberculosis risk in funeral home employees. *J Occup Environ Med* May 1998:497-503.

Kerfoot EJ. Formaldehyde vapor emission study in embalming rooms. *The Director* 1972:42.

Kerfoot EJ, Mooney TF. Formaldehyde and paraformaldehyde study in funeral homes. *Am Ind Hygiene Assoc J* 1975;36:533-537.

McDonald L. Blood exposure and protection in funeral homes. *Am J Infect Control* August 1989:193-195.

McKenna MT, Hutton M, Cauthen G, et al. The association between occupation and tuberculosis. *Am J Resp Crit Care Med* 1996;154:587-596.

Nethercott JR, Holness DL. Contact dermatitis in funeral service workers. *Contact Dermatitis* 1988;18;263-267.

State of Minnesota. Minnesota Rule Chapter 5206.0400, Subpart 5. *Employee Right-To-Know Standards.* Minneapolis, MN: Department of Labor and Industry, 1995.

Turner S, Kunches L, Gordon K, et al. Occupational exposure to human immunodeficiency virus (HIV) and hepatitis B virus (HBV) among embalmers: A pilot seroprevalence study. *Am J Pub Health* October 1989:1425-1426.

Williams TM, Levine RJ, Blunden PB. Exposure of embalmers to formaldehyde and other chemicals. *American Industrial Hygiene Asso. Journal* 1984;45:172-176.

APPENDIX 1

▶ HAZARDOUS CHEMICALS

The following three examples represent chemicals commonly used in the preparation room. Synonyms, dilution limits, and health effects come from an material safety data sheet (MSDS) directory, which is available to the public on the Internet, at the University of California, one of many sites that offer MSDSs. The term "MSDS" or the specific chemical name should be used when doing a search. A complete list of hazardous chemicals may be obtained by contacting the National Funeral Directors Association, 13625 Bishop's Drive, Brookfield, WI 53005 for its publication, *Hazard Communication Program.* It is important to understand that the severity of the health effects listed for the chemicals will depend on the amount of material in the product, the frequency and duration of your exposure, and your individual susceptibility. Some states with their own OSHA programs have replaced the Federal Hazard Communication Rule with an Employee Right-to-Know Rule. For example, the State of Minnesota recognizes 1025 hazardous chemicals and provides a list of these chemicals in its Employee Right-to-Know Rule.

▶ EXAMPLES OF HAZARDOUS CHEMICALS

Formaldehyde. (formic aldehyde; paraform; formol; formalin (methanol-free); fyde; formalith; methanal; methyl aldehyde; methylene glycol; methylene oxide; tetraoxymethalene; oxomethane; oxymethylene; when in aqueous solution, the term formalin is often used.)

OSHA Action	OSHA TWA (PEL)	OSHA STEL
Level: 0.5 ppm	0.75 ppm	2 ppm

Health Effects: Ingestion. Acute Exposure—Liquids containing 10 to 40% formaldehyde cause severe irritation and inflammation of the mouth, the throat, and the stomach. Severe stomach pains will follow ingestion with possible loss of consciousness and death. Ingestion of dilute formaldehyde solutions (0.03–0.04%) may cause discomfort in the stomach and the pharynx.

Health Effects: Eye Contact. Acute Exposure—Formaldehyde solutions splashed in the eye can cause injuries ranging from transient discomfort to severe, permanent corneal clouding and loss of vision. The severity of the effect depends on the concentration of formaldehyde in the solution and whether or not the eyes are flushed with water immediately after exposure.

Note: The perception of formaldehyde by odor and eye irritation becomes less sensitive with time as one adapts to its use. This can lead to overexposure, if a worker is relying on formaldehyde's warning properties to alert him or her to potential overexposure.

Chronic Exposure—permanent corneal clouding and loss of vision.

Health Effects: Skin Contact. Acute Exposure—Formalin is a severe skin irritant and a sensitizer. Contact with formalin causes white discoloration, smarting, drying, cracking, and scaling. Prolonged and repeated contact can cause numbness and a hardening or tanning of the skin. Previously exposed persons may react to future exposure with an allergic eczematous dermatitis or hives.

Chronic Exposure—a hardening and tanning of the skin. Sensitive persons can develop an allergic eczematous dermatitis and hives.

Health Effects: Inhalation. Acute Exposure—formaldehyde is highly irritating to the upper respiratory tract and eyes. Concentrations of 0.5 to 2.0 ppm may irritate the eyes, nose, and throat of some individuals. Concentrations of 3 to 5 ppm also cause tearing of the eyes and are intolerable to some persons. Concentrations of 10 to 20 ppm cause difficulty in breathing, burning of the nose and throat, cough, and heavy tearing of the eyes; and concentrations of 25 to 30 ppm causes severe respiratory tract injury leading to pulmonary edema and pneumonitis. A concentration of 100 ppm is immediately dangerous to life and health. Deaths from accidental exposure to high concentrations of formaldehyde have been reported.

Chronic Exposure—Formaldehyde exposure has been associated with cancers of the lung, nasopharynx and oropharynx, and nasal passages. Prolonged or repeated exposure to formaldehyde may result in respiratory impairment. Rats exposed to formaldehyde at 2 ppm developed benign nasal tumors and changes of the cell structure in the nose as well as inflamed mucous membranes of the nose. Structural changes in the epithelial cells in the human nose have also been observed. Some persons have developed asthma or bronchitis following the exposure to formaldehyde, most often as the result of an accidental spill involving a single exposure to a high concentration of formaldehyde.

Incompatibilities: Strong oxidizing agents, caustics, strong alkalies, isocyanates, anhydrides, oxides, and inorganic acids. Formaldehyde reacts with hydrochloric acid to form the potent carcinogen, bis-chloromethyl ether. Formaldehyde reacts with nitrogen dioxide, nitromethane, perchloric acid and aniline, or peroxyformic acid to yield explosive compounds. A violent reaction occurs when formaldehyde is mixed with strong oxidizers. Oxygen from the air can oxidize formaldehyde to formic acid, especially when heated. Formic acid is corrosive.

Found in: Embalming adhesive gel, feature builder, embalming spray, sanitizing embalming spray, preservative cream, arterial embalming chemicals, preservative/disinfectant gel, supplemental embalming gel, accessory embalming chemical, incision sealer, preinjection chemicals, bleaching agents, cavity embalming fluid/gel.

Phenol (benzenol; carbolic acid; hydroxybenzene; monohydroxybenzene; monophenol; oxybenzene; phenic acid; phenyl alcohol; phenyl hydrate; phenyl hydroxide; phenylic acid; phenylic alcohol)

OSHA TWA (PEL)	ACGIH TWA (PEL)
for skin: 5 ppm	for skin: 5 ppm
NIOSH-recommended	NIOSH-recommended
TWA (PEL): 5 ppm	ceiling: 15.6 ppm

Health Effects: Ingestion. Acute Exposure—Inhalation may cause severe irritation of the mucous membranes, profuse sweating, headache, intense thirst, nausea and vomiting, abdominal pain, diarrhea, salivation, cyanosis, tinnitus, twitching, tremors, and convulsions. The central nervous system may initially be stimulated followed by severe, profound depression progressing to coma. The heart rate may increase, then become slow and irregular. The blood pressure may increase slightly and then fall markedly with dyspnea and fall in body temperature. Stertorous breathing, mucous rales, and frothing at the mouth and nose may indicate the presence of pulmonary edema that may be followed by pneumonia. Methemoglobinemia and hemolysis have been reported occasionally. Death may occur from respiratory, circulatory, or cardiac failure. If death is not immediate, jaundice and oliguria or anuria may occur. Ingestion of 250 ppm is immediately dangerous to life or health.

Chronic Exposure—Symptoms of chronic phenol poisoning may include vomiting, difficulty swallowing, ptyalism, diarrhea, anorexia, headache, vertigo, muscle weakness and pain, mental disturbances, dark or smoky urine, and possibly skin eruptions. Extensive damage to the liver and kidneys may be fatal. Hind limb paralysis has been reported in animals. Pathologic findings, in animals repeatedly exposed to phenol vapors, include extensive necrosis of the myocardium, acute lobular pneumonia, vascular damage, and liver and kidney damage.

Health Effects: Skin Contact. Acute Exposure—Contact with 0.5% solutions may cause local anesthesia, 1% solutions sometimes cause skin necrosis, and 10% solutions may cause burns. Phenol burns may be severe, but painless due to damage to nerve endings. The skin may turn white, and later yellowish-brown and may be deeply eroded and scarred. Gangrene may occur at the site of contact. Vapors and liquid may be readily absorbed through the skin to cause systemic effects as detailed in acute inhalation exposure. There have been several reports of cardiac arrhythmias associated with application of solutions of phenol, hexachlorophene, and croton oil to the skin. Profound coma and death have been reported to occur within 10 minutes following skin contact. Pathologic findings included congestion of the lungs, liver, spleen, and kidneys.

Chronic Exposure—Prolonged exposure may cause a blue or brownish discoloration of the tendons over the knuckles of the hands, dermatitis, vitiligo, and rarely, skin sensitization. Symptoms of chronic phenol poisoning may occur as detailed as under chronic inhalation exposure. Evaluated by Registry of Toxic Effects of Chemical Substances (RTECS) as producing carcinogenic and neoplastic tumors in mice.

Health Effects: Eye Contact. Acute Exposure—Phenol vapors have caused marked irritation from brief, intermittent industrial exposure to 48 ppm. Concentrated liquid or solid may cause severe irritation with redness, pain, and blurred vision. Concentrated phenol in human eyes has caused chemotic conjunctiva, hypesthetic, white cornea, edematous eyelids, and severe iritis. In some cases, the eyelids have been so severely damaged that they required plastic surgery. The final visual results have varied from complete recovery, to partial recovery, to blindness and loss of the eye. Crystalline or concentrated aqueous phenol on rabbit eyes causes almost instantaneous white opacification of the corneal epithelium. Eight hours later, the cornea was anesthetic, the surface ulcerated, and the stroma opaque. Five weeks later, entropion, scarring of the conjunctiva, and opacity of the cornea occurred.

Chronic Exposure—Repeated or prolonged exposure to phenol vapors may cause conjunctivitis and has caused gray discoloration of the sclera with brown spots near the insertion of the rectus muscle tendon.

Health Effects: Ingestion. Acute Exposure—Ingestion may cause immediate intense burning of the mouth and the throat, white or brownish stains and areas of necrosis on the lips and in the mouth and esophagus, marked abdominal pain, pale face, and contracted or dilated pupils. Systemic effects may occur as detailed under acute inhalation exposure. The approximate lethal dose in humans is 140 mg/kg.

Chronic Exposure—Persons ingesting phenol-contaminated well water experienced diarrhea, dark urine, and sores and burning in the mouth. Other symptoms of chronic phenol poisoning may occur as detailed under chronic inhalation exposure. Administration of phenol in drinking water to rats for three generations produced stunted growth at 7000 ppm over two generations; offspring of rats given 10,000 ppm died; at 12,000 ppm animals did not reproduce. Other reproductive effects have also been reported in animals.

Incompatibilities: *Alkalies:* acetaldehyde; aluminum and alloys; aluminum chloride plus nitrobenzene; 1,3-butadiene; boron trifluoride; diethyl etherate; calcium hypochlorite; formaldehyde; lead and alloys; magnesium and alloys; metals and alloys; oxidizers (strong); peroxodisulfuric acid; peroxomonosulfuric acid; plastics; rubber; sodium nitrate; trifluoroacetic acid; sodium nitrite; zinc and alloys.

Found in: Embalming cauterant; embalming chemical disinfectant; cavity embalming fluid/gel, preservative/disinfectant gel; accessory embalming chemical.

Glutaraldehyde (1,5-pentanedial)

OSHA PEL: 0.2 ppm   ACGIH TLV: 0.2 ppm

Health Effects: Inhalation. Acute Exposure—Irritation, headaches, may cause nose and throat irritation and burning, difficulty in breathing.
Chronic Exposure—None known.

Health Effects: Ingestion. Acute Exposure—May cause nausea, vomiting, and systemic illness.
Chronic Exposure—None known.

Health Effects: Skin Contact. Acute Exposure—Sensitization dermatitis.
Chronic Exposure—None known.

Health Effects: Eye Contact. Acute Exposure—Loss of vision.
Chronic Exposure—None known.
Incompatibilities: Strong oxidizing agent.

Found In: Arterial, cavity, and accessory embalming fluids; humectant; tissue filler; disinfectant and preservative gels.

▶ OTHER DANGEROUS CHEMICALS USED IN THE FUNERAL PROFESSION

The following is a sample listing of commonly used chemicals found in the compounding of products used in the preparation room. Each of these toxic chemicals is explained in more detail on the MSDS that accompanies the product.

Acetone (2-propanone; dimethylformaldehyde; dimethyl ketone; beta-ketopropane; methyl ketone; propanone; pyroacetic ether)—A narcotic in high concentrations which can cause skin irritation. Prolonged inhalation can cause headache, dryness, and throat irritation. A dangerous fire risk when exposed to heat, flame, or oxidizers. Found in: accessory embalming chemicals, external sealing composition, lip tint, solvents, and sealants.

Alkyl dimethylbenzyl ammonium chloride—This material belongs to the chemical family called quaternary ammonium compounds. It is a skin and eye irritant, has moderate-to-high oral toxicity, and is moderately toxic via skin absorption. Found in: cold disinfectant, embalming spray, and embalming cauterants.

Amaranth (trisodium salt of 1-[4-sulfo-1-naphthylazo]-2-naphthol-3, 6-disulfonic acid)—Formerly known as red dye #2, this member of the azo dye family is a suspected human carcinogen. It is no longer acceptable in food, drugs, or cosmetics. Found in: coloring powder for arterial fluids.

Amitrole (2-amino-1,2,4-triazole)—Moderate-to-low oral toxicity. Listed by International Agency for Research on Cancer (IARC) and National Toxicology Program (NTP) as a possible carcinogen. Found in: cavity fluid.

Ammonia—Causes nose and throat irritation; may cause bronchial spasm, chest pain, pulmonary edema, and skin burns. Incompatible with hypochlorite (household bleach) that is often used to disinfect the preparation area after embalming. Found in: cleaning agents used to neutralize formaldehyde.

2-Butoxyethanol (butyl Cellosolve, ethylene glycol monobutyl ether)—Mildly irritating to skin, and can be absorbed through contact. It is a strong respiratory and eye irritant, and exposure may result in transient corneal clouding; repeated overexposure can cause fatigue, headache, nausea, and tremors. It is a moderate fire risk, which will react with oxidizers. Found in: arterial embalming chemicals.

Camphor—High-to-moderate ingestion hazard. Local exposure may cause irritation. Found in: embalming fluid.

Carbon tetrachloride (tetrachloromethane)—Can cause depression, nausea, vomiting, and local skin irritation; prolonged exposure and absorption through the skin could produce liver and kidney failure. Found in: organic solvents.

Chlorine salts (hypochlorites)—Chlorine salts produce chlorinated vapor causing moderate-to-severe skin and eye irritations, tissue damage, and moderate-to-severe respiratory irritation. They are strong oxidizers and are highly reactive, and can be a serious fire risk when exposed to reducing agents (acids) or petroleum derivatives. Found in: embalming deodorant, bleach, and disinfectants.

Chloroform (trichloromethane)—Formerly used as an anesthetic, chloroform causes depression and skin and eye irritation; prolonged exposure can lead to cardiac and respiratory arrest or paralysis; chronic exposure may cause liver damage. Listed in IARC and NTP as a possible carcinogen. Found in: accessory embalming chemical sealant.

Cresol (2-hydroxy-4-methylphenol)—The health effects are similar to those of phenol, but not as severe. It is corrosive to skin, eyes, and mucous membranes; capable of causing burns at point of contact; and can be absorbed through the skin. Chronic low-level exposure can cause skin rash and discoloration, gastrointestinal disturbances, nervous system disturbances, and kidney and liver damage. It is a moderate fire hazard that can react vigorously with oxidizing materials. Found in: disinfectant and accessory embalming chemicals.

Diethanolamine—A severe eye irritant and mild skin irritant which is moderately toxic through ingestion. It can react with oxidizers. Found in: humectant and arterial embalming fluid.

Diethylene glycol—A skin and eye irritant which is highly toxic through inhalation. It can react with oxidizers. Found in: arterial and cavity embalming fluids.

Dimethylformamide—A strong irritant to skin and other tissues, it is readily absorbed through the skin. Inhalation or skin contact can cause gastrointestinal disturbances, facial flushing, elevated blood pressure, central nervous system (CNS) disorders, and liver and kidney damage. It is a moderate fire risk which can be an explosion hazard when exposed to flame. Dimethylformamide is reactive with a variety of halogenated materials and organics. Found in: solvents.

Ethyl acetate—Irritates the eyes, gums, skin, and respiratory tract. Repeated overexposure can cause conjunctivitis and corneal clouding; high concentrations can result in congestion of the liver and kidneys. Ethyl acetate is a dangerous fire risk. Found in: embalming cosmetic spray, cavity fluid, sanitizing spray, and sealing lacquer.

Ethyl alcohol (denatured ethanol, SD alcohol)—Ethyl alcohol is generally not considered an occupational health hazard, but its flammability makes it a safety hazard. The terms "SDA" or "SD alcohol," mean "specially denatured alcohol." SDA is ethyl alcohol to which another substance, such as *tert*-butyl alcohol, has been added to make it unfit for human consumption. Found in: cavity fluid, cosmetics.

EDTA (ethylenediaminetetraacetic acid)—EDTA is found in a variety of products as either tetrasodium or disodium salt. Both react chemically to bind calcium, which inhibits the blood clotting mechanism. EDTA is a skin irritant, causing dryness and cracking. Found in: arterial fluids, preinjection fluids, co-injection fluids, cavity fluids.

Ethylene dichloride (1,2-dichloroethene or 1,1-dichloroethene)—A strong irritant to skin and eyes which is toxic via inhalation and skin absorption. Ethylene dichloride is listed in IARC as a possible carcinogen. It is a dangerous fire risk. Found in: embalming fluid and cavity fluid.

Ethylene glycol (1,2-ethanediol)—Moderately irritating to skin, eyes, and mucous membranes; very toxic through inhalation, producing depression and damage to blood-forming organs. Ethylene glycol does not readily vaporize at room temperature, and inhalation would be likely only by heating or mechanical action (aerosolization). Ingestion can lead to respiratory, renal, and cardiac failure. Brain damage may also result. Chronic exposure can cause anorexia, decreased urinary output, and involuntary rapid eye movement. Ethylene glycol is combustible and can react violently with certain acids and oxidizers. Found in: arterial and cavity embalming chemicals, external embalming seal, tissue surface embalming seal, anticoagulant/clot remover, and water correctives.

Ethylene glycol monomethyl ether (methyl Cellosolve)—Moderately toxic via inhalation, ingestion, and skin absorption. May cause conjunctivitis, transient corneal clouding, and upper respiratory tract irritation. Found in: cosmetics.

Formic acid (methanoic acid)—Corrosive to skin, eyes, and mucous membranes. Formic acid has a moderate-to-high oral toxicity, and can be absorbed through the skin. It is a moderate fire risk. Found in: supplemental embalming chemicals and bleaching agents.

Hexylene glycol (2,4-hexanediol)—An eye, skin, and mucous membrane irritant which is moderately toxic through inhalation and ingestion. Large oral doses can have a narcotic effect. A low fire risk, hexylene glycol can react with oxidizers. Found in: arterial embalming fluid.

Isobutane (2-methylpropane)—While otherwise practically nontoxic, the inhalation of isobutane can cause suffocation. A dangerous fire risk when exposed to heat, flame, or oxidizers. Found in: aerosol propellants, cosmetics, insecticides, and deodorants.

Isopropyl alcohol (2-propanol)—An eye, nose, and throat irritant , in high concentration, it causes: mild narcotic effects, corneal burn, and eye damage. Drying to the skin, isopropyl alcohol is moderately toxic via ingestion. Ingestion or inhalation of heavy vapor concentrations can cause flushing and CNS depression. As little as 100 mL can be fatal if ingested. It is a dangerous fire risk and a moderate explosion risk when exposed to heat, flame, or oxidizers. Found in: cavity and accessory embalming fluids, feature builder, cosmetics, color concentrate, fungal inhibitors, preinjection chemicals, liquid embalming cosmetics and sprays, tissue filler, supplemental embalming gels, aerosol deodorant, sealing lacquers, and solvent thinners.

Methyl alcohol (wood alcohol, methanol)—A skin, eye, and respiratory tract irritant which is moderately toxic via inhalation, and moderately to highly toxic through ingestion. The main target is the CNS, but it also affects the eyes, optic nerve, and possibly the retina. Overexposure can cause depression, sight impairment, weakness, and gastrointestinal disturbances. Severe overexposure can result in cardiac depression. Because methyl alcohol is metabolized slowly, sufficient daily intake can lead to cumulative exposure symptoms. Methyl alcohol is a dangerous fire and explosion risk when exposed to heat, flame, and oxidizers. Found in: arterial, cavity, and accessory embalming fluids and gels; cleaning and disinfecting fluids, gels and solvents; tissue fillers; embalming cauterants; bleaching agents; cosmetics; and color concentrates.

Methyl ethyl ketone (2-butanone)—Repeated exposure can cause skin irritation and inflammation; vapors can produce eye, nose, and throat irritation. Methyl ethyl ketone is highly volatile and a narcotic by inhalation, affecting both the CNS and the peripheral nerves. Methyl ethyl ketone can react violently with aldehydes and acids. It is a dangerous fire risk and moderate explosion risk when exposed to heat, spark, or flame. Found in: embalming cosmetic spray, sealing lacquer, and thinners.

Methylene chloride (dichloromethane)—High oral toxicity, very dangerous to the eyes, causing corrosion of eye tissue. Because it vaporizes readily, inhalation is an important hazard, resulting in CNS depression, headache, dizziness, nausea, vomiting, and a feeling of intoxication. The material can also irritate the respiratory tract, cause liver damage, and exacerbate coronary artery disease. Chronic exposure can cause skin, CNS, and liver damage. The material is a suspected human carcinogen. The body metabolizes methylene chloride into carbon monoxide, lowering the blood's ability to

carry oxygen. The problem is intensified for smokers and those with anemia or related conditions. Found in: external embalming sealants, aerosol insecticides and deodorizers, cosmetic sprays, and solvents.

Mineral spirits (naphtha, hexane and heptane distillates)—Moderately toxic via ingestion and moderately irritating to skin, eyes, and mucous membranes, the mist is highly irritating to the respiratory tract. Symptoms of overexposure often resemble drunkenness. Chronic overexposure can lead to photosensitivity, headache, nausea, dizziness, indigestion, and lack of appetite. Mineral spirits are incompatible with strong oxidizers and are a highly dangerous fire risk when exposed to heat, flame, or spark. Found in: liquid embalming cosmetics and sprays, and organic solvents.

Molding plaster (calcium sulfate, gypsum, plaster of Paris)—Generally considered a nuisance dust, although prolonged or repeated exposures can induce lung disease. Found in: cavity desiccant and embalming powders.

Nitrocellulose—A dangerous fire and explosion hazard when in dry form. Less flammable when wet. Found in: feature builder and sealing lacquer.

Orthodichlorobenzene (1,2-dichlorobenzene)—Moderately toxic via inhalation and ingestion; irritating to skin, eyes, and upper respiratory tract. Acute exposure can induce narcotic symptoms. Repeated or prolonged skin contact with liquid can cause burns. Chronic exposure may cause lung, liver, and kidney damage. It is a moderate fire risk when exposed to heat or flame and can react violently with oxidizing materials. Found in: cavity and supplemental embalming chemicals and gels, and bleaching agents.

Oxalic acid (ethanedioic acid)—Highly irritating and caustic to skin. Damage is characterized by cracks, fissures, slow-healing ulcerations, blue skin, and yellowish, brittle nails. Highly irritating to tissues via ingestion. Can cause corrosion of mucous membranes, severe gastrointestinal disturbances, and acute poisoning. The major effects of inhalation of dusts and mists are corrosion and ulceration of the nose and the throat, severe eye irritation, nosebleed, headache, and nervousness. Chronic exposure can cause upper respiratory and gastrointestinal disturbances, urinary disorders, gradual weight loss, and nervous system disturbances. Found in: embalming adhesive gels.

Paradichlorobenzene (1,4-dichlorobenzene)—Moderately toxic via inhalation; symptoms include irritation of skin, eyes, and upper respiratory tract. Prolonged or chronic skin exposure can cause burns. In liquid form, it can be absorbed through the skin. Chronic exposure can cause liver, kidney, and lung damage. It is a moderate fire risk, and incompatible with oxidizers. Found in: deodorizing powders.

Paraformaldehyde—Can produce formaldehyde when heated. Paraformaldehyde has moderate oral toxicity and low dermal toxicity. It is a moderate fire risk and can react with oxidizers. Found in: embalming/deodorizing powders, sealing powders, cavity desiccants, and hardening compounds.

Paratertiary pentyl phenol (p-tert-amyl phenol)—A skin and eye irritant; it is moderately toxic through skin contact and ingestion, and is slightly flammable. Found in: cavity embalming solutions, disinfectant sprays, antiseptic soaps, and bleaching agents.

Propane—Propane can cause suffocation and at very high concentrations can cause CNS depression. It is a dangerous fire and explosion risk when exposed to heat, flame, or oxidizers. Found in: propellants, aerosol embalming sealants, cosmetic sprays, and insecticide/miticide sprays.

Propylene glycol (1,2-propanetriol, 1,3-propanetriol)—A skin and eye irritant. Found in: cavity embalming fluid.

Quartz (crystalline silicon dioxide)—Prolonged, repeated exposure to quartz can lead to lung disease characterized by shortness of breath and a troublesome, unproductive cough. Quartz can react violently with certain fluorine-containing compounds. Found in: finishing powder.

Quaternary ammonium compounds—Skin and eye irritant; a common cause of skin inflammation; highly toxic via ingestion; symptoms include nausea, vomiting, possible convulsions, and collapse. Found in: disinfectants, cavity and accessory embalming fluids.

Sodium hypochlorite—Strongly irritating and corrosive to tissues. A strong oxidizing agent that will react violently with organic acids and formaldehyde. It is moderately toxic via inhalation and ingestion. Found in: household bleach and other bleaching agents.

Sodium pentachlorophenate—Widely used as a fungicide and disinfectant, the material has high toxicity via inhalation and ingestion and is highly irritating to the skin. Found in: arterial embalming chemicals.

Talc—Mainly regarded as a nuisance dust, prolonged or repeated exposure may lead to lung disease although the mechanism of inducement is unclear. Found in: drying powder.

Toluene (1,2-dimethylbenzene)—Skin, eye, and respiratory tract irritant. Prolonged or repeated contact can cause drying of skin. Overexposure can produce narcotic effects, depression, headache, dizziness, nausea, fatigue, lack of coordination, and a burning sensation of the skin. Acute poisoning, however, is rare. It is a dangerous fire risk when exposed to heat, spark, or flame. Found in: external embalming sealers, lip cosmetics and cosmetic sprays, sealing lacquer, solvents, and thinners.

Trichloroethane (1,1,2-trichloroethane)—A moderate skin and eye irritant causing inflammation and producing CNS depression, dizziness, drowsiness, incoordination, and psychological disturbances. Trichloroethane can also cause gastrointestinal disturbances and irregular heartbeat. High doses can have a narcotic effect and cause heart failure. Found in: cleaning solvents, sanitizing embalming sprays, aerosol lanolin skin creams, and cosmetics.

Trichloroethylene—A strong eye and skin irritant which can be absorbed through contact. Overexposure can cause CNS depression, headache, dizziness, tremors, nausea, vomiting, fatigue, and irregular heartbeat. Symptoms may resemble those of alcohol intoxication. Addiction and weakness in the extremities have been reported. Chronic exposure can damage the liver and other organs. Found in: cleaning solvents.

APPENDIX 2

▶ MATERIAL SAFETY DATA SHEET TERMINOLOGY

Action level—That level at which certain actions must occur. In the Formaldehyde Standard, the level at which periodic monitoring for formaldehyde becomes necessary and at which medical surveillance becomes necessary.

Acute effect—Adverse effect on a human or an animal which has severe symptoms developing rapidly and coming quickly to a crisis. Also see "chronic effect."

ACGIH—American Conference of Governmental Industrial Hygienists is an organization of professional personnel in governmental agencies or educational institutions who are employed in occupational safety and health programs.

Chronic effect—An adverse effect on a human or an animal body, with symptoms which develop slowly over a long period of time or which recur frequently. Also see "acute effect."

Hazardous chemical—Any chemical whose presence or use is a physical hazard or a health hazard.

HCS—Hazard Communication Standard is an OSHA regulation issued under 29 CFR Part 1910. 1200.

Health hazard—A chemical for which there is significant evidence, based on at least one study conducted in accordance with established scientific principles, that acute or chronic health effects may occur in exposed employees. The term "health hazard" includes chemicals which are carcinogens, slightly or highly toxic agents, reproductive toxins, irritants, corrosives, sensitizers, hepatotoxins, nephrotoxins, neurotoxins, agents which act on the hematopoietic system, and agents that damage the lungs, skin, eyes, or mucous membranes.

MSDS (Material Safety Data Sheet)—Any data sheet that contains information required under many state regulations and Federal Regulations, Title 29, Part 1910.1200 (g), regarding the physical, chemical, and hazardous properties of a substance or mixture.

NIOSH—National Institute for Occupational Safety and Health, U.S. Public Health Service, U.S. Department of Health and Human Services (DHHS). Among other activities, NIOSH tests and certifies respiratory protective devices and air sampling detector tubes, recommends occupational exposure limits for various substances, and assists OSHA and MSHA in occupational safety and health investigations and research.

PEL—Permissible exposure limit is an exposure limit established by OSHA's regulatory authority. It may be a time-weighted average (TWA) limit or a maximum concentration exposure limit.

STEL—Short-term exposure limit (ACGIH terminology).

TWA—Time-weighted average exposure is the airborne concentration of a material to which a person is exposed, averaged over the total exposure time, generally the total workday (8 to 12 hours).

CHAPTER 4

THE PREPARATION ROOM

CHAPTER OBJECTIVES

▶ Preparation room design
▶ Preparation room equipment
▶ Preparation room requirements
▶ Instruments
▶ Preparation room supplies

Each funeral establishment may have a preparation room or funeral homes with several branch operations may have the embalming done at one location. A newer concept is the independent centralized embalming facility. These centralized embalming centers are shared by several funeral homes in a community. Where central facilities are used, funeral establishments can maintain a **holding room** for cosmetizing, dressing, and casketing the bodies after they have been delivered from the embalming center. Some states require that each funeral facility maintains a preparation room even if a central embalming facility is used.

▶ OBJECTIVES

The primary purpose of a well-designed and organized preparation room is to provide a safe and comfortable workplace. It should also be available to serve as a public relations tool if a community group wishes to tour the funeral establishment. A tour that does not include the preparation room can only serve to heighten unfounded suspicions and misconceptions concerning the embalming process.

In planning remodeling or new construction, emphasis should be placed on making the area functional and efficient. A layout that saves a few steps can save many working hours in the course of a year. A door planned to be just barely wide enough to accommodate the removal cot or a casket can be a source of annoyance, inconvenience, and irritation long after the small extra cost of a slightly wider door is forgotten. This room needs to be a clean, comfortable, and efficient workplace.

▶ PREPARATION ROOM CONSIDERATIONS

General Rules

1. Preparation room is kept strictly private during body preparation. Persons admitted should be limited to:
   a. Licensees and registered trainees.
   b. Those authorized by the family.
   c. Those authorized by state statute or rules and regulations.
2. Limited authorized persons can be in the room when preparation work is not being performed:
   a. Maintenance employees.
   b. Hairdresser, cosmetologist, barber, persons with other responsibilities.
   c. Staff members for dressing and casketing remains.
3. Identify the room by signage:
   a. Strictly private area.
   b. Occupational Safety and Health Administration (OSHA) warnings.
4. Secure the preparation room:
   a. State regulations may require security locks.
   b. Establish a security plan for the handling of the remains of high-profile persons.
   c. Inventory and label personal effects.
   d. Preparation room should not be located so that it becomes a passage to other building areas.
5. Maintain the dignity of the remains. Be sure that:
   a. The body is properly identified.
   b. The remains are covered.
   c. A modesty cloth is used during preparation.

6. Maintain highest moral standards.
   a. Keep body covered as practical.
   b. Guard loose talk and remarks.
   c. Repeat nothing outside of preparation room.
   d. Disclose no confidential facts as to age, condition of the body, deformities, or diseases causing death.
7. Maintain a clean and healthy environment.
   a. Properly dispose of clothing of the deceased: (1) launder and return to the family; or (2) destroy after proper authorization.
   b. Proper disposition of all waste (see Chapter 3): Statutes, rules, and regulations vary for individual states.
   c. Be sure ventilation, heating, and cooling systems work properly.
   d. Maintain all mechanical apparatus so no leakage occurs.
   e. Perform and document regular maintenance and cleaning of the preparation room.
8. Maintain an adequate supply of chemicals and sundries necessary for preparation work, restorative, and cosmetology treatments.
9. Maintain an adequate number of tables and positioning devices; this will help to keep movement of bodies minimal.
10. Document through the use of a decedent care report each deceased human body that comes into the custody of the facility.

▶ REGULATIONS

Funeral home facilities are governed by a variety of laws and regulations from federal, state, and local agencies because they are public places of business and employ workers in a workplace. A brief review of the major sources of regulations governing the preparation room environment follows, and throughout this chapter, reference is made generally to standard requirements. Funeral home owners are advised to consult experts in the legal and construction fields to be certain that their facilities, planned or existing, conform to all local requirements.

OSHA Requirements
The federal OSHA prescribes in detail the physical and environmental requirements that employers must meet to provide a safe workplace. These requirements are enforced through workplace inspections, warnings, and citations. In the event of failure to correct continual noncompliance or serious violations, substantial fines are levied. A well-known example is the Hazard Communication Standard.

Lesser known requirements have to do with the necessity for an adjacent shower and locker facility, electrical grounding, ramp and stair-step angles and heights, and a host of other areas of concern to the worker. Caution should be exercised to be certain that **all** OSHA requirements are being met in the workplace.

Four areas of OSHA directly impact the funeral service practitioner: (1) OSHA General Rule; (2) Hazard Communication Standard; (3) Formaldehyde Standard; and (4) Blood-borne Pathogen Standard (see Chapter 3).

"Right to Know" Laws
An emerging area of legislation on the local and state levels is "right to know" legislation. This is directed at employers and requires them to post information warning employees of chemicals that may be hazardous or harmful to their health and well-being. Firms in locales that have enacted such legislation may have to meet these requirements as well as those of OSHA.

Building Permits
All construction of any magnitude requires that a building permit be obtained from local authorities. The application procedures usually require that detailed plans and specifications be submitted regarding plumbing, electrical, and other construction materials to ensure that all materials and construction meet certain minimum standards. A competent architect, contractor, or both should be consulted prior to permit application in a particular locale.

State Codes and Local Ordinances
State boards of health and mortuary science have enacted regulations governing the minimum standards for preparation rooms. The Board of Embalmers and Funeral Directors of Ohio is an excellent example of state rules and regulations setting the minimum facility and equipment standards for the preparation or embalming room.

Ohio. Chapter 4717-1-16. "If embalming will take place at the funeral home, the funeral home shall maintain on the premises a preparation room which shall be:

■ adequately equipped
■ maintained in a sanitary manner for the preservation and care of dead human bodies.

Such rooms shall:

■ contain only articles, facilities, and instruments necessary for the preparation of dead human bodies for burial or final disposition
■ be kept in a clean and sanitary condition

■ shall be used only for the care and preparation of **dead human bodies**

The minimal requirements for the preparation or embalming room shall be as follows:

1. Sanitary floor (cement or tile preferred).
2. All instruments and appliances used in the embalming of a dead human body shall be thoroughly cleansed and sterilized using an appropriate disinfectant immediately at the conclusion of each individual case.
3. Running hot and cold water with a lavatory sink for personal hygiene.
4. Exhaust fan and intake vent, permanently installed and operable with the capacity to change the air in the room **fifteen times each hour**.
5. Sanitary plumbing connected with sewer, cesspool, septic tank, or other department of health approved system.
6. Porcelain, stainless steel, metal-lined, or fiberglass operating table.
7. All opening windows and outside doors shall be adequately screened and shielded from outside viewing.
8. All hydro-aspirators shall be equipped with at least one air breaker.
9. Containers for refuse, trash, and soiled linens shall be adequately covered or sealed at all times.
10. First-aid kit and eyewash.
11. The embalming or preparation room shall be strictly private. A "private" sign shall be posted on the door(s) entering the preparation room. No one shall be allowed therein while the body is being embalmed except the licensed embalmers, licensed funeral directors, apprentices, officials in discharge of their duties, and other authorized persons.
12. All waste materials, refuse, used bandages, and cotton shall be destroyed in accordance with all applicable OSHA and EPA regulations.
13. Every person, while engaged in actually embalming a dead human body, shall be attired in a clean and sanitary smock or gown covering the person from the neck to below the knees and shall wear impervious rubber gloves, and shall wear any and all items required under any applicable OSHA regulations.
14. All bodies in the preparation room should be treated with proper care and dignity and should be properly covered at all times.
15. Ingress and egress of the preparation room must be situated so that functions in the funeral home will not impede or interfere with entering or exiting said room.
16. Sufficient emergency lighting.

HOLDING ROOM. The state of Ohio has also set rules for a "holding room." A "holding room" is not used for embalming. Its use would include:

■ cosmetic, restorative treatment, and dressing of embalmed bodies received from a central embalming facility or shipped from another location
■ preparation of bodies for identification without embalming
■ storage of embalmed or unembalmed bodies
■ cavity embalming which may include aspiration or reaspiration of a body

The rule is as follows, "If embalming will not take place at the funeral home, the funeral home shall maintain on the premises a **holding room** which shall be adequately equipped and maintained in a sanitary manner for the holding of dead human bodies. Such holding room shall be kept in a clean and sanitary manner and used only for the holding and storage of **dead human bodies.** The minimum requirements for the holding room shall be as follows:

1. Sanitary floor;
2. Running hot and cold water with a lavatory sink for personal hygiene;
3. All opening windows and outside doors shall be adequately screened and shielded from outside viewing;
4. Containers for refuse, trash, and soiled linens shall be adequately covered or sealed at all times;
5. The holding room shall be strictly private. A "Private" sign shall be posted on the door(s) entering the room. No one shall be allowed therein while the body is being held except the licensed embalmers, licensed funeral directors, apprentices, officials in discharge of their duties, and other authorized persons;
6. All bodies in the holding room should be treated with proper care and dignity and should be properly covered at all times;
7. Ingress and egress of the holding room must be situated so that functions in the funeral home will not impede or interfere with entering or exiting said room.

If the holding room is equipped with a hydro-aspirator or electric aspirator, the aspirator shall be equipped with at least one air breaker."

Extensive planning and consultation are required in advance of any construction in the funeral home in general and the preparation room in particular. There are several national architectural firms that specialize in the design and construction of funeral facilities. Funeral home owners, as business people serving the public and employing people in the workplace, have special obligations that must be met. Individual state statutes, rules, and regulations along with local city, and county ordinances must be consulted for up-to-date compliance with respect to the preparation room, holding room, and refrigeration facilities.

The funeral home or embalming facility may wish to have its own set of regulations. These might include such items as (1) persons who may have egress to the room; (2) cleaning schedules; (3) scheduled disposition of medical and non-medical waste; (4) responsibility for stocking and ordering inventory; (5) machine maintenance schedule; (6) protocols for disinfecting and cleaning of instruments, drains and machines.

► PREPARATION ROOM LOCATION

Basement
The basement is often where space is most readily available, although frequently this is not the most desirable site. Ceiling height is the most common difficulty in this area because of overhead pipes as well as heating and air conditioning ducts. Sometimes, pipes and ducts may be diverted, run between floor joists, or sometimes concealed in wall cabinets. Lighting fixtures may also be kept from lessening head room if they are recessed between floor joists.

Plumbing can present vexing questions if sewer drains are substantially above floor level. Ventilation and air conditioning are more costly in basement areas. Stairs can be a considerable inconvenience—even a hazard. An elevator, lift, or ramp may offer a solution here.

A wet basement might be the greatest single deterrent to using this area. Normal dampness is rather easily handled by a dehumidifier, and it is essential that this be done.

First or Second Floor
The first floor is usually the most logical and least costly location of a preparation room if ample space is available. Natural daylight is normally available to create more pleasant working conditions; however, other considerations now arise. Access to the room should be from a non-public area. If the room is adjacent to a public area, such as the selection room, adequate soundproofing is extremely important. If this is impractical or impossible, a flashing light should be installed in the preparation room to alert staff members that a family is in the next room. Odor control and proper exhaust venting must be provided. Those who work in a funeral home become accustomed to certain odors that would be obvious and objectionable to a visitor.

If the installation of an elevator is feasible in a two-story building, the second floor may well be the best of the several alternatives. More natural light is available, and ventilation is less expensive and more effective. Normally, a second-floor room is completely removed from the public areas. Here again, sound levels must be considered. Plumbing may be non-existent in the immediate area, but totally new plumbing may be reasonable considering the other advantages to be gained.

► PREPARATION ROOM SIZE

The size requirement of the preparation room is of critical importance in determining the location. A room that is too large can necessitate extra steps and encourage use of the surplus space for storage. Many problems can be forestalled by partitioning a part of the area for planned storage. Allow adequate work space but keep all equipment, instruments, and supplies readily accessible.

The firm that conducts as many as 100 funerals annually should find one permanent table ample. A folding table will serve in an emergency and can double as a dressing table when required. An area 120 to 150 square feet for this room should be considered a minimum. This should allow for ample cabinets and counter space, assuming the room is not an unusual shape and that it does not have more than one or two doors opening into it. When locating plumbing for the table, keep in mind the need to allow ample passage for the removal cot and for a casket, if casketing is to be done in the preparation room. Doors and corridors leading to the room must also be of ample width, especially if turning corners is required.

A firm anticipating 100 to 150 funerals per year should try to provide a bit larger area if at all possible. One table would normally still be adequate, but the extra folding table is essential.

A firm contemplating 150 to 350 funerals annually should provide a minimum area of approximately 400 square feet and two completely equipped tables. A firm doing a larger volume should seriously consider a separate dressing room where hairdressing and cosmetizing may be done.

Some considerations when remodeling or building new might include

- Once volume of use is determined, keep the space where the embalming operation will be performed as small as is practical.
- Minimum operating spaces saves steps.
- Minimum operating spaces are easier to keep sanitary.
- Minimum operating spaces are easier to ventilate, heat, and cool.
- Keep instruments, fluids, and sundries in convenient locations within the area of operation; storage spaces should be placed so bending is not necessary.

Figure 4–1. A, B. Flooring plans showing use of the "station or booth concept." (*Continued*)

■ Lifting devices should be used for moving bodies.

■ Adequate tables will decrease the necessity to move bodies; ideally, once the body is placed on a preparation table, it should not have to be moved until it is placed in a casket, shipping container, or on a cot.

■ Floors, countertops, and all flat surfaces should be constructed of materials that can easily be sanitized.

The **"station" or "booth"** concept in embalming room design uses one or more fully equipped small operating areas (within a large preparation room) where the embalming is performed. The room space adjacent to the embalming stations is where restorative work, cos-

metizing, hairdressing, dressing, and casketing of the remains are performed. The small operating stations are more private and, because of their size, easily sanitized and cleaned. The number of preparations performed per year determines the number of stations that should be constructed. One station for each 150 preparations has been suggested. The following floor plans #1 (Fig. 4–1A) and #2 (Fig. 4–1B) show the use of the "station concept." Floor plan #3 (Fig. 4–1C) is suggested for a central embalming facility or an embalming facility within a large funeral establishment. Note that this plan includes a covered delivery and receiving area, walk-in cooler for storage, crematory facility, "station" preparation area, dressing and casketing areas, and an employee restroom, shower, and changing area.

Figure 4–1. (*Continued*) **C.** Flooring plan suggested for central embalming facility or an embalming facility within a large funeral establishment.

► PHYSICAL DESIGN

Discuss the requirements with an architect for a new building or when remodeling. Show the architect the existing equipment and describe the movement made in the room. Consider plumbing needs. Plumbing costs should not always be the overriding determining factor.

Maneuverability within the finished room is tremendously important. When the tentative location for the table(s) is set, mentally go through the motions of getting the removal cot and the casket into the room. Once the general plan seems satisfactory, draw the room to scale with all equipment in place and think again about all the movements that must take place in the finished room.

Storage Cabinets and Countertops

Next, consider storage cabinets. Although space should be provided for working quantities of supplies, the preparation room should not double as a storeroom.

Ready-made base cabinets are generally 24 inches deep. Obviously, these would normally be the least costly. Depending on the size and shape of the room, however, custom cabinets may be a necessity. They could be 18 or 12 inches deep, if space is very limited. If the space is such that cabinet depth is not a problem but counter length is limited, it might be desirable to use a stock 24-inch cabinet and hold it out from the wall to permit a 30-inch deep countertop. The vacant space behind the cabinets might be used for water pipes or electrical wiring.

Table Arrangements

There are virtually as many table arrangements as there are sizes and shapes of rooms; however, two are the most common and popular.

Conventional Parallel Table Plan. The conventional parallel table plan is a perfectly functional layout, although it may not be the best choice because the exhaust system,

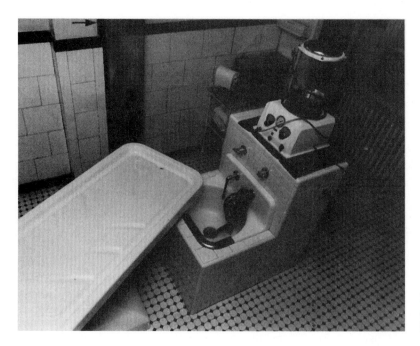

Figure 4–2. Island preparation design. Note the duct for exhaust that pulls fumes to the floor, away from the embalmer.

depending on where it is placed, may draw odors past the embalmers. With this plan, caution must be taken against making the waste sink a part of the cabinet line. This makes the sink and surrounding areas more difficult to clean. Instead, mount the sink on the face of the base cabinets or on the floor, leaving some clearance between the sink and cabinet.

The "island" cabinet (Fig. 4–2) gives the embalmer freedom to pass completely around the table without stepping over hoses and electric cords. No part of the wall storage cabinets is obstructed. All plumbing connections are within the cabinet and readily accessible if a problem should arise.

Two-Table Room Arrangement. If a sufficiently large square or rectangular room is available, the two-table room arrangement is preferred. It provides two completely separate work areas, allows maximum flexibility in movement within the room, and generally does not interfere with doors.

Flooring. After the location of the preparation room in the building and the layout of the room itself have been considered, perhaps the first specific aspect of the room that should be discussed is the floor.

The floor must withstand very heavy traffic and considerable static weight. If selected carelessly, it can harbor infectious organisms, cause anything on wheels to roll toward low spots, cause glare, and create difficult working conditions or perhaps require recovering or even structural repair sooner than it should. The architect must be made fully aware of the weights this floor will hold and, therefore, the amount of structural support necessary. Flooring should be resistant to scuff marks

and stains. Dyes in embalming fluids should be easily removed. Light-colored flooring puts more brightness in the work area. A matte finish to the floor is more desirable than a glossy finish. The matte finish produces less glare, shows fewer scuff marks, and is easier to maintain than a glossy finish.

Basement Preparation Room

It is essential that the proper base be laid for any cement floor. There should be a thick stone bed covered by vinyl vapor barrier sheeting underneath the cement. A small ditch should be constructed around the outside, with ample leach lines to feed into the ditch in case water does start to collect. The cost of a small sump pump might well be worthwhile. Located in an out-of-the-way spot, it would pick up and discharge any water accumulation. Building codes should be consulted.

If the preparation room is located in a basement with a cement floor, it is best to cover it with something; standing on cement is uncomfortable. Building a wood floor over the cement is a common answer to this problem. If the wood floor were built directly on top of the concrete, moisture would cause it to rot. Therefore, various methods are used to raise the wood floor and leave an air space between it and the concrete. In addition to preventing rot, the space acts as an excellent sound absorber. Any wood floor needs to be covered with a non-absorbent material.

It is also important to have enough floor joists and a thick enough wood subfloor to support the heavy concentrated weight the floor will bear. Try to anticipate locations for desired electrical and plumbing lines before closing up the floor.

First or Second Floor Preparation Room

When building a preparation room on the first or second floor, the architect should again be cautioned about the loads that the floor must support. An embalming table can weigh 300 or 400 pounds and that, plus the weight of a subject, could create a low spot on an insufficiently supported floor. The floor's sinking, in turn, can cause cracking of tiles or other floor coverings. Over a span of 12 feet, a normal floor (without a bearing wall) could use 2 × 10-inch timbers on 16-inch centers for floor joists; however, a preparation room with 2 × 12-inch timbers on 12-inch centers is preferred. Alternatively, to keep timber height uniform with that of adjoining rooms, the 2 × 10-inch timbers on 16-inch centers should be doubled.

▶ FLOOR COVERING

Terrazo Floor

A terrazo floor is one sort that might be considered for this application. It is a natural polished floor that is very durable and easy to maintain. Terrazzo is very hard and, therefore, tiring to stand on for extended periods. Also, it is slippery when wet. This problem can be overcome with the use of rubber mats.

Clay and Ceramic Tile

Clay and ceramic tile are both excellent choices. The size of such tiles makes a very important difference. The large 4 × 4-inch tiles with a slight roundness on the top make a natural recess or ditch for the grout fill as well as for dirt and accumulated wax. Some 1 × 1-inch tiles are also rounded and create the same difficulties. There are, however, flat 1 × 1-inch tiles and these are good. Any cleaning implement, from a hand sponge to an electric scrub brush machine, will make contact at all points and leave the floor completely clean. Remember that liquids will be spilled occasionally. A floor of glazed ceramic tiles would become slippery and such tiles should be avoided.

Vinyl Tile

Vinyl tile is, for good reason, probably the type of flooring most commonly chosen. It is very resilient, so it is comfortable to stand on for several hours. It is attractive and sold in many colors and patterns, so it can easily be color coordinated with any room. The three basic types of vinyl flooring are no-waxing sheet vinyl, homogeneous vinyl tile, and vinyl-asbestos tile.

Vinyl flooring is intended for home use and if it is selected for a preparation room, it is very necessary to purchase tile rated to withstand a load limit in excess of 100 pounds per square inch. When using sheet vinyl, have the flooring cut; so it can extend several inches up the walls; this seals the seams where the wall and floor come together.

Asphalt Tile

Asphalt tile is made of resin asphalt compounds and asbestos fibers, it is very hard and brittle. Asbestos fibers are no longer used in these products. Of all tile floors, it is the least expensive per square foot. It is easy to install, too! However, it must be used on cement or on an exceptionally strong floor that will not "work" (move) at all. Asphalt tile becomes increasingly brittle with age and new tiles will not have the aged appearance of those around them, making repaired areas very visible. This type of floor needs to be well waxed to ensure long life in the preparation room.

Epoxy

Epoxy is usually used directly over a cement floor. A layer of epoxy is spread over the floor and then chips of color (supplied with the epoxy) are often sprinkled onto it. The epoxy flooring should be finished in a rough coat fashion to prevent slippage. When the epoxy sets, several coats of clear plastic are applied. The number of coats (and the quality of the particular brand chosen) determines the durability of the floor. Epoxy coverings can also be used over old tile, wood, and other types of floors, but preparation of the old surface must be extremely thorough. Finally, these preparations can also be used on all surfaces. Epoxy floors are seamless, so it is an easy surface to disinfect.

Paint

Paint, of course, is the least expensive floor covering of all. But it will not stand up under wear and it is especially susceptible to damage from chemicals, so spillage is a real problem. An oil-based enamel paint is recommended.

▶ WINDOWS, DOORS, CEILINGS, AND WALLS

Windows, doors, and ceilings all function to some degree to control sound, light (Fig. 4–3), and odors.

Windows

The first factor influencing the selection of a window is the location of the preparation room in the building. If the preparation room is built in the basement, there will probably be a need to augment the natural ventilation available with some system of forced air. Aside from the obvious odor problems, the natural summer dampness in most parts of the country is a problem in a basement. Windows can be an available source for fresh incoming air when mechanical exhaust systems are running.

Privacy must always be ensured in the preparation room. In a basement location, frosted glass is usually necessary. Wire reinforcement in the glass is often essential in city areas because of vandalism. Frosted jalousie

Figure 4–3. Preparation room lights. **A.** Adequate lighting. Note the number of electrical outlets available. **B.** Adjustable cosmetic lights.

windows afford privacy while permitting air flow and can be a good choice. The inverted awning-type window ensures privacy when the window is open.

There are other considerations in selecting windows for first and upper floors. Movements within the room should not be visible as silhouettes or shadows on the window. When work must be done at night, heavy drapes are suggested as well as rolling floor screens or folding screens. At street level, windows can be protected from view by shrubbery or a louvered fence. Use inside or outside the building of materials that substantially decrease the volume of air flow possible through the windows should be avoided. Access to fresh air is important.

One of the best sources of light if architecture permits is the glass block wall; however, additional windows then become necessary for ventilation. If the preparation room is located on the top floor and is wedged between other buildings, restricting light and air flow from regular windows, plastic dome skylights should be considered. This sort of window also allows full use of wall space. Ventilation is aided as warm air rises rapidly to the ceiling and through the skylight under most weather conditions.

Doors

Some state rules now require that preparation room doors be locked. This would be a good rule for all establishments to follow. Many funeral establishments use touchpad locking devices. This eliminates the need for keys, and the codes can be periodically changed.

Unless an architect is made aware that caskets will be taken through the door, she or he might well specify a conventional 30-inch door. **A 3-foot opening should be an absolute minimum. The narrower the corridor or passageway from which the room is to be entered, the wider the door should be to permit turning.** In addition to width, the direction in which the door opens is very significant. If a normal hung door might create problems, perhaps a "pocket" or recessed sliding door might be the answer. Should there be a structural reason that this is not practical, double-hinged doors folding to the right or left may be required.

The doors in the preparation room should be of high quality. Pre-hung doors are an excellent choice because they are of good quality and also save time in installation. To some extent, the size of the entrance and the area to which that entrance leads determine the type of door needed. If the door leads to an adjoining garage, the insurance company or building code will probably call for a metal-covered door. In selection of an interior door, choices include doors with solid cores, hollow cores, solid fresco cores, solid wood staved cores, solid wood flake cores, or lead shield cores. All are available with different odor and sound control properties.

Advise the architect that all doors must be wide enough so that a stretcher or casket can easily pass through, and that the stretcher or casket may need to be turned at various angles to move it into or from a hallway or around some wall or other obstacle on one side of the door or the other. This warning has been previously mentioned but bears repeating. **Improper door size is one of the most common errors in preparation room planning**. The minimum width of the door should be at least 36 to 40 inches.

Ceilings

Ceilings can present a real problem, more so in renovation than in new construction, and, in particular, if the preparation room is in the basement. Frequently, the basement location means a low ceiling made lower by water pipes, heating ducts, and electrical lines. If consideration is being given to renovate such a ceiling to better insulate for sound, for the sake of appearance or for sanitation reasons, it must first be determined if there is sufficient height below the pipes, ducts, and electrical lines to construct a ceiling. If there is not enough height in the room or a room is being designed for a new building, be sure that at least 4 inches of sound insulation material is used, and the contractor allows complete and easy access to all pipes, valves, and electrical connections.

New "hung" or suspended ceilings can be an excellent choice if sufficient height is available. The large tiles provide easy access to everything above. Repainting or even replacing old ceiling tiles is a fairly inexpensive way to brighten up the room every few years.

Many suspended ceilings are available as complete systems, incorporating light fixtures and ventilation systems as well as the tile. Such systems, which disperse air through large areas of the ceiling, are especially suited to delivering large quantities of air at considerable temperature differentials with minimal draft and noise. Most of these systems require at least $15\frac{1}{2}$ inches of hanging height.

Johns–Manville offers acoustical tile specially treated with antibacterial finish and bacteriostatic core. Tests have shown that the finish reduces bacterial population on the surface by 90% in 6 hours, and the bacteriostatic core does not support bacterial proliferation. For ceilings full of pipes or ducts, remember to clean the tops of these regularly with a good disinfectant.

Many funeral homes are created from old residences, and this usually means plaster ceilings. If the ceiling is in good condition, a coat of paint will make it look excellent again. If the plaster is at all loose, do not add ceiling material to it. Pull off the old ceiling, or at least all that is loose. Fur out the old base to align the new ceiling correctly.

The material of the various suspended ceilings should be checked for fire-retardant qualities. Ratings are given by most manufacturers in their data booklets.

Simple painting may not be sufficient to save an old ceiling, but the "hung" ceiling may not be a good choice because of height limitations. A new ceiling of three-eighths-inch plasterboard properly nailed with the new, better-gripping plasterboard nails and correctly taped can give years of service. Acrylic enamel paint would make it an easy ceiling to wash. **A white ceiling is a must. It gives the advantage of reflected light, and as accumulation of dirt is readily apparent on white, it is easy to make sure the ceiling is kept clean and sanitary**.

Another good ceiling material is one of the high-gloss finish hardboards. Marlite is a good example.

Walls

As with ceilings, walls should be selected with careful concern for the ease with which they can be kept sanitary (Fig. 4–4). Late in 1974, California enacted new

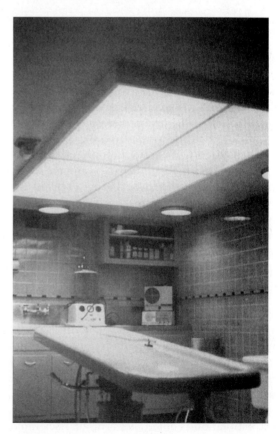

Figure 4–4. Walls tiled from the floor to the ceiling. The ceiling is soundproof.

regulations specifying sanitary requirements not only for preparation rooms but also for storage rooms (where bodies are held awaiting disposition). If a new wall is to be created, the material and method of construction are, in part, determined by the sort of room that will be on the other side. If that room is to be used by the public (as an arrangement or smoking room), then the wall must be insulated against noise and odor. Never plan an employee bedroom or kitchen next to a preparation room. Control of odor and bacteria is a constant worry.

A possible covering or finish for any wall of concrete is glazed masonry block. This comes in many sizes, styles, and colors and is easy to keep clean. The contractor must see to it that the mason keeps the grout joints smooth and close to flush with the tile surfaces for ease of cleaning. A poured concrete wall can be spray-painted after imperfections are plastered. Many plain and multicolored epoxy paints are available for use over any concrete surface. These surfaces should be finished with a clear glaze.

Modern adhesives make it possible to use ceramic tile on wallboard, which creates an excellent looking, durable wall. When dry wallboard is used by itself, it should be taped and surfaced carefully and sealed with good washable enamel. Plasterboard will absorb moisture, so it must be kept an inch or two from the floor and a cove base used. In a basement or damp area, set plasterboard considerably away from the outer wall. Acrylic and latex enamel paints will seal and protect plaster, drywall, and natural wood. It will also render them impervious to liquids, gases, and microbes.

Marlite wallboard is used extensively and is available in many colors with matching moldings. Marlite is one of the easiest walls to maintain, as are Formica surfaced cabinets. Reinforced fiberglass panels are available, which are a highly sanitary material. It is always good to make panels in this type of wall removable for easy access to wiring and other equipment located inside the wall.

Many choose to use tile of some sort only part of the way up the wall and paint or wallpaper above that. This is fine, provided that good, washable paint or paper is used. A flexible vinyl floor covering can also be used on a wall if there is a solid base surface to which it may be glued.

Sound Insulation

Sound insulation should not be overlooked. If the room is below, above, or adjacent to public areas the sounds of instruments dropping or machines in operation will certainly be unwelcome in those areas. Many companies make special-density cellulose fiber structural board that can be used in ceilings, walls, and floors to deaden sound. The use of such material in preparation room construction is highly recommended.

Figure 4–5. A floor water supply for the preparation table.

▶ PLUMBING

As with all facets of preparation room planning, to avoid later difficulties with plumbing, work closely with the architect and describe all the work that goes on in the area so that all fixtures, waste lines, and other equipment can be properly located. In case of blockages, all cleanout points in waste lines should be conveniently accessible (Fig. 4–5). Addition of a fixture not initially planned will probably not be easy.

Water pipe is like electrical service wire in that the larger the diameter of the pipe or wire, the more water or current will flow through it. Today, copper is usually used for water pipe because it does not easily corrode or rust. Another very convenient material to work with is polyvinyl chloride for both supply and drain. It is approved by many communities for residential use, but restrictions may be enforced for commercial applications.

The feed line after the water meter is normally three-fourth to 1 inch in diameter. The supply lines to the preparation room should be at least three-fourth inch in diameter. This size allows enough volume to operate waste sink flushometers properly and creates a good vacuum in a hydroaspirator. Some embalmers find that the vacuum is not great enough in their aspirators unless they run both hot and cold water through a dual mixing faucet. This lack of suction could be the result of very small feed pipes or old, galvanized pipes.

> A good reason to have removable panels and ceiling tiles in strategic areas (so that access to plumbing and electrical wiring is convenient) is that of changing municipal codes. If there is a question of compliance with a plumbing code, it will be possible to make changes without ripping out the walls.

The second major plumbing consideration deals with codes. Having discussed bringing in an adequate water supply, the subject of disposal of waste water must be considered. How wastes are handled is a major concern. Codes and regulations change as knowledge of good sanitation procedures increases.

Backflow

Backflow is the unwanted reverse flow of liquids in a piping system. It can be caused by back-siphonage, back-pressure, or a combination of both. Back-siphonage is due to a vacuum or partial vacuum in the water supply system. It is caused by **ordinary gravity**—when water supply is lost and a fixture that is elevated is opened, allowing air into the system, water will (by gravity) reverse flow; **undersized piping**—high-velocity water traveling through undersized piping can cause an aspirator effect and draw water out of branch pipes causing a partial vacuum and a reverse flow; and **vacuum**—pumping water from the supply system creates a pressure drop or a negative pressure in the system, or a break in the main or

excessive usage at a lower level in the system can also be a cause.

Many water departments now require a backflow prevention (one-way) valve at the point at which the water enters the funeral home from the street. The installation of these devices is favored where the water enters the preparation room (not just the funeral home) on both hot and cold lines. In this way, the public within the funeral home, as well as the community, are protected from accidentally contaminated water.

In the early 1970, the state of Connecticut started a program requiring the use of back-flow prevention devices. Since then, additions to these regulations now require special faucets to be used with hydroaspirators, which must be equipped with vacuum breakers. These faucets are made for industrial use as in commercial laundries. The fixture is dull in finish and has a vacuum breaker built into the top of the spout.

Electric Aspirator. The trocar is attached via the hose on the right side of the impeller casing. The hose coming off the left side leads directly to the top of the flush sink. The small tube of the top of the impeller casing draws water from the bulb that is attached to the water faucet. The water faucet attachment has two water supplies— one to the bulb to keep the impeller lubricated when no aspirant is flowing through the trocar, and one of the opposite side (with an attached hose) for water to be supplied for other purposes. The impeller casing has three screws that allow for removal of the impeller for replacement or drying (Fig. 4–6A).

Hydroaspirator with Vacuum Breakers. The hydroaspirator is attached to a water faucet over a flush sink. A

Figure 4–6. A. Electric aspirator. **B.** Hydroaspirator.

Figure 4–7. Vacuum breakers.

clear plastic hose connects the aspirator and trocar. The level near the bottom of the aspirator allows for clean water flow from the hose or for aspiration (suction) if the lever is vertically aligned with the aspirator (Figs. 4–6B; 4–7; 4–8; 4–9).

One consideration is to put vacuum breakers into the hot and cold supply lines for the preparation room rather than on each faucet. A siphon-breaking device or backflow preventer is a rather simple mechanism that is attached to a threaded faucet before the hydroaspirator is mounted. It combines a check valve and air vents. When water forces open the check valve, the air vents are automatically closed. If water pressure drops, the check valve closes automatically and the air vents are opened,

preventing any backflow into the supply line. The air vents break any built-up vacuum. This inexpensive but effective device is available through most preparation room suppliers.

Backflow and siphonage are very real hazards in funeral homes, especially if the volume and pressure of the water entering the building are not great enough to adequately supply all outlets in the building. For example, if the pressure is barely adequate for aspiration, flushing a toilet or starting a washing machine can cause such a drop in pressure at the aspirator faucet that a vacuum results, drawing waste materials into the waterline.

Because of the serious nature of backflow problems, OSHA has addressed the problem nationally.

Figure 4–8. Hydroaspiration in a visible position.

Figure 4–9. A. Flush drain. **B.** Floor drain.

Subpart J of the Occupational Safety and Health Act pertains to general environmental controls. Paragraph 1910.141(b)(2)(ii) contains the following statement: "Construction of nonpotable water systems carrying any other nonpotable substance shall be such as to prevent backflow or back siphonage into a potable water system.*

In discussing placement of hydroaspirators, it is important to remember that the aspirator should not be attached to a faucet in a sink in such a way that it is below the top of the sink walls (Fig. 4–8). This means that the operator cannot see the aspirator. The aspirator, therefore, should be at least 2 inches above the rim of the sink. Large, clear, plastic tubing can be attached to the aspirator so the embalmer can see the materials being aspirated, this will also help to avoid splashing. Another problem with hydroaspirators can occur during aspiration of tissue particles. These can become lodged in the aspirator throat and block it, causing the operator to inject water into the body via the trocar.

---

*This revision was published in **Federal Register.** 1973;38:10930.

Drains

No discussion of preparation room plumbing would be complete without a discussion of drains. In planning the location of drains, remember that the drain pipe must have a downward slope of one-fourth-inch over every foot of length from point of entry into the room to the point of exit. Commercial sealed sump pumps can be installed to lift wastes. Also, where codes allow, flush-up toilets may be used (Fig. 4–9A). Such toilets need a minimum of 40-pounds psi of pressure sustained at 4 gallons per minute for a 10-foot lift.

A central floor drain surrounded by a slope is inconvenient. Church trucks and cots can wobble, roll, and cause damage. A floor drain in an out-of-the-way corner surrounded by a small area of slope avoids these problems (Fig. 4–9B). Waste drains must be vented to flow properly. A drain in a basement floor, in an area with a high water table, must have a one-way flap installed to prevent backup. Also, in areas where sewers are not available and septic tanks are used, remember to check codes to determine minimum distances between septic tank systems and wells for water.

Figure 4–10. A. Wide porcelain utility sink. **B.** Stainless steel utility sink.

Water Supply

Most codes require hot as well as cold water in the preparation room. Certain states even set a minimum temperature requirement of 130°F or 145°F. OSHA requires that all steam and hot water pipes be insulated when it is possible for an employee to come in contact with the pipes. It is not always convenient to insulate. One possible alternative for pipes leading to freestanding sinks is to enclose them in a cabinet.

Convenient water service to the embalming table, the embalming machine, and the sinks can save much time and many steps. The table is the work center. Water can be fed to it either from an overhead supply or directly from service sinks. If the table is permanently located, a supply line can be placed under the head area, coming up from the floor or dropping from the ceiling. The overhead service is really handy for washing the remains and shampooing and rinsing the hair.

Sinks

There are many alternatives from which to choose in selecting a waste sink for the embalming table (Figs. 4–8 and 4–9A). A sink that permits good floor maintenance should be selected. Flushable sinks, whether floor standing or wall-hung, are the most sanitary. The flush valve incorporates a vacuum breaker. A minimum of 20-pounds psi is required at the valve while flushing.

Hand sinks should be located conveniently for the operator and need not be too large. Remembering the need for sanitation, controls should be selected that do not require handling of faucets. There are controls for knee operation, foot operation, and elbow or forearm

operation. A gooseneck faucet facilitates the filling of large bottles and pails (Fig. 4–10A).

Sinks can have surfaces of china, enamel on pressed steel, or stainless steel. Stainless steel is popular but harder to keep clean looking. A bottle or instrument dropped in a stainless sink makes an awful racket! Flush-surface hand sinks in countertops are even easier to maintain than wall-mounted ones. If plans call for a separate dressing room, the cosmetician and hair-dresser should have their own sink.

▶ VENTILATION

No discussion of the embalming environment is complete without a thorough and cautionary discourse on the subject of ventilation and the necessity to protect the embalmer. Adequate ventilation is essential. A preparation room should have 12 to 20 air exchanges per hour; 15 changes are recommended.

Formaldehyde

Formaldehyde is irritating to work with, for this reason alone proper ventilation is absolutely necessary.

Formaldehyde gas may cause severe irritation to the mucous membrane of the respiratory tract and eyes. Morrill reported sensory irritation (itching of eyes, dry and sore throat, increased thirst, and disturbed sleep) in paper-process workers at 0.9 to 1.6 ppm formaldehyde. Bourne and Seferian reported from another occupational setting intense irritation of eyes, nose, and throat at levels ranging from 0.13 to 0.45 ppm. More recent studies by Kerfoot and Mooney and Moore and Ogrodnik* conducted in funeral homes indicate that concentrations from 0.25 to 1.39 ppm evoke numerous complaints of upper respiratory tract and eye irritation and headache among embalmers. Schoenber and Mitchell report that acute exposure to formaldehyde phenolic resin vapors at levels around 0.4 to 0.8 ppm causes lacrimation and irritation of the upper as well as the lower respiratory tract. The levels at which serious inflammation of the bronchi and lower respiratory tract would occur in humans are unknown; inhalation of high levels, however, has caused chemical pneumonitis, pulmonary edema, and death.

Emerging technology and thought in the design and construction of preparation rooms reflect the recognition that **because formaldehyde is heavier than air, exhaust systems located at or near floor level, when combined with the introduction of uncontaminated air from the ceiling level, are an efficient method of ventilation**. In addition, such systems have the added advantage of drawing fumes and contaminants down and away from the operator's face during the embalming procedure. **The key to the creation of an embalming environment protective of the embalmer's health and comfort is air flow and adequacy of ventilation**.

The number and location of windows and doors are obviously components of the total ventilation system. Cross-ventilation (which requires windows on opposite walls) is highly desirable and should be designed into every preparation room if at all possible.

If there is sufficient height in the room to install a hung ceiling, install one that will dispense air through large areas in the ceilings. These have the ability to deliver large quantities of air at considerable temperature differentials with minimal draft and noise.

Many preparation rooms are equipped with the familiar kitchen exhaust hood. When it is installed over the waste sink at a height of about 4 feet, air is drawn out slightly above table level. Because the hood is located over the waste sink, unpleasant odors are kept away from the operator. **In choosing the location of the exhaust, care should always be taken so that air flows away from the operator**. Calculations should also be obtained from a ventilation engineer to determine the number of room air changes per hour created by the system.

The grill on the exhaust fan, and on all other grills in the room, should be easily removable for cleaning. Grills are often loaded with dust "kitties," and this environment is a perfect site for proliferation of bacteria. Be careful when planning an exhaust vent that goes directly from the preparation room to the roof. The architect may not realize that such a vent, located too near

---

*See Selected Readings for complete Kerfoot and Mooney Study and Moore and Ogrodnik studies.

a roof-mounted air conditioner, could cause foul odors and pathogens to return through the air conditioner's intake vent.

Basement preparation rooms are the toughest to ventilate properly. One major problem in some areas of the country is the stagnant, humid air that can make a basement very unpleasant during the summer. Mold can start developing unless a dehumidifier is installed.

The possibility of drafts creating dehydration should be considered carefully in laying out the preparation room. Several new preparation rooms have required expensive redesign and reinstallation of ventilation systems because the first few cases embalmed were so seriously dehydrated by drafts.

Air Conditioning

Although there are many different air conditioning units to choose from, the size of the room in cubic feet and the desired number of room air changes per hour determine the size of the unit needed. If the entire funeral home is air conditioned by the same unit, there must be independent controls for the preparation room. Odors must not reach the main air flow serving the funeral home. Many times, a separate preparation room "zone," controlled manually, is recommended.

The wall or window unit is also adaptable for cooling the preparation room. Such units pull in cool fresh air from outdoors. If properly balanced with the exhaust system, a "once through" ventilation system can be created and used during the embalming operation.

▶ PREPARATION ROOM EQUIPMENT

Refrigeration units since the mid-1970s, when the Federal FTC Rule required permission for embalming, there has been a rise in the number of funeral facilities having refrigeration units. These can range in size from a unit holding two bodies to a walk-in room which can hold 50 or more deceased human remains. The purpose of these cooling units is to slow the postmortem changes in the deceased body in particular decomposition.

Refrigeration temperature ranges from 35°F to 45°F. The State Board of Pennsylvania mandates that the temperature must be maintained between 35°F and 40°F.

The cooling unit should be locked by key or touch pad. A log should be kept with the following information: name of deceased, date, time, and employee who placed the deceased into or removed the deceased from the cooler. For large coolers, this log should include the location of the deceased within the cooler. A cleaning schedule needs to be maintained for the cooler and any spills of biohazard liquids needs to be immediately cleaned. Floors and body trays must be frequently disinfected and washed. Bio-hazard bins within or outside the cooler will provide a place for disposal of soiled laundry or soiled cleanup materials. For walk-in coolers, a composite floor with floor drains is necessary. Sufficient lighting should be provided within the cooling unit.

All decedents placed into the cooler need to have an identification attached to the body and the body bag. Human remains need to be positioned in a supine position with shoulders and head elevated. They should be within a body bag or covered with sheeting. Unembalmed bodies should be sprayed with a topical disinfectant, any purge material removed from the face and neck and a light coating of massage cream placed on the face and neck before being placed into the cooler.

Body Lifts

Lifting devices are essential. Their use can include movement of the deceased from the removal cot to the embalming table; removal from the embalming table to a dressing table or placement within a casket; removal of shipped-in remains from the shipping container to the dressing table; placement of decedent into a shipping container. As much lifting as possible should be done by mechanical devices.

Body Transfer Board

These thin, smooth, flat polyethylene boards, are strong, non-absorbent, and easily cleaned. Placed under the body, they can be used to move the body from the removal cot to other tables in the preparation room for embalming or refrigeration storage. They can also be used to move bodies between embalming tables to dressing or storage tables.

Tables

Embalming tables are available with stainless-steel, porcelain or stain-resistant fiberglass tops and cast iron, steel, or aluminum bases. These bases may have a hydraulic or ratchet-type raising, lowering, or tilting mechanism. They all have a drain channel around each side, with a drain hole at the foot end. Most stainless-steel tables have wheels, whereas the older porcelain tables have a swivel-action base (Fig. 4–11). "Body bridges" can be used with the stainless-steel and fiberglass tables; they elevate the body above the table making the entire table a drain channel. Thus, drainage is easily flushed away from the body and the embalmer.

At the completion of the embalming, the body may be transferred from the embalming table to a dressing table. Dressing tables usually have a laminated plastic top and an aluminum frame. The frame has wheels, is adjustable in height, and perhaps can fold in the middle. There is no drain channel or hole in a dressing table as in the embalming table.

Injection Apparatus

Most arterial embalming is done using electric machines for the injection of arterial solution. To be complete, however, several older mechanical methods are considered in this discussion. These devices are generally used today when the electronic machines are not working or when there is an electrical failure. Basically, six devices can be used to inject arterial solution: (1) gravity; (2) bulb syringe; (3) combination of gravity and bulb syringe; (4) hand pump; (5) air pressure machine; and (6) centrifugal pump.

Gravity Injection (Historical). The arterial solution is poured into a large glass percolator that has a delivery hose attached to the bottom of the bowl. The device is then elevated above the body and the solution flows into the arterial system. Approximately, one-half (0.43) pound of pressure is developed for each foot of height the device is raised above the injection point (for every 28 inches of height, 1 pound of pressure is created). Because of height restrictions in most preparation rooms, pressure is limited with gravity injection. This method of injection is still widely used for injection of bodies that will be used for anatomical dissection. Gravity embalming provides a slow, steady method of injection that allows the body to accept the embalming solution at a slower rate allowing more of the arterial solution to be retained by the body tissues (Fig. 4–12).

Bulb Syringe (Historical). This hand-held and hand-operated device consists of a rubber bulb with hoses attached to either end. A one-way valve in the device allows for this pump to operate. One hose is dropped into a container of embalming solution. Arterial solution flows into the bulb when the device is relaxed. Once the bulb is full, squeezing the bulb forces the arterial solution into the delivery hose and into the body. It is important to remember that the solution actually passes through the bulb syringe. Pressures are unknown and it does require the use of one hand. As pressure builds within the body, the bulb syringe becomes more difficult to squeeze (Fig. 4–13).

Combination Gravity and Bulb Syringe (Historical). In this method of injection, the delivery hose from the gravity percolator connects to the bulb syringe. The body can be embalmed by the gravity method, but pressures and rate of flow can be increased periodically by squeezing on the bulb syringe. The combination produces a greater pressure and rate of flow of the arterial solution.

Hand Pump (Historical). This hand-held device is a pump with two slip-hubs to which hoses can be attached. One hub delivers air to create pressure; the other hub creates a vacuum. Arterial solution does **not** flow

Figure 4–11. A. Hydraulic, porcelain preparation table. Note the elevated central portion and ribs to drain fluids away from the body. **B.** Hydraulic, stainless steel embalming table shown with body "bridges." (**Courtesy of Ferno-Washington, Inc., Wilmington, Ohio**.)

through the hand pump. The arterial solution is placed in a jar and the lid is sealed into position. Air pumped by the hand pump enters through the hose leading from the hand pump to the jar. A delivery hose, which drops to the bottom of the jar, then carries the solution out of the jar and into the body. A careful check is necessary to be certain that air is not injected into the body if all the arterial solution is injected. By attaching the air hose to the other hub of the hand pump, air can be withdrawn from the jar and; thus, a vacuum created within the jar. A trocar can be attached to the free end of a hose which is attached by a gooseneck inserted into the jar lid. The aspirated contents will flow into the jar. No aspirated material passes through the handpump.

Air Pressure Machine (Historical). The air pressure machine (Fig. 4–14) operates just like the hand pump, but because it is motorized, it relieves the embalmer from having to physically operate the device. The air pressure machine, like the hand pump, can be adapted to aspiration. Embalming solution and aspirated materials **do not** flow through the machine. The machine provides only air pressure or a vacuum. The delivery hose from the machine is attached to a reinforced plastic jar or metal pressure tank. The jar is the source of arterial solution, and also it will be the container into which aspirated materials will collect. This device can be very dangerous and pressures must be carefully observed. Some will produce pressures and vacuum up to 30 psi. This method

Figure 4–14. Air pressure machines may be used for injection or aspiration.

Figure 4-12. Gravity injector.

A

B

Figure 4–13. A. Bulb syringe—injection only. **B.** Hand pump—injection or aspiration.

of injection is still widely used in Great Britain and Europe.

Centrifugal Pump. Because the centrifugal pump is the most widely accepted method of injecting arterial solution today, a more extensive explanation is given for this mechanical pump (Fig. 4–15). The centrifugal pump embalming machine is a self-contained device. Over the years, a wide variety of machines, each with special features, have been available. Some even contain a separate system similar to an air pressure machine for aspiration. Most of these machines have large-volume tanks, a few of which hold as much as 3½ gallons of solution. With the motorized force pump, a constant preset pressure can be maintained in addition to the preset rate of flow of arterial solution into the body. It is always recommended that pressure be adjusted prior to arterial injection. The rate of flow can be determined once the arterial injection begins.

During the embalming, it may become necessary to reset pressure and rate of flow to establish a good distribution of the embalming solution. The pressure ranges in the motorized force pump can be very great. Some machines are capable of producing up to 200 pounds of pressure. In some machines, the motorized centrifugal pump runs at a constant speed. In others, the speed can be varied, and in yet other machines, two separate motors operating at different speeds are available. Many of these machines can produce a pulsating injection of fluid into the body.

Several terms must be explained at this point. **Pressure** is the force required to distribute the embalming solution throughout the body. The **rate of flow** is the amount of embalming solution that enters the body in a given period and is measured in ounces per minute. **Potential pressure** is the pressure reading on the gauge in the centrifugal machine, indicating the pressure in the delivery line of the machine with the rate-of-flow valve closed or the arterial tubing clamped shut.

"15" - *Potential Pressure* - Rate of Flow Closed

"10" - *Actual Pressure* - Rate of Flow Open

"5" - *Differential Pressure* - The Rate of Flow

Figure 4–15. Centrifugal pump. **A.** Potential pressure (15), rate of flow closed. **B.** Actual pressure (10) rate of flow open. **C.** Differential pressure (5) or rate of flow.

Differential pressure is the difference between the potential pressure reading and the actual pressure reading; this is an indicator of the **rate of flow. Actual pressure** is the reading on the pressure gauge on the centrifugal pump when the rate-of-flow valve is open and the arterial solution is entering the body.

In the example described in Figure 4–15, with the rate-of-flow valve **closed,** the potential pressure is 15-pounds psi. The differential pressure is 5 and the actual pressure when the rate of flow valve is open is 10. If it were open until the gauge dropped to 5 actual pounds, the differential would be 10, or it can be said that the rate of flow would be twice as fast as the previous setting. The differential reading indicates the amount of resistance in the body, in the arterial cannula, and in the tube running from the machine to the cannula. The differential is also an important indicator of the rate of flow. Flow rate gauges may also be added to the centrifugal machine.

There has been much misunderstanding in regard to the pressure that may exist inside the body as a result of the injection of solution. The mere fact that a pressure gauge reading on the device used for injection indicates a given pressure at which the fluid is leaving the machine does not necessarily mean that this pressure exists within the body. To determine what the pressure reading on the gauge really means, take a look at the schematic diagrams (Figs. 4–16 and 4–17) showing the internal structure of an embalming machine, with four different flow paths shown as "filled" tubes (solid black) numbered from 1 to 4.

Liquid flows from the "well" beneath the tank to the pump from which it follows either path 1 or 2 or both paths (Fig. 4–16). Path 1 represents the bypass flow from

Path No. 1

Path No. 2

Figure 4–16. Pressure paths 1 and 2.

EMBALMING MACHINE
TANK

PUMP

FLOW
GAGE

FLOW
CONTROL
VALVE   PRESSURE
GAGE   PRESSURE
VALVE

Path No. 3

EMBALMING MACHINE
TANK

PUMP

FLOW
GAGE

FLOW
CONTROL
VALVE   PRESSURE
GAGE   PRESSURE
VALVE

Path No. 4

Figure 4–17. Pressure paths 3 and 4.

Figure 4–18. Centrifugal embalming machine. These machines are available with or without pulsation.

the pump back to the tank. As the pump functions at a steady and continuous capacity, it is necessary to provide such bypass when injection of fluid at a slow rate is desired. Otherwise, the full force of the pump pressure could not be controlled to permit such low injection rates. Path 2 is the flow from the pump to the intermediate line just prior to the outlet line.

The intermediate line contains the rate-of-flow control valve and the pressure control valve. As may be surmised, the pressure control valve determines how much fluid will be returned to the tank via path 3 (Fig. 4–17), which constitutes a second bypass in the system. If, for example, a maximum pressure is set at the pressure valve control, very little, if any, liquid will flow through path 3. The needle valve in the pressure control valve actually cuts off fluid flow to that bypass and so the fluid is forced, then, to flow on to the outlet.

As the fluid proceeds to the outlet, the rate-of-flow control valve will determine how much will be delivered

to the arterial tube outlet indicated by path 4. When pressure, as regulated by the rate-of-flow control valve, is drastically reduced so that only a small trickle of fluid is delivered, then high pressures can readily be registered on the pressure gauge. This does not mean, as can be readily realized, that the fluid is leaving the arterial tube under **that** much pressure!

In other words, with liquid flow paths 3 and 4 cut off by reducing the rate of flow and cutting off the bypass of fluid beyond the pressure control valve (causing high pressures to be registered), fluid can then leave the pump in large quantities only through path 1, which is the bypass back to the tank. It should be remembered that regardless of the amount of pressure being used or how fast the rate of flow might be, the pump **always** operates at the same speed and its output is **always** the same. With this knowledge in mind, safety features in the nature of the bypass are included in pressure machines. The pressure reading on the gauge merely indicates the amount of resistance being offered to the flow of the liquid **within** the confines of the machine. Continual use of "high" pressure places a heavy load on the motor and pump and, most often, this is not necessary (Fig. 4–18).

▶ INSTRUMENTATION

An embalming chemical supply catalog lists many instruments, most of which come in a variety of sizes and modifications. Actually, very few instruments are needed in the preparation of the unautopsied or autopsied body. Most instruments have several uses and this helps to limit the number needed. Unlike a surgical procedure,

Figure 4–19. Aneurysm needle.

embalming is not performed under sterile conditions, so instruments can be reused during the embalming process. Most instruments are constructed of steel and plated with nickel or chrome for protection against rust or chemical agents. They are chemically treated to be heat resistant and durable.

General Instruments

Aneurysm Needle. A blunt instrument (Fig. 4–19), the aneurysm needle, is used for tissue dissection for determining the location and elevation of arteries and veins. The aneurysm needle has an "eye" in the hook portion of the instrument, which could be used for passing ligatures around a vessel. An **aneurysm hook** is similar but has a sharp pointed tip. Most embalmers prefer to work with the blunt instrument.

Bistoury Knife. The bistoury knife is a curved cutting instrument that cuts from the inside outward (Fig. 4–20). Some embalmers prefer this type of instrument for opening arteries and veins. It can also be used for the excision of tissues.

Hemostat (Locking Forceps). A wide variety of hemostats are available. The hemostat can be used to clamp leaking vessels. A modification is the **arterial hemostat**, which is used to hold the arterial tube in an artery. The ends of hemostats may be curved or straight, serrated or smooth, or plain or rat-toothed. **Dressing forceps** are very long hemostats. They can be used for packing orifices or handling contaminated bandage dressings (Figs. 4–21 to 4–23).

Scalpel. The scalpel is a sharp cutting instrument used for making incisions (Fig. 4–24). It can be purchased with a permanent blade, or the handles can be purchased and disposable blades used. OSHA regulations requires a **sharps container** for the disposition of scalpel and razor blades, These puncture proof containers come in a variety of sizes.

Figure 4–20. Bistoury knife.

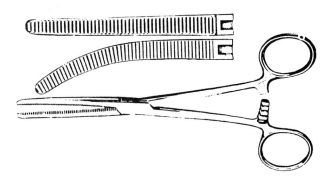

Figure 4–21. Serrated edges.

Scissors. Scissors are used for cutting. Like the bistoury knife and scalpel, scissors can also be used to open arteries and veins (Fig. 4–25). There is an **arterial scissors** (Fig. 4–25D) manufactured for opening vessels. Scissors vary in length, and their tips may be straight or curved, or pointed or blunt. The blunt side should be used against the skin surface of the body. **Bandage scissors** (Fig. 4–25E) have a very large blunt end to help protect the skin from being cut.

Separator. The separator is used to keep vessels elevated above the incision. This instrument can be made of hard rubber, bone, or metal. Often, the handle of an aneurysm needle is designed to function as a separator (Fig. 4–26).

Suture Needles. A variety of suture needles are available (Fig. 4–27). The large **postmortem needles** (Fig. 4–27A,B) are used to close autopsy incisions as well as incisions made to raise vessels for injection. These needles are half or double curved. The three-eighth-inch **circle needle** is used for more delicate suturing. The needle eye may be the patented type called a "spring eye" for "self"-threading. The edges can be smooth or cutting (Fig. 4–27C). The half-curved **Loopuypt needle** (Fig. 4–27E) is designed to better grip the instrument.

Figure 4–22. Arterial hemostat.

Figure 4–24. Scalpel.

Figure 4–23. Dressing forceps.

A

B

C

D

D

Figure 4–25. A–E. Various types of scissors.

Figure 4–26. Separator.

Figure 4–27. Miscellaneous types of suture needles. **A.** Postmortem half-curved suture needles. **B.** Postmortem double-curved suture needles. **C.** Three-eighths-inch circle needles with "spring eye." **D.** Half-curved suture needles. **E.** Loopuypt needles.

Figure 4–28. Forceps. **A.** Angular springs. **B.** Straight spring.

Spring Forceps. The spring forceps is an instrument used for grasping and holding tissues. The limbs may be straight, curved, or angular (Fig. 4–28). Angular spring forceps are used as a drainage instrument, generally in the internal jugular vein. The tips of forceps may be serrated, smooth, or rat-toothed. Most embalmers use several types and lengths of spring forceps. This instrument is available in a large variety of lengths.

Suture Thread. Suture thread is sold by the twist or cord, three cord being thinner than five or seven cord. Suture thread is available in nylon, cotton, and linen. Some embalmers prefer that it be waxed. Dental floss can also be used for suturing.

Injection Instruments

Arterial Tubes. There are many types, lengths, and sizes of arterial injection tubes: those small enough for injection of infants and distal arteries, such as the radial and ulnar arteries in the adult, and those large enough for injection of the large carotid arteries. Carotid tubes are short and very large in diameter. The hub of an arterial tube can be a **threaded** type (Fig. 4–29A), to which a stopcock can be attached, or a **slip-type,** to which the delivery hose from the machine can be directly attached. The tube itself can be curved or straight. Luer-Lok (Fig. 4–29C) arterial tubes were developed for high-pressure injection. These tubes attach to a connector on the delivery hose much the same as a hypodermic needle attaches to a syringe.

Stopcock. The stopcock is used to attach the delivery hose from the injection device to the arterial tube (Fig. 4–30A). Luer-Lok stopcocks are used for arterial tubes

with Luer-Lok attachments (Fig. 4–30B). The stopcock can be used to maintain and stop the flow of fluid into the arterial tube.

Y Tube. The Y tube was developed for the embalming of autopsied bodies. It allows the embalmer to embalm both legs or arms or sides of the head at the same time (Fig. 4–31). Double Y tubes have been developed that allow for injection of four body regions at the same time.

Hypovalve Trocar. The hypovalve trocar is designed for hypodermic treatments (Fig. 4–32). It is **not** used for aspiration but rather for injection.

Drainage Instruments

Drain Tube. The drain tube is a metal cylinder with a cleaning rod designed to be inserted into a vein (Fig. 4–33). Drain tubes are always inserted **toward** the heart. They help to keep the vein expanded and can be closed to build circulatory pressure. The stirring rod can be used to fragment large clots. There are many sizes. Jugular drain tubes are generally very large in diameter and short; axillary drain tubes are often slightly curved; infant drain tubes can be used for small vessels such as the femoral and iliac in the infant. A hose can easily be attached to the drainage outlet so the blood drained can easily be controlled or collected and disinfected.

Angular Spring Forceps. These angular forceps have a working length of $2\frac{1}{2}$ to 7 inches. They are inserted much like the drain tube into a vein and directed toward the heart. They allow clots to be grasped and pulled from within a vein.

Figure 4–29. A. Curved threaded arterial tubes. **B.** Straight threaded arterial tubes. **C.** Luer-Lok.

Figure 4–30. Stopcocks. **A.** Stopcock used to attach the delivery hose from the injection device to the arterial tube. **B.** Luer-Lok stopcock used for arterial tubes with Luer-Lok attachments.

Figure 4–31. A Y tube used for embalming autopsied bodies.

Figure 4–32. Hypovalve trocar. Designed for hypodermic treatments. Used for injection, not aspiration.

Figure 4–33. Drain tubes can be used to build circulatory pressure.

Figure 4–34. Iliac drain tube. This long tube is designed to be inserted into the external iliac vein.

Figure 4–35. Groove director. Used to expand a vein to help guide a drain tube or drainage device into the vein.

Figure 4–36. Autopsy aspirator. The many openings guard against clogging during aspiration of either blood or arterial fluid from the cavities of autopsied bodies.

Iliac Drain Tube. The iliac drain tube is a long drain tube designed to be inserted into the external iliac vein and the tip is directed into the right atrium of the heart (Fig. 4–34). These tubes may be soft rubber, plastic, or metal.

Grooved Director. The grooved director is used to expand a vein to help guide a drain tube or drainage device such as angular spring forceps into a vein for drainage (Fig. 4–35).

Aspirating Instruments

Autopsy Aspirator. An autopsy aspirator has many openings so as to be "non-clogging." It is used to aspirate blood and arterial fluid from the cavities of autopsied bodies (Fig. 4–36).

Hydroaspirator. The hydroaspirator is an aspirating device that creates a vacuum when water is run through the mechanism (Fig. 4–37). Most hydroaspirators are equipped with a vacuum breaker so aspirated material flowing through the device does not enter the water supply should there occur a sudden drop in water pressure.

Nasal Tube Aspirator. The nasal tube aspirator attaches to the aspirating hose. It is designed to be inserted into the nostril or throat for limited aspiration of the nasal passage or the throat (Fig. 4–38).

Trocar. The trocar is a long hollow needle. The length and the diameter of this instrument are quite variable (Fig. 4–39). The points are threaded so they may be changed when dull. The handle may be threaded or have a slip hub. Infant trocars are short and small in diameter. They may also be used for hypodermic injection treatments. The standard trocar is used to aspirate and inject body cavities.

Cavity Fluid Injector. The cavity fluid injector screws onto the cavity fluid bottles. When the device is inverted, cavity fluid flows through the trocar into the body cavities (Fig. 4–40).

Trocar Button. A threaded plastic screw used for closing trocar punctures, the trocar button may also be used to close small punctures, surgical drain openings, and intravenous line punctures. They are available in several sizes (Fig. 4–41).

Trocar Button Applicator. The trocar button applicator is used to insert the trocar button (Fig. 4–42).

Feature Setting Devices

Eyecaps. Eyecaps are plastic disks inserted under the eyelids. They keep the eyelids closed and prevent the eyes from sinking into the orbit (Fig. 4–43).

Figure 4–37. Hydroaspirator. This aspirating device creates a vacuum when water is run through the mechanism.

Figure 4–38. Nasal tube aspirator. Attaches to the aspirating hose. Designed for nasal insertion.

Figure 4–39. Trocar. A long hollow needle with threaded points that can be changed.

Figure 4–40. Cavity fluid injector. Screws onto cavity fluid bottles.

Figure 4–41. Trocar button. Threaded plastic screw used for closing trocar punctures.

Figure 4–42. Trocar button applicator. Used to insert the trocar button.

Figure 4–43. Eyecaps.

Figure 4–44. Mouth formers.

Mouth Formers. Mouth formers are plastic or metal devices used to replace the teeth when the natural teeth or dentures are absent (Fig. 4–44).

Needle Injector. A needle injector is used to insert a "barb" into the mandible and maxilla to hold the lower jaw in a closed position. Several types of handles are available which can make the device easier to use. An electric version is also available (Fig. 4–45).

Positioning Devices

Positioning devices enable the embalmer to properly position the head, arms, hands, and feet of the deceased.

Most are constructed of metal, hard rubber, or plastic. Embalmers often employ specially cut blocks of wood to elevate shoulders, arms, and feet. These devices should be properly painted with a water-resistant paint so they can be cleaned after each use.

Head Rests. Headrests can be used to elevate the head and neck. They can be used to support the arms and raise the feet. A head rest can also be placed under the thigh area to help steady bodies with severe spinal curvature or an arthritic condition (Fig. 4–46).

Figure 4–45. Needle injector.

Figure 4-46. Headrests.

Arm and Hand Rests. Arm and hand rests consist of two curved metal arm holders attached by an adjustable strap. The strap rests across the body while the arms are secured in the arm holder. It is designed to fit bodies of different size and retain both arms and hands in a desirable position.

Shoulder, Body, and Foot Rests. Rests of plastic or metal blocks are used to raise shoulders, feet, or buttocks off the table.

▶ PLASTIC UNDERGARMENTS

Plastic garments can be used to protect clothing from conditions such as ulcerations, gangrene, or burnt tissue. They help to control leakage from the tissue donor body, autopsied body or the condition of edema. Those most frequently used include: pants, coveralls, stockings, sleeves, Capri garments and unionalls. With the exception of sleeves, all of those listed come in a variety of sizes. Powdered deodorants and preservatives may be placed within the garment to control odor and absorb any leakage. The coverall covers the trunk of the body from the upper thigh to the armpit. The unionall covers the entire body except for the hands, neck, and head areas (Fig. 4–47). The Capri garment combines pants and stockings.

UNIONALL　　**STOCKINGS**　　**COVERALLS**

CAPRI PANTS　　**SLEEVES**　　**PANTS**　　**SHIRT JACKETS**

Figure 4-47. Plastic undergarments.

► CONCEPTS FOR STUDY AND DISCUSSION

1. List all the instruments you may need to use in the embalming of a non-autopsied body. List all the instruments you may need to use in the embalming of an autopsied body.
2. Discuss the disadvantages of a basement preparation room.
3. Discuss the proper locations for an exhaust system in the preparation room.
4. How does the hand pump differ from the bulb syringe?
5. With reference to the centrifugal injection machine, explain the terms potential pressure, actual pressure, and differential pressure.
6. Review the statutes, rules, and regulations your state has concerning the preparation room.

► BIBLIOGRAPHY

Bourne H, Seferian S. Formaldehyde in wrinkle-proof apparel processes: Tears for my lady. *Ind Med Surg* 1959;28:232.

Hendrick DJ, Lane DJ. Occupational formalin asthma. *Br J Ind Med* 1977;34:11.

Johnson P. NIOSH. Health Hazard Evaluation Determination Report HE 79-146-670, March 1980.

Kerfoot E, Mooney T. Formaldehyde and paraformaldehyde study in funeral homes. *Am Ind Hyg Assoc J* 1975;36:533.

Moore LL, Ogrodnik EC. Occupational exposure to formaldehyde in mortuaries. *J Environ Health* 1986;49(1):32-35.

Morrill E. Formaldehyde exposure from paper process solved by air sampling and current studies. *Air Cond Heat Vent* 1961;58:94.

Porter JAH. Acute respiratory distress following formalin inhalation. *Lancet* 1975;2:876.

Proctor NH, Hughes JP. *Chemical Hazards of the Workplace.* Philadelphia, PA: JB Lippincott, 1978:272.

Riccobono PX. *Current Report: Bureau of National Affairs.* October 1979:471.

Sakula A. Formalin asthma in hospital laboratory staff. *Lancet* 1975;2:876.

Schoenber J, Mitchell C. Airway disease caused by phenolic (phenol–formaldehyde) resin exposure. *Arch Environ Health* 1975;30:575.

U.S. Department of Labor. *Occupational Safety and Health Standards (OSHA) for General Industry.* January 1978.

USDHEW/PHS/HRA. *Minimum Requirements of Construction and Equipment for Hospitals and Medical Facilities.* National Technical Information Service, DHEW Publication No. (HRA) 74-4000, September 1974.

Whitaker L. The preparation room. *Dodge Mag,* The Dodge Company, Cambridge, MA. 1997–1998;89(2)-90(3).

CHAPTER 5

DEATH—AGONAL AND POSTMORTEM CHANGES

CHAPTER OBJECTIVES

▶ Death—agonal changes
▶ Postmortem physical changes
▶ Postmortem chemical changes
▶ Signs and tests of death

Death is a process and not a moment in time. During the process there is a series of physical and chemical changes, starting before the medicolegal time of death and continuing afterward. In the sequence of death there is a point of irreversibility that can generally be diagnosed by physicians. When this point is reached, nothing more can be done to restore intelligent life.

Because most deaths in the United States occur in an institutional setting, the pronouncement of death is typically the responsibility of persons who have the legal certification and authority to make a determination that death has, in fact, occurred. There are those times, however, where death may occur someplace other than an institution. In such cases, funeral home personnel may be among the first to arrive at a death scene. As such, it is important that they understand and honor the medicolegal relationships that exist in the jurisdiction where the death has occurred.

From a layperson's perspective, death might be thought of as the point at which an individual "draws his last breath." In reality, there is a sequence of steps leading up to that point, and a series of changes associated with the steps. In higher biological organisms, such as humans, these changes result in a cessation of integrated tissue and organ functions. As a result, there is a loss of heartbeat, cessation of spontaneous breathing, and absence of brain activity (*Stedman's Medical Dictionary*, 1995, p. 443). The process takes place in a sequence of steps which can be described as an expanding inability of the body to sustain the physiologic and metabolic processes that are necessary for life. The period of time over which the steps occur is known as the **agonal period**.

The agonal period might be quite short, as would be the case in an accident where death resulted from sudden, fatal injuries. Or, the process might take place over an extended period of time, as would be the case in a death caused by chronic illness. Whether the agonal period is long or short, at a given point in the process, the body can no longer function as a whole organism.

▶ PROGRESSION OF SOMATIC DEATH

Agonal refers to death or dying (*Taber's Cyclopedic Medical Dictionary*, 2001, p. 58). During the agonal period the body is said to be **moribund**, a dying condition, or dying (*Taber's Cyclopedic Medical Dictionary*, 2001, p. 1377). Physical observations that can be made during the dying process include **death rattle** and **death struggle**. Death rattle is a respiratory gurgling or rattling in the throat of a dying person, caused by the loss of the cough reflex and the accumulation of mucous (*Stedman's Medical Dictionary*, 1995, p. 444).

Death struggle is the semiconvulsive twitches that often occur before death.

The agonal period occurs prior to the point in the process where the body loses its ability to sustain vital physiologic and metabolic activities. Once the body loses its ability to sustain physiologic and metabolic activity, **somatic death** occurs. Somatic death is defined as the death of the entire body (*Stedman's Medical Dictionary*, 1995, p. 444). It proceeds in an orderly progression from clinical death to brain death, then to biological death, and finally to postmortem cellular death.

Clinical death occurs when spontaneous respiration and heartbeat cease. It is during this time that the person can be resuscitated and, therefore, this is the reversible phase of the somatic death process. If respiration and heartbeat are not reestablished, **brain death** will result. **Biological death** refers to the period in the process where simple life processes of the various organs and tissues of the body begin to cease. When biological death occurs, respiration and circulation cannot be restored.

Even after the process of dying has begun, however, there may still be a store of oxygen, nutrients, and other vital elements at the cellular level. Individual cells can sustain metabolic activity by utilizing available stores of essential elements. At some point, individual cells will use up stored elements, or will be overcome by autolytic processes, and die. This is **postmortem cellular death**. Cells that are more specialized and/or active will react more quickly to the decrease of oxygen or nutrients. The progression of cellular death can thus continue for a number of hours after somatic death, as shown in these examples:

Brain and nervous system cells	5 min
Muscle cells	3 h
Cornea cells	6 h
Blood cells	6 h

It is worth noting that cellular death also occurs in the body as part of normal biological processes and as a result of disease processes.

ANTEMORTEM PERIOD

Cellular death
Necrobiosis
Necrosis

STAGES OF DEATH

Agonal period
Somatic death
Clinical death
Brain death
Biological death
Postmortem cellular death

The accompanying chart presents an order of occurrence for the changes that take place in the body before death (**antemortem period**) and as death is progressing. The terms are defined as follows:

- **Necrobiosis** refers to the physiologic, or natural, death of cells as they complete their life cycles.
- **Necrosis** refers to the pathologic death of body cells as a result of disease processes (e.g., gangrene or decubitus ulcers).
- **Clinical death** occurs when spontaneous respiration and heartbeat irreversibly cease.
- **Brain death** occurs in a sequence of events that are a function of time without oxygen. The first part of the brain to die, usually in 5 or 6 minutes, is the cerebral cortex. Next the midbrain dies, followed by the brain stem.
- **Biological death** is the irreversible phase of somatic death and represents the cessation of simple body processes. The organs no longer function.
- **Postmortem cellular death** is the process during which individual cells die. It may take a matter of hours depending on numerous variables.

▶ CHANGES DURING THE AGONAL PERIOD

As the process of death progresses, there are changes that take place in the body. These changes are of great importance to embalmers because, in their variations, they contribute to multiple complications that must be addressed by embalming procedures and techniques. The changes that occur in the death process will, to an extent, dictate what procedures and techniques are appropriate for a given case. Therefore, it is important that embalmers recognize and understand death as a process.

As medical science has brought new therapies and treatments to medicine, the potential for an extended agonal period has been increased. As a result, the embalmer is more likely to encounter cases where: (1) disease processes have had longer to work on the body; (2) secondary infections have increased in the body; and (3) drug therapies have dramatically affected the tissue conditions and the chemical balance of the body.

Agonal period changes can be categorized according to their effect on the: (1) temperature of the body; (2) ability of the body to circulate blood; (3) moisture content of the tissues; and (4) translocation of microorganisms within the body.

Temperature Changes

Two thermal changes can occur during the agonal period. **Agonal algor** is a cooling or decrease of the body temperature prior to death. This is often seen in the death of elderly patients, especially when death occurs slowly. The metabolism has slowed in these individuals and, no doubt, the circulatory system has slowed. **Agonal fever** is an increase of the body temperature just prior to death. This is often seen in persons with infection, toxemia, or certain types of poisoning. Frequently, elevated temperature can stimulate microbial growth.

Circulatory Changes

Three circulatory changes are possible in the agonal period. **Agonal hypostasis** is the settling of blood into the dependent tissues of the body. It occurs as a result of the slowing of circulation just prior to death, which allows the force of gravity to overcome the force of circulation. **Agonal coagulation** occurs as the circulation of blood slows and the formed elements of the blood begin to clot and congeal. **Agonal capillary expansion** is the opening of the pores in the walls of the capillaries. It occurs as the body attempts to get more oxygen to the tissues and the cells.

SIGNS OF DEATH

The presence of death might be manifested by the changes that have taken place in the body. The signs of death might include

1. Cessation of respiration
2. Cessation of circulation
3. Muscular flaccidity
4. Changes in the eye, including:
   a. Clouding of the cornea
   b. Loss of luster of the conjunctiva
   c. Flattening of the eyeball
   d. Dilated and unresponsive pupils
5. Postmortem lividity
6. Rigor mortis
7. Algor mortis
8. Decomposition

From American Board of Funeral Service Education: *Embalming Syllabus*, Portland, ME: American Board of Funeral Service Education; 2001:11, with permission.

Moisture Changes

Two changes in tissue moisture are possible during the agonal period. **Agonal edema** is an increase in the amount of moisture, or fluids, in the tissues and the body cavities. It may result from disease processes or from agonal capillary expansion. **Agonal dehydration** is a decrease in the amount of moisture, or fluids, in the tissues and the body cavities. It may result from disease processes or from agonal capillary expansion.

The relationship between agonal edema and agonal dehydration can be thought of in terms of shifts in the balance and location of body moisture. The tissue fluids that flow or gravitate to other places in the body will create a shift in the moisture balance. Thus, one area may become edematous while another will become dehydrated. In agonal capillary expansion, the increased size of the openings in the capillary walls, while intended to allow more oxygen into the tissues, also allows fluids to flow out of the capillaries and into the intercellular spaces. This movement of fluids constitutes a shift in the moisture balance by which the greater amounts of moisture flow to the intercellular spaces while the moisture within the capillary will be reduced.

Translocation of Microorganisms

Translocation is the movement of microorganisms from one area of the body to another. It occurs as organisms normally confined to a specific area of the body by natural body defenses are able to move as the body loses its ability to keep them in check. The movement may be the result of the organism: (1) having natural motility; (2) entering the blood stream and circulating to other parts of the body; or (3) gravitating to other parts of the body during hypostasis or shifts in tissue moisture.

▶ POSTMORTEM CHANGES

In the period between death and embalming the composition and condition of the body continues to change (Table 5–1). Generally, unless there are some intervening variables, the nature and extent of the changes will be greater if the time between death and embalming is longer. The embalming process is intended to retard, interrupt, or reverse the changes. For that reason embalmers tend to prefer having all legal and professional requirements satisfied in a timely fashion so that they can begin the embalming process as soon after death as possible. If the time lapse between death and embalming is too long, there may be complications severe enough to affect the successful outcome of the embalming process. These postmortem changes are classified as physical changes and chemical changes (Fig. 5–1).

Physical changes are brought about by the forces of nature. The forces of nature act on the body in such a way as to create changes in the physical state of the body or body tissues. These physical changes, however, do not create chemical by-products or change the chemical composition of the body. The force of gravity, for example, may move blood from one place to another in the body. No new products are formed by this movement. The blood merely changes physical location.

A **chemical change** is brought about by chemical activity. As a result, new substances are formed. For example, there are autolytic processes taking place in the body during the postmortem period. These processes

TABLE 5–1. POSTMORTEM PHYSICAL AND CHEMICAL CHANGES

Change	Classification	Description
Algor mortis	Physical	Cooling of the body to the temperature of the surrounding environment
Dehydration	Physical	Loss of moisture from the surface of the body to the surrounding atmosphere
Hypostasis	Physical	Gravitation of blood and body fluids to dependent areas of the body
Livor mortis	Physical	Postmortem intravascular blood discoloration brought about by the presence of blood in the dependent surface vessels of the body
Increase in blood viscosity	Physical	Thickening of the blood after death caused primarily by the loss of the liquid portion of the blood to the tissue spaces
Endogenous invasion of microorganisms	Physical	Relocation of microorganisms in the body as a result of the cessation of natural and metabolic activities which, in life, keep the organisms in check
Postmortem caloricity	Chemical	Temporary rise in body temperature after death
Change in body pH	Chemical	Change in body tissues from slightly alkaline in life (pH 7.38–7.40) to acid (pH 6.0–5.5) during rigor, then a return to alkaline in decomposition
Rigor mortis	Chemical	Temporary postmortem stiffening of body muscles by natural body processes
Postmortem stain	Chemical	Extravascular color change brought about by hemolysis where liberated hematin seeps through the capillary walls and into the body tissues; this type of stain cannot be removed by arterial injection and venous drainage
Decomposition	Chemical	Separation of compounds into simpler substances by the action of bacterial and/or autolytic enzymes

are largely dependent on autolytic enzymes, which break tissues by stimulating chemical reactions between substances found in the tissues. As existing substances react chemically with one another, new chemical compositions are formed.

Postmortem Physical Changes

The postmortem physical changes include (1) algor mortis, (2) hypostasis, (3) livor mortis, (4) dehydration, (5) increased viscosity of the blood, and (6) endogenous invasion of microorganisms (Table 5–2). These changes are brought about by the stoppage of blood circulation, gravity, and surface evaporations.

Algor Mortis. Algor mortis is the postmortem cooling of the body. Generally, the temperature of the surrounding

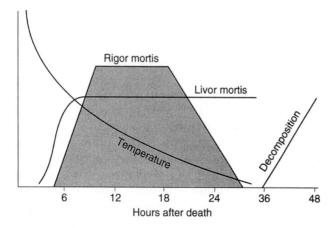

Figure 5–1. Principal postmortem changes.

environment is cooler than the temperature of the body and, over time, the temperature of the body will cool to the temperature of the surrounding environment. The rate at which a body will cool depends on a number of variables. Factors within the body itself are called **intrinsic factors** and those in the surrounding environment are called **extrinsic factors** (Fig. 5–2).

Intrinsic factors include (1) the ratio of surface area of the body to body mass, (2) body temperature at the time of death, and (3) combinations of the effects of the ratio of surface area to body mass and body temperature at the time of death.

In life, a portion of body heat is lost to conduction, radiation, and convection as the blood circulates through the superficial vessels of the skin. The blood is warmed again as it circulates back through the body's internal organs. A larger body will have more surface area to lose body heat, but that potential to lose heat can be offset by body mass. A smaller body will have less surface area to lose body heat and would therefore require less body mass to offset the loss of heat. In death, there is no opportunity for the blood to regain the lost heat because there is no circulation. Therefore, if a body has a larger surface area from which heat can be lost, its temperature will decrease more rapidly, unless there is something to offset the potential to lose heat. Here again, heat loss can be offset by body mass. In short, a body with more mass will be better insulated against heat loss and will, therefore, cool at a slower rate. Infants, for example, are more likely to cool faster because, among other factors, they have a higher ratio of surface area as compared with their body mass (Walter, 1989).

TABLE 5–2. EMBALMING SIGNIFICANCE OF POSTMORTEM PHYSICAL CHANGES

Algor mortis	Slows the onset of rigor mortis and decomposition
	Helps to keep blood in a liquid state
	Can increase the degree of livor mortis and postmortem stain
Hypostasis	Responsible for livor mortis
	Hemolysis can later cause postmortem stain
	Increases tissue moisture in dependent tissues
Livor mortis	Discoloration can vary from slight reddish hue to almost black, depending on blood volume and viscosity
	Intravascular so it can be cleared
	Can be "set" as a stain if excessively strong uncoordinated embalming solution is injected
	Can help to expand the capillaries
	If it clears during arterial injection, it can be used as a sign of fluid distribution
Dehydration	May be gravitated or massaged from an area
	Accompanied by increased blood viscosity
	Can create a "temporary" postmortem edema in the tissues
	Darkens skin surface and cannot be bleached
	Causes wrinkling and shriveling of features
	If extreme enough, can retard decomposition
	If extreme enough, can preserve the body
Increase in blood viscosity	Thickened blood and coagulation
	Increased resistance of arterial injections
	Hampers drainage
Endogenous invasion of microorganisms	Pathologic danger to the embalmer
	Promotes and aids decomposition

If the body temperature is elevated at the time of death, it will take longer for the body to cool to the temperature of the surrounding environment because the temperature will simply have farther to drop. Body temperature can elevate because of increased metabolic activity, the presence of fever, or an inability of the body to regulate its temperature. Likewise, low body temperature at the time of death will influence the length of time for the body to cool to reach a point of equilibrium with the surrounding environment. Body temperature can decrease as a result of exposure to cold or an inability of the body to regulate its temperature.

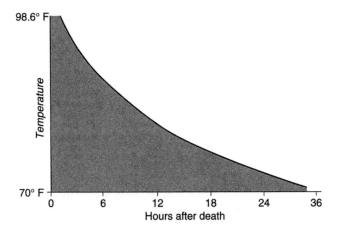

Figure 5–2. Algor mortis versus time.

Rapid cooling of the body by refrigeration or natural means helps to slow the onset of rigor mortis, slow the onset of decomposition, and keep the blood in a liquid state. These are all advantageous for embalming. A body that has been cooled rapidly will, however, be more likely to have discoloration from livor mortis and postmortem staining.

Extrinsic factors that affect postmortem cooling of the body include (1) body coverings and (2) the surrounding environment. Body coverings include clothing or other coverings that protect the skin from direct exposure to the environment. In addition to providing added insulation, an external covering will also retard or prevent heat loss that results from conduction, radiation, and convection.

The surrounding environment itself will affect the rate at which a body loses heat. A body submerged in 70°F water, for example, would lose heat more rapidly than in 70°F air temperature, because water would conduct heat away from the body more quickly than air.

Hypostasis. Hypostasis is a process by which blood settles, as a result of gravitational movement within the vessels, to the dependent, or lower parts of the body. The dependent part(s) of the body would be those parts closer to the ground. The designation of dependent part(s) would change depending on the position of the body. For example, if a body were lying on its back, the

Figure 5–3. Dark areas show livor mortis and postmortem stain. The light-colored area on the back shows contact pallor where the body is rested against the table.

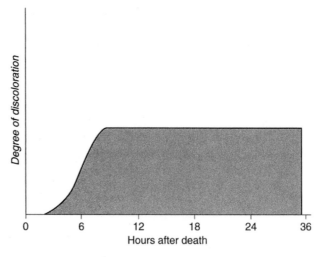

Figure 5–4. Livor mortis.

tissues of the back of the body (trunk, neck, legs, etc.) would be the areas where blood settled. If a person were sitting upright, blood would gravitate to the hips, legs, and feet.

It is also important to note that the gravitational movement of the blood can be effected by constrictions, ligatures, or other factors that would impede free movement of the blood within the vessels. **Contact pallor** refers to the areas where blood movement has been inhibited. It is most obvious in areas where the body has been in contact with a surface. The weight of the body pressing against the capillary beds prevents the blood from settling into the area. Although the surrounding area may be discolored, the area in contact with the surface will stay quite pale (Fig. 5–3).

Thinner, or less viscous, blood will tend to flow with less resistance and will thus gravitate to dependent parts of the body more readily. The factors that affect the viscosity of the blood will therefore influence the speed at which postmortem hypostasis takes place. Possible factors include refrigeration, medication, and disease processes. Conversely, factors that thicken, or increase viscosity, will slow the rate at which postmortem hypostasis takes place. Possible factors include heat, medication, and disease processes.

The embalming significance of hypostasis lies in the postmortem discolorations that potentially result from the gravitational movement of blood. In embalming terminology, hypostasis describes the process by which blood gravitates to the dependent parts of the body. Hypostasis is the term for the process, not for the discoloration.

Livor Mortis. The settling of blood brings about a discoloration that appears within 1/2 to 2 hours after death

(*Stedman's Medical Dictionary,* 1995, p. 990). In embalming terminology, this discoloration is called livor mortis. Livor mortis is a postmortem intravascular blood discoloration that occurs as a result of hypostasis. It is also known as **postmortem lividity** or **cadaveric lividity.** The discoloration may first be noticed as dull reddish patches. As it becomes more established it can take on a deep reddish-blue appearance. Livor mortis is categorized as an intravascular discoloration, meaning that it occurs within the blood vascular system and can be reduced or removed during the embalming process as embalming solution flushes the pooled blood from the area (Fig. 5–4).

Two factors play an important role in the degree of intensity of livor mortis: blood volume and blood viscosity. In cases where excessive bleeding has taken place, either internally or externally, there will be less blood available to pool. This may reduce the instance or intensity of livor mortis. Likewise, if blood is thicker and not readily subject to gravitation, the appearance of livor mortis may be effected (Table 5–3).

Dehydration. The loss of water from body tissues and fluids by surface evaporation is called dehydration. There are two basic factors at work in postmortem loss of body moisture: **surface evaporation** and **gravitation or hypostasis** of blood and body fluids.

Surface evaporation results from the passage of air or air currents over the surface of the body. It is to the embalmer's advantage to have the body covered or in some way protected against the effects of the air currents.

Gravitation or hypostasis of the blood and body fluids is the physical movement of body fluids to dependent regions of the body. The higher areas where the liquids move from are likely to become dehydrated. Conversely, the lower areas where the liquids are flowing to may become engorged, a condition called **postmortem edema.**

TABLE 5–3. EMBALMING CONSIDERATIONS AND BLOOD DISCOLORATIONS

Antemortem Hypostasis	Postmortem Hypostasis —Time→	Livor mortis —Time→	Postmortem Stain —Embalming→	Formaldehyde Gray
Occurs prior to death or during the agonal period	Begins at death	Seen as soon as blood fills superficial vessels; begins approximately 20 min after death; depends on p.m./a.m. hypostasis	Normally occurs approximately 6 h after death; cause of death and blood chemistry vary rate	Occurs after embalming
Intravascular	Intravascular	Intravascular	Extravascular	Intravascular or extravascular
Movement of blood to dependent tissues[a]	Movement of blood to dependent tissues[a]	p.m. blood discoloration as a result of p.m./a.m. hypostasis	p.m. blood discoloration as a result of hemolysis	Embalming discoloration
a.m. physical change	p.m. physical change	p.m. physical change	p.m. chemical change	—
	Speed depends on blood viscosity	Color varies with blood volume and viscosity and the amount of O₂ in blood	May occur prior to, during, or after arterial fluid injection	Seen after arterial fluid injection
a.m.	p.m.	p.m.	p.m.	p.m.
—	—	Pressed on skin clears	Pressed on skin does NOT clear	Seen as a gray stain
—	—	Removed by blood drainage	Not removed by blood drainage	Methemoglobin HCHO + blood
—	Arterial injection stops progress	Arterial injection (mild) clears/with drainage	Strong solutions bleach and "set" livor as stain	—
	Speeded by cooling of body, low blood viscosity	Speeded by cooling, blood "thinners," low blood viscosity, CO deaths	Speeded by cooling, rapid red blood cell hemolysis, CO deaths	Speeded by poor drainage

p.m., postmortem; a.m., antemortem.
[a]Dependent body area varies with body position.

A third factor also works in conjunction with the gravitation of liquids, **imbibition**. Imbibition is the ability of the cells to draw moisture from the surrounding area into themselves. The areas where the liquids move to can become edematous (e.g., postmortem edema).

As dehydration occurs, the blood will become increasingly viscous. Eventually the formed elements of the blood will stick together in clumps, a process that creates what is referred to as **sludge**. Obviously, sludge does not lend itself to establishing good drainage during arterial embalming.

Dehydration will bring about surface discolorations ranging from a yellow into the browns and, finally, black. In addition to being very hard to the touch and discolored, dehydrated tissue is also shriveled and wrinkled. Dehydration is a postmortem physical change that occurs before embalming, but can also be increased by embalming and can continue after embalming (Fig. 5–5).

Increase in Blood Viscosity. Viscosity refers to the thickness of a liquid. The blood is composed of two portions: (1) a "solid" portion made up of the various groups

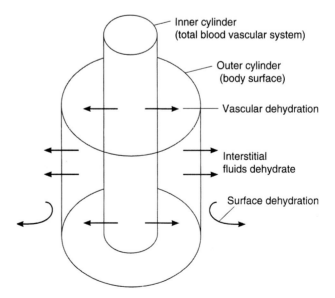

Figure 5–5. Total vascular system and the effects of dehydration.

of blood cells and (2) a "liquid" portion in which the cells are suspended. After death, blood has a tendency to increase in viscosity and thicken. This thickening is brought about by the dehydration of the body. As the tissues lose moisture to the surrounding air, the liquid portion of the blood begins to move through the capillary walls into the tissue spaces. Given enough time and the proper conditions, this liquid could leave the body by surface evaporation. The remaining blood begins to thicken as a result of a gradual loss of the liquid or serum portion of the blood.

As a result of this thickening, the blood cells begin to stick together, and if this occurs in the arterial system, the agglutinated blood will eventually clog small arteries during arterial injection. On the venous side, blood drainage will be difficult. Not only is dehydration responsible for the thickening of blood, but gravity alone tends to "drain off" the liquid portion of the blood, leaving behind a more viscous blood.

If this thickening occurs fast enough it will diminish the degree of discoloration created by livor mortis, because the blood will not move as fast into the dependent tissues. What generally happens is the blood settles into the dependent tissues first; then the blood increases in viscosity.

Endogenous Invasion (Translocation) of Microorganisms

Following somatic or functional death, normally structurally intact epithelial, fascial and other tissue barriers undergo a loss of structural integrity and permit the body wide translocation and distribution of systemic microflora and create alternate body fluid and body tissue reservoir sites of host contamination. All body fluids and body tissues may become reservoirs of infectious agents within a relatively short postmortem interval.*

Endogenous invasion of cerebrospinal fluid by bacterial agents associated with the colon occurs within 4 to 6 hours of death. *The colon, designated as the postmortem origin of "indicator" organisms recovered from extraintestinal sampling sites, seems to be the primary source of many of the translocated microbial agents.* The isolation of "indicator" organisms as well as nonindicator organisms from such sampling sites as the left ventricle of the heart, the lungs, the urinary bladder, and the cisterna cerebellomedullaris indicates the extent to which microbial agents of low, moderate, and high virulence can translocate within a relatively brief postmortem interval of 4 to 8 hours. The postmortem multiplication of systemic and translocated recoverable microbial agents may begin within 4 hours of somatic death and reach peak

densities of 3.0 to 3.5 × 10⁶ organisms per milliliter of body fluid or per gram of body tissue within a 24- to 30-hour postmortem interval.*

Postmortem factors contributing to the translocation of endogenous microflora include (1) chemical and physical changes, (2) movement and positional changes of the body, (3) passive recirculation of blood from contaminated body sites, (4) thrombus fragmentation and relocation, and (5) the inherent true mobility of many of the intestinal bacilli. The relocated organisms may exit from body openings, natural and other, and contaminate adjacent animate and inanimate surfaces. They may also become airborne particulates in the form of aerosols (droplet infection particle) or dried particles (droplet nuclei), expanding the potential spread of biological hazards.

For the embalmer, the most troublesome organism that could translocate and cause very definite postmortem problems is **Clostridium perfringens.** This tissue gas-producing anaerobic bacillus is responsible for true tissue gas. Its presence throughout the body after death can bring about immediate embalming and preservation problems. Within just 1 or 2 hours of death, if this organism is present in the tissues, it can produce gases that distend the tissues to the point where viewing the body might be impossible. Of all the agonal changes, the problems that can arise from the translocation of *C. perfringens* are most critical to the embalmer.

Postmortem Chemical Changes

The postmortem chemical changes include **postmortem caloricity, postmortem stain, shift in pH, rigor mortis, decomposition** (Table 5–4).

Postmortem Caloricity. Metabolism is defined as the sum of all the chemical reactions that occur within a cell. It is dependent on oxygen. There are two phases to metabolism: (1) **anabolism**, the building phase and (2) **catabolism**, the breakdown phase that releases heat and energy. After death occurs, the cells may still have a supply of oxygen and, therefore, metabolism will continue. The continuation of metabolism after death will create heat and may be responsible for the elevated postmortem temperature known as postmortem caloricity.

Postmortem Stain. Postmortem stain is the extravascular blood discoloration brought about by the hemolysis of blood. After death, the blood gravitates into the vessels of the dependent areas of the body. The pooling of blood in the dependent areas of the body results in an intravascular discoloration called livor mortis. Over time, the red blood cells of the pooled blood begin to break down. The breakdown or hemolysis of red blood

---

*See Selected Readings, "Summary of Guidelines Submitted to OSHA from the National Funeral Directors Association Committee on Infectious Disease," 1989.

*See the Selected Readings section for the complete Rose and Hockett reprint.

TABLE 5–4. EMBALMING SIGNIFICANCE OF POSTMORTEM CHEMICAL CHANGES

Rigor mortis	Creates extravascular resistance
	Makes positioning the body more difficult
	Makes posing features more difficult
	May contribute to tissue distention during arterial injection
	Increases demand for preservative
	Reduces the absorption of preservative
	pH change affects chemical reaction of embalming solution
	May contribute to uneven (splotchy) coloration if arterial dye is used
	May create a false sign of preservation
Postmortem stain	Extravascular discoloration that generally cannot be removed by arterial injection alone
	May result in gray discoloration when reacting with embalming chemicals
	Sign of delay between death and embalming
	Indicates an increased demand for preservative
Postmortem caloricity	Speeds the rigor mortis cycle
	Speeds decomposition
Shifts in pH	Interferes with arterial solution reactions
	May result in "splotching" of dye on the skin surface
Decomposition	May cause poor distribution of embalming solution
	Tissues may easily distend during arterial injection
	Increased demand for preservatives
	May be manifested by discoloration, odor, skin-slip, gases in cavities and tissues, purge

cells begins approximately 6 to 10 hours after death. The onset of hemolysis occurs faster in some bodies, most frequently in persons who died from carbon monoxide poisoning or in bodies that have been refrigerated (Fig. 5–6).

Each red blood cell contains several million hemoglobin molecules. Hemolysis releases the hemoglobin, which rapidly decomposes into globin and heme. The heme then passes through the walls and pores of the capillaries and moves into the tissue spaces where

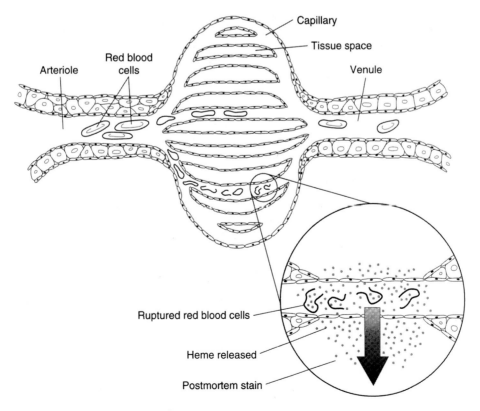

Figure 5–6. Postmortem stain.

it stains the tissues a reddish color. This reddish stain is permanently fixed, because it is now extravascular.

Tardieu spots are extravascular blood discolorations which cannot be removed by arterial injection and blood drainage. They appear in the **same dependent areas** as livor mortis and postmortem stain and can be found with either condition. These are small petechia hemorrhages and sometimes larger purpura patches of discoloration which have resulted from the rupture of small vessels and/or capillaries. They generally are seen 18 to 24 hours following the death. These discolorations are very common in asphyxial or slow deaths (DiMaio and DiMaio, 2001, p. 24).

Shift in Body pH. In chemistry, degrees of acidity or alkalinity of a substance are expressed in pH values. The neutral point, where a solution would be neither acid nor alkaline, is pH 7. Increasing acidity is expressed as a number less than 7 and increasing alkalinity as a number greater than 7. Maximum acidity is pH 0 and maximum alkalinity is pH 14. Because each unit on the scale represents a logarithm, there is a 10-fold difference between each unit (*Taber's Cyclopedic Medical Dictionary*, 2001, p. 1636).

Normal pH for a body is approximately 7.4. After death there is a drop in pH of the blood and tissue fluid into the acid range (approximately 3 hours after death). The body remains acidic during rigor mortis and then gradually, as the decomposition process advances, the body becomes increasingly alkaline.

During life, the carbohydrates (glycogen) stored in the liver and muscles are broken down to pyruvic and lactic acid by the oxygen present. Normally, this pyruvic acid is oxidized to carbon dioxide, water, and energy. The energy, in turn, is used to build up the adenosine triphosphate (ATP) of the body by converting adenosine diphosphate and adenosine monophosphate to ATP. The oxygen present in life prevents the buildup of lactic acid by oxidizing it to carbon dioxide and water. After death occurs, the oxygen is gradually used up, and the lactic acid is no longer inhibited and begins to accumulate in the muscle tissues. This buildup of acid occurs during the first hours after death (approximately the first 3 hours). This cycle is closely and directly related to the cycle of rigor mortis. The pH will drop to an acid level of approximately 6.0 and has been recorded as low as 5.5.

As a result of the acid buildup in the tissues, conditions become right for the breakdown of the soft proteins of the body. Later, as the protein breaks down, there is a gradual buildup in the tissues of nitrogen products such as ammonia and amines. The ammonia, which is basic, neutralizes the acids present in the tissues from carbohydrate breakdown. As the body contains much more protein than carbohydrates, the ammonia products gradually begin to build to a point where the pH of the tissues becomes basic (or alkaline). During decomposition the tissues are found to have an alkaline pH.

Rigor Mortis. Rigor mortis is the postmortem stiffening of muscles by natural processes. This condition affects only the muscles, and usually all of the muscles of the body are affected. Once the condition passes, it does not recur. Usually, the muscles are relaxed as death occurs. This is called **primary flaccidity**. If the body is embalmed while the muscles are flaccid, the proteins will react well with the preservative and tissue fixation will occur. If the body is embalmed while rigor is fully developed, the stiffness of the muscles will impede distribution. The proteins of the muscles are tightly bound together so they are less reactive. Within 36 to 72 hours, rigor mortis passes naturally from an unembalmed body. This is called **secondary flaccidity**. In this phase, there will be a greater demand for preservative because muscle protein has been broken down to some extent. Rigor results from the body's inability to resynthesize ATP that causes the muscle proteins to lock together and form an insoluble protein. Rigor marks the end of muscle cell life and is generally observed in the average body 2 to 4 hours after death (Fig. 5–7). The minimum temperature at which it occurs is 32°F. Its ideal temperature for occurrence is 98°F to 100°F. It is halted if the body temperature would be elevated above 120°F and if the body was exposed to temperatures below 32°F (American Board of Funeral Service Education, 2008).

"Rigor when it develops involves all the muscles at the same time and at the same rate. However, it becomes most evident in the smaller muscles" (DiMaio and DiMaio, 2001, p. 27). So it is first demonstrated in small muscles such as the jaw and gradually it becomes evident in large muscle groups. Thus it appears to begin in the involuntary muscles of the eye, then moves to the jaw and face, neck, upper extremities, trunk, and lower

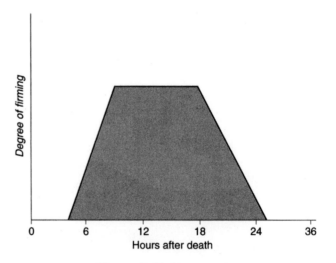

Figure 5–7. Rigor mortis.

extremities. This directional occurrence of rigor mortis from the face to the feet is known as Nysten's law. This law is named after Pierre Nysten (1774–1817) who was a French pediatrician (*Taber's Cyclopedic Medical Dictionary*, p. 1487).

Rigor mortis can be forcibly broken by flexing, bending, rotating, and massaging the joints and muscles. Once broken, rigor does not redevelop. A condition which may be mistaken for rigor is called cold stiffening; it is due to solidification of body fats and tissues when the body is exposed to cold temperatures.

Cadaveric spasm, which is a sudden involuntary movement or convulsion brought about by involuntary muscular contractions, may also be associated with rigor mortis (*Taber's Cyclopedic Medical Dictionary*, p. 1895). If rigor mortis occurs irregularly in the different muscles, it can cause movements in the limbs, which are known as cadaveric spasms (*Stedman's Medical Dictionary*, p. 1640).

Decomposition. The three major biochemicals in the body are proteins, carbohydrates, and lipids. Of the three, proteins are most important from the standpoint of structure and function. Proteins are the principle component in connective tissue, tendons, cartilage, ligaments, skin, hair, and nails. They are responsible for body movements by the action of contractile proteins found in the muscles. They play a number of other roles in body function and can be described as essential elements to the living body (Fig. 5–8).

Proteins are also an essential element from the standpoint of embalming because successful embalming is achieved by establishing cross-linkages between proteins of the body and proteins of microorganisms. Proteins are large molecules that contain elements of carbon, hydrogen, oxygen, and nitrogen. The chemical bond that links two proteins together is called a **peptide bond** or **peptide linkage**. It is possible for many proteins to link together. During decomposition, the protein chains break down. If the breakdown is caused by catalytic enzymes, the enzymes are called **proteases**.

AUTOLYSIS. In human remains the enzymes of decomposition have two different sources: saprophytic bacteria and lysosomes. These bacteria are normal residents of the human digestive tract. After death, they translocate and increase in number by using dead organic matter for their nutrition. Aerobic bacteria may also enter the body through the respiratory tract. They deplete the tissues of oxygen, producing chemical conditions favorable for anaerobic organisms, most of which originate in the intestinal tract.

In addition to bacterially caused decompositions, living cells have their own self-destruct mechanisms. During life, organelles called lysosomes contain the digestive enzymes of a cell. As the pH changes from alkaline to acidic, the membranes surrounding the lysosomes rupture. As the cells' own digestive enzymes are released, they digest the surrounding cellular material. This process is called **autolysis,** which means cell self-decomposition. The products of autolysis are amino acids, sugars, fatty acids, and glycerol. These substances are sources of food and energy for microorganisms. Therefore, autolysis also favors microbial destructive action on human remains.

Hydrolysis has been called the single most important factor in the initiation of decomposition. It is a chemical reaction in which the chemical bonds of a substance are split by the addition or taking up of water (*Taber's Cyclopedic Medical Dictionary*, p. 1014). The result of this reaction is the formation of simpler compounds which have water's hydrogen ion (H^1) and hydroxyl ion (^2OH) on either side of the chemical bond (*Stedman's Medical Dictionary*, p. 817). When hydrolysis occurs, water is broken apart, another compound is broken apart, and new products are formed. The process requires (1) water, (2) catalysts, and (3) compounds with which to react. Hydrolysis is the first chemical reaction in the putrefactive process. During hydrolysis large protein molecules are broken down into smaller fragments called **proteoses**, **peptones**, and **polypeptides**. These intermediates are a good food source for bacteria, which increase dramatically during putrefaction. As degradation continues, the final products are amino acids.

These amino acids undergo further chemical changes. Amines, carbon dioxide, and water are some of the products. **Amines** are organic compounds that are considered to be derivatives of ammonia. Amines such as skatole, indole, cadaverine, and putrescine are alkaline substances that have a foul odor. They are commonly called **ptomaines**.

Protein decomposition is known as **putrefaction**. Some authorities restrict the term putrefaction to the

Figure 5–8. Decomposition.

decomposition of proteins by **anaerobic bacteria** (those able to live without oxygen) and use the term **decay** for the decomposition of proteins by **aerobic bacteria** (those that need oxygen to live).

Water is abundant in the human body and is therefore present and available for hydrolysis during life and after death. Hydrolysis requires the presence of a **catalyst**, which is a substance that influences the rate of a chemical reaction, without itself becoming part of the products of the reaction. Enzymes found within cells act as catalysts. After death, tissues become slightly acid. This shift in pH causes the lysosomes within the cells to rupture. Lysosomes are cell inclusions that contain digestive enzymes. In the presence of water, the released enzymes begin to digest the carbohydrates, fats, and proteins of the cell. The end products of the hydrolysis of the proteins are amino acids. As proteins hydrolyze, the resulting products make more and more sites available for union with the preservative. It can be stated then that hydrolytic processes greatly increase the preservative demand of the body tissues. The presence of amino acids increases formaldehyde demand because there are more sites available for a union with formaldehyde. Carbohydrates are reduced to monosaccharides (simple sugars) and fats are reduced to fatty acids and glycerine.

The rate at which hydrolysis occurs is speeded by heat and slowed by a cold environment. A mild acid pH can also stimulate hydrolysis. As the process continues, more and more nitrogen end products are produced. This causes the pH to shift to an alkaline condition. The alkaline (or basic) condition now provides an excellent medium for bacterial growth. With this growth of bacteria the process of putrefaction greatly increases.

CATALYSTS. In the previous discussion of the types of decomposition reactions, it was shown that catalysts were needed for chemical reactions to take place. A **catalyst** is a substance that speeds up the rate of a chemical reaction without itself being permanently altered in the reaction. Inasmuch as decomposition is a chemical change, the presence of catalysts is needed in addition to the reactants. In every chemical reaction there is a **transition state,** where chemical bonds of reactants are broken and new chemical bonds are formed. At this point in a reaction, there is a higher level of energy needed. That boost of energy is provided by the catalyst. Enzymes serve as catalysts. Enzymes are also proteins and are therefore influenced by temperature and pH.

It is known that there are temperature fluctuations related to the agonal period and to the period between cellular death and embalming. It is also known that after death, the pH of the body changes from its normal 7.4 to a more acidic pH. As the body becomes somewhat acidic, it also becomes a favorable environment for microorganisms to multiply and contribute to decomposition. As the process continues, the pH of the body shifts back to alkaline, which is an excellent environment for enzymes to accelerate decomposition.

DECOMPOSITION OF CARBOHYDRATES. The breakdown of carbohydrates does not have any significant effect on embalming. Carbohydrates are stored in the body as glycogen (a polymer of glucose). The process by which glucose breaks down is called **fermentation.** We say, therefore, that fermentation is the bacterial decomposition of carbohydrates under aerobic conditions. The products of this breakdown of carbohydrates are organic acids, but they are not produced in sufficient quantity or strength to alter the overall alkaline environment that exists in a decomposing body and do not produce any foul odors. The final products of the breakdown are carbon dioxide and water.

DECOMPOSITION OF LIPIDS. Body fats are broken down by hydrolysis that occurs in the presence of enzymes called lipase. The products of this breakdown are glycerol and fatty acids. These by-products do not significantly affect the embalming operations because they do not change the alkaline environment, nor do they give off any bad odors.

Of note to embalmers is the formation of a compound called **adipocere**, commonly known as "grave wax." Adipocere is thought to be composed of fatty acids and appears in bodies that have been dead for an extended period of time (3 months or longer).

DECOMPOSITION ORDER. Decomposition proceeds at different rates in various body areas.

Cells, tissues, and organs that contain high levels of moisture and autolytic and bacterial enzymes break down before similar structures that contain less water and autolytic and bacterial enzymes. The optimum temperature for decomposition is 98°F. The process is greatly slowed or stopped at temperatures below 32°F or above 120°F (American Board of Funeral Service Education, 2008).

Order of decomposition of the body compounds:

1. Carbohydrates
2. Soft proteins
3. Fats
4. Hard proteins
5. Bones

The vascular system is one of the last organ systems to decompose. Even in advanced decomposition it would be possible to inject some preservative chemicals in an attempt to slow decomposition and control odor.

Figure 5–9. Partial decomposition. Both hypodermic and arterial embalming treatments were used. Note the discolorations.

SIGNS OF DECOMPOSITION. There are five classic signs of decomposition: *color, odor, skin slip, gases,* and *purge.* Decomposition in the dead human body is not a uniform process. It may be present in one location and absent in another. Decomposition can also be present without all five "signs" being present at the same time. For example, a body may evidence decomposition by skin slip and color changes but exhibit no abdominal gases or purge.

COLOR CHANGE. The first external color change that occurs in the unembalmed body is a greenish discoloration over the right lower quadrant of the abdomen. This discoloration is caused by the combination of hydrogen sulfide (a product of putrefaction) with hemoglobin from the blood (Fig. 5–9). In many bodies this discoloration follows the surface outline of the large intestine, which is located just beneath the abdominal wall. The abdomen as a whole gradually discolors and the chest, neck, and upper thighs are affected in time.

The blood trapped in the superficial vessels gradually breaks down, staining the surrounding tissues. The outline of the veins on the surface of the skin is easily detected. This purplish brown discoloration of the superficial veins is most pronounced in the veins of the shoulder, upper chest, lower abdomen, and groin. An early discoloration that occurs as a result of the hemolysis or breakdown of red blood cells is postmortem stain.

ODOR. As the proteins of the body decompose, putrefactive odors become apparent. This odor is caused by foul-smelling amines, mercaptans, and hydrogen sulfide.

DESQUAMATION (SKIN SLIP). The outer layers of the skin weaken because the deeper skin layers are undergoing autolysis. Hydrolysis of collagen and elastin causes the superficial skin to be pulled away easily from the deeper skin layers. As decomposition progresses, accumulations of gases and liquids can separate layers of skin, forming

---

Taphonomy is the scientific study of decomposition. It is a complex subject comprised of many aspects and variable factors. In 1981, Dr. William Bass established the first Forensic Anthropology Center at the University of Tennessee, Knoxville. This facility has become known as the "body farm." Today there are five such research facilities in the United States. One of the purposes was to study decomposition rates of human remains for crime scene investigation.

The environment and surroundings play a major role influencing the rate of decomposition. Bodies that lay in full exposure to sunlight will decompose faster than those submerged in cool water or buried beneath the soil. Scientists studying rates of decomposition have established categories to describe the conditions of a deceased body when found.. Embalmers should have an understanding of decomposition rates and decomposition changes. The following chart gives a brief summary of decomposition rates and changes.

Category Title and Time	Stage	Changes
Category 1. Fresh: 1–6 days	1	putrid odor, lividity, rigor mild
	2	abdominal green, hemolysis intense rigor → rigor passed desquamation, dehydration of features and fingers
	3	hemolysis, tissues soften, desquamation
Category 2. Bloat: 7 to 23 days	4	body swelling begins, head and Face discolored, marbling of Superficial veins bullae or blebbing on the skin surface
	5	moderate swelling; head and trunk discolored
	6	maximum body swelling
Category 3. Destruction/Active Decay 24 to 50	7	gasses released, soft tissues putrefied total breakdown of the blood
	8	partially skeletonized, adipocere, mummification
Category 4. Dry/Skeleton 51–64	9	skeleton with ligaments
	10	skeleton with no soft tissues

blisters. The blisters, which can become quite large, contain a putrid-smelling, gassy, watery, blood-stained fluid. If the blisters are touched or disturbed, the skin easily slips away; thus the term "skin slip." When the skin is pulled away a shiny, pink, moist surface is exposed. Gradually, this moist area dehydrates, turns brown, and becomes slightly firm to the touch.

GASES. As decomposition progresses, gases begin to form in the viscera. This formation of gas generally starts in the stomach and intestines. Later, gases form in the body tissues. The gas causes the abdominal cavity to swell, and later the body tissues become distended. Gases in the tissues can actually be moved by the application of pressure. This movement is called crepitation. As the gas moves through the tissues it can be felt and may actually make a crackling sound. Weakened areas such as the eyelids, scrotum, and breasts easily distend with gases. In time, eyelids, cheeks, and lips distend and the tongue protrudes.

PURGE. Purge is defined as the evacuation of gases, liquids, and semisolids from a natural body orifice. In decomposition, purge is generally caused by the buildup of pressure from gas formed in the abdomen. The pressure forces gases, liquids, and semisolids along the path of least resistance, which is usually toward a natural body orifice. The purge from the stomach is generally a foul-smelling liquid that resembles the appearance of coffee grounds. Purge from the lungs is generally described as frothy, and if blood appears in this purge it may retain its red color. Stomach and lung purge will usually exit from the mouth and nose.

▶ TESTS OF DEATH

Although generally not the professional or legal responsibility of the embalmer, there are circumstances where an embalmer might benefit from knowledge of how medical personnel make a determination that death has occurred. Inasmuch as the legal requirements of death certification call for medical verification from a physician, it follows that tests for death would be conducted by a physician. However, it is also true that a physician may not necessarily view the body before certifying the medical cause of death, and therefore, the tests for death can also be performed by a properly trained individual.

Expert Tests
Expert tests require certain training and skills of the person who administers the test. Any procedure used to prove a sign of death that is conducted by a person or persons who are legally certified and authorized to do so would be categorized as an expert test. Expert tests will, as a rule, be conducted or reviewed by a physician. Examples include:

- **Stethoscope**—an instrument used to mediate sounds produced in the body. This instrument would be used to listen for sounds of respiration or cardiac activity (*Taber's Cyclopedic Medical Dictionary*, 2001, p. 2055).
- **Ophthalmoscope**—an instrument used to examine the interior of the eye, especially the retina. This instrument would be used to examine the blood vessels in the retina for signs of circulating blood. Because it is a light source, it could also be used to detect responses in the pupils of the eyes (*Taber's Cyclopedic Medical Dictionary*, 2001, p. 1510).
- **Electroencephalogram (EEG)**—a record of the electrical activity of the brain (*Taber's Cyclopedic Medical Dictionary*, 2001, p. 675).
- **Electrocardiogram (ECG, EKG)**—a record of the electrical activity of the heart (*Taber's Cyclopedic Medical Dictionary*, 2001, pp. 672, 748).
- **Evoked response**—method of testing the function of certain sense organs, even if the subject is unconscious or uncooperative. For example, in a living patient, an **auditory evoked response** will appear on an electroencephalograph if sound reaches the brain. If there is no evoked response, the technician may conclude that sound did not reach the brain (*The Merck Manual of Diagnosis and Therapy*, 1982). Brain death would be one reason for the absence of an evoked response.

Inexpert Tests
There are situations where individuals may want to check to see if death has occurred where the equipment or expertise required for expert tests is not available. When such a test is used, it is called an **inexpert test**. Inexpert tests include:

- **Ligature test**—a finger is ligated with string or a rubber band. If the ligation causes swelling or discoloration, it indicates that circulation of blood is still occurring.
- **Ammonia injection test**—a small amount of ammonia is injected subcutaneously. If there is a reddish reaction in the skin, it indicates that life is present.
- **Pulse**—digital pressure to check for pulse beat.
- **Listening for respiration or heart beat**—placing your ear over the chest of the individual.

► CONCEPTS FOR STUDY AND DISCUSSION

1. Make a list of body and environmental conditions which would speed the decomposition of a dead human body. Make a list of body and environmental conditions which would slow the decomposition of a dead human body.
2. Discuss agonal changes and how they change the physical and chemical makeup of the body.
3. What factors can speed or slow the establishment of livor mortis?
4. Discuss the signs of decomposition.
5. Discuss the process of hypostasis and explain how the progression of events leads to livor mortis and postmortem stain.
6. Discuss the pH changes that occur in the dead human body after death.
7. Discuss postmortem physical and chemical changes and how they change the makeup and condition of the body.

► BIBLIOGRAPHY

American Board of Funeral Service Education, *Course Content Syllabus: Embalmings*, Portland, ME: American Board of Funeral Service Education, 2008: 12–14.

American Board of Funeral Service Education, *Embalming Syllabus*, Portland, ME: American Board of Funeral Service Education, 2001:14.

DiMaio DJ, DiMaio VJ. *Forensic Pathology*, 2nd ed. Boca Raton, FL:CRC Press, 2001.

Stedman's Medical Dictionary, 26th ed. Baltimore: Williams & Wilkins, 1995.

Taber's Cyclopedic Medical Dictionary, 19th ed. Philadelphia: Davis, 2001.

The Merck Manual of Diagnosis and Therapy. Rahway, NJ: Merck, Sharp & Dohme, 1982:1941.

Walter JB. *Pathology of Human Disease*. Philadelphia: Lea & Febiger, 1989:327.

CHAPTER 6

EMBALMING CHEMICALS

CHAPTER OBJECTIVES

▶ Types of embalming chemicals
▶ Vascular and cavity fluids
▶ Chemical components of vascular and cavity fluids
▶ Purposes of chemical components
▶ Preservative action on body tissues

Funeral service professionals are concerned about the safety of the work environment as well as the quality of the earth's land, air, and water resources. Manufacturers of embalming chemicals are raising the safety standards by formulating newer and safer sanitizing, preservative, supplemental, and accessory embalming products. These formulations are safer to use, less toxic, and hazardous to the embalmer and to the environment. Ongoing studies remain inconclusive as to the carcinogenic properties of a number of embalming chemicals, formaldehyde being the most important.

The embalmer's exposure to various chemicals has been greatly reduced by the employment of safer handling standards. At this point in time (2011) formaldehyde, depending on the investigative agency is considered a carcinogen, or a probable carcinogen, and is gradually being replaced by non-formaldehyde preservatives in various embalming formulations. While these newer formulations effectively sanitize they provide only a very temporary preservation of the deceased human body. This chapter introduces some of these newer non-formaldehyde preservatives.

A work environment with sufficient ventilation, properly located exhaust and incoming air ducts—a minimum of 15 air changes per hour—greatly reduces exposure to the hazardous effects of embalming chemicals.

▶ PRECAUTIONS

Embalming chemicals are packaged in concentrated form. The embalmer dilutes the preservative and supplemental fluids. Cavity fluids, accessory chemicals, bleaching agents, solvents, osmotic gels, and powders are used in their concentrated form. Most of these chemicals are toxic and hazardous if they contact living tissue either by inhalation or skin contact. At the very least, these chemicals are irritating to living tissue. Contact dermatitis is a commonly reported skin malady. Containers should always be safely stored, tightly sealed, and handled only when proper protective equipment (PPE) is worn and ventilation systems are operational. Any chemical spills or accidents should be immediately attended by following Occupational Safety and Health Association (OSHA) guidelines and the written spill plan of the funeral facility.

▶ FORMULATIONS AND CHEMICAL COMPONENTS

Six general chemical groups provide the basic components of the various embalming formulations (Fig. 6–1):

1. Preservatives
2. Disinfectants (germicides)
3. Modifying agents
   a. Buffers
   b. Anticoagulants (water conditioning agents)
   c. Surfactants (wetting agents, surface tension reducers, penetrating agents or surface active agents)
   d. Humectants
4. Dyes (coloring agents)
   a. Cosmetic (active)
   b. Non-cosmetic (inactive)

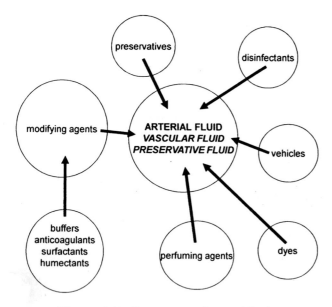

Figure 6–1. Components of arterial fluid.

5. Perfuming agents (masking agents)
6. Vehicles

These chemicals are combined in various concentrations to produce vascular (preservative) embalming fluids, cavity fluids, supplemental embalming fluids, and some accessory chemicals used in the preparation of the dead human body. Five of the previously listed groups of chemicals are added to the concentrated embalming fluid in order to control the adverse effects of the main preservative chemical (usually formaldehyde), to maintain stability of the fluid, and to lengthen its shelf life. The functions of these various chemicals can be understood by looking at the following terms that are associated with embalming chemicals and fluids:

- **Arterial (embalming, vascular, or preservative) fluid**—the concentrated, preservative embalming chemical that will be diluted with water to form the arterial solution for injection into the arterial system during vascular embalming
- **Arterial solution (embalming solution, primary dilution)**—the in-use solution composed of the concentrated embalming fluid diluted with water and other additive (supplemental) chemicals for injection into the body
- **Cavity fluid**—concentrated embalming chemicals, which are injected into the cavities of the body following aspiration in cavity embalming. This chemical can also be used for surface and hypodermic embalming
- **Supplemental fluid**—fluid injected for purposes other than preservation and disinfection. Some are injected before the preservative solution; others are injected with the preservative solution

(preinjection and coinjection fluids; water corrective fluid)
- **Accessory chemicals**—a group of chemicals used in addition to vascular and cavity embalming fluids; most are applied to the body surface (gels and powders)
- **Special purpose fluids**—fluids designed for use with special body conditions such as jaundice or bodies requiring a high preservative demand as seen in bodies with renal failure, extensive burns, or decomposition.

▶ HISTORICAL: ESTABLISHMENT OF MINIMUM STANDARDS

To understand the significance of the preservative chemical in an embalming fluid, it is helpful to look briefly at the establishment of minimum standards for disinfection of remains from a historical viewpoint.

After the turn of the 20th century (approximately 1906), when formaldehyde became a widely used component of embalming fluids, various state health departments required that a minimum amount of formaldehyde be used to embalm bodies for them to be considered disinfected. This established a standard amount of formaldehyde to be incorporated into the formulations. At that time a minimum amount of embalming solution was to be used in the preparation of bodies dead from noninfectious diseases as well as those dead from infectious and contagious diseases. The minimum standard established was not less than the following: 1 gallon of 14% of a 40% solution of formaldehyde (5.6%) for every 100 pounds of body weight for "normal cases" and 1 gallon of this same strength for every 75 pounds of body weight for infectious and contagious disease cases.

In these early years, the manufacturers of embalming fluid sold it with the water already added. (The fluid was sold by the half gallon ready for injection.) Later, because of the costs involved in bottling, packing, and shipping, it was decided to omit as much of the water as possible and sell the concentrated solution in pint bottles. To maintain the required minimum standards established by state laws, each pint bottle had to contain at least 8.96 oz of 40% formaldehyde and the same proportion of other chemicals. It must be kept in mind that formaldehyde acts harshly on body tissues, does not distribute or diffuse well, dehydrates, and darkens and grays body tissues. The use of strong embalming solutions (approximately 5.75%) was enforced in the years immediately following the influenza pandemics of 1918 and 1919. To overcome the adverse effects of formaldehyde on the body, a variety of supplemental fluids, such as blood solvents (later known as preinjection solutions), were developed; coinjection and jaundice fluids were developed and in use as early as 1910. It would not be until the development of penetrating agents and machine injection in the mid- to late 1930s that milder arterial solutions would be employed; the standard until the early 1970s would be 1 to 1.5% solution strength. This was quite sufficient to produce firming. The suggested standard using these milder solutions since the mid-1930s has been to use 1 gallon of arterial solution for every 50 pounds of body weight. It was not until the early 1970s that research demonstrated that a minimum of at least a 2% formaldehyde-based arterial solution was necessary to disinfect body tissues effectively. In the near future it is expected that formaldehyde and phenol-based preservative fluids will be replaced with fluids containing preservatives and disinfecting elements that do not have the adverse effects of the preservatives currently in use. The "50 pound rule" is of little value today as a standard, for so often extreme conditions are seen, with edema, delayed preparation, decomposition, systemic infections, low protein levels, liver and kidney failure, that using a 1% solution at a volume of 1 gallon for every 50 pounds of body weight may be inadequate. The conditions of the body, the degree of firmness desired by the embalmer, and the length of time between death and disposition must be the determining factors in selecting an arterial fluid and the strength and volume at which it must be injected.

▶ GENERAL CHEMICAL PRINCIPLES OF EMBALMING FLUIDS

Commercial embalming fluids are composed of various chemicals and the same chemicals, when used in different concentrations, may produce different effects. This means each individual chemical component has a specific function to perform. Each reacts according to its own concentration, distribution, diffusion, and individual activity.

Among the main chemicals common to almost all embalming preservative solutions are formaldehyde and methyl alcohol. The remaining substances used in embalming solutions vary immensely.

Just as important as the need to replace equipment at frequent intervals and to maintain the proper facilities with which to manufacture and compound chemical solutions is the need to improve and make changes in the general nature of formulations. These changes are occasioned by developments in the technical fields. Suppliers make use of such developments and adapt them into existing products or design new products containing them. This factor makes it unlikely that two different "brands" of fluid will have a similar composition. The continuing investigations and studies conducted by the technical staffs of fluid manufacturers who maintain research laboratories also often result in attention being devoted to some particular compound that produces an innovative effect when blended with special chemicals.

Today, the many commercially available chemical preservative solutions differ with respect to the following factors: pH of the solution; type of buffer materials used to maintain pH; grade of formalin used; type of alcohol; surfactants (anionic, nonionic, or cationic); anticoagulants; modifiers; and physical features such as specific gravity and surface tension.

In brief, the "20-index" fluid made by one manufacturer today can be expected to be chemically different in composition and even to produce different embalming results from that produced by another firm.

There is no general agreement on what constitutes a "standard" embalming fluid. Embalmers show varying preferences in the type of results they desire. Some require a fast-acting fluid with little or no internal cosmetic effect, whereas others desire such a fluid to produce an internal cosmetic effect. In other instances, a mild to moderately firming fluid that produces a noticeable coloring is preferred. An important factor for consideration is the effect of pathologic conditions on the fluid injected and vice versa. Finally, the chemical preservation solution may produce different results when applied to different cases.

▶ GREEN OR NATURAL BURIAL FLUIDS

Formaldehyde replacements are slowly coming onto the market. This has been driven by the "Green" or "Natural" burial movement along with studies which have labeled formaldehyde as carcinogenic. Fluid manufacturers would like to produce a product not needing an OSHA MSDS sheet! These fluids provide some disinfectant and preservative properties. The temporary preservation being 3 to 5 days in length, to possibly a week or longer. Some are environmentally safe, biodegradable, and of a non-toxic nature. Most do not produce tissue firmness. Composition includes oil ingredients derived from gums and resins of plants including a variety of spices. They are antiseptic in nature and they can precipitate and coagulate proteins. Certain alcohols have been found to be good vehicles for these temporary preservatives; in addition, these alcohols are capable of adding and retaining moisture as well as precipitating and coagulating protein. Embalming chemical manufacturers are revisiting ingredients used in formulations for preservation prior to the discovery of formaldehyde. A popular preservative in the 18th and 19th century was "rectified spirits" which was simply re-distilled wine or brandy! Various spices have been used all throughout the history of embalming, dating as far back as the Egyptians. Reference for their use is found in the Bible.

► CHEMICAL COMPONENTS OF EMBALMING FLUIDS

Preservatives

Generally speaking, the chemical compounds classified under "preservative or fixative chemicals" are the agents in the chemical preservative solution which react with proteins. Such compounds change a protein from a state in which it is easily decomposed to a state in which it will endure and not undergo putrefaction for a delayed period of time. Reaction of a preservative and a protein changes the nature of the protein molecule. Aldehydes, for example, react with various forms of nitrogen found in proteins. The products of such reactions are an altered protein structure and water.

Formalin (37% formaldehyde), as the commercial source of formaldehyde, is still the most commonly used chemical for this purpose. Other examples are paraformaldehyde, formaldehyde polymerization products or formaldehyde "donors," light aldehydes, glyoxal, glutaraldehyde, phenol, phenolic derivatives, and some alcohols.

Formaldehyde and Formaldehyde-Type Preservatives.
Formaldehyde was discovered in 1859 by the Russian scientist Alexander Butlerov (1828–1886). Nine years later, German scientist Wilhelm VonHofmann conclusively identified formaldehyde and found a reliable way to make it through the oxidation of menthol with air using a metal catalyst. This basic process is still today in the manufacture of formaldehyde. Annually in the United States formaldehyde production exceeds five million metric tons. The Formaldehyde Council Incorporated (FCI), located in Arlington, Virginia, is the science and advocacy center for the formaldehyde industry in the United States.*

Formaldehyde is everywhere, it is produced in the atmosphere by lightning, it is essential to the working of the human body, it is used in making vaccines and in home construction materials (paneling, particle, and fiberboard). Cooking of certain vegetables such as cabbage and Brussels sprouts produces formaldehyde. Formaldehyde is used to de-caffeinate coffee, add permanent-press qualities to clothing and draperies, and to make buttons.

Formaldehyde, however, is also a known toxin, some individuals experience sensitivity to even low levels of formaldehyde. Acute exposure may include watery eyes, a burning sensation of the eyes, irritation of the nose and throat, coughing, wheezing, nausea, and skin irritation. In 1987, the OSHA established the Formaldehyde Rule. (OSHA 29CFR1910.1048) Since the 1980s

various organizations including the National Cancer Institute (NCI) have investigated the long-term exposure effects of formaldehyde upon workers—especially occupations such as anatomists, pathologists, embalmers, and laboratory workers. NCI has suspected formaldehyde to be a causative agent of leukemia and to yield a definite increase in the risk of various types of cancers. In 1987 the Environmental Protection Agency (EPA) classified formaldehyde as a probable carcinogen but nonetheless a carcinogen for nasal sinus cancer, nasopharyngeal cancer, and a possible causative agent of leukemia. The International Agency for Research on Cancer (IARC) since June of 2004 has classified formaldehyde as a carcinogen.

A study among embalmers exposed to formaldehyde by the NCI released in October 2009 showed, "the number of years of embalming practice and related formaldehyde exposures in the funeral industry was associated with statistically significantly increased mortality from myeloid leukemia and associations with brain cancer were unclear."* The agency concluded there was a considerable amount of missing data and further studies were warranted. Formaldehyde studies continue to be inconclusive because so many factors are variable: short- and long-term length of exposure, efficiency of ventilating systems in preparation rooms, personal protective equipment worn, type and strengths of chemicals used, and accuracy of reporting. What appears to be lacking is the biological mechanism of formaldehyde as a leukemogen.

Formaldehyde is a colorless gas at ambient temperature. It has a strong, irritating odor and is very soluble in water. The commercial source of formaldehyde is an aqueous solution of the gas dissolved in water called formalin.

FORMALIN. Formaldehyde is generally available as formalin, an aqueous solution containing 37% formaldehyde gas by mass in water, or in water and methyl alcohol. The solution has a density slightly greater than water and corresponds to a solution that is 40% formaldehyde by volume. The National Formulary (NF) [formerly United States Pharmacopoeia (USP)] grade of formalin contains an average of 7% methyl alcohol, 37.0% minimum—37.3% maximum formaldehyde, and the remainder water. The alcohol present in the solution acts as an antipolymerant by stabilizing the formaldehyde so that it will not precipitate.

The 37% by mass (40% by volume) solution is the regular product of commerce. There are available, however, certain solutions that contain 40, 55, and even

---

*www.formadehyde.org

*A study is summarized in The Director, May 2010, Page 57, Vol 82, No.5, Brookfield, WI

70% by mass formaldehyde in alcohol. The last two concentrations mentioned are subject to precipitation. The precipitate is **paraformaldehyde**, a solid form of formaldehyde. The formaldehyde that drops out of solution to the bottom of the container is not available for chemical reaction and results in a weaker concentration of formaldehyde in the top layers of the solution than at the bottom. In other words, the concentration of formaldehyde throughout the solution is not uniform.

For many years the word **index** was generally understood to be the percentage strength of concentrated embalming fluid and referred to the amount of absolute formaldehyde gas by volume present. It should be understood that the reference was to formaldehyde gas and not to formalin, which is the 40% (by volume) solution of formaldehyde. The former Embalming Chemical Manufacturers Association (ECMA) and the schools and colleges of mortuary science have generally agreed on the following definition of index: "An embalming fluid will be said to have formaldehyde index, N, when 100 mL of fluid, at normal room temperature, contain N grams of formaldehyde gas." Thus, a 20-index product contains 20 g of formaldehyde gas per 100 mL of concentrated fluid. The word **index**, therefore, identifies only the absolute formaldehyde gas present in any given product. It is not a measure of the total aldehyde concentration present. **Index refers only to the amount of formaldehyde gas present**.

The chemistry of formaldehyde is a very specialized and complicated field of study. The disinfectant properties of formaldehyde, which depend on its concentration, have been extensively studied. It is classified as a high-level (8% formaldehyde plus 70% alcohol) or intermediate-to-high level (4% to 8% formaldehyde in water) disinfectant. Formaldehyde has a broad spectrum of action on microorganisms. It destroys putrefactive organisms when carried by a proper vehicle that permits it to penetrate these organisms. It preserves tissues by forming new chemical compounds with the tissues. The new compounds that are formed are stable and unfit as food for organisms. An interesting comparison is

> The buttons on your coat, the comb on your dresser, and many other things you may commonly use are made of formaldehyde and phenol or carbolic acid, as it is commonly known. Either formaldehyde or carbolic acid would injure you severely if taken into your mouth. You may, however, with impunity hold a button from your coat in your mouth because it differs definitely from either of its components. In other words, it is a resin.

This statement describes the action of formaldehyde on albuminous materials. New resins are formed that are neither formaldehyde nor albumin. These resins may be hard resins, soft resins, or semihard resins, depending on the control chemicals (modifying or plasticizing materials) used in combination with the formaldehyde.

Formaldehyde acts quickly on the particular area with which it is in contact. The more formaldehyde there is in a certain area, the greater the action on the tissues in that area. The closer the tissue to the formaldehyde, the greater the action on it. This action takes up more formaldehyde than may be needed for preservation, possibly leaving little or no formaldehyde for the more remote tissue areas.

To use an analogy, the preceding action of formaldehyde on tissue may be compared with the action of a sponge in water. The sponge absorbs or takes up water depending on how much water there is to begin with and also depending on how long the sponge is permitted to remain in contact with the water.

If an embalming solution is hurried through the circulatory system as the result of too much pressure and excessive drainage, some tissue areas will receive little or no formaldehyde. This, in turn, causes "soft spots" to develop. Such areas result when tissue does not receive a sufficient amount of formaldehyde to preserve them. There is also the possibility that a localized tissue area, because of some pathologic condition, may be undergoing decomposition. Thus, the free amines produced by the decomposition may absorb more than their usual share of formaldehyde so that little formaldehyde is left for remote parts. This situation is further exacerbated when an average of only 2 gallons of solution is injected. In such a case it is possible that an insufficient amount of formaldehyde is used to achieve thorough preservation of the body tissues.

There are **disadvantages** to the use of formaldehyde as a preservative in embalming fluids: it rapidly coagulates the blood, converts the tissues to a gray hue when it mixes with blood not removed from the body, fixes discolorations, dehydrates tissues, constricts capillaries, and deteriorates with age, can be oxidized to formic acid, and can be decomposed to an alcohol and organic salt in a strongly alkaline pH. It has an unpleasant odor and is very irritating to the embalmer. In addition many studies have been done on the carcinogenic nature of formaldehyde. Some support it being a carcinogen, while others lead to its classification as a suspected carcinogen.

However, the **advantages** of formaldehyde as a preservative in embalming fluids outweigh the disadvantages. The advantages include the following. Formaldehyde is 100% organic, it is broken down by sunlight and in the soil it is broken down by bacteria and nitrogen. Formaldehyde is inexpensive, bactericidal, and inhibits the growth of yeasts and molds. It rapidly destroys autolytic enzymes and rapidly acts on the body proteins converting them to insoluble resins thereby inhibiting tissue decomposition. Only a small percentage of formaldehyde is needed to act on a large amount of protein; it produces rapid fixation, which aids in positioning the dead human body and also indicates that preservation is taking place. It is estimated that as little as 8 oz of formaldehyde is necessary to temporarily preserve the average human-deceased body. Finally, formaldehyde deodorizes the body amines formed during putrefaction.

PARAFORMALDEHYDE. Paraformaldehyde is a polymer of formaldehyde. It is a white, powdery solid containing from 85% to 99% formaldehyde. The NF grade of paraformaldehyde contains 95% formaldehyde. Paraformaldehyde is generally prepared from water solutions of formaldehyde by processes involving evaporation and distillation until concentration to a point at which solidification or precipitation takes place. This form of formaldehyde is used where powdered preparations are involved, such as in hardening compounds or other powdered preparations used for "dusting" the body walls and viscera.

TRIOXANE. Another polymer of formaldehyde is trioxane (trioxymethylene), a colorless crystalline material with an odor resembling that of chloroform. This material is sometimes incorporated into formulations to act as an accessory preservative. It is rather costly when compared with other forms of formaldehyde and, therefore, is too expensive to warrant its extensive use for embalming purposes.

OTHER ALDEHYDES. Some lower or "light" aldehydes have been proposed for use in embalming preparations and some are occasionally found in modern embalming fluids. Examples of these are acetaldehyde, propionaldehyde, and pyruvic aldehyde (methylglyoxal). Among the higher aldehydes found in embalming fluids are furfural and benzaldehyde. The important requirement of an aldehyde is that it possesses denaturing and cross-linking properties that enable it to produce a firm tissue.

CONDENSATION PRODUCTS (FORMALDEHYDE "DONOR" COMPOUNDS, FORMALDEHYDE REACTION PRODUCTS). Aliphatic nitrohydroxy compounds are formed as the result of a condensation reaction between nitroparaffins (nitromethane, nitroethane, etc.) and certain aldehydes. Compounds of this type, in the presence of the proper catalyst (such as potassium carbonate), give off formaldehyde at a slow rate. When in solution, such formaldehyde condensation products exhibit an acid pH and need the alkaline catalyst to release the formaldehyde.

Other types of formaldehyde "donor" compounds are the methylol derivatives of hydantoin. These also liberate formaldehyde at a slow rate. Both types are used in low-odor or "fumeless" products. These complex organic substances make it possible to formulate fluids that are pleasant to use, because they do not give off noxious, irritating fumes. The formaldehyde is released after being distributed to all soft tissue areas where the usual preservative action is exerted. The disadvantage in using such materials is twofold: they have a slow reaction rate and are very expensive.

Dialdehydes. In addition to the previously discussed aldehydes, chemical compounds also exist that contain two-aldehyde functional groups in the same molecule; hence, they are called dialdehydes. As far back as 1941, several firms in this industry investigated the possibility of using the then-known dialdehyde compounds available on a commercial scale. The principal dialdehyde and probably the only one available at that time in large commercial quantities and at an economical price, that made its use in embalming formulations feasible was glyoxal, the lowest member of the dialdehydes. On November 2, 1943, a patent (US Patent 2333182) was granted relating to the use of glyoxal in embalming fluid formulations.

GLYOXAL. Glyoxal is available commercially as a 30% yellowish, aqueous solution containing small amounts of ethylene glycol, glycolic acid, formic acid, and formaldehyde. It is also available as a special 40% clear solution. Because it contains a chromophore group, glyoxal solution tends to stain tissue yellow. This feature limits the use of glyoxal mainly to cavity fluid formulations, especially because its optimal pH range of activity is about 9 to 10.

GLUTARALDEHYDE. In the early 1950s, a method was developed that made it possible to manufacture the five-carbon, straight-chain dialdehyde glutaraldehyde in commercial quantities. Glutaraldehyde was first employed as an embalming and fixative agent in early 1955 and was subsequently patented for use in embalming preparations. When used for such purposes, it is commercially supplied as a stable 2.5% aqueous solution that has a mild odor and a light color. Glutaraldehyde reacts through crosslinking to insolubilize both protein and polyhydroxy compounds. The pH of the commercial solution is 3.0 to 4.0 and the specific gravity is 1.058 to 1.068. While still used in the United States, glutaraldehyde is not permitted for use in embalming formulations in Europe and Great Britain.

An interesting feature of glutaraldehyde is that, unlike other aldehydes, it is capable of reacting with protein structures over a wide pH range. This is an important advantage for an aldehyde in embalming, because after death, tissue pH varies in different parts of the body and as time elapses between death and embalming.

In their pure forms both glyoxal and glutaraldehyde are liquids at ambient temperature, whereas formaldehyde is a gas.

In combining with proteins and tissue, glutaraldehyde changes the nature of the proteins, makes them unsuitable as food for bacteria, and makes them resistant to decomposition changes. At the same time less moisture is removed from the tissues as the result of the chemical reaction between glutaraldehyde and proteins than when formaldehyde is used. In addition, glutaraldehyde used as a disinfecting agent is effective against most microorganisms including viruses and spores making it many times more effective as a disinfectant than formaldehyde.

Phenol. Phenol (C_6H_5OH), also known as carbolic acid, is classified as a preservative as well as, a germicide. Phenol was one of the most commonly found components of both arterial and cavity fluids manufactured in the "early" days of the fluid industry. Today, it is used chiefly in cavity fluid formulations. Phenol is a coal-tar derivative that is a colorless crystalline solid. Upon exposure to strong light or metallic contamination, it darkens and assumes an amber or reddish brown appearance when in solution. The potency of phenol is not impaired to any great extent when such change occurs.

Phenol penetrates the skin very readily and is very rapidly absorbed by protein structures. Phenol and phenolic derivatives are good germicides. In addition, they assist formaldehyde in forming insoluble resins with albumins. Generally, their use in embalming fluids is confined to cavity fluids because they tend to produce a "putty gray" tissue. Phenol is also used in the formulations used to embalm cadavers for medical schools. In addition to its preservative and germicidal qualities, it is a mold inhibitor. Formulations containing phenol are often used as bleaching agents to lighten discolorations on the skin surface. The solution either is applied as an external pack or is injected subcutaneously with a hypodermic syringe. Phenol is corrosive to living tissue and special care needs to be taken to protect the eyes and the skin of the embalmer.

USES FOR CONCENTRATED PHENOL SOLUTIONS IN EMBALMING

▶ Preservative
▶ Germicide and fungicide
▶ Bleaching agent
▶ Cautery agent
▶ Reducing agent
▶ Drying agent

It is unfortunate that the most powerful germicides among the phenols are not water soluble. Some of the halogenated phenols found in embalming formulations include **ortho**-phenylphenol, **para**-chloro-**meta**-cresol, dichloro-**ortho**-phenylphenol, tribromothymol, and sodium salts of these and other phenol-related chemicals.

Sometimes the expression **triple-base fluid** is used. This refers to a fluid containing phenol, methyl alcohol, and formaldehyde. A "double-base" fluid presumably is one containing formaldehyde and methyl alcohol, or formaldehyde and phenol, or methyl alcohol and phenol. Commercial fluids almost always contain phenols in combination with formaldehyde and methyl alcohol. The presence of the latter two compounds improves the bacteria-killing power of phenols. They generally do not produce readily detectable firmness of tissue such as that produced by aldehydes.

Salts. Various salts have been used in embalming products since the early days of embalming. Among the more commonly used compounds are potassium acetate, sodium nitrate, and some salts of aluminum. The salts of the heavy metals are not used, as after 1906, many states prohibited their use in embalming compositions.

How Preservatives Work

The study of biochemistry is a very complex subject and is beyond the scope of this textbook. The intent of this section on preservation is to give a brief explanation of how the main types of chemicals preserve tissue. In order for this to be accomplished the make-up of amino acids and proteins is briefly described in the following paragraph.

The embalming process is primarily directed toward the proteins of the body It is in the cross-linking of proteins both those of the body and of microorganisms that disinfection and preservation are achieved.

An amino acid is an organic compound that contains both an amino (NH_2) group and a carboxyl (COOH) group. There are 20 amino acids that are necessary for the growth and metabolism of human body. When two or more amino acids are joined together a polypeptide is formed. These compounds are the building blocks of proteins. The site where the amine group of one peptide and the carboxylic acid of another peptide join is called the peptide bond or peptide linkage. These 20 different amino acids are linked in a specific sequence in chains up to thousands of units to form proteins. Since amino acids are the building blocks of proteins, they are also found as end products of protein breakdown (decomposition). Owing to the fact that amino acids contain NH_2 they can also be preserved or cross-linked.

$$\underset{\text{Amino acid}}{\overset{O}{\underset{\text{HO}-\text{C}}{\parallel}}-\overset{R}{\underset{|}{\text{CH}}}-\overset{H}{\underset{|}{\text{N}}}-\text{H}} + \underset{\text{Formaldehyde}}{\overset{O}{\underset{\text{H}-\text{C}}{\parallel}}-\text{H}} \longrightarrow \underset{\text{Fixed amino acid}}{\overset{O}{\underset{\text{HO}-\text{C}}{\parallel}}-\overset{R}{\underset{|}{\text{CH}}}-\text{N}=\overset{H}{\underset{|}{\text{C}}}-\text{H}} + \underset{\text{Water}}{\text{H}_2\text{O}}$$

Amino acid   +   Formaldehyde ⟶ Fixed amino acid   + Water

OR

$$\underset{\text{Amino acid}}{\overset{O}{\underset{\text{HO}-\text{C}}{\parallel}}-\overset{R}{\underset{|}{\text{CH}}}-\overset{H}{\underset{|}{\text{N}}}-\text{H}} + \underset{\text{Formalin}}{2\text{OH}-\text{CH}_2-\text{OH}} \longrightarrow \underset{\text{Fixed amino acid}}{\overset{O}{\underset{\text{HO}-\text{C}}{\parallel}}-\overset{R}{\underset{|}{\text{CH}}}-\overset{\text{CH}_2-\text{OH}}{\underset{|}{\text{N}}}-\text{CH}_2-\text{OH}} + 2\text{H}_2\text{O}$$

Amino acid   +   Formalin   ⟶   Fixed amino acid   +   Water

Figure 6–2. Cross-linking of proteins by formaldehyde.

Action of Preservative Compounds or "Mechanisms[†]". There are several compounds that affect preservation of proteins. These compounds or chemicals include **aldehydes, phenol** and its derivatives, **alcohols, acids**, and **salts**.

FORMALDEHYDE. Methanal, methyl aldehyde, methylene oxide, formic aldehyde, oxymethylene; HCHO is the line formula; CH_2O is the molecular formula; structurally $H_2C=O$; formaldehyde achieves preservation by cross-linking proteins at the peptide linkage. Other terms used to describe this include fixating, denaturing, and coagulating of protein. This concept is easily demonstrated by the cooking of an egg. The egg white is a liquid upon starting and turns white becoming semi-solid as heat is applied. The protein in the egg is denatured or coagulated. Denaturing protein during the embalming process is done by inserting a methylene bridge ($-CH_2-$) between the nitrogens in the amino groups of adjacent proteins. One of the properties of formaldehyde is that it combines with water to form methylene glycol, which is the source for the methylene bridge. The oxygen atom in formaldehyde links to a hydrogen atom from each of the two amino groups to form water. It should be mentioned that proteins by their very nature attract and hold water molecules between the various amine, RNH_2, and carboxylic acid, COOH, groups found throughout their structure. Proteins in living tissue are coiled and folded in order to perform a specific function. Embalming causes these folds and coils to be undone and or cross linked thus denaturing the protein. When the preservative reacts with the amine and acid portions of these folds, it releases the water molecules that were attracted by the partial polarity of the amino acids, hence the dehydrating effect of formaldehyde on tissue. In addition to the dehydration of tissue, the loss of water normally found in and around the proteins causes a gelling or coagulation of the protein producing the firm feel of embalmed tissue (Fig. 6–2).

Disinfection and inactivation of proteolytic enzymes is achieved by the same mechanism as most bacteria/enzymes have or are protein in nature.

PHENOL. aka carbolic acid, hydroxybenzene; line formula C_6H_5OH. Phenol is a crystalline solid at room temperature, very soluble in water, and it is weakly acidic.

Phenol does not preserve by cross linking the protein as formaldehyde does. It preserves by penetrating the phospholipid bi-layer of the cell (bacterial cells as well) and then dissociating in the cytoplasm of the cell. The dissociation of the acidic hydrogen causes the negative charge that is left on the benzene ring to become delocalized. In this delocalized form, phenol inhibits further decomposition of proteins and inactivates proteolytic enzymes as well as destroying bacteria.

ALCOHOLS. One carbon-methyl alcohol, methanol, wood alcohol, two carbon-ethyl alcohol or ethanol, and three carbon-propyl alcohol or propanol and its isomer iso-propyl alcohol preserve tissue and disinfect in a manner similar to phenol. However, the hydroxyl groups, OH, in these alcohols do not dissociate or produce an acidic hydrogen. The destruction of proteolytic enzymes and proteins is achieved by removing the water in the cell, which is necessary for normal metabolism to take place.

SALTS. Salts preserve by desiccation. Salts pull the water out of the cells depriving them of the water needed for normal metabolism. This type of preservation does not usually produce viewable results as sought by modern embalming.

One of the main forces that allow tissue to be preserved and bacteria to be disinfected is the formation of water or removal of water from the substance that is being preserved. While the mechanisms that affect this change in the proteins differ, the end result is similar; that is the proteins are rendered unsuitable as food for bacteria and or resistant to decomposition, both putrefactive and saprophytic[*].

Germicides

An important purpose of embalming is the sanitizing of the tissues of the body. Germicides are incorporated into **arterial fluids, some coinjection fluids, cavity fluids, and**

[†]Chemical mechanisms refer to the manner in which electrons and atoms transfer or move in chemical reactions.

*Prepared by David G. Hicks and Paul Cimiluca ; Cincinnati College of Mortuary Science; Cincinnati, Ohio, 2010.

surface disinfectants. The embalmer uses the surface sanitizing agents when treating the nasal and oral cavities as well as the surface of the body and, in the case of the autopsied body, the surface walls of the abdominal, thoracic, pelvic, and cranial cavities.

Germicides kill or render incapable of reproduction disease-causing microorganisms. As these microbes are made of proteins and the enzymes that they make are protein in nature, most of the preservative chemicals act as germicides. Formaldehyde, phenol, and phenolic derivatives are germicidal. Glutaraldehyde in an alkaline pH is particularly effective. Quaternary ammonium compounds such as Roccal and zephiran chloride are good examples of germicides incorporated into cavity fluids.

Quaternary Ammonium Compounds. These materials are used chiefly for their germicidal and deodorizing qualities. They consist of mixtures of alkyl radicals from C_8H_{17} to $C_{18}H_{37}$, that is, high–molecular-weight alkyl dimethyl benzyl ammonium chlorides. Aqueous solutions are usually neutral (pH 7). These compounds are compatible neither with the wetting agents used in arterial fluids nor with many of the coloring materials incorporated into such fluids. Consequently, their use is restricted to cavity fluids and specialty formulations used for cold sterilization of instruments, linens, gowns, clothing, and other items; cleaning agents for mold proofing remains; and deodorant sprays.

Modifying Agents

Modifying agents control the rate of action of the main preservative chemicals of embalming formulations. Many preservatives, when used alone, exert adverse effects that interfere with good embalming results. For example, formaldehyde (when used alone) is so harsh and astringent that it sears the walls of the small capillaries and prevents diffusion of the preservation solution to remote soft tissue areas. It is necessary to control the rate of fixation so that the firming action is delayed long enough to permit thorough saturation of tissue cells. When the hardening effect of the aldehyde is delayed, the more uniform distribution of the coloring or staining agent is made possible. Buffers, humectants, water conditioners, and inorganic salts usually control the rate of chemical action, modify the adverse color reaction produced by the preservative chemical in the tissues, and control capillary restriction or other undesirable results produced by the preservative materials.

1. **Buffers.** Agents that serve to control the acid–base balance of fluid and tissues.
2. **Humectants.** Agents that help to control tissue moisture balance.
3. **Anticoagulants (water conditioning agents).**

4. **Surfactants (wetting agents, surface tension reducers, penetrating agents or Surface active agents)**

It should be pointed out that many chemicals in the preceding list serve similar functions. Many buffers can also act as water conditioners and anticoagulants. In addition, some of these chemicals are also inorganic salts and contribute to the osmotic qualities of the embalming solution. Even humectants can play a role in influencing osmotic quality. Because certain chemicals have multiple uses in embalming solutions, specific chemicals appear under different headings. For example, in a discussion of the anticoagulants, buffers are also reviewed.

Buffers. Buffers are employed in embalming fluids to stabilize the acid–base balance of the fluid. These pH stabilizers not only help to maintain the acid–base balance of the fluid, but, in addition, assist in stabilizing the pH of the tissues where the embalming fluid reacts with the cellular proteins. The tissues of the body after death contain varying levels of acids or bases. Normal body pH is about 7.38 to 7.4 after death, and through the rigor mortis cycle the tissues will have an acid pH as a result of carbohydrate breakdown. After the rigor cycle, the tissues become basic as a result of protein breakdown. These reactions are not uniform throughout the body, so tissues will vary in pH depending on rigor mortis and decomposition cycles. In addition, the cause of death can influence tissue pH. Buffers play a very important role in providing good pH medium for the reaction of preservative with body proteins.

Many of the compounds used as anticoagulants serve as buffer pairs. Examples are borates, carbonates, phosphates, and salts of ethylenediaminetetraacetic acid (EDTA).

BORATES. In a report released by the Public Health Service in 1915, it was found that **borax** (sodium borate) was a good, efficient stabilizer of formalin, providing a desired degree of alkalinity that rendered formalin stable for long periods. It has been found to reduce the hardening and graying actions of formaldehyde. Depending on the specific type of formulation and other compounds present, in addition to borax, boric acid may also be added to certain embalming formulations. Formulations containing a well-balanced mixture of borates have been found to keep formaldehyde stable beyond 2 years. The loss in formaldehyde strength in such instances is insignificant.

CARBONATES. Sodium carbonate is used alone or in combination with borates to modify the action of formaldehyde on tissue. Magnesium carbonate is also used sometimes and may be added to the formalin prior to combination with the other chemicals in a formulation. From all indications it would appear that carbonates are not as efficient as borates in preventing the deterioration of formalin over long periods.

In a **Report and Review of Research in Embalming and Embalming Fluids** by the Minnesota State Department of Health, N.C. Pervier and F. Lloyd Hansen of the University of Minnesota studied the tissue reaction to injections of formaldehyde at various pH values. These investigators found that addition of a strong base, such as sodium hydroxide, improved tissue coloring; however, the high concentration of sodium hydroxide used caused deterioration of the preservative. When they injected formaldehyde solutions containing 1%, 2%, and 3% acid (HCl), the tissue tended to assume a putty-gray coloration. Since pH extremes are detrimental to formaldehyde, today, most arterial fluids are found to be slightly alkaline (with a pH of 7.2–7.4).

Humectants. Humectants are described as having a coating action; they wrap around the formaldehyde molecule and thus keep the formaldehyde from making direct contact with albuminous material until the tissues are thoroughly saturated and bathed with the preservative solution. The formaldehyde is under shackles for a time, and as it travels through the capillaries and to the tissue cells it gradually sheds its shackles and, on release, acts on the albuminous material. Humectants bring about cellular hydration. The addition of humectant compounds to embalming fluids assists in making the tissue more flexible and rubbery. In some instances such materials are also called plasticizing agents because of their pliable effects. These compounds include glycerine, sorbitol, glycols, and other polyhydroxy alcohols. Cosmetic oils, lanolin, and its derivatives are also used for their emollient properties.

GLYCERINE. A by-product of the manufacture of soap, glycerine can be classified as an alcohol. It has also been produced synthetically from petroleum products. Although glycerine is not itself a germicide and has no preservative qualities, it does increase the germ-killing power of other chemicals, probably because it is an excellent solvent for disinfecting chemicals; its good solvent ability makes it an efficient carrier for the chemicals. Glycerine is also a good lubricator and is hygroscopic, which means it has affinity for moisture. If retained in the tissues, it helps to prevent dehydration.

SORBITOL AND THE GLYCOLS. Sorbitol is probably used more extensively today in embalming fluids than is glycerine. Chemically, it has a straight chain of six carbon atoms and six hydroxyl groups, whereas glycerine has three carbon atoms and three hydroxyl groups in its structure. Commercially, sorbitol is generally available as a 70% aqueous solution. An important characteristic of sorbitol is that it loses water at a slower rate than glycerine, and consequently, for controlling the rate of moisture loss, it is more efficient than glycerine. One disadvantage of sorbitol solutions is that at very low temperatures, sorbitol precipitates from solution. Different types of glycols (mainly propylene, ethylene, and diethylene) are also found in embalming preparations. Sometimes, these materials are used alone with formaldehyde; in other instances, they may be incorporated into a formulation already containing either glycerine, sorbitol, or both.

Ethylene glycol is a colorless, syrupy liquid with very little odor. It is readily soluble in water. Because of its hygroscopic properties it is used as a moisture-retaining and softening material.

Propylene glycol is reported to be superior to glycerine as a general solvent and inhibitor of mold growth. Like ethylene glycol, it is colorless, odorless, and completely soluble in water.

EMULSIFIED OILS. Materials such as lanolin and silicon are not in themselves water soluble, but certain fractions or derivatives are used that can easily be dispersed in aqueous solutions. It is the purpose of these materials in embalming fluid to mitigate the drying effect of the preservative agents. Highly penetrative oils of the oleate and palmitate types are also employed to help reduce the drying effect of aldehydes. Use of such materials requires an emulsion system that is able to maintain the formulation in a stable and uniform state over a long period.

GUMS—VEGETABLE AND SYNTHETIC. The use of vegetable and synthetic gums is generally prompted by the need to restore moisture to tissue or to maintain the normal appearance of tissue when the subject is to be held for a period of time prior to burial. These materials, when added to water, swell and retain moisture as the gum molecule is distributed to the soft tissue areas. Because of their molecular size, the gums, on taking up moisture, are actually trapped in the capillary bed and aid both in restoring moisture to the area and in filling out the tissues to overcome the emaciated appearance.

As these materials are large molecular entities they are generally added to the arterial embalming solution after the initial injection has been made and all surface discolorations have been cleared. Use of such compounds prior to complete removal of blood from the tissues may interfere with proper distribution of the injected preservative solution. Examples of vegetable gums include **karaya** and **tragacanth.** The synthetic gums are generally formed from cellulose and have varying composition.

Inorganic Salts

The inorganic salts used in embalming fluids serve a variety of functions. They can act as buffers, anticoagulants, preservatives, germicides, and water conditioners. Their use is quite simple in that they can be dissolved in the limited space of the 16-oz standard bottle of concentrated embalming fluid. By controlling the amount of inorganic salts used, the fluid remains balanced, as some of the salts do not "settle out" of the concentrated fluid. A role for salts in any solution is their ability to control the osmotic qualities. This is true in embalming fluid. Once the embalming solution reaches the capillary beds, it is very important that the solution be able to pass through the microscopic pores of the capillaries and thus enter the tissue spaces. It is a role of the inorganic salts to maintain an osmotic quality of the embalming solution that helps to draw fluid from the capillaries into the tissue spaces. Likewise, special fluids are used on bodies whose tissues are saturated with edema. These "special-purpose" fluids, when mixed according to the manufacturer's directions, actually draw the excess tissue moisture (edema) from the tissues back into the capillaries, from which it can then be removed by the drainage process. It is the osmotic qualities of those "special-purpose" fluids that bring about the dehydration of these bodies (see Chapter 21).

Anticoagulants (Water Conditioners or Softeners). Anticoagulants are an important component of embalming fluids, especially arterial fluids, because they are used to maintain blood in a liquid state and thereby make it easy to remove from the circulatory system.

When blood collects in the capillary bed in the dependent parts of the body after death, it has a tendency to thicken and clot very easily. In some cases, as in death from pneumonia, the blood tends to clot more readily. The volume of circulating blood tends to decrease when high fever precedes death, and the blood becomes more viscous and clots more readily after circulation stops.

It is therefore necessary to include, in an embalming fluid, chemicals that maintain blood in a liquid state so that it is easily displaced from the body. Such chemicals inhibit or stop the clotting of blood. Claims are often made that such materials also "liquefy" clotted blood, but it is not likely that this happens.

The compounds that are used for this purpose must be chemically compatible with, or inert toward, other intimately blended components of the formulation. The materials that are employed as anticoagulants also function as "water softeners" or "water conditioners"; however, products specially designed for that purpose are commercially available and are sold for use as additives or supplemental chemicals with the arterial solution. The products known as water "softeners" or water "conditioners" are used for one or all of four reasons.

First, such products are intended to be used as aids to improve drainage by keeping blood in a liquid state during the embalming operation and softening the framework of clotted material so that it readily breaks up into smaller pieces.

Second, by reducing the hardness of water, such materials enhance the function of the arterial fluid. The interfering chemicals such as calcium, magnesium, and iron actually prevent the preservative chemicals present in arterial fluids from performing their intended function of penetrating soft tissues to achieve preservation.

Third, experience and experimental work have indicated that the dyes used in embalming fluids produce the best internal cosmetic effect under slightly alkaline conditions. The arterial fluids cannot be compounded to stay on the alkaline side of the pH scale because aldehydes, especially formaldehyde, undergo breakdown and lose strength when kept under alkaline conditions for long periods. Consequently, the alkaline conditions must be created at the time the solution is going to be used. During such short periods, alkaline pH does not adversely affect the preservative chemicals. Addition of water softeners ("clot-dispersing products") to the embalming solution prepared for injection produces a most desirable alkaline condition. Such materials enhance the coloring properties and action of dyes by increasing their intensity.

Fourth, investigations have definitely shown that most aldehydes (and formaldehyde in particular) function better as fixative or firming agents under slightly alkaline conditions. But, as pointed out in the preceding paragraph, aldehydes cannot remain under alkaline conditions more than a couple of weeks (even less) without losing their effectiveness. Therefore, the alkaline conditions must be created more or less "on the spot" at the time the fluid is used. This is where the specially designed additive products come into play. Greater firmness is attained by progressive action where such materials are used along with the arterial fluid.

Often, it is claimed that a certain arterial fluid contains all of the materials necessary to reduce to zero hardness the water used in preparing the embalming solution. Because of the preservative materials that must be incorporated into the arterial fluid formulation (in addition to wetting agents, modifiers, coloring agents, perfuming materials, etc.), however, there is a limit to the amount of anticlotting and water-softening compounds that can be added to the formula. If sufficient amounts of such compounds were to be added to the regular arterial fluids to achieve the results expected from and produced by "water softeners," the chemical and physical balance of the formulation would be adversely affected. If this balance is adversely affected several things may happen:

- There may be interference with proper penetration and diffusion of the preservative solution.
- There may be interference with the drainage qualities of the embalming solution.
- By disruption of the chemical balance of the solution, addition of the extra amounts of anticlotting and water-softening chemicals to the arterial fluid formula could cause a gradual reduction of the formaldehyde strength of the fluid.

Consequently, embalming fluid manufacturers supply, as separate supplemental products, "water softeners and conditioners" that are added to the embalming solution prepared for injection. This procedure enables the embalmer to use as much material as the case may require for proper and effective water- and clot-softening action.

The compounds in this class of embalming chemicals include those usually found in buffer systems. As has been pointed out previously, the degree of acidity or alkalinity of the medium in which a chemical reaction takes place influences, to a great extent, the chemical reaction that takes place between compounds and substances. During life, blood and body tissues have a pH in the range of 7.2 to 7.4. After death, however, tissue pH varies greatly. Also, the pH of the body tissues at the time of embalming depends on the time that has lapsed since death. An embalming formulation containing the proper buffer mixture will perform uniformly because the buffer mixture will neutralize excess acidity or alkalinity and, thus, facilitate the action in a given pH range.

It is also necessary to maintain an embalming formulation at a given pH if it is to be retained for a long shelf life. Some chemicals that are used are stable only in certain pH ranges and so buffer agents must be employed to keep constant the acid–base balance of the solution. This ensures against deterioration and breakdown of the chemical compounds. For example, earlier it was stated that formaldehyde is not stable at high pH, that is, under alkaline conditions, over long periods. When embalming fluid is compounded, the manufacturer must try to anticipate the shelf life of the product so that the fluid is as effective the day it is used as the day it was compounded. A formaldehyde index on a fluid bottle label is maintained only through the proper chemical balance of the formulation, which also includes proper acid–base control of the solution.

Another important factor is that as the prepared embalming solution diffuses through the circulatory system, it comes into contact with tissues that may well be at different pH values. The acid–base balance of the tissues should also be so controlled and maintained by the buffer so that the fluid performs under the best pH conditions.

Many preservative chemicals when used alone exert adverse effects that interfere with the achievement of good embalming results. For example, formaldehyde when used alone is so harsh and astringent that it sears the walls of the small capillaries and prevents diffusion of the preservative solution to remote soft tissue areas. Consequently, it is necessary to control the action of the formaldehyde so that the fixation of tissue (firming action) is delayed sufficiently to permit thorough bathing of tissue cells. By delaying the hardening action of formaldehyde, uniform distribution of the coloring or staining agent is also possible. It can be said that these modifying agents also enhance the internal cosmetic effect.

BORATES. In addition to its function as a stabilizer of formaldehyde, sodium borate also serves to prevent or reduce coagulation. Sodium borate (borax, sodium tetraborate, or pyroborate) is a white crystalline powder that is readily soluble in a mixture of water and glycerine. Boric acid is a white powder that is often used in combination with borax.

EDTA. The sodium salts of EDTA are very effective sequestering or chelating agents, which means that they very readily combine with calcium ions to prevent blood coagulation and also to remove hardness chemicals from the water supply. Generally, these materials are not found in arterial fluids. These agents are alkaline and are not compatible with the other compounds in embalming fluids over a long shelf life. Such materials are used most advantageously as separate formulations; that is, in the form of supplemental or accessory chemicals that are added to the embalming solution at the time of use.

OTHER MATERIALS. Among the other compounds often used as anticlotting materials are magnesium sulfate (Epsom salts), sodium chloride, sodium sulfate, and sodium phosphates. At one time or another, these compounds have been recommended for use in capillary wash solutions, and some are still used in arterial fluid formulations. This class of chemicals also contains some of the materials employed in buffer systems to maintain a constant pH in a fluid formulation. These are used in combination with those mentioned earlier.

Surfactants (Wetting Agents). Probably one of the greatest developments that has occurred in the chemistry and physics of embalming since the discovery of formaldehyde is the principle of removing body liquids by lowering their surface tension. It is necessary, before complete circulation may take place in the body, to remove the liquid that is held in the capillaries. Capillary attraction, or the force that attracts and holds liquid in the capillary tubes, is the result of surface tension. If the surface tension of the liquid in these tiny tubes is lowered, the liquid easily loosens and flows out.

Much has been said and written about the important role and use of surfactants (**surface-active agents, tension breakers, tension reducers**) in embalming formulations. Actually, there is no industry that has not investigated these compounds and found them adaptable for a variety of uses. The chemical structure of surfactants is rather complex: one part of the molecule has a strong attraction or affinity for water, whereas the other part of the molecule dislikes water. This latter part of the molecule has an affinity for nonaqueous liquids. Such a complicated molecular makeup functions to lower or reduce the surface tension of the solution to which the surfactant is added. In a water-and-oil mixture the surfactant destroys the surface tension of the components so that the oily mixture is more easily dispersible in water. Other materials are made "water soluble" in a similar manner.

It should also be remembered that each cell in the soft tissues of the body is surrounded by a film of body liquid mostly water in composition. For easy, rapid penetration of the cell, this surface film must be dispersed. Such chemical substances, then, are used in embalming fluids for three reasons.

First, by lowering the surface tension of the preservative solution (the embalming solution), surfactants aid or cause the embalming solution to flow more readily and rapidly through the capillaries so that **all** of the millions of tissue cells are literally bathed by the embalming solution and, thus, thoroughly preserved. Naturally, the technique of injecting the solution and draining employed by the embalmer can assist or handicap the function of the surfactant. The process of moving the solution through the body being embalmed is a technique that should be planned and controlled by the embalmer to ensure that a sufficient amount of preservative chemicals is uniformly distributed throughout the body. It is also important that some of the normal moisture lost during embalming be replaced to safeguard against dehydration.

Second, by reducing the capillary attraction (which is a phenomenon of surface tension) of blood and body liquids, surfactants cause the almost immediate clearing of blood from the capillaries. Surface tension is reduced, and the liquid more readily moves and flows out the capillary bed and through the venous drainage system. Since two things cannot occupy the same space at the same time, the capillaries must be emptied of blood before injected solution can flow through them to reach the tissues of the body. Only the solutions that pass by osmosis through the capillary walls into the intercellular spaces have any chance of being absorbed by the tissue cells. The embalmer must help the solution reach the tissues by employing the necessary physical manipulation such as massage and intermittent or restricted type of drainage.

Third, by increasing the ability of the solution to filter through the semipermeable capillary walls in a uniform manner, it is possible to incorporate coloring agents into the solution and obtain a normal appearance internally (Fig. 6–3).

Surface Tension and Embalming Solutions. Solids, liquids, and gases are all made up of molecules arranged in characteristic patterns depending on the material being studied. These molecules have an affinity or attraction for one another. Again, depending on the materials under study, this degree of molecular attraction differs. For example, the attractive force is greater between water molecules than it is between alcohol molecules. At 20° C, the surface tension of water is 72.75 dynes per centimeter, and for methyl alcohol it is 22.61 dynes per centimeter. (Note: a dyne is the force required to accelerate a 1 gram mass 1 centimeter per second.) Thus, water has a surface tension value more than three times that of methyl alcohol and penetrates much more slowly. In other words, the lower the surface tension value, the faster the rate of penetration by the liquid substance.

The surface tension of water is lowered by the addition of surfactants. Wetting or penetrating chemicals tend to destroy the bonds or attractive forces that normally exist between water molecules so that they seemingly break away from each other. The net effect of such physiochemical action is to cause liquids to diffuse and penetrate more readily through cellular tissue.

Surface tension is also defined as the contractive forces that cause liquids to assume the shape in which they have the least surface, that is, a sphere. Wetting agents reduce this contractive force.

In embalming solutions, the addition of surfactants in proper concentrations produces better penetration of the preservative chemicals in a more uniform manner. This enables the preservative solution to more readily displace the body fluids from all cellular tissue and replace them to achieve the embalming function. Also, coloring agents are uniformly distributed through the use of surfactants. The even diffusion of such agents throughout the soft tissues results in a more natural color and appearance.

Surface tension changes with the variations in temperature. As the temperature rises, the surface tension value of a solution decreases. In embalming, this means that if warm water is used to prepare the solutions for

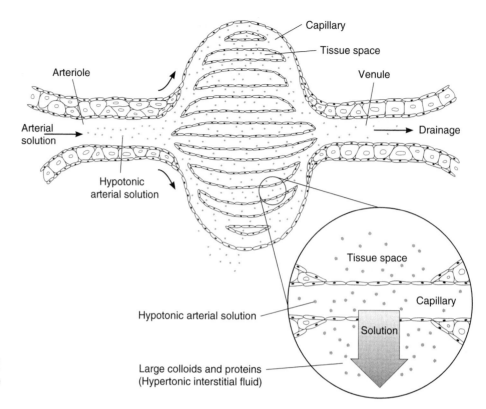

Figure 6–3. Movement of arterial solution from the capillaries into the tissue spaces.

injection, the resultant solution may be expected to penetrate more rapidly because of the lowered surface tension value. Also keep in mind that the chemical reaction between the preservative chemicals and the tissues will take place more rapidly as a result of using warm water. The fixative or firming action will also occur faster than usual.

Surfactants also increase the germicidal activity of chemical solutions. It is believed that this is due to an increased speed of penetration into the bacterial cells as a result of the lowering the surface tension of the solution.

Surfactants and Surface Tension. From the preceding discussion it might appear that the embalmer could easily make his or her embalming technique more efficient by simply adding an extra surfactant to the embalming solution. This is not true. Surfactants function best in very low concentrations and must be carefully selected by experienced chemists with respect to the other substances present in the formulation. It is necessary to determine compatibilities among all the components of an embalming fluid and the surfactant, and the amount of surfactant to use to produce a properly well-balanced chemical formulation. Addition of extra surfactant to an embalming solution may result in excessive drainage as well as oversaturation of tissue.

The following considerations, which must be thoroughly explored by the chemist in evaluating specific applications for any given surfactant, serve to illustrate the complex nature of such chemicals. The discussion is by no means complete.

Surface-active agents are generally classified into three groups: anionic, cationic, and nonionic. In brief, if the surfactant molecule tends to ionize, then it is either anionic or cationic. If it does not ionize in solution, it is nonionic.

Surfactants such as soap, alkyl sulfonates, alkyl aryl sulfonates, salts of thioalcohols, and oils are **anionic**. These compounds are compatible with other anionic and nonionic agents. They are not normally compatible with and are frequently precipitated from solutions by cationic materials and by certain inorganic cations such as aluminum, calcium, and magnesium.

An example of **cationic** surfactants is the quaternary ammonia compounds. The principal disadvantage of these compounds is that they are inactivated by anionic substances such as soap which is routinely applied to the external surface of the body.

Nonionic surfactants do not ionize in solution, but owe their surface activity and water solubility or dispersibility to nonionized polar groups within the molecule, such as hydroxyl or ether linkages. Ethylene oxide condensation products with amides and fatty acids belong to this group (specific examples are the Atlas "Tweens" and "Spans").

In actual chemical formulating practice, the result to be achieved by the end product must be kept in mind in deciding the type of surfactant to employ. Most generally, a blend of such materials is incorporated into embalming fluids to achieve the results mentioned at the beginning of this discussion.

Dyes (Coloring Agents)

The coloring materials used in modern embalming fluids generally are employed for the purpose of producing an internal cosmetic effect that closely simulates the natural coloring of tissues. Such materials have high staining qualities and as they diffuse to the superficial tissue areas from the circulatory system, they impart color to the tissue. Usually, a blend of coloring materials, ranging from straw or amber to brilliant red, is used. The type of dye used depends to great extent on the pH of the arterial fluid. Dyes that color tissues are called **active dyes**. Those that merely lend color to the fluid in the bottle are **inactive dyes**.

Active dyes are usually a blend of dyes, mainly coal–tar derivatives. Red dyes of various shades and degrees of intensity are usually blended in an attempt to restore a natural color to the tissues. The coloring materials selected for use in any given embalming fluid formulation depend to a great extent on the pH of the solution. Examples include eosin, erythrosine, ponceau, fluorescein, amaranth, and carmine.

Types of Coloring Agents. Coloring materials may be placed into two classes.

Natural coloring agents are vegetable colors such as cudbear, carmine, and cochineal. **Cudbear** is a purplish red powder prepared from lichens by maceration in dilute ammonia and caustic soda and fermentation. **Carmine** is an aluminum and calcium salt of carminic acid. **Cochineal** is a red-coloring matter consisting of the dried bodies of the female insects of **Coccus cacti**. The coloring principle is carminic acid, $C_{22}H_{20}O_{13}$. This class of dyes is not generally incorporated into modern solutions.

Synthetic coloring agents are the coloring materials used in modern fluids and are mainly coal–tar derivatives. They are economical to use and are the most permanent if they are chemically compatible with the other substances in the fluid. Many different types and shades are available under rather confusing diversified commercial names and chemical nomenclature. For better solubility, most of the coal–tar dyes are supplied as sodium or potassium salts of the synthetic coloring matter. These materials then may be said to be dyes of alkali metal salts that have been reacted with coal–tar compounds. Several dyes are available.

- **Eosin**   Known as tetrabromofluorescein, $C_{20}H_8Br_4O_5$; red crystalline powder
- **Erythrosine** Brown powder that forms cherry red solutions in water; known chemically as the sodium salt of iodeosin, $C_{20}H_6I_4Na_2O_5$, FD&C No.3
- **Ponceau**   Dark red powder that is soluble in water and acid solutions; forms a cherry red solution and is a naphthol disulfonate compound
- **Amaranth**   Coal–tar azo dye, $C_{20}H_{11}N_2Na_3O_{10}S_3$, that forms a dark red-brown color in water but is only slightly soluble in alcohol. FD&C No. 2

Other synthetic dyes include croceine scarlet, rhodamine, rose bengal, acid fuchsin, and toluidine red.

COLORING MATERIALS IN EMBALMING FLUIDS. Coloring materials in use today in embalming fluids belong to a group known as biological stains, as such materials are used in clinical laboratories to stain different types of tissue for study under the microscope. The coloring agents used in fluids must be stable in the presence of formaldehyde, must be water soluble, should impart a natural flesh color to the tissues, and should have high tinctorial or staining qualities so that small amounts can produce the desired color. This last requirement is important because arterial fluids are diluted before use.

The coal–tar dyes possess the requirements of a coloring agent for use in embalming fluids. Molecularly they are fine enough to diffuse evenly and uniformly through tissue cells. As soon as surfactants (wetting agents) began to be used in embalming solutions, it was found possible to add staining materials to the formulations because wetting agents diffused the dye very effectively. The specific material that is to be used in any given formulation must be carefully selected, as some dyes produce different coloring effects at different pH values and different extents of dilution.

Natural color materials such as the vegetable dyes are considered too unstable for use in embalming fluids. Some have good color-fast features but do not diffuse evenly because of their large molecular structures.

Newer environmentally friendly non-toxic formaldehyde-free embalming fluids contain such dyes as erythrosine (FD&C Red 3) because it is biodegradable. This type of dye would be usable if the body were to be buried in a strictly Green Cemetery.

Perfuming Materials (Masking Agents, Deodorants)

Generally, deodorants or perfuming agents are selected not only for their power in covering harsh chemicals but also for the pleasant odor they impart to a solution. By blending special synthetic essential oils with the harsh preservative chemicals in a formulation, the harshness or "raw" odor of the solution is reduced and replaced to some extent by a more pleasing scent.

Floral compounds such as wisteria, rose, and lilac types, along with nondescript essential oils and aromatic esters, are used quite extensively in embalming formulations because of their strong aroma. This property makes it possible to cover objectionable fumes during brief exposures. Such materials are made water soluble through the medium of nonionic surfactants.

If the formulation does not contain a high concentration of formaldehyde or other irritating chemicals, it is possible to use synthetic compounds that give off odors resembling spices (clove, cinnamon), fruit (strawberry, peach, etc.), mint (spearmint, peppermint, menthol), and many other aromas designed by the essential oil chemist. Sassafras, oil of wintergreen (methyl salicylate), and benzaldehyde have been among some of the more commonly used materials for this purpose.

Occasionally, use of high concentrations of perfuming and masking agents in chemical solutions is made in an attempt to hide high concentrations of formaldehyde, especially in so-called fumeless fluids. Usually, the scent of the perfuming agent is immediately detected, while the presence of the formaldehyde remains in the background. The individual finally becomes aware of the formaldehyde as a result of a pinching sensation in the nose; the delayed awareness manifests in the form of an explosive effect with a resultant shortness of breath. The individual does not realize how much fumes are present until too late. Unfortunately, there are products still advertised as "fumeless" or "odorless" when, in reality, they are not. The true low-odor type of product is based on the use of "donor" compounds that release the aldehyde when contact with tissue so that a minimum amount of gas is released to bother the user.

The essential oils used in embalming fluids are selected on the basis of their stability in the presence of preservative chemicals and their ability to remain in solution when water is added. Some essential oils possess antiseptic properties but this usually is not why they are used in embalming formulations.

Vehicles (Diluents)

The active preservatives and other compounds in the formulation must be dissolved in a common solvent. As water is an essential part of tissue, its use in embalming solutions facilitates the diffusion and penetration of the active preservative components of fluids. The vehicle (sometimes called "carrier") must be a solvent or mixture of solvents that keeps the active substances in a stable and uniform state during transport through the circulatory system to all parts of the body.

To maintain the proper density and osmotic activity, that is, the proper chemical and physical balance of the formulation, the vehicle or diluent may include glycerine, sorbitol, glycols, or alcohols in addition to water. Quite often, a special solvent may be used as part of an innovation to dissolve or keep in solution any special "new" compound.

▶ CONCEPTS FOR DISCUSSION

1. Using the Internet, search for the various uses of formaldehyde; studies of formaldehyde as a carcinogen.
2. Research recent funeral service journals, fluid company catalogues, and the internet and describe the composition of the various green or natural embalming fluids. Make a list of their advantages and disadvantages.
3. List advantages and disadvantages of embalming with formaldehyde.
4. Describe the difference of embalming with formaldehyde and glutaraldehyde.
5. What is the purpose of modifying agents in embalming fluids?
6. Discuss the following statement: The function of anticoagulants is to dissolve blood clots.
7. Briefly outline how formaldehyde acts on body proteins to bring about preservation.
8. Anticoagulants are sometimes referred to as water conditioners. How do they condition the water?
9. What is the role of surface tension in the embalming process?
10. Differentiate among cationic, anionic, and nonionic surfactants.
11. What is the difference between active and inactive dyes?
12. What is meant by a vehicle in embalming fluids and what is its purpose?

▶ FURTHER READINGS

Block SM, ed. *Disinfection, Sterilization, and Preservation*, 5th ed. Philadelphia: Lippincott Williams & Williams, 2001.

Dorn JM, Hopkins BM. *Thanatochemistry, A Survey of General, Organic, and Biochemistry for Funeral Service Professionals*, 3rd ed. Upper Saddle River, NJ: Prentice Hall, 2010.

Eckles College of Mortuary Science, Inc. *Modern Mortuary Science*, 4th ed. Philadelphia: Westbrook, 1958:206.

Encyclopedia of Industrial Chemical Analysis, Vol. 12. *Embalming Chemicals*. New York, NY: Wiley, 1971.

Champion Co. "Enigma: Champion's Fourth Generation Chemostasis Infusion Chemicals: Embalming Redefined for the 21st Century". In: *Champion Expanding Encyclopedia of Mortuary Practices*, No. 657. Springfield, OH: Champion Co., 2009.

Formaldehyde Council Inc., www.formaldehyde.org.

Champion Co. "General chemical principles of embalming fluids". In *Expanding Encyclopedia of Mortuary Practice*, Nos. 365–371. Springfield, OH: Champion Co., 1966.

Dodge Co. Green Embalming: A Paradigm Shift". In *Dodge Magazine*, Vol.103 No.1, Cambridge, MA: Dodge Co., Winter 2011.

Dodge Co. "In Search of the Perfect Embalming Chemical". In *Dodge Magazine*, Vol. 102 No.4. Cambridge, MA: Dodge Co., 2010.

New Jersey State Funeral Directors Assn. "Putting Alternative Preservatives to the Test". In *The Forum*, Vol.76, No. 3, Wall, NJ: New Jersey State Funeral Directors Assn., January 2010.

New Jersey State Funeral Directors Assn. "The Future of Formaldehyde". In *The Forum*, Vol. 75, No. 3, Wall, NJ: New Jersey State Funeral Directors Assn., January 2009.

Walker J. *Formaldehyde*, 3rd ed. ACS Monograph No. 159. New York, NY: Reinhold, 1964.

CHAPTER 7

USE OF EMBALMING CHEMICALS

CHAPTER OBJECTIVES

▶ Safe work practices
▶ Arterial fluids
▶ Supplemental arterial fluids
▶ Cavity Fluids
▶ Special purpose arterial fluids
▶ Accessory embalming chemicals

This chapter examines the selection and use of the various embalming chemicals: (1) arterial preservative fluids, (2) supplemental vascular fluids, (3) cavity fluids, and (4) accessory embalming chemicals.

The arterial and cavity fluids are usually sold in America in concentrated form in 16-oz (pint) plastic bottles. The preservative arterial fluids are diluted with water and/or supplemental arterial chemicals. Cavity fluids are used undiluted.

The arterial fluid labels, or the literature which accompanies them, will recommend dilutions and often total volume of arterial solutions which should be injected for specific body conditions. **These are only guidelines.** The embalmer must make the final determinations as to (1) type of arterial fluid(s) to use, (2) strength of the arterial solution, and (3) volume of arterial solution to inject. The strength and volume of the initial arterial solution is determined by the **preembalming analysis.** Subsequent solution strength and volume is determined **during** the arterial injection of the body.

The embalmer must (1) be able to analyze the body conditions along with the length of time between embalming and disposition of the body, (2) evaluate what embalming fluids to employ, and (3) properly use the chemicals in necessary strengths and volume to meet the preservative demands of the deceased human body. It is more accurate to say that embalming is more about critical thinking and problem solving than following "recipes."

▶ WORK PRACTICE CONTROLS IN THE USE OF CHEMICALS

The embalmer handles various chemicals during preparation of the body. Care should be taken in the handling of all these chemicals, even such seemingly harmless products as talcum and drying powders. Some general guidelines that apply to the handling of embalming chemicals include the following.

1. *Wear eye protection when handling embalming chemicals.* Safety goggles, a face shield, or some type of protective eye covering should be used at all times. Some industrial hygienists recommend wearing both safety goggles and a face shield. Formaldehyde, if splashed into the eye, is a severe irritant. Flush immediately with cool running water. An embalmer working with a chemical containing phenol (carbolic acid) or concentrated phenol should be certain that his or her eyes and skin are protected. Phenol can cause severe burns. Whenever this chemical is accidentally splashed into the open eye, seek medical help immediately.
2. *Wear protective clothing during embalming.* Many embalming fluids contain dyes that leave permanent stains on clothing.
3. *Wear gloves when working with embalming chemicals.* Some individuals can develop a sensitivity to the chemical agents in embalming fluids.

These sensitivities can cause skin irritations and eruptions similar to allergic reactions. Formaldehyde has a tendency to dry the hands of the embalmer. This drying (after several days) can lead to cracking of the skin. Broken skin is an avenue for the entrance of pathogenic microbial agents. Formaldehyde is also an irritant to the skin and, if concentrated enough, such as in cavity fluids, can cause an inflammation of the skin.

4. *If chemicals are splashed or spilled onto the skin, flush the areas with cold running water.*
5. *When using chemicals, be certain that ventilation systems are in operation and, if necessary, wear a mask.* Formaldehyde fumes can be quite irritating and exposure to these fumes should be kept to a minimum. Care should also be taken in the handling of solvents used in mortuary cosmetology. Whenever embalming powders or cosmetic powders are in use, be certain that rooms are well ventilated. Particulate matter from these powders is respirable and many of the small particulates in these powders are not exhaled but retained in the lungs.
6. *Dilute any spillage immediately with cool water.* Formaldehyde can be neutralized by applying a small amount of household ammonia to the spill. Any sponges or rags used in cleaning these spills should be flushed with cold water. If necessary, leave the room until the fumes decrease to a level at which working in the room to clean up the spill can be tolerated.
7. *Do NOT use formaldehyde-based chemicals as an antiseptic.* These chemicals are not for use on living tissue.
8. *Keep chemical material safety data sheets available as well as chemical manufacturers' first-aid information.*
9. *Be certain that bottles that are destroyed have first been flushed out with water.*
10. *Keep machine tanks and fluid bottles covered and capped at all times to help reduce fumes.*
11. *Be certain that formaldehyde is removed from the area as much as possible before working with disinfectants containing strong oxidizers, for example, sodium hypochlorite (laundry bleach). Studies have shown that there is a possibility that bis(chloromethyl) ether, a carcinogen, may be formed when formaldehyde reacts with bleach. It should be noted that the conditions necessary for this reaction to occur are unlikely to exist in the typical preparation room.*
12. *Pour fluid into an embalming machine tank already filled with water rather than filling the machine with water after fluid is first placed in the tank (Fig. 7–1).*

Figure 7–1. Pouring the arterial fluid into the machine tank after it has been filled with water reduces formaldehyde exposure. Keep the machines covered by using the lid.

▶ FORMALDEHYDE BEST MANAGEMENT PRACTICES

Formaldehyde continues to be the primary preservative incorporated in most arterial fluids. Formaldehyde is toxic and care must be taken when handling products containing this chemical. The following recommendations, drafted in 2009, by the National Funeral Directors Association, are for work practices for products containing formaldehyde; however, these practices can be applied to **all toxic chemicals** used in the preparation room.

The National Funeral Directors Association (NFDA) has issued these Formaldehyde Best Management Practices (BMP's) at a time when there are new appraisals about the health hazards associated with formaldehyde. In 2009 the International Agency for Research on Cancer (IARC) found sufficient evidence to conclude that formaldehyde exposure may cause leukemia, a disease of the bone marrow and blood. The National Cancer Institute (NCI) is reassessing the cancer risk from formaldehyde exposure to funeral directors and others, and domestic and international agencies are reconsidering the health and safety risks associated with formaldehyde. The U.S. Congress is investigating the health effects from the exposure of Hurricane Katrina trailer residents. Thus, in the face of formaldehyde's new scrutiny and the absence of definitive and conclusive scientific results, NFDA believes it is important to protect its members by keeping them informed about formaldehyde and its potential risks. This is a working document first drafted and approved in 2009 and last up-dated in August 2010.

1.0 Ensure adequate and effective ventilation in the preparation room.

2.0 Select and use the proper embalming product in considering the environmental, health and safety characteristics of the product and the condition of the remains.

3.0 Take precautions in the preparation room to limit formaldehyde exposure and emissions during routine embalmings.

4.0 Observe special precautions to limit formaldehyde exposure and emissions when embalming organ procurement cases and autopsied remains, as such embalmings may increase the embalmer's formaldehyde exposure risk.

5.0 Be familiar with and follow federal, state and local environmental, OSHA and health requirements that apply when embalming is performed.

1.0 Ensure adequate and effective ventilation in the preparation room.

Preparation room ventilation is the **single most important factor** in reducing health risks associated with formaldehyde exposure. Make sure that the ventilation system in the preparation room is properly designed and operating effectively. An effective ventilation system assures that as much formaldehyde as possible is drawn away from the embalmer's breathing zone. Consult a Heating, Ventilating and Air Conditioning (HVAC) professional to assess and maintain the ventilation system, and the heating and cooling needs of the work area.

1.1 Have no fewer than 15 air changes per hour in the preparation room.

The appropriate air change rate for the space will be dependent upon site specific factors, such as the configuration of the preparation room and the nature of the funeral home's business, including the number of daily embalmings and whether more than one embalming table is used simultaneously for embalming. A minimum of 15 air changes per hour indicates that preparation room air will be changed approximately every four minutes. Scientific studies show that preparation room activities that have the greatest formaldehyde generation rate usually have a duration of four to five minutes.*

1.2 Employ a local exhaust ventilation (LEV) system for added capture of formaldehyde emissions.

LEV systems are commonly used in a wide variety of industrial settings, typically at low cost, to enhance room ventilation systems. A LEV system, to be effective in a preparation room, must capture formaldehyde emissions, before those emissions enter the breathing zone of the embalmer. A LEV system is especially useful for any funeral home that engages in osmotic embalming for cases with poor circulation, organ and tissue procurement cases and autopsied remains.

1.3 Provide a source of fresh, clean air that prevents excessive negative pressure and improves quality in the preparation room.

Air introduced into the space should be equal to or greater than the volume of air exhausted from the space and drawn from a source free of contaminants.

Embalming room air should never be recycled or re-used.

1.4 Establish a standard operating procedure for ventilation system activation whenever an individual is in the preparation room.

To ensure use of the ventilation system, wire the ventilation system's activation to the preparation room's light switch.

1.5 Vent waste air from the preparation room HVAC system to the outdoors.

The ventilation discharge should be located above ground level, away from human receptors and free of any obstruction that would impede the airflow.

Because formaldehyde is heavier than air, locate the discharge vent **below and away** from the breathing zone of the embalmer.

1.6 Monitor the effectiveness of the preparation room HVAC system no less than annually.

A properly functioning HVAC system is the key to eliminating the risk of formaldehyde exposure in the workplace. To ensure that formaldehyde exposure does not exceed acceptable limits, conduct and document exposure monitoring annually, more frequently than OSHA requirements,* through the use of a formaldehyde exposure monitoring device. Consult an HVAC professional

---

*Refer to *www.state.nj.us/health/surv/documents/fuhomevent.pdf* for information on calculating and confirming air changes per hour in your preparation room. See NFDA, *Formaldehyde Vapor Reduction in the*

Funeral Home Preparation Room – Recommendations for Effective Preparation Room Ventilation, August 2010.

*Be sure to follow OSHA formaldehyde exposure monitoring requirements, which necessitate monitoring anytime there is a significant change in the preparation room, such as the installation of new equipment, a change in the ventilation system itself, a renovation of the preparation room, the introduction of a new chemical product containing formaldehyde, the introduction of new procedures, an increase in the number of preparations conducted or when a new embalmer is assigned and begins work in the preparation room.

regularly to ensure effective working of the funeral home's ventilation system.

1.7 Do not use ozone generators.

Scientific studies show that at concentrations below public health standards, ozone generators do not remove or even reduce formaldehyde. The U.S. EPA has issued a warning based on peer-reviewed, scientifically supported findings against the use of ozone generators because ozone, like formaldehyde, may cause serious health effects.

2.0 Select and use the proper embalming product considering the condition of the remains.

2.1 Make a practice of using the least concentrated solution and reserving the most highly concentrated solution for the most difficult cases.

The art and science of embalming requires selection of the proper product in view of the condition of the remains.

2.2 Substitute environmentally friendly products for traditional embalming products.

Discuss product options with the funeral home's chemical supplier. Funeral service suppliers might be able to provide environmentally friendly, less toxic embalming products. Consider using formaldehyde-free products.

2.3 When mixing embalming solutions, always add arterial fluids to water.

Studies indicate that bursts of formaldehyde from mixing solutions pose risk for the embalmer. Do not add water to arterial fluid. This simple change in procedure will greatly reduce the embalmers exposure to emissions from products containing formaldehyde. Start with the smallest amount of arterial fluid in the embalming solution product; more arterial fluid can be added later.

3.0 Take precautions in the preparation room to limit formaldehyde exposure and emissions during routine embalmings.

3.1 Institute work practices to avoid formaldehyde spills and if spills occur, clean spills of formaldehyde immediately.

Spills of formaldehyde have been shown to be a significant source of formaldehyde emissions. Chemical pillows and other chemicals are commercially available from industry suppliers for spill response. Ammonia serves as an inexpensive and effective neutralizer to formaldehyde. However, be sure to use a product containing a material that either permanently absorbs or destroys the formaldehyde

3.2 Always keep the lid on the embalming machine.

The embalming machine lid should be removed only when water and embalming flu-ids are added to the machine. The lid is designed to reduce emissions from the embalming solution in the machine.

3.3 If embalming wastewater is discharged into a sink, always use a sink cover to limit splashing and exposure.

Covering an embalming waste sink with Plexiglas or other appropriate material will prevent splashes and aerosols from entering the embalmer's work area.

3.4 Use all appropriate personal protective equipment to avoid skin and eye contact with formaldehyde-containing products (and any chemical products of any type.)

Make the switch from latex to nitrile gloves. Nitrile has high chemical resistance against formaldehyde without the failure rate of latex.

3.5 Limit exposure to formaldehyde and blood-borne pathogens through the use of a drain tube.

Run the drain tube (via a connection hose) from the remains to the end of the table, away from the embalmer, into the sink or discharge opening.

3.6 Follow the funeral home's written 30-day cleaning, decontamination and inspection schedule to ensure proper functioning of eyewash stations and emergency showers.

Emergency equipment must be tested to ensure that it will function properly when it is needed. Prepare a written policy that establishes a routine inspection procedure implemented every 30 days to test the functioning of eye wash stations and emergency showers.

4.0 Observe special precautions to limit formaldehyde exposure and emissions when embalming organ procurement cases and autopsied remains, as such embalmings may increase the embalmer's formaldehyde exposure risk.

4.1 Employees may elect to use a properly fitted respirator, even when measured exposure limits do not exceed OSHA standards.

Employees may elect to use a respirator even when exposure limits do not exceed OSHA standards. If this is the case, the funeral home must obtain a medical evaluation of each employee who wishes to use a respirator, even though a full OSHA-mandated respiratory program is not required.

4.2 Carefully monitor and restrict the use, to the greatest extent possible, of the most highly concentrated formaldehyde products, such as osmotic gels, hardening compounds and disinfecting sprays.

Studies have indicated that the use of compounds containing high concentrations of formaldehyde contribute significant amounts of formaldehyde to preparation room air. For that reason, the use of these compounds should be limited and other alternatives investigated.

5.0 Be familiar with and follow all federal, state and local environmental, OSHA and health requirements that apply when embalming is performed. Various environmental, OSHA and health requirements apply when an embalming is performed. Often, product selection will govern the application of these requirements. Periodically review and re-evaluate the products used in the preparation of remains. Know the constituents of the products and the requirements that these constituents make applicable. Determine whether your locality has a mechanical code or other requirements that apply to ventilation systems.

▶ PRESERVATIVE VASCULAR FLUIDS

A **preservative vascular fluid** is the concentrated embalming fluid that contains the following types of chemicals—preservatives, germicides, vehicles, dyes, perfuming, and modifying agents. This concentrated **arterial fluid** is added to water to form the **arterial solution** called the **primary dilution.**

A **preinjection fluid** is a **supplemental fluid** that may be injected **before** the injection of the preservative arterial solution. Its purpose is to expand the vascular system, promote drainage, and prepare the tissues for reception of the preservative arterial solution. A **Coinjection fluid** is a **supplemental fluid** that is mixed and injected along with the arterial solution. The coinjection fluid is designed to enhance the distribution and effectiveness of the arterial solution.

The following terms describe some of the qualities of the various fluids (Table 7-1).

Preservative Formaldehyde Arterial Fluids

1. Index
   a. *Strong:* those fluids with a formaldehyde index in the range 26 to 36
   b. *Medium:* those fluids with a formaldehyde index in the range 16 to 25
   c. *Low:* those fluids with a formaldehyde index in the range 5 to 15
2. Color
   a. *Noncosmetic:* those fluids that contain little or no active dye and do not color the tissues
   b. *Cosmetic:* those fluids that contain an active dye that colors the tissues
3. Firming speed
   a. *Fast-firming:* those fluids buffered to firm tissues rapidly

TABLE 7–1. VARIOUS ARTERIAL CHEMICALS USED IN EMBALMING

Aldehyde-Based Vascular Fluid (Preservative)	Supplemental Fluid
Index	Preinjection
Strong	Coinjection (standard)
Medium	Internal bleach
Low	Tissue gas
Nonformaldehyde	Edema corrective
Color	Germicide booster
Noncosmetic	Humectant (restorative)
Cosmetic	Water corrective
Reds	Dyes
Suntan	Pink tints
Firming speed	Suntan tints
Fast	
Slow	
Firmness	
Low	
Medium	
Strong	
Antidehydrant	
Humectant	
Nonhumectant	
Special purpose	
Jaundice	
High index	
Dehydrating	
Nondehydrating	
Tissue gas	
Infants	

   b. *Slow-firming:* those fluids buffered to firm body tissues slowly
4. Degree of firmness
   a. *Soft:* those fluids that are buffered and contain chemicals to control the preservative reaction to produce very little firming of the tissues.
   b. *Mild:* those fluids that are buffered and contain chemicals to control the preservative reaction to produce a medium firming of the tissues.
   c. *Hard:* those fluids that are buffered and contain chemicals to control the preservative reaction to produce very definite and hard firming of the tissues.
5. Moisturizing qualities
   a. *Humectants:* those fluids that contain large amounts of chemicals that act to add and retain tissue moisture.
   b. *Nonhumectants:* those fluids that do not contain chemicals that add or retain moisture.

Special-Purpose Arterial Fluids

1. *Jaundice fluids:* those fluids compounded to cover or remove the discoloration of jaundice.
2. *High-index special-purpose fluids:* a group of chemicals with indices usually greater than 30, used in the preparation of extreme cases, such as bodies with edema, those dead from renal failure, bodies dead for a long time, and bodies evidencing decomposition.
    a. *Dehydrating:* fluids compounded to bring about dehydration of the body tissues.
    b. *Nondehydrating:* fluids compounded to contain large amounts of preservatives but controlled so as not to dehydrate tissues.
3. *Tissue gas fluids:* fluids designed to arrest and control the causative agent (*Clostridium perfringens*) of tissue gas.

Preservative Nonformaldehyde Arterial Fluids

1. These contain nonformaldehyde preservatives; should be biodegradable
2. These are nontoxic and nonhazardous to the embalmer
3. These produce little or no firming of the body tissues
4. These provide a temporary preservation of the body
5. Some may be environmental friendly and usable by Green and Natural Burial groups

▶ ARTERIAL FLUID DILUTION

The mixture of arterial fluid with water and/or supplemental fluids is called the **primary dilution.** In the tissue spaces, the arterial solution is further diluted; this is called the **secondary dilution.** Fluid manufacturers generally make dilution recommendations. These recommendations are placed on the bottle label or printed in a technical manual. For the experienced embalmer, the proper use of any embalming chemical comes with its use over time. Through the use of the chemical, the embalmer observes its reaction on body conditions and at what strengths the chemical can be used to achieve the results desired by the embalmer. Most manufacturers also state that, if desired results are not being achieved, the judgment of the embalmer determines how the dilutions should be changed.

To obtain optimum results, the arterial chemicals, strength and volume of the arterial solutions, and the techniques for arterial injection and drainage need to vary somewhat with each body. **Each deceased human body has its own preservative demand.** This demand is determined by the (1) physical conditions of the body,

(2) body protein, (3) antemortem pathological conditions, (4) antemortem effects of drugs and chemotherapy, and (5) the postmortem conditions which are present. This **preembalming analysis** of the body establishes the arterial fluids to be used and the strength of the arterial solutions.

After arterial injection has begun, the embalmer needs to determine the strength and volume of subsequent arterial solutions to adequately distribute the solution to all body areas and meet the preservative demands of the body. Some embalmers prefer that the body tissues be extremely firm, whereas others prefer skin textures to be less firm and more natural to the touch. Arterial dilutions may need to be adjusted to achieve this desired result.

Labels often contain information pertaining to one general body condition, such as moisture content. Others may include a specific condition (e.g., recommended dilutions for decomposing bodies, frozen bodies, bodies dead from renal failure, or infants). Some may contain a minimum dilution at which to begin injection. Speaking in general terms, in the preparation of the unautopsied, "average body" milder solutions are used to begin the embalming because this will assist in the clearing of intravascular blood discolorations. Subsequent injections can be increased in strength to achieve desired firmness and disinfection of the tissues. Contrast that with a body in which a condition such as renal failure, generalized edema, or early signs of decomposition may be present, and there is a necessity to begin and continue with a very strong arterial solution. **The analogy of arterial fluid could be likened to the prescribing of medicine in which not every type or dosage of a drug will react on each patient and each condition in the same manner.**

Fluid labels may contain an **index** number. Index is defined as *the amount of formaldehyde, measured in grams, dissolved in 100 mL of solution.* Some manufacturers do not use the term "index" as a measurement of the overall capability of a fluid to preserve a body. One reason is that index is only a measure of formaldehyde. Often, a combination of preservatives will be used in an arterial fluid formulation; therefore, other preservative factors are present in the formulation. To determine the strength of a primary dilution using the index factor, a very simple equation can be employed. This formula has four factors:

$$\text{Index} \times \text{volume of fluid} = \text{strength of solution} \times \text{total volume}$$
$$c \times v = c' \times v'$$

To prepare a 2% arterial solution using a 25-index fluid, it is necessary to know how much fluid is needed to make a 1-gallon solution of 2% strength.

TABLE 7–2. PREPARATION OF VARIOUS PERCENTAGE ALDEHYDE "IN USE" SOLUTIONS[a]

Concentration Rate per Gallon (oz)	% Aldehyde in Concentrate (Index)				
	15	20	25	30	35
4	0.47	0.625	0.78	0.94	1.10
5	0.59	0.18	0.98	1.17	1.38
6	0.70	0.94	1.17	1.41	1.64
7	0.82	1.10	1.37	1.64	1.91
8	0.93	1.25	1.56	1.88	2.19
9	1.05	1.41	1.76	2.11	2.46
10	1.17	1.56	1.95	2.34	2.73
11	1.29	1.72	2.15	2.59	3.01
12	1.41	1.86	2.34	2.81	3.28
13	1.52	2.03	2.54	3.05	3.55
14	1.64	2.19	2.73	3.28	3.83
15	1.76	2.34	2.93	3.52	4.10
16	1.88	2.50	3.13	3.75	4.38
17	1.99	2.66	3.32	3.98	4.65
18	2.11	2.81	3.52	4.22	4.92
19	2.23	2.97	3.71	4.45	5.20
20	2.34	3.13	3.91	4.69	5.47
21	2.46	3.18	4.10	4.92	5.74
22	2.58	3.44	4.30	5.16	6.02
23	2.70	3.59	4.49	5.39	6.29
24	2.81	3.15	4.69	5.63	6.56
25	2.93	3.91	4.88	5.86	6.84
26	3.05	4.06	5.01	6.09	7.11
27	3.16	4.22	5.27	6.33	7.38
28	3.28	4.38	5.47	6.56	7.66
29	3.40	4.53	5.66	6.80	7.92
30	3.52	4.69	5.86	7.03	8.20

[a]Fluid ounces × index ÷ by 128 (oz/gal) = % aldehyde in solution.
Source: Courtesy of Champion Co., Springfield, Ohio.

Since 1 gallon is 128 oz

$$25 \times x = 2\% \times 128 \text{ oz of total solution}$$
$$25x = 256$$
$$x = \frac{256}{25}$$
$$x = 10.2 \text{ oz of arterial fluid}$$

Approximately 10 oz of arterial fluid and 118 oz of water would be needed to make 1 gallon of 2% strength arterial solution.

Using the label directions, determine the strength of the arterial solution when 7 oz of fluid and one full gallon of water are used (Table 7–2).

$$25 \times 7 = x \times 135 (128 \text{ oz of water and 7 oz of fluid of fluid})$$
$$175 = 135x$$
$$x = \frac{175}{135} \quad \text{or} \quad x = 1.29\%$$

Quantity of Arterial Solution

The average 160-pound unautopsied body contains approximately 10 pints (one-and-a-half gallons) of blood. During the embalming of the body, this blood is replaced with the arterial solution; a portion of the arterial solution will remain in the vascular system and a necessary portion is needed to move into the tissue spaces to preserve the body cells and tissues. Drainage taken during arterial injection contains blood, tissue fluid, and arterial solution. It is estimated that as much as 55% of the arterial solution can be lost in the drainage (see, **Selected Readings: The Measurement of Formaldehyde Retention in the Tissues of Embalmed Bodies**). It is the arterial solution that remains within the body that preserves and sanitizes. A review of a number of embalming care reports shows that 3 to 4 gallons of the proper strength of arterial solution are generally sufficient for the embalming of this "average" deceased body. These are bodies without edema, renal failure, or signs of decomposition.

The "50-pound rule" is an old rule but it is still found on the labels of some arterial fluids. It simply states that 1 gallon of properly prepared arterial solution should be injected for each 50 pounds of body weight. This was a guideline used for many years. It rather complies with the preceding paragraph. However, today with the overuse of medications, all too often edema is present or multiple system failure occurred prior to death or there have been extensive delays between the death and the embalming. These situations call for stronger arterial solutions and often in greater volume than 1 gallon for every 50 pounds of body weight.

▶ PRESERVATIVE DEMAND: ARTERIAL SOLUTION STRENGTH AND VOLUME

A sufficient quantity of arterial solution at the proper strength needs to be injected. Medications used over a long period of time may have had effects, which increase the demand for fluid. Examples include

- the effect of the drug on the preservative solution
- the damage the drug has done to the body proteins
- the damage done to specific organs such as the liver and the kidneys, causing retention of wastes such as ammonia and urea in the tissues
- the damage done to the cell membrane—a possible condition in which it is difficult for fluids to pass through the cell membranes.

Consider these points in determining the strength and amount of fluid to inject:

- time between death and preparation
- time between preparation and disposition

- moisture content of the body
- renal failure and the buildup of nitrogenous **wastes** in the body
- liver failure and the buildup of toxic wastes in the body tissues
- weight of the body
- amount of adipose tissue versus muscular tissues accounting for body weight
- protein levels of the body
- progress of the postmortem physical and chemical changes, especially the stages of decomposition and rigor mortis
- nature of death—sudden heart attack versus wasting disease; use of life-support systems for many weeks
- chemotherapy and medications given to the individual.

▶ GENERAL GUIDELINES FOR ARTERIAL SOLUTION STRENGTH AND VOLUME

"Embalming the unautopsied body: Inject a sufficient volume (quantity), of arterial solution at a strength (quality) necessary to meet the preservative demands of the body; using a pressure and rate of flow so as to distribute the solution to all body regions causing the solution to diffuse to the tissues and cells without noticeable distension or dehydration. Body regions can vary: some regions may receive insufficient solution while other areas may receive too much. Some body regions may have a higher preservative demand because of disease processes. This may necessitate a separate injection (multi-point) possibly using a different strength of arterial solution."

General Guidelines:

1. General "rules"
   a. The arterial solution must be strong enough to meet the preservative (formaldehyde) demands of the body.
   b. Begin with a mild solution and then increase strength once distribution is established.
   c. If you dilute a high index fluid to make a mild or "very mild" solution, you not only dilute the preservative, for example, formaldehyde but also dilute all of the modifying agents.
2. Preferences of the embalmer: embalming is an **art** and a **science.** Some embalmers or funeral homes want the bodies to have a natural feel; others prefer that the bodies be very firm to the touch. If we embalmed all bodies by **science,** they might all look like anatomical subjects!

3. The "average body" contains about 10 pints of blood. By injecting 3 to 4 gallons of solution, this more than displaces the blood and fills the vascular system and tissue spaces. It is estimated that as much as 50% of injected arterial solution can be lost through drainage.
4. **Manufacturer's recommendations:** Some fluid companies will give dilution directions. These directions may be based on one of the following:
   a. First gallon strength, for example, 4 to 6 oz; subsequent dilutions at 6 to 10 oz based on the body needs **or** minimum, medium, and maximum ounces at which the fluid can be used.
   b. The 50-pound rule—based on body weight.
   c. Body moisture conditions; dilutions for no edema; mild and intense edema.
   d. Specific fluids for specific body conditions, for example, jaundice, decomposition, renal failure, trauma, refrigerated, edema, and frozen bodies.
   e. Strength will be based on the "clearing of the blood discolorations"; the rule here is inject "mild solutions" first, followed by stronger solutions.
   f. Manufacturers will state that the embalmer must use sufficient fluid and solution to achieve the embalmer's desired results.
5. Dr. Jerome F. Frederick—1968: Average body = 160 pounds; contains 10,700 g of protein; needs 470 g of formaldehyde which equals three bottles of a 30-index fluid (see **Selected Readings: The Mathematics of Embalming Chemistry**).
6. Rendon/Rose Hockett guidelines: 2% strength arterial solution; volume: 3 to 4 gallons or the 50-pound rule (see **Selected Readings**).
7. Armed services rules: viewable remains, 2 to 3% formaldehyde = equal parts of humectant; nonviewable remains, minimum of 3% solution (see **Selected Readings**).
8. Waterless embalming: two bottles arterial; two bottles water conditioner; two bottles coinjection; one bottle humectant.

▶ WATERLESS EMBALMING

Waterless embalming is a concept that has been discussed among embalmers and in funeral service literature for many years. It has seen more frequent use since the mid-1970s, when more bodies exhibited edema and tissues that were difficult to firm, as the result of chemotherapy and the extensive use of drugs. It is based on the theory that "water does not preserve!" A waterless solution is composed of an arterial fluid not diluted with water but rather **diluted with** supplemental fluids such as coinjection, humectants, and water-corrective fluids.

The phrase "waterless" is somewhat deceptive for almost all embalming chemicals contain a certain amount of water in their formulations. The water is used as a solvent for some of the chemicals. The phrase "waterless" simply means that no water is added by the embalmer.

Example: 16 oz of a preservative arterial fluid mixed with 48 oz of a coinjection, 48 oz of water corrective, and 16 oz of humectant—to make a gallon of solution. Second and subsequent injections could contain 16 oz of a preservative arterial fluid, 16 oz of humectant, 16 oz of water conditioner, and 16 oz of coinjection to make half-gallon solutions.

Waterless embalming provides maximum preservation using a minimum amount of arterial solution. This may be very valuable when swelling of tissues is a concern to the embalmer. If desired little or no drainage can be taken when a waterless solution is employed. Several examples include:

- Facial trauma
- Bodies exhibiting decomposition
- Septic bodies
- Refrigerated bodies
- Frozen bodies
- Bodies with tissue gas
- Gangrene in a localized area
- Edema in a localized area
- Highly infectious and/or contagious bodies
- Bodies needing to be re-embalmed

Arterial Solution pH

The pH of the arterial solution is determined by the fluid manufacturer. This is not an element of the fluid that the embalmer determines. Most arterial fluids are buffered to be slightly alkaline in pH, approximately 7.2 to 7.4. At this pH, the fluid reaction is stable, dyes in the fluid work well, and the tissues do not exhibit a tendency to turn gray.

Some fluids are buffered to rapidly react. When using these fluids, the embalmer must be certain that a sufficient volume of fluid has been injected. Because these fluids cause rapid firming of the body, there is a tendency to use an insufficient amount of solution.

With all embalming, after surface blood discolorations have been cleared, intermittent drainage can be employed. Inject a sufficient quantity of solution, making every effort to **retain** as much solution as possible within the body.

Arterial Fluid Temperature

The best instructions to follow in diluting arterial fluids are the manufacturer's recommendations. Most companies state on the label what temperature of water to employ. The majority of fluids are diluted with room temperature water. Only in special cases, such as in the treatment of tissue gas or decomposition, it is recommended that fluids be diluted with warm water. When in doubt, use water at room temperature to dilute the fluid.

Density/Specific Gravity

Certain solid chemical substances known as salts play an important role in determining the characteristics of the different embalming fluids and in controlling, to a large extent, the reactions between the cellular tissues and the chemical solution. When salt is dissolved in water, it is possible to form solutions of different concentrations depending on the amount of salt added to the water. The more salt (solute) added to the water (solvent), the more concentrated the solution becomes. In other words, the strength of the solution actually indicates how much solute is present. The amount of solute in a solution has a direct effect on the density of the solution.

Density is defined as mass per unit volume and is expressed in such units as grams per cubic centimeter. Thus, it can be seen how density relates to the concentration of the solute in the solution. Often, it is desirable to compare the density of a given substance with the density of water. This ratio is called **specific gravity.** If a substance has a specific gravity of 1.5, it means that compared with the density of water, the substance is 1.5 times as dense. Again, as with density, the specific gravity of a solution varies with concentration.

In solutions used in medicine, either the density or the salt concentration of a solution is frequently compared with that of blood. If a solution contains less of a dissolved substance than is found in blood, it is said to be **hypotonic.** If it contains a greater quantity of a dissolved substance than is found in the blood, it is said to be **hypertonic.**

During embalming, blood and other body liquids are eventually replaced with the chemical preservative solution, which changes the nature of tissue. Such change resists decomposition. The penetration of such solution into all soft tissue areas should be thorough to achieve complete preservation and produce the best results.

It has been found that a solution that is slightly hypotonic to blood and body fluids produces the best embalming results. A review of the scientific principle involved will show why this is so.

In part **A** of the accompanying diagram, a membranous bag, such as from a section of animal intestine that is "semipermeable," that is, permeable to some materials

Semi-Permeable Membrane   10% Salt Solution NaCl

Hypertonic Solution

Distilled Water (Hypotonic)

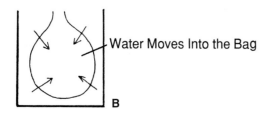

Water Moves Into the Bag

but not to others, is placed in a container of distilled water. The bag contains a 10% salt solution. In part **B**, it is observed to increase in volume. This demonstrates that water has passed into the bag. Now, it will be interesting to reduce this observation to a simple explanation.

The distilled water, being "hypotonic" (i.e., of **less** density), passes to the inside of the bag, which contains the more highly concentrated solution (i.e., of **higher** density). The solution in the bag in diagram **A**, then, is hypertonic to the distilled water. What is the importance of all this to the embalming operation and to embalming fluids?

It is known that a solution will penetrate to the side or region containing the more dense solution; this fact is used in compounding fluids and in establishing the proper concentrations to use in embalming. When diluted according to the recommended usage, the resultant solution is slightly hypotonic to blood and body liquids. If less of the concentrated fluid is used, then the resultant solution may be more hypotonic than desired for proper embalming results. The tissues tend to become "waterlogged," which eventually results in skin slip (desquamation) because of the lack of sufficient preservative material.

On the other hand, if too much concentrated fluid is used, according to the preceding principle, a hypertonic solution results, and it will have the effect of removing too much moisture. This, of course, causes excessive dehydration. In some instances, the embalmer may want to make use of this principle to remove excess moisture from tissue areas, such as in dropsical or edematous cases. The "special" fluids designed for such purposes incorporate this principle.

Briefly, then, an embalming solution that is less dense (i.e., hypotonic) than the tissue liquids will flow rapidly through the capillary walls into the soft tissue areas. If the solution is designed so that it has a greater density (i.e., hypertonic) than the tissue liquids, it will draw tissue liquid through the capillary wall into the circulatory system and away from the soft tissue areas.

Osmotic Qualities

For the average or "normal" body, in which there is no edema or dehydration, the arterial solution should be hypotonic in its osmotic composition. This is generally achieved by following the manufacturer's dilution instructions. When the solution is hypotonic to the body tissues, the fluid moves from the capillary vessels into the tissue spaces. If these solutions were hypertonic, tissue fluids would move from the tissue space into the capillary vessels, thus causing dehydration and lack of arterial fluid in the tissues.

There are instances when hypertonic solutions are desired. This type of solution is generally used when embalming bodies with skeletal edema (edema of the limbs). These solutions help to move the excess water from the tissue into the capillary vessels by increasing the osmotic permeability of the cell membranes. From there, the water can be removed through drainage. Some embalmers add Epsom salts to the arterial solutions to create these hypertonic dehydrating solutions. The high-index special-purpose fluids, when diluted in a certain manner, create dehydrating hypertonic solutions.

▶ SPECIAL-PURPOSE ARTERIAL FLUIDS

High-Index Fluids

These preservative arterial fluids have a formaldehyde index of 28 to 36. Such fluids are designed for use in the preparation of difficult-to-embalm bodies. In addition, these fluids have two other uses. First, some embalmers use these fluids for routine preparations. Second, these fluids can be used to fortify or increase the firming and preservative qualities of regular arterial solutions.

Example. An embalmer mixes a solution of arterial fluid using a 22-index fluid and uses 8 oz to the gallon for the solution. If firming of the body seems not to be happening, in the second and subsequent gallons, several ounces of the high-index fluid will be added to the solution to increase the preservative strength of the solution.

Solutions are always mixed from mild to strong, not the reverse. If there is to be a change in solution strength, embalming solutions are always increased in strength.

The following statement from the Dodge Chemical Company regarding one of its special-purpose high-index fluids explains well the use of this chemical:

The more severe the conditions of the body, the stronger the primary solution should be. When little drainage is anticipated, stronger concentrations and less total volume of solution should be used. When normal drainage is achieved, the volume of solution to be used will be governed by the size, weight, and conditions of the body. In general, in treating bodies of "difficult" types, a good rule to follow is: more rather than less chemical—and less rather than more water. Water will not preserve nor will it arrest putrefaction—but it will create swelling and distension.

There are situations in which the use of high-index fluid is advised, such as for bodies

- dead for extended periods of time
- that have been frozen or extended refrigeration
- that have undergone extensive treatments with drugs
- that have been institutionalized
- with traumatic injuries for which restorative treatments will be needed
- with evidence of decomposition
- with gangrenous limbs
- that are difficult to firm
- with skeletal edema
- dead from renal failure
- with bloodstream infections
- with tissue gas present
- obese bodies

Some companies produce two types of high-index fluids: **dehydrating** and **nondehydrating.** The nondehydrating fluid is designed to deliver a strong formaldehyde and preservative action with a minimum of dehydration. As with other arterial fluids, it is best to follow the dilutions recommended by the manufacturer. Most of the high-index fluids, when used as a "booster" fluid, work well with standard arterial fluids of other companies. Because of the problems encountered with delayed embalming and the wide use of drug therapy today, *this arterial fluid should always be kept on hand in the preparation room.*

Jaundice Fluids

A second special-purpose preservative arterial fluid is jaundice fluid. Jaundice fluids are used not only to preserve the body but also to hide or rid the body of mild jaundice or to prevent the jaundice color from changing to green. These fluids are most effective on the body that has only a mild jaundice discoloration as opposed to bodies with deep jaundice discoloration. These fluids do little to remove deep discoloration.

Bleaching Fluids. Bleaching fluids oxidize the discoloration. The chemicals employed in the formulations include peroxides, citric acid, and phenols. These chemicals are usually employed in an alcohol medium.

Coupling Compound System. The coupling compound system combines a chemical with the bile pigment to decolorize the pigment. A preinjection coupling compound (e.g., a diazo agent in a nonacidic medium) is injected first. The aldehyde arterial injection follows. The system is complex, time consuming, and not always reliable.

Chemical Adduct System. In the chemical adduct system, a chemical is combined with formaldehyde; later, the formaldehyde is slowly released.

A final caution with regard to jaundice fluids; manufactures directions should be followed. When using a jaundice fluid, do *not* mix this fluid with other arterial fluids or preinjection fluids, unless the directions accompanying the jaundice fluid call for the use of a preinjection fluid. If a preinjection fluid is recommended, it would, no doubt, be best to use the preinjection fluid manufactured by the same company that made the jaundice fluid.

Tissue Gas Fluid

A variety of fluids have been manufactured by chemical companies to treat the condition known as tissue gas. This condition is caused by *C. perfringens*, an anaerobic spore forming bacterium. It is important that the directions for these fluids be carefully followed.

Nonformaldehyde Preservative Arterial Fluids

Environmental issues and the probable carcinogenic qualities of formaldehyde have been leading to a development of arterial fluids using preservatives other than formaldehyde. Some of these fluids contain preservatives, modifying agents, and dyes that are nontoxic, nonhazardous, and biodegradable. Such fluids can be used for the temporary preservation of bodies being buried in "Green" or "Natural" cemeteries.

Other formaldehyde-free fluids contain chemicals that are not biodegradable and can be considered hazardous to the embalmer or the environment. They do provide a temporary preservation of the body but they cannot be used for bodies that are to be buried in strict Green Cemeteries.

These fluids may produce little or no firming of the body tissues. As indicated, the preservation of the body is very temporary. **Manufacturer's directions for use should be strictly followed.**

► SUPPLEMENTAL FLUIDS

Preinjection Fluid

A preinjection fluid is injected into the body before the preservative arterial solution is injected. These fluids were first used because the early arterial fluids were so strong and harsh that they caused difficulty in clearing the blood from the capillaries and veins. The preinjection fluid (also called a **primary injection fluid** or **capillary wash**) was designed to clear the blood vascular system of the blood prior to injection of the preservative solution.

Today, arterial fluids contain a number of modifying agents that allow the arterial solutions to distribute and diffuse uniformly. For this reason, many embalmers do not use preinjection fluids. Others, however, still feel the necessity to flush the vascular system with a preinjection solution. This helps to improve distribution and drainage, clear blood discolorations, adjusts the pH of the tissues which helps to reduce graying of the tissues, reduces blood coagulation, and reduces harsh effects that may be caused by preservatives such as formaldehyde. Two factors are necessary to obtain the best results with this chemical: (1) a sufficient quantity should be injected and (2) some time should be allowed for the chemical to work properly.

Manufacturer's instructions will give dilutions and amount of chemical to inject. These fluids have little or no preservative and it is possible to waterlog the tissues, with improper use.

Some preinjection fluids contain small amounts of preservatives. For this reason, some embalmers use these chemicals to embalm infants and children; however, **it is preferable that standard preservative arterial fluid be used for the preparation of infants and children.** The embalmer may wish to use a preinjection solution only to assist in preparing the circulatory system for the preservative arterial solution.

Preinjection treatment is generally used only on unautopsied bodies and not for treatment on autopsied bodies in which each body area is separately injected. Also note that preinjection fluids contain little or no active dye to color the tissues.

In embalming bodies where there has been any great time delay between death and embalming or where the embalmer feels circulation may be difficult to establish, preinjection fluids should be avoided. A preinjection fluid can loosen clots in the venous system and, thus, make them easier to remove. This, in turn, improves blood drainage. If there is any clotting in the arterial system, preinjection fluids can loosen these clots as well. They will be carried by the fluid to smaller arteries where they can easily block circulation channels. Preinjection fluid works best when it is used on bodies that the embalmer feels circulation will be very good.

The following statements have been compiled from several different fluid company catalogs and contain descriptions of different preinjection fluids. Reading these may help the student, in particular, to understand the purpose of these fluids.

Examples

Fluid A promotes drainage and capillary circulation. *Many bodies present the challenge of a highly complex residual body chemistry. The extent and identification of this chemistry are not always known.* Fluid A is proven to be the embalmer's best and most direct approach to the control of adverse residual body chemistry. Fluid A is unmatched in its scope for body conditioning, and its use prevents complications.

Fluid B is a very fine primary injection fluid. It conditions the arterial system and expands the small arterioles and venules to make the subsequent arterial injections more effective and complete. Research has shown that an alkaline condition of the tissues is desirable to retain their natural color (acid brings on an ashen gray appearance), and yet, a strongly alkaline solution tends to waterlog the body. The bonus feature of Fluid B is a *touch of preservative* effect. It has been found that a low index of formaldehyde in a *slightly alkaline* primary injection fluid is the complete answer, actually making the tissues more receptive to later contact with preservative chemicals. *One of Fluid B's most important functions is to establish the proper pH in the circulatory system and adjacent tissues to promote constantly uniform results in all cases.*

Coinjection Fluid

An arterial fluid and a coinjection fluid should combine to form a homogenous solution that can be distributed and diffused throughout the body. As for the amount to use, remember that the manufacturer's labels are the best guide.

Most coinjection fluids are used in an amount equal to the amount of concentrated arterial fluid. Or, half as much coinjection fluid as concentrated arterial solution is used. Generally, the amount of coinjection fluid should never exceed the amount of concentrated arterial fluid. When too much coinjection fluid is used (plus the use of water softeners), it has a tendency to distribute unevenly and the dyes have a tendency to "blotch." When in doubt, a good rule is to use equal amounts of coinjection fluid and concentrated arterial fluid.

When should a coinjection fluid be used? This chemical, unlike a preinjection chemical, can be employed with every preparation. It assists in distributing and diffusing the arterial solution and helps to control and enhance the arterial fluid. In some special conditions, embalmers use the coinjection fluid as the diluent, for example, in the technique of "rapid tissue fixation." Some individuals also practice waterless embalming. In this process, the coinjection fluid takes the place of water in the arterial solution.

Examples

Fluid ABC *acts with all arterial fluids.* A few ounces added to the arterial solution will ensure the creation of an unparalleled naturalness. In addition, it will practically eliminate the possibility of dehydration and feature shrinkage, no matter how long the interval between the embalming and interment. *Distribution and diffusion will be increased to a pronounced degree,* drainage will be more copious, preservation will be more permanent, and the skin will have the same velvety freshness it had in life. Fluid ABC is indispensable in every operation in which a standard arterial fluid is used. It is especially effective in emaciated subjects, infants and the aged, and in all situations in which pathologic or climatic conditions necessitate the use of a stronger than normal arterial solution. Fluid E diffuses unhindered through the capillary walls and all internal membranes to enter every tissue cell and combine with the cellular protoplasm. It creates a permanent, waxy, moisture-retaining shield, the presence of which can be detected by the velvety texture of the skin.

Fluid DEF is a *dual-purpose fluid* for addition to each arterial injection. In action, it *softens and lubricates blood clots.* At the same time, it conditions and *reduces water hardness to zero,* with an overall improvement in embalming results. It is not a blood solvent, nor is it a preservative. It does, however, contribute importantly to the solution of any drainage problem. It breaks down clots so that they may be removed by way of the drain tube. To date, there is no known chemical that can be used effectively to dissolve a blood clot totally without having, at the same time, an adverse effect on the circulatory system.

Water Corrective Fluid

Water corrective chemicals can be added (used as a coinjection fluid) to all embalming solutions when water is used as a vehicle. This means that a water conditioner can be added to a preembalming solution as well as to a preservative solution. It is best to follow the manufacturer's guidelines as to the amount to use. Generally, only a few ounces are used for each gallon of solution. Overuse of this chemical can cause blotching of fluid dyes. Details as to the purposes of this chemical can be reviewed in Chapter 6 of this text. Some embalmers use water corrective chemicals for all injections; others rarely or never use this product. In areas of the country where water is exceptionally hard, its use can be most valuable.

Water corrective chemicals can also be used as vehicles for "waterless" embalming solutions. Here, one or more bottles of chemical can be used to dilute the arterial fluid. Water conditioners can also be used for removing salts and other solidified chemicals from the embalming machine. Generally, 8 oz or more can be added to warm water to flush and clean the machine.

Dyes

Dye is used in arterial solutions for several reasons. Inactive dyes merely color the arterial fluid. Active dyes serve several functions:

1. They act as a tracer so that the location of the arterial fluid can be noted in areas of the body, a sign of arterial fluid distribution.
2. They help restore the natural color of the skin, which changes when blood is drained from the tissues.
3. They help to prevent the body from darkening as a result of reaction with the blood, which remains within the body after the embalming.

Dye can be used in all arterial solutions injected or only in the final gallon of solution. There are two main objections to the use of additional dye throughout the embalming operation: (1) the tissues will be overstained and create a cosmetic problem and (2) the embalmer, seeing the dye in the superficial tissue, may tend to underembalm the body.

The amount of dye to add again depends on the fluid manufacturer. Follow the directions on the label and then add or cut back to suit individual preference. For some dyes, only several drops are required per gallon, whereas for other dyes, several ounces are required.

Humectant (Restorative) Fluid

The separately purchased humectant is really a coinjection fluid. The reason for this is quite simple. The humectant is added and injected along with the arterial fluid. Some embalmers use humectants only when the body is dehydrated. Others add extra humectant to all arterial solutions when embalming a body with normal moisture to prevent dehydration. The amount of humectant added to each gallon of solution should follow the manufacturer's directions. Humectants hydrate and add moisture to the tissues and they also prevent tissue dehydration.

Some humectants are colloids, and these viscous colloid mixtures, when injected into the arterial system, have a tendency to draw moisture **out of the tissues** and into the capillaries. If additional humectants are used and solutions are injected into the body with continuous drainage, evidence of dehydration can be seen in such areas as the lips, fingers, and backs of the hands. Most embalmers, when adding humectants to the arterial solution, use intermittent drainage. In this manner, the humectant is held in the capillaries and tissue spaces and does not draw moisture from the tissues.

For a severely emaciated body, some embalmers add a large amount of humectant to the final gallon injected.

In addition, they close off the drainage, causing the facial tissues to distend, restoring them to their natural contour. If this technique is employed, a close watch must be kept on the facial features; gross distention of such areas as the tissues around the eyes can cause more problems.

Edema Reducing Fluid

Edema corrective coinjection chemicals reduce tissues swollen with edema. Manufacturer's instructions should be strictly followed. The amount of chemical to use will depend on the severity of the edema. The corrective chemical is added to the preservative arterial solution as a coinjection fluid. It can be very effective in reducing swollen facial tissues, which often accompany vascular or heart surgery.

The edema corrective chemical changes the osmotic qualities of the embalming solution and draws the edema from the tissue spaces back into the venous drainage. Best results are obtained when a region, such as the head, is separately injected using the corrective treatment. Massage and elevation of the affected area also help to remove the swollen condition. If too much chemical is used, areas such as the facial tissues or hands can become dehydrated. This can produce dark discoloring of the tissues and wrinkles.

Tissue Gas Coinjection Fluid

Tissue gas coinjection fluids are germicidal and act on the microbe responsible for tissues gas formation, *C. perfringens*. This coinjection fluid is usually added to an arterial solution. Strictly follow the manufacturer's directions for use.

Internal Bleach and Stain Remover

This supplemental chemical is added to the arterial solution to lighten blood or decomposition discolorations when they are present on the face or hands.

▶ CAVITY FLUID

As the name indicates, cavity fluid is injected into the body cavities. Routinely, cavity fluid is injected into the thoracic, abdominal, and pelvic cavities. In some special cases, the cranial cavity can also be treated by injecting some fluid via a large needle or infant trocar into the cranial cavity.

Depending on the size of the body, 32 (or two bottles) to 48 oz (or more) of cavity fluid are distributed via the trocar over the viscera of the thoracic, abdominal, and pelvic cavities. The principal component of these fluids is preservative. Obviously, there is little need for dyes, anticoagulants, or humectants in these fluids.

Cavity fluid *preserves*, *disinfects*, and *deodorizes* organs of the cavities, contents of the hollow viscera, and walls of the cavities. There are, however, other uses for cavity fluids:

- Preservation of viscera removed at an autopsy.
- As a surface compress to help treat tissues not reached by arterial profusion.
- Injection via hypodermic needle or trocar into tissues that lack sufficient arterial preservation.
- As a surface compress on lesions and pathologic conditions to dry and deodorize.
- As an arterial fluid in the preparation of difficult cases such as advanced decomposition, tissue gas, and jaundice. Use only those cavity chemicals recommended by the manufacturer for arterial injection; not all cavity chemicals can be injected arterially.
- As a surface treatment for gangrenous and dropsical limbs to help dry and preserve the tissues.
- To bleach blood discolorations.
- To dry tissues when excisions have been performed.
- For surface preservation of fetal remains.

Fumeless Cavity Fluids

Because formaldehyde is the principal component of most cavity fluids, working with these chemicals can be very difficult because of the pungent odor produced by formaldehyde. Fumeless fluids, particularly cavity fluids, are produced by many manufacturers. There are three ways in which fumeless fluids can be produced: (1) covering the formaldehyde with a perfuming- or masking-type deodorant, (2) substituting other preservatives for formaldehyde (a good example would be the use of phenol), or (3) using formaldehyde donor compounds (these compounds do not release the formaldehyde until it is in contact with the tissues). A problem with the first method, perfuming the formaldehyde, is that the embalmer can breathe these fumes with little irritation at the time but later notices that large amounts of formaldehyde have been inhaled. The second method is good and is used by many manufacturers, but other preservatives lack the penetrating qualities of formaldehyde. The last method is used mainly in the production of arterial fluids. Its cost is prohibitive in the formulation of most cavity fluids.

▶ ACCESSORY EMBALMING CHEMICALS

Accessory chemicals are those used to treat the dead human body for purposes other than arterial embalming or cavity treatment. They include autopsy gels, concentrated cautery chemicals, hardening compounds, concentrated preservative powder, concentrated deodorant powder, concentrated disinfectant powder, mold inhibitors, powdered sealing agents, cream or "putty" sealing agents, and surface sealing agents.

Autopsy (Surface) Gels

These surface preservative gels are available in two viscosities: a gel that is thin and can be poured and a more viscous gel that can easily be applied by brush to surfaces. Preservative gels are used in several ways. They may be

- poured over the viscera returned from an autopsy in the plastic bag in which the viscera have been placed.
- applied to the surface of viscera in partial autopsies.
- used as a preservative in the orbital area after enucleation.
- applied to the walls of cavities and surfaces, such as the cranial cavity and calvarium in autopsied bodies.
- applied as a surface preservative to pathologic conditions such as decubitus ulcerations and gangrenous or necrotic areas.
- applied as a disinfectant and as an odor reducer.
- applied to surface areas of the body that the embalmer feels have received insufficient arterial fluid.
- used to bleach discolored areas such as ecchymoses and postmortem stains.
- used to preserve, cauterize, and deodorize burned tissues.
- used to pack the anal orifice and colostomy opening.

Preservative gels are designed as surface or osmotic preservatives. These adhering and penetrating gels not only preserve tissues but also bleach blood and decomposition discolorations. In addition, they eliminate odors when applied to pathologic conditions such as gangrene or decubitus ulcerations.

As with most preservative chemicals, care should be taken to use these gels in a well-ventilated embalming room and with proper protective covering worn. When the gels are applied to an external surface, they should be covered with cotton or plastic. This improves the effectiveness of the gel in addition to reducing the fumes.

Each manufacturer recommends the length of time the gels should remain on a surface to be most effective. Several hours would be a good rule. The embalmer can check from time to time on the working action of the gel. When the gels are applied to necrotic areas (as on the legs), plastic stockings should be placed on the body and the gel should not be removed. The same is true for application over decubitus ulcerations. The compresses should be left in place and plastic garments such as pants or coveralls should be placed on the body.

Cautery Chemicals

Cauterizing chemicals are liquids that are basically phenol (carbolic acid). Those sold through embalming manufacturers contain about 2 to 5% of phenol. It should be emphasized that whenever these chemicals are used, the embalmer must wear eye protection. Unlike most embalming chemicals that irritate the eyes, carbolic acid can actually burn and scar eye tissue. Gloves must be worn when handling phenol.

A cautery chemical can be applied to the areas where the skin has been removed, for example, abrasions, skin slip, blisters that have been opened, and burned areas. Phenol is a rapid-acting cautery agent and dries these areas in minutes. Phenol can be used as a surface bleach (applied as a pack) or injected by hypodermic needle subcutaneously. Phenol is a reducing and constricting agent. It can be injected into swollen areas such as black eyes or hematomas and allowed to remain for a time. When external pressure is placed on the swollen area, some of the phenol is forced from the area along with some of the liquids responsible for the swelling. In addition to the above, cautery chemicals are good germicides.

Tissue Builder

A tissue builder is a chemical injected by hypodermic syringe and needle **after** arterial embalming. It is injected into sunken areas of the face and hands to help restore their natural contour when the body exhibits a great loss of weight. Individual features such as the lips or the fingers can also be treated with this chemical. Once injected beneath the skin, it can be spread through the tissues by finger pressure. It is important to not overfill an area; it is almost impossible to remove the tissue builder once it is injected. Tissue builder contains nitrocellulose and several types of alcohols.

Solvents

The embalmer uses three solvents in various embalming treatments. A **general solvent** is used for cleansing of the skin surface, usually the face and the hands. Most of these solvents can also be used for cleansing of the scalp and hair. They are useful in removing cosmetics from the hair, eyelashes, and eyebrows. Older formulations contained chemicals such as trichloroethylene or acetone. Newer products are free of these chemicals and less toxic to the embalmer. A **tissue builder solvent** (methyl alcohol) is used to clean hypodermic syringes and needles that have been used for the injection of tissue builder. Some embalmers like to store syringes with a few milliliters of solvent in them. Anytime a syringe is used, it should be flushed with this solvent before another chemical is used. A third solvent found in the preparation room is finger nail polish remover, primarily **acetone.**

Hardening and Autopsy Compounds

These compounds are blends of powdered chemicals. They dry moist tissue. In addition, some hardening compounds contain powdered preservatives, disinfectants, and deodorants. The primary use of this embalming chemical is in treatment of the cavities of the autopsied body. The powdered compound can also be used to treat the viscera returned after an autopsy. A hardening compound is often used in the plastic garments placed on bodies with burned tissue, decubitus ulcerations, or edema. Some of the chemicals used in these compounds are

- plaster of paris (dehydrating agent)
- paraformaldehyde (preservative, disinfectant)
- aluminum chloride and alum (dehydrating agent, disinfectant, preservative)
- wood powder (cellulose, very fine sawdust), whiting (calcium carbonate), and clays (moisture absorbing chemicals)

Chemical manufacturers have made an effort to develop "dustless" hardening compounds for the safety of the embalmer. Bentonite is an absorbent, heavier particulate clay that creates little dust. When embalming powders are used, the room should be well ventilated and a mask and goggles should be worn. Every effort should be made to reduce the inhalation of any particulate. Consult the Kerfoot studies in *Selected Readings* for the dangers caused by embalming powders.

The hardening compounds are not as effective preservatives and disinfectants as the autopsy gels. The gels have a much greater penetrating ability.

> Minimum amounts of autopsy and hardening compounds should be used when the body is to be cremated. These powders are not reduced by the cremation process, so their presence increases the amount of cremated remains. The cremated remains and the powders cannot be separated. This can make the need for a larger urn necessary.

Autopsy compounds are similar to **hardening compounds.** Autopsy compounds absorb excess moisture, preserve, firm, and sanitize tissues. They are specifically formulated for use on the exposed tissues of the cavities and walls of autopsied bodies. These compounds can also be used on bodies in which areas of skin have been removed for donation. To reduce dust, paraformaldehyde has been replaced by some manufacturers, with formaldehyde releasing preservative chemicals such as hydroxymethyl-5 or 5-dimethylhydantoin.

Embalming Preservative Powder

As the name indicates, embalming powder is designed to preserve tissue. The fumes this powder generates help to preserve and disinfect tissues. Many contain *para*-dichlorobenzene crystals, which arrest mildew and mold. Paraformaldehyde is the chief ingredient of these powdered preservatives. Some embalming powders also serve as deodorants and disinfectants. They do not have the absorbent and drying qualities of a hardening compound. The embalming powder can assist in preservation of the walls and organs of autopsied bodies if placed directly on burned or decomposing tissue. These powders can also be used for preservation of stillborn infants and can be applied to cancerous tissues, bedsores, and mutilated body parts. They help to preserve the tissues and control odors that may be present.

Embalming powder can also be put into the plastic garments placed on limbs with edema. When bodies are to be shipped to a distant point for interment, embalming powder can be placed in the casket to help control mildews or molds. These powders also help to control maggots and vermin.

The labels of embalming powders should be consulted since some are preservatives, whereas others are merely disinfectants and deodorants. It would be helpful to purchase an embalming powder that serves all three purposes.

Mold Inhibitors

Mold retarding chemicals are applied topically. They generally contain phenol or thymol. Mold retardants can be purchased in a prepared form and sprayed or painted on the surface of the body before placing it in storage. Refrigeration can retard mold growth but not stop it; in fact, some molds thrive best at cool temperatures. If mold is present, it can be scraped from the skin surface and a phenol mold retardant painted over the area to inhibit further growth. Mold becomes a problem when bodies must be kept for extended time periods. Of course, warm and moist environments encourage its growth.

Sealing Agents

Sealing agents are used to prevent leakage from sutured incisions. The agent is placed in the incised area during suturing. If any moisture develops within the incision, these agents absorb that moisture and are converted into a gelatinous material that helps to prevent leakage from the sutures. Two types of powder have been used for many years; more recently, a cream or "puttylike" material has been used.

The "putty" sealing agent can be used in various restorative procedures such as restoration of enucleated eyes, as a base for deep wound restorations, as a substitute for tissue builder, and to fill in sunken temple areas in autopsied bodies. It can be applied with a spatula or a specially designed injector.

Sealing agents are also surface glues. These help to prevent leakage from sutured tissues. Surface glues can be applied with a brush or can be purchased as a spray. Many of these agents can be directly covered with mortuary cosmetics when they are used in restorative work. Surface sealing agents work best on dry tissue surfaces.

Supplemental Addendum

Supplements embalming chemicals also include germicidal soaps and detergents, contact embalming liquids and sprays, orifice and topical disinfectants, and formaldehyde absorbent chemicals.

▶ KEY TERMS AND CONCEPTS FOR STUDY AND DISCUSSION

1. Define the following terms:
   Arterial fluid
   Coinjection fluid
   Hypertonic solution
   Hypotonic solution
   Osmosis
   Preinjection fluid
   Primary dilution
   Secondary dilution.
2. List and define four special-purpose arterial fluids.
3. Define a "waterless" embalming solution and give several examples where this type of solution may be helpful in establishing thorough preservation.
4. Give five purposes for a preinjection fluid.
5. List eight criteria that help the embalmer to determine the type, strength, and volume of arterial fluid.
6. List several purposes for addition of an active dye to arterial fluid.
7. Give several uses for autopsy gels.
8. You are designing a new preparation room. Describe in detail the ventilation system you would install in this new room.
9. Give several uses for cavity fluid.
10. How many ounces of a 25-index arterial fluid must be used to prepare a 1-gallon 2.0% strength arterial solution? To prepare a 1.5% strength solution? To prepare a 3.0% strength solution?
11. If 8 oz of a 20-index arterial fluid is used to prepare a 1-gallon solution of arterial fluid, what will be the strength of this solution? If 12 oz of arterial fluid was used? If 6 oz of arterial fluid was used?
12. How much water must be added to make a 2.0% arterial solution if 6 oz of a 20-index fluid is used? If you desire to make a 1.5% solution? If you desire to make a 3.0% solution?

▶ BIBLIOGRAPHY

Bedino JH. Enigma: Champion's fourth generation chemostasis infusion chemicals: Embalming redefined for the 21st century. In: *The Champion Expanding Encyclopedia of Mortuary Practices*, No. 657. Springfield, OH: Champion Co., 2009.

Dorn JM, Hopkins BM. *Thanatochemistry, a Survey of General, Organic, and Biochemistry for Funeral Service Professionals*, 3rd ed. Upper Saddle River, NJ: Prentice Hall, 2010.

Frigid Fluid Co, Funeral Home Catalog, www.frigidfluidco.com, Northlake, IL. 2004.

Jack Adams. Waterless embalming—a valuable technique. In: *Dodge Magazine,* Vol. 102 No. 2. Cambridge, MA: Dodge Co., 2010.

James Bedino. Waterless embalming—an investigation. In: *The Champion Expanding Encyclopedia*, Nos. 619–620. Springfield, OH: Champion Co., 1993:2490-2497.

Leandro Rendon. General chemical principles of embalming fluids. In: *The Champion Expanding Encyclopedia*, Nos. 365–371. Springfield, OH: Champion Co., 1966:1478-1504.

Mathews MC. *Embalming Chemistry Note Outline.* Minneapolis, MN: University of Minnesota, 1998.

Pervier NC. *Textbook of Chemistry for Embalmers.* Minneapolis, MN: University of Minnesota, 1961.

Pierce Chemicals; Royal Bond. www.piercechemical.com. Dallas, TX. 2009.

Putting alternative preservatives to the test. In: *The Forum,* Vol. 76, No. 3.

Wall, NJ: New Jersey State Funeral Directors Assn. January 2010.

CHAPTER 8

ANATOMICAL CONSIDERATIONS

CHAPTER OBJECTIVES

▶ Embalming injection and drainage sites
▶ Vessels used for arterial injection and drainage
▶ Vessel extents, linear and anatomical guides
▶ Relationship of arteries, veins, and surrounding anatomical structures
▶ Vessels of the body trunk cavities

It is essential that the embalmer possesses a sound understanding of and familiarity with the human body to efficiently approach and solve embalming problems. This chapter emphasizes those areas of anatomy most concerned with the embalming process. The orientation is strictly anatomical and space in the text is not consumed with considerations of the functional significance of any structure.

Before one can conceptualize the internal anatomy of the body, he or she must first be familiar with surface features and the manner in which they relate to underlying structures. A thorough knowledge of surface anatomy permits one not only to make appropriate skin incisions but also to anticipate which structures will appear when the incisions are made.

A portion of this chapter is devoted to the fundamentals of surface anatomy as it relates to underlying musculoskeletal and visceral structures. As a complete treatment of these topics is well beyond the scope of this text, this discussion is limited to those aspects of greatest importance to the embalmer.

All descriptions used throughout the text assume that the body is in the anatomical position: the subject is standing erect, the arms of the subject are at the sides with the palms of the hands facing the observer, the feet are together, and the subject is facing the observer.

The embalmer should have a detailed understanding of the blood vascular system. For each of the major vessels used in embalming, the anatomical guide, linear guide, and anatomical extent (limit) of each artery are given.

An **anatomical guide** is a method of locating a structure, such as an artery or a vein, by reference to an adjacent known or prominent structure. A **linear guide** is a line drawn or visualized on the surface of the skin to represent the approximate location of some deeper-lying structure. The **anatomical limit** is the point of origin and point of termination of a structure in relation to adjacent structures.

Because the blood in the veins flows in the *direction opposite* that of blood in the arteries, the anatomical limit and the linear guide for the veins would be the *opposite* of those of the respective artery. The anatomical guides for the arteries and the veins would be the same.

▶ COMMON CAROTID ARTERY AND INTERNAL JUGULAR VEIN

Surface Features and Landmarks

Surface features of the neck that the embalmer should be able to locate and describe are the clavicle, mandible, angle of the jaw, mastoid process of the temporal bone, hyoid bone, sternum, sternoclavicular articulation, suprasternal notch, and thyroid cartilage of the larynx. The embalmer should also be familiar with one muscle, the **sternocleidomastoid muscle (SCM).** In addition, the location of the external jugular vein should be recognized. Underlying the skin in this area is a thin, delicate cutaneous muscle (a muscle of facial expression) called the **platysma,** the presence of which is indicated by the shallow, transverse wrinkles of the neck.

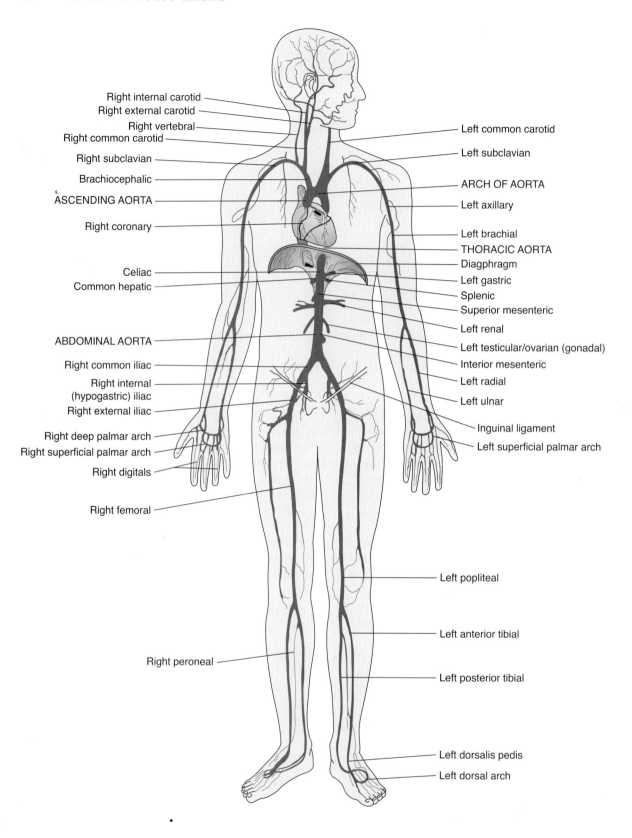

Right internal carotid
Right external carotid
Right vertebral
Right common carotid
Right subclavian
Brachiocephalic
ASCENDING AORTA
Right coronary
Celiac
Common hepatic
ABDOMINAL AORTA
Right common iliac
Right internal
(hypogastric) iliac
Right external iliac
Right deep palmar arch
Right superficial palmar arch
Right digitals
Right femoral
Right peroneal

Left common carotid
Left subclavian
ARCH OF AORTA
Left axillary
Left brachial
THORACIC AORTA
Diagphragm
Left gastric
Splenic
Superior mesenteric
Left renal
Left testicular/ovarian (gonadal)
Interior mesenteric
Left radial
Left ulnar
Inguinal ligament
Left superficial palmar arch
Left popliteal
Left anterior tibial
Left posterior tibial
Left dorsalis pedis
Left dorsal arch

Consider first the anterior triangle of the neck. Draw an imaginary line along the midline of the neck between the tip of the mandible and the sternum. Extend this line superiorly along the anterior border of the SCM and then anteriorly along the lower margin of the body of the mandible. These three lines and their anatomical parallels describe the **anterior triangle.** In the midline, one can palpate (feel), from above downward, the hyoid bone and the thyroid and cricoid cartilages. The external carotid artery and several of its branches are located in the anterior triangle. Here, these vessels are relatively superficial, being covered only by skin and subcutaneous tissue.

Anterior Triangle of the Neck

The skin over the anterior triangle is thin and underlaid by the thin, cutaneous platysma muscle. This muscle acts to alter the contour of the skin of the neck in much the same manner that the muscles of facial expression modify the appearance of the face. The significance of the muscle to the embalmer is that most structures of importance in the embalming process lie beneath the plane of this muscle. With the skin and platysma incised and reflected, the contents of the anterior triangle and the surrounding area are brought into view.

The SCM is a useful guide to the anterior triangle. Attached to the mastoid process of the temporal bone and the manubrium of the sternum, the muscle courses obliquely along the side of the neck. On the muscle surface, one can identify the external jugular vein together with some of its tributaries. The external jugular and the internal jugular veins cannot be confused because of the relationship of the former to the outer surface of the SCM.

Lying posterior and roughly parallel with the SCM muscle are the carotid sheath and its contents. The sheath is an investment of fascia that extends up into the neck and contains within it the common carotid (medial) artery, the internal jugular vein (lateral), and the vagus nerve (between the artery and the vein). The lower portion of the sheath is crossed anteriorly by the central tendon of the omohyoid muscle. Identification of this muscle can guide the embalmer to the underlying carotid sheath and provide confidence that the operation has not progressed too deep.

If the sheath is incised, the upper portion of the internal jugular vein and the common carotid artery become visible. The vein lies lateral to and partially overlaps the artery. A few variable tributaries of the internal jugular vein may be seen crossing the carotid artery in this area. The vagus nerve (cranial nerve X) can be identified between and posterior to the two vessels within the sheath.

In the upper portion of the anterior triangle, the common carotid artery divides into internal and external carotid arteries and several branches of the latter

Figure 8–1. Linear and anatomical guides for the common carotid artery.

may be identified here. The internal carotid, of course, has no branches until it enters the cranium.

Common Carotid Artery

Linear Guide. Draw or visualize a line on the surface of the skin from a point over the respective sternoclavicular articulation to a point over the anterior surface of the base of the respective earlobes.

Anatomical Guide. The right and the left common carotid arteries are located posterior to the medial border of the SCM, on their respective sides of the neck (Fig. 8–1).

Anatomical Limit. The right common carotid begins at the level of the right sternoclavicular articulation and extends to the superior border of the thyroid cartilage. The left common carotid begins at the level of the second costal cartilage and extends to the superior border of the thyroid cartilage.

Origins. The right common carotid is a terminal branch of the brachiocephalic artery. The left common carotid is a branch off the arch of the aorta.

Branches. There are no branches of the right common carotid, except the terminal bifurcation into the right internal and external carotid arteries. The left common carotid also has no branches, except the terminal bifurcation into the left internal and external carotid arteries.

Branches of the Right and Left External Carotid Arteries. Ascending pharyngeal, superior thyroid, lingual, facial,* occipital, posterior auricular, maxillary, superficial temporal (Fig. 8–2; also see Fig. 9–4).

---

*To raise the facial artery for injection, the incision is made along the inferior border of the mandible just anterior to the angle of the jaw.

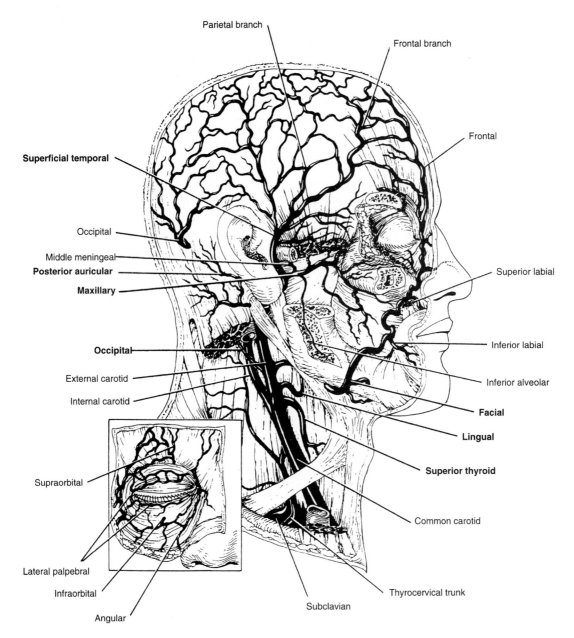

Figure 8–2. Cross-section of the head and the neck. Branches of the external carotid artery are shown in bold type.

Branches of the Right and Left Internal Carotid Arteries. Branches arising within the carotid canal, in addition to ophthalmic, anterior cerebral, middle cerebral, posterior communicating, and choroidal branches.

Relationship of the Common Carotid to the Internal Jugular Vein. The internal jugular vein lies lateral and superficial to the common carotid artery.

Contents of the Carotid Sheath. Internal jugular vein (lateral to artery), vagus nerve (between and posterior to artery and vein), common carotid artery (medial to vein) (Fig. 8–3).

▶ THE AXILLA—SURFACE ANATOMY

When the arm is extended (or abducted), conceptualization of the axilla is easy. Think of a truncated pyramid: four walls, a base, and an apex that has been made flat and parallel with the base. Surface landmarks of the axillary region are the ribs and intercostal muscles and the anterior and posterior axillary folds. The most obvious boundaries of the axilla are its anterior and posterior walls, which comprise the anterior and posterior axillary folds. The anterior fold can be identified by grasping (with one hand) the mass of tissue on the anterior surface of the axilla on the contralateral side of the body.

Figure 8–3. Right common carotid artery and internal jugular vein. The artery lies medial to the vein.

Most of the substance of this fold consists of the pectoralis, major muscle with contributions from the pectoralis minor, and the subclavius muscles.

The posterior axillary fold can be identified by grasping (with one hand) the tissue mass on the posterior side of the axilla on the contralateral side of the body. This fold consists of the latissimus dorsi, subscapularis, and teres major muscles. The medial axillary wall consists of ribs 2 through 6 and their intercostal muscles, covered externally by the serratus anterior muscle. The ribs can usually be palpated even if they are not visible on the chest surface.

The serratus anterior muscle also contributes to the medial wall but is visible as a surface feature only in lean, muscular subjects. The shaft of the humerus makes up a portion of the lateral wall, and although it cannot be seen, it is easily palpated.

The biceps brachii and coracobrachialis muscles also contribute to the lateral wall. The former is discernible in virtually all subjects, whereas the latter is clearly defined only in lean, muscular subjects. The apex of the axilla is an opening called the **cervicoaxillary canal,** which transmits structures from the neck into the arm and is bounded by three bony points of interest: the clavicle, the scapula, and the first rib. The cervicoaxillary canal is an important point of interest to the embalmer, particularly in autopsied bodies. Of the three landmarks that demarcate this canal, only the first rib is difficult to palpate. The base of the axilla is closed with dome-shaped fascia and skin on which the axillary hair is found.

Familiarity with the surface features of the axilla guides one to the important axillary contents, including the axillary artery and its six branches, the axillary vein, and the many elements of the brachial plexus. The ax-

illary sheath invests the major structures that leave the neck and pass through the cervicoaxillary canal to enter the axilla. On opening the axillary sheath, the first structure encountered is the axillary vein. If the extremity is abducted, the vein comes to lie over the axillary artery and partially obscures it.

The six typical branches of the axillary artery are fairly consistent and the axillary artery is relatively large. Identification of the artery within the sheath may prove difficult because of the many nerves of the brachial plexus that surround and partially obscure the artery. There are three large nerve cords of the brachial plexus: medial, lateral, and posterior. They are grouped around the middle portion of the axillary artery in positions corresponding to their names.

Within the axilla, the nerve cords and some of the terminal branches form specific anatomical relationships with the axillary artery, making access to the artery sometimes awkward. These are large nerves in some cases, and care must be taken to avoid confusing elements of the plexus with the axillary artery. Careful inspection and the knowledge that the nerves surround the artery will remove any confusion. *Approach to the axilla is made through an incision along the midaxillary line.*

Axillary Artery

Linear Guide.. Draw or visualize a line on the surface of the skin from a point over or through the center of the base of the axillary space to a point over or through the center of the lateral border of the base of the axillary space. This line is parallel to the long axis of the abducted arm.

Anatomical Guide. The axillary artery is located just behind the medial border of the coracobrachialis muscle.

Anatomical Limit. The axillary artery extends from a point beginning at the lateral border of the first rib to the inferior border of the tendon of the teres major muscle (Fig. 8–4).

Origin. The axillary artery is a continuation of the subclavian artery.

Branches. Highest (supreme) thoracic artery, thoracoacromial artery, lateral thoracic artery, subscapular artery, anterior humeral circumflex artery, posterior humeral circumflex artery.

Relationship of the Axillary Artery to the Axillary Vein. The axillary artery is located lateral and deep to the axillary vein.

Figure 8–4. The axillary space is outlined and the location of the coracobrachialis muscle illustrated.

Incision for Raising the Axillary Vessels. The incision is made along the anterior margin of the hairline of the axilla with the arm abducted.

Brachial Artery

Linear Guide. Draw or visualize a line on the surface of the skin from a point over the center of the lateral border of the base of the axillary space to a point approximately 1 inch below and in front of the elbow joint.

Anatomical Guide. The brachial artery lies in the bicipital groove at the posterior margin of the medial border of the belly of the biceps brachii muscle.

Anatomical Limit. The brachial artery extends from a point beginning at the inferior border of the tendon of the teres major muscle to a point inferior to the antecubital fossa (Fig. 8–5).

Origin. The brachial artery is a continuation of the axillary artery.

Relationship of the Brachial Artery and the Basilic Vein. The accompanying basilic vein is located medial and superficial to the brachial artery.

Location of the Incision. The brachial artery is usually raised by an incision made along the upper one-third of the linear guide.

▶ DISTAL FOREARM

The distal forearm is the area in which the radial and ulnar arteries can be approached should they need to be raised for injection (Fig. 8–6). The radial artery lies on the lateral side of the forearm and the ulnar artery on

Figure 8–5. Linear guide, anatomical guide, and suggested incision location for the brachial artery.

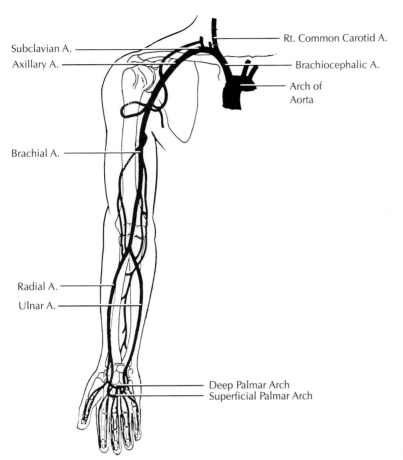

Subclavian A.

Axillary A.

Brachial A.

Radial A.

Ulnar A.

Rt. Common Carotid A.

Brachiocephalic A.

Arch of
Aorta

Deep Palmar Arch
Superficial Palmar Arch

Figure 8–6. Arteries of the distal forearm.

the medial side. The distal forearm permits easy access to the radial artery. Surface features of importance here are the styloid process of the radius and the tendon of the flexor carpi radialis muscle. In the interval between these two structures lies the radial artery on the anterior surface of the styloid.

A pulse may be obtained here easily in the living subject. The styloid is the most distal and lateral bony structure in the forearm, and just medial to this, one can palpate the tendon of flexor carpi radialis. In the distal region, the fleshy bellies of the muscles tend to yield to long, usually well-defined tendons. Here, a layering of the musculature is evident. In the most superficial layer are four muscles, including the pronator teres, flexor carpi radialis, flexor carpi ulnaris, and palmaris longus. Only the tendon of the pronator teres does not reach the distal forearm.

The second layer consists of one muscle with four tendons, one each leading to digits 2 through 5. This muscle is the flexor digitorum superficialis. The three muscles in the deep group are the flexor digitorum profundus, the flexor pollicis longus, and the pronator quadratus. Of these three, only the pronator has no long

tendon. Some of these tendons are useful guides to the radial and ulnar arteries.

Consider first the identification of the radial artery. An additional muscle, the brachioradialis, must be introduced here. This muscle is seen partially in the flexor compartment of the forearm. It is, nevertheless, an extensor muscle. In the proximal forearm, the radial artery is overlaid by the brachioradialis muscle but at no point is the artery crossed by this or any other muscle. This situation keeps the radial artery superficial and permits easy access to it at any point along its course in the forearm. In the middle and distal forearms, the radial artery lies medial to the brachioradialis and lateral to the flexor carpi radialis. Its course is described by a line drawn from the middle of the cubital fossa to the medial side of the radial styloid process. It is easiest to approach the artery with an incision in the distal two-thirds of the forearm along this line.

The ulnar artery is located on the medial side of the distal forearm. It lies between the tendon of the flexor carpi ulnaris muscle and the tendons of the flexor digitorum superficialis muscle. Here, it will always be found traveling with the ulnar nerve, with which it should not be confused. Together with the venae comitantes, the nerve and artery will be found in a connective tissue sheath from which the vessels must be freed before beginning injection.

The course of the ulnar artery is indicated by a line curving medially from the midpoint of the cubital fossa to the pisiform bone in the wrist. An incision along the distal one-third of this line permits access to the flexor carpi ulnaris muscle, which is then reflected medially to expose the ulnar artery.

Radial Artery

Linear Guide. Draw or visualize a line on the surface of the skin of the forearm from the center of the antecubital fossa to the center of the base of the index finger.

Anatomical Guide. The radial artery lies just lateral to the tendon of the flexor carpiradialis muscle and just medial to the tendon of the brachioradialis muscle.

Anatomical Limit. The radial artery extends from a point approximately 1 inch below and in front of the bend of the elbow to a point over the base of the thumb (thenar eminence).

Origin. The radial artery originates at the bifurcation of the brachial artery.

Relationship of the Radial Artery and the Vena Comitantes. Two small veins (venae comitantes) lie on either side of the artery. They may be helpful in locating the artery, for they generally contain some blood.

Ulnar Artery

Linear Guide. Draw or visualize a line on the surface of the skin from the center of the antecubital fossa on the forearm to a point between the fourth and fifth fingers.

Anatomical Guide. The ulnar artery lies just lateral to the tendon of the flexor carpi ulnaris muscle. (It lies between the tendons of the flexor carpi ulnaris and flexor digitorum superficialis.)

Anatomical Limit. The ulnar artery extends from a point approximately 1 inch below and in front of the bend of the elbow to a point over the pisiform bone (hypothenar eminence).

Origin. The ulnar artery originates at the bifurcation of the brachial artery.

Relationship of the Ulnar Artery to the Venae Comitantes. Two small veins (venae comitantes) lie on either side of the artery. They can be useful in locating the artery, for they generally contain some blood.

▶ ARTERIES OF THE BODY TRUNK

Table 8–1 outlines the arteries of the body trunk and their branches (Fig. 8–7).

In embalming infants, the ascending aorta (as it leaves the heart) or abdominal aorta can be used for injection points. A midsternal incision is used for the ascending aorta. An incision from the xiphoid process directed downward and to the left of the midline is used to raise the abdominal aorta.

In the adult, where partial autopsies have been performed or visceral organs are donated without autopsy, the abdominal or thoracic aorta can be used as a point of arterial injection.

External Iliac Artery and Vein

The use of the external iliac artery and vein as a site for arterial injection and blood drainage should be mentioned (Fig. 8–8). The external iliac artery is a continuation of the common iliac artery. (The common iliac is one of the terminal branches of the abdominal aorta.). The external iliac artery extends to a point under the center of the inguinal ligament. The artery lies exactly at this ligament lateral to the external iliac vein.

In the autopsied body, this artery is used for the injection of the lower extremities. Injecting the external iliac artery rather than the common iliac in the autopsied body eliminates the need to clamp off the internal iliac artery (which usually has been cut during the removal of the pelvic organs). In the unautopsied body, when the body is very obese, the femoral vessels are located very deep and are hard to work with; however, the external iliac artery, where it passes under the inguinal ligament, is quite superficial, and this can be a good location if there is a need to use this vessel in the unautopsied obese body.

Because insertion of an artery tube into the femoral artery (directed toward the upper area of the body) actually places the tip of the tube into the external iliac artery, the term *iliofemoral* is used by many embalmers to indicate the use of the vessels at a site near the inguinal ligament.

▶ INGUINAL REGION

The inguinal region is an area below the inguinal ligament in which the femoral vessels may be approached for injection and drainage. As a rule, the subcutaneous tissue in the thigh masks underlying soft tissue structures, so the embalmer must rely on bony landmarks in this area. Fortunately, the anterior superior spine of the ilium and pubic tubercle are easily identified. These two bony processes serve as attachments for the inguinal ligament. The positions of the underlying femoral vessels can be identified if the operator begins by placing the

TABLE 8–1. ARTERIES OF THE BODY TRUNK

Artery	Description	Branches
Ascending aorta	Originates at the left ventricle; at its beginning, the aortic semilunar valve should close, thus creating the pathway for arterial solution distribution	Right coronary artery Left coronary artery
Arch of the aorta	Center of arterial solution distribution	Brachiocephalic artery Left common carotid artery Left subclavian artery
Right subclavian	Begins at the right sternoclavicular articulation and extends to the lateral border of the first rib; in the complete autopsy (with neck organs removed), the branches need to be clamped	Vertebral artery Internal thoracic artery Inferior thyroid
Left subclavian	Begins at the level of the left second costal cartilage and extends to the lateral border of the first rib	
Descending thoracic aorta		Its branches include nine pairs of thoracic intercostal arteries

Descending abdominal aorta	Extends from the diaphragm to the lower border of the fourth lumbar vertebra	Parietal
		  Inferior phrenic
		  Superior suprarenals
		  Lumbar
		  Middle sacral
		Visceral (unpaired)
		  Celiac axis
		  Superior mesenteric
		  Inferior mesenteric
		Visceral (paired)
		  Middle suprarenals
		  Renals
		  Internal spermatic (male), ovarian (female)
		  Common iliacs (terminal)

thumb of the left hand on the subject's right anterior superior iliac spine and the left middle finger on the subject's right pubic tubercle. If the operator's left index finger is now allowed to bisect the interval between his or her thumb and middle finger (i.e., bisect the inguinal ligament), the tip of the index finger will indicate the approximate position of the femoral vessels in the thigh. The procedure can be repeated on the subject's left side using the operator's right hand. The incision to raise the vessel can be made on the linear guide.

▶ FEMORAL TRIANGLE

The inguinal ligament serves as the base for this triangle whose two sides consist of the medial border of the sartorius and the lateral border of the adductor longus muscles (Fig. 8–9). In addition to skin and subcutaneous tissue covering the triangle, the roof consists of a dense sheet of fascia, the fascia lata, which attaches firmly to the inguinal ligament and encircles the thigh. This roof must be incised to expose the boundaries and contents of the triangle.

Lying on the surface of the fascia lata is the great saphenous vein that has coursed up the medial aspect of the thigh all the way from the foot. The operator should not mistake the great saphenous for the femoral vein. This potential mistake can be avoided simply by remembering anatomic relationships. **If the vein in question is lying on the surface of the dense, white fascia lata and if the fascia lata has not yet been incised, then the vein must be the great saphenous or one of its tributaries.**

If the great saphenous is followed, it disappears through an opening in the fascia lata called the "fossa ovalis." This opening is not so glamorous, as some textbooks would have one believe. Rather, there is a hiatus in the fascia lata and the great saphenous insinuates itself through the fascia and empties directly into the femoral vein. So, it is clear that identification of the great saphenous will lead directly to the femoral vein near the base of the femoral triangle. Around the hiatus one is likely to encounter inguinal lymph nodes, which may have to be resected.

When the roof of the triangle is incised and reflected, the contents and borders come into view. The femoral vessels are contained within the femoral sheath,

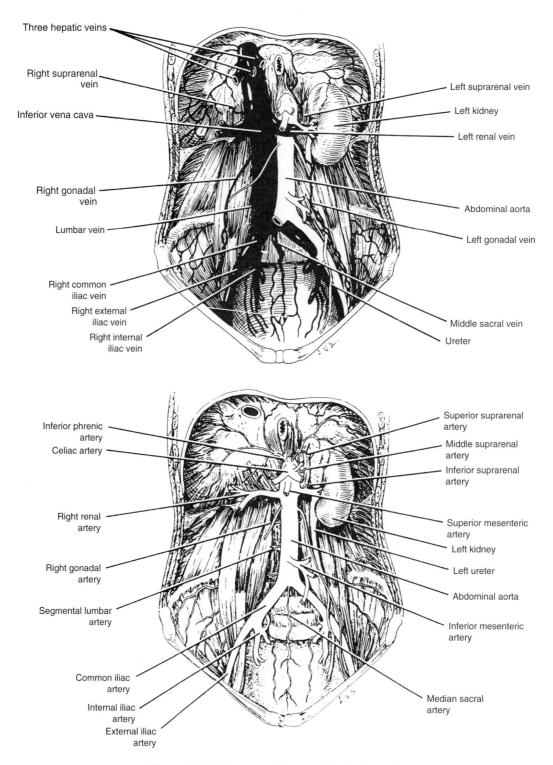

Figure 8–7. Arteries and veins of the body trunk.

which is a continuation into the thigh of abdominal wall and pelvic fascias. The sheath is subdivided into three compartments which, from lateral to medial, contain the femoral artery, femoral vein, and lymphatic vessels and nodes. The most medial compartment is designated the femoral canal and is the site of femoral hernias. There-

fore, a femoral hernia is always situated medial to the femoral vein. This relationship is an important one to remember if preparing a subject whose inguinal region is distorted (such as with a hernia).

To gain access to the femoral vessels, open each of the other two compartments separately. An incision

Figure 8–8. Incision location for left external iliac vessels. The linear guides are also shown.

in the sheath over each vessel will cause the artery and vein to be delivered easily. At the base of the triangle, the artery lies slightly anterior and lateral to the femoral vein and its position may be identified at the midpoint of the inguinal ligament. The vessels are best approached 1 to 2 inches from the base of the triangle, where they lie side by side and are easily accessible.

As the vessels approach the apex of the triangle, their relationship shifts to an anteroposterior one so that the femoral artery, femoral vein, deep femoral vein, and deep femoral artery lie one in front of the other, making access to most of them somewhat difficult.

The most lateral structure at the base of the femoral triangle is the femoral nerve, which lies outside the femoral sheath. This very substantial nerve and its many branches should not be confused with the adjacent femoral artery because the nerve lies without the sheath.

The floor of the triangle is entirely muscular and different authors consider that either two or three muscles constitute the floor. Laterally, the iliopsoas muscle emerges beneath the inguinal ligament. Just medial to this lies the pectineus muscle. Certainly, these two mus-

cles contribute to the floor of the triangle. The disagreement comes about as a result of whether the medial or lateral border of the adductor longus muscle is considered to be the medial boundary of the triangle. The distinction is academic but in this text the adductor longus is treated as part of the floor for the following reason. The triangle is easily visualized in terms of the number 3. There are three borders: the inguinal ligament, the sartorius muscle, and the adductor longus muscle. Basically, three structures are contained within the triangle: the femoral nerve, the femoral artery, and the femoral vein. Each of these has branches or tributaries, but three major structures are present. Finally, if the adductor longus is considered to be a part of the floor, there are three muscles in the floor: the iliopsoas, the pectineus, and the adductor longus.

At the apex of the femoral triangle, the femoral vessels, but not the femoral nerve, enter the subsartorial or adductor canal. Recognizing the relationships of the femoral artery and vein at the triangle apex facilitates the understanding of the anatomical relationships of these vessels after they emerge from the adductor canal and enter the popliteal fossa or space.

Femoral Artery

Linear Guide. Draw or visualize a line on the surface of the skin of the thigh from the center of the inguinal ligament to the center of the medial prominence of the knee (medial condyle of the femur).

Anatomical Guide. The femoral artery passes through the center of the femoral triangle and is bounded laterally by the sartorius muscle (its medial border) and medially by the adductor longus muscle.

Anatomical Limit. The femoral artery extends from a point behind the center of the inguinal ligament to the opening in the adductor magnus muscle (Fig. 8–10).

Origin. The femoral artery is a continuation of the external iliac artery.

Figure 8–9. Femoral triangle showing the linear guide for the femoral vessels.

Figure 8–10. Right femoral artery with arterial tubes.

Branches. Superficial epigastric, superficial circumflex iliac, external pudendal, profunda femoris.

Relationship of the Femoral Artery and Vein. The femoral artery lies lateral and superficial to the femoral vein.

Popliteal Fossa

On the posterior aspect of the knee, two sets of tendons and two fleshy muscle heads can be identified. This describes the popliteal fossa as a trapezoid and can be subdivided into an upper femoral and a lower tibial triangle.

The femoral triangle (not to be confused with the femoral triangle in the inguinal region) is bounded laterally by the long and short heads of the biceps femoris and medially by the tendons of the semimembranosus and semitendinosus muscles. The tibial triangle is limited medially and laterally by the diverging medial and lateral fleshy heads of the gastrocnemius muscle and, to a lesser extent, by the plantaris muscle laterally. The base of each triangle is an imaginary line drawn through the middle of the joint. These surface landmarks serve as guides to the underlying popliteal vessels within the boundaries of the space.

The muscular boards of this fossa are overlaid by a roof of deep fascia, subcutaneous tissue, and skin. Intrusion into this space provides access to the popliteal vessels for injection and drainage. After recognizing and dispatching minor vascular and nervous branches external to the deep fascia, the fascia is incised to gain access to the vessels. The major contents of the space include the tibial and peroneal nerves (from the sciatic) and their branches, the popliteal vein and its tributaries, the popliteal artery and its branches, and a good deal of fat and lymphatic tissue.

As the space is approached posteriorly, the first structures to be encountered are the tibial and peroneal nerves. The tibial nerve is the larger of the two and is located directly in the midline. The common peroneal nerve, on the other hand, leaves the sciatic nerve at about midthigh and courses down the lateral aspect of the popliteal space.

With the tibial nerve retracted, the popliteal vein comes into view, lying superficial (posterior) to the *popliteal artery, which is the deepest (most anterior) structure in the fossa.* Remember that this relationship was established as these vessels entered the adductor canal. The vessels are bound together by connective tissue, which must be loosened and reflected to gain access to the vessels. Several branches and tributaries of the vessels are also found in the fossa, but these need not be identified by name here.

Deep (anterior) to the popliteal artery, the floor of the fossa is formed by the lower end of the femur and a portion of the capsule surrounding the knee joint.

Linear Guide. Draw or visualize a line on the surface of the skin from the center of the superior border of the popliteal space parallel to the long axis of the lower extremity to the center of the inferior border of the popliteal space.

Anatomical Guide. The popliteal vessels are located between the popliteal surface of the femur and the oblique popliteal ligament.

Anatomical Limit. The popliteal artery extends from a point beginning at the opening of the adductor magnus muscle to the lower border of the popliteus muscle.

Origin. The popliteal artery is a continuation of the femoral artery.

Branches. There are five pairs of genicular arteries, and five muscular branches.

Relationship of the Popliteal Artery and Vein. The vein lies posterior and medial to the artery. Because of the location of these vessels, the vein can also be described as lying superficial to the artery.

▶ DISTAL LEG

In the distal leg, the superficiality of the anterior tibial artery makes it easily accessible as an injection site. The popliteal artery ends by dividing into two terminal branches: the anterior tibial artery and the posterior tibial artery. The branches begin at the lower border of the popliteus muscle. In the distal portion of the leg, the

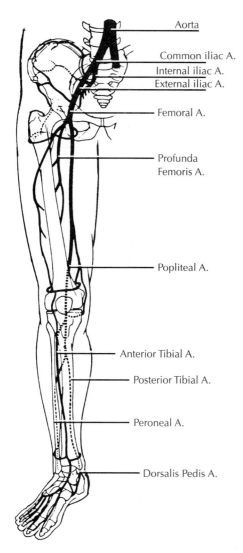

Figure 8–11. Arteries of the distal leg.

Anterior and Posterior Tibial Arteries

Linear Guide. Anterior Tibial Artery: Draw or visualize a line from the lateral border of the patella to the anterior surface of the ankle joint. *Posterior Tibial Artery:* Draw or visualize a line on the surface of the skin from the center of the popliteal space to a point midway between the medial malleolus and the calcaneus bone.

Anatomical Guide. Anterior Tibial Artery: The anterior tibial vessels are located in a groove between the tibialis anterior muscle and the tendon of the extensor hallucis longus muscle. *Posterior Tibial Artery:* The posterior tibial vessels are located between the posterior border of the tibia and the calcaneus tendon.

Anatomical Limit. Anterior Tibial Artery: The anterior tibial artery extends from a point beginning at the inferior border of the popliteus muscle to a point in front of the middle of the ankle joint on the respective sides. *Posterior Tibial Artery:* The posterior tibial artery extends from a point beginning at the inferior border of the popliteus muscle to a point over and between the medial malleolus and the calcaneus of the respective foot.

Branches and Tributaries of the Vessels. Anterior Tibial Vessels, Posterior Tibial Vessels: right and left peroneal branches, right and left dorsalis pedis arteries.

▶ FOOT

Tendons passing onto the dorsum of the foot from the leg pass posterior to and are restrained by two thickenings of fascia, the superior and inferior extensor retinacula, which lie anterior to the ankle. In addition, the anterior tibial artery and the deep peroneal nerve also pass deep to these retinacula. Only inconsequential superficial nerves and veins lie superficial to these retinacula.

Skin on the dorsum of the foot is thin and loosely applied. The subcutaneous tissue permits easy visualization of the venous network, which is so prominent here.

Tendons of two extrinsic muscles of the foot, the extensor hallucis longus and the extensor digitorum longus, are easily identified as they pass to the great toe and digits 2 through 5, respectively. The dorsalis pedis artery is situated in the interosseous spaces between the tendon of extensor hallucis longus and the first tendon of extensor digitorum longus as it passes to the second digit. An incision made from a point midway between the medial and lateral malleoli to the interosseous space will provide access to the dorsalis pedis artery.

Linear Guide (Dorsalis Pedis Artery). Draw or visualize a line from the center of the anterior surface of the ankle joint to a point between the first and second toes.

arteries become superficial and can be used as points of injection for the foot. Injection could also be made toward the head to embalm the distal leg and thigh (Fig. 8–11).

The anterior tibial artery is the smaller of the terminal branches of the popliteal artery. As it approaches the distal portion of the leg, it becomes very superficial. It can be raised by making an incision just above the ankle, just lateral to the crest of the tibia. In front of the ankle joint, the anterior tibial artery now becomes the dorsalis pedis artery.

The posterior tibial artery is also one of the terminal branches of the popliteal artery and passes posteriorly and medially down the leg. In the area between the medial malleolus and the calcaneus bone, the artery can be raised by the embalmer for injection of the foot. The artery terminates by dividing into the medial and lateral plantar arteries.

► CONCLUSIONS

The anatomy of several potential injection sites has been considered. More than just vascular anatomy has been presented with the hope that complete familiarity with the anatomy of these regions will facilitate the work of the practitioner. Being aware of the anatomy peripheral to the blood vessels at an injection site and having a solid command of anatomical relationships in these areas should make the embalmer more comfortable with and more confident in his or her operations.

► CONCEPTS FOR STUDY AND DISCUSSION

1. Describe the anatomical position.
2. Define anatomical guide, linear guide, and anatomical limit.
3. Give the anatomical limits of the right and the left common carotid arteries.
4. Give the linear guide and the anatomical guide for the common carotid artery.
5. Give the anatomical guide for the facial artery.
6. List the eight branches of the external carotid artery and the areas they supply.
7. Give the bony boundaries of the cervicoaxillary canal.
8. Give the linear and anatomical guides and anatomical limits for the axillary and brachial arteries.
9. Describe the relationship of the internal jugular vein to the common carotid artery and the relationship of the axillary vein to the axillary artery.
10. Give the extent of the axillary artery.
11. Give the linear and anatomical guide for the radial and ulnar arteries.
12. List the branches, from right to left, of the arch of the aorta and the visceral and parietal branches of the abdominal aorta.
13. Give the anatomical and linear guides and the anatomical limits for the femoral artery.
14. Describe the relationship of the femoral artery to the femoral vein.
15. Give the linear guides for the popliteal artery, anterior tibial artery, posterior tibial artery, and dorsalis pedis artery.

CHAPTER 9

EMBALMING VESSEL SITES AND SELECTIONS

CHAPTER OBJECTIVES

▶ Selection of vessels for injection
▶ Selection of vessels for drainage
▶ Suggested techniques for raising vessels
▶ Vascular injection procedures

There are several anatomical locations where arteries and veins may be elevated for the arterial embalming of the dead human body. One of the major objectives of making a preembalming analysis of the body is the selection of vessels to employ for injection and drainage.

The proper selection of vessels should produce the most satisfactory results. This selection is based on various intrinsic and extrinsic factors. Embalming analysis is not simply a preembalming evaluation. During injection of the body, it may become necessary to select other vessels for injection and drainage. Analysis is necessary throughout the entire process.

▶ VASCULAR INJECTION PROCEDURES

One-Point Injection
An artery and a vein at one location are used for injection and drainage (e.g., injection from the right common carotid artery and drainage from the right internal jugular vein, or injection from the right femoral artery and drainage from the right femoral vein).

Split Injection
The injection is made in an artery at one location and the drainage occurs from a vein at another location (e.g., injection of the right common carotid artery and drainage from the right femoral vein, or injection from the right femoral artery and drainage from the right internal jugular vein).

Restricted Cervical Injection
Both right and left common carotid arteries are raised; tubes are placed into each of the arteries and directed toward the head. A tube is inserted toward the trunk of the body, either in the right or the left artery. The inferior portion of the other artery is tied off. Drainage is generally taken from the right internal jugular vein. Some embalmers prefer to open and drain from both the right and the left internal jugular veins if the face is badly discolored. During downward injection (toward the trunk), the arterial tubes directed toward the head **remain open**.

Multipoint Injection
Multipoint injection is vascular injection from two or more arteries (e.g., injection is begun from the right femoral artery but the embalming solution does not distribute to the left leg or the left arm; subsequently, the left femoral and the left brachial arteries are raised and injected.)

Six-Point Injection (Sectional Embalming)
In the unautopsied body, six arteries are raised that will separately inject the head and the limbs, for example, each "section" or body "region": right and left common carotid arteries, right and left axillary (or brachial) arteries, and right and left femoral (or external iliac) arteries. Drainage can be taken from each location or from one location such as the right internal jugular vein. The body trunk can be embalmed by injection of any one of these six arteries **toward the trunk**.

> With the unautopsied body, this can become a 12-point injection for the tube at each location can be turned and injection made toward the trunk of the body. This can be beneficial with bodies where arterial injection to the tissues of the trunk of the body was poor; a good example would be bodies which exhibit early decomposition.

In the autopsied body, a six-point injection may include injection of the right and left common carotid arteries to embalm the head, right and left subclavian (axillary or brachial) arteries to embalm the upper extremity, and right and left common iliac (external iliac or femoral) arteries to embalm the lower extremity.

▶ VESSEL SELECTION

Two of the most important objectives in making the embalming analysis of the body are the selection of an artery (or arteries) for injection of arterial solution and the selection of a vein for drainage.

In the **unautopsied** body, the arteries most frequently used for embalming are the common carotid, femoral, and the axillary arteries. Because of the value of using an accompanying vein for drainage, the **femoral** and the **common carotid** vessels are preferred to the axillary artery.

Once injection of the body is begun, the embalmer needs to continually ask two questions:

1. What areas of body **are** receiving arterial solution? What areas of body **are not** receiving arterial solution?
2. Has an area received sufficient arterial solution?

There needs to be constant **observation → evaluation → implementation → results.** This four-step method is used during the embalming analysis **before**, **during**, and **after** arterial injection.

Example: If a one-point or a restricted cervical injection plan is used by the embalmer after a sufficient quantity of arterial solution has been injected (perhaps 1 gallon), the embalmer must evaluate what areas of the body **are** receiving arterial solution and what areas **are not** receiving arterial solution. Various embalming techniques can be used in an attempt to stimulate the flow of the solution into the body areas where the solution is lacking. Once the embalmer is satisfied that all body regions have sufficient arterial solution, those areas where there is insufficient solution can be separately injected by multipoint embalming. With multipoint embalming, an evaluation must also be made; if the preservative is not reaching all areas of a body region, perhaps more distant arteries can be raised and injected (e.g., the axillary artery may have been raised to inject the right arm;

if solution is not entering the hand, the radial or ulnar artery can be raised and injected). After multipoint injection, an evaluation must again be made. If there is still insufficient solution in an area, supplemental methods of embalming (e.g., hypodermic or surface compresses) must be used.

A similar protocol of working from major arteries that supply large regions, to smaller arteries that supply localized body areas, and finally the possible use of supplemental embalming treatments, is utilized in the embalming of the **autopsied** body.

To summarize, a pattern of vessel selection, injection, and observation is as follows:

> - ▶ Select artery for injection of the body and a vein for drainage
> - ▶ Inject
> - ▶ Observe and evaluate
> - ▶ If an area does not have enough arterial solution, raise an artery that directly supplies that area
> - ▶ Inject from this second artery
> - ▶ Observe and evaluate
> - ▶ If needed, use supplemental embalming treatments, hypodermic and surface compresses or gels

General Considerations

Most embalmers are right-handed and find working on the right side of the body much easier. If the internal jugular vein is to be used for drainage, the right internal jugular vein leads directly into the right atrium of the heart; drainage instruments are much easier and more effective when inserted into the right internal jugular vein. Selecting the left common carotid or left femoral vessels for one-point injection sites would afford the same advantages.

Selection of an injection site and vascular injection procedure involves two criteria: (1) factors concerning the vessels and (2) general body conditions.

Situations in which it may be necessary to locate severed or cut portions of arteries to inject arterial solution include (1) bodies where extensive autopsies have been performed, (2) bodies where partial autopsies have been performed, (3) bodies from which one or more organs and/or tissues for transplantation have been removed, and, (4) bodies with traumatic injuries.

Arteries, veins, and nerves tend to be grouped together in their routes through the body. It is essential that the embalmer be able to distinguish between these structures (Table 9–1).

Nerves have a silvery appearance and, when examined with the naked eye, show striations along their surface. When cut, they have no lumen or opening and

TABLE 9–1. COMPARISON OF ARTERIES, VEINS, AND NERVES

Artery	Vein	Nerve
Lumen	Lumen	Solid structure
Creamy white	Bluish when filled with blood	Silvery white
Thick walls are demonstrated when artery is rolled between two fingers; edges of the artery are easily felt	When vein is rolled between two fingers, walls collapse and edges are not felt	Solid structure is demonstrated when nerve is rolled between two fingers
Vasa vasorum may be seen on surface	Vasa vasorum not visible	Vasa vasorum not visible
Remains open when cut	Collapses when cut	Solid when cut; ends tend to fray
Generally empty of blood	Generally some blood or clotted material present	No blood present

their cut edges take on a frayed appearance similar to the frayed cut ends of a rope.

Veins are thinner than arteries. They contain valves, which arteries do not, but like arteries, when cut they do have an opening or lumen. When their sides are cut, veins collapse, creating a funnel effect.

Arteries have very thick walls as compared with healthy veins. Arteries are creamy white in appearance, and often, small vessels called the **vasa vasorum** can be seen over the artery surface (especially in arteries exhibiting arteriosclerosis). The most distinguishing feature of an artery is that if it is cut, **the lumen remains open** and very pronounced. The walls of the artery, unlike those of the vein, do not collapse. The common carotid arteries are quite elastic and can easily be stretched after dissection and cleaning. The femoral arteries are more muscular and not as elastic as the carotids.

It is most important that the embalmer should be familiar with the location of arteries in relationship to their accompanying veins.

▶ SELECTING AN ARTERY AS AN INJECTION POINT

The selection of an artery or arteries for embalming is based on conditions of the individual artery and conditions of the body with respect to these questions:

1. How superficial or deep is the artery?
2. What structures surround the artery?
3. How close to the aorta is the artery?
4. What is the diametric size of the artery?
5. Can the body be positioned properly if this artery is used?
6. Will incisions for the artery be on an exposed body area?
7. Can drainage be taken from the vein which accompanies the artery?
8. If arterial clotting is present, in what direction will these clots be moved during injection?
9. How much arteriosclerosis is present in the artery at the injection site?

Other factors governing the selection of an artery or arteries for injection include the following:

1. Age of the deceased
2. Sex of the individual with respect to the type of clothing which will be worn
3. Weight
4. Fat distribution
5. Disfigurations present (e.g., arthritic conditions, tumors, or scar tissue)
6. Diseases present
7. Edema, localized or generalized
8. Location of obstructions or congestion, possibly creating discolorations or a lack of preservative solution flow to a body region
9. Trauma present from mutilation, accident, or surgery
10. Vascular interruptions from organ and/or tissue donation
11. Medicolegal requirements with regard to autopsies; preparation for medical schools; preparation for international shipping; preparation under military contracts; requirements of a coroner or medical examiner.
12. Cause of death
13. Manner of death

In addition to these variables, two nonvariable guidelines must be considered: (1) Prepare each body with the assumption that the body is dead from an infectious and contagious disease; (2) prepare each body with the assumption that final disposition and viewing will be delayed.

With respect to size (diameter) of an artery, of the four choices for an injection point, the common carotid artery is the largest, because it is nearest to the heart. The femoral (or external iliac) is the second in size, and the axillary artery is the smallest in diameter. Any artery could be used as an injection site to inject the entire body, but the use of a small vessel such as the radial or ulnar to embalm the entire body allows for a very slow rate of flow of arterial solution. It could also be difficult to build sufficient pressure in the arterial system to properly distribute and diffuse the arterial solution. The larger, more elastic arteries such as the common carotid and the femoral allow for use of the higher pressures and greater rates of flow necessary to achieve uniform distribution of the arterial solution.

As for the accessibility of the artery, deep-seated vessels within the thorax or the abdomen are very difficult to use for injection of the adult body. In infants and children, these vessels can be considered, for they are easier to reach. In the unautopsied adult body, vessels near the surface of the skin and with few branches can easily be raised to the surface of the incision. The common carotid arteries do not have branches (except their terminals) and can easily be raised to the skin surface. Likewise, the femoral arteries and the external iliac arteries (at the inguinal ligament) are not held tightly in position by large numbers of branches.

The accompanying vein is one of the most important factors in selecting an injection site. Can this vein be used for drainage? The common carotid artery is accompanied by the large internal jugular vein. On the right side of the neck, this vein leads directly into the right atrium of the heart, and the right atrium is the center of drainage. The femoral artery is also accompanied by a large vein that may be used for drainage.

The size of the artery, its accessibility, and, finally, the possibility of draining from the accompanying vein must be considered in selecting an artery for injection. As previously stated, in the unautopsied adult body, this choice is among four vessels: (1) the common carotid artery, (2) the right and left common carotid arteries, (3) the femoral artery (or external iliac if raised at the inguinal ligament), and (4) the axillary artery (or brachial artery).

The second group of factors used in the selection of vessels for an injection site includes these body conditions:

1. Age of the body
   a. In the infant, additional vessels may be considered for injection such as the ascending aorta or the abdominal aorta.
   b. With respect to infants, the size of the artery may be the factor that determines which vessel can be used. The common carotid is the largest. A set of small infant arterial tubes should always be available.
   c. In the elderly, many times the femoral vessel is found to be sclerotic; the common carotid artery is rarely found to exhibit arteriosclerosis.
2. Weight of the body
   a. In obese bodies, the femoral artery is found quite deep in the upper thigh. Its depth should not preclude its possible use. If the vessel must be raised, it should be raised at the inguinal ligament, or the external iliac artery can be used. At this location, the vessel is the most superficial.
   b. Drainage is also a factor to consider with obese bodies. The internal jugular vein affords the best clearing of the body, especially the tissues of the face. Keep in mind that the weight of the viscera in heavy bodies provides resistance to the flow of arterial solution as well as resistance to drainage.
   c. In obese bodies, large quantities of arterial solution are needed to adequately preserve the body. To avoid distension of facial tissues, it is best to select the right and the left common carotid arteries, which would be raised at the start of embalming.

   The best approach to embalming obese bodies is to raise both the right and left common carotid arteries (restricted cervical injection) and use the right internal jugular vein for drainage. In this manner, large volumes (often of a strong solution) can be injected into the trunk areas without overinjecting the head and the face. Restricted cervical injection allows the use of higher injection pressures and greater rates of flow.
   d. With very thin bodies, care should be taken to minimize any destruction of the sternocleidomastoid muscle of the neck. All other factors taken into consideration, use of the femoral vessels, if possible, might prove advantageous in the preparation of these bodies.
3. Disease conditions
   a. A condition such as arthritis may necessitate the avoidance of certain body areas; legs can be in the fetal position in the elderly or in bodies that have suffered from certain brain tumors, making use of the femoral vessel quite difficult (see Fig. 11–8).
   b. A goiter condition in the neck may make use of the carotid artery and the jugular vein difficult, because the vessels will be pushed out of their normal location.
   c. Tumors or swollen lymph nodes in the neck, groin, or axillary area should be avoided for injection.
   d. Burned tissues should be avoided if possible; leakage will be a problem and suturing will be difficult.
   e. When edema is present in an area such as the upper thigh, raising a vessel should be avoided in this area; closure (suturing) may be difficult and leakage a problem. When edema is generalized (anasarca), large quantities of arterial solution must be injected. Here, it would be best to use restricted cervical injection, raising

both the right and left common carotid arteries. This allows the embalmer to inject large quantities of arterial solution. Many times, these arterial solutions are very strong. The restricted cervical injection allows the use of large amounts of fluid to saturate other body areas without overinjecting the face. A separate, milder solution can then be used for injection of the head.

f. A **ruptured aortic aneurysm** often dictates that additional arteries may need to be injected. Often, some circulation can be established in these conditions. In the majority, there is direct loss of all arterial fluid to the abdominal cavity, necessitating six-point injection of the body and treatment of the trunk walls, buttocks, and shoulders by hypodermic embalming.

g. When **scar tissue** is seen in a location where a vessel is to be raised (such as the upper inguinal area), no doubt, surgery has been performed. Scar tissue beneath the skin can be very difficult to work within raising vessels, and it may be wise, if possible, to use another vessel.

h. **Gangrene,** particularly in the lower extremities, indicates that the deceased suffered from a poor blood supply into the affected limb(s) or the presence of a clot in an artery or a vein. Most often, that poor blood supply is the result of arteriosclerosis. For example, if the foot or lower leg evidences gangrene, or a recent amputation has occurred, the femoral vessel should be avoided as the primary injection point. Use of the carotid arteries is advised, because generally, little arteriosclerosis is associated with these vessels.

4. Interruption of the vascular system
   a. *Mutilation or trauma:* Traumatic death can result in severed arteries. These conditions must be individually evaluated by the embalmer; arteries exposed as a result of the trauma may be considered as sites for injection. Also, standard points of injection such as the common carotid can be used and the severed arteries clamped during arterial injection. Secondary points of injection will, no doubt, be required.
   b. *Ulcerations:* Ruptured vessels can be the result of ulcerations. If this occurs in the stomach, there will be a great loss of blood during the agonal period. If sufficient arterial solution is lost during injection, the embalmer must select multipoints of injection to treat those areas of the body not reached by arterial solution.

When arterial solution is evidenced in purge from the mouth or the nose during arterial injection and there is still blood drainage, continue to inject arterial solution and evaluate the distribution of the solution.

When arterial solution is evidenced in purge from the nose or the mouth during arterial injection and there is no blood drainage, it would be wise to discontinue injection, evaluate the distribution of solution, and sectionally treat, by arterial injection, those areas not reached by sufficient arterial solution.

c. *Autopsies:* Partial autopsies must be evaluated by the embalmer as to the selection of arteries for injection. For example, if the viscera were removed only from the **abdominal cavity,** the portions of the body above the diaphragm could be embalmed by (1) injecting from the thoracic aorta upward and (2) injecting from the right common carotid and ligating the thoracic aorta. Even after a complete autopsy, there can be a choice of vessels depending on the lengths of vessels left by the dissecting pathologist. For example, the subclavian artery or perhaps the axillary artery can be used to inject the arm. If the external iliac arteries have been cut under the inguinal ligament, the femoral vessels may have to be injected. In some autopsies, the entire arch of the aorta may be present and most of the upper areas of the body can be injected from the branches of the arch.

d. *Organ and tissue donation:* There needs to be a careful evaluation of the arterial system when organs or tissues have been recovered for transplant. Disruption of the arterial system by organ or tissue removal will often require multipoint arterial injection and extensive use of surface and hypodermic embalming treatments.

e. Ruptured aortic aneurysm (see above).

5. Clotting
   If an embalmer feels that clots may be present in the arterial system, particularly in the aorta, the femoral artery should **not** be used as the starting point for injection. The best choice in this situation is to begin the injection of the arterial solution from the common carotid, because if any coagula do break loose, it is better that this material be directed toward the legs. If the femoral artery is used, the coagula could be pushed up into the common carotid arteries or the axillary vessels. These arteries supply body areas that will

be viewed. Clotting may be suspected in bodies that have been dead for long periods, in deaths from systemic infections and febrile disease, and in bodies of persons who were bedfast for long periods.

When the embalmer suspects that the blood vascular system is heavily clotted or that distribution of arterial solution will be difficult, the best vessel to use in beginning the arterial injection is the common carotid artery, and drainage should be taken from the right internal jugular vein. An even better method is to raise both common carotid arteries at the beginning of the embalming (restricted cervical injection). As the head is thus separately embalmed, the embalmer maintains control over solution distribution into the facial tissues.

6. Facial tissue distension
The possibility of distension of the facial tissues during injection exists in (1) bodies dead for long periods of time; (2) bodies with facial trauma, and (3) bodies that have been frozen or in refrigeration for extended periods of time. Use of restricted cervical injection would best control the amount of arterial solution entering the facial tissues in the unautopsied body.

7. Facial discolorations
Intense livor mortis and possibly postmortem stain are frequently seen when bodies have died from congestive heart failure or pneumonia. Any postmortem condition, in which the head is dependent to the heart, can increase this discoloration. Obese bodies when the shoulders and head have not been elevated will exhibit intense livor mortis. Postmortem refrigeration and the antemortem use of blood thinners can contribute to facial livor mortis, when the head is in a dependent position.

In the preparation of these bodies, this intense discoloration necessitates elevation of the shoulders and head. The right internal jugular vein is the best choice for drainage. It may be necessary to open and drain both right and left internal jugular veins. Clearing of these tissues is also assisted by direct injection of arterial solution into the head, which is best achieved by raising and injecting the right and left common carotid arteries.

8. Volume and strength of arterial solution
In the unautopsied body, stronger solutions may be necessary if (1) there is a long delay between the death and the embalming, (2) the body shows evidence of decomposition, (3) death was due to uremic poisoning or burns, and (4) skeletal edema is present. To avoid running excessive amounts of solution through the facial tissues, restricted cervical injection is recommended.

9. Medicolegal requirements
These examples illustrate specific requirements in selection of an injection site:
a. An embalmer preparing a body under orders from the military services may be instructed to follow military standards for the choice of vessels for injection.
b. Some hospitals allow arterial embalming prior to autopsy; in such situations, the hospital may have preference as to the vessels to use for injection of the body.
c. Some medical schools may allow embalming and a funeral service before the body is taken by the medical school. Specific vessels may be necessitated by the medical school for the embalming of the body.

▶ MULTIPOINT INJECTION SITES

When arterial embalming solution has failed to distribute to a particular area, or if the embalmer feels that an insufficient amount of arterial solution is present in a body area, the first consideration should be the direct arterial injection of that area. **The injections here all involve treatment of the head or appendages.** If there is insufficient arterial solution in any area of the **trunk portion** of the body, these areas are best treated by hypodermic injection of the area rather than by arterial treatment.

Three methods of embalming can be used to treat body areas that have not received enough arterial solution: (1) arterial embalming, (2) hypodermic embalming, and (3) surface embalming.

Multipoint injection of the head or limbs could include injection of one or more of the following arteries in the **head,** the right and left common carotid and the right and left facial arteries; in the **arms,** the left or right axillary, brachial, radial, or ulnar artery; and in the **legs,** the left or right external iliac, femoral, popliteal, anterior tibial, or posterior tibial artery. As part of the ongoing embalming analysis, the embalmer must determine what additional injections are necessary to properly arterially embalm the areas where additional solution is needed.

Example 1. Suppose the starting injection site was the right femoral artery. Assume that there is no arterial solution in the entire left arm. Methods to stimulate the flow of the arterial solution into the arm have been unsuccessful. It is presumed that a clot or coagulum that was present in the abdominal aorta has been freed and has moved into the left subclavian artery. Now, the embalmer must select a secondary injection site. It is almost certain that the left axillary or brachial artery may be used. Injection from this point should establish distribution of solution down the arm and into the hand.

Example 2. Using the same set of circumstances as in Example 1, assume that arterial solution reaches only as far down the left arm as the elbow. Now, the embalmer must decide whether the radial or ulnar artery (or both) should be raised, the hand injected, and then the arterial tube reversed and some solution injected back toward the elbow.

Example 3. Assume that a body has been embalmed using the right common carotid artery for injection. Drainage was taken from the right internal jugular vein. After arterial embalming, it is felt that the right leg does not have enough arterial solution. The embalmer raises the right femoral artery to inject the leg. Drainage can be taken from (1) the right internal jugular vein, (2) the right femoral vein, or (3) the heart (during aspiration).

▶ ELEVATION OF VESSELS

After selecting an injection site, the embalmer elevates the vessels to the skin surface, places ligature under the vessels, and opens and inserts tubes into the artery for arterial solution injection and a drainage device into a selected vein for drainage.

After injection of the arterial solution, the embalmer evaluates the body to determine whether any further injection is necessary for regions that may have received an inadequate amount of preservative. If such areas are found, sectional injection sites are selected and an artery or arteries raised for direct injection into the areas needing additional solution.

This section of the chapter involves the general protocol for raising vessels. Later, the specific locations for incisions and the protocol for raising vessels with respect to the individual artery selected are examined.

1. Select instruments and prepare ligatures for the vessels to be used. Be certain that arterial tubes, especially very small tubes, are clear and working before inserting them into an artery.
2. Locate vessels and their respective sites for skin incision by the linear guide on the surface of the skin.
3. Generally, make incisions where the vessels are nearest the skin surface.
4. In the dissection for the vessels, remember that muscles do **not** have to be cut to locate arteries, veins, and nerves. These run in groups **between** the muscles. The only muscle that may have to be divided for locating vessels is the sternocleidomastoid muscle.

5. Make an incision through the skin. Use blunt dissection through the superficial and deep fascia. Locate the vessels on the basis of their anatomical guides and surrounding structures. Raise each vessel to the surface of the incision and place ligatures loosely around each vessel raised.

Example. When the internal jugular vein and the common carotid artery are raised, the vein is the superficial vessel. After a ligature is placed around the vein, it is pulled laterally. The artery can easily be located on the medial side of the vein, a little deeper than the vein. The common carotid artery is described as being **medial** and **deep** in its relationship to the internal jugular vein.

6. The order in which vessels are raised varies, depending on the relationship of the artery to the vein. Two general rules should be remembered:
   a. *When both the artery and the vein are to be used (as in a one-point injection), always raise the superficial vessel first.*
   b. *When both the artery and the vein are to be used at the same location* (as in a one-point injection), **always insert instruments** (arterial tube or drainage instrument) **into the deepest vessel first**.

Example. When raising the right internal jugular vein and the right common carotid artery, raise the vein **first,** because it is the most superficial. Pull the vein laterally, raise the **deeper** common carotid artery to the surface, open the artery, insert the arterial tubes, return to the vein, open the vein, and insert the drainage instrument.

7. Make an incision into the artery, insert the arterial tube, and tighten the ligature to secure the tube into place.
8. Always use arterial tubes slightly smaller than the lumen of the artery into which they are to be inserted. **Do not** force arterial tubes into arteries.
9. If clotted material is present in an **artery,** especially in the common carotid artery, attempt to gently remove this material.
10. Arteriosclerosis does not always mean that it cannot be used for injection. Starting from the incision, find the "softest" portion of the exposed artery. Some forms of arteriosclerosis actually form a "wall" around the lumen. Open the sclerotic artery—observe if there is a small lumen pushed to one side of the artery into which a small arterial tube can be inserted.
11. If an artery is accidentally broken (arteries remain open and do not collapse), merely locate the two open ends and attach a hemostat to

each. Carefully apply new ligatures and insert arterial tubes.

▶ INSTRUMENTS AND LIGATURES

To raise an artery for injection and a vein for drainage, the following instruments may be used:

Instrument	Use
Scalpel	Making the incision; opening the artery or the vein
Double-point scissors	Making the incision; preparing ligatures; opening the artery or vein
Aneurysm needle	Dissecting fat and fascia; elevating vessels at surface
Bone separator	Elevating vessels at skin surface
Arterial tubes	For insertion into the artery for injection of fluid
Drainage tube	For insertion into the vein for drainage control
Angular spring forceps	For insertion into the vein for drainage control (in lieu of a drainage tube)
Straight spring forceps	Passing ligatures around the vessels
Grooved director	Assisting in expansion of the vein for insertion of the drainage device

This list represents the minimum number of instruments. Various other instruments can also be used. These include arterial hemostats (for holding the arterial tubes in place within the artery; this is of great help in autopsy preparation), ligature passers, arterial scissors, and retractors. Ligatures for securing the arterial and drain tubes are generally linen or cotton thread. The cotton is somewhat thicker and softer and many embalmers prefer it.

Cut ligatures long enough so that you can get a good grip on the string to make a very secure tie. A length of 8 to 12 inches is comfortable to work with.

▶ VESSELS USED FOR ARTERIAL EMBALMING

The arteries discussed in this chapter from the standpoint of injection site are the common carotid artery, femoral artery, external iliac artery, axillary artery, brachial artery, popliteal artery, radial artery, ulnar artery, facial artery, abdominal aorta, thoracic aorta, anterior tibial artery, and posterior tibial artery. With respect to these arteries, the area supplied, the considerations for their use, precautions, locations for incisions

for raising the vessels, and the protocol for raising the vessels and inserting instruments when both the artery and the vein are being used for an injection and drainage site are discussed.

Also discussed (along with the accompanying artery) is the use for drainage of the internal jugular vein, femoral vein, external iliac vein, axillary vein, and inferior vena cava. The location and use of the right atrium of the heart as a drainage point are included in the discussion. Because the incisions for the veins are the same as those for the arteries, the student is asked to refer to the artery incisions.

Common Carotid Artery

To be accurate in the discussion of this vessel, consideration is given to the use of a one-point injection, but there follows a discussion of **restricted cervical injection,** which employs both right and left common carotid arteries.

The common carotid artery is the largest vessel the embalmer can raise from a superficial point in a body region outside the trunk area. The incision is made in the inferior portion of the neck. This large artery is closely situated near the **arch of the aorta,** which is the central distribution point for arterial fluid. The common carotid artery can well be described as the "best choice" for injection of the body, especially if there has been any time delay between death and preparation or if vascular difficulties are anticipated.

1. Regions supplied
   a. If the injection is directed superiorly, the head and the face are embalmed.
   b. If the injection is directed inferiorly, the opposite side of the face and the head are embalmed as are the trunk and appendages.
2. Considerations
   a. It is very large in diameter.
   b. It has no branches except the terminal branches, so it is easily raised to the skin surface.
   c. It is very elastic.
   d. It is rarely found to be sclerotic.
   e. It supplies fluid directly to the head.
   f. It is situated close to the arch of the aorta.
   g. It is accompanied by a very large vein that can be used for drainage.
   h. Arterial coagula are pushed away from the head.
3. Precautions
   a. The head may be overinjected.
   b. If leakage occurs, it may be seen.
   c. Some types of instruments, if improperly used, may mark the side of the face or jaw line.
   d. The incisions may be visible with some types of clothing.

4. Incisions for the common carotid and the internal jugular vein
   a. *Supraclavicular* (anterior lateral): The incision is made on the clavicle (collar bone) from a point near the sternoclavicular articulation and is directed laterally.
   b. *Anterior vertical* (parallel): The incision is made from a point near the sternoclavicular articulation and is directed upward on the sternocleidomastoid muscle.
   c. *Posterior vertical* (parallel): The incision is made posterior to the sternocleidomastoid muscle, 2 inches below the lobe of the ear, and is directed downward toward the base of the neck.
   d. *Anterior horizontal*: The incision is made at the base of the neck from a point on the sternocleidomastoid muscle and is directed posteriorly.
   e. *Flap incision (semilunar)*: This incision is used by the operator when it is necessary to raise the vessels on both the right and left sides for injection or drainage. The incision extends from a point lateral and slightly superior to the sternoclavicular articulation and is directed downward on the upper chest wall, across and upward to a similar location on the opposite side. The pattern may be either a U or an inverted C in shape.
   f. *Strap line*: This incision is adaptable to the embalming of females. The incision is made approximately 2 inches lateral to the base of the neck on the line where the strap of the undergarments crosses the shoulder (Fig. 9–1).

5. Suggested protocol for raising the common carotid artery and the accompanying internal jugular vein
   a. Take a position **at the head of the embalming table.**
   b. Turn the head of the body in the **direction opposite** that of the vessels being raised (i.e., if the right common carotid is being raised, turn the head to the left).
   c. Place a shoulder block under the shoulders and lower the head of the body on the head block.
   d. Make the incision. Dissect through (or cut through) the platysma muscle and the superficial fat and fascia.
   e. The sternocleidomastoid muscle will exhibit an area where its fibers part at the clavicle (it looks like a triangle).
   f. Raise the **internal jugular vein:** Put a ligature around the vein and pull it laterally.
   g. Go **medial and deep** and locate the common carotid and bring it to the surface; put two

A

B

Figure 9–1. A. Anterior vertical, posterior vertical, and strap line incisions. **B.** Supraclavicular, semilunar, and anterior horizontal incisions.

strings around the artery; open the artery; insert arterial tubes superiorly and inferiorly; secure them with a tight ligature.
   h. Return to the vein; open the vein and insert a drainage instrument (Fig. 9–2).

6. Protocol if the internal jugular vein is collapsed (and cannot be easily identified).
   a. Make the proper incision.
   b. Take a position at the **head of the table.**
   c. Elevate the shoulders and lower the head.
   d. Turn the head in the direction opposite that of the vessels being raised.
   e. Palpate the common carotid artery after dissection.
   f. Bring the artery to the surface and insert arterial tubes into the artery.
   g. Begin arterial injection.
   h. When vein becomes dilated, elevate it to the surface and ligate.

Figure 9–2. A. Point at which an anterior parallel incision is made. **B.** The (superficial) internal jugular vein is raised first. **C.** A ligature is placed around the vein and it is pulled laterally. **D.** With the vein pulled laterally, the artery, which is medial and deep to the vein, is raised.

E

F

Figure 9–2. (*Continued*) **E.** Arterial tubes are placed into the common carotid and secured with ligatures. **F.** The operator elevates the vein and inserts a drainage instrument toward the heart. Note the suggested position of the operator throughout this procedure.

Internal Jugular Vein

The right internal jugular vein is in direct line with the right atrium of the heart. The right atrium is the central point of blood drainage in the dead human body. The left internal jugular, although a very large vein, does not lead directly into the right atrium. Instead, it joins with the left subclavian vein to form the left brachiocephalic vein, which crosses to the right side of the chest, joins with the opposite brachiocephalic vein, and forms the superior vena cava. For this reason, the right internal jugular vein is preferred as a drainage site.

1. Considerations
   a. The vein is very large.
   b. There is direct drainage from the face and the head.
   c. It is accompanied by the common carotid artery, which can be used for injection.
   d. The right internal jugular vein leads directly through the right brachiocephalic and superior vena cava into the right atrium, allowing easy removal of clotted material that may be present.

2. Precautions
   a. Leakage may be visible.
   b. Drainage instruments, if improperly used, may mark the face.
   c. The incision may be visible with some clothing.

Because of its size, its location with respect to the right atrium of the heart, and its ability to directly drain the head, the right internal jugular vein certainly must be considered as one of the best possible sites for drainage during arterial injection.

An excellent method of embalming involves raising **both** the right and left common carotid arteries at the beginning of the embalming process. This method of embalming, **restricted cervical injection**, most effectively controls arterial solution entering the head and the face (Fig. 9–3). The procedures are as follows:

1. Raise the right common carotid artery and the right internal jugular vein.
2. Insert an arterial tube into the right common carotid artery directed toward the head. Insert a

Figure 9–3. Restricted cervical injection affords control over the amount and strength of solution entering the facial tissues.

second tube into the artery directed toward the trunk. **Be certain to keep the stopcock OPEN on the tube directed toward the head.**

3. Insert a drainage device into the right internal jugular vein.

4. Raise the left common carotid artery only. **Insert a tube into the artery directed toward the head and leave the stopcock OPEN.** Tie off the lower portion of the artery.

The following are some advantages to use of the restricted cervical injection:

- The arteries are large.
- Carotids are very elastic and have no branches, so they are easy to elevate.
- The arteries are accompanied by the largest veins.
- The arteries are rarely sclerotic.
- Clots or coagula present in the arterial system will be pushed away from the head area.
- Solution is supplied directly to the head.
- This injection allows the best control over the amount of arterial solution entering the head.
- Two strengths of arterial solution can be used: one for the trunk and another for the head.
- Two rates of flow can be used: one for the trunk and a second for the head.
- Two pressures can be used: one for the head and another for the trunk.
- Large volumes of solution can be run through the trunk without overinjecting the head.

Features may be set after the trunk is embalmed and aspirated if purging took place during injection.

Facial Artery

The facial artery can be used in two situations: in bodies that have been autopsied and the common carotid and portions of the external carotid removed and in bodies with clotting or sclerosis of the carotid artery, most frequently found in persons who have suffered from an extracerebral stroke.

The facial artery supplies arterial solution to the soft tissues of the face, the upper and lower lips, the mouth area, the side of the nose, and the medial tissues of the face and some portions of the lower eyelid. The artery is smaller than the carotid or femoral and requires a very small arterial tube (see Fig. 8–2).

In life, the facial artery can be felt pulsating by touching the inferior margin of the mandible just in front of the angle of the jaw. It is in this same location that a small incision is made to raise the artery. Fibers of the platysma muscle have to be opened, and by moving the aneurysm needle along the inferior margin of the mandible, the embalmer can find the artery. This incision is best closed with super glue (Fig. 9–4).

Axillary Artery

The axillary artery is a continuation of the subclavian artery. It begins at the lateral border of the first rib after passing through the **cervicoaxillary canal**. (This canal is bounded by the first rib, clavicle, and scapula.) This vessel can be used to embalm the entire body.

During the early years of embalming, when much work was done at the residence of the deceased, this vessel was preferred. The head received a large amount of solution, and the incision itself was easily hidden from view. It was a very "clean" artery to employ for injection,

Figure 9–4. Left facial artery.

and drainage was generally taken directly from the right side of the heart by use of a trocar. Early arterial solutions were quite strong, so large volumes were not injected. The small volume would quickly clear the head when injection was from the axillary.

Today, the axillary artery is used principally as a secondary point of injection where there is insufficient arterial solution in the arm or hand. The axillary vein is relatively small and may not allow easy access for the passage of clotted materials.

1. Regions supplied
   a. If the arterial tube is directed toward the hand, the axillary supplies fluid directly to the arm and hand.
   b. If the tube is directed toward the body, the entire body can be embalmed from this location.
2. Considerations
   a. Arterial solution flows directly into the arm and hand.
   b. The artery is close to the face.
   c. The vessels are superficial.
   d. The artery is close to the center of arterial solution distribution.
3. Precautions
   a. The arm must be extended, especially if the vein is to be used for drainage.
   b. The artery is small for injection of the whole body.
   c. The artery is accompanied by a vein that is small for drainage.
   d. There exists the danger of overinjecting the facial tissues.
   e. There are numerous branches and, often, anomalies.
4. Incision for the axillary artery and vein
   a. The arm should be extended (abducted) a little less than 90 degrees from the body. The incision is made parallel to the linear guide. Many embalmers make this incision along the anterior margin of the hairline of the axilla.
5. Suggested protocol for raising the axillary artery and vein

   When the arm is abducted, the artery will be found slightly anterior and deep to the axillary vein and the brachial plexus. The vein can be described as being located medial and superficial to the axillary artery (Fig. 9–5).
   a. Abduct (extend) the arm and rest the distal portion of the arm on the hip of the embalmer. Try not to abduct the arm beyond 90 degrees, as this tends to compress the structures in the arm.
   b. Make the incision along the anterior margin of the hairline.
   c. Begin the dissection and first locate the axillary vein. This will be a superficial vessel.
   d. Place a ligature around the vein and pull the vein away from the incision and downward.
   e. Go "above" and "behind" the vein to locate the artery.
   f. Pass two ligatures around the artery.
   g. Incise the artery and place arterial tubes into the vessel.
   h. Return to the vein, pass a second ligature around the vein, and open the vein and insert a drainage tube or forceps toward the heart.

Brachial Artery

The brachial artery supplies fluid directly to the arm and the hand. If the tube is directed toward the body, the artery is large enough that the entire body can be embalmed from this point, but because of the small size of the brachial artery, injection would be quite slow and it would be very difficult to build effective arterial pressure. Drainage from the accompanying basilic vein is difficult, as this vein is quite small.

The incision for the brachial artery may be made anywhere along the upper half of the linear guide. The proximal third is preferred. Many embalmers make this incision approximately 1 inch above and parallel to the linear guide. To raise the artery, the arm should be abducted.

Radial Artery

The radial artery supplies solution directly to the thumb side of the hand. It is quite superficial and may easily be palpated through the skin in the area of the wrist. The incision is made parallel to the artery directly on the linear guide, approximately 1 inch above the base of the thumb (Fig. 9–6).

Ulnar Artery

The ulnar artery supplies arterial solution directly to the medial side of the hand. The incision is made parallel to the vessel directly over the linear guide. Generally, the incision should terminate approximately 1 inch above the pisiform bone (Fig. 9 7).

There are times when injection of the axillary or brachial artery alone will establish adequate flow of solution into the arm and the hand. With heavy clotting, however, it is necessary to raise and inject both the radial and the ulnar arteries to adequately embalm the hand. Also, a tube may be directed toward the arm from the radial or ulnar artery in an attempt to inject more solution into the arm area.

If there is difficulty clearing the hand, the embalmer may try injecting only the radial artery. When this is done, digital pressure should be placed on the ulnar artery. By application of such pressure, short-circuiting

Figure 9–5. A. Location of incision used for raising the axillary artery. This particular incision raises the axillary artery where it becomes the brachial artery. **B.** The artery lies deep (behind) to the vein. **C.** Ligatures are passed around the artery. **D.** An arterial tube is inserted to demonstrate how the arm would be injected.

of the solution will not occur and more solution will flow into both sides of the hand.

Some embalmers also raise the brachial artery in the area of the antecubital fossa, where the artery divides into the radial and ulnar arteries. The arterial tube can be directed into each of these arteries from this point, avoiding an incision in the wrist area, which may be a difficult area to tightly suture, especially if edema is present.

Femoral Artery

The second, most frequently used set of vessels for arterial embalming comprises the femoral artery and the femoral vein. The artery is located superficial and lateral

to the femoral vein. Because it is a continuation of the external iliac artery and vein, this set of vessels is often referred to as the iliofemoral vessels.

1. Regions supplied
   a. When the injection is directed toward the foot, the artery directly supplies solution to the leg and the foot.
   b. When a tube is directed toward the head, the artery supplies arterial solution to the opposite leg as well as the remainder of the body.
2. Considerations
   a. The artery is large.
   b. The incision is not visible.

Figure 9–6. Left radial artery.

c. Both sides of the head may receive an even distribution of solution (especially important if dyes are used with the arterial solution).

d. The artery is accompanied by a large vein, which can be used for drainage.

e. With the proper instruments, it can be a "clean" method of embalming; no solution or blood will pass under the body.

f. The head and arms can be posed without having to be further manipulated after embalming.

Figure 9–7. Right ulnar artery.

3. Precautions

a. The most frequent reason for inability to use the femoral artery as an injection point is the presence of arteriosclerosis in the artery.

b. In obese bodies, the vessels may be very deep.

c. There is no control over the solution entering the head, especially when large volumes of solution must be injected or when strong solutions are used.

d. Coagula in the arterial system can be pushed into the vessels that supply the arms or the head, areas that will be viewed.

e. Large branches might be mistaken for the femoral artery.

4. Incision for the femoral artery and vein

a. This incision is made over the linear guide for the artery beginning at a point slightly medial to the center of a line drawn between the anterior superior iliac spine and the pubic symphysis. Some embalmers prefer to make the incision directly over the inguinal ligament; others prefer to make the incision an inch or more inferior to the inguinal ligament. The external iliac vessels at the inguinal ligament become the femoral vessels. The external iliac artery lies lateral and slightly superficial to the external iliac vein at the inguinal ligament. The acronym VAN can be used: the Vein is the most medial structure, then comes the Artery, and the most lateral structure is the Nerve.

5. Suggested protocol for raising the femoral artery and vein

a. Stand at the right or the left side of the table.

b. Make the incision parallel to the vessels, on the linear guide through the skin and the superficial fascia.

c. Dissect superficial fat and fascia bluntly. Observe the great saphenous vein, which is quite superficial.

d. Locate the sartorius muscle. The vessels are found along the medial side of this muscle.

e. Locate the femoral artery and dissect the artery free. Place a ligature around the superior and the inferior portions of the dissected artery.

f. Pull the artery laterally (toward the embalmer) and dissect medially and deeper to free the femoral vein.

g. Clean off the vein, being careful not to rupture it. Also, be careful around the tributaries, which may be full of blood. Bring the vein to the surface and pass one ligature around each end of the dissected portions of the vein.

h. Make an incision into the vein and insert the drainage device, tube, or forceps toward the heart. Tie the tube into the vein. (Keep the vein ligatures on the medial side of the thigh and the artery ligatures on the lateral side of the thigh.)

i. Bring the artery to the surface of the incision. Incise the artery and insert one arterial tube directed toward the head and a second tube directed down the leg. Secure both with the ligatures (Fig. 9–8).

Femoral Vein

The femoral vein may be used as a drainage point. The vein is large, and because of its location the incision will not be seen. Because of its location, the femoral vein is assisted by gravity in draining blood from the body.

1. Considerations
   a. The vein is large.
   b. With tubing attached to a drain tube, it can be a very clean method of drainage; water and blood need not come down over the table and under the body.
2. Precautions
   a. The weight of the viscera can restrict drainage from the upper portions of the body.
   b. Abdominal pressure from gases or ascites can exert pressure on the vein and restrict drainage.

A

B

C

D

Figure 9–8. A. The femoral artery and veins are raised. **B.** The artery lies just lateral to the sartorius muscle. **C.** The femoral artery is superficial and slightly lateral to the vein. **D.** Ligatures are passed beneath the artery and it is pulled laterally, toward the embalmer.

E

F

G

Figure 9–8. (*Continued*) **E.** The femoral vein is raised; it is medial and deep to the artery. **F.** Ligatures are passed around the vein and a drain tube is inserted toward the heart. **G.** Arterial tubes are placed in the artery.

c. In obese bodies, the vein is very deep.
d. Many tributaries flow into the femoral vein, and care must be taken not to rupture any of them.
e. Clots in the right atrium and the upper areas of the vascular system may be difficult to remove.
f. Pressure on the heart from hydrothorax (as frequently seen in deaths from pneumonia) may make it difficult to establish good drainage from the right atrium and the large veins of the head and the arms.

Popliteal Artery

The popliteal artery is used as a secondary injection site when solution has not reached the area of the leg below the knee. Because of the inconvenient location of this artery, it is generally used only in special circumstances.

Examples include severance of arteries from traumatic mutilation of the leg or bone removal for transplant.

Most tissues of the body are best preserved and more uniformly preserved by arterial injection. As the legs will not be viewed, other methods of embalming can be used, including surface and hypodermic embalming. **FIRST,** attempt to inject the legs using the external iliac or the femoral artery.

As previously stated, the popliteal artery is generally used only when there has been an interruption of the arterial pathway, as in accidents or mutilations. The limbs of the arthritic body may be in such a position that the femoral vessels cannot be used, and, because of the "swayed" position of the legs, the popliteal artery may be easy to work with.

Two incisions can be used: (1) The body may be turned and the incision made down the center of the popliteal space, parallel to the artery. (2) If the body is

Figure 9–9. Incision location (optional) for the left popliteal artery.

Figure 9–10. Right anterior tibial artery, lateral to the crest of the tibia.

not turned, the knee can be slightly flexed and a longitudinal incision made along the posterior–medial aspect of the lower third of the thigh, actually just superior to the popliteal space (Fig. 9–9). Because of the location of the artery and the size of the vessels, the accompanying vein is not used as a drainage site.

Anterior and Posterior Tibial Arteries

The anterior and tibial arteries supply arterial solution directly to the portion of the leg below the knee and into the foot. Unlike the superficial radial and ulnar arteries, which supply the distal portion of the arm and the hand, these arteries are deeper, making them more difficult to locate and to bring to the surface of the incisions. In addition, the skin covering the distal portion of the leg is very tight, making suture of the incisions very difficult. When suturing is difficult, leakage can become a problem.

With regard to arteriosclerosis, it would be most impractical to attempt to raise and inject the tibial arteries when the femoral artery is affected by arteriosclerosis, especially if gangrene or necrosis is present in the foot or in the distal portion of the leg. Treatment, when the latter conditions are present, is best accomplished by hypodermic treatment of the leg with cavity fluid; the leg should be painted with preservative autopsy gel and a plastic stocking containing embalming powder placed on the limb.

The incision for raising the anterior tibial artery is made along the lateral margin of the inferior third of the crest of the tibia. In the distal portion of the leg, it lies at the superficial margin of the tibia. By using the aneurysm needle to dissect down along the tibia, the embalmer can locate the artery (Fig. 9–10).

The incision for the posterior tibial artery is made midway between the medial malleolus and the large calcaneous tendon.

Abdominal Aorta and Thoracic Aorta

The abdominal aorta and thoracic aorta are large vessels very deeply seated in the abdominal and thoracic cavities. They lie in the center of the body and can be found on the anterior surface of the spinal column. The thoracic or abdominal aorta may be used for injection after complete or partial autopsy or organ donation and in infants.

The thoracic or abdominal aorta may become a vessel for injection in certain bodies where an incision has been made from which the vessels can be dissected and identified. Such bodies might include those dying following recent surgery; bodies in which partial autopsies have been performed, or the bodies of organ donors. Drainage may be taken from a vein that the embalmer raises such as the femoral or internal jugular vein. Drainage may also be taken directly from the inferior or superior vena cava. Use of the aorta for injection and the vena cava for drainage is determined by the amount of exposure of these vessels created by the partial autopsy or organ removal.

In the unautopsied infant, the abdominal aorta can be exposed by making an incision to the left of the midline, beginning a few inches below the xiphoid process of the sternum and extending over the abdominal wall approximately 4 inches in length. The greater omentum is thus exposed. It can be reflected upward, and the small intestines can be pushed aside or lifted out of the abdominal cavity to expose the abdominal aorta

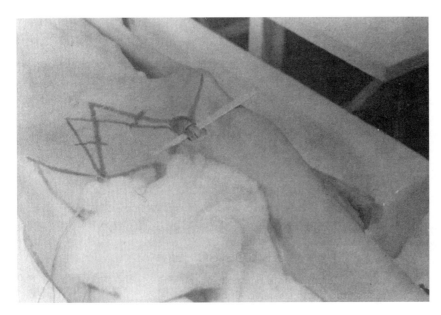

Figure 9–11. Linear guides and incision location for raising the left external iliac artery and vein. The artery is lateral to the vein at the inguinal ligament.

and the inferior vena cava resting on the spinal column in the midline of the abdomen.*

The thoracic aorta in the infant can be exposed by making a midline incision down the center of the sternum. Because the sternum is quite soft, a sharp scalpel can be used to divide it. The sternum is retracted and held in this opened position. The pericardium of the heart is now exposed and can be cut open with a pair of surgical scissors. After the pericardium is opened, the right auricle, the little ear-like appendage at the top right side of the heart, can be cut open and used as a site for drainage. If the heart is moved to the right, the descending thoracic aorta can be exposed as well as the arch of the aorta above it. The aorta can be opened and a tube inserted for injection (see Chapter 16).

External Iliac Artery

For considerations on the use of the external iliac artery, see section Femoral Artery, above. The incision is made over the inguinal ligament (Fig. 9–11). Because the external iliac artery passes beneath the inguinal ligament, it lies on the lateral side of the external iliac vein. If the leg is injected from this point, in the autopsied body, the artery supplies solution to the lower extremity and the anterior abdominal wall.

Internal Iliac Artery

The internal iliac artery is a branch of the common iliac artery that runs medially into the pelvic cavity. In the autopsied body, injection of this artery supplies

embalming solution to the gluteal muscles and the peroneal regions.

Inferior Vena Cava

For completeness, at this point, the inferior vena cava is discussed as a drainage point. This site can be used for drainage when a partial autopsy has been performed. If the contents of the thorax have been removed, the abdominal viscera and lower extremities can be injected (1) through the abdominal aorta or (2) by clamping off the aorta and injecting the femoral artery. With either point of injection, drainage can be taken directly from the remnants of the inferior vena cava. The inferior vena cava is located to the right of the abdominal aorta at the posterior portion of the diaphragm.

If the contents of the abdominal cavity have been removed in a partial autopsy, the thoracic viscera, the head, and the arms can be injected from the descending thoracic aorta. Or, the aorta can be clamped closed and the upper portions of the body injected from the carotid or axillary vessels. Drainage can easily be taken directly from the remnants of the inferior vena cava.

When drainage is taken from the inferior vena cava, it is not necessary to place a drainage device in the vein. To create intermittent drainage, the inferior vena cava can be closed shut with a hemostat. A large piece of cotton can also be held over the vena cava with a gloved hand.

Right Atrium of the Heart

When drainage is difficult to establish, the right side of the heart may be pierced with a trocar for drainage. The trocar is inserted into the right side of the heart and should be placed in the right atrium. Piercing of the

---

*These procedures should be used only when absolutely no other methods would produce satisfactory results, and when used, be certain that proper permission has been obtained.

heart should not begin until one-half to one full gallon of arterial solution has been injected.

To drain from the right side of the heart, the trocar is inserted through the abdominal wall at the standard point of entry (2 inches to the left and 2 inches above the umbilicus). The trocar is directed into the mediastinum area and intersects a line extending from the lobe of the **right** ear to the **left** anterior superior iliac spine. Actually, if the trocar is simply directed toward the right ear lobe, the point should pass into the right side of the heart. The aspirator can be stopped at this point and the drainage established by a gravity system.

It is wise to attach clear plastic tubing to the trocar so that further movement of the trocar can be **stopped** immediately after it enters the heart. This very old method for removing blood during arterial injection was used when bodies were embalmed at the residence of the deceased.

► MAKING THE INCISION INTO THE ARTERY AND VEIN

To open the artery or the vein, a scissors or scalpel may be used, depending on the preference of the embalmer. In the method most commonly employed to open the artery or the vein, the embalmer simply makes a **transverse** cut into the vessel from the edge of the vessel to the center or just slightly beyond the center. Cutting too far may weaken the vessel enough that it will break into two pieces.

Very elastic arteries such as the carotid and the axillary arteries can easily be stretched to the surface of the incision. With arteries such as the femoral, when some sclerosis is present, raising the vessel to the skin surface can create great tension on the artery. Care should be taken in opening sclerotic vessels to avoid breaking the vessel. As soon as you observe the lumen in this type of vessel, cut no further.

A longitudinal incision may also be used to open vessels. Most embalmers prefer to elevate these vessels on a bone separator. Using a scalpel, cut a longitudinal incision in the center of the vessel running parallel to the vessel. Most embalmers prefer to use a scalpel; however, double-point scissors can also be used. The longitudinal incision is not recommended for opening sclerotic arteries. Many embalmers use this incision for veins, for it provides a large opening for drainage instruments. Two arterial tubes may be placed into position using this incision for the artery.

A combination of transverse and longitudinal incision is preferred by many embalmers, especially for opening veins. It is also most helpful when a drainage tube is to be inserted, because it permits drainage from the opposite end of the vein. A wedge can also be cut

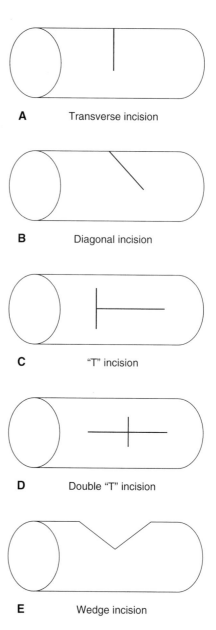

Figure 9–12. A. Transverse incision. **B.** Diagonal incision. **C.** "T" incision. **D.** Double "T" incision. **E.** Wedge incision.

into an artery or a vein with double-point scissors or a scalpel. This method is not recommended for sclerotic arteries (Fig. 9–12).

► CONCEPTS FOR STUDY AND DISCUSSION

1. Explain each of the following methods of injection:
   a. Multipoint injection
   b. Sectional embalming
   c. Restricted cervical injection
   d. One-point injection
   e. Six-point injection
   f. Split injection

2. Differentiate between arteries, veins, and nerves.

3. List the 12 major factors to consider in choosing an artery for injection and a vein for drainage.

4. List several advantages to use of the common carotid artery as a vessel for injection.

5. List the steps for raising and inserting instruments into the common carotid artery and the internal jugular vein.

6. List six incisions that can be used to raise the common carotid artery.

7. List the advantages to use of the restricted cervical method of injection.

8. Describe the relationship of the common carotid artery to the internal jugular vein.

9. Describe the relationship of the femoral artery to the femoral vein.

10. Describe the relationship of the axillary artery to the axillary vein.

11. Give the steps for raising and inserting instruments into the femoral artery and vein.

12. Describe where the incisions are made for raising the radial and ulnar arteries.

13. Describe several incisions that can be used to open an artery for insertion of the arterial tube.

14. List the incisions that can be used to raise and inject the popliteal artery.

▶ BIBLIOGRAPHY

American Board of Funeral Service Education, *Course Content Syllabus,* St. Joseph, Missouri: American Board of Funeral Service Education, 2008.

CHAPTER 10

EMBALMING ANALYSIS

CHAPTER OBJECTIVES

► Variable factors of embalming analysis
► Variable embalming treatments
► Pre-embalming considerations
► Embalming considerations
► Post-embalming considerations

No single chapter in any embalming textbook or classroom lecture could cover the subject of embalming analysis. The **embalming analysis** includes those analytical observations of the deceased human body, by the embalmer, **before**, **during**, and **following** the arterial embalming of the body. The observations of the conditions of the body determine the treatments necessary to create and maintain the body in a well-preserved condition while maintaining a presentable appearance. The analysis incorporates relevant factors from the disciplines of anatomy, pathology, microbiology, chemistry, restorative art, and of course embalming. Monitoring the body must continue until either final disposition or release of custody of the body to another funeral establishment. **The analysis, monitoring, and the embalming techniques used need to be fully documented in an Embalming Care Report and kept as a permanent record.**

► PREVIOUS SYSTEMS OF ANALYSIS

Older embalming textbooks describe hundreds of diseases, poisons, and traumatic modes of death and the embalming treatment for each. The treatment, however, only concerned the specific pathological or traumatic problem. No consideration was given to any other factors such as the time between death and preparation, postmortem changes, etc.

In the late 1950s, a "typing of bodies" analysis was developed. Bodies were classified by conditions of the body rather than by a specific cause of death. Professor Ray E. Slocum of The Dodge Company published a very complete system of "body types" based primarily on the time between death and preparation, and the degree to which postmortem changes had occurred. Separate categories were established for bodies with jaundice and for infants. In all, Professor Slocum established six categories, and with each category, he described a specific formulation of chemicals necessary for the preparation of the body. This "recipe" method might be fine for one embalming chemical company, but there are many manufacturers of embalming chemicals, and formulations and fluids vary from company to company.

The Slocum method of body typing, or **pre-embalming observation,** is the approach most embalmers take in determining what embalming techniques to employ. It would be too difficult to approach each body by the specific disease or effects produced by a specific drug.

Medicine took a radical change in the early to mid-1960s with the extensive development and use of medications. Now, the embalmer has to be concerned with the cause of the death, effects of the medications, and the postmortem body changes. Often, the conditions created by the medications become the primary concern in the embalming analysis. It combines the **effects** of disease and medications.

► PRESENT DAY METHODOLOGY

The observable conditions of the body combined with information concerning the death provide the data necessary for the embalmer to devise the treatments necessary for the embalming of the body and maintaining the embalmed body. This analysis of the body is done within three time periods: *before, during,* and *after* embalming. The analysis follows four simple steps:

1. observation and evaluation
2. proposed method(s) of treatment
3. implementation
4. observation of results.

The analysis of the body using these steps lets the **body** primarily tell the embalmer what needs to be done in each time period to obtain the objectives of temporary preservation, sanitation, and achieving and maintaining an acceptable appearance of the deceased.

Communication

Communication is most important between the embalmer—the arranging funeral director—and the family of the deceased. It is important for the embalmer to know if visible tumors or long-standing discolorations or scars need to be removed or altered. If the face is emaciated or swollen, what are the expectations of the family with respect to restoration? If hair has been shaved from the head or lost due to chemotherapy, what does the family wish to be done for replacement? The embalmer often needs direction for shaving the facial hair of the deceased male or how a beard or moustache is to be trimmed. In the preparation of a deceased female, the embalmer needs to be informed of hairstyle, facial cosmetics, eye treatments, lipstick color, and fingernail polish, which the family requests. In addition, at the start of the embalming, it is helpful if the embalmer knows the location and date of the disposition of the body.

Just as important, the arranging funeral director needs to know the condition of the body with respect to height and weight, so properly sized clothing and casket can be selected. The funeral director also needs to know the condition of the remains, if death was traumatic, or if postmortem procedures were performed such as autopsy, organ and/or tissue donation. The funeral director also needs to know what extra time may be required for the preparation of the deceased when some of the previously mentioned conditions are present. This is important so that a satisfactory time can be set for viewing of the deceased that is accommodating for the family, funeral home and the embalmer.

General Embalming Analysis Factors and Embalming Treatments

The following is a list of embalming analysis factors that help the embalmer "to read the body" and to formulate the various embalming techniques.

- body conditions, including age, weight, musculature, body build

- immediate cause and manner of death
- effects of disease and/or trauma
- effects of drugs and medical treatments
- postmortem physical and chemical changes
- postmortem procedures: refrigeration; autopsy; organ/tissue recovery
- postmortem interval between death and embalming
- post-embalming: time between preparation and disposition.

The preceding general list of analysis factors allows the embalmer to select the proper techniques for the embalming of the body. A general list of embalming techniques (which can be performed in different ways) would include

- positioning of the body
- method of mouth and eye closure
- treatments for visible antemortem swellings that need to be reduced
- treatments for removing or altering visible antemortem discolorations
- techniques to use to raise sunken or emaciated facial tissues
- vessels for injection and drainage
- strength of the embalming solution
- volume of the embalming solution
- injection pressure and rate of flow
- necessary supplemental embalming treatments
- delayed or immediate cavity treatment following arterial injection.

The correct embalming treatment is dictated by the **conditions of the body** and not solely by the cause of death. Very few causes of death determine the embalming technique. Three examples could include death from a contagious or infectious disease, death from a ruptured aortic aneurysm, and death from renal failure.

In making an embalming analysis, three important guidelines should always be considered:

1. *The body must be SEEN at all stages of preparation to make the embalming analysis.*
2. *Prepare each body as if the deceased were dead from an infectious and highly contagious disease.*
   a. This is the premise for using Universal Precautions.
   b. Doing so sets a standard for embalming solution quality and quantity.
   c. Following this procedure sets a standard for disinfection practices with regard to the body and the preparation room environment.
3. *Prepare each body as if the disposition (with viewing) of the deceased will be delayed.*
   a. Doing so sets a standard for embalming chemical quality and quantity.

b. Following this procedure sets a standard for embalming thoroughness.

Extrinsic and Intrinsic Factors

The 2008 embalming committee of the American Board of Funeral Service Education lists the following **variable factors** to be considered in making an analysis of the body. These factors are given consideration throughout this text:

1. intrinsic factors
   a. cause and manner of death
   b. body conditions
      (1) pathological conditions
      (2) microbial influence
      (3) moisture content
      (4) thermal influences (fever)
      (5) nitrogenous waste products
      (6) weight
      (7) gas in tissues and/or cavities
      (8) age
   c. presence or absence of discolorations
   d. postmortem physical changes
   e. postmortem chemical changes
   f. effects of pharmaceutical agents
   g. illegal drugs
2. extrinsic factors
   a. environmental
      (1) atmospheric conditions
      (2) thermal influences
      (3) microbial influences
      (4) vermin
   b. time intervals
      (1) time between death and embalming
      (2) time between embalming and disposition
   c. The embalmer
      (1) firmness of the tissues of the embalmed body
      (2) personal preference for injection and drainage sites
      (3) personal preference for setting features
      (4) personal preference for positioning head and hands
      (5) time preference for cavity treatment.

▶ EMBALMING ANALYSIS, PART I: PRE-EMBALMING ANALYSIS

Embalmers consider four major factors in making a pre-embalming analysis: (1) general conditions of the body; (2) effects produced by disease processes; (3) effects produced by drugs or surgical procedures; and (4) effects of the postmortem period between death and embalming. In effect, the embalmer must learn to "read" the conditions of the body.

The embalmer must be concerned with the **conditions** of the body he or she can see, touch, or even smell. Most often, the embalmer does not know, at the time of the embalming, the cause of death or the medications which have been administered. It is also in this phase that treatments must be considered for antemortem conditions produced by trauma or surgery; postmortem events such as refrigeration, autopsy, organ and tissue recovery; and the postmortem changes that have occurred in the body.

MOST COMMON EMBALMING VARIABLES

Arterial injection site(s)
Venous drainage site(s)
Fluids for arterial embalming
Strength and volume of arterial solution
Injection pressure and rate of flow
Method of mouth and eye closure

▶ ADDITIONAL PRE-EMBALMING INFORMATION

Additional information may be obtained from the following sources. This information along with the conditions presented by the body will contribute to the pre-embalming analysis and the treatments necessary for the care of the deceased.

1. Certificate of death.
2. Infectious or contagious conditions of the deceased provided by the medical facility.
3. Information concerning the location and date for viewing and final disposition of the deceased. This could involve the shipping of the body to another funeral establishment or to a foreign country.
4. Shipping to a location outside of the United States may require specific embalming treatments and preparation of specific forms.
5. Specific family requests such as removal or alteration of: (1) a deceased man's facial hair; (2) longstanding scars or tumors; (3) medical device removal; and (4) cosmetic treatments.

General Intrinsic Body Conditions

The general intrinsic conditions of the body include age, body weight and build, musculature, protein level, and general skin condition.

Age

CHILD OR INFANT.   Arteries and veins will be much smaller than in the adult; specially sized instruments are needed for injection and drainage. Milder solutions may be needed (but preservative demands must determine solution strengths). A needle injector may not be usable for mouth closure. Positioning will vary from that for an adult.

ELDERLY.   Arteriosclerosis may eliminate the use of the femoral artery as an injection point. Absence of teeth and dentures may create problems in setting features. Suturing may be needed for mouth closure if the jawbone has atrophied.

Weight

EMACIATED.   Solution strengths may need to be reduced. Dehydration may create problems with eye closure and mouth closure.

OBESE.   Femoral vessels may be too deep to use for injection. Very large quantities of arterial solution will be needed. The internal jugular vein will afford the best drainage site. Restricted cervical injection will best control arterial solution entering facial tissues. There will be positioning problems.

Musculature.   In the healthy adult with firm skin and well-developed musculature, the embalmer can expect the embalming solution to result in very good firming of the body tissues. If there is a delay between death and preparation, this body can be expected to display intense rigor mortis, making it difficult to establish good distribution of the solution. Where bodies are wasted from disease and the musculature is not well developed and the skin is loose, the embalmer can expect little or no firming of the limbs from the embalming solution; swelling is expected if large volumes of mild solutions are injected. Senile, loose, flabby tissue does not assimilate the arterial solution as well as healthy, firm tissues.

Disease Processes and the Cause of Death.   The cause of death may not be known at the time of embalming; however, the embalmer can observe the effects that diseases have had on the body. For example, **jaundice** may be caused by the effect of drugs on the liver or red blood cells, obstruction of the bile duct, hepatitis, cancer of the liver, and hemolysis of red blood cells. It is the condition of jaundice that concerns the embalmer, not the disease that caused this condition.

The following excerpts, from an article written by Murray Shor (1972) of the American Academy of Funeral Service, illustrate how the same disease can produce different conditions in different persons. (Remember that it is not the cause of death or the disease but the **conditions** produced by the disease in the body that should concern the embalmer.)

> Let us begin by examining a very common disease and cause of death today—cancer. This pathological condition may attack and be confined to the stomach. In such an event, the patient would not be able to retain foods, either liquid or solid, for weeks just prior to death. He actually might die of starvation although the primary cause of death would be cancer of the stomach.

Primary Condition Unimportant

The embalmer now is presented with a thin, emaciated, dehydrated subject. The primary condition in the stomach is of little significance to him.

Consider next another patient with the same basic disease—cancer. In this subject, the malignancy is of the liver or the right suprarenal gland. The attendant enlargement of these structures bears down upon and obstructs the cisterna chyli, the lymph collecting station of the abdomen and lower extremities. This prevents the lymph from returning to the venous system from these areas. All of the parts drained by this system will become edematous and ascites will develop.

The primary cause of death in both examples is cancer. In one case, we have a subject with edema, ascites, and anasarca; in the other, an emaciated, dehydrated subject. We should also note here that many other diseases can cause the above-described conditions. (If we learn to treat the conditions, we will treat them successfully—regardless of the cause of death.)

Let me illustrate this further. In incompetence of the right atrioventricular valve of the heart, the valve fails to close efficiently. During the diastole, blood will regurgitate from the right ventricle to the right atrium. This, of course, reduces the amount of blood the right atrium can receive from the inferior vena cava. In turn, the amount of blood the vena cava receives from its tributaries is minimized. The resulting venous congestion in the lower venous system increases transudation of plasma and results again in edema and ascites. Whether the excess fluid is a result of cancer of the viscera or damage to the heart valves, the embalming treatment is the same.

Same Basic Treatment

By the same token, emaciation, whether caused by cancer of the stomach, actual starvation, or pulmonary tuberculosis, requires the same basic embalming treatment.

Further inquiry into cancer shows that obstruction to the passage of bile into the intestinal tract can lead to the very common embalming problem—jaundice. This condition also can be caused by obstruction of the common bile duct—a disease not usually related to cancer. Here again, it is the symptoms and not the disease that pose an embalming problem.

A disease that is as common as cancer and can produce as varied a group of postmortem conditions is arteriosclerosis. Depending on the vessel or vessels involved, we can get a wide range of different embalming problems.

For example, let us consider renal arteriosclerosis. Here, the blood vessels carrying blood to the kidneys are impaired. As a result, the kidneys diminish in size and efficiency. Nitrogenous wastes and urea instead of passing out of the body via kidney and other excretory organs will remain in the bloodstream and tissue spaces. The result will be uremia, cachexia, and possibly edema and ascites, as in some cancers. Arteriosclerosis can affect the vessels of the brain, causing a **stroke** which, in turn, can lead to other abnormalities. One of these is long-term **paralysis** of the extremities with the attendant atrophy and vasoconstriction. Another is long periods of confinement to bed, with the often attendant **decubitus ulcers**. A third is **immediate death** with **no special embalming problems**.

Again, the decubitus ulcers and the atrophied parts can stem from any other disease that confines the patient to bed for extended periods of time. In all these situations, the resulting conditions cause much greater embalming problems than the disease that led to them. The embalmer must not overlook the fact that any two or three of the diseases discussed here can and do coexist. So can each disease exist in two or more forms. Therefore, a patient can die with stomach and liver cancer. A patient can have liver cancer and renal or cerebral arteriosclerosis. In reality, then, **an embalmer should ask, "What conditions exist?" rather than "Of what did the subject die?"**

The reader should not construe this article to mean that the author discourages the study of pathology. It is intended, rather, to encourage the student to correlate his studies of pathology with embalming. It is incumbent upon him to learn the embalming treatments for the basic postmortem conditions that create problems. If the conditions are identified and properly treated, the embalming procedure will succeed regardless of the disease that caused the condition.

Drug Treatments and Surgical Procedures

Since the 1960s, there has been an increase in the therapeutic use of drugs. Like the hundreds of diseases and their effects on the body, it would be impossible for the embalmer to embalm a body using chemical formulations designed to combat the effects of a specific drug. Most often, a patient is given combinations of drugs, often over a long period. A drug does not always produce the same effects in each person. Here again, it is impor-

tant that the embalmer have an understanding of the possible effects of drugs and of the fact that embalming problems often stem from the long usage of drug therapy. The embalmer must treat the conditions that can be observed in the dead human body and **not** the effects of a specific medication.

Some effects of the long-term use of medications, which can affect the embalming of the body, include: (1) jaundice; (2) discolorations such as purpura and ecchymosis; (3) edema; (4) difficulty in establishing tissue firmness; (5) loss of hair (alopecia); (6) internal bleeding; (7) renal failure causing an increase in nitrogenous wastes in the tissues; (8) changes in the walls of cells making it more difficult for preservatives to act on body proteins; and (9) swelling of facial tissues (steroids).

Chemotherapeutic Agents are Toxic. The one axiom that can be universally applied to **all** chemotherapeutic agents is that they are **toxic**. Cellular changes occur when they are used, no matter which drug is administered. Even the relatively innocuous aspirin pill has its effects. Drugs have an effect on the skin, circulatory system, liver, and kidneys. Such changes may be comparatively minor in nature, limited to slight discolorations that respond readily to cosmetic treatment. But when they assume major proportions such as acute jaundice or saturate the body tissues with uremic poisons, the fixative action of the preservative chemicals contained in the arterial solutions used is seriously impaired (Table 10–1, Fig. 10–1).

Figure 10–1. Loss of cranial hair but growth of facial hair, and emaciation in this female is the result of extensive chemotherapy. Alopecia.

TABLE 10–1. EMBALMING COMPLICATIONS CREATED BY EXTENSIVE DRUG THERAPIES

Complication	Result
Immediate allergic reaction to the drug	Tissues appear swollen
	Discolored skin surface
	Possible skin eruptions
Liver failure	Edema (ascites); edema of lower extremities
	Increase in ammonia in the tissues (neutralizes formaldehyde)
	Purges caused by rupture of esophageal veins
	Gastrointestinal bleeding; fluid loss; possible purge
	Hair loss
	Jaundice
Renal failure	Increase in ammonia in the tissues
	Edema of tissues
	Gastrointestinal bleeding
	Pulmonary edema
	Congestive heart failure
	Discoloration of the skin (sallow color)
	Uremic pruritus of the skin
Damage to blood vessels	Skin hemorrhage (ecchymosis, purpural hemorrhage)
Damage to the walls	Breakdown of the skin; skin-slip often present
Clot formation (poor circulation of embalming fluids)	Breakage during arterial injection (causes discolorations)
Loss of cranial hair	
Growth of facial hair and hair on the forehead on women and children	
Creation of resistant strains of microbes	Disinfection treatment more difficult
	Exposure of embalmer to drug-resistant microbes
Cell membranes become less permeable	Creates "solid" edema that cannot be removed
	Makes passage of arterial solution into cell very difficult
Killing one type of microbe can stimulate growth of other types	Antibiotics used to kill bacteria give fungal organisms a chance to multiply
Jaundice	Breakdown of the red blood cell
	Liver failure
Congestive heart failure	Edema
	Drainage difficulties
	Facial discolorations
Scaling of skin (seen on facial tissues and between fingers)	Death of the superficial cells
Difficult tissue firming	Protein degeneration
	Ammonia buildup in the tissues which neutralizes formaldehyde
	Presence of edema

Blood Thinners. Drugs that thin the blood in life will often reduce postmortem blood clotting in the vascular system. Reduced postmortem clotting will improve distribution and subsequent diffusion of the arterial solution.

Bodies that exhibit a mid-line scar over the sternum no doubt in life had open heart surgery, valve repair or vascular by-pass, most of these persons take some form of anti-coagulant or blood thinning medication. Keeping the blood thin will increase postmortem hypostasis of the blood and intense livor mortis in the dependent tissues. Expansion of the veins in the distal arm will be noted when the arms are lowered to the sides of the body.

These indicators inform the embalmer that good distribution of the embalming solution can be expected.

Surgery. In making a pre-embalming analysis, choice of embalming technique may be greatly influenced by whether death occurred during or immediately after surgery. Surgery could be the primary factor in an analysis, as illustrated in the following examples.

HEART SURGERY OR AORTIC REPAIR. During these procedures, the heart may be stopped for a period during which an artificial means of life support is used. Frequently, if death occurs during or shortly after this type of surgery, the face and neck are grossly distended with edema. Repair of an abdominal aneurysm may not always be successful, and the interruption in circulation will necessitate sectional arterial injection.

ABDOMINAL SURGERY. Abdominal surgery on the bowel can result in peritonitis. There can be intense distension of the abdomen and bloodstream infection. These conditions require the use of a strong, well-coordinated arterial solution.

Whenever death follows surgery, there exists the potential for leakage from arteries and veins involved in the surgical procedure. The embalmer should use dyes to indicate the distribution of arterial solution. It may be necessary to inject a greater volume of arterial solution to compensate for solution that may be lost to the abdominal or thoracic cavities.

All surgical bodies should undergo thorough cavity treatment. The formation of tissue gas is always a possibility. Be certain a liberal amount of undiluted cavity fluid is injected into the area where the surgery was performed. It is also a good precaution to inject some undiluted cavity fluid into the tissues surrounding the surgical incision. Recent surgical incisions should be resutured before cavity aspiration and injection. It is most important in surgical deaths to reaspirate and possibly reinject the cavities.

Time: Postmortem Interval Between Death and Embalming

Pre-embalming analysis includes observation and evaluation of those changes that can occur during the postmortem interval between death and embalming. These conditions often can take precedence over the conditions created by disease, drugs, or the general conditions of the body.

For example, a person dies of cancer and is very emaciated and jaundiced because of the effects of drugs on the liver, and the body is not discovered in its residence for 2 days. If the weather is warm or a furnace is running, the postmortem changes, such as rigor mortis, stain, and decomposition, will determine the treatments that the embalmer must employ to preserve, sanitize, and restore the body.

As a general rule, best results are obtained when embalming is done as soon as possible following the death. Three postmortem conditions that interfere most with good distribution of the arterial solution are blood coagulation, rigor mortis, and decomposition. Embalming the body before these changes are established helps to produce better results.

If there is to be a delay between death and preparation, refrigeration will help to slow the onset of some postmortem changes. Cooling of the body helps to slow postmortem blood coagulation, the onset of rigor mor-

tis and decomposition. Refrigeration, however, can create its own problems depending on how long it is used. In time refrigeration can create dehydration, increase blood viscosity and postmortem edema, intense livor mortis and postmortem stain. Refrigeration can also create false signs of preserved tissue by the solidification of fats in the subcutaneous tissues and producing a "reddish" hue to the skin resembling dyes used in the embalming fluids. These conditions need to be carefully noted when making a pre-embalming analysis. The embalmer must also keep in mind that many bodies released from a coroner or medical examiner's office were kept first in a warm environment—possibly for a long period—and then placed under refrigeration. Those postmortem changes which occurred before refrigeration may still remain. Table 10–2 summarizes these changes and lists some of the embalming concerns they can create.

► EMBALMING ANALYSIS, PART II: DURING ARTERIAL INJECTION OF THE BODY

The second part of the analysis is an evaluation of the treatments begun in the preparation of the body. When a problem is encountered, the embalmer must decide what new approach to take to solve the problem. **During this phase of analysis, after the injection of each gallon of arterial solution, the embalmer needs to re-evaluate the distribution, diffusion, and effect the arterial solution has produced.** The following are some of the concerns of the embalmer:

1. What areas of the body are receiving arterial solution? This can be noted by the presence of fluid dyes in the tissues and the clearing of intravascular discolorations such as livor mortis.
2. What areas are not receiving arterial solution? Dyes will not be present and livor mortis, if present, will not be cleared; no firmness will be present.
3. What can be done to stimulate the flow of arterial solution into areas not receiving solution?
   a. Massage along the arterial route that supplies fluid to the area.
   b. Increase the pressure of the solution being injected.
   c. Increase the rate of flow of the solution being injected.
   d. Lower, raise, or manipulate the body area.
   e. Close off the drainage to increase the intravascular pressure.
4. What areas must receive sectional arterial injection? Areas that did not receive solution even after massage and changes in injection protocol must be injected separately.

TABLE 10–2. POSTMORTEM PHYSICAL AND CHEMICAL CHANGES

Change	Embalming Significance
Physical	
Algor mortis	Slows onset of rigor and decomposition
	Keeps blood in a liquid state; aids drainage
Dehydration	Increases the viscosity of the blood; sludge forms
	Partly responsible for postmortem edema; increasing preservative demands
	Darkens surface areas; cannot be bleached
	Eyelids and lids will separate; lips wrinkle; fingers wrinkle
	Could retard decomposition if severe enough
Hypostasis	Responsible for livor mortis and eventual postmortem stain
	Increases tissue moisture in dependent tissue areas
Livor mortis	Varies in intensity from slight redness to black depending on volume and viscosity of the blood
	Intravascular discoloration; can be cleared
	Can be set as a stain if too strong an uncoordinated arterial solution is used
	Keeps capillaries expanded; can work as an aid to distribution
Increase in blood viscosity	If it clears **by itself** it could serve as a sign of arterial solution distribution
	Sludge is created; intravascular resistance
	Postmortem edema can accompany problem
	Blood removal becomes difficult; distribution can be poor
Translocation of microbes	Speeds decomposition in various body regions
Chemical	
Rigor mortis	Extravascular resistance
	Positioning difficult; features may be hard to pose
	pH not conducive for good fluid reactions
	Tissues swell easily
	False sign of preservation (fixation)
	After passage, firming is difficult
	Decomposition is usually minimal when present
	Increases preservative demand
Decomposition	Color changes; odor present; purges; skin-slip; gases
	Poor distribution of solutions
	Increased preservative demand
	Rapid swelling in affected tissue areas
Postmortem stain	Extra-vascular; cannot be removed; may be bleached
	Generally seen after the sixth hour; delayed problems
	Increased preservative demand
	False indication of fluid dyes
	Will turn gray after embalming; cosmetic problem
Postmortem caloricity	Sets off the rigor and decomposition cycles
Shift in the body pH	Interferes with fluid reactions
	Dyes can splotch

5. Has the body as a whole received sufficient arterial solution and has the solution been of sufficient strength?
   a. A high-index arterial fluid can be injected or added to the remaining arterial solution to boost the preservative qualities of the solution.
   b. If there is doubt as to the amount of solution, inject additional amounts as long as there is no distension of the neck or facial tissues; inject until preservation is well established.
6. Has sufficient arterial solution been retained by the body? The most important portion of the so-lution being injected is that which **remains** in the body to preserve the tissues after blood and surface discolorations clear; intermittent drainage can be used to help the tissues retain more embalming solution. It has been estimated that more than 50% of the drainage is arterial solution. **See Selected Readings,** The Measurement of Formaldehyde Retention in the Tissues of Embalmed Bodies.
7. Is the arterial solution having too much of a dehydrating effect on the tissues? A humectant coinjection fluid can be added.

8. Should additional fluid dye be added for internal coloring of the tissues? Additional dyes may be added throughout the embalming procedure.

9. If purge begins from the mouth or nose, what is its origin and cause? Let the purge continue during the arterial injection **unless** the purge is arterial solution. If the purge is arterial solution and drainage **continues, inject** additional arterial solution to make up for the preservative lost in the purge. If the purge is arterial solution and there is **no** drainage, it can be assumed there is a major rupture in the vascular system. Evaluate the amount of tissues embalmed and consider multipoint injections.

10. Are the tissues firming? This will depend on several factors; in conditions such as **renal failure, emaciation, edema,** and **wasting degenerative diseases,** firming may be very difficult to establish; poor firming can also be a result of the type of arterial fluid being used. (Some fluids have a slow firming action and others produce less firming of body tissues.) If there is doubt as to the preservative needs of the tissues, the arterial solution can be increased in strength either by preparing a new solution using a higher-index fluid or by using more concentrated fluid per gallon. A high-index fluid can be added to boost the strength of the solution being injected.

11. Does another site need to be selected for drainage? Example – when injecting and draining from the right femoral artery and vein, should there be little drainage and the face and neck begin to discolor and veins of the neck become prominent. These changes indicate the internal jugular vein(s) needs to be opened and drainage taken from a location above the heart.

TO INCREASE ARTERIAL SOLUTION STRENGTH

1. Prepare a solution using a higher-index arterial fluid.
2. Add a higher-index arterial fluid to the present solution.
3. Add more concentrated arterial fluid to the present solution.

► EMBALMING ANALYSIS, PART III: EVALUATION OF THE BODY AFTER ARTERIAL EMBALMING

Post-embalming Monitoring and Treatments

Finally, in the process of **monitoring** the body while in the custody of the funeral home, the embalmer needs to check on a daily basis for any adverse changes. These changes could include the presence of gas in the tissues or cavities, odor, purge, change in color in visible areas, skin slip, maggots, etc.

When an embalmed body has been received from another funeral establishment, an evaluation must be made of all body areas. Some of the following treatments may be necessary: (1) reinjection of a particular body area; (2) supplemental preservative treatments; (3) cavity reaspiration and reinjection; and (4) mouth and eyes opened and reset. Embalming analysis is an ongoing process from the beginning of the embalming until disposition of the body.

In this third phase of analysis, an evaluation of the preservation of the body is necessary. The primary, and if necessary, multi-point injections have been completed. Areas that are still lacking solution must now be treated using the supplemental preservative treatments of hypodermic injection or surface embalming. Some of the following considerations are evaluated during this third phase of the analysis:

1. What body areas have not received arterial solution after primary and multi-point injections are completed?
   a. Look for the absence of fluid dyes, little or no firming of the tissues, and the presence of intravascular discolorations.
   b. Treatment now must be hypodermic injection of the area or surface embalming or a combination of both.

2. Should cavity embalming be done immediately after arterial injection or delayed several hours?
   a. This may depend on the time at which the body must be ready for viewing.
   b. In thin, emaciated bodies, an attempt may have been made to fill out the tissues with a humectant—restorative coinjection; this chemical should be given time to ensure the tissues are firmed before aspiration is done.
   c. If a body is dead from an infectious disease, the embalmer may wish to delay aspiration to help ensure that any blood removed in the aspirated material will have time to mix with the arterial solution injected. With these bodies, some embalmers inject a bottle of cavity fluid and wait several hours **before** aspirating; this helps to ensure disinfection of the aspirated materials.

3. Are the features set properly?
   a. Be certain that the mouth is dry. Remove moist cotton and replace it with dry cotton if purge developed during embalming or if

moisture leaked from the method of mouth closure where the skin was broken.

b. Lips and eyelids must not be moist if they are to be glued.

c. If the eyelids seem soft, cotton can be used for eye closure, and a drop of cavity fluid can be placed on the cotton to make an internal compress before adhesive is applied to the eyelids.

d. If residual air is present in the mouth after gluing, the lips can be cracked open or limited aspiration of the thorax can be done to remove the air.

4. What if purge developed during embalming?

a. Be certain the nose is tightly repacked and the mouth has been dried of any purge material.

b. Purge may be aspirated from the throat and nasal passages using a nasal tube aspirator.

c. Anal purge can be corrected after cavity embalming; force as much of the fecal material from the orifice; pack the anal orifice with cotton saturated with cavity fluid, phenol cautery fluid, or a chemical solution used for treatment of skin lesions. It may be necessary to use a purse string suture around the anal orifice to ensure no further purge. Pants and coveralls or a diaper can be used to protect clothing from any further purge.

5. Is the body well groomed? Nails and hands should be cleaned, hands cupped, and fingers together.

6. Are the body and hair clean and dried? The body must be turned on its side to check for clots or debris that were not cleaned away. Turning the body allows it to be dried on all sides.

7. Have decubitus ulcerations been treated? Compresses should be removed from decubitus ulcerations or skin lesions and replaced with clean compresses and fresh chemical or embalming powder. Plastic stockings, pants, or coveralls can be placed on the body to hold the compresses in position.

8. Is there any leakage? Intravenous line punctures leak after arterial injection and even after cavity embalming. They should be properly sealed with a trocar button or superglue.

9. Are tracheotomy and colostomy openings closed? A purse string suture can be used to close these openings. They should be packed with a cautery chemical and cotton. The tracheotomy can also be filled with some incision seal powder. These openings should be covered with glue and cotton after the suturing is completed.

10. Are incisions sutured? Sutures should be tight and not seeping. If leakage is present the sutures should be removed and the incision resutured.

These 10 items represent the type of evaluation necessary during the third and final stage of embalming analysis.

Table 10–3 is by no means complete but serves to illustrate some of the variables considered by the embalmer in choosing treatments to achieve good sanitation, preservation, and restoration of the body.

▶ POST-EMBALMING MONITORING

During the time the embalmed body is in the custody of the funeral establishment, it is necessary to daily monitor the body to note any adverse changes (Table 10–4). Several examples of these changes are as follows:

- *Dehydration.* It is possible that dehydration can be caused by: (1) embalming chemicals within the body, (2) gravitation of tissue fluids from the face and neck, or (3) environmental loss of moisture due to air conditioning or heating. The results of dehydration can be a darkening of the skin, a "sunken" look to the face, as well as wrinkled and separated lips and eyelids.

- *Purge.* This condition is caused by a buildup of gases in the abdominal and thoracic cavities. It needs immediate correction. In addition to aspirating the cavities, it may be necessary to open and dry the mouth and reset the mouth.

- *Odor.* This condition may be caused by gasses accumulating in the cavities, and it may be necessary to reaspirate and reinject the cavities. Early decomposition may be evidenced. Depending on the time remaining until disposition, reembalming may be necessary. Odors may be temporarily covered by the use of plastic garments and absorbent embalming powders.

- *Leakage.* The source of leakage may be edema or possibly an embalming incision that was not sutured. The source needs to be identified and the soiled garments removed, dried, or replaced. Plastic garments may be necessary to contain or control any further problems.

- *Softening of visible tissues.* This condition can create discoloring of the tissues or possible blebs and skin-slip. The extent of the problem needs to be evaluated and either arterial, hypodermic or surface embalming corrections need to be utilized.

- *Tissue gas.* Swelling of the tissues may be evidenced in addition to crepitation when the

TABLE 10–3. EMBALMING TECHNIQUE VARIABLES

Description	Variation
Setting of features	Before embalming, during embalming, after embalming
Method of mouth closure	Needle injector, muscular suture, mandibular suture, dental tie
Method of denture replacement	Cotton, mouth former, kapoc, "pose" material
Method of eye closure	Cotton, eyecaps
Time for raising vessels	Before setting features, after setting features
Artery for primary injection	Right common carotid, right femoral, right axillary
Vein for drainage	Right internal jugular, right femoral, right axillary, heart
Method of injection/drainage	One-point, split injection, restricted cervical, six-point
Method of drainage	Continuous, intermittent, alternate
Drainage instrument	Drainage tube, angular spring forceps, trocar for heart drainage
Body treated with pre-injection	Used, not used
Arterial fluid strength	Low index, medium index, high index
Arterial solution injected	Mild fluid solution, moderate fluid solution, strong solution
Coinjection fluid	Used, not used
Fluid dye	Used, not used
Fluid dye color	Pink, tan
Use of fluid dye	Mixed with all solutions used, used only in last gallon of solution
Humectant coinjection	Used, not used
Time usage of humectant	Used in all solutions, used in final gallon only
Arterial solution strength	Same used for all solutions injected, mild followed by stronger
Pressure for injection	Low (2–10 pounds), medium (10–20 pounds), high (20 or more pounds)
Rate of flow	Very slow (5–10 ounces), medium (10–15 ounces), fast (more than 15 ounces)
Change of pressure	Not changed during injection; begin low then increase
Change of rate of flow	Not changed during injection; begin slow then increase
Volume of solution injected	Based on weight, edema, time dead, firming of tissues, other
Method of aspiration	Hydroaspirator, electric aspirator, air pressure
Time of aspiration	Immediately after arterial injection, delayed
Reaspiration	Performed, not performed
Method of trocar closure	Trocar button, sutured
Method of cavity fluid injection	Gravity injector, via embalming machine
Cavity fluid reinjected	Done, not done, done only if gases are present
Signs of fluid distribution	Fluid dye, clearing of livor, firming, combinations
Features glued after embalming	Performed, not performed
Type of glue used for features	Rubber-based glue, superglue
Treatment for lack of fluid	Local arterial injection, surface compress, hypodermic injection

tissues are touched. Other signs of this condition could include the formation of blebs, skin-slip, and odor. This condition may require a reembalming of the body.

These are just a few of the problems that may occur during the time between preparation of the body and disposition. If some problems keep occurring, the embalming staff should be informed that changes in embalming techniques may be necessary.

▶ SOME GENERALIZATIONS

Whenever it is felt that circulation is going to be a problem because of pathology (arteriosclerosis), time delay since death, and other factors, the first choice should be the common carotid artery and internal jugular vein.

If the preceding conditions exist and it is necessary to run large volumes of solution or very strong solutions into the trunk regions, use the restricted cervical injection.

Whenever facial or neck swelling is anticipated or observed, use the restricted cervical injection.

After injecting a strong solution, never inject weaker solutions into the same area; always inject **mild solutions** first, after which **stronger solutions** can be injected.

After livor and other intravascular discolorations are cleared, the best response is obtained with average or mild solution. After intravascular discolorations are cleared, solution strengths can be increased. At this time, some form of restricted drainage can be safely used (e.g., intermittent or alternate drainage).

TABLE 10–4. BODY CONDITIONS AND EMBALMING TREATMENTS

Condition	Treatment
Normal body; some livor; dead less than 6 h; no edema; no chemotherapy	Any vessel for injection and drainage, pre-injection; mild to moderate solutions (3–5 gallons, will vary with body size); set tissue to desired firmness
Extensive livor of facial areas; dead less than 6 h; no extreme pathology	Clear discolorations with a mild to moderate solution; jugular and common carotid recommended; step-up strength to set to desired firmness
Postmortem stain present; body in or out of rigor; dead more than 6 h	Begin with strong coordinated arterial solutions; continue to increase after circulation is established; restricted cervical injection; slow injection; dye for tracer; section injection where needed; hypodermic and surface treatments where needed
Decomposition evident	Restricted cervical injection; strong coordinated solutions; dye for tracer; sectional/hypodermic and surface treatments where needed
Bodies refrigerated more than 12 h; some rigor; livor	Solution stronger than average; avoid pre-injection; dye tracer; circulation problems expected; restricted cervical injection
Jaundice; no edema; yellow	Jaundice fluid; mild solutions (however, must meet preservative demands); femoral vessels if possible, may respond to preinjection; dye for counterstain
Jaundice green	Cannot be cleared; solution strength based on preservative demands; plenty of dye to counterstain
Generalized edema of body	Start with solution a little above normal strength; continue to increase; if circulation is poor increase to very strong solutions
Localized edema	Treat general embalming based on condition of the tissues; separate sectional embalming of area with edema; hypodermic and surface treatments
Extra-vascular discolorations from chemotherapy or pathology	Use solutions based on size of body, length of time dead, etc.; treat the discoloration when on hands and face with hypodermic and surface treatments
Autopsied; dead less than 12 h	Moderate solutions; increase if needed to achieve desired firmness
Autopsied; dead more than 12 h; refrigerated	Solutions stronger than normal; dyes for tracing; restricted drainage to help achieve circulation; higher pressure may be needed
Death from second-degree burns	Begin with strong solutions; use dye for tracer; death will be related to uremia; may need 100% fluid; do the same if autopsied
Localized gangrene/ischemia/possible diabetic	Strong solutions when circulation problems are anticipated; bacterial complications can exist in these bodies; hypodermic/sectional and surface treatments to areas affected; dye for arterial tracing
Frozen bodies	Strong solutions; dye for tracer; restricted cervical injection
Emaciated with edema	Mild to strong solutions depending on circulation (it should be greater than good); again if edema is localized, sectional embalming
Emaciated	Mild solutions in large volume; add humectants to last injection; restricted drainage
Generalized edema with jaundice	Always treat for preservation first; moderate to strong solutions; dye for tracer; inject until edema is treated
Trauma of face/black eyes/lacerations/ restorative work needed infants/children with no pathological complications	Restricted cervical injection if not autopsied; strong solutions; dye for tracer vessels (iliac/carotid/aorta) if not autopsied; standard arterial fluid; inject strength and volume as needed; based on weight and body conditions; dye for tracing
Dehydrated bodies not dead very long	Mild solutions; restricted drainage; humectants in last injection
Bodies with chemotherapy, some edema; skin hemorrhage; expect fixation problems	Use restricted cervical injection; strong solutions into trunk areas; dye for tracing; may help force fluid into tissue spaces
Eye enucleation/no other remarks	To control solution entering head, use restricted cervical injection when body not autopsied; use a stronger than normal solution; do not pre-inject
Contagious disease	Use solutions a little stronger than normal (2–3%); run plenty of volume; avoid personal contact with "first" drainage; run volume and increased strengths depending on other body conditions (i.e., weight/edema)
Obese	Begin with a slightly stronger than normal solution; after blood discolorations clear, strength may continue to be increased; first, vessel choice common carotid/jugular; second, choice external iliac
Arteriosclerosis noticed when raising a common carotid	Stronger than normal solutions; high pulsating pressure; dye for tracer; sectional; hypodermic and surface treatments
Arteriosclerosis seen when raising femoral as first vessel	Go to common carotid and jugular; use a solution a little stronger than normal; inject based on other body conditions

▶ CONCEPTS FOR STUDY AND DISCUSSION

1. Define embalming analysis, intrinsic factors, and extrinsic factors.
2. List the three time periods of embalming analysis.
3. Explain the purpose of embalming analysis.
4. Describe the four categories of information used in embalming analysis.
5. Discuss why the conditions present in the body are more important in an embalming analysis than the actual cause of death.
6. List several effects brought about by long-term drug therapy.
7. List postmortem physical changes and chemical changes.
8. If a body purges during visitation, how would you explain what has happened to the family? What corrections are necessary?
9. What precautions can be taken to prevent purge during the embalming of the body?
10. How would you reembalm a body where tissue gas has developed during the time of viewing?

▶ BIBLIOGRAPHY

Chemotherapy and embalming results. In: *Champion Expanding Encyclopedia*. Springfield, OH: Champion Chemical Co., 1986: No. 570.

Embalming Course Content Syllabus. Portland, Maine: American Board of Funeral Service Education, , April 2001.

Frederick JF. *Effects of Chemotherapeutic Agents*. Boston, MA: Dodge Chemical Co., 1968.

Shor M. Knowledge of effect of disease simplifies embalming. *Casket and Sunnyside* September 1960.

Shor M. Conditions of the body dictate the proper embalming treatment. *Casket and Sunnyside* November 1972.

Slocum RE. *Pre-embalming Considerations*. Boston, MA: Dodge Chemical Co., 1958.

CHAPTER 11

PREPARATION OF THE BODY PRIOR TO ARTERIAL INJECTION

CHAPTER OBJECTIVES

▶ General pre-embalming treatments
▶ Shaving and grooming
▶ Setting facial features
▶ Treatments for pathological conditions
▶ Treatments for invasive medical devices

The embalming of the dead human body can be divided into three time periods, each containing procedures that are best performed within the specified period. The primary reason is that the preservative fluid used for embalming coagulates the proteins of the body, which firms the tissues, making their position difficult to change.

THREE TIME PERIODS

Pre-arterial injection	Period prior to the injection of the arterial solution
Arterial injection	Period during which arterial solution is injected into the body
Post-arterial injection	Period after the arterial injection

In each period specific procedures are carried out. They all culminate in the completely embalmed body. In Chapter 1, complete chronologies for embalming autopsied and unautopsied bodies are detailed.

Analysis of the body is performed during each period using four steps: (1) observation, (2) analysis of the observation, (3) implementation of a plan of treatment, and (4) observation of the results.

Body conditions and the skill of the operator may influence the period during which certain procedures are performed. For example, stomach or lung purge may dictate that the mouth be closed and set **after** arterial embalming, once the cavity aspiration has been completed. This can be done using the **restricted cervical method of injection.** Likewise, the mouth is usually sealed with an adhesive in the post-embalming period but, if there is a problem of "buck" teeth, it may be necessary to glue the lips **prior** to the injection of the arterial solution to achieve good mouth closure. The embalmer must learn to be flexible in technique, relying on the conditions of the body to dictate the order of embalming procedures.

The embalmer should devote full attention to the observation of solution distribution during the injection of the embalming solution. Attention should also be given to drainage and techniques to improve arterial solution circulation to all areas of the body. During the injection phase of the embalming, the embalmer should employ as many techniques as possible to ensure **retention** of the arterial solution and minimize any tissue swelling (Fig. 11–1).

▶ DOCUMENTATION AND ARRANGEMENTS

Before the embalming process begins, the embalmer must verify that permission has been given for embalming the body. State law will dictate who has the rights to give this permission and whether the permission can be oral or must be in written. Signatures should be obtained, for identification of the deceased and

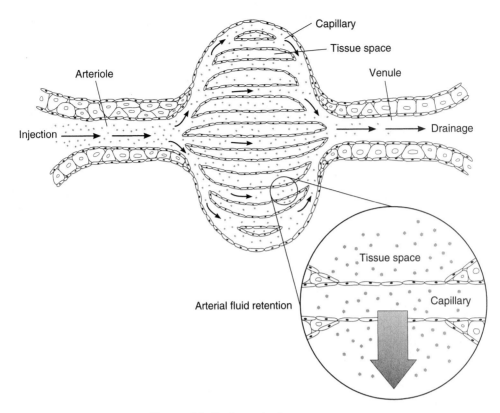

Figure 11-1. Arterial solution retention.

restorative work, when necessary. **At least one of the identification tags on the body (if available) should become a part of the permanent file.** Photographs given by the family or taken by the funeral home need to be labeled and kept secure. In addition, the Federal Trade Commission requires specific disclosures to the person arranging the funeral as to the price for embalming services and statements as to when embalming is not necessary for final disposition. All the documentation pertaining to the body including the permission for embalming, positive identification, decedent care report, clothing, and personal effects inventory should become part of the permanent file of the deceased.

A clear understanding of the embalming between the person making the arrangements and the funeral director is important. Embalming is the most acceptable means by which family and public can view the deceased over a period of time. Preparation of the remains can take time and funeral arrangements should allow for a proper amount of time to prepare the remains. This is especially important when tissues and organs have been donated, autopsies have been performed, death is by trauma, when the body is to be shipped to or has been received from another city, or when restorative work is necessary.

The arranging funeral director should be aware of the postmortem condition of the deceased. This includes but is not limited to body weight and height, swollen or emaciated facial features, visible injuries from trauma, visible pathological growths or discolorations, visible surgical incisions, condition of the hair, and discolorations such as jaundice or postmortem stain. Particularly the facial hair of the deceased male should be noticed, i.e., moustache, goatee, and beard.

There are families today who may wish to view the body without standard arterial and cavity embalming. Their request may be for a very limited period—hours instead of days. Refrigeration or minimum embalming treatments may be requested. Some families may have interest in "Green" or "Natural" burial where formaldehyde-based chemicals cannot be used—this may necessitate the use of biodegradable preservatives with very limited preservation or stabilization of the body by refrigeration or the use of ice. In these situations there should be a clear understanding between the arranging party and the funeral director. Proper documents need to be executed and signed.

▶ PRELIMINARY PREPARATION

In the time period before arterial injection, the embalming process begins when the deceased is transferred from the removal cot or refrigeration storage to the preparation table. **Whenever possible deceased human bodies should always be transferred or moved**

using mechanical lifting devices. The body should be temporarily centered on the table with the head as near as possible to the upper end of the table.

Clothing, sheeting, and/or the body bag should be sprayed with a topical disinfectant. This serves to sanitize and deodorize these articles. Standing at the side of the embalming table, embalmers can gently roll the body toward them by placing their hands on the shoulder and the hip of the deceased (Fig. 11–2A). After the body is slightly turned, the sheets may be pushed beneath the center of the body. (This is also a way to re-

move clothing.) Next, the embalmer rolls the body back to the supine position. Finally the embalmer moves to the opposite side of the body, repeats the rolling process, and thus removes the sheeting that enveloped the body.

In moving a wrapped body, the embalmer should always **pull,** NOT **push,** the body. For example, transfer of the body from the removal cot to the embalming table can be accomplished in three steps: (1) placing the removal cot next to the embalming table; (2) standing on the opposite side of the embalming table and reaching across the table to the deceased on the removal cot; and (3) pulling the legs of the deceased onto the table first, then the portions of the sheet that envelop the trunk and shoulders (Fig. 11–2B). If the body has been placed on a plastic "body-board" it is easy to pull the board along with the body onto the preparation table.

A

B

Figure 11–2. A. Turn the body by gripping the shoulder (upper arm) and the hip. **B.** The embalmer can easily move a body by placing one hand under the neck and one under the thigh and pulling the body toward him or her. Placing a sheet beneath the body makes the transfer between tables much easier.

GUIDELINES FOR LIFTING OR MOVING

Preparation

▶ Evaluate the situation

▶ When moving a body from a cot to a table or from an embalming table to a dressing table be certain wheels are locked on one of the devices

▶ Get help if you think more than one person needs to make the transfer

Technique

▶ If it is necessary to lift the body stand with feet apart with them even with your shoulders

▶ Stand close to the body — when elevated keep body being lifted close to your body

▶ When lifting — squat down — keep back straight — lift with your legs

Never twist, turn or bend back when lifting — change direction with your feet

When moving a body from a cot to a table or from one table to another, place: (1) a sheet, or (2) a Teflon-like moving board, under the body. Always pull the body from one table to another, but DO NOT try to push the body

Know your limits

▶ Do not attempt to move or lift if the object is too heavy

▶ Team for heavy lifting but have good communication with the team member as you move

---

It is easier to position the body on the embalming table while the deceased is wrapped or partially clothed. After clothes have been removed, the deceased can be moved more easily if the embalming table was first moistened with water. Clothing should be removed without cutting whenever possible, labeled and properly stored for dry cleaning, and returned to the family. Very soiled clothing and underclothing should be disposed of in a sanitary manner. All clothing should be checked for valuables. Rings, jewelry, and other valuables should be documented and securely stored until they can be returned to the family. Some embalmers protect the rings on the deceased by placing adhesive tape around the ring finger. Others prefer to place a piece of string or gauze around the ring and tie the loose ends of the string to the wrist if it is to be left on the body during embalming. Glasses, jewelry, watches, and religious articles should be removed during embalming.

▶ PRIMARY DISINFECTION OF THE BODY

After the sheeting or clothing has been removed and the body is placed in the center of the table, the surface and orifices of the body are treated with a topical disinfectant.* The surface disinfectant should be sprayed onto the body with particular attention to all body orifices. Follow manufacturer's instructions as to contact time. A droplet-type spray is preferred over pressurized sprays, which lose too much of the disinfectant to the surrounding air and can then be inhaled by the embalmer. Pressurized sprays also have the tendency to convert the surface microbes on the body into airborne microbes.

Disinfection of the body should also include the destruction of body lice or mites (scabies). If scabies is suspected, a commercial pediculicide should be applied to the skin and the hair of the deceased. The embalmer should carefully handle these bodies so that the insects do not infest the skin of the embalmer. Carefully check for fly eggs or maggots, especially in the months of summer or in the warm climates. Fly eggs appear as yellowish clusters in the corners of the eyes, nostrils, or ears or within the mouth. If present, these eggs can develop into the eating larval stage known as maggots in 24 hours. Great care should be taken to remove all eggs. If the larval stage has begun, a mortuary larvicide can be used.

Maggots eat even embalmed tissue, so it is very important to remove and destroy them. To prevent flies from depositing eggs, keep the body covered. Nostrils can be packed in the months of summer and small pieces of cotton can be placed in the nostrils (extending outside the nostril) when the body is left in the preparation room or is shipped. In the months of summer, some funeral homes make a habit of covering the face of the body at night. Outside windows and doors of the prepa-

ration room should be screened. In addition, insecticides should be used if flies are present in the preparation room. Once fly eggs develop into the larval stage, the problem becomes very difficult, if not impossible, to control.

▶ WASHING THE BODY

The body should be thoroughly washed with warm water and a germicidal soap. Special attention should be given to the areas to be viewed—the face and hands. These areas must be free of all debris for good cosmetic application after the embalming. If the skin of the hands, particularly between the fingers, is scaly, a solvent such as a dry hair shampoo can be used to remove the scaling skin. This condition can also be found on the forehead and the parts of the face. This scale must be removed if cosmetics are to be applied. It is also useful to apply massage cream to these areas and wipe the cream away with a cloth after it has been worked into the pores of the skin. After thorough washing and rinsing, the body should be dried with toweling. Use disposable items in these procedures, for they can be destroyed and will not have to be laundered. Manipulation during washing and drying the body also helps to relieve rigor mortis.

When sodium hypochlorite (Bleach) is used in the solution for washing the body, it is important that the chemical be washed away with water before any contact is made with formaldehyde. Sodium hypochlorite and formaldehyde can be combined to produce a toxic and carcinogenic product.

The fingernails should be cleaned using soap, water, and a nail brush in the preembalming period. It is much easier to remove debris under the nails at this time (great care should be taken not to break the skin if an instrument is used to clean the nails). Any stains on the fingers or the nails can be removed with a solvent. Nail polish can be removed with a commercial remover or acetone. Trimming and brushing the nails greatly helps to clean the fingers and nails.

▶ CARING FOR THE HAIR

The hair can be washed at the beginning and at the end of embalming. Note the following points:

1. Wash the hair with warm water and a good germicidal soap; a commercial shampoo may also be used.
2. Washing the hair should deodorize the hair.
3. Hair rinses may be used to help untangle long hair. These products usually assist in deodorizing and styling the hair.

---

*Disinfectants are discussed in detail in Chapter 3.

4. Blow-drying helps to style the hair, for both men and women.
5. When in doubt as to the method of styling the hair, comb or brush it straight back.
6. When hair is very thin and has a tendency to fall out, dry it before combing or brushing and avoid as much brushing or combing as possible.
7. Use cool water to remove blood from the hair.
8. If lice or mites are suspected, apply a commercial pediculicide before washing. Follow instructions for the use of this chemical.
9. When dandruff or scaling of the skin is present (often seen when therapeutic drugs have been used for longer periods), several washings may be necessary. The hair can also be washed with the "dry wash" solvent shampoos.
10. Do not comb curly hair when wet; knead the hair with a towel while blow-drying. This helps to retain the curl.
11. Braids should be combed out prior to shampooing.

(See Selected Readings: Professional Hair Care for Human Remains)

▶ SHAVING THE BODY

After topically sanitizing the body, washing and drying the hair and body surfaces, packing the mouth and nasal orifices, and temporarily positioning the body, the embalmer can shave the body. Facial hair should be removed from all bodies—men, women, and children (see next paragraph). The nostrils should also be trimmed at this time. Shaving the body not only improves the appearance of the deceased but greatly assists in the application of cosmetics to facial tissues. If hair were to remain on the face, cosmetics (whether creams, liquids, or powders) would stick to the hair, making the appearance of the deceased quite unnatural.

Permission and directions should be obtained from the family with respect to the facial hair on a deceased male. It is much easier to remove a mustache or beard before arterial injection. If there is doubt about shaving and the family cannot be consulted, embalm the body and shave later. This process is more difficult, but it is much easier to shave the body after embalming than restore a beard or mustache.

The administration of therapeutic drugs often induces growth of facial hair on women and children. Drug therapy and some pathological conditions can even induce hair growth on the forehead. In women and children, this facial hair is easily removed by lightly passing a safety razor over the facial tissues. Shaving the forehead can be very difficult. Shaving lather should be applied and great care should be taken not to nick the skin. After shaving the forehead, apply massage cream.

Note the following points during shaving the face:

1. Use a good, sharp blade; more than one blade may be needed to shave some bodies.
2. Use a double-edged safety razor, single stainless razor, or straight edge razor.
3. Apply warm water to the face with a washcloth first.
4. Use shaving cream to lather the face.
5. When there is doubt about the length of sideburns, mustache, or beard, consult the family. If they cannot be reached, these areas can always be shaved after arterial embalming.
6. When using a new blade, it is wise to begin shaving on the left side of the face or in the neck area to slightly dull the blade.
7. Shave in the direction of hair growth; bodies vary, and sometimes shaving must be directed against or perpendicular to the growth.
8. Use small, short, repeated strokes over an area to achieve the closest shave; an area can be shaved repeatedly or (as stated in item No. 7) from one or several different directions (Fig. 11–3).
9. Clean the razor frequently with warm water.
10. Try to shave an area without lifting the razor off the face; apply pressure on the razor and "slide" the razor over the area being shaved.
11. Use a small piece of cotton or washcloth (gauze or cheesecloth) to pull the skin taut and make an even area for shaving; this is helpful in shaving the area immediately under the mandible and the upper neck area.
12. After shaving, wash the face with a washcloth and warm water; a thin layer of massage cream may be applied.

Razor abrasions are areas of the face where small pieces of flesh have been removed. Application of massage cream helps to prevent the area from dehydrating and turning brown. During arterial injection, arterial solution may leak through these nicked areas. It may be necessary to place a very small piece of wax over these areas **after** cosmetics have been applied. This prevents the areas from further drying and showing through the cosmetic, especially when alcohol-type transparent cosmetics are used. If necessary, an opaque cosmetic can be used to hide the discoloration.

If a beard or mustache or the face in general must be shaved after arterial injection, lather the face with a very moist, warm lather. Use a sharp, new blade in the razor. To avoid nicking the tissue, shave in small areas

A

B

Figure 11–3. A. Slide the razor over the face, shaving in the direction of beard growth. **B.** The best results are achieved by shaving from several directions.

and keep applying lather to the area being shaved. When completed, apply a thin film of massage cream.*

In shaving a beard, many embalmers first trim off the longer hair of the beard with shears or hair clippers. This process is not necessary; the beard can be shaved without the preliminary clipping. Shaving should be di-

rected from the cheek areas downward over the face. Heavy growth may necessitate the use of several blades.

After the body has been shaved, massage cream may be applied. Some embalmers prefer that a light application of this cream be made after the features are set; others prefer to apply massage cream after embalming; some do not apply cream at all because of the type of cosmetic they will use. Massage cream has several uses:

1. It protects the face and hands from surface dehydration.
2. It prevents broken skin areas such as razor abrasions from dehydrating and turning dark brown.
3. It acts as a lubricant when the face is massaged to break up rigor mortis.
4. It is an excellent skin cleanser.
5. It provides a lubricating base that can be used for massaging the facial tissues, neck, and hands during arterial injection.
6. It protects areas of the face from damage if stomach purge from the mouth or nose occurs.
7. It provides a base for cream cosmetics.

There are two types of massage creams. One, the type generally sold by mortuary companies, has a greasy feel. The second is a face or hand cream that has a water base. After application, the cream can hardly be felt. The grease type may be more useful if the embalmer requires massage cream for use with mortuary cosmetics. In addition to creams that can be applied by hand, several spray anti-dehydrants are available; these are basically silicone or lanolin sprays; baby oil can also be applied by brush to the face and hands. Whether a cream or spray, it need not be applied heavily. A very small amount adequately serves to protect the skin areas to which it is applied.

▶ RELIEVING RIGOR

The embalmer manipulates the limbs while undressing, washing, and drying the body to relieve rigor mortis if present. Rigor mortis may be responsible for the body being in a very undesirable position. It is necessary to remove the rigor by firmly manipulating the muscles.

When limbs are **flexed, rotated, bent,** and **massaged** to relieve rigor, capillaries can become torn. This can lead to swelling during arterial injection. Avoid excessive exercise of the muscles in relieving rigor mortis. Relieving the rigor helps not only in positioning the body but also in removing extravascular resistance in the circulatory system. Relief of the rigor may result in better arterial solution distribution and also better drainage. A routine procedure for relieving rigor mortis is as follows:

1. Firmly rotate the neck from side to side.
2. Flex the head.

---

*Shaving with an electric razor after vascular embalming and over a dry face is effectively used by some embalmers.

3. Push the lower jaw up to begin to relieve the rigor in the muscles of the jaw. Repeat this several times. If the mouth is firmly closed begin by pushing the mandible upward; then firmly push on the chin to attempt to open the mouth. Massage the temporalis and the masseter muscles on the sides of the face. This may help open the mouth.

4. Flex the arm several times, then extend it. Finally, rotate the arm at the shoulder.

5. Grasp the fingers as a group on the palm side of the hand and attempt to extend all the fingers at the same time.

6. Grasp the foot and rotate it inward. Repeat several times. Attempt to flex the legs at the knee. Raise and lower the legs several times.

▶ POSITIONING THE BODY

The objective of preembalming positioning is to make the body appear comfortable and restful in later repose in the casket. Preservative arterial solution generally firms the muscles in the position in which the embalmer places the body prior to arterial embalming. It can be difficult to reposition the body after embalming. The position of the body as it rests on the embalming table should approximate the desired position of the body when casketed. Three position levels are desired: (1) the highest level should be the head, (2) the middle level should be the anterior thoracic wall (chest), and (3) the lowest level should be the anterior abdominal wall (abdomen) (Fig. 11–4).

The body should be placed in a supine position in the center of the embalming table with the head located near the top of the table. This position allows adequate room for positioning devices for the head and arms. The

Figure 11–4. The three levels of position: head, chest, and abdomen.

carotid vessels can then be raised by the embalmer standing at the head of the table.

Establish the levels of positioning. Rest the buttocks on the table (or on a **body bridge**) to establish the abdominal level. Next, place a body bridge under the shoulders. Elevation of the head and shoulders helps to promote drainage from the head and neck areas. A variety of positioning devices can be used for shoulder supports. Some embalmers prefer that the support elevates the shoulders as much as 4 in. off the table. Additional head support would then be needed for the head rest. The chest and the head are so elevated to prevent blood that remains in the heart after embalming from gravitating into the neck and facial tissues and graying these tissues. This discoloration is often referred to as **formaldehyde gray**.

Elevating the shoulders also helps to dry the body; air can easily pass under a large area of the back. This elevation helps to keep any water on the table from contacting the skin of the back and the neck. It is easier to clean under the body. If the body is obese, a higher shoulder elevation will be needed to establish the three levels of positioning by raising the head and chest above the abdomen. In positioning the obese body, the higher shoulder support allows the embalmer to slightly lower the height of the head. By doing so, the chin can be pushed forward and thus elevated, creating some visible neck area. The neck will appear a little thinner when the chin is pushed upward.

If facial swelling from edema is present, elevation of the head and the shoulders can be very important in draining the edema from the tissues of the face and the neck. At the conclusion of the aspiration phase of cavity embalming as an **operative aid,** a trocar can be passed under the clavicles channeling the neck tissues; this establishes routes for the drainage of edema into the thoracic cavity. As a **manual aid,** a pneumatic cuff or elastic bandage can be applied to the external tissues of the neck to assist in the removal of edema (or swollen tissues).

Shoulders are elevated to: (1) assist drainage, (2) keep water off larger areas of the back and shoulders, (3) prevent gravitation of blood into facial tissues after embalming, (4) assist in drying the body by allowing air to pass beneath the body, (5) assist in draining edema from the facial and neck tissues, and (6) position the head and chest higher than the abdomen.

If a problem should arise because of crippling of the limbs (the body cannot lie in an even supine position), a head block can be placed under one of the upper thighs (Fig. 11–5). This block prevents the body from turning from side to side. If placed under the left thigh, the block assists in turning the entire body slightly to the right.

The head is adjusted on the headrest **after** the shoulders have been elevated. If the shoulders had to

Figure 11-5. Blocking the thigh assists in the positioning of some bodies.

Figure 11-6. A sheet or towel can help in positioning hands and fingers.

be elevated greatly, the headrest will need additional elevation. Placing a folded towel between the head and the headrest may be sufficient to elevate the head to the desired position. The head should be slightly tilted to the right about 15 degrees. In some localities, the head is positioned straight without any turn. Custom, of course, dictates such protocol.

With obese persons the chin should be slightly elevated. This makes the neck look a little thinner and somewhat visible. In positioning obese persons it may be helpful to leave the head straight. Turning the head can make the neck and jowl area look swollen and distended. Elevating the left shoulder in the casket turns the entire body slightly to the right. Should there be disfiguration on the left side of the face or if some of the hair has had to be shaved for surgical purposes, leaving the head straight can help to keep these problems from being seen.

Prior to the start of the injection of arterial solution, the hands should be placed on the embalming table or even lowered over the table. This forces the blood in the veins of the arms to gravitate into the capillaries of the hands and may expand these tiny vessels. Once the embalmer sees that fluid is being distributed into the arms and hands, then elevate the hands and place them on the abdominal wall. The elbows should be elevated off the embalming table with either a head block or an arm positioning device. Raising the elbows prevents them from interfering with the drainage of blood or water that may be passing along the drains on either side of the table. The elbows should be kept close to the sides of the body.

Custom may dictate the position in which the hands are to be placed. To help hold the hands in a cupped position and in proper place during embalming, a sheet

or large towel can be mounded and the hands placed on top (Fig. 11–6).

Care should be taken to ensure that the fingers remain together (do not separate) and are slightly cupped. A large ball of cotton can be placed in the palm to cup the fingers, and masking tape or gauze can be used to keep fingers together during embalming. A drop of super adhesive (superglue) between the fingers may be valuable in keeping fingers together.

The embalmer must also properly position legs and feet (Fig. 11–7). The feet should be placed as close together as possible. During the embalming process, some embalmers prefer not only to place the feet together but also to elevate them. At this time, note any unusual size problems pertaining to the length of the body.

If the body is quite obese the straight distance between the elbows should be measured. It is important with overweight bodies to position the arms so that the elbows are as close as possible to the upper area of the abdominal wall. This can save inches in the casket and avoid the use of an oversized casket. Turning the body slightly when it is placed into the casket will also help reduce body width.

If length is a problem, an oversized casket should be ordered. Keeping the feet together and flexing the toes save a little space. Flexing the legs as well as omitting shoes may also help. Oversized caskets may mean that an oversized vault is needed or that the casket cannot be placed in a crypt or a shipping container. In positioning the body, every effort should be made to use a standard-sized casket.

Caskets are available in the following dimensions: several casket companies now specialize in oversized

A

B

Figure 11–7. A. One pose in which hands, arms, and the blanket may be positioned. **B.** Straight legs and feet allow shoes to be shown, resting on the casket foot pillow.

caskets of varying lengths and widths and can, if necessary, build to custom dimensions.

Metal	Standard	6 ft 7 in.	×	24 in.
	Oversized	6 ft 9 in.	×	26 in.
			×	28 in.
			×	31 in.
Wood	Standard	6 ft 3 in.	×	22 in.
	Oversized	6 ft 6 in.	×	24 in.
			×	26 in.
			×	28 in.

▶ POSITIONING PROBLEMS

A stroke, paralytic condition, or arthritis may contribute to the distorted positions of the extremities (Fig. 11–8). Often the arms are drawn up on the chest and the hands are tightly clenched. In addition, there may be severe spinal curvature. When the spine is curved extra elevation of the head is necessary. A head block placed under a thigh helps to keep the body level. It may even be necessary to place straps around the body and table to hold the body in the correct position. Limbs can be gently forced, but if it appears that ligaments or skin will be torn, leave the limbs in their position.

A **manual aid,** such as splinting and wrapping a limb, can be used to position a limb. The **operative aid** of cutting tendons should only be used when absolutely necessary. When the legs are drawn up, as in the fetal position, injection and drainage may be accomplished from the carotid location. Every attempt should be made to obtain good solution distribution, so the iliac or femoral vessels do not have to be raised and injected. After casketing, disfigured arthritic hands can be partly hidden from view by placing the casket blanket around the hands. This procedure and how they will be handled should be explained to the family prior to viewing.

Autopsied bodies present several positioning problems. If the spine is removed, it is very difficult, but very necessary, to place a shoulder block beneath the shoulders. The neck and shoulders have to be lifted to place the support under the shoulders. Some embalmers force a pointed wooden dowel into the foramen magnum at the base of the skull. This dowel extends down into the spinal area of the neck and prevents the head from easily turning from side to side. Once the body is casketed, a wedge of cotton can be placed under the ear to help

Figure 11–8. Severe arthritis of the lower limbs.

hold the head in proper position. Rigor mortis may or may not be present in autopsied bodies. If present in the arms, it should be relieved as much as possible. Attempt to keep the arms in the proper position during and immediately after injection.

After autopsy, sutures are completed and the body is washed and dried. It may be necessary to use strips of sheets to tie the arms into proper position. This is very important when the body is to be shipped to another funeral director. Do not let the arms lie at the sides of the body. Be certain they are properly positioned and, if necessary, tie them into position. These ties will later be removed when the body is dressed.

▶ SETTING THE FEATURES

Generally, the features are set in the preembalming period. After the tissues are embalmed it may be difficult to align the tissues to obtain the desired expression. Features can be temporarily set when purge is expected. In this manner the mouth can be dried and the throat packed after the body has been aspirated.

Mouth closure and **lip closure** are two distinct procedures. Mouth closure raises and holds the lower jaw into position; lip closure brings and holds together the mucous membranes of the lips.

Mouth Closure Sequence
1. Relieve the rigor mortis present.
2. Disinfect the oral and nasal cavities and swab them clean.
3. If applicable, remove and clean dentures.
4. Pack the throat area.
5. If applicable, replace dentures.
6. Close the mouth to observe the natural bite.
7. Secure the mandible by one of the methods of mouth closure.
8. Place the lips in a desired position, attempting to make the line of mouth closure at the level of the inferior margin of the upper teeth.
9. Embalm the body.
10. Check the mouth for moisture or purge material.
11. Seal the mouth.

One of the four conditions exists when the mouth is set: (1) natural teeth are present; (2) natural teeth are present but several are missing; (3) dentures are present (complete set—well fitting, lower denture only—no upper denture, upper denture only—no lower denture, old and very loose fitting dentures, new ill-fitting dentures, partial plates); and (4) neither dentures or natural teeth are present.

Dentures are personal property and many hospitals and nursing homes return them to the family with the belongings. Funeral directors should make every effort to instruct institutions to keep the dentures with the body. When death occurs at home, the persons removing the body should ask for the dentures. It is possible to open the mouth after embalming and insert dentures, but this task can be very time consuming and often difficult if a hard-firming arterial solution has been used.

The embalmer should relieve the rigor mortis before disinfecting the mouth. The mouth can then be cleaned and dried. If purge is present, a nasal tube aspirator can be used to aspirate purge material. Following aspiration again disinfect the mouth and nasal cavity. The throat and nasal cavities can be packed with cotton to help control purge and odor arising from the stomach or lungs. Some embalmers prefer to cover the cotton with massage cream so that the cotton does not draw purge material from the stomach or the lungs, as a wick would do.

Many problems may be encountered in setting the mouth. The expression of the deceased is one of the most criticized areas of the embalming process. A picture of the deceased, if available, may be helpful in determining the correct expression. The lips should be examined:

- Remove loose skin or scabs or any debris with massage cream, solvent, or warm water.
- Fever blisters—open and drain.
- Tight scabs—loosen with massage cream or remove with a scalpel; or leave and later glue to opposing lip to conceal the scab.
- Observe the "weather line" (the line between the moist and dry portions of each red lip) to determine the thickness of the lips.
- **NORM**. The upper mucous membrane is generally longer and thinner than the lower mucous membrane. (The mucous membranes are the "red" portions of the lips.)

A rare problem today is "buck teeth" or dental prognathism. A simple method can be used to correct this condition:

1. Secure the jaw closed using one of the methods of mouth closure.
2. Place a strip of cotton over the lower teeth. This helps to push the lower lip forward.
3. Using rubber-based lip glue, secure the upper and lower lips together (super adhesive or superglue may also be used).
4. Embalm the body.
5. Reopen the mouth to be certain there is no purge or air in the mouth; then reglue the lips (Fig. 11–9).

Figure 11–9. A. Preembalming treatment for buck teeth. **B.** Place a strip of cotton over the lower teeth to project the lower lip. **C.** Application of glue. **D.** End result.

The use of a super adhesive greatly facilitates the procedure. If there is a condition that warrants removal of the teeth or showing the teeth, the family should be consulted.

Securing the Mandible for Mouth Closure

Method 1: Needle Injector. A widely used method of mouth closure today involves the needle injector. A pin

with an attached wire is driven, by a hand or electrical operated needle injector device, into the center of the maxilla, and a similar pin with a wire attached is driven into the mandible in an opposing position (Fig. 11–10). The two wires are then twisted together to hold the mandible in position. The pin inserted into the maxilla should be placed at the center where the two maxillae fuse. This is called the **nasal spine.** Here, the bone is generally quite strong.

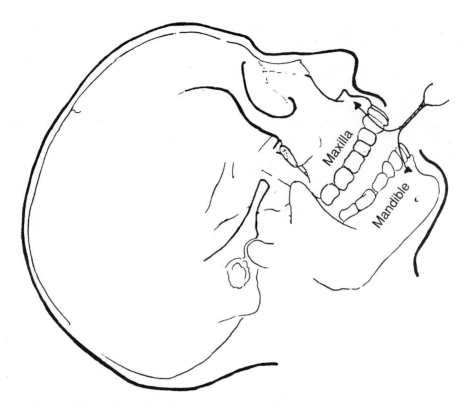

Figure 11–10. Needle barbs are inserted into the mandible and maxilla.

If dentures are to be used, it may be wise to insert the teeth before the wire pins are driven into the maxilla and mandible. Most upper dentures at their center have a small notch, and the pin can be driven into the bone at the location of this notch. Some denture wearers exhibit an atrophy of the maxilla and mandible; other bodies exhibit a condition where these bones have become diseased and are very porous. In both instances, it may be difficult, if not impossible, to use the needle injector to close the mouth. Suturing is then necessary. The embalmer can try various points along these bones to locate a solid point for the pins to be placed. The needle injector should be held at a right angle to the bone.

If the bones have been fractured, as often occurs in automobile accidents, four needle injector wires can be used. Place one on the either side of the fracture so that two pins are inserted into the mandible. Then, insert two pins into the maxillae. The wires can then be **crossed,** making a ×, and thus the fractured bones can be aligned.

It is important when inserting the pins into the bones that near the point where the skin from the mouth attaches to the gums, the skin be "torn" or pulled over the heads of the pins. This gives the fleshy portion of the lips better contact. Often, when bodies are shipped from another location and the lips are parted, all that needs to be done is to open the mouth and lift the skin over the pin heads to obtain good contact of the mucous membranes.

Method 2: Muscular Suture. In a muscular suture, a variety of needles and suture threads may be used:

1. Open the mouth and raise the upper lip.* Insert the threaded needle at a point where the upper lip joins the maxilla under the left nostril. The needle should slide along the bone and enter the left nostril. Draw the threaded needle out of the left nostril. (By keeping the needle against the maxilla, a "pull" will not be noticed.)
2. Pass the needle through the septum of the nose. Keep the needle as close to the bone as possible. Direct the needle into the right nostril and pull the needle and thread from the right nostril.
3. Insert the needle into the base of the right nostril, keeping the needle against the maxilla. Push the needle into the area where the skin of the upper lip joins the maxilla.
4. Place the lower denture into the mouth first, then place the upper denture. If the denture is not available, fill the mouth with cotton or use a denture replacement.

*Order is optional; suturing may begin with the mandible or maxilla.

5. Pull the lower lip out and insert the needle on the right side of the mandible at a point where the lower lip joins the gum. Be certain to keep the needle against the bone. Make a very wide stitch exiting the needle on the left side of the mandible in the same position where the lower lip joins the gum.

6. Tying the two free ends of the string together pulls the jaw up into position where the two mucous membranes will come into contact (Fig. 11–11).

The primary disadvantage of this method of mouth closure is that a pucker might result at the top of the chin that can easily be seen. Keeping all sutures close to the bones helps to relieve this problem.

Sublingual Suture

This method of mouth closure is similar to the Muscular Suture (see: Method 2 above). The lower suture to raise the mandible is made **behind the lower teeth** with a curved needle. Pass the needle, from right to left, through the musculature and tissues (lingual frenulum) which extend from the posterior surface of the tongue to the floor of the mouth. The needle is then passed up and over the front of the maxilla and through the septum of the nose, as described in Method 2. The jaw is raised to a desired height and the two ends of ligature are tied together. This method eliminates any "pucker" or pull on the visible areas of the chin.

Method 3: Mandibular Suture. Mandibular suture is identical to muscular suture except that instead of placing the suture in the musculature of the chin, it is passed around the mandible.

1. Open the mouth and insert the needle at the center of the mouth at the base of the tongue behind the lower teeth at a point where the floor of the mouth joins the gum. Push the needle downward, exiting the point where the base of the chin joins the submandibular area.

2. Reinsert the needle into the same small hole at the base of the chin and pass the needle upward just in front of the center of the mandible, where the lip attaches to the gum. Now, the suture has passed completely **around** the mandible. By pulling on both ends of the suture the string will "saw" itself through the soft tissues until it reaches the mandible. The small hole can be covered with a small piece of wax after cosmetics are applied. It should not prove to be a leakage problem. If it does, place a drop of super adhesive on the area.

3. If dentures are used, insert the lower dentures at this point and tie the two ends of the suture together. In this manner, the lower dentures are tied into position. This is an excellent manner for securing loose-fitting dentures.

4. Insert the upper dentures if they are being used.

5. Pass the threaded needle into the left nostril as in the muscular method of mouth closure.

6. Complete the suture by tying both the free ends of the suture together (Fig. 11–12). A bow may be tied in case an adjustment needs to be made.

This method of mouth closure is excellent to use when the body is to be shipped to another funeral home. It ensures that the mouth will not open during transport.

Method 4: Dental Tie. To use the dental tie of mouth closure the deceased must have natural teeth on both the mandible and the maxilla. A thin thread or dental floss is tied around the base of one tooth in the upper jaw and one tooth in the lower jaw. The two strings are then tied together to hold the jaw in position. Opposing incisor teeth are generally used, but any of the front teeth can be used. It would be too difficult to use the molars. In addition to securing normal mouth closure the dental tie helps to align a fractured jaw. Several dental ties can be used to align a jaw (Fig. 11–13).

A variation of the dental tie: tie a ligature around a tooth on the lower jaw. Thread a needle with the one end of the ligature and pass the needle up through the septum of the nose (as in the musculature suture). Raise the jaw to the desired height and tie the end of the ligature attached to the tooth to the end of the ligature which was passed through the septum of the nose.

Method 5: Drill and Wire. A small hole is drilled through the mandible and a similar hole is drilled through an opposing point on the maxilla. A small wire is passed through the holes and the wire is secured to hold the jaw in position. In lieu of a wire, thread can be passed through the holes with a suture needle. This method has been used over the years to align jaws that have been fractured. Be certain that the drill being used is properly grounded and that care is taken not to cut the fleshy portion of the lips.

Method 6: Chin Rest (Historical). The chin rest consists of two small prongs that are inserted into the nostrils. Attached to the two prongs is a sliding support, which can be placed under the chin to hold the chin in the desired position. This method of mouth closure is very

Figure 11–11. A–E. Muscular suture for mouth closure.

Figure 11–12. A–D. Mandibular suture for mouth closure.

old and depended on the harsh, very firm reaction obtained with early embalming fluids. These fluids rapidly and rigidly firmed the tissues. After the tissues of the face and jaw firmed, the device was removed.

Method 7: Gluing the Lips. This method of mouth closure is generally limited to infants and children. The lips are sealed prior to arterial injection. After the fluid has firmed the body, the lips can be reopened and the mouth is dried and checked for air or purge material and then resealed. This method is not recommended for adults.

Modeling the Mouth

Raising and securing the mandible in position are the first steps in the process of mouth closure. Once the lips have been brought into contact the embalmer must create a pleasing and acceptable form. The curvature across the mouth and lips is described as **horseshoe shaped**.

Natural teeth, when present, create the foundation. It is helpful to place some cotton over the molar teeth to slightly fill out the posterior area of the cheek. This is necessary when the body is emaciated. Gravity tends to result in some sagging of the cheek area. Placing cotton or mortuary putty over the area of the molar teeth helps

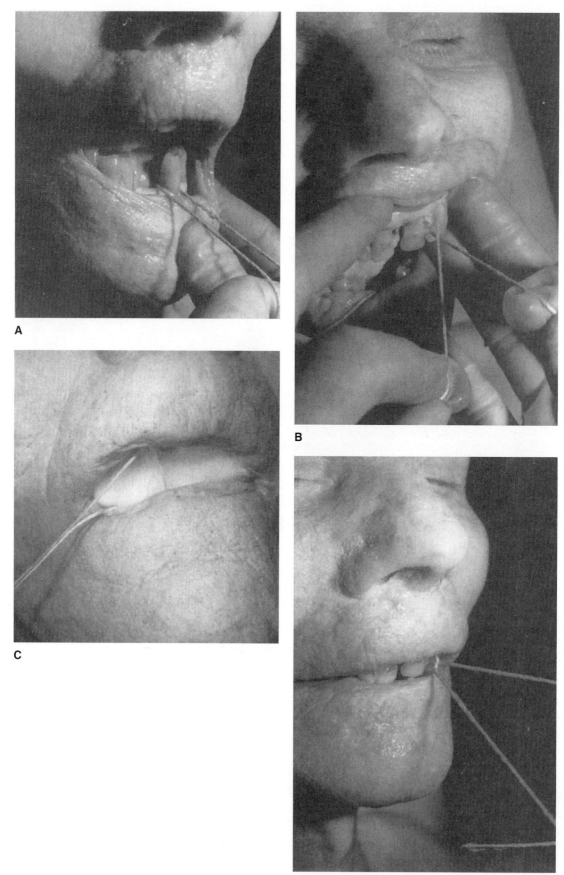

Figure 11-13. A-D. Dental tie.

fill out the area and to slightly lift the tissues into their normal position.

When natural teeth are present but several are missing, cotton, mortuary putty (mastic), kapok, or nonabsorbent cotton is used to fill in the missing teeth after the mouth closure is secured. This helps to give an even curvature to the mouth.

When all natural teeth are missing and no dentures are present, pack the throat and oral cavity. Secure the jaws into position using one of the methods of mouth closure. A mouth former can be placed over the jaw bones, but if a mouth former is used, it should be placed over the jaws prior to securing mouth closure. The needle injector wires or the suture thread helps to hold the mouth former in position. Some formers have holes through which the needle injector wires or the suture thread can be passed to hold the former in place. These formers come in a variety of materials such as plastic, cardboard, or metal, and can be trimmed to fit securely. If more support is needed to replace the missing teeth cotton, webbing-cotton or mortuary putty (mastic) can be placed over the mouth former. If a mouth former is not used cotton, kapok, webbed-cotton, or mortuary putty can be substituted.

If cotton is used to replace missing dentures, use long strips. **Remember the horseshoe curvature of the mandible and the maxillae.** The cotton should be placed in such a manner that a small portion covers the mandible and the maxillae, the same way a denture does. Always model the upper integumentary lip first. Some embalmers prefer to wet the cotton strips they use to model the mouth. Squeeze out the excess water and place the cotton strips. This prevents the cotton from sinking. If mortuary putty is used as a dental replacement, inject it using a long nozzle injector. The mouth can easily be molded to obtain the horseshoe curvature (Fig. 11–14).

Figure 11–14. Bilateral view of face. Note the curvature of the mouth.

When there are dentures but no natural teeth, insert the dentures prior to using the needle injector. The dentures should be cleaned and disinfected. Cotton placed on the tongue can help to hold the dentures in position. The mandibular suture method of mouth closure can be used to tie the lower denture into position. If dentures do not fit well, attempt to use the upper denture. The upper denture gives the best foundation for the curvature of the mouth. It can be held in position by placing cotton or mortuary putty in the area normally occupied by the lower denture. If the denture is new and does not appear to fit, do not use it. When placing dentures in the mouth, **always insert the lower denture first. After it is in position insert the upper denture.** In most people, the line of mouth closure (where the two mucous membranes meet) is located at the inferior margin of the upper teeth. So, establishing the curvature of the upper integumentary lip is the key to a natural appearance.

There are occasions when rigor is so intense that the jaws cannot be opened. It is still wise to use some form of mouth closure. In these instances, if dentures are in the mouth, it is impossible to remove them for cleaning. Spray a disinfectant into the mouth and dry and clean the buccal cavity with cotton swabs.

Positioning and Closing the Lips

After the mouth has been closed, and, if necessary the cheeks padded, the line of closure should be established. In the bilateral view of the mouth (looking from the chin upward) the horseshoe curvature of the mouth is easily observed. By keeping this curvature in mind, the embalmer avoids making the mouth look flat and straight. The center of the mouth should give the most forward projection. Try to obtain some depth at the corners. **The mouth is convex in curvature from corner to corner.** The line of closure is along the inferior margin of the upper teeth. Inserting a small amount of cotton high on the maxillae, on a line from the corner of the mouth to the center of the closed eye, helps to raise the area surrounding the corner (angulus oris eminence) (Fig. 11–15).

This angulus oris eminence (the area surrounding the corner of the mouth) can be reinstated with tissue builder after arterial embalming. The upper red lip (mucous membrane) is usually thinner and longer than the lower red lip. This appearance can later be produced when cosmetics are applied. The weather line (the line between the moist and dry portions of each red lip) helps to determine the thickness of each red lip. Remove any debris on the lips prior to embalming. To hold the lips in position during embalming the following products can be used (see Fig. 11–15): lip seal creams (very thick massage creams), petroleum jelly, rubber-based eye and lip glue (for gluing the lips). A super-adhesive should only be used for the most difficult situations.

Figure 11–15. Lines of closure for positioning the lips. Various closure profiles are shown.

Application of a thick cream to the lips during embalming to hold them in position also helps to smooth wrinkles on the lips. Natural wrinkles or lines in the mucous membranes are vertical, but lines from dehydration are horizontal. Place a very thin film of lip cream on each lip, and then bring the lips into contact. They tend to slightly pull away from each other. In doing so, the horizontal wrinkles will be removed. After embalming, wrinkled lips can be corrected by gluing, tissue building, or waxing. These same three methods can be used if the lips are slightly separated after embalming (Fig. 11–16). Some embalmers find it helpful to keep the lips **slightly separated** during arterial injection. This allows the mucous membranes to round out and prevents the lip closure from presenting a tight or pursed look.

If the lips are glued **prior** to embalming, they should be opened **after** embalming to be certain there has been no arterial fluid or blood leakage into the mouth during injection and that no purge material is present. Air from the lungs can be forced into the mouth during aspiration of the body and, if present, needs to be released. The lips can then be glued again after the buccal cavity is cleaned and dried.

Eye Closure

In establishing the line of eye closure, the upper eyelid (superior palpebra) forms two-thirds of the closed eye; the lower eyelid (inferior palpebra) forms one-third of the closed eye. The line of closure is located in the inferior one-third of the **eye orbit**. The line of closure is not leveled. As a result the inner corner of the line of closure (inner canthus) is slightly superior to the outer corner of the eye (outer canthus).

Figure 11–16. Good mouth closure.

The general procedure for eye closure is as follows:

1. Closure of the eyelids is generally done prior to arterial injection. If necessary, it is easier to close the eyes than the mouth after the body has been embalmed.

2. The eyes can be cleaned with moist cotton. Like all areas of the body, the eyes should be sanitized using a topical nonastringent disinfectant. Conjunctivitis and herpes infections of the eye could be communicable to the embalmer. Great care is advised with any discharges—even tearing—from the eyes of a body dead from Creutzfeldt–Jacob disease. In addition to cleaning the surface and corners of the eyes, clean and align the lashes.

3. Cleaning the eyes also helps to relieve rigor mortis in the muscles of the eyelids. If the face is emaciated or dehydrated, the eyelids may have to be stretched slightly to establish closure. This can be done by placing the smooth handle of an instrument such as a pair of forceps or an aneurysm needle under the eyelid and gently stretching the lids.

4. To help establish the anterior projection of the closed eye and to keep the lids closed, use an eye cap or cotton. These are inserted under the lids. Care should be taken to close the small inner corner of the eye (the inner canthus). If not closed, this area dehydrates, resulting in a brown discoloration which can be quite noticeable.

    a. *Eye cap.* These plastic or metal disks are approximately the size of the anterior portion of the eyeball. They are generally perforated, and the small perforated projections help to hold the lids closed. The convex shape of the cap helps to maintain the convex curvature of the closed eye. The cap itself prevents the eye and lids from sinking into the orbit should the body begin to dehydrate. Should the eyes be sunken, use several caps or two caps with mortuary putty or a piece of cotton sandwiched between to elevate the closed eyelids.

    b. *Cotton.* Cotton may be placed under the closed eyelids to keep the lids closed, elevate the lids, and establish the convexity of the closed eye. A piece of cotton about the size and thickness of a nickel can be used. Lift the upper lid and insert the cotton under the upper eyelid with an aneurysm handle or forceps. Lift the upper eyelid over the cotton and place it in its proper position. Evert the lower eyelids and insert the cotton into the area covered by the lower eyelid. Lift the lower eyelid into position.

After arterial injection if the eyelids do not seem to contain enough preservative solution, several drops of cavity fluid can be placed on the cotton used for eye closure **under** the lids. The lids should then be glued. This will make a preservative pack under the eyelids. Preservation should always be the first concern (Fig. 11–17).

Difficult Eye Closure. In cases of extreme emaciation, postmortem dehydration, or if the fluids have been extracted from the eye globe during autopsy, the eyes can be sunken and the eyeball itself dehydrated. Sometimes the eyeball can be rounded by the direct injection of tissue builder into the eye globe. To bring the eyelids together the lids may need to be exercised and stretched to secure closure. After stretching the lids, preembalming gluing of the lids may be helpful. The lids should **abut** but not overlap. In these difficult closures, however, overlapping may be necessary, and if the lids must be overlapped an attempt should be made to show some of the lower eyelid.

To control dehydration some embalmers place massage cream or a thick holding or staying cream on the cotton or eye caps under the lids. Cotton can also be saturated with an anti-dehydrant chemical and placed under the lids as a method of eye closure. The difficulty in using massage cream under the eyelids is that a solvent has to be used to clean the cream from the line of closure if the lids are to be glued. **Difficult closures can easily be corrected by using super adhesive to hold the lids together**.

Embalmed remains which are received by a funeral home may exhibit a separation of the eyelids. Superglue is helpful when the eyelids have separated during

Figure 11–17. A–E. Eye closure with cotton.

transport from another funeral home. Exercise the lids with an instrument under the eyelids then reset the lids with cotton or an eye cap and glue the lids together.

▶ PACKING THE BODY ORFICES

A topical disinfectant should be sprayed over the outer surfaces of the anal and the vaginal orifices. Cotton packing saturated with phenol solution, undiluted cavity fluid, or autopsy gel should be placed into the vaginal and the anal orifices. Some embalmers prefer to do this after embalming, because they prefer that any discharges from these orifices be allowed to exit the body during embalming. After arterial and cavity embalming, the orifices are tightly packed and the body is washed.

The ears should be cleaned and packed. The throat and nasal cavities would be packed during the setting of the features.

▶ TREATMENT OF INVASIVE DEVICES

The following invasive devices may be treated by the embalmer before, during, or after embalming. As indicated, several of these conditions must be treated during the preembalming period. Any medical device which in any way marks the face should be immediately removed; the facial tissues should be cleaned, disinfected, and a light coating of massage cream should be applied. This is especially necessary when there may be a delay between the arrival of the body at the embalming facility and the embalming of the body. **All invasive devices which are removed should be disinfected and placed in a biohazard waste container.**

Pacemaker (Internal or Implantable) See chapter 2 Fig. 2–3d

These devices contain three elements, a pulse generator, battery (generally lithium iodide), and one or several long wire leads. The pacemaker is often implanted in a subcutaneous pocket below the clavicle. It can be palpated beneath the skin—often a slight bulge denotes the device. The leads are passed transvenously through the subclavian or cephalic vein. The leads can interfere with drainage if the internal jugular vein is used for drainage.

If the body is to be cremated the pacemaker must be removed. If the body is not to be cremated permission should be given for the removal—if removed, the device should be returned to a medical facility or buried with the body. The device can be removed either before or following embalming. Often the pacemaker can be reached through the carotid incision used for embalming. Otherwise, an incision can be made over the device and the pocket is opened and the device is removed.

Surgical Incisions

Check the suture to see if the healing process has begun. If the sutures are recent, the area can be disinfected at this time and cauterized with a surface pack or the margins can be injected with a phenol cautery or cavity fluid. Temporary metal sutures can be removed with a hemostat **after arterial injection,** and the surgical incision can be tightly sutured using a baseball suture. Incision seal powder can be placed within the incision to ensure against leakage. Glue can later be placed over the surface of the suture after the body has been washed and dried. If the incision is in a visible area, super adhesive or a restorative suture may be necessary. The small metal "staples" can be removed by grasping them in their center with a hemostat; then move the hemostat from side to side to allow the small, bent metal edge embedded in the skin surface to be freed.

Feeding and Air Passageway Tubes

Tubes that enter the mouth or the nostrils should be removed in the preembalming period. These tubes, if left in place for any time, can mark the corners of the mouth or nose (Fig. 11–18). When the tubes have been in the patient's mouth or nose for several weeks, the surrounding skin may be destroyed. Massage of these areas during arterial injection may help to restore them to their normal contour. After embalming, it may be necessary to use restorative wax or tissue builder to restore these areas.

Abdominal Feeding Tubes See chapter 2 Fig. 2–3c

A feeding tube may also be inserted into the stomach through a small incision in the abdominal wall. These tubes can be removed before or after arterial embalming. The area of the abdomen should be disinfected. A small piece of cotton saturated with phenol, autopsy gel, or undiluted cavity fluid can be inserted into the abdominal opening after the tube is withdrawn or cut. A small

Figure 11–18. Air passageway tube.

purse-string suture can be used to close the abdominal opening. A large trocar button can also be used if the opening is small enough.

Surgical Drains

Surgical drains can be removed before or after arterial embalming. Drain openings should be packed with cotton saturated with phenol, autopsy gel, or undiluted cavity fluid. A small purse-string suture or large trocar button is used to close the opening. This should be done prior to cavity embalming.

Intravenous Catheters

Any tubing placed into the circulatory system, whether an artery or a vein, should remain in place until the arterial embalming is completed. These invasive devices did not hamper circulation during life, and leaving them in place will not interfere with arterial injection or blood drainage. They can be removed after arterial and cavity embalming is completed. When these tubes are removed from the areas that will not be seen after the body is dressed, their openings can be enlarged with a scalpel and a trocar button can be inserted to prevent leakage. Super adhesive can also be applied to these openings, especially in visible areas such as the back of the hands or the neck.

Tracheotomy Tubes

Tracheotomy tubes should be removed in the preembalming period and the area should be disinfected. Some cotton saturated with a disinfectant or cautery agent can be placed in the opening to disinfect the respiratory passages. Close these openings **after** arterial embalming. Should any purge develop in the lungs or stomach, this opening in the base of the neck provides an outlet for the purge material. The tracheotomy opening should be closed **before** aspiration and injection of the cavities. The embalmer may encounter two types of tracheotomies: with the older tracheotomy the skin around the opening contains a great amount of scar tissue. It is not possible to close the opening with a purse-string suture. Pack this type of tracheotomy with cotton and incision seal powder (or mortuary putty) to the surface level of the skin; then place glue over the opening. With the recent tracheotomy there is little or no scar tissue around the opening. After packing with cotton and incision seal powder, a small purse-string suture can be made to close the opening.

Colostomy

The colostomy bag and the surrounding abdominal wall area should be disinfected. The colostomy sleeve and bag can be removed either before or following arterial embalming. Insert the cotton saturated with phenol solution, undiluted cavity fluid, or autopsy gel into the abdominal opening. Sometimes a portion of the stoma is exposed. Apply the cotton to this portion of the bowel and use the cotton to gently push the bowel into the abdominal cavity. Close the opening with a purse-string suture. Surface glue and cotton can be applied to prevent any leakage. The bag and its contents (which were removed) should be deodorized and disinfected by pouring some undiluted cavity fluid into the bag. The bag and its contents should be placed in a biohazard container.

Urinary Catheter

A catheter can be inserted into the urinary tract through the urethra or the abdominal wall. It can be removed prior to arterial embalming. Cut the small side vent with scissors to allow the dilated balloon located within the bladder to collapse. Then pull the catheter from the body: if the catheter was inserted through the abdominal wall, a small purse-string suture or large trocar button can be used to close the opening. In females, the urethra can be packed with the cotton saturated with cavity fluid, autopsy gel, or a phenol cautery chemical after the catheter is removed. Be certain to dispose the catheter in a biohazard container.

▶ CASTS AND ORTHOPEDIC DEVICES

Most embalmers remove a cast if possible, an exception being casts on the legs. If the entire leg is in a cast, it may be very difficult to remove it and, of course, the cast would not be visible after the body is dressed. The difficulty involved in leaving a cast in place is that the embalmer cannot ensure that embalming solution was distributed to the area covered by the cast. If a leg case is to remain, it must be protected from drainage during the embalming; it can be elevated and covered with plastic.

There are two types of casts: plaster and fiberglass. Both must be sawed open. Often the fiberglass, if thin enough, can be cut open. Some arm casts can even be pulled off the body. A vibrating cast-cutting saw can be used to remove the cast. Casts should be removed prior to arterial embalming.

Orthopedic devices usually involve a system of metal rods attached to bone. The rods do penetrate the skin. These devices can be removed by loosening any fastenings by which the rods are held into position. The rods themselves usually can be unscrewed from the bone. These devices can be removed either before or after arterial embalming.

▶ GENERAL PREEMBALMING TREATMENTS

Most of the treatments that follow employ concentrated solutions that contain either formaldehyde or phenol. Personal protective equipment should be worn when handling these chemicals. When formaldehyde, phenol, bleaching surface compresses, or surface preservative gels are used, cover them with plastic to: (1) control odor, (2) prevent evaporation, and (3) prevent inhalation of toxic fumes by the embalmer.

Hypodermic syringes should always be cleaned with tissue builder solvent. The needle and the syringe should be flushed with tissue builder solvent; 10 cm^3 of the solvent can remain in the syringe with needle attached for storage. A 17-gage needle works well for most of these treatments. When injecting the face with any of the chemicals listed, the point of entry, when possible, should be **inside the mouth** or a hidden point of entry should be used, since unlike tissue builder, these chemicals can leak. Injection of the backs of the hands can be done by entering the hypodermic needle **between** the fingers. Some leakage can be expected, this should stop in a short period of time. If there is a problem, these points can be sealed with superglue.

Visible Discoloration—Livor Mortis, Postmortem Stain, Ecchymosis, Purpura

Discolorations of the face, arms, and hands should be carefully examined before arterial injection. Livor mortis and postmortem stain usually involve large areas such as an entire face, side of the face, or entire hand. Livor mortis is an intravascular blood discoloration; postmortem stain is extravascular. Stain cannot be cleared by arterial injection but can be bleached to a lighter color. Livor can be distinguished from stain by pressing on the discoloration, if the discoloration lightens and the imprint of the fingers can be seen, this is a good test; the discoloration is intravascular and can be cleared. Livor can also be removed from an area by elevating the affected tissues. Livor and stain can occur in the same tissues— livor precedes stain. Refrigeration, blood thinners, and carbon monoxide all speed hypostasis of the blood and the resulting livor mortis and postmortem stain.

Elevation of the shoulders and head will prevent the occurrence of livor mortis or if present, promote its removal from the facial tissues.

Ecchymosis and purpura are localized antemortem, extravascular blood discolorations. These conditions are frequently seen on the backs of the hands. The discolorations cannot be removed but can be bleached. The treatments that follow will bleach and ensure good preservation of the affected areas. Optional treatments include:

1. Subcutaneous hypodermic injection using a phenol bleaching chemical (or undiluted cavity fluid) **before** arterial injection.
2. Subcutaneous hypodermic injection using a phenol bleaching chemical (or cavity fluid) **after** arterial injection.

3. Application of a surface preservative gel or compress of a bleaching solution **before, during,** and **following** arterial injection.
4. A combination of surface and hypodermic treatments **either** before or following arterial injection.

(Note: the embalmer has the choice of performing these treatments either **before or after** arterial injection. This choice may be determined by the recommendation of the chemical manufacturer or by the preference of the embalmer.)

Skin Lesions and Ulcerations

As the embalmer undresses, disinfects, washes, and dries the body, observe any rashes, lesions, infected areas, decubitus ulcers, and skin cancers. After cleansing the body, the embalmer should begin treatment of these areas immediately to: (1) disinfect the affected area, (2) preserve the tissues surrounding the lesion, (3) dry the tissues, and (4) deodorize the tissues. These areas should be of concern to the embalmer for the following reasons:

1. They can be a source of contamination to the embalmer, e.g., staph infections and herpes infections.
2. The area can be necrotic and the decomposition of the superficial and deep tissues may already be in progress.
3. Blood supply to the actual necrotic and infected tissues may be poor so there will be little or no contact between the injected arterial solution and the diseased tissue.
4. Odors may be present and if tissues are left untreated, the odor may be noticed even after embalming, dressing, and casketing.
5. Necrotic tissue can contain anaerobic gas bacillus microbes that can produce gas gangrene.

A common example of necrotic and infected tissue is the decubitus ulcer (pressure or bed sore). These ulcerations result from the limited circulation into the areas where there has been pressure contact, usually with the bedding. Staph infections create necrotic tissue that can involve the greater portion of the hip, buttocks, or shoulder. These areas and any area of infection (e.g., pustules) should be sprayed with a topical disinfectant. If one is not available, the area can be swabbed with undiluted chlorine bleach, undiluted cavity fluid, or a cautery chemical.

If the ulcerated area is covered with a bandage, saturate the bandage with undiluted cavity fluid or undiluted phenol cautery solution. Later, remove the bandage and inject hypodermically the necrotic tissue with undiluted cavity fluid or cautery solution. If there are no bandages, place a compress of cotton saturated with undiluted cavity chemical, undiluted phenol cautery solution, or autopsy gel over the area during embalming.* This helps to control odors, to preserve the necrotic tissue, and to destroy any microbes and their products that may be present. Hypodermic treatment of the walls of these lesions after embalming is very important, as gas bacillus (**Clostridium perfringens**), a source of tissue gas, may be present.

After embalming and treatment by hypodermic injection and fresh surface preservatives, cotton compresses with embalming powder can be applied to the area. These treatments sanitize and deodorize the affected tissues. Plastic goods such as coveralls, Capri garment, pants, sleeves, or stockings can be placed over the treated area. If the hip or the buttocks is affected, a large diaper can be made with sheeting or an adult disposable diaper can be used.

Lacerations and Fractures

A **laceration** is defined as a jagged tear in the skin. In the preembalming period, a laceration should be cleaned of any blood or dirt present. This is easily done with germicidal soap and cool water. After the edges of the laceration are cleaned, the torn skin should be aligned. Several small bridge sutures (using dental floss) can be placed along the laceration to hold the edges in position during embalming. If the laceration is in an area of the body that will be seen, some massage cream can be placed around the area after the bridge sutures are in place. This protects the good skin. If the laceration is in a body area that will not be viewed **after arterial injection,** the laceration can be sewn with a baseball suture, using incision seal powder within the laceration to prevent leakage. During embalming, arterial solution may escape from the laceration. After embalming, dry the laceration, treat the edges with a hypodermic injection of phenol cautery solution, and then either suture or glue them closed. Some embalmers prefer to place a compress of undiluted cavity fluid or autopsy gel over the lacerated tissues during embalming to ensure good preservation of the torn tissues.†

When bones are fractured (Fig. 11–19), the embalmer is able to observe the distortion by touch or sight. Make every attempt to align all bones, especially facial bones, in the preembalming period. If skull bones or facial bones are fractured, small incisions may have to be made to realign them.

Abrasions

An **abrasion** is defined as "skin rubbed off." The embalmer encounters two types of abrasions:

---

*Cover with plastic to control odor and fumes and to prevent the chemical from dehydrating.
†Cover with plastic to contain fumes.

Figure 11–19. Compound fracture of the radius.

- **Dry Abrasion**—Dry abrasions are the abraded areas that have dehydrated. The area resembles a scab. The tissue is dark brown to black, very rough, and firm to the touch. This is a cosmetic problem and can be covered with an opaque cosmetic or waxed after embalming.
- **Moist Abrasions**—Moist abrasions are the abraded areas that are moist to the touch; some bruising may be present.

In the preembalming period, for abrasions located on the visible areas of the body (face, head, neck, arms, or hands), clean the affected area as some blood may be present. Moist abrasions can be covered with a compress of undiluted cavity fluid, phenol cautery solution, or autopsy gel. During embalming, arterial solution may pass through the abraded tissues. After embalming, the objective should be to dry these abrasions so the tissues **will become sealed.** A hair dryer can be used to dry moist abrasions. **Cosmetics, wax, and some glues can only be applied to dry tissues.**

Skin-Slip, Torn Skin, Blisters, Pustules, and Scabs

The preembalming treatment, when skin-slip, torn skin, scabs, or similar conditions are present, starts with the application of a topical disinfectant. All loose skin should be carefully removed (Fig. 11–20). Blisters and pustules need to be opened and drained. After cleaning all debris, the nude flesh can be coated using: (1) a surface preservative gel and (2) surface pack of undiluted cavity fluid or phenol compound. This establishes good preservation and will help to start drying the nude skin. In visible areas such as face and hands, surrounding good tissues need to be protected by applying a light coating of massage cream. During arterial injection these surface treatments can remain in place. Arterial fluid may seep through the affected areas. After embalming remove surface chemicals and air dry the nude tissues.

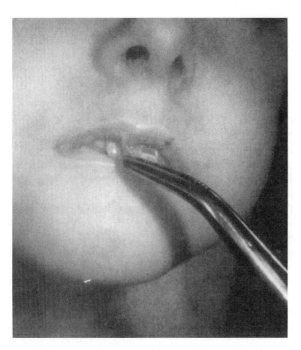

Figure 11–20. Fever blister being removed.

These areas will discolor, but they can then be treated with an opaque cosmetic if they are in a visible location.

Gases

During undressing, disinfecting, and cleaning of the body, the embalmer should determine if gas is present in the cavities or body tissues. There are three sources of gas in the dead human body. When gases are present in the tissues, distension and swelling may also occur. The gas can be felt by moving the fingers over the tissues. Pressing on the tissues feels as if they were stuffed with cellophane tissue. This movement may also produce a crackling sound, called **crepitation**. There is only one way to remove gas from tissues. The tissues must be opened and the gas must be allowed to escape.

Subcutaneous Emphysema: Gas or Air in the Tissues. Subcutaneous emphysema originates from a penetration or tearing into the pleural cavities or lung tissues. When gas is detected in the tissues and neither odor nor skin-slip is present, examine the body for punctures that may have been made into the lungs, recent tracheotomy, or fracture of the clavicle, sternum, or ribs. Subcutaneous emphysema can be widespread in a body.

Gas from Decomposition. If there has been a time delay, signs of decomposition may be present, as may discoloration, odor, purge, skin-slip, and gas. This gas can accumulate in the viscera, body cavities, or skeletal tissues.

True Tissue Gas. The source of this gas is Welch's bacillus (*C. perfringens*). It is an anaerobic spore former and thrives on dead necrotic tissue. The microbe can be passed from body to body through contaminated cutting instruments. A very strong odor of decomposed tissue may exhibit. The condition continues to increase and may begin in the agonal and postmortem periods. Because it spreads so rapidly and is so hard to control, viewing of the body may be impossible. Its presence should immediately be recognized and appropriate steps should be taken to control it. Use extreme care to disinfect all cutting instruments used in the embalming. Disposable scalpel blades should be removed and placed in an OSHA-approved sharps disposal unit and the trocar immersed in concentrated arterial solution using a coinjection chemical specifically designed for bodies with "true tissue gas."

In the preembalming period, a great concern can be distension of the abdomen. Severe distension may restrict the flow of arterial solution and the drainage of blood. The abdomen should be punctured and the gas be allowed to escape. Release of the gas may be accomplished by one of the following:

1. Make a puncture with a scalpel approximately at the standard point of trocar entry—2 in. to the left and 2 in. above the umbilicus. This in itself may allow enough gas to escape that sufficient pressure will be relieved.
2. Insert a trocar at the standard point of entry and, keeping the point high over the viscera, attempt to relieve the gases.
3. Make a small 3 to 4 in. incision over the abdominal wall, possibly opening some of the intestinal viscera, to allow gas to escape.
4. Make an opening with a scalpel on the abdominal wall and insert a "pointless" trocar or large drain tube.

If the facial tissues and the upper chest areas evidence the presence of gas, it would be advantageous to raise both common carotid arteries for injection. The half-moon incision, running from the center of the right clavicle to the center of the left clavicle, is useful. This incision allows gases to escape. Gases already present in the face can be channeled, after embalming, pressure is applied to the distended areas and the gas is forced to exit through these incisions.

It is important that the embalmer should determine the type of gas present. True tissue gas is very rare, but it is most difficult to control. The gas most frequently seen is subcutaneous emphysema. This is generally found when a rib has been fractured during the administration of cardiopulmonary resuscitation (CPR). Table 11–1 outlines the characteristics of these gases.

TABLE 11–1. GASES CAUSING DISTENSION

Type	Source	Characteristics	Treatments
Subcutaneous emphysema	Puncture of lung or pleural sac; seen in CPR treatments; puncture wounds to thorax; rib fractures; tracheotomy	No odor; no skin-slip; no blebs; gas can be extreme, present even in toes; can create intense swelling; rises to highest body areas	Gas will escape through incisions; establish good arterial preservation; channel tissues after arterial injection to release gases
True tissue gas	Anaerobic bacteria; *C. perfringens*	Very strong odor of decomposition; skin-slip; skin blebs; the condition and amount of gas increase with time; spore-forming bacteria may be passed by cutting instruments to other bodies	Use of special "tissue gas" arterial solutions; localized hypodermic injection of cavity fluid; channel tissues to release gases
Gas gangrene	Anaerobic bacteria; *C. perfringens*	Foul odor; infection	Strong arterial solutions; local hypodermic injection of cavity chemical
Decomposition	Bacterial breakdown of body tissues; autolytic breakdown of body tissues	Odor may be present, skin-slip in time; color changes; purging	Proper strong chemical in sufficient amounts by arterial injection; hypodermic and surface treatments; channel to release gases
Air from embalming apparatus	Air injected by embalming machine (air-pressure machines and hand pumps are in limited use today)	First evidence in eyelids; no odors; no skin-slip; amount would depend on injection time—most would be minimal	If distension is caused, channel after arterial injection to release gases

Ascites

When the abdomen is tightly distended, the embalmer should determine if the distension is caused by gas or edema. Often, simply the insertion of the trocar into the upper areas of the abdomen can determine the difference. If there is generalized edema of the tissues and tortuous veins are visible over the abdominal wall, the presence of edema in the abdomen (ascites) can be expected. If the abdomen is very tense some of this fluid should be removed prior to arterial injection, for it will create a resistance to the flow of arterial solution and interfere with blood drainage.

Not all the ascitic fluids need to be removed, only enough to relieve the intense pressure in the abdomen. An easy method is to insert a trocar, not at the standard point of trocar entry but at a point a little lower on the abdominal wall in the area of the right or left inguinal area. This lower point allows the ascitic fluid to drain from the cavity by gravity. Insert the trocar, keeping the point directed under the anterior abdominal wall. This instrument can be left in this position during the entire embalming. Drain enough of the edema to relieve the intense pressure. Placing a hand on the abdominal wall and applying slight pressure can assist in drainage of the edema. Attaching tubing to the trocar can provide

a direct drainage of ascitic fluid directly into the sewer system or into a container where it can be disinfected. Edema within the abdominal cavity does NOT dilute the arterial solution but it WILL DILUTE the cavity fluid.

► CONCEPTS FOR STUDY AND DISCUSSION

1. Using the Internet, expand upon the rules you would want your employees to follow when lifting and removing a body from a residence.
2. Draw and label the entire area of the face known as the mouth—this extends from the base of the nose to the top of the chin. Describe in detail the mucous membranes "in the norm".
3. List several uses of massage cream.
4. Name the three levels of positioning the body.
5. List several reasons for placing a support beneath the shoulders.
6. List several methods of mouth closure.
7. What is the difference between lip closure and mouth closure?
8. In the norm, how does the upper mucous membrane differ from the lower?
9. How can preembalming purge be treated?

10. Make a list of all the treatments you can perform before the arterial injection of the body.

▶ BIBLIOGRAPHY

Embalming Course Content Syllabus. Portland, ME: American Board of Funeral Service Education, 2008.

From Alpha to Omega in the Preparation Room, 4th ed. Dallas, TX: Professional Training Schools, 1999.

Mayer JS. *Restorative Art,* 13th ed. Dallas, TX: Professional Training Schools, 1993.

Restorative Art Course Content Syllabus. Portland, ME: American Board of Funeral Service Education, 1998.

Thomas CL. *Taber's Cyclopedic Medical Dictionary,* 19th ed. Philadelphia: F.A. Davis, 2001.

CHAPTER 12

INJECTION AND DRAINAGE TECHNIQUES

CHAPTER OBJECTIVES

- ▶ Safe work practices
- ▶ Arterial solution distribution
- ▶ Injection techniques
- ▶ Drainage
- ▶ Drainage techniques

During arterial embalming of the body, four processes take place **at the same time:** (1) **injection** of the arterial solution at a set rate of flow and pressure from the machine; (2) **distribution** of the embalming solution through the blood vascular system; (3) **diffusion** of the embalming solution from the blood vascular system (capillaries) to the cells and tissues; and (4) **drainage** of the contents of the blood vascular system, including some of the fluids of the tissues, and a portion of the embalming solution.

When all four of these processes are successful, a sufficient amount of embalming solution is delivered to the tissues to achieve a uniform preservation and sanitation of the body tissues without distension. In addition, these processes remove intravascular discolorations, color the tissues, and establish the proper moisture balance in the tissues, so that dehydration or overly moist tissue is not a problem.

Injection involves not only the pressurized injecting apparatus but also the equally important artery (or arteries) used for the delivery of the arterial solution and the vein (or veins) used for drainage. In the unautopsied body, the ideal artery for injection is the largest artery, the aorta. Its location, however, makes the aorta an impractical choice. The best location for drainage is the right atrium of the heart, but again, its location within the thoracic cavity makes it an impractical choice. Therefore, the vessels used for injection and drainage should be as close as possible to both the aorta and the right atrium.

▶ WORK AND ENGINEERING CONTROLS

Work practice and engineering controls are those work procedures and building mechanisms that reduce the exposure levels to formaldehyde and other hazardous chemical vapors during the embalming of the body. Some examples include the following items:

1. Adequate and properly operating air exchange system.
   a. The exhaust ventilation should draw fumes **away** from the embalmer.
   b. There needs to be a good supply of incoming clean, fresh air.
2. Prevent spillage of chemicals.
   a. Gently mix embalming solutions and avoid splashing.
   b. Keep the rate-of-flow valve on the embalming machine closed or stopcocks on arterial tubes closed to prevent leakage, before and after injection, or when the delivery hose is being moved between injection sites.
3. Keep embalming machines in good repair.
   a. No leakage from within the machine apparatus.
   b. No leakage where hose attachments are made to machine or arterial tube.
4. Rinse fluid bottles and empty into the arterial solution.
5. Cap all chemical bottles.

6. Keep a lid on the embalming machine reservoir.
7. Use continuous aspiration of body cavities during the injection of the autopsied body.
8. Clamp all accessible leaking arteries during the injection of the autopsied body.
9. Restrict drainage as much as possible after blood discolorations have cleared
   a. Helps to retain embalming solution within the body.
   b. Lowers the volume of chemicals placed into the waste system.
10. Use closed drainage.
    a. Attach tubing to the drain tube.
    b. Direct heart drainage with trocar.
11. Cover the waste sink to avoid splashing and aerosolization.
12. Use moving water to immediately remove drainage from the embalming table.
13. Avoid high water pressure to avoid splashing.

These controls combined with personal protective attire and equipment will greatly reduce exposure to chemicals or their vapors. Refer Chapter 3 for a discussion of personal protective equipment.

► ARTERIES FOR INJECTION/VEINS FOR DRAINAGE

Arteries are used for injection of the arterial solution, because, unlike some of the long veins of the body, they **do not** have valves. When arterial solution is injected "down" the leg, the drainage is returned "up" the leg through the veins. In life, blood flows back to the heart. In embalming, drainage flows in a similar direction, toward the heart. This direction of drainage flow makes the **right atrium** of the heart the center of drainage.

The embalming solution, injected into an artery, does not enter the chambers of the heart. The **aortic-semilunar valve closes** as the arterial solution fills the ascending aorta and the arch of the aorta. The central point of arterial solution distribution is said to be the **arch of the aorta**.

► INJECTION TECHNIQUES

Embalming of the unautopsied body begins when the embalmer selects a suitable artery or combination of arteries (as in restricted cervical injection) from which the arterial solution can be distributed throughout the **entire body**. Should injection of the embalming solution from this injection site fail to distribute the fluid to all areas of the body, other arteries must be raised and injected.

Embalming analysis continues throughout the embalming process. In the preembalming period, an artery and a vein are selected for the primary injection and drainage sites. During arterial injection the embalmer will note which regions of the body are **not** receiving arterial solution. A decision must then be made to select another injection point to embalm the region of the body lacking arterial solution. The following are vascular injection procedures:

One-point injection	Injection and drainage from one site
Split injection/ drainage	Injection from one site and drainage from another site
Multi-point injection	Injection at two or more sites
Restricted cervical	Injection of both common carotid arteries
Six-point injection	Injection of the right and left common carotid, axillary (subclavian/brachial) and femoral (common/external iliac) arteries

One-point Injection

In single-point injection, one location is used for **both** injection and drainage, requiring only one incision to be made. The most frequently used one-point injection sites are the right common carotid artery and accompanying internal jugular vein, and the right femoral artery and accompanying vein.* The axillary (or brachial) artery and vein is least used. **Years ago, when most embalming was performed at the residence of the deceased and a minimum amount of very concentrated fluid was injected, the axillary, no doubt, was the most frequently used artery because the head could easily be cleared of discoloration, and drainage could easily be collected from this site or by drainage from the right atrium of the heart. Also, the incision would not be seen by the family after the preparation.**

CRITERIA FOR SELECTION OF AN ARTERY AS AN INJECTION SITE

1. Size (diameter) of the artery
2. Practicality of drainage from the accompanying vein
3. Depth of the location of the artery
4. Flexibility of the artery because of its branches
5. Effect on posing the body
6. Incision location if leakage is a possibility (if edema is in the area of the artery)
7. Proximity of the vessel to the arch of the aorta

---

*Reference is made to Chapters 8 and 9 concerning the advantages and disadvantages of each artery and vein as a point for injection or drainage. The left vessels could also be used.

CRITERIA FOR SELECTION OF A VEIN FOR DRAINAGE

1. Size (diameter) of the vein
2. Proximity to the right atrium of the heart
3. Discolorations of the face and neck (blood)
4. Ease with which vein can be brought to the surface because of tributaries
5. Depth of vein

Often embalming necessitates the use of large volumes of embalming solution. The internal jugular or femoral vein allows for better drainage than the small axillary or basilic veins. Good drainage is essential when a large amount of solution is being injected. Some embalmers prefer to drain from each injection site when sectional embalming is performed in the unautopsied body; others prefer a central site such as those just mentioned.

There are three major injection sites: the common carotid, femoral (external iliac), and axillary (brachial) arteries. These arteries are large in size (especially the femoral and common carotid) and they are located as close to the aorta as is possible in the unautopsied body. An arterial tube comparable to the size of the artery is recommended (when arteriosclerosis is not a concern) for maximum rate of flow of the embalming solution. The diameter of the arterial tube determines to a great degree the volume and velocity of embalming solution injected in any given time period and under any given pressure. Procedures for such an injection from the three major sites are as follows:

Figure 12–1. Single-point injection and drainage from the right femoral artery and vein. Note the concurrent disinfection of the instruments. A hose is attached to collect drainage from the drain tube, closed system of drainage.

RIGHT FEMORAL ARTERY AND VEIN

1. Insert a drainage tube **directed toward the heart** into the femoral vein
2. Insert an arterial tube directed toward the right foot into the femoral artery
3. Insert an arterial tube directed toward the trunk (head) of the body
4. Inject the right leg first
5. Inject the trunk, arms, and head

Note: See Figure 12–1

RIGHT COMMON CAROTID INTERNAL JUGULAR VEIN

1. Insert an arterial tube into the right common carotid artery directed downward toward the trunk of the body
2. Insert an arterial tube into the right common carotid artery directed upward toward the right side of the face, leaving the stopcock **open**
3. Insert a drainage instrument into the right internal jugular vein **directed toward the heart**
4. **Inject** the trunk of the body; several gallons of solution are required for the adult body
5. Inject sufficient solution up the right side of the head

RIGHT AXILLARY ARTERY AND VEIN

1. Insert an arterial tube into the axillary artery directed toward the right hand
2. Insert an arterial tube into the right axillary artery directed toward the trunk and the head of the body
3. Insert a drainage instrument in the axillary vein directed toward the heart
4. Inject the head and the trunk first
5. Inject the right arm

Note: See Figure 12–2A.

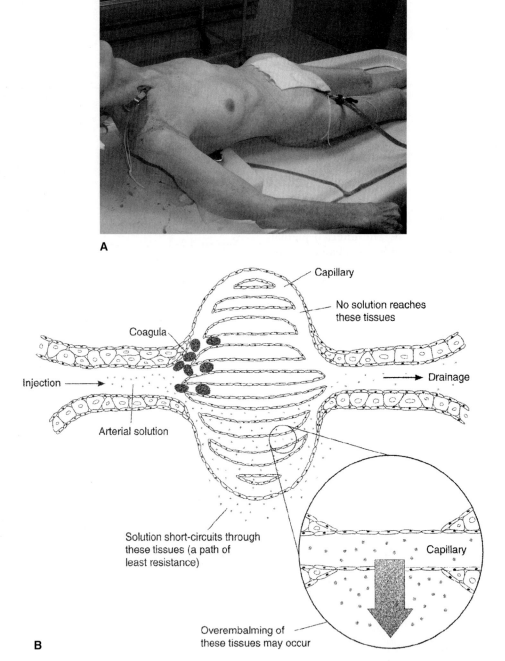

Figure 12–2. A. Split-injection. Femoral artery injected, drainage from right internal jugular vein. **B.** The greatest disadvantage of the one-point method of injection and drainage is the short-circuiting of arterial solution. Solution has a tendency to find direct routes from the arterioles to the venules in the region around the injection site. This can account for overembalming of the area near the injection site and loss of a large amount of arterial solution through the drainage.

Short-circuiting of Arterial Solution. A disadvantage of any injection and drainage from the same point is the short-circuiting and loss of the arterial solution. The solution has a tendency to find direct routes from the arterioles to the venules or through only portions of the capillaries in the region around the injection site and thus spills into the drainage. This can account for overembalming of the area near the injection site and loss of a great amount of arterial solution through the drainage.

Fluids Follow the Path of Least Resistance. Quite often the skin area is the path of least resistance, for the skin has a greater amount of capillaries than deeper body tissues. The skin areas surrounding the injection and drainage points frequently receive a greater volume of solution (Fig. 12–2B). Embalming in which only the skin and the superficial portions of the body and not the deeper tissues receive solution has been referred to as **shell embalming**. Massage, manipulation, and restriction of drainage all help to reduce shell embalming and encourage movement of arterial solution into the muscles and deep tissues.

Coagula in the Arterial System Can Easily be Pushed into Minute Arterial Tributaries. The solution then seeks out paths of least resistance and quickly finds its way into the venous system. Once there, it can easily be removed at the drainage site. Unrestricted drainage also contributes to the short-circuiting problem (Fig. 12–2B).

Split Injection/Drainage

Split injection is the injection of solution from one site and the drainage taken from another location. This method reduces short-circuiting of the solution and attempts to establish a more even distribution of the arterial solution. The most frequently used combination of vessels in the split injection method is the right internal jugular vein (drainage) and the right femoral artery (injection). **What starts out as a one-point injection can lead to split injection if drainage is difficult to establish. An example would be if the embalmer begins with a one-point injection using the femoral vessels, but soon finds difficulties with the drainage. Raising the internal jugular vein generally solves the drainage problem.** Examples of split injection include the following:

RIGHT FEMORAL ARTERY, RIGHT INTERNAL JUGULAR VEIN

1. Insert a drainage instrument into the right internal jugular vein directed toward the heart
2. Insert an arterial tube into the right femoral artery directed toward the right foot
3. Insert an arterial tube into the right femoral artery directed toward the trunk and head of the body
4. Inject the right leg and foot first; drainage is taken from the jugular
5. Inject the trunk and head of the body, drainage is taken from the jugular

---

RIGHT COMMON CAROTID ARTERY, RIGHT FEMORAL VEIN

1. Insert a drainage instrument into the right femoral vein directed toward the heart
2. Insert an arterial tube into the right common carotid artery directed toward the right side of the head
3. Insert an arterial tube into the right common carotid artery directed toward the trunk of the body
4. Inject down the right common carotid artery first to embalm the trunk of the body and left side of the face; drainage is taken from the femoral vein
5. Inject the right side of the head; drainage is taken from the femoral vein

---

Multi-point Injection

Multi-point injection is the injection from two or more arteries. Multi-point injection is used when the arterial solution does not evenly distribute to the entire body. An example would be injection of the body from a one-point site using the femoral artery and vein. If the solution did not enter the left arm, the left axillary (brachial) artery can be used to inject the arm. If the fluid still does not reach the hand, the radial or ulnar arteries can be raised to inject the hand.

Six-point Injection

This method of injection can be used as the primary injection technique. If the embalmer is preparing a body dead for a long period and anticipates poor solution distribution and possibly tissue distension, he or she can **begin** the embalming using sectional injection. The embalmer would raise several arteries for injection; drainage is taken from each injection location **or** from one drainage point.

A **six-point injection** is a sectional injection. It involves the injection of six arteries, the right and left common carotids, right and left subclavian (axillary or brachial) arteries, and the right and left femoral (common, external iliac) arteries. The six-point injection is used in the preparation of most autopsied bodies. It can also be used in the preparation of the unautopsied body. Preparation of bodies of members of the armed services and bodies being shipped to some foreign countries may require a six-point injection with multi-point drainage.

The sectional procedure ensures thorough distribution throughout a body region. This type of injection allows different solution strengths to be used in different body regions. A suggested procedure for the **six-point injection** follows:

1. Raise the right internal jugular vein and insert a drainage instrument directed toward the heart.

2. Raise the right common carotid artery and insert an arterial tube directed toward the trunk of the body. Also insert a tube directed toward the right side of the head.

3. Raise the left common carotid and insert a tube directed toward the left side of the head. Tie off the lower portion of the artery.

4. Raise the right axillary (or brachial) artery and insert an arterial tube directed toward the right hand. Tie off the upper part of the artery.

5. Raise the left axillary (or brachial) artery and insert a tube directed toward the left hand. Tie off the upper part of the artery.

6. Raise the right femoral artery and insert an arterial tube directed toward the right foot. Tie off the upper portion of the artery.

7. Raise the left femoral artery and insert an arterial tube directed toward the left foot. Tie off the upper portion of the artery.

8. Inject in the following order: right leg, left leg, right arm, left arm, trunk of the body (inject down the right common carotid), left side of the head, and right side of the head.

9. Drainage can be taken from the right internal jugular vein for all body areas injected, or drainage may be taken from each accompanying vein.

10. The body may be aspirated before injecting the head, if purge has been a problem.

Some embalmers refer to a 12-point injection. This is a six-point injection but arterial solution is injected both toward the head and the limbs as well as toward the trunk of the body.

CONDITIONS THAT MAY REQUIRE MULTIPOINT INJECTION

1. When a body area does not receive arterial solution
2. Bodies dead for long time periods
3. Bodies that show evidence of decomposition
4. Death caused by a ruptured aortic aneurysm
5. Bodies dead of highly contagious diseases involving the blood vascular system (this method of injection maximizes tissue saturation with embalming chemicals)
6. When disposition of the body is to be delayed
7. When required by military or shipping regulations
8. When a one-point injection has been used but embalming solution purge develops and drainage stops (distribution cannot be observed)
9. Bodies with generalized edema
10. Bodies that are difficult to firm
11. Bodies that exhibit poor peripheral circulation
12. Bodies that exhibit poor distribution after a one-point injection is completed
13. Bodies with true tissue gas
14. Body or area of the body needing to be reembalmed **after** cavity embalming has been done
15. Autopsied bodies
16. Organ and/or tissue donors

Restricted Cervical Injection*

In restricted cervical injection, both common carotid arteries are raised so that the head can be separately injected (Fig. 12–3). This injection method is the standard practice in many funeral establishments.

1. Raise the right common carotid artery and insert an arterial tube directed toward the trunk of the body. Insert an arterial tube directed toward the right side of the head and **leave the stopcock open.**

2. Insert a drainage instrument into the right internal jugular vein directed toward the heart.

3. Raise the left common carotid artery and insert an arterial tube directed toward the left side of the head; **tie off the lower portion of the left common carotid artery and leave the stopcock open**.

4. Inject the trunk of the body **first**; drainage is taken from the right internal jugular vein. (Solution entering the head by collateral circulation exits through the two open stopcocks. Only the trunk of the body is embalmed.)

5. Inject the left side of the head.

6. Inject the right side of the head.

Restricted cervical injection can be a routine embalming technique, with the difficulties encountered in embalming today (time delays, poor distribution as a result of vascular clotting, edema, and difficulty in firming as a result of drug therapy). Hence, more embalmers are using restricted cervical injection as their primary injection method.

The restricted cervical method of injection affords the **greatest control** over entry of arterial solution into the head. Because the tubes that are directed upward are left open while the trunk is injected, any solution that does reach the face and head via the collateral circulation **exits** the carotid arteries through the open arterial tubes.

---

*Much of this information was supplied by David G. Williams, Pittsburgh, Pennsylvania.

Figure 12–3. Restricted cervical injection.

The restricted cervical injection is recommended in several situations.

"Normal" Unautopsied Body. This technique allows the embalmer to control the amount of arterial solution entering the head. It allows large volumes of fluid, increased pressures, and faster rates of flow to be used for embalming the body trunk and the limbs without over injection of the head and the face. A separate solution can be prepared for injection of the head and the face.

Bodies with Facial Trauma. With restricted cervical injection a minimum volume of a very strong solution can be injected into the head to preserve and firm tissues with a minimum amount of tissue distension.

Bodies in Which Facial Distension Is Anticipated. Delayed embalming, refrigerated, frozen, and bodies exhibiting early signs of decomposition are all examples where the face can easily swell during arterial injection. Restricted cervical injection allows the trunk to be saturated with large amounts of strong solution, while the head and facial tissues are injected separately to control distension.

Bodies in Which Eye Enucleation Has Been Performed. Restricted cervical injection allows complete control over the strength, amount of solution, pressure, and rate of flow of arterial solution entering the facial tissues and thus helps to control distension of the eyelids.

Bodies with Generalized Edema. A large volume of solution can be injected into the trunk areas. Frequently, if facial tissues are not edematous, a milder solution can be used for injection of the head to prevent distension and/or dehydration of the tissues.

Difficult-to-Firm Bodies. With many of the drugs used today protein levels in the body can be low. Restricted

cervical injection allows the embalmer to inject large quantities of preservative solutions without overembalming the facial tissues.

Bodies with Distribution Problems. Restricted cervical injection allows the use of high pressures and high rates of flow without distending the facial tissues.

Bodies with a High Formaldehyde Demand. Burned bodies and bodies dead from renal failure require large amounts of preservative. Restricted cervical injection allows the embalmer to inject strong solutions of special-purpose high-index fluids without overembalming the facial tissues.

Bodies in Which Purge Is Expected. In a body that purges prior to arterial injection, the purge often continues during the embalming process. Examples include bodies with esophageal varices (as in alcoholism); bodies that suffered pneumonia, tuberculosis of the lungs, and ulcerations of the upper digestive organs; and bodies that show decomposition changes. Restricted cervical injection allows the embalmer to embalm the limbs and the trunk areas, then **aspirate the body,** set the features, and embalm the head. This eliminates the necessity to reset the features if purge occurs.

Jaundiced Bodies. The head can be embalmed with a jaundice fluid preparation or other jaundice treatment. Restricted cervical injection allows thorough distribution of the solution to the facial tissues. The remainder of the body can be injected using arterial solutions suitable to the body conditions. First inject the body, then inject the head and the face.

ADVANTAGES TO THE USE OF RESTRICTED CERVICAL INJECTION

1. Amount of arterial solution entering the facial tissues can be controlled
2. Large volumes of arterial solution can be injected into the trunk without overinjecting the head and the face
3. Two solution strengths can be used: one for the trunk and the limbs and another for the head and the face
4. Arterial coagula, if present in the aorta, are pushed toward the lower extremities
5. Different pressures can be used to inject the head and the trunk
6. Different rates of flow can be used to inject the trunk and the head
7. The trunk can be injected first and the body can be aspirated to stop purging; the features can be set **after aspirating,** and then the head can be injected last
8. The **instant tissue fixation** technique can be employed for trauma and decomposition cases
9. For jaundiced bodies, only the head is treated with jaundice fluids

ADVANTAGES TO USE OF THESE VESSELS FOR RESTRICTED CERVICAL INJECTION

1. Arteriosclerosis is rarely seen in the carotid arteries; they are very large vessels and very elastic
2. The common carotid arteries have no branches (except their terminal branches) and thus are easily raised to the surface
3. Clots present in the right or left carotid artery can be identified and removed
4. The carotid arteries allow direct injection of the head and facial tissues
5. The carotid arteries are accompanied by the large internal jugular veins, which directly drain the head and the face

▶ INSTANT TISSUE FIXATION

Instant tissue fixation is an embalming technique that makes use of restricted cervical injection. This embalming technique is used for the injection of the head (although other body areas can be similarly treated) with a limited amount of very strong arterial solution. Some examples of when it is used would include:

- Early decomposition when facial swelling is anticipated.
- When facial trauma is present.
- When facial tissues must be dried and firm for restorative treatments.
- When facial excisions are necessary, cancers, etc.
- Reembalming of the face.

Vessels
Both right and left common carotid arteries are raised and usually drainage is taken from the right internal jugular vein. In this method of injection, very little drainage is taken as only a minimal amount of arterial solution is injected.

Solution Strength
A very strong arterial solution is prepared, and in some cases, a waterless solution can be used. One solution suggested contains 16 oz of a high-index arterial fluid (25-index or above), 16 oz of a coinjection chemical, 16 oz of water, and 1 to 1½ oz of arterial fluid dye. This solution is designed to immediately preserve, dry, and firm the tissues.

Pressure
The solution is mixed in the machine. When a centrifugal injection machine is used, the pressure with the rate of flow valve **off** should be set at 20 lb or above.

Method of Injection
Connect the injection hose to the arterial tube in the left common carotid artery. Be certain that the arterial tubes used are as large as the arteries allow. Turn the machine **on** with the rate-of-flow valve **closed**. Set the pressure at 20 lb. Once the hose is connected, open the rate-of-flow valve a full turn and immediately turn it **off**. This creates a "pulse" type of fluid flow. The solution is injected in a strong spurt, under high pressure, for only a moment. Repeatedly turn the rate-of-flow valve on and off until sufficient solution has been injected. Only a minimum amount of solution is needed because of its strength. The dye will indicate the presence of the solution in the tissues. In addition, the dye helps to prevent graying of the tissues. Next, the right side of the head is injected in the same manner. High pressure is used, but the rate-of-flow valve is turned on and off for only a moment each time. The purpose of this method of embalming is to inject a very strong but minimal amount of preservative solution. Thus, maximum preservation is achieved with a minimum of tissue distension (Fig. 12–4).

Figure 12–4. Facial tissues embalmed using the instant tissue fixation technique prior to the removal of a cancerous tumor of the right cheek.

▶ VARIATIONS OF INJECTION TECHNIQUES

The autopsied body presents its own injection problems. When the body has undergone a complete autopsy, generally a six-point (sectional) injection is used; each body extremity is embalmed separately.

After surgeries, partial autopsies, or when organs have been removed for donation, direct access and use of the abdominal or thoracic aorta as an injection site becomes a possibility.

Traumatic injuries may result in the severance of vessels. It may become necessary to inject severed arteries to preserve a body extremity. Arteries when cut or severed will remain open—the lumen of the vessel can be seen—this can be helpful in locating a vessel for injection.

▶ DRAINAGE

As stated at the beginning of this chapter, four processes occur at the same time in the embalming of the body: (1) injection of the solution, (2) distribution of the solution, (3) diffusion of the solution, and (4) drainage. Distribution and diffusion of arterial solution are discussed in Chapter 13.

the lymphatics. These lymphatics have valves similar to those of veins and contain lymph nodes along their routes. Their fluid eventually enters the blood vascular system by flowing into the thoracic and the right lymphatic ducts. The thoracic duct empties lymph into the junction of the left subclavian vein and the left internal jugular vein. The lymph from the right lymphatic channel empties into the junction of the right subclavian vein and the right internal jugular vein

In life, the lymph is composed of the fluids that pass from the blood through the walls of the capillaries. Here it is called tissue or interstitial fluid. More fluid enters the interstitial spaces from the blood than is directly reabsorbed back into the bloodstream by the capillaries. This excess fluid is drained by the lymph system. Once the interstitial fluid enters the lymph capillaries it is called lymph. At the time of death these lymph channels can be the site of large numbers of microbes. The lymph system is part of the defense system for protecting the body from pathological microbes. Embalming solution will diffuse from the interstitial spaces into the lymph channels. Massage and manipulation of the body during injection combined with the use of restricted drainage help to move embalming fluid throughout the lymph system

Embalming solution can be diffused through the lymphatics in the following order: lymphatic capillary → lymphatic vessel → lymph nodes → lymph vessels → lymphatic trunk → subclavian veins

LYMPHATIC CIRCULATION

The lymphatic vessels originate as blind-end tubes called lymph capillaries (Fig. 12–5). These tubes are located in the spaces between the cells. The lymph capillaries are larger and more permeable than the blood capillaries. They converge to form lymph channels called

Drainage is brought about by displacement. As the arterial solution fills the vascular system the contents of the vascular system are displaced. There are 5 to 6 qt of blood in the vascular system of the average body. This accounts for approximately 8% of the body weight. At death, there is generally a wave contraction of the arterial system. This contraction forces the greatest volume

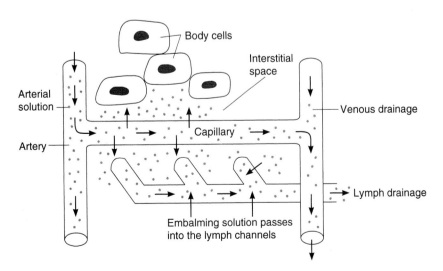

Figure 12–5. Drainage consists of blood, interstitial fluid, embalming solution, and lymphatic fluid.

of blood into the capillary and the venous portions of the blood vascular system.

It has been estimated that after death, 85% of the blood is found in the capillaries, 10% in the veins, and 5% in the arteries. Amounts of blood in the vascular system vary depending on the cause and the manner of death. In addition, the blood will gravitate (postmortem hypostasis) into the dependent body regions over time. This engorges the dependent capillaries with blood (livor mortis) and leaves the less-dependent tissues free of most of the blood.

Contents of Drainage

Drainage is composed of blood and blood clots, interstitial fluid, lymphatic fluid, and embalming solution. As arterial solution flows into the capillary, a portion of the solution passes through the walls of the capillary and is retained by the body. This retained preservative is the portion of the embalming solution that preserves, sanitizes, moisturizes, and colors the body tissues. Some of the embalming solution moves through the capillaries, into the venules and veins, and exits as part of the drainage. It has been estimated that 50% or more of the drainage taken during embalming is actually embalming solution.

The color and consistency of the drainage change during the injection in the body. During injection of the first gallon of embalming solution, drainage contains more blood than for subsequent injections. As the blood in the vascular system is gradually displaced and replaced with embalming solution, the drainage lightens in color and becomes thinner. The initial drainage is the most dangerous; however, all drainage should be carefully controlled and splashing should be avoided. Embalming the body raised on "body bridges" allows the drainage to fall onto the preparation table where it can be washed into the sanitary sewer system. Closed drainage (a clear plastic hose attached to a drain tube and the open end placed in the sanitary drain) will not expose the embalmer to the contents of the drainage.

As the embalming solution passes through the capillaries, some of the interstitial fluid in the tissue spaces is drawn into the capillaries by osmosis because of the high concentration of the embalming solution, especially when strong arterial solutions are used. Some interstitial fluid will also enter the drainage through the lymphatic system. Dehydration can result when too much interstitial fluid is removed. In bodies with skeletal edema, this is how the edema is removed from the tissue spaces.

Drainage can then be said to consist of blood, venous blood coagula, interstitial fluid, and arterial solution (Fig. 12–6). Bacteria and microbial agents and their products that have entered the blood vascular system before or after death are also removed in the drainage. In bodies with skeletal edema, the edematous fluid may

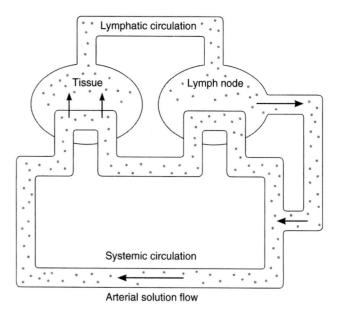

Figure 12–6. Lymphatic and systemic circulation.

be part of the drainage. Venous coagula are included in the contents of the drainage. Several types of clotted materials present in the drainage; however, all clotted materials come from the **veins** or from a heart chamber. It is impossible for any arterial coagula to pass through the capillary beds and enter the venous side of the circulatory system. The following coagula can be identified:

- **Postmortem coagula**—These coagula are not actual clots, but simply blood inclusions that have congealed and stuck together; they can be large and dark.
- **Postmortem clots**—These clots are multicolored. The bottom portion of the clot is dark, for it was formed by red blood cells that gravitated to the dependent part of a vessel. The clear layer on the top of the clot is a jelly-like layer of fibrin.
- **Antemortem clots**—Clots such as thrombosis form in layers—a layer of platelets, followed by a layer of fibrin, followed by another layer of platelets, and so on.

The viscosity of the blood can vary depending on the cause of death and the time between death and embalming. As the body gradually dehydrates after death, the viscosity of the blood increases. Bodies that have been refrigerated for very short periods after death, have been administered anticoagulant drugs such as heparin or dicumarol, or have died from carbon monoxide poisoning, exhibit low blood viscosity.

The volume of drainage is not equal to the volume of embalming solution injected. A large portion of the blood vascular system, particularly the arteries, is empty at death. This entire area must be filled, which accounts for the delay often noted between the start of the injection and the start of the drainage. At the conclusion of the embalming, the arterial system is filled; some of the injected solution is found in the capillaries and the veins, and some has passed through the capillaries to be retained by the tissues and the cells.

In some bodies, there will be little or no drainage.

> As long as the solution is distributing and there is no swelling or discolorations in the tissues, drainage need not be a concern

Sometimes there is little to drain, as illustrated in these examples:

1. In cases of esophageal varices and ruptured ulcerations of the digestive tract (blood has been lost to the lumen of the esophagus, stomach, or intestines), drainage actually occurs within the intestinal tract.
2. Accidental death could cause the spleen or other internal organ to rupture; blood is lost from these sites and drainage also occurs at these ruptures.
3. Traumatic death may result in a large loss of blood outside the body. This hemorrhage decreases the volume of blood available for drainage.
4. Insertion of the drainage tube into the femoral or external iliac vein may tear the vein, allowing drainage to flow into the abdominal cavity.
5. When a preinjection embalming solution is used, a portion of the blood is removed. At the time of arterial solution injection, there is less blood to drain.
6. Pathological lesions such as with tuberculosis may account for a blood loss in life and will create an internal site of drainage at the time of arterial solution injection.
7. Bloodstream infections frequently cause extensive clotting, and anemic diseases reduce blood volume; these factors contribute to poor distribution and low drainage volume.

Often in bodies in which hemorrhage into the digestive tract or abdominal cavity occurred prior to death, there may be a gradual swelling of the abdomen as the arterial solution is injected because some of the drainage (and arterial solution) will fill the digestive tract or abdominal cavity. This drainage can later be removed with a trocar. Likewise, hemorrhage into the stomach, esophagus, or lung tissues can result in a purge during injection. The purge will take the form of drainage. It is actually possible to drain from the mouth if a stomach ulcer has ruptured large veins! Aspiration can later remove these fluids. Some medications cause gastrointestinal bleeding. If this bleeding was intense, a major portion of the drainage may flow into the intestinal tract during arterial injection.

The bodies just described may demonstrate two forms of drainage: internal, into a cavity or hollow organ, and external, through the drainage tube or exit as purge.

Good drainage may be expected under the following conditions:

1. The interval between death and preparation is short; the body retains some heat.
2. The body shows early evidence of livor mortis, indicating that the blood has a low viscosity and can easily be moved.
3. Death was not the result of a febrile disease or a bloodstream infection.
4. Skeletal edema is present.
5. The body is jaundiced.
6. The person had been treated with blood thinners or anticoagulants (e.g., heparin, dicumarol, aspirin), resulting in low blood viscosity.
7. The body was refrigerated shortly after death but not for a long period.
8. Death was due to carbon monoxide poisoning.

Purpose of Drainage

The bodies used for dissection are often embalmed but not drained and most are swollen to the point where they could not be viewed for funeral purposes. Bodies dead for long periods of time can be slowly embalmed without draining and are often suitable for viewing. Drainage is taken for a number of reasons:

1. *To make room for the arterial solution.* Distension would result without removal of some of the blood (especially today, when 3 to 5 gal of preservative solution is injected into the average body).
2. *To reduce a secondary dilution of the arterial fluid.* The blood in the capillaries along with the interstitial fluids can dilute the embalming solution.
3. *To remove intravascular blood discolorations.* Livor mortis is a postmortem intravascular blood discoloration. Discolorations such as carbon monoxide and capillary congestion are antemortem blood discolorations. Injection of arterial solution accompanied by blood drainage should greatly reduce or remove these discolorations.
4. *To remove a tissue that rapidly decomposes.* Blood is a liquid tissue that rapidly decomposes after death, and decomposition of the blood can result in discolorations, odors, and formation of gas.
5. *To remove an element that speeds decomposition.* Blood, a portion of which is liquid, can hasten hydrolysis and the decomposition of the body tissues. Moisture is needed for decomposition and blood can provide that medium.
6. *To remove bacteria present in the blood.* With some diseases, the microbes normally found in the

intestine can translocate to the bloodstream. After death, this translocation greatly increases. Removal of blood as drainage helps to reduce microbial agents in the body.

7. *To prevent discolorations.* When the blood in the body (hemoglobin) mixes with the formaldehyde of the arterial solution methyl-hemoglobin can form, which produces a gray color in the tissues (formaldehyde gray).

8. *To reduce swollen tissues.* When pitting edema is present in the skeletal tissues, it is possible to remove some of the edematous fluid via the blood drainage from the body.

Drainage, from some bodies, is most important in clearing very pronounced discolorations, especially when the face, the neck, and the hands are affected. **If a primary purpose for drainage must be stated, it would be that the drainage makes room for the arterial solution so it can be evenly distributed to all tissues of the body with a minimum distension.**

Center of Drainage

The center of drainage in the dead human body is the right atrium of the heart (Fig. 12–7). The superior vena cava returns blood to this chamber from the head and

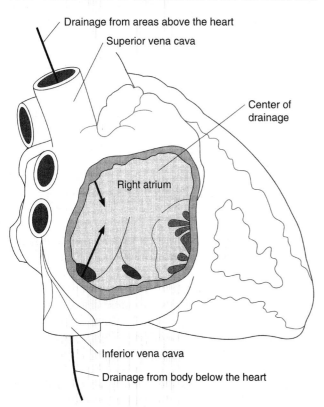

Figure 12–7 labels:
- Drainage from areas above the heart
- Superior vena cava
- Center of drainage
- Right atrium
- Inferior vena cava
- Drainage from body below the heart

Figure 12–7. The center of drainage in the dead human body is the right atrium of the heart. The superior vena cava returns blood to this chamber from the head and the upper extremities. The inferior vena cava returns blood from the visceral organs, trunk, and legs.

the upper extremities. The inferior vena cava returns blood from the visceral organs, trunk, and legs. If the internal jugular vein is used as a drainage point, all blood from the lower extremities and visceral organs must pass through the right atrium to be drained. Likewise, if drainage is to be taken from the femoral vein, blood from the arms and the head must pass through the right atrium. After death, the blood in the right atrium frequently congeals. This condition warrants drainage from the right internal jugular vein where an instrument, such as angular spring forceps, can be placed directly into the right atrium to fragment this coagulum.

Above and Below Heart Drainage

Some embalmers also use two locations for drainage. A second drainage point is often used when the femoral vein is used as the beginning injection and drainage point. If there is a blockage in the inferior vena cava, right atrium or the jugular veins, the neck and the face can begin to discolor. The veins of the neck and possibly the tissues of the neck can distend. The right internal jugular vein should be raised and opened as a second drainage site.

> Drainage instruments are inserted into the vein and directed toward the heart

Drainage Sites

The primary drainage site is the location from which drainage is first taken. In the unautopsied body, the veins most commonly used for drainage are the right internal jugular vein, the femoral vein, or the external iliac vein.

Axillary and basilic veins can be used, but their small size and the need to extend the arm make these veins an impractical choice. **Any vein can be used for drainage whether it is large or small or on the right or left side of the body.** In unusual circumstances, even the external jugular vein can be used if the internal jugular vein is obstructed by a cancerous growth or a large attached thrombosis.

> A broken vein can still be used as a drainage site; if an instrument such as angular forceps cannot be inserted, a groove director may be used. Following injection the area can be dried and the ends of the broken vein are ligated

Should a vein tear while it is being raised, the following steps can be taken to attempt to place an instrument in the portion of the vein leading to the heart:

1. Force as much blood from the vein as possible.
2. Clean the area using an absorbent material.

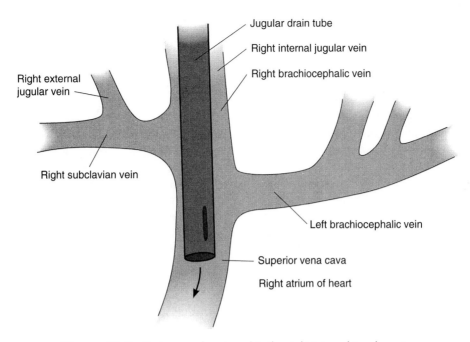

Figure 12–8. Drainage tube placed in the right internal jugular vein.

3. Observe where blood is seeping from the broken portion of the vein.
4. Clamp an edge of the wall of the broken vein with a small serrated or rat-toothed hemostat, or place the hemostat across the entire broken portion of the vein.
5. Gently insert a drainage device toward the heart; if the vein has been torn into two pieces, do not remove the hemostat.
6. After embalming, pass ligatures and tie off the severed ends of the vein (holding them with hemostats).

In Chapter 9, the advantages and the disadvantages of the various veins for drainage are discussed, as are the incision locations and the relationships of veins to arteries. The internal jugular vein is the most valuable drainage point. It is the largest systemic vein that can be raised in the unautopsied body. The right internal jugular vein leads directly into the right atrium of the heart. Figure 12–8 illustrates why the **right** and not the left internal jugular vein is most frequently used for drainage. Should there be a complication with the right internal jugular vein, the left can be used, but note that the vein turns to the right, often making insertion of a drainage instrument difficult.

Direct Heart Drainage*
The right atrium of the heart can be directly drained using a trocar (Fig. 12–9). This very old method of

drainage was often used when embalming was performed at the residence of the deceased. The drainage could be conveniently collected in bottles, which could be taken back to the funeral parlor to be emptied.

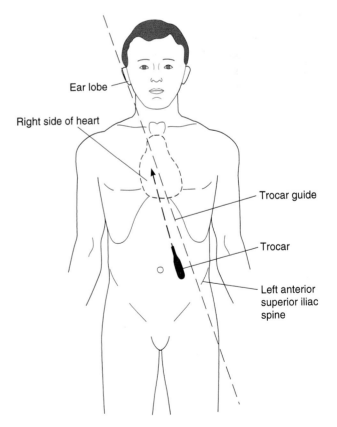

Figure 12–9. Direct heart drainage.

---

*This method is not intended for use as a primary drainage technique but only in special situations where a vein cannot be used for drainage.

To drain directly from the right atrium of the heart, start by injecting approximately 1½ to 1 gal of embalming solution to fill the vascular system. To drain the heart, insert the trocar at approximately the standard point of entry, 2 in. to the left and 2 in. above the umbilicus. Draw an imaginary line across the body connecting the **left** anterior superior iliac spine and the lobe of the **right** ear. Direct the trocar toward a point where this line crosses the right side of the sternum. This point is approximately at the level of the sternum where the fourth rib joins the sternum. Be certain to keep the trocar slightly to the right of the sternum. The trocar point should be kept in the anterior portion of the mediastinum. If there is sufficient pressure in the right atrium, simply placing the trocar in the heart chamber should be sufficient to start drainage. The trocar can be attached to the hydroaspirator.

Do not turn the hydroaspirator on to full suction; half is quite sufficient. Insert the trocar with the hydroaspirator running. As soon as the heart is pierced, the hydroaspirator can be turned off. Most hydroaspirators are lower than the height of the embalming table, so a natural gravity system is established. It is important that a plastic hose be used on the trocar, for the embalmer can then see immediately when the right side of the heart has been punctured.

If the embalmer is unfamiliar with this technique of drainage, it can easily be practiced. Begin cavity aspiration by aspirating the right side of the heart first. The embalmer need not pierce only the right atrium with the trocar; the right ventricle can also be pierced. There should be sufficient pressure in the right side of the heart that the suction of the aspirator on the trocar can open the right atrioventricular valve and, in this manner, drain the right atrium. Should the trocar puncture the ascending aorta or the arch, sufficient embalming solution may be lost to necessitate a six-point injection.

Drainage Instrumentation

A large variety of drainage devices are available. The most standard drainage instruments are the drain tube and the angular spring forceps. **Drainage instruments are inserted into veins and directed toward the heart.** Some embalmers prefer to lubricate these devices with massage cream to facilitate their entry into the vein. Drain tubes contain a plunger rod, which can also be lubricated with massage cream. After each use, drain tubes should be disassembled, flushed with water, cleaned and disinfected.

The **groove director** is used to assist in the insertion of a drainage tube or forceps into the vein. The groove director is inserted into the vein first. Once it is in place, the drainage instrument is slid along the grooved portion of the instrument. The grooved portion should face the lumen of the vein.

Many times, a drainage tube cannot be fully inserted into the vein; it should not be forced. As long as a portion of the tube can be inserted, it will keep the vein expanded. Changing the position of the tube in the vein often assists with the drainage. Tubes should be tied into a vein, but loosely enough so that their position can be changed.

Drainage tubes come in a variety of lengths and diameters. Those for use in the internal jugular vein (Fig. 12–10) are very large in diameter and short in length. Axillary drain tubes are long and slightly curved for insertion into the axillary vein. Axillary drain tubes are not very large in diameter. A variety of drainage tubes are made for the femoral vein; they come in a wide range of diameters and lengths. One type of iliac drain tube

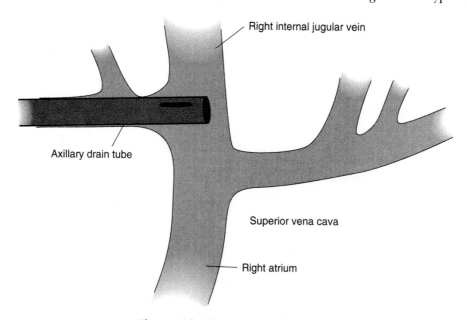

Figure 12–10. Drainage tube insert.

is designed to be inserted into the external iliac vein, and the tip of the tube reaches into the right atrium of the heart; they are approximately 20 in. in length and made of plastic, metal, or rubber. Drainage tubes, with very small diameters, are also available for embalming unautopsied infants.

Advantages of the drain tube	Disadvantages of the drain tube
The tube keeps the vein expanded	The size of the opening is limited to the diameter of the tube
The "stirring" rod helps to fragment coagula	The tube can block the opposite portion of the vein. The tube can block other veins
Drainage can be shut off to build intravascular pressure	Coagula cannot be grasped
	The tube may mark the face or interfere with positioning of the head
Closed drainage technique can be used	The tube can easily be pushed through the vein into a body cavity

Angular spring forceps can be used to assist drainage from any vein.

Advantages of the angular spring forceps for jugular drainage	Disadvantages of the angular spring forceps
It provides a very large opening for the drainage	It may have to be removed to close the vein for intermittent drainage
The head can be positioned to the right	Drainage may splatter
The forceps does not mark the face	Embalmer's contact with the drainage is increased
Coagula can be grasped	
It does not block other venous tributaries	

The angular spring forceps is convenient to use for drainage from the right internal jugular vein. It **does not block** drainage from the left in nominate vein, right subclavian vein, or upper portion of the right internal jugular vein. These tributaries can be blocked if the jugular drain tube is used. It provides a wide opening for the passage of coagula and it allows the right side of the head to drain. Large masses of coagula can be broken and easily removed from the superior vena cava and the right atrium. The head can easily be positioned without the forceps marking the side of the face.

Methods of Drainage

Many embalmers use a combination of drainage methods. They begin the injection using continuous drainage and then restrict the drainage (using intermittent drainage) after the blood discolorations clear. **There are three basic types of drainage in relationship to arterial injection.**

METHODS OF DRAINAGE IN RELATION TO INJECTION

Alternate
Concurrent
Intermittent

Alternate Drainage. In alternate drainage, the arterial solution is never injected while drainage is being taken. A quart or two of the arterial solution is injected; then the arterial injection is stopped and venous drainage commences. This is allowed to continue until drainage subsides; then the drainage instrument is closed. The process is then repeated. Injection and drainage are alternated until the embalming is completed. Because 1 or 2 qt of fluid is constantly injected into a confined system, it is believed that a more uniform pressure is developed in all parts of the body. More complete distribution of arterial solution is achieved and more complete drainage results. Fluid diffusion is enhanced, for pressure filtration is increased. This method increases preparation time and care must be taken to avoid distension.

Concurrent (Continuous). In concurrent drainage, injection and drainage are allowed to proceed at the same time throughout the embalming.

Distension is possible with any method of drainage or injection. As soon as distension is evident, stop injection

Because of the open drainage, it may be difficult to attain a pressure sufficient to saturate tissues throughout the body. Clots (in the venous system) may not be dislodged when the concurrent method is used. Fluid will follow the path of least resistance and more embalming solution may be lost to the drainage. This method of drainage may dehydrate and wrinkle body tissues. It has value in the preparation of bodies with high moisture content to the tissues (edema), for which dehydration is encouraged.

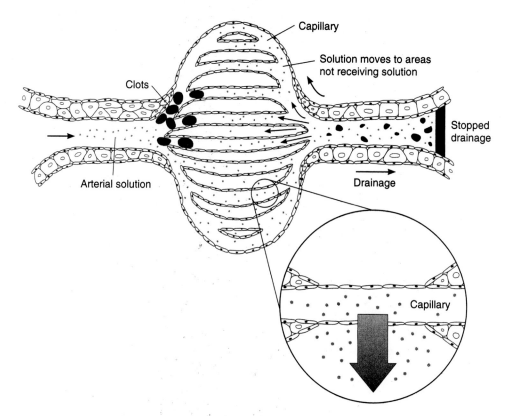

Figure 12-11. Intermittent drainage.

Intermittent Drainage (Fig. 12–11). In this process, the injection of the embalming solution continues throughout the embalming and the drainage is shut off for selected short periods. Some embalmers stop drainage until a particular amount of solution is injected (1 or 2 qt); others stop drainage until surface veins are raised. It is important that surface intravascular blood discolorations clear before intermittent drainage is begun. This method is less time consuming than the alternate method, encourages fluid distribution and pressure filtration, helps to prevent short-circuiting of the embalming solution and its loss to the drainage, and promotes retention of the embalming solution by the tissues. Intermittent drainage helps the body to retain tissue fluid (which provides a proper moisture balance) and is recommended when colloidal fluids such as humectants or restorative fluids are used to slightly distend emaciated tissues.

Techniques for Improving Drainage

Drainage (1) makes room for the arterial solution in the vascular system, (2) allows for a thorough distribution of the embalming solution, (3) prevents distension of the body tissues, and (4) prevents adverse discolorations. Creation of good drainage can be done in two periods, prior to injection of the preservative solution and during injection of the preservative solution.

Preembalming techniques include the following:

- *Selection of a large vein.* Preference is generally the internal jugular or the femoral, or external iliac vein.
- *Selection of a large drainage instrument.* An angular spring forceps or drainage tube is used.
- *Injection of a preinjection fluid.* Follow the manufacturer's dilution of the chemical and volume of the chemical injected. If a preinjection chemical is not used, a mild arterial solution can be injected to clear blood discolorations and establish circulation.
- *Removal of extravascular pressure such as gas and fluids in the abdomen.*

The following techniques are included during injection:

- Use of drainage devices to fragment clots.
- Use of massage and pressure applied over the heart and/or liver to move venous clots.
- Increase in the rate of solution injection or increase in the pressure of the solution being injected.
- Intermittent and alternate forms of drainage techniques.
- Selection of another drainage site if necessary.

Disinfection of the Drainage

The initial or first drainage taken presents the greatest risk to the embalmer when the cause of death was bloodborne infection (acquired immunodeficiency syndrome, hepatitis, or bloodstream sepsis). At present, the Occupational Safety and Health Administration permits bulk blood, suction, and aspirated fluids to be carefully drained into a sanitary sewer system. Drainage consists of blood, interstitial fluids, lymph, and arterial solution. The arterial solution in the drainage will to some degree sanitize the blood and body fluid portions of the drainage. By draining into a sewage system, the drainage also become highly diluted by the addition of running and flushing water.

To minimize contact as blood is being drained, tubing may be attached to the drain tube. This creates a **closed drainage system**. The tubing can be placed directly into a sewage drain. The closed drain system also allows the drainage to be easily collected. In deaths from highly infectious and or contagious diseases—for example, Creutzfeldt–Jacob disease, human immunodeficiency virus, and hepatitis—drained blood can be disinfected by collecting the drainage in a container and adding at least $1\frac{1}{2}$ gal of "fresh" undiluted sodium hypochlorite (household bleach). Cover the container and let the solution stand for a minimum of 1 hour. The waste can then be very carefully poured into the drain being very careful to avoid splashing. Flush the drain with running water for 10 minutes.

Closed Drainage Technique. Another technique in preventing blood contamination for the embalming of bodies dead from highly infectious and/or contagious disease is to take very little or no drainage. This technique involves the injection of a very strong arterial solution (e.g., waterless) at a very slow rate of flow. Aspiration should be delayed as long as possible to allow the embalming solution to diffuse to all regions of the body. If the face discolors to avoid graying of the tissues, a very limited drainage can be taken or drainage can be taken directly from the right atrium of the heart by using the trocar.

Some embalmers recommend injecting as much arterial solution as possible prior to draining into bodies dead from contagious disease and, several minutes later, beginning the drainage. This interval allows some mixing of the blood and the embalming solution.

▶ CONCEPTS FOR STUDY AND DISCUSSION

1. Select vessels for injection and drainage of a morbidly obese, unautopsied body. Defend the selection you have made by explaining the advantages of using your selection.

2. List the advantages of using restricted cervical injection.
3. List the contents of drainage.
4. List the purposes for drainage.
5. List several techniques for stimulating drainage.
6. Complete the following distribution problems:

Embalming Solution Tracing Problems

ONE-POINT INJECTION AND DRAINAGE

Skeletal tissues	Trace arterial solution from the femoral artery (tube directed downward) to the right great toe; drain from the right femoral vein
Skeletal tissues	Trace arterial solution from the right femoral artery to the left side of the upper lip; drain from the right femoral vein
Visceral tissues	Trace arterial solution from the right femoral artery to the fundus of the stomach; drain from the right femoral vein

SPLIT INJECTION AND DRAINAGE

Skeletal tissues	Trace arterial solution from the right femoral artery to the right great toe; drain from the right internal jugular
Skeletal tissues	Trace arterial solution from the right common carotid to the left upper lip; drain from the right femoral vein
Visceral tissues	Trace arterial solution from the right common carotid to the appendix; drain from the right femoral vein

RESTRICTED CERVICAL INJECTION

Skeletal tissues	Inject the right common carotid down to reach the left lower lip; drain from the right internal jugular
Skeletal tissues	Inject the right common carotid down to reach the right upper lip (with the stopcock directed upward closed); drain from the right internal jugular
Visceral tissues	Inject down the right common carotid to the tissues of the left lung; drain from the right internal jugular

► BIBLIOGRAPHY

Collison K. Creutzfeldt-Jakob disease—fact and fiction: Part 2. *The Dodge Magazine.* January 2002; 94(1).

Investigating factors relating to fluid retention during embalming, Parts I and II. In *Champion Expanding Encyclopedia*, Nos. 499 and 500. Springfield, OH: Champion Chemical Co., August/September 1979:2013–2020.

Johnson EC. A study of arterial pressure during embalming. In *The Champion Expanding Encyclopedia.* Springfield, OH: Champion Chemical Co., 1981:2081–2084.

Kroshus J, McConnell J, Bardole J. The measurement of formaldehyde retention in the tissues of embalmed bodies. *Director.* March/April 1983:10–12.

Mechanics of proper drainage. In *Champion Expanding Encyclopedia*, No. 442. Springfield, OH: Champion Chemical Co., November/December 1973:1785–1788.

Removal of blood via the heart. In *Champion Expanding Encyclopedia.* Springfield, OH: Champion Chemical Co.; May 1976:1885–1888.

Shor M. An examination into methods old and new of achieving greatest possible venous drainage, *Casket and Sunnyside.* July 1964:20.

CHAPTER 13

DISTRIBUTION AND DIFFUSION OF ARTERIAL SOLUTION

CHAPTER OBJECTIVES

► Arterial solution distribution
► Arterial solution diffusion
► Extravascular and intravascular resistances
► Injection pressure and rate of flow
► Signs of arterial solution distribution

Arterial embalming could also be called "capillary embalming." The capillaries, the smallest blood vessels of the body, link the injected embalming solution with the cells of the body. The embalming solution that passes from the capillaries to the tissues comes into contact with the proteins of the cells. The preservatives in the solution stabilize the proteins and create a condition of temporary preservation. This chapter discusses the movement of arterial solution through the blood vascular (intravascular) and interstitial (extravascular) systems of the body. On reaching the capillaries, the embalming solution, by a series of passive physical transport systems, moves to the cells of the body.* The movement of embalming solution from the intravascular to the extravascular location is called **fluid diffusion**. The remainder of the embalming solution, which passes into the venous system of the body, helps to remove the blood and the intravascular blood discolorations. Drainage, which exits a vein during arterial injection, is made up of blood, tissue fluids, lymph, and some of the arterial solution.

The ability of the embalmer to retain as much preservative within the body as possible without visible distension of the tissues is a key factor in thoroughly preserving and sanitizing the body.

While vascular embalming should be thought of as a **unified process**, this process can be divided into **four** divisions: (1) **Delivery of the arterial solution** from the em-

balming machine through the connecting tubing and arterial tube into the artery. (2) **Distribution of arterial solution** is the movement of arterial solution from the point of injection throughout the arterial system and into the capillaries (perfusion). (3) **Diffusion of arterial solution** is the movement of arterial solution from inside the vascular system (intravascular) through the walls of the capillaries to the tissue spaces (extravascular). (4) **Drainage**, the discharge or withdrawal of blood and blood clots, embalming solution, and interstitial and lymphatic fluids from the body during vascular embalming. The drainage is taken from a body vein.

From this simple diagram, it is seen that the preservative solution delivery, distribution, diffusion, and drainage occur at the same time once the vascular system has been filled with sufficient embalming solution. These processes work similarly to a lawn sprinkler or soaker hose. Arterial solution fills the vascular system, much like water fills the hose to reach the sprinkler. Some of the arterial solution flows through the walls and pores of the capillaries into the tissue spaces, as water passes through the holes in the sprinkler to reach the grass. The major difference is that all the water is sprayed out of the sprinkler. In embalming, a portion of the arterial solution stays inside the capillaries and flows into the veins to be removed as drainage.

The material drained during embalming of the body is a mixture of blood, arterial solution, and interstitial fluid. It has been demonstrated that as much as 50% of the drainage can be arterial solution. Because the

---

*Passive transport systems require no energy by the cell to operate.

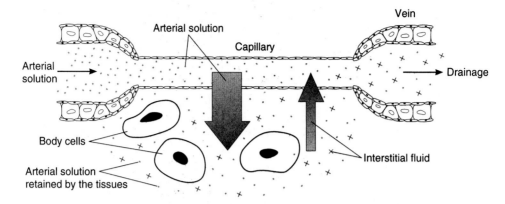

Figure 13–1. Drainage and retention of arterial solution.

vascular system is **not a closed** system, the arterial solution is allowed to pass through the walls and small pores of the capillaries to enter the interstitial spaces (Fig. 13–1). In these tissue spaces, a fluid surrounds and bathes the cells of the body. In life, this tissue fluid serves to transport the nutrients and oxygen carried by the blood to the cells, as the blood remains in the blood vascular system and does not have direct contact with the cells. The tissue fluid also carries the wastes of cell metabolism to the blood vascular system, where they are carried to the organs of the body that dispose of these wastes.

In the embalming of a body that has been dead a long time and in which decomposition has begun, injection can result in the immediate swelling of tissues. This swelling occurs because the capillary walls (only one cell in thickness), after being decomposed, can no longer hold arterial solution. Arterial solution thus flows from the large arteries into the small arterioles and then directly into the interstitial spaces. As almost all the arterial solution enters the interstitial spaces, the tissues become distended. In embalming this type of body, it is important to inject a strong arterial solution, so that the maximum amount of preservation is achieved with minimum tissue distension. This is particularly important for the face and hands if the body is to be presentable for viewing.

A similar process occurs in arterial embalming. Arterial solution flows through the arteries into the capillaries. A portion of the solution leaves the capillaries and passes into the fluid in the tissue spaces. Eventually it moves to and enters the cells and makes contact with the cell proteins. In this manner, the cells of the body are preserved or embalmed. The embalming solution that passes through the pores or walls of the capillaries and eventually embalms the cells is the **retained arterial solution**. It is this retained arterial solution that stabilizes the body proteins and brings about the temporary preservation of the dead human body.

The arterial solution that remains in the capillaries and is pushed ahead into the venules and veins and is eventually drained from the body serves only to clear the vascular system of blood. This solution can embalm only the walls of the vascular system. The vascular system is extensive and the preservation of arteries, capillaries, and veins would, no doubt, diminish decomposition of the body. Nevertheless, muscle cells and connective tissue cells account for the bulk of the body, and their preservation is essential if decomposition is to be halted and a thorough and extended preservation of the body achieved.

Drainage is a combination of **blood**, **arterial solution**, **interstitial fluids**, and **lymphatic fluids**. It is easy to see how blood and embalming solution are elements of the drainage, but interstitial fluid becomes part of the drainage through two routes. In living bodies, excess interstitial fluid is carried away from the spaces between the cells by the lymph system. This system empties into certain large veins of the body. In the embalming process, some embalming solution diffuses into the interstitial fluid and is removed by the lymph system. Even more importantly, embalming solution is present in the capillaries, and as it moves through the capillaries it draws some tissue fluid with it into the drainage. This explains why dehydration often occurs in areas such as the lips and the fingers during injection—more tissue fluid is being removed than is being replaced by embalming solution.

Arterial embalming involves both physical and chemical applications. Filling the arterial system by forced injection with some apparatus that pushes solution into the body under pressure involves physical procedures. Control of the drainage is a physical process. Some of the injected solution is forced through the walls of the capillaries simply by the physical process of filtration.

The arterial fluid is chemical in nature. When properly diluted, it makes a homogeneous solution that is

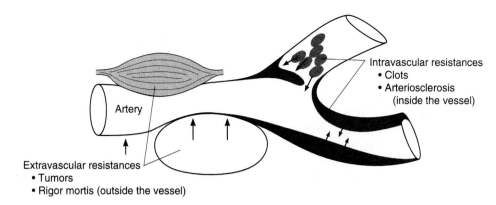

Figure 13–2. Extravascular resistance outside and intravascular resistance within the vessel.

described as hypotonic. Through the physical processes of osmosis and dialysis, this hypotonic solution passes from the capillaries into the interstitial spaces. The preservatives in the solution chemically combine with the proteins in the body cells and the protein in microorganisms and their products to form new compounds and alter the proteins in such a manner that the tissues are preserved and sanitized.

▶ ARTERIAL SOLUTION INJECTION

Arterial embalming begins with the injection of a preservative solution, under pressure, into an artery of the body.* Arterial (vascular) embalming can be defined as the injection of a suitable arterial (embalming) solution, under pressure, into the blood vascular system to accomplish **temporary preservation**, **sanitation**, and **restoration** of the dead human body. The solution moves from the arteries to the capillaries and then passes through the capillaries to come into contact with the body cells. A portion of the embalming solution remains in the capillaries to remove the blood and its products from the vascular system in the form of drainage. This drainage is taken from a vein of the body.

It is necessary to inject an embalming solution under pressure. The early embalming injection apparatus was simply a container of the arterial solution elevated above the body to create the pressure needed to distribute the solution throughout the body. The body offers resistance to the injection of the solution. As the solution is injected into the vascular system by way of an artery, the resistances are described in relationship to the vascular system. Resistances within the blood vessels are called **intravascular resistances**; resistances outside the blood vessels are called **extravascular resistances** (Fig. 13–2).

Resistances affect the arterial solution distribution. Poor or good distribution of the arterial solution results in poor or good diffusion of the embalming solution, respectively. Pressurized injection is needed to overcome the resistances that interfere with arterial solution distribution. As embalming solution travels from the large central trunk of the arterial system (the aorta) into the arterial branches (arterioles and capillaries), the diameter of the arterial system actually **expands** because of the innumerable branches of the vessels. The injection pressure needed to force the solution through the narrow arteries **decreases** by the time the solution reaches the capillaries. Pressurized injection is also responsible for a portion of the **diffusion** of the arterial solution.

The arterial solution at the microcirculatory level can take three routes: (1) A portion flows through the capillaries, where some of the embalming solution passes through the walls of the capillaries to embalm the tissues. (2) The portion that remains in the capillaries flows on to the venules. This embalming solution helps to remove the blood from the capillaries and the veins and eventually exits as drainage. (3) The remaining embalming solution flows through direct connections that link arterioles and venules. It eventually exits as drainage.

Intravascular pressure (IVP), which brings about pressure filtration that moves the embalming solution from the capillaries into the interstitial spaces, is created by the pressure from the machine and the expansion of the elastic arteries. This pressure effects embalming solution filtration through the walls of the capillaries. Pressure filtration is one of the major processes by which embalming solution enters the tissue spaces. IVP also remains with the embalming solution that flows into the venous system. This is what helps to create the small (approximately one-half pound) pressure that the drainage exhibits. No doubt, a lot of the drainage pressure is brought about by arterial solution flowing directly through connecting routes—directly from arterioles to venules and not passing through the capillary routes.

---

*Some embalmers may prefer to begin the arterial embalming (of the unautopsied body) by injecting a preinjection arterial solution.

During life, some capillaries remain devoid of blood as a result of vasoconstriction. Also, some areas of the body are engorged with blood because of the activity of the body, which causes vasodilation. For example, in a person who is running, more blood is concentrated in the muscles being used rather than in those muscles not being used. At death, the vascular system relaxes and thus increases its capacity. As a result, the embalmer can inject a large volume of solution without causing immediate distension of the tissues or drainage.

The drainage from the average body generally amounts to one-half or less of the total volume of arterial solution injected. It is the intent of the embalmer that 50% or more of the arterial solution injected be retained by the body for the embalming of cells and tissues. The embalmer must make every attempt to promote even distribution of the embalming solution throughout the body and to have the tissues retain as much embalming solution as possible. An old rule was to inject 1 gallon of a sufficient strength of embalming solution for every 50 pounds of body weight. Today, it is necessary to rely on the **embalming analysis** and the **response** of the body tissues as the solution is injected, to determine the amount of solution that needs to be injected and the needed strength of the solution. Observation and evaluation will also determine if multipoint injection is needed to reach all body areas with the preservative solution.

Extravascular and intravascular resistances are responsible for nonuniformity in distribution of the embalming solution. The diameters of the artery, the arterial tube, and the delivery hose from the machine to the arterial tube all produce resistance. As a point for injection, the artery with the largest diameter, generally the common carotid or the femoral artery, should be selected. An arterial tube of appropriate size should be inserted into the artery. The arterial tube should not damage the inner wall of an artery.

▶ INTRAVASCULAR RESISTANCE

Intravascular resistances can be caused either by narrowing or obstruction of the lumen of a vessel. This narrowing or obstruction is brought about by conditions found either within the lumen of the vessel or within the walls of the vessel. The **lumen** can be **obstructed** by blood, antemortem emboli, antemortem thrombi, and postmortem coagula and thrombi.

As the embalming solution flows from the aorta into the narrowing branches of the arterial tree, the lumen of the arteries also narrows. A coagulum that is loosened and moved along with the solution will eventually clog a small distributing artery. Arterial coagulum could never be reduced to a size where it could pass through arterioles and capillaries. When a coagulum reaches an arterial branch through which it can move no farther,

distribution of solution beyond this point is stopped. The only way tissues beyond this point can receive embalming solution is through the collateral circulation.

Intravascular resistance resulting from **narrowing of the lumen** can be caused by arteriosclerosis, most frequently seen in the arteries of the lower extremities; vasoconstriction, frequently seen on one side of the body as a result of a stroke; arteritis, brought about by inflammation of the artery; and intravascular rigor mortis, postmortem narrowing caused by rigor mortis of the smooth muscles in the arterial walls. Unlike extravascular resistance, the embalmer can do little to remove intravascular resistance (Fig. 13–3).

▶ EMBALMING PROCEDURES FOR INTRAVASCULAR PROBLEMS

The following embalming techniques can be used when intravascular problems are anticipated:

1. Use sufficient pressure and rate of flow to uniformly distribute the arterial solution. A slow rate of flow can help to prevent coagula in the arteries from floating free and clogging smaller branch arteries. Once circulation is established, a faster rate of flow can be used.
2. If arterial coagula are anticipated (i.e., bodies dead for long periods, gangrene evidenced in distal limbs, and death from infections) inject from the right common carotid artery (or restricted cervical injection). This pushes arterial coagula away from the arteries that supply the head and arms (the areas to be viewed). The legs can be injected separately, if necessary, or treated by hypodermic and/or surface embalming.
3. Avoid using a sclerotic artery for injection. The common carotid is rarely sclerotic, whereas the femoral and iliac arteries are frequently sclerotic.
4. Use the largest artery possible for the primary injection point. This is usually the common carotid, external iliac, or femoral artery.
5. Use an arterial tube of proper size, so that it will not damage the walls of the artery.

▶ EXTRAVASCULAR RESISTANCE

Extravascular resistance is pressure placed on the outside of a blood vessel. This pressure is sufficient to collapse or partially collapse the lumen of the vessel. The embalmer is better able to reduce or remove extravascular resistance than intravascular resistance. Therefore, the following discussion of extravascular resistances includes techniques that can be used to reduce or remove the pressures that these resistances place on blood vessels.

A
B

Figure 13–3. A. Example of clots in the aorta. **B.** Example of arterial clotting. (*Courtesy of Debra A. Goethals, Chicago, IL.*)

Rigor Mortis

The postmortem stiffening of the voluntary skeletal muscles is a strong extravascular resistance. Rigor mortis is not a uniform condition. It may be present in some muscles and absent in others. This can cause a very uneven distribution of arterial solution. Embalming prior to or during the onset of rigor is generally recommended. When rigor is present, gentle but very firm manipulation and massage of the muscles helps to reduce the rigor. The massage and manipulation can be done prior to and during arterial injection. During the injection of the first gallon of arterial solution, firm massage and exercise of the extremities can be very important in establishing good distribution. Massage should be done especially along the arterial routes (e.g., axilla, wrist, sides of fingers, groin, and popliteal space).

Gas in the Cavities

Decomposition gases in the abdominal cavity can exert enough pressure to push the large abdominal aorta and inferior vena cava against the spinal column, thus causing these vessels to narrow or collapse. Most frequently, this pressure can be removed at the beginning of the em-

balming by puncturing the abdominal wall with a trocar or scalpel and releasing some of the gasses. It may also be necessary to puncture some of the large and small intestines. This can easily be done without fear of interrupting the circulation.

Expansion of the Hollow Viscera During Injection

Too rapid an injection of arterial solution, especially in bodies dead for long periods, can result in expansion of the hollow visceral organs. This expansion causes the abdomen to swell and places sufficient pressure on the aorta and vena cava so as to collapse their lumens. Stomach purge often accompanies this abdominal distension. Insert a trocar into the abdominal cavity, keeping the point just beneath the anterior abdominal wall, and puncture some of the distended intestines.

Tumors and Swollen Lymph Nodes

These distended growths and organs can place pressure on the blood vascular system, creating distribution and drainage problems. Sectional injection may be necessary. A higher injection pressure and pulsation may help to obtain good distribution. Massage and manipulation may also help to encourage solution distribution and drainage.

Ascites and Hydrothorax

Enough fluid may accumulate in the thoracic and abdominal cavities to interfere with blood drainage and arterial solution distribution. Drainage from several sites may be necessary. The ascites can be removed or relieved by inserting a trocar into the abdominal cavity or inserting a drainage tube through a puncture made in the abdominal wall.

Contact Pressure

Portions of the body that push against the embalming table or against positioning devices (such as shoulder blocks) may not receive enough arterial solution. Contact pressure can restrict the flow of solution into the shoulders, buttocks, and backs of the legs. During embalming, these areas should be manipulated and massaged to relieve the pressure from the contact with the embalming table.

Visceral Weight

In all bodies, abdominal viscera create some resistance. In obese bodies, however, there can be sufficient visceral weight on the large vessels in the abdomen to restrict drainage and possibly solution distribution. Higher pressures, pulsation, and a more rapid rate of flow may help to overcome this resistance. Manipulation and massage of the abdominal area may also assist distribution and drainage.

Bandages

An elastic bandage or any bandage wound around an extremity should be removed prior to arterial injection. Such bandages can disrupt drainage from the hands and feet. During injection, even a patient identification band can be a source of vascular resistance.

Skeletal Edema

Skeletal edema can be intense enough that it exerts extravascular resistance to the distribution of embalming solution as well as a resistance to blood drainage. Numerous conditions, from pathological disorders to drug treatments, can bring this about (Fig. 13–4). These intense edemas are frequently seen postoperatively, particularly after open heart or vascular surgery. Higher injection pressures, pulsation, manipulation, and massage assist in distribution and drainage. Sectional vascular embalming may be necessary.

Inflammation

Inflamed tissue can swell to the extent that vascular constriction results. Higher injection pressures, pulsation, and massage may assist in distributing arterial solution

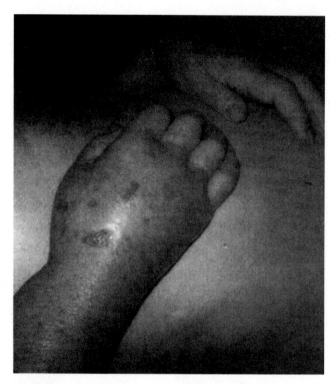

Figure 13–4. A right hand and arm distended with edema.

into these body areas. Sectional vascular and hypodermic embalming may be necessary.

▶ COMBINED RESISTANCE

Extravascular and intravascular resistances rarely exist in and of themselves. In embalming the "average" body, a combination of resistances is found. For example, in embalming a 62-year-old man who died from a myocardial infarction, resistances might originate from rigor mortis (because of delay between death and preparation), arteriosclerosis (some degree of sclerosis can be found), contact pressure (possible in every body), and blood in the dependent portions of the vascular system.

These four sources of resistance demonstrate that even in a sudden death, vascular resistances are present that can restrict good arterial distribution and blood drainage. In the preceding example, the rigor may be intense enough that distribution is reduced to the point where sectional embalming is required. If the person had been taking an anticoagulant, the blood may remain in a liquid form and postmortem clotting would be diminished. Thus, arterial distribution and blood drainage would be much better.

At the time of death, invasive treatments and drugs administered could cause extensive ecchymoses on the backs of the hands or extreme antemortem subcutaneous emphysema, resulting in gross distension of the tissues of the neck and face. Delays between death and preparation greatly increase the amount of postmortem coagula in the vessels.

All these hypothetical factors demonstrate that the embalmer must prepare each body on the basis of the conditions exhibited by the individual body. The embalming analysis must be based upon the individual body conditions. As the embalming progresses, further analysis must be made as to the extent of arterial distribution, volume of drainage, clearing of discolorations, amount of tissue distension, degree of firming, and any new conditions that arise.

▶ NEED FOR RESISTANCE

Resistance is not a totally negative factor in arterial embalming. If there were total resistance on the arteries, no distribution could take place. If there was total resistance on the veins, drainage would not be possible and distension of the tissues would result. In embalming any body, a certain amount of resistance is found throughout the vascular system. The injection pressure is greatest on the arterial side of the capillaries. This pressure overcomes arterial resistances and helps to distribute the embalming solution. The resistance in the capillaries and on the venous side of the capillaries slows the embalming solution and helps to hold it within the capillaries, giving the solution an opportunity to diffuse (to pass from the capillary to the interstitial spaces). This brings about a more even distribution of the embalming solution, because it reduces short-circuiting of the embalming solution; and helps the tissues to retain more embalming solution, for it allows for better filtration of the embalming solution into the tissues.

If there were no resistance, the embalming solution would pass directly through the capillaries and into the drainage. To illustrate the problems that arise when there is little or no resistance, take the case of a person who dies from a ruptured aneurysm of the abdominal aorta. Some solution may be distributed, but most of the embalming solution will follow the path of least resistance through the torn artery and fill the abdominal cavity.

During injection and drainage of the body, most embalmers create resistance to effect better penetration of the embalming solution and reduction of the loss of solution. Intermittent or alternate methods of drainage are used. The solution is injected against a closed drainage system, which creates the resistance. In addition, some embalmers inject the last one-fourth to one-half gallon of embalming solution with the vein used for drainage tied off. Aspiration can be delayed several hours. This technique helps the capillaries to hold the embalming solution and gives the solution time to diffuse.

Figure 13–5. A. No resistance. **B.** Total or great resistance. **C.** Movable resistance.

Figure 13–5 illustrates the need for some degree of resistance. Figure 13–5A shows little or no resistance. The solution rushes through the tissues, resulting in tissue dehydration. Filtration is reduced, solution can easily short circuit, and the evenness of distribution is reduced.

Figure 13–5B demonstrates total resistance, perhaps a situation in which there is very extensive blood clotting. Once the system is filled, tissue distension becomes a major problem and uniformity of distribution is reduced.

Figure 13–5C represents a movable resistance, such as liquid blood in the venules and veins or the use of intermittent drainage. Blood removal is more complete, distribution is more uniform, and, most important, more embalming solution is retained by the body with a minimum of tissue distension.

▶ PATHS OF LEAST RESISTANCE

When vascular resistances are present in a body, the arterial embalming solution generally distributes to those areas where little or no resistance exists. As a result, certain body areas receive too much solution and others do not receive enough. Three questions must be asked: (1)

Is the embalming solution flowing into the blood vascular system? (2) What body areas are and what areas **are not** receiving embalming solution? (3) Has a body area received **sufficient** arterial solution?

Three indicators can be used to tell if arterial solution is being distributed throughout the vascular system:

1. A decrease in the solution volume in the tank of the embalming machine.

2. When the rate-of-flow valve is opened on the centrifugal injection machine, there should be a drop on the pressure gauge. This drop is the **differential pressure**. Greater the drop, the greater the rate of flow. The differential reading of 10 in Figure 13–6B indicates that the embalming solution is being injected twice as fast as it would if the differential reading were 5 (Fig. 13–6A). The fact that the dial dropped to 5 or 10 from the reading of 15 when the rate-of-flow valve was closed indicates that solution is entering the body. As the solution fills the vascular system, the dial reading may rise. This shows that more resistance is being created by the filling

Rate of Flow Closed
Pressure 15
Rate of Flow Opened
Pressure 10
Differential of 5

A

Rate of Flow Closed
Pressure 15
Rate of Flow Opened
Pressure 5
Differential 10

B

Figure 13–6. Pressure–flow differentials. **A.** Slower rate of flow. **B.** Faster rate of flow.

of the vascular system. To keep the rate of flow at the original speed, the pressure or the rate of flow has to be increased.

Example. The machine is turned on with the rate-of-flow valve (or the stopcock) turned off. (**No** solution is entering the body.) The pressure is set at 20 pounds. The rate-of-flow valve is now opened and the dial drops to 15 pounds. The differential reading is 5. After a gallon and a half is injected, the needle on the dial rises to 18. This indicates the system has been filled and more resistance is being encountered. To establish the original rate of flow, try to open the rate-of-flow valve so the needle drops to 15. If this does not happen, increase the pressure to 23 pounds. If the dial remains at 18 the differential is again 5, and this was the original rate of flow. Differential "pressure" is a good indicator of the resistance in the body. (**It may also indicate that an arterial tube is clogged. The tube should always be checked prior to use to be certain it is clean.**)

3. There should be drainage if the solution is entering the body and making the proper circuit through the arteries, capillaries, and veins.

Once it has been determined that the arterial solution is entering the body at a rate of flow and pressure that do not cause distension, the embalmer must determine which body regions are receiving arterial solution and which areas are not. A group of indicators known as the **signs of arterial solution distribution and diffusion** help to make this determination. Most of these indicators, such as the presence of fluid dye in the tissues, demonstrate only the presence of embalming solution in skin regions.

The dermis, the deep layer of the skin, is very vascular and offers little resistance to the flow of embalming solution, as the solution flows rapidly and easily into the surface areas of the body. The embalmer can easily detect the presence of embalming solution in the skin. Concern must be given to the deep tissues and the muscles. It is very important that solution distribute to these body tissues, which offer more resistance. To achieve this deeper penetration of solution, the drainage can be restricted and massage must be very firm. Penetrating agents in the arterial solution also promote the passage of solution into the deeper tissues.

The skin areas offer little resistance to the flow of solution; also, some localized areas can receive large amounts of arterial solution. These areas are generally in the vicinity of the artery injected. Solutions will establish pathways where they quickly pass through a group of capillaries near the artery being injected. The solution then passes rapidly into the drainage. This frequently happens when injection and drainage occur at the same location. This short-circuiting reduces the total volume of solution available for saturation of other body areas.

Many direct connections exist between arterioles and venules in the microcirculation of the blood. Here, again, is a route that offers little resistance to the flow of fluid. Embalming solution can rapidly pass from the arterial system to the veins without distributing to the tissues. Restricting the drainage can reduce the amount of arterial solution lost in these direct routes.

Once the embalmer determines that solution is entering the body and where it is within the body, it must be determined which body areas have received sufficient solution. **There is no one positive test for determining if a body area has sufficient arterial solution**. If there is any doubt about solution distribution, the embalmer should raise an artery that supplies the area and make a separate injection. Hypodermic or surface embalming may be necessary. With local injections, it may be wise to increase the strength of the injected chemical to help ensure good preservation. It is better to slightly overembalm an area than to risk the chance that an inadequate amount of preservative has reached the area.

▶ INJECTION PRESSURE AND RATE OF FLOW

Injection pressure is needed to overcome intravascular and extravascular resistances. The pressure needed is created by the injection apparatus (embalming machine); it can be as simple as a gravity percolator or as complex as some of the centrifugal pumps (Fig. 13–7).

Injection pressure is the amount of pressure produced by an injection device to overcome initial resistance within the vascular system.

Figure 13–7. Rate-of-flow meter.

Rate of flow is the amount of embalming solution injected in a given period, or the speed at which the embalming solution enters the body. The rate of flow is generally measured in ounces per minute.

Injection pressure and rate of flow are related, but not identical. Of the two, the rate of flow is the factor of most concern to the embalmer. The ideal rate of flow can be as much arterial solution as the body can accept as long as (1) the solution is evenly distributed throughout as much of the body as possible, and (2) there is little or no distension of the tissues. The ideal pressure is the amount needed to establish this rate of flow.

By the use of a centrifugal pump, it is possible to have a set pressure with the rate-of-flow valve closed. It is then possible to open the rate-of-flow valve to a certain point and establish the desired rate of flow. **In the use of a centrifugal pump injector, it is recommended that the pressure be set with the rate-of-flow valve closed**. The pressure set with the rate-of-flow valve closed is called the **potential pressure**. When the rate-of-flow valve is opened the resultant pressure reading is called the **actual pressure**. The difference between actual pressure and potential pressure is the rate of flow or the **differential pressure**.

There are many theories as to the amount of pressure and rate of flow that should be used. Keep in mind that these factors vary in different ways:

1. *From body to body.* Bodies injected shortly after death when rigor is not present can be injected much faster than bodies that have been dead for a long period of time with rigor fully established. A low pressure can be used to establish a high rate of flow in a recently deceased body.

2. *In different body areas.* Fluids always follow the path of least resistance. Areas such as the skin and vascular visceral organs and glandular tissues easily accept fluid. Resistance is greater in tissues where arteriosclerosis is present in the arteries or in body areas where blood has clotted or coagulated in the vessels.

3. *As embalming proceeds.* As embalming proceeds, resistance increases: (a) when vessels are empty and the solution rapidly enters (after the vessels fill, more resistance is created); (b) when the preservative in the solution acts on the capillaries, allowing less solution to flow into the tissue spaces (more solution will then be directed into the drainage); (c) when the tissue spaces become filled to capacity with arterial solution; and (d) when arterial clots move and block small arteries and venous coagula are hardened by the preservative solution, making them more difficult to remove.

It can easily be seen that the needed pressure and rate of flow can vary from body to body and at different times in the embalming process.

After death, and depending on the cause of death, large arteries may collapse because the volume of circulating blood has decreased. Increase in the pressure or rate of flow may well promote filling of the vessels and start good distribution. When this has been accomplished, the amount of pressure can be reduced. The pressure used at that time should be sufficient to maintain a rate of injection that is slightly greater than the amount of drainage. (On the average, the total drainage will equal approximately one-half of the total volume of solution injected.)

FACTORS THAT MUST BE DETERMINED BY THE EMBALMING ANALYSIS

1. Method of mouth closure
2. Vessels for injection and drainage
3. Strength of the embalming solution
4. Volume of the embalming solution
5. Injection pressure
6. Injection rate of flow

Note: These factors will vary by the individual body and can vary in different areas of the same body.

Ideal pressure is then defined as the pressure needed to overcome the vascular resistances of the body to distribute the embalming solution to all body areas.

The **ideal rate of flow** is defined as the rate of flow needed to achieve uniform distribution of the embalming solution without distension of the tissues.

There are two strong schools of thought on injection rate. Some embalmers prefer a low pressure and a rapid rate of flow. (**Note:** Injection machines have been developed on this idea of low pressure but high rates of flow.) Other embalmers feel a high pressure but a very slow rate of flow is ideal. One study has suggested a moderate rate of injection for the **average unautopsied** body as a rate of 1 gallon of solution over a 10- to 15-minute time period. They have recommended a pressure of 2 to 10 pounds to achieve this rate of flow.* Coagula are found in the arteries as well as in the veins. Using slower rates of injection may help to keep these coagula from moving to smaller distal arteries where the vessel would become blocked and diminish or completely stop the distribution of arterial solution from that point.

Not all bodies can be injected within the same set time at the same rate of flow and injection pressures. As soon as distension is evident, injection should be stopped. The injection pressure can be reduced, the rate of flow can be reduced, or sectional embalming can be done. Likewise, if arterial solution is not entering some areas of the body, the rate of flow can be increased, the pressure can be increased, or sectional embalming may be necessary.

These three factors combined: sufficient pressure, adequate rate of flow, and a restricted drainage (e.g., intermittent type) should produce the following results: a removal of blood from the main and collateral circulation; saturation of the soft tissues with the injected arterial solution; a buildup of IVP; restoring of moisture to the tissues, if a proper solution is injected; a retention of a sufficient amount of arterial solution within the tissues to provide sufficient preservation without tissue distension.

For the injected embalming solution to accomplish its function of preservation, it must reach and penetrate **all** tissue areas. Merely flushing the solution through the blood vascular system and out the drain tube does not achieve the intended purpose. It requires time for the preservative solution to diffuse out of the capillaries and penetrate, and saturate tissues.

Clinical studies have demonstrated that as much as 50 to 55% of the embalming solution can be lost through the drainage, regardless if a high or a low pressure is used for embalming. Techniques such as restricted drainage may help to retain more embalming solution within the body.†

The foregoing would be true under "ideal" conditions. The **ideal rate of flow** and the **ideal pressure** will vary from body to body. The "ideal" values of these two factors is the pressure necessary and the rate of flow necessary to overcome the resistances and evenly distribute the preservative solution throughout the entire body, while at the same time the body retains as much of the preservative solution as possible without distension or dehydration of the body tissues.

▶ CENTER OF ARTERIAL SOLUTION DISTRIBUTION

The ascending aorta and the arch of the aorta are the center of arterial distribution. The arch is a continuation of the ascending aorta and gives off three large branches from its superior surface. From right to left, these are the

---

*See Selected Readings: Guidelines Submitted to OSHA from the National Funeral Directors Association *Committee* on Infectious Diseases (Summer 1989).

†Kroshus J, McConnell J. The measurement of formaldehyde retention in the tissues of embalmed bodies. *Director* March/April 1983; 10–12 (See Selected Readings).

brachiocephalic artery, which supplies the right side of the head and right arm; the left common carotid artery, which supplies the left side of the head and face; and the left subclavian artery, which supplies the left arm. The arch continues as the descending thoracic aorta through which the embalming solution is distributed to all other parts of the body.

The arch of the aorta is a continuation of the **ascending aorta**, which begins at the left ventricle. The embalming solution is injected into the arteries of the body because of the valve at the beginning of the ascending aorta called the **aortic semilunar valve**. This valve is situated between the left ventricle of the heart and the ascending aorta. As embalming solution is injected, the ascending aorta fills and causes the aortic semilunar valve to close (Fig. 13–8). Once it is closed, the arteries of the body can begin to fill with the embalming solution. If the valve fails to close, or leaks, the left ventricle fills with embalming solution. If this happens, the cusps of the left atrioventricular (bicuspid) valve close, allowing the arteries of the body to fill.

If, for some reason, both the aortic semilunar valve and the bicuspid valve fail to close (solution injected under too much pressure), arterial solution will flow to the lungs through the pulmonary veins, which could create a purge. The solution might flow into the right ventricle through the pulmonary artery, and from the right ventricle to the right atrium, from which it would exit through the drainage.

▶ SIGNS OF ARTERIAL SOLUTION DISTRIBUTION AND DIFFUSION

There are a number of indicators which can be used to tell if the arterial solution is present in an area. In addition to the presence of the solution, there needs to be a sufficient amount of the solution; and the solution needs to be at a strength where the tissues will be stabilized. Most of the signs of distribution and diffusion are surface indicators.

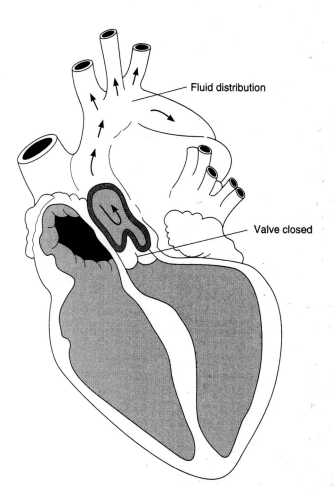

Figure 13–8. Arch of the aorta, ascending aorta, and the closed semilunar valve.

SIGNS OF ARTERIAL SOLUTION DISTRIBUTION

▶ Fluid dye
▶ Distension of superficial blood vessels
▶ Blood drainage
▶ Clearing of intravascular blood discolorations

SIGNS OF ARTERIAL SOLUTION DIFFUSION

▶ Dye in the tissues
▶ Firming of the tissues
▶ Loss of skin elasticity (beginning firming)
▶ Drying of the tissues
▶ Rounding of fingertips, lips, and toes
▶ Mottling of the tissues (bleaching)
▶ Fluorescent dye observed using "black light"

Dyes

The most reliable sign of arterial distribution and diffusion is the presence of an active fluid dye in the tissues of the skin. As active fluid dyes stain the tissues, they act not only as a sign of solution distribution, but also clearly demonstrate solution diffusion. The dyes help to prevent formaldehyde gray and provide an excellent internal cosmetic. They are available in pink and suntan.

Figure 13–9. Livor mortis starting to clear in the legs.

Many arterial fluids contain active dye, but additional dyes may be added separately to the arterial solution.

Fluorescent Dye
A coinjection arterial chemical that contains a fluorescent dye that cannot be seen without the use of a "black light" is available for injection with the preservative arterial solution. When the lights of the embalming room are extinguished and a "black light" is held over the body, areas of the body in which the coinjection fluorescent dye is present glow a bluish white. It is important to remember that fluid dyes indicate only surface profusion of the embalming solution.

Clearing of Intravascular Blood Discoloration
It is most important that the livor mortis be observed prior to the injection of arterial solution (Fig. 13–9). Livor is generally found in the dependent body areas. The fingertips and nailbeds should be carefully inspected. Depending on the cause of death and the position of the body, livor may be present even in the face. If this blood discoloration is pushed on, it should lighten, indicating that the blood present is still in the vascular system. During injection, the livor mortis should be removed. Many times, the "breaking up" of large areas of livor mortis can easily be observed. Massage can help to stimulate the flow of the arterial fluid into an area and the resultant "clearing" of the livor mortis.

Distension of Small Surface Vessels
When fluid reaches certain body areas such as the hands, feet, or temple of the face, small vessels can often be observed by their distension. It should be pointed out that gravitated blood can also cause the veins to rise when hands are placed on the embalming table. Gas in the cavities can cause small vessels to distend. Observe vessel areas (e.g., temples, backs of hands) prior to and during arterial injection to be certain any distension of the vessel(s) is brought about by arterial injection.

Loss of Skin Elasticity
As the solution begins to firm the tissues, skin areas exhibit a loss of elasticity. When the skin is gathered and gently pulled upward, it slowly settles back into proper position.

Firming (Fixation) of the Tissues
Rigor mortis can easily be mistaken for firming of the tissues by the arterial solution. It is most important that in making the preembalming analysis of the body, the **presence of rigor** be noted. Some bodies exhibit little or no firming after good embalming. Most bodies exhibit some degree of firming depending on the amount and strength of embalming chemical injected. Firming, although not a fool-proof sign of embalmed tissue, is nevertheless an indicator that most embalmers rely on as a sign of arterial distribution. Some embalming chemicals are designed to produce tissues that are only slightly firm or that exhibit no firming. Different embalming chemicals can also affect the degree and speed of tissue firming.

Drying of the Tissues
As arterial solution reacts with the tissues to the skin, the surface of the body dries slightly. Areas not reached by the embalming solution often appear shiny and somewhat moist to the touch. This is not a very reliable sign of distribution and should **not** be relied on as an accurate indicator.

Bleaching of the Tissues
Some arterial fluids produce a mottled effect of the skin when the solution is present. This mottled coloring is caused by the bleaching quality of some arterial fluids. Dyes in the embalming solution, however, can mask this bleaching effect. Bleaching is not a reliable sign of arterial fluid distribution.

Blood Drainage
The presence of blood drainage indicates that embalming solution is being distributed to the tissues and organs of the body. It does not, however, indicate what specific areas of the body are receiving arterial solution. As a sign of distribution, it does not account for short-circuiting of arterial solution. Some body areas might be receiving too much and other body areas might not be receiving any solution. Excellent preservation can be accomplished in some bodies with little or no drainage. Restricting the drainage can often help in the distribution of the arterial solution.

Rounding of Fingers, Lips, and Toes

With some embalming formulations, the tips of the fingers, lips and toes slightly plump or "round-out" when reached by the arterial solution. Depending on the method of drainage and the strength of the embalming solution, the reverse can happen; these areas can wrinkle when fluid reaches them as a result of dehydration. It is an unreliable test of distribution.

> Most embalmers use several signs of distribution to ensure that a sufficient amount of arterial solution has reached a body area. The most reliable in the preceding list are dyes, clearing of intravascular blood discolorations, and firming of tissues. Dyes may be difficult to observe in persons with dark swarthy complexions and darker African-Americans. For clearing of livor mortis and the presence of dye observe the palms of the hands, bottoms of the feet and beds of the fingernails. When observation of dye is difficult, look for rounding out of lips, nose, and fingertips. Dyes will also help to prevent darker skinned bodies from taking on a "grayness" to the skin.

▶ OBSERVATIONS PRIOR TO INJECTION

Several signs of arterial solution distribution and diffusion can be confused with several postmortem changes. It is important that the embalmer note these changes prior to injection, so they are not mistaken as a sign of arterial distribution.

Observe for the Presence or Absence of Livor Mortis in All Body Areas Prior to the Start of the Arterial Injection

Examine the nailbeds. Some degree of livor is generally present. In some bodies, however, depending on the position of the hands, the livor may gravitate from the fingers and hands. If this were not noted at the start of the embalming, the **absence** of the livor could be mistaken for clearing of the livor by the arterial injection.

Note the Degree of Rigor Mortis Present in the Tissues

An attempt should always be made to relieve the rigor prior to injection. This is not always possible in areas such as the legs or jaw. Rigor can easily be mistaken for firming of the tissues by the arterial solution.

Observe the Distension of Veins or Small Arteries

Veins on the backs of the hands can be distended before arterial solution is injected as a result of gravitation of the blood. Gases in the cavities or conditions such as ascites or hydrothorax can put pressure on the diaphragm and heart and cause small vessels to fill with blood. This distension or its absence should be noted prior to arterial injection.

Note any Discoloration of the Skin

Skin of refrigerated or frozen bodies or bodies dead from carbon monoxide poisoning may have a pinkish hue. It is important to note this discoloration (resulting from hemolysis) prior to arterial injection. The pink hue from hemolysis can be mistaken for the presence of arterial solution dye in the tissues.

Check for Firmness of the Tissues

Tissues of bodies placed in refrigeration, as many are done today, not only appear to be embalmed (hemolysis) but also feel slightly firm, as does embalmed tissue. This firming is due to the slight firming of subcutaneous fatty tissues as a result of the refrigeration. This condition should be noted with refrigerated bodies, so it is not mistaken for distribution and firming by the arterial solution.

▶ IMPROVING ARTERIAL SOLUTION DISTRIBUTION

Several mechanical (or physical) procedures improve the distribution of the arterial solution. The embalmer may also use a combination of these procedures. **During the injection of the first gallon of arterial solution, firm massage and exercise of the extremities can be very important in establishing good distribution.**

1. Increase the rate of flow of the arterial solution being injected.
2. Increase the pressure of the arterial solution being injected.
3. Inject the arterial solution using pulsation.
4. Restrict the drainage; use intermittent drainage and the alternate method of drainage.
5. Massage the body. Massage should be firm, not merely rubbing the surface of the body. Massage should be directed along the arterial routes (e.g., if solution is not entering the legs, massage should first be concentrated on the inguinal areas).
6. Inject an adequate volume of embalming solution. Often, when large volumes of embalming solution are injected, body areas that received little or no arterial solution during the early part of the embalming receive solution after 2 or 3 gallons have been injected.
7. Relieve extreme abdominal extravascular pressures caused by gas or abdominal edema (ascites). A trocar can be entered from the left

Figure 13–10. The hands are lowered to facilitate circulation.

inguinal area keeping the point under the anterior abdominal wall; the transverse colon can be pierced to relieve gas; if edema is present, some of the fluid can be drained.

8. If distribution of the solution appears to be happening but there is little drainage, selection of another drainage site may improve not only the drainage but also the distribution of the solution.

Treatments for specific areas may also be applied. For **facial tissues**, massage the neck where the common carotid arteries are located. For the **arms**, lower them to the sides or over the embalming table; massage should first be concentrated in the axilla (Fig. 13–10). For the **fingers**, massage the radial and ulnar artery areas of the forearm and then massage the sides of the fingers (where the vessels are located); pressure can also be applied to the nail beds. For the **legs**, massage the inguinal areas over the femoral arteries, flex the legs, and turn the foot inward; this helps to "squeeze" the muscles of the legs.

Massage can attract arterial solution to an area. Areas such as the lips and eyelids often respond well to massage (when it is needed). Squeezing the lips can attract solution into the labial tissues. Care should be taken that swelling or dehydration (wrinkles) does not result.

Body areas that receive no solution or inadequate amounts of arterial solution should be injected separately. If distribution is still a problem, restricting drainage from the limb, massaging, increasing the pressure or rate of flow of injection, or using pulsation with higher pressures may all help to distribute solution into a particular body area.

A preservative solution must enter a body **region or area** before it can reach a **specific location**. Arterial solution cannot enter the fingers if it is not entering the arm.

> When doubt exists as to whether a body area has received any or an adequate amount of arterial solution, raise the artery that supplies the area and separately inject the area.

▶ DIFFUSION OF THE EMBALMING SOLUTION

One of the keys to arterial embalming is arterial fluid **diffusion**. Fluid diffusion can be defined as the passage of some elements of the injected embalming solutions from within the capillary (intravascular) to the tissue spaces (extravascular). The capillary network of the blood vascular system is so vast that a pin can hardly be inserted into the living skin without rupturing a sufficient number of these smallest of blood vessels to cause bleeding (Fig. 13–11).

Capillaries are the smallest blood vessels. They link the smallest arteries (arterioles) to the smallest veins (venules). They are actually the extensions of the inner linings of these larger vessels. Their walls are composed of endothelium, which lines the entire vascular system and is made up of flat, single-layered cells called **squamous epithelium**. These very thin-walled cells form the semipermeable membranes through which substances in the blood must pass to reach the body cells.

In the living body, the blood does not have direct contact with body cells. All of the cells (e.g., muscle cells, nerve cells) are surrounded by a liquid called interstitial (tissue) fluid. Blood nutrients and oxygen must pass through the walls of the capillaries and into the interstitial fluid. These products diffuse through the tissue fluid to reach the body cells. This same movement occurs in embalming. The arterial solution must pass from within the capillary, through the walls of the capillary, into the interstitial fluid, and finally to the body cells. It must then enter the cells of the body and react with the protoplasm protein. The preservative will also act on the proteins in the membranes surrounding the cells.

▶ METHODS OF ARTERIAL SOLUTION DIFFUSION

At the beginning of this chapter, it was stated that "arterial embalming could actually be called capillary embalming." It is at the capillary level that most embalming begins. (Additionally, the lining of the blood vascular

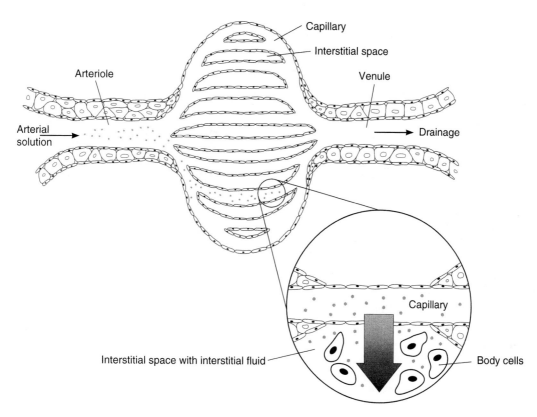

Figure 13–11. Diffusion of the embalming solution.

system is disinfected and preserved as the embalming solution passes through the vessels.) From the capillaries, embalming solution moves to the interstitial fluid that surrounds each cell. The solution makes contact with proteins in the interstitial fluid, proteins in the cell membranes, and proteins in the cytoplasm of the cell.

In the living cell, **active transport,** is one method by which nutrients pass into the cell, through the cell membrane, and wastes are removed from the cell. This method of transport depends upon energy produced by the living cell. This system of transport does not function in the dead human body.

Physical (or passive) transport mechanisms are responsible for the movement of embalming solution from within the capillaries to the tissue spaces. The energy needed to move the solution through the walls of the capillary originates from a nonliving mechanism. Passive mechanisms can move materials through dead cell membranes (capillaries). The major passive (or physical) transport processes for the movement of embalming solutions are pressure filtration, osmosis, and dialysis.

Pressure Filtration

Pressure filtration caused by IVP is one of the most important passive transport systems for the passage of embalming solution from the capillary to tissue fluid. In

this process, both the solute and solvent portions of the embalming solution pass into the interstitial fluid. Penetrating agents (wetting agents, surface tension reducers, or surfactants) in the concentrated embalming fluid lower its surface tension. The reduction of surface tension makes the embalming solution "wetter," and it can more easily pass through the minute pores and the cell membranes of the capillaries.

IVP places enough pressure on the embalming solution to force it through the pores between the cells of the capillary walls. This is similar to the effect of a lawn soaker hose. Some of the solution enters the tissue spaces to mix with the interstitial fluid. The embalming solution that remains in the capillary pushes on to remove the blood and exits as part of the drainage.

In the agonal period, respiration can become difficult and shallow. Sufficient oxygen is not delivered to the blood. As a defense mechanism, the pores between the cells of the capillaries expand in an attempt to get more oxygen. It is theorized that at death the capillaries are permeable, for their pores are still expanded. As a result, embalming solution can easily be filtered (or pushed) through these pores (caused by IVP). In some bodies, the capillaries may have begun to decompose. The injected solution can now easily flow through the broken capillaries into the tissue spaces.

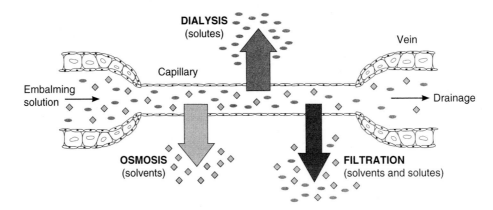

Figure 13–12. Summary of solution diffusion: pressure filtration, osmosis, and dialysis.

When this happens, the body tissues easily distend. This is seen in bodies that have been dead for long periods. These bodies easily swell and there is little or no drainage.

Likewise, when the limbs are exercised to break up rigor mortis, many capillaries may be torn. The muscle tissues can rapidly swell on injection and, again, drainage is minimal. In bodies in which decomposition is evident or rigor is present, stronger solutions should be used so preservation can be achieved with a minimal amount of solution. This keeps swelling at a minimum. Pressure filtration is, no doubt, one of the primary mechanisms by which embalming solution comes into contact with the interstitial spaces and fluids (Fig. 13–12).

Osmosis

Osmosis is a passive transport mechanism involved with liquid (or solvent) movement. It involves the passage of a solvent (such as water) through a semipermeable membrane from a dilute to a concentrated solution. Embalming solutions are more dilute (or less dense) than the interstitial fluids that surround the body cells. The interstitial fluids and the embalming solution are separated by the walls of the capillaries, which are semipermeable. Some of the chemical compounds found in the interstitial fluid cannot move through the capillary walls into the blood vascular system. The more dilute solution, in this case the embalming solution, is described as hypotonic, meaning it is more dilute or less dense than the interstitial fluid. For example, in mixing a 1-gallon solution of embalming solution, assume that 8 ounces of concentrated fluid is added to 120 ounces of water; for every ounce of embalming fluid, 15 ounces of water is used as a dilutant.

Some of the hypotonic embalming solution will easily pass through the walls and minute pores of the capillary to enter the interstitial spaces and mix with the interstitial fluid. It will then travel through the interstitial fluid and come into contact with the cells. Again, the

process of osmosis will occur. This time the mixture of interstitial fluid and embalming solution will pass through the cell membrane and the preservatives will enter the cytoplasm of the cell. All along this route, contact of the preservative solution is made with proteins whether they are in the walls of the capillaries, in the interstitial fluid, in the membranes of the cells, or in the cytoplasm of the cell. New substances are being produced from the reaction between the protein and the preservative. In this manner, the process of preservation occurs.

When the directions are not followed and embalming solutions are made too weak (too dilute), these solutions will rapidly pass through the capillaries into the tissue fluids. Not only can swelling occur, but inadequate preservation also results. These tissues become "waterlogged" with the weak solution, and the process of decomposition can actually be accelerated. A reverse condition can be created by mixing solutions that are too concentrated. These concentrated solutions can cause the moisture in the interstitial fluid to move into the capillaries, bringing about dehydration. In conditions such as edema, a more concentrated (or dense) embalming solution can be used.

When the embalmer dilutes the concentrated arterial fluid with water, this dilution is called **primary dilution**. In addition to water, coinjection fluid may also be used as a diluent in addition to such chemicals as humectant and water softener. These solutions are described as being hypotonic for embalming the average body under normal moisture conditions. They allow some moisture to be added to the tissues and assist in retaining tissue moisture.

Within the tissue spaces, where the interstitial fluid is present, dilution of the arterial fluid continues. This dilution of the embalming solution that occurs in the tissues of the body is called the **secondary dilution**. The moisture found in the tissues dilutes the fluid. In addition, the fluid that remains in the capillaries and exits with the drainage is also diluted by the liquid portion of the blood. The secondary dilution of the fluid can be very great in bodies with skeletal edema.

In making an embalming analysis, the embalmer must evaluate the moisture conditions of the body. Are the tissues dehydrated? Are the tissues moist as a result of edema? Or are the tissues normal? On the basis of these observations, the primary dilution is prepared. On the labels of embalming fluid, most chemical manufacturers indicate the number of ounces of concentrated fluid to use per gallon based on the moisture content of the body.

Dialysis

The third method of passive transport by which the embalming solution passes from the capillaries to the cells is dialysis. Dialysis is the diffusion of the dissolved crystalloid solutes of a solution through a semipermeable membrane. Interstitial fluid, cytoplasm of the body cells, and embalming solutions are composed primarily of the solvent water. Dissolved in these solutions are very small solutes called **crystalloids** and very large solutes called **colloids**.

The embalming solution in the capillary is separated from the interstitial fluid by the semipermeable membrane of the capillary wall. The cytoplasm within the cell is separated from the interstitial fluid by the semipermeable **cell membrane**. In dialysis, small crystalloids can diffuse through the semipermeable membranes, but large colloids in the solutions cannot. Water is the primary solvent in embalming solutions; alcohols and glycerine are other examples. The solutes in embalming fluids are various crystalloids such as salts, preservatives, and germicides and colloids (humectants). Interstitial fluid comprises the solvent water and various crystalloid salts and colloids (proteins, enzymes, etc.). Crystalloids in the embalming solution can diffuse through the capillary semipermeable membrane into the interstitial fluid. These preservatives, germicides, dyes, and so on then spread through the interstitial fluid and again pass through the cell membrane to enter the cytoplasm of the cell.

To repeat, dialysis is the diffusion of crystalloids across a semipermeable membrane that is impermeable to colloids. It is the process of separating crystalloids (smaller particles) from colloids (larger particles) by the difference in their rates of diffusion through a semipermeable membrane.

► MOVEMENT OF EMBALMING SOLUTIONS FROM OUTSIDE THE CAPILLARIES TO INSIDE THE CELLS

Fluid diffusion was defined as the movement of embalming solution from within the capillary (intravascular) to the interstitial fluid (extravascular). Embalming solution does not stop moving once it leaves the capillary and enters the interstitial space to mix with the interstitial fluid. The interstitial fluid (intercellular or tissue fluid) is a viscous solution similar to the cytoplasm found inside the cells of the body. It contains inorganic chemicals, proteins, carbohydrates, and lipids dissolved in water. This fluid surrounds the cells of the body and is the connection between the blood vascular system (capillaries) and the body cells. Embalming solution must pass from the capillaries into the interstitial fluid, spread through the interstitial fluid, and finally enter the cells of the body (Fig. 13–13). Once inside the body cells, the embalming solution again diffuses to come into contact with all portions of the cell.

The concentrated embalming elements are spread through the interstitial fluid by the passive transport systems called **diffusion** and **filtration gravitation**. Passage of embalming solution into the body cells is brought about by the passive transport systems of **adsorption, osmosis**, and **dialysis**.

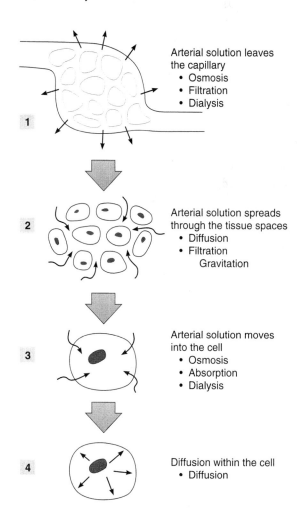

1. Arterial solution leaves the capillary
   • Osmosis
   • Filtration
   • Dialysis

2. Arterial solution spreads through the tissue spaces
   • Diffusion
   • Filtration Gravitation

3. Arterial solution moves into the cell
   • Osmosis
   • Absorption
   • Dialysis

4. Diffusion within the cell
   • Diffusion

Figure 13–13. Movement of embalming solution from outside the capillaries to inside the cells.

Diffusion

Diffusion means scattering or spreading. Small particles such as molecules are always moving in all directions. For example, place a drop of fluid dye into a gallon of water and let the solution of dye and water set without stirring. In a short period, the entire gallon of water is slightly and evenly colored by the dye. The concentrated drop of dye has spread through the water. Diffusion occurs from a region of high concentration to a region of lower concentration. In a similar manner, once the embalming solution passes into the interstitial fluid, it spreads (or diffuses) through the interstitial fluid to come into contact with the cells of the body. By the processes of dialysis, adsorption, and osmosis, it passes into the cell and, once in the cell, spreads through the cytoplasm by diffusion.

Adsorption

The cytoplasm of the body cells is composed of a continuous aqueous solution (cytosol) with all the organelles (except the nucleus) suspended in it. The fluid inside the cells of the body is called a **colloidal dispersion**. The large colloid molecules, because of their large surface area, tend to **adsorb** molecules. Colloidal dispersions in cells adsorb molecules from the surrounding interstitial tissue fluids. In this manner, some of the embalming solution present in the interstitial fluid is adsorbed into the body cells.

Gravity Filtration

Gravity filtration is the extravascular settling of embalming solution by gravitational force into the dependent areas of the body. This passive transport system helps to move embalming solution throughout the interstitial fluid. In the embalmed body, gravity filtration is responsible for the movement of embalming solution into the dependent tissues—lower back, buttocks, and backs of arms, legs, and shoulders. It may be of some value in moving embalming solution into those areas that are in contact with the embalming table. This slow movement continues for some time after the injection of solution. This is **not** a gravitation of fluids through the vascular system. It is extravascular movement of the solution through the interstitial fluid.

Summary

Passive transport systems require some amount of time to work. Pressurized injection, the penetrating agents found in the arterial fluids, and pressure filtration constitute the primary transport system for the movement of arterial solution from the capillaries to the tissue spaces. Osmosis, dialysis, gravitation filtration, and diffusion all take longer. Many embalmers prefer a delay between injection and cavity aspiration. In addition to a delay, many embalmers prefer to inject the last half-gallon of arterial solution with the drainage closed. This method allows a maximum filtration pressure to be established. The delay after injection can be 1 or 2 hours. Some embalmers feel that several hours are needed. There should be some interval between injection and aspiration, even if it is only the time in which incisions are sewn and the body washed and dried. This interval gives the solutions an opportunity to fully penetrate the capillaries.

▶ CONCEPTS FOR STUDY AND DISCUSSION

1. Define the following terms, which pertain to the arterial solution moving from the machine to the cells of the body:
   Absorption
   Adsorption
   Arterial fluid
   Arterial solution
   Arterial solution diffusion
   Arterial solution distribution
   Capillary
   Center of arterial solution distribution
   Crystalloid
   Dialysis
   Diffusion
   Gravity filtration
   Hypertonic solution
   Hypotonic solution
   Interstitial fluid
   Osmosis
   Passive transport system
   Pressure filtration
   Primary dilution
   Retained embalming solution
   Secondary dilution
   Semipermeable membrane
   Solute
   Solvent
2. Discuss the movement of arterial solution from the machine to an individual body cell.
3. Why would the ascending aorta and the arch of the aorta be considered the "center of arterial solution distribution"?
4. Why is some resistance valuable to drainage?
5. Discuss fluid dilutions for the normal (moisture content) body; emaciated and dehydrated body; body with skeletal edema; and body with ascites and/or hydrothorax but no skeletal edema.
6. Discuss several false signs of arterial solution distribution to a body area.

▶ BIBLIOGRAPHY

Anthony CP. *Textbook of Anatomy and Physiology.* St. Louis, MO: CV Mosby, 1979:40–53.

Arnow LE. *Introduction to Physiological and Pathological Chemistry.* St. Louis, MO: CV Mosby; 1976:66–73.

Dhonau CO. *The ABCs of Pressure and Distribution, File 86.* Cincinnati, OH: Cincinnati College of Embalming.

Dhonau CO. *Manual of Case Analysis,* 2nd ed. Cincinnati, OH: Embalming Book Co., 1928.

Frederick JF. The mathematics of embalming chemistry, Parts I and II. *The Dodge Magazine* October–November 1968.

Johnson EC. A study of arterial pressure during embalming. In *Champion Expanding Encyclopedia.* Springfield, OH: Champion Chemical Co., 1981:2081–2084.

Kroshus J, McConnell J, Bardole J. The measurement of formaldehyde retention in the tissues of embalmed bodies. *Director* March/April 1983:10–12.

Zweifach BW. The microcirculation of the blood. *Scientific American* January 1959.

CHAPTER 14

CAVITY EMBALMING

CHAPTER OBJECTIVES

▶ Purposes for cavity embalming
▶ Body cavities and contents
▶ Trocar guides
▶ Sequences: aspiration–injection–reaspiration

The oldest methods of embalming, dating back to the Egyptians, included treatment of the viscera. Until the "modern era" of embalming, most embalming techniques involved not only removal of the viscera (evisceration) from the thoracic and abdominal cavities, but also removal of the brain from the cranial cavity. Embalmers using these early embalming processes recognized the difficulty in preserving the body if some method of visceral treatment was not practiced. With the introduction and use of the "trocar" toward the end of the nineteenth century, embalmers began to move away from a direct incision approach to preserve and sanitize the contents of the body cavities.*

There is a need to continue the preservation and sanitation process after arterial embalming.

1. Purulent materials, blood, and edematous fluids within the body cavities, along with possibly unembalmed tissues, continue to decompose and remain an excellent medium for bacterial growth. Untreated microbes can become a source of gases and odor and can create a possible purge from an external body orifice.
2. The **contents** of the hollow visceral organs (stomach, intestines, urinary bladder) are not reached by the arterial solution.

3. There is no way of knowing if the walls and tissues of the visceral organs have received the arterial solution.

The aspiration procedure and subsequent perfusion with cavity fluid are designed to reach the substances and microbes found in the spaces within the thoracic, abdominopelvic, and sometimes cranial cavities. In addition to these substances, those materials found within the hollow viscera and portions of the visceral organs themselves that are not reached by arterial injection are treated in the process of cavity embalming.

Cavity embalming—**not a visible procedure**—is normally a two-step process: aspiration of the cavities and their contents followed by the injection of a strong preservative/disinfectant chemical. This process takes place **after** the arterial embalming. Often, depending on the condition of the body, the process involves subsequent steps of reaspiration and reinjection of the cavities.

There may be occasions when cavity treatment is **not** employed in preparation of the body, for example, when the body is bequeathed to a medical school (where the school permits vascular preparation of the body for viewing by the family and public), and when a hospital allows the body to be arterially embalmed prior to a postmortem examination (autopsy).

There are also situations in which arterial embalming is not possible. Cavity embalming, along with surface and hypodermic embalming, would be the principal means of preserving and sanitizing the remains. These

---

*Inventor of trocar: Samuel Rogers, U.S. Patent No. 207551, New York City, August 27, 1878.

cases include badly decomposed and badly burned bodies.

▶ CHRONOLOGY OF CAVITY TREATMENT

1. Arterial embalming
    a. Limited treatment of the abdominal cavity prior to or during arterial injection if the abdominal wall is very tense
        (1) Drainage of edema from the abdominal cavity if ascites exists
        (2) Removal of gases if the abdomen is tightly distended with gas
    b. Limited aspiration of the thorax if subcutaneous emphysema is present
2. Aspiration of the cavities
    a. Time of treatment
        (1) Immediately after arterial injection
        (2) Several hours after arterial injection
    b. Suggested order of aspiration
        (1) Thoracic cavity and its contents
        (2) Abdominal cavity and its contents
        (3) Pelvic cavity and its contents
3. Injection of cavity chemicals into the body cavities
4. Closure of the trocar point of entry
5. Washing and drying of the body
6. Possible reaspiration
7. Possible reinjection

Not all microorganisms die with the host. Many survive and multiply for a period of time after somatic and cellular death. During the agonal period and then the postmortem period following somatic death, microbes from the hollow intestinal organs enter the bloodstream and lymph channels where they translocate to the skeletal tissues and interstitial fluids. In tissues not reached by arterial treatments, the decomposition cycle can occur and produce undesired effects. Cavity treatment destroys microbes and inactivates the media on which these microbes can grow and multiply.

Cavity embalming treats: (1) the **contents** of the hollow viscera (Table 14–1); (2) the **walls** of the visceral organs not embalmed by arterial injection; (3) and the **contents** of the spaces between the visceral organs and the walls of the cavities.

The contents of the **hollow** portions of the viscera are not perfused during arterial injection. Materials within these spaces continue to decompose if untreated, and the resulting products of decomposition may cause **odors, gas formation, and possibly purge.** The gases may move into the skeletal tissues and cause distension of viewable areas such as the face and hands.

It is impossible to determine which visceral organs did or did not receive arterial solution. The embalmer

TABLE 14–1. CONTENTS OF THE HOLLOW VISCERA THAT MUST BE TREATED

Organ	Contents to Be Aspirated or Treated
Lungs, trachea, bronchi	Blood, edema, purulent material, gases
Stomach	Hydrochloric acid, undigested food, blood, gases
Small intestine	Gases, undigested foods, partially digested foods, blood
Large intestine	Gases, fecal material, blood
Urinary bladder	Urine, pustular material, blood
Gallbladder	Bile
Pelvis of the kidney	Urine, pustular material, blood
Heart	Blood
Inferior vena cava, portal veins	Blood

cannot look at these organs for signs of arterial distribution, so cavity embalming serves to **ensure** that the walls and parenchyma of the hollow viscera and the stroma and parenchyma of the solid organs are embalmed.

The solid organs treated by cavity embalming are the pancreas, spleen, kidneys, liver, and lungs. If cranial cavity treatment is performed, the solid brain and brain stem will also undergo aspiration and injection of a preservative solution.

Undigested or partially digested foodstuffs within the stomach and small intestines, as well as the gases and liquids resulting from the breakdown of these materials, are removed by the aspiration process. Those not removed are treated by the injection of cavity fluid (Table 14–2). If these materials are not removed or treated, gases could form, placing sufficient pressure on the stomach and diaphragm to create purge from the oral or nasal cavities.

Note: The liquids in these cavities not only **decompose.** Some of these liquids also serve as **media for bacteria** and as a **diluent** for cavity chemicals.

Purge from the **mouth** originates from either the contents of the **lungs**, the contents of the **stomach**, or the throat area (esophageal veins that hemorrhage) (Table 14–3).

TABLE 14–2. CAVITY CONTENTS THAT MUST BE TREATED

Cavity	Material to Be Treated
Thoracic	Blood, edema, purulent material, gases
Pericardial	Blood, edema
Abdominal	Blood, edema, purulent material, gases
Pelvic	Blood, edema, purulent material, gases
Cranial	Blood, edema, gases

TABLE 14–3. DESCRIPTION OF PURGE

Source	Orifice	Description
Stomach	Nose/mouth	Liquids, semisolids, dark brown "coffee ground" appearance; odor; acid pH
Lungs	Nose/mouth	Frothy; any blood present is red in color, little odor
Brain	Nose/ear/eyelids	Gases can move into tissues of the eye, fractures can cause blood to purge from the ears, creamy white semisolid brain matter may exit through a fracture or the nasal passage

Purge from the **nose** can also originate from the lungs, stomach, or throat. If fecal material is not removed or treated by cavity chemicals, it can cause sufficient gases to form within the abdomen to cause a lung purge (by pressure on the diaphragm) or stomach purge. In addition, purge from the **anal orifice** is quite possible. Rectal hemorrhage can be a source of bloody purge from the anal orifice.

Cranial purge is very rare. Gases within the cranial cavity can spread into the facial tissues through the various foramina that lead from the cranial cavity to the soft facial tissues. Generally, a liquid or semisolid purge from the cranial cavity is the result of a fracture of the temporal bone. The point of exit of the purge is the ear. If gas, in the cranial cavity, is of sufficient pressure, the eyes and eyelids can become distended.

In some diseases, infections of the brain or meninges may lead to formation of gases or edema in the cranial cavity. Hemorrhages from a stroke can also cause blood and edema to accumulate in the cranial cavity. In bodies in which decomposition is advanced, sufficient pressure may be present to cause a purge from the cranial cavity.

Foramina in the area of the **eye**, which serve as pathways for gas that affects the eye and surrounding tissues, include the optic foramen, superior orbital fissure, inferior orbital fissure, infraorbital foramen, supraorbital foramen, anterior ethmoidal foramen, and posterior ethmoidal foramen.

In certain preparations, such as after recent cranial surgery (gunshot or trauma to the head) or advanced decomposition, aspiration and injection of a few ounces of cavity fluid into the cranial cavity may prevent the buildup of gas in the cranial cavity. The point at which the aspirating device is introduced into the cranium is discussed later in this chapter.

It is not necessary to aspirate the brain of an adult who suffered from hydrocephalus. The bones at this time in life are ossified and the condition should present little problem in embalming.

Some embalmers routinely aspirate and inject the cranial cavity on every body. There is a very heavy arterial supply to the brain through both the internal carotid arteries and the vertebral arteries. In the majority of embalmings, these routes should supply sufficient arterial solution to the brain and even to the cerebrospinal fluid.

In preparation of the unautopsied stillborn child or infant, the embalmer should consider the need for cranial treatment. The stillborn or infant brain can decompose very rapidly. Carefully evaluate the presence of gases in the tissues around the eyes and give consideration to the time between death and preparation. It may be most advantageous in these preparations to at least inject some cavity fluid into the cranial cavity with a large hypodermic needle.

▶ INSTRUMENTATION AND EQUIPMENT REQUIRED

A pointed trocar, tubing, a device to create a suction or vacuum, are the items needed to accomplish the process of aspiration. After aspiration, a gravity cavity injector or other injection device is connected with tubing to the trocar to inject the disinfectant/preservative chemicals. To close the opening in the body wall, a needle and ligature or trocar button and inserter are used. A disinfection tray is needed for cleaning and disinfecting the trocar (see Chapter 4).

Instruments Used to Create a Vacuum

Hydroaspirator. The hydroaspirator is installed on a cold water line, preferably over a flush sink; when the water is turned on, a vacuum is created. Proper operation of the equipment depends on the water pressure of the water line. A vacuum breaker is normally a part of the hydroaspirator and protects against a backflow into the water line. Local ordinance directives for proper installation of the aspirator may require other vacuum breakers at different heights above the water level of the receptacle into which the aspirant flows.

A few ounces of material such as blood passing through the water of the hydroaspirator can give the appearance of a very large quantity of material. Although it is helpful to observe the material passing through the hydroaspirator, it is more important to observe the material being withdrawn from the body at a position near the trocar. A piece of plastic or glass tubing can be inserted into a portion of the tubing used for aspiration. Clear tubing can be used so the aspirated material can be observed. Some trocars have a glass portion in the handle that allows the material flowing through the trocar to be observed.

Hydroaspirators can become clogged with small pieces of solid or semisolid material. There is a distinct sound change when this happens. Water then **reverses** and flows into the tubing, trocar, and body cavity. The hydroaspirator should be shut off immediately and the hose removed from the trocar. An attempt should be made to "flush" the material from the hydroaspirator. If this is unsuccessful, the hydroaspirator may be disassembled and the material removed from the inside of the device.

Electric Aspirator. An electric aspirator contains an electric motor with an encased impeller on the shaft. The impeller creates the suction. A small-diameter water line may be attached to the encasement for lubrication of the impeller. The electric aspirator is perhaps more expensive and requires more maintenance than the hydroaspirator. The electric aspirator may be the preferred device in funeral homes where there is low water pressure. An attachment to the electric aspirator allows the embalmer to add a disinfectant solution to the materials being aspirated.

Hand Pump (Historical). A dual-purpose piece of equipment, the hand pump, permits removal of air or forces air into an enclosed airtight container. Drawing the air out of the container creates suction and is used for aspiration. In the past, a glass jar with a "gooseneck" and the hand pump were commonly used. The "gooseneck" is the rubber stopper that makes the jar airtight. The stopper has two openings for two hose attachments. One hose allows air movement out of the jar, and the second hose leads to a trocar. This method is little used today.

Air Pressure Machine (Historical). The air pressure machine operates on the same principle as the hand pump. The machine has two outlets. One creates a vacuum; the other can be used to force air into a jar. Again, a "gooseneck" is employed. The concentrated aspirated material is collected in the jar. Care should be taken to use jars specially made for aspiration, as there is a danger of glass implosion. The contents of the jar can be poured into the sewer line, or, if the embalmer desires to disinfect the contents, they can be treated in the jar prior to being released into the sewer system.

Instruments Used in Aspiration

Trocar. A trocar is a long hollow needle (metal tube) with a removable sharp point that is available in varying lengths and bores. Whetstones or other sharpening devices can be used to keep the points honed, or the point can be replaced. The trocar is used to pierce the wall of the abdomen and the walls of the internal organs in the thoracic and abdominal cavities. The trocar, attached to the suction device, is used to withdraw the contents of the organs and residual fluid that has pooled in the cavities.

The trocar is also used to introduce the disinfectant/preservative solution over and into the internal organs.

An 18-inch-long, $5/16$-inch-bore trocar is used in aspiration of the abdominal and thoracic cavities of the adult body. Opening the cavities after the trocar has been used would reveal all the organs in their **proper positions**. The embalmer would have to examine the viscera for the **pierce marks** made by the trocar, as these punctures close.

The **infant trocar** is approximately 12 inches in length and about $1/4$ inch in diameter. It is used in cavity treatment of infants and children. Many embalmers also use it for hypodermic injection of preservative chemicals into areas of the limbs or trunk not reached by arterial embalming.

Complete disinfection/sterilization of the trocar is important. Microorganisms have been carelessly transferred from one body to another via the trocar. Trays of sufficient size and length for the trocar are needed whether the chemical or autoclave method of sterilization is used. For example, after its use in a body with true tissue gas, an improperly cleaned trocar can harbor the spore-forming microorganism **Clostridium perfringens**.

Tubing. Clear plastic or rubber tubing 6 to 8 feet in length and $3/8$ to $1/2$ inch in diameter is needed to connect the trocar to aspiration devices. The wall of the tubing must be thick enough to preclude collapse as the suction is generated. Clear or semi-clear tubing permits visual examination of the material being removed and aids in determining which organ or space is being aspirated.

Nasal Tube Aspirator. A 10-inch, 90-degree curved metal tube with a $3/16$-inch bore, the nasal tube aspirator is designed for aspiration of the nasal/oral cavity. It is placed through the nasal opening or between the lips. The primary problem in the use of this instrument is the diameter of its opening. Even a small semisolid particle can easily clog this instrument.

Autopsy Aspirator. The autopsy aspirator is an 8- to 10-inch-long, $3/8$-inch-bore metal tube. A collector is attached to one end and a hose to the other. This equipment is used for aspiration of the cavities of the autopsied body, and has a number of openings to prevent clogging of the instrument. The aspirator can be set to operate while the body is being embalmed. The non-clogging feature is designed to free the embalmer's hands so constant attention is not needed.

▶ VISCERAL ANATOMY

The embalmer should constantly be aware of the internal structures he or she is attempting to preserve. Although comprehensive treatment of the internal anatomy is beyond the scope of this textbook, it is appropriate to include here limited descriptions of internal soft tissue structures to provide the embalmer with a quick reference source should he or she encounter a simple anatomical question or problem.

Cranium

The interior of the cranial vault comprises anterior, middle, and posterior cranial fossae in which portions of the brain and brainstem are located. The frontal lobes of the cerebrum rest on that portion of the skull floor created by the anterior cranial fossa. The temporal lobes, hypothalamus, and midbrain cover the floor of the middle fossa. The large, posterior fossa houses the medulla, pons, and entire cerebellum.

Thorax

Although the lungs are properly described as contents of the thorax, their apices extend above the level of the first rib into the neck. The right lung comprises three lobes and the left lung two lobes, although this is subject to some variation. The left lung is further characterized by the presence of a cardiac notch or impression to accommodate the ventricles of the heart. Medially, both lung surfaces relate to the contents of the mediastinum and contain the hilar structures, that is, the pulmonary vessels and the main-stem bronchi. Inferiorly, the lungs are related to the diaphragmatic pleura and the diaphragm.

The heart is positioned retrosternally in the middle mediastinum and extends from the second intercostal space inferiorly to the fifth. The lateral cardiac margins extend beyond the lateral margins of the body of the sternum. The great vessels arise from the base of the heart at the level of the second intercostal space, behind the upper portion of the body and the manubrium of the sternum.

Abdomen

The majority of abdominal viscera consist of some part of the digestive apparatus, which is mainly tubular with some modifications and specializations of this basic structure in various locations. As the straight-tubed esophagus passes through the diaphragm and enters the abdomen, it quickly gives rise to the stomach. The remainder of the alimentary or digestive tube, in order, consists of the duodenum, jejunum, ileum (small intestine), cecum, ascending colon, transverse colon, descending colon, sigmoid colon, rectum (large intestine), and anus. Organs that facilitate digestion include the gallbladder, liver, and pancreas.

A rather peripatetic organ, the stomach is one whose location varies with changes in the position and orientation of the body. It is, therefore, difficult to describe specific relationships of the stomach. Similarly, the shape of this organ is dependent on the amount and type of food-stuffs contained therein as well as the extent to which the digestive process has progressed. A "typical" stomach possesses greater and lesser curvatures, a fundic region that extends above the level at which the esophagus enters, and a pyloric region at the junction of the stomach and the duodenum.

The small intestine is divided into three segments—continuing from the stomach, the C-shaped **duodenum** is the first part of the small intestine, about 10 inches in length and is the shortest part of the small intestine. It merges to become the second part of the small intestine, the **jejunum**, approximately 8 feet in length; the jejunum merges into the third portion of the small intestine called the **ileum** and measures approximately 12 feet in length and terminates at the cecum of the large intestine. These organs occupy much of the abdomen and both are suspended by a fan-shaped mesentery from the posterior body wall.

The large intestine can be distinguished grossly from the small bowel by: (1) its larger diameter; (2) the presence of three longitudinal strips of muscle, the taenia coli, (3) sacculations or pouches called haustra; (4) and fatty appendages called epiploic appendices, none of which is found on the small intestine.

A diverticulum, the **cecum**, marks the beginning of the large intestine and extends inferiorly beyond the level at which the ileum joins the ascending colon. The cecum is situated in the right iliac and hypogastric regions. Opening from it is the vermiform appendix. Extending superiorly from the cecum is the retroperitoneal **ascending colon**, which continues to the right colic or hepatic flexure, inferior to the liver in the right lumbar region. Here, the colon turns sharply to the left in the umbilical region, as the **transverse colon**. This is a freely movable portion of the large bowel, suspended by the transverse mesocolon from the posterior body wall and extending to the left colic or splenic flexure in the left hypochondriac and lumbar regions. Here, the colon again becomes retroperitoneal and descends to the level of the iliac crest as the **descending colon**. In the left iliac region, the descending colon forms the **sigmoid colon** which is once again freely movable, being suspended by the sigmoid mesocolon. Anterior to the third sacral vertebra, the sigmoid colon gives way to the **rectum**.

The largest glandular organ in the body is the liver, which develops as an outgrowth of the digestive tract and retains a functional and anatomical relationship with it. It rests primarily in the right hypochondriac and epigastric regions. The upper surface of the liver is higher on the right than on the left. The upper surface rests against the inferior surface of the diaphragm from which it is suspended by the coronary ligaments. On the inferior surface of the liver is the gallbladder, whose cystic duct is joined by the common hepatic duct from the liver to form the common bile duct that empties the duodenum.

The gallbladder and the lower portion of the right lobe of the liver lie anterior to the right hepatic flexure in the right lumbar region.

The pancreas lies cradled in the C-shaped duodenum and extends across the midline from the right to the left at about the level of the second lumbar vertebra. The major subdivisions of the pancreas include the head, neck, body, and tail. The main duct of the pancreas typically joins the common bile duct immediately as they both enter the duodenum.

The remaining unpaired organ in the abdomen is the spleen, which is located in the left hypochondriac region. Lying in the umbilical left and right lumbar regions are the usually paired kidneys. These lie along the posterior body wall, with the right slightly lower than the left because of encroachment by the large right lobe of the liver. Both kidneys lie at the level of the umbilicus and both are retroperitoneal. In its own separate capsule at the superior pole of each kidney is a suprarenal gland.

Pelvis

Internal pelvic viscera in the male include the prostate gland, seminal vesicles, urinary bladder, and rectum. The last structure was already discussed. The prostate gland is situated at the base of the urinary bladder, surrounding the prostatic or initial portion of the male urethra.

The urinary bladder is situated behind the pubic symphysis in the midline and its shape and size are dependent on the volume of urine contained within it. This muscular, distensible structure receives urine from the kidneys via the paired ureters, which open posterolaterally into the bladder.

In the female, the urinary bladder occupies a position similar to that in the male but is separated from the rectum by the intervening uterus and its adnexa. In addition to the uterus and bladder, other visceral structures in the female pelvis include the ovaries, uterine tubes, and vagina. The muscular unpaired uterus is positioned in the midline and is supported by a double layer of peritoneum called broad ligament. The uterus is divided into several parts including the fundus, body, and cervix.

Through the cervix, the cavity of the uterus communicates with the vagina, which is a distensible tube, flattened anteroposteriorly. The uterine tubes communicate with the opening directly into the abdominal cavity and the uterine cavity. The abdominal cavity, therefore, opens to the external environment via the uterine tubes, the cavity of the uterus, the cavity of the cervix, and the vagina. The paired ovaries are located on the posterior aspect of the broad ligament on either side of the uterus. The uterus, tubes, and ovaries are supported by an elaborate system of "ligaments" derived from reflections of the peritoneum.

▶ TOPOGRAPHICAL DIVISIONS OF THE ABDOMEN

The following topographical systems of dividing the abdomen serve to give the practitioner an approximate location of the various abdominal organs. The embalmer should have a thorough knowledge of the location of the visceral organs. This understanding is important: (1) in the process of cavity embalming; (2) when one or more organs have been removed for transplant; (3) and when partial autopsies have been performed. In addition, the embalmer needs to have a good understanding of the relationship of the vascular system to the visceral organs.

Contents of the Abdomen: Nine-Region Method

To establish the nine abdominal regions (Table 14–4), extend two **vertical** lines upward from a point midway

TABLE 14–4. THE NINE ABDOMINAL REGIONS

Right Hypochondriac	Epigastric	Left Hypochondriac
Part of the liver Part of right kidney Greater omentum Coils of small intestine Gallbladder	Stomach including cardiac and pyloric openings Portion of liver Duodenum, pancreas Suprarenal glands and parts of kidneys Greater omentum	Part of liver Stomach, fundus, and cardiac regions Spleen Tail of pancreas Left colic splenic flexure Part of left kidney Greater omentum
Right Lumbar	Umbilical	Left Lumbar
Lower portion of liver Ascending colon Part of right kidney Coils of small intestine Greater omentum Right colic (hepatic) flexure	Transverse colon Part of body kidneys Part of duodenum Coils of small intestine Greater omentum Bifurcation of the abdominal aorta and inferior vena cava	Part of left kidney Descending colon Coils of small intestine Greater omentum
Right Inguinal (Iliac)	Hypogastric	Left Inguinal (Iliac)
Cecum, appendix Part of ascending colon Coils of small intestine Greater omentum	Bladder in adults if distended Uterus during pregnancy Coils of small intestine Greater omentum	Part of descending colon Sigmoid colon Coils of small intestine Greater omentum

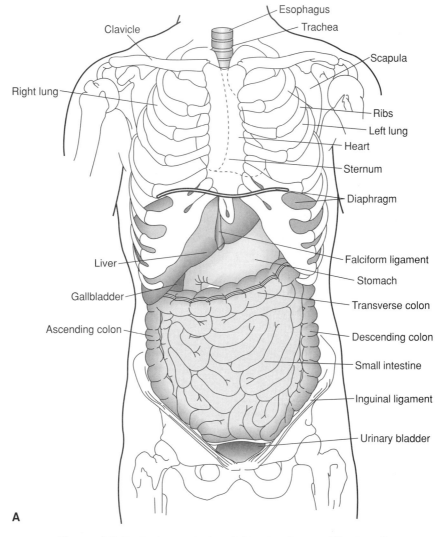

Clavicle

Right lung

Liver

Gallbladder

Ascending colon

Esophagus

Trachea

Scapula

Ribs

Left lung

Heart

Sternum

Diaphragm

Falciform ligament

Stomach

Transverse colon

Descending colon

Small intestine

Inguinal ligament

Urinary bladder

A

Figure 14–1. A. Anatomical and directional terms. (*Continued*)

between the anterior superior iliac spine and the symphysis pubis. Draw two **horizontal** lines. Join the upper line to the lowest point of the costal margin on each side, at the level of the inferior margin of the tenth costal cartilage. Join the lower horizontal line to the tubercles on the respective iliac crests (Fig. 14–1).

Contents of the Abdomen: Quadrant Method

There is a second method of dividing the abdomen into regions and that is the **four-region plan**. A **horizontal** line is drawn from left to right through the **umbilicus**. A **vertical** line is drawn down the midline of the body. This establishes upper right and left quadrants and lower right and left quadrants (Fig. 14–2).

Trocar Guides

The efficiency of using the trocar to pierce the internal organs and aspirate their contents is enhanced by the use of trocar guides. **The main guides are to reach the stomach, cecum, urinary bladder, and the heart**. The guides, all originate at the common insertion point—2 inches to the left and 2 inches superior to the navel. The point of the trocar is inserted into the abdomen and kept close to the anterior abdominal wall until the specific organ is reached.

Guide for the Right Side of the Heart. Direct the trocar to intersect a line drawn from the left anterior—superior iliac spine and the right earlobe. After the trocar has passed through the diaphragm, depress the point and enter the heart (Fig. 14–3).

Guide for the Stomach. Direct the trocar point toward the intersection of the fifth intercostal space and the left midaxillary line (established by extending a line from the center of the medial base of the axillary space inferiorly along the rib cage); continue until the trocar enters the stomach (Fig. 14–3).

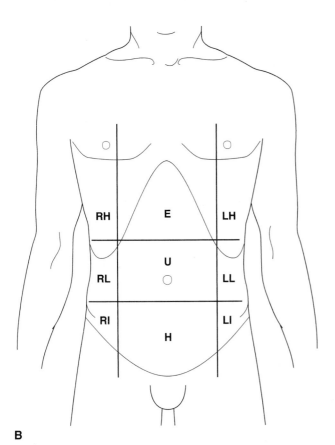

B

Figure 14–1. (*Continued*) **B**. The nine regions of the abdomen. RH, right hypochondriac; E, epigastric; LH, left hypochondriac; RL, right lumbar; U, umbilical; LL, left lumbar; RI, right inguinal; H, hypogastric; LI, left inguinal.

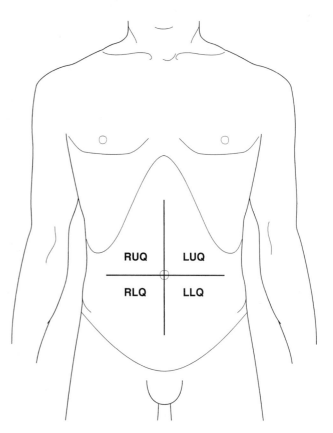

Figure 14–2. Division of the abdomen into quadrants. RUQ (LUQ), right (left) upper quadrant; RLQ (LLQ), right (left) lower quadrant.

Guide for the Cecum. Direct the trocar toward a point one-fourth of the distance from the right anterior-superior iliac spine to the pubic symphysis; keep the point of the trocar well up near the abdominal wall until within 4 inches of the right anterior-superior iliac spine; then dip the point 2 inches and insert it forward into the colon (see Fig. 14–3).

Trocar Guide for the Urinary Bladder. Keep the point up near the abdominal wall directing the trocar to the median line of the pubic bone (symphysis pubis) until the point touches the bone. Retract the trocar slightly, depress the point slightly, and insert into the urinary bladder.

▶ PARTIAL ASPIRATION PRIOR TO OR DURING ARTERIAL TREATMENT

Cavity embalming, complete aspiration and injection of cavity fluids, **follows** arterial injection and drainage. There is one exception to this rule: When the abdomen is tightly distended with gas or edema, this pressure should be relieved **prior to or during** arterial injection.

The presence of fluid (as in ascites) or gas in the abdomen can be great enough to act as an **extravascular resistance**. This resistance may also interfere with drainage. Drainage may be difficult to establish until this extravascular pressure is relieved.

Two methods can be employed: First, using a scalpel, puncture the abdomen at the standard point of trocar entry 2 inches left and 2 inches superior to the umbilicus. Insert a trocar or blunt instrument such as a large drain tube into the cavity and release the gases or edema. It may be more useful to make this puncture in the lower area of the abdomen in the right or left inguinal area or the hypogastric region of the abdomen. From this point, edema will be able to gravitate easier from the abdomen, and if gases are the trouble, it may be easier to pierce the **transverse colon** with a trocar from this more distant point (Fig. 14–4).

Second, using a scalpel, make a small incision in the abdominal wall. Dissect into the abdominal cavity. A portion of the large intestine can be incised if gas is the problem; edema drainage can be taken from the opening. Cover this opening with cotton or gauze saturated with a disinfectant so that microbial agents are not released into the air.

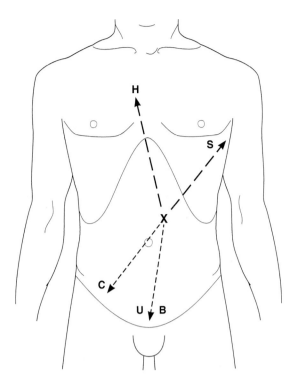

Figure 14–3. Trocar guides. S, stomach; C, cecum; UB, urinary bladder; H, heart; X, insertion point.

The first method using the trocar is much cleaner and will be found to be generally more effective in relieving abdominal pressure (gas or edema) prior to or during arterial injection.

▶ ANTEMORTEM SUBCUTANEOUS EMPHYSEMA

A condition where there is a noticeable amount of gas in the tissues **prior to embalming** is antemortem subcutaneous emphysema. Many times, the facial tissues will be quite distended, the tongue will protrude, gases may be felt all along the thoracic walls, and, in the male, the scrotum may be distended with gas.

If there is no odor and if there are no signs of decomposition, palpate for a broken rib or examine the body for a puncture wound to the thorax or a very recent tracheotomy opening. Look for large needle punctures over the skin of the rib cage. This condition is brought about by a rupture or by the puncturing or tearing of the pleural sac of the lung. Air was forced into the tissues as the person struggled to breathe air. If the condition is severe enough, try and remove some of this gas **prior to arterial embalming**.

Insert the trocar into the abdomen at the standard point of entry, then direct the point through the diaphragm, keeping the point just under the rib cage so as not to damage any of the large vessels. This should help to relieve some of the gases. Likewise, using a carotid incision will help to relieve gases from the neck tissues. Removal of these gases can be better accomplished by channeling and/or lancing the tissues after the arterial injection is completed.

▶ TIME PERIOD FOR CAVITY TREATMENT

There are two periods during which cavity aspiration and injection can take place: (1) immediately following arterial injection; and (2) several hours following arterial injection. This time delay will allow the intravascular pressure to assist the diffusion of the arterial solution from the capillaries into the interstitial spaces. Some embalmers inject the last quarter gallon of arterial solution with the drainage closed, being careful to remove the arterial tubes and drainage devices quickly and to tie off the vessels so as much pressure as possible remains within the vascular system.

Begin aspirating **prior to suturing incisions that were made for the arterial injection**. Aspiration takes the pressure off the vascular system and thus decreases the possibility of leakage from the incision should some small vessels leak.

Some embalmers do not perform the cavity embalming until the time of dressing and casketing, while others perform the cavity embalming immediately at the

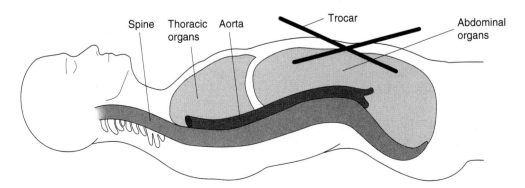

Figure 14–4. Trocar levels to relieve abdominal distension from edema (ascites) or gases.

conclusion of the arterial embalming. The theory of aspiration shortly after arterial injection has the following advantages:

1. Large numbers of microbes that can easily multiply and accelerate decomposition are removed as soon as possible.
2. Removal of the microbes prevents the possibility of translocation of the microbes to the skeletal tissues.
3. Removal of these microbes prevents or minimizes the possible production of gases that could cause purge.
4. Immediate aspiration removes materials that could purge if sufficient gases were generated during the delay.
5. Removal of the contents of the hollow viscera and cavities eliminates a bacterial medium.
6. **Most important**, removal of blood from the heart, liver, and large veins helps to prevent blood discolorations and the condition of "embalmer's gray," caused by blood not removed during arterial injection.
7. If there has been some distension of the neck or facial tissues during arterial injection, immediate aspiration decreases the swelling. This is often seen in bodies dead from pneumonia when hydrothorax is present.

The second theory is to have a long delay prior to aspirating the body. Some embalmers delay aspirating for 8 to 12 hours. The theory is to allow a maximum time for the arterial solution to penetrate into the tissue spaces and into the walls of the visceral organs. This will then make the walls easier to pierce with the trocar when the aspirating is done. If a humectant coinjection or a humectant restorative "to fill out" emaciated tissue has been used, some chemical manufacturers suggest that the last half gallon be injected with the vein ligated and a delay made between arterial injection and aspiration. This delay gives the tissues of the face time to firm in a "filled-out" condition.

▶ ASPIRATION TECHNIQUE BY TROCAR

The standard point of trocar entry is located 2 inches to the left of and 2 inches superior to the umbilicus. This point is used for the standard trocar; from it, the embalmer is able to reach all areas of the thoracic, abdominal, and pelvic cavities. The trocar should also be able to reach above the clavicle into the base of the neck. A second reason for using this point, especially with infants and children, is that the liver is on the right side of the body. At the location where the trocar is inserted, it is easier to move the instrument from point to point.

If it were inserted on the right side, the trocar would be entangled in the solid tissues of the liver.

During the aspiration of the cavities, the trocar can be withdrawn enough to let air pass through the instrument. This helps to "clean out" materials in the tubing and the instrument. Some embalmers withdraw the trocar several times during aspiration and plunge it into a container of water to flush out the tubing and trocar.

An orderly method of aspiration should be employed. Gases are usually found in the anterior portions of the abdominal and thoracic cavities. Liquids gravitate to the posterior portions of the cavities. If each cavity is "fanned" from right to left, most of the viscera are pierced. This "fanning" can be done in about three levels of depth.

Begin by inserting the trocar and aspirating the most anterior portions of the cavity. Then progress from right to left within the middle portion of the cavity, and finally from right to left through the deepest portions of the cavity. Treat both abdominal and thoracic cavities in this manner.

▶ RECENT SURGERY OR ORGAN REMOVAL

If the deceased was an organ donor or died during the course of an operation and no autopsy was performed, the surgical incision or the incision used to remove the organ(s) may or may not have been loosely closed by the hospital. For such bodies, the following protocol simplifies treatment of the cavities:

1. Disinfect the surgical incision with a **phenol solution**.
2. Arterially embalm the body.
3. Remove loose sutures, surgical staples, and so on, and open the incision.
4. Swab the edges of the incision with a phenol solution.
5. Suture closed the incision using a tight baseball suture. If possible, use sufficient quantities of incision seal powder.
6. **Aspirate the cavities and inject cavity fluid.**

> Any surgical drainage openings should be closed by suture or trocar button **prior** to aspiration of the cavities.

▶ PARTIAL AUTOPSIES AND ORGAN DONATIONS

After a partial autopsy on an adult, the unautopsied cavity can be difficult to treat from the cavity that has been opened. It is much simpler to treat the walls of the autopsied cavity by hypodermic treatment and painting with autopsy gel. Fill the cavity with an absorbent material and saturate the material with a cavity fluid. Suture the cavity closed. **Now treat the unautopsied cavity** by aspirating the cavity and its visceral contents. Inject a sufficient quantity of cavity fluid.

▶ DIRECT INCISION METHOD

In the treatment of bodies that have recent surgical incisions or from which organs were removed after death, resuturing followed by aspiration and injection with the trocar is recommended.

An alternate method can be used where a body cavity (or cavities) has been opened by surgery or a partial autopsy or removal of a donated organ. **The direct incision method** uses this incision to lance and drain the various organs and aspirate the cavity. Cavity fluid can be injected after the body is resutured. This method is unsanitary and can be time consuming. Often, there is no access to both the abdominal and thoracic cavities.

▶ ORDER OF TREATMENT

There is no specific order of treatment, but the embalmer should proceed in an orderly fashion in treating the cavities to ensure that no areas are missed. Years ago, some instructors taught that each organ should be separately treated. That is, the stomach was aspirated (with one puncture) and then, without removing the trocar, the stomach was filled with cavity fluid. The embalmer then moved on to treat another organ until all hollow viscera and cavities had been embalmed.

A suggested order might be **thoracic** cavity, abdominal cavity, and pelvic cavity. Likewise, when injecting cavity fluid, inject the thoracic cavity first, then the abdominal and pelvic cavities.

▶ ASPIRATION OF THE THORACIC CAVITY

At the standard point of entry, direct the trocar into the thoracic cavity. A good point at which to begin aspiration is the right side of the heart, using the trocar guide as an imaginary line running from the left anterior superior iliac spine to the lobe of the right ear. Intersect this line with the trocar in the mediastinal area. This technique also provides practice for those occasions on which the trocar may have to be used as a drainage instrument (which will have to be inserted into the right atrium of the heart). Next, aspirate the anterior chambers of the right and left pleural cavities. Direct the trocar a little lower and pierce the central portions of the lungs and the heart.

> Observe what is being aspirated. Clear tubing is a help. Remember, the hydroaspirator may be 10 feet away from the body. Look through clear tubing at what is being immediately removed from the body.

Finally, aspirate the deep areas of the pleural cavities. If hydrothorax is present, edematous liquids will be found, often in great quantities. Be certain that the trocar is directed to either side of the vertebral column where the great vessels enter and leave the lungs. This also aspirates the bronchial tubes leading to the trachea.

▶ ASPIRATION OF THE ABDOMINAL CAVITY

After aspiration of the thorax, the trocar can be withdrawn and the stomach aspirated. Use the trocar guide. Move the trocar toward a point established along the **left** midaxillary line, at about the level of the fifth intercostal space. As the trocar moves toward this point, it should pierce the stomach.

Several passages can be made through the stomach wall. Aspiration not only **removes** gases, liquids, and semisolids from the organs, but also **pierces** the viscera so that cavity fluid can better penetrate the visceral organs. Next, the cecum and bladder can be aspirated again using the trocar guides.

In similar "fanning" movements, aspirate the entire abdominal cavity again. Try to establish three levels. Remember, gases, when they can move, will be in the anterior portions and liquids in the posterior portions of the cavities.

In aspiration of the abdomen, the small intestines and the greater omentum have a tendency to cling tightly to the small holes located in the point and shaft of the trocar. For this reason, it is best to keep the instrument in constant motion, except when a large amount of liquid such as edema in bodies with ascites is being drained. Removing the trocar from time to time helps to prevent clogging of these small holes.

Pay special attention to the posterior of the liver. It is here that the great vessels enter and leave this organ. The liver is very difficult to preserve. Therefore, numerous passes with the trocar should be made through the solid portions of this organ. Also, give special attention to the large intestine, especially the **transverse colon**. Check the previous charts to observe the location of this intestinal organ. The large intestine, especially the transverse portion, should be thoroughly pierced to allow the escape of gases and to assist later in penetration of the cavity fluid.

To assist the trocar in piercing the abdominal organs, place external pressure on the abdominal wall. Do this with a gloved hand. Hold the trocar with one hand

and apply the pressure with the other. Apply pressure gently on the abdominal wall. To facilitate passage of the trocar through the coils of the small intestine, in addition to applying pressure on the abdomen, pass the trocar to a bony part such as the ilium or pubic bone. In this way, the point of the trocar will pass through the intestine rather than push it aside or slip around it.

Another method that can be used in aspirating the **abdomen** and inferior portion of the thorax is to insert the trocar in the center of the right or left inguinal region of the abdomen. Long passes can be made with the trocar, which will pass through the lumen of the intestines as the point forges ahead through the diaphragm. Many embalmers feel they can better pierce the large and small intestine from this point of trocar entry.

▶ TREATMENT OF THE MALE GENITALIA

After aspiration of the pelvic and abdominal cavities of the male, the trocar need **not** be inserted into the scrotum to aspirate this organ. Cavity fluid should, however, be injected into the shaft of the penis and the scrotum if these organs appear not to have received arterial solution.

To enter the scrotum, direct the point of the trocar to the most anterior portion of the symphysis pubis. Draw back slightly on the trocar and direct the point over the top of the symphysis pubis into the scrotum. In cases of hydrocele, edema of the scrotum, make several such passages into the scrotum. Be careful not to puncture the organ. Then, with a cloth placed around the scrotum, much of the water can be forced into the pelvic cavity. Later, undiluted cavity fluid can be injected into the scrotum.

Another condition less frequently encountered is a hernia involving the scrotum. A portion of the intestines moves into the scrotum. This condition can be severe enough to make dressing the body difficult. The trocar should be directed into the scrotum to pierce the loops of the intestine and remove as much of the content as possible. Later, this area should be injected with cavity fluid. The embalmer can also use the trocar to pull the intestine back into the abdominal cavity. This is slowly accomplished by pulling on the intestine with the point of the trocar. Gradually, the intestine can be manipulated into the abdominal cavity. This will make dressing of the body much easier.

▶ CRANIAL ASPIRATION

The point of entry in cranial aspiration is the right or left nostril. A small trocar is introduced into the nostril and pushed through the **cribriform plate of the ethmoid bone**. At this point, the instrument enters the anterior portion of the cranial cavity (Fig. 14–5). It is not possible to move the trocar into the posterior portion of the cavity; therefore, any gases present must be removed from this anterior position.

Inject only a few ounces of concentrated cavity fluid. This is done by using a hypodermic syringe with a long needle. After injection, tightly pack the nostril with cotton to prevent leakage.

▶ INJECTION OF CAVITY CHEMICALS

After the complete aspiration of the thoracic and abdominal cavities, preservative/disinfectant cavity chemicals are placed within the cavities over the viscera. **Concentrated cavity fluid** is always used. In cases of hydrothorax or ascites or where blood has escaped during arterial injection or during aspiration of the organs, the fluids—blood and edema—dilute the cavity fluid.

The volume of chemical is determined by the mass of tissues to be treated, which is estimated on the basis of body size and weight. On the average, for a body weighing 150 pounds, 16 ounces of undiluted cavity chemical is used for each (thoracic, abdominal, and pelvic) cavity. Larger bodies may require considerably more chemical. Smaller bodies, such as infants, require less.

Prior to cavity chemical injection, it is necessary to wash and flush the trocar thoroughly. All organic materials must be flushed from the trocar if concentrated cavity fluid is to pass through the instrument. The undiluted cavity chemical may be injected by two methods: gravity injector and machine injection. The gravity injector is attached directly to the 16-ounce bottle of cavity fluid. A hose connects the injector to the trocar. The higher the bottle is raised, the faster the fluid flows into the body. A small opening on the side of the gravity injector allows air to flow into the cavity fluid bottle. By placing a finger over this opening, the embalmer stops the flow of cavity fluid. This can be done when the trocar must be withdrawn to change its position within a body cavity. After use, the gravity injector, tubing, and trocar should be rinsed with cold water to disperse all the cavity fluid. The trocar can then be immersed in a cold liquid sterilant.

In machine injection, three bottles of cavity fluid are placed in the tank of the embalming machine. The delivery hose is then connected directly to the trocar. Pressure and rate of flow should both be set very low. The tubing alone can hold several ounces of cavity fluid. Following injection, make certain that the cavity chemical is thoroughly rinsed from the machine. Wash the machine with warm water and ammonia and then run fresh cold water through it.

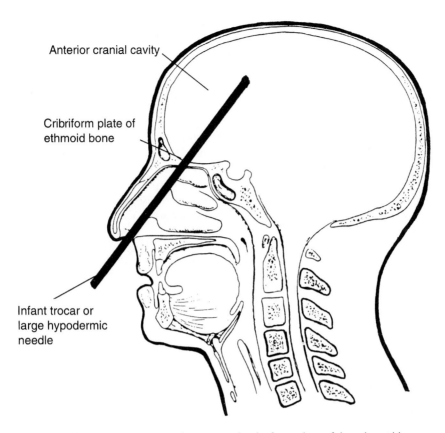

Anterior cranial cavity

Cribriform plate of
ethmoid bone

Infant trocar or
large hypodermic
needle

Figure 14–5. Anterior cranial cavity and cribriform plate of the ethmoid bone.

The chemicals are sprayed or made to flow over the **anterior surface** of the viscera close to the anterior wall of the thoracic and abdominal cavities. The cavity chemicals gravitate through the openings in the viscera made by the trocar and are absorbed by or rest on the posterior surface of the cavity walls.

After the cavity fluid is injected, some embalmers make several passes with the trocar through the abdomen and thorax to release gases that may have been displaced to the surface of the cavities. This movement of the trocar helps to distribute the cavity fluid. Cover the open end of the trocar with a cloth saturated with disinfectant so formaldehyde fumes and/or body gases are not released into the air.

After the trocar puncture has been closed and during the post-embalming washing and drying of the body, **turn the body on its sides** not only to wash and dry the back and sides of the body, but also to distribute the cavity fluid and bring any trapped gases to the surface of the cavities.

The cavity chemicals should be kept in the body and not be allowed to spill or run onto the surface of the abdominal wall. Use a wet cloth to wrap the trocar and cover the opening in the body as the fluids are injected. If cavity chemicals accidentally flow onto the surface of the body, immediately flush with cold running water.

It is possible to inject cavity fluid into the trachea or esophagus. If the nasal passages or throat have not been tightly packed with cotton when the features were set, this fluid can exit when the body is turned to be dried after it is washed. Limited aspiration can be done with the nasal tube aspirator after the body is placed into a supine position. The nasal passages can be tightly repacked with cotton. Open the lips and, using dry cotton, make certain all the liquid is dried from the mouth. If the embalmer feels that cavity fluid purge may be a problem during dressing and casketing, reaspirate the thoracic cavity at this time, giving special emphasis to the posterior of the neck, where the trachea and esophagus are located. Packing the throat and nasal passages with an abundant amount of cotton prior to embalming can help reduce the chance of cavity fluid purge.

▶ CLOSURE OF THE ABDOMINAL OPENING

To complete the aspiration procedure, the opening in the body wall is closed. Several methods can be used. Each embalmer uses his or her own preferred method. The plastic, threaded trocar button provides complete closure and is easily removed if further aspiration and reinjection are necessary later.

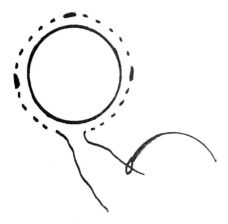

Figure 14–6. Pursestring suture.

Two sutures are commonly used to close the trocar opening: the **pursestring** (Fig. 14–6) and the **"N" or reverse stitch**. Sutures offer the advantage of a complete closure. A bow can be used to secure the suture. It can easily be opened if reaspiration is necessary. To minimize exposure to any fluid that may leak from the abdominal opening, if the embalmer plans to suture the opening closed, place the stitch after aspiration, just before the cavity fluid is injected. After injection, pull the suture tight to close the opening.

The barrel of the trocar can enlarge the abdominal opening if there is poor integrity to the abdominal skin to a size where a trocar button would be impossible to use. This condition necessitates the use of sutures for closure.

Some embalmers do not close the trocar openings but allow them to remain open for the escape of any gases. If this is done, the opening should be covered with cotton and the cotton covered with plastic to prevent any soilage of the clothing. This technique is not recommended when the body is being shipped.

▶ REASPIRATION/REINJECTION

Several hours, following the embalming of the body, it may be necessary to again aspirate the body cavities. This is called **reaspiration**. In most circumstances, this is sufficient treatment. However, if an abundant amount of gas appears to be present in the cavities or if the trocar indicates to the embalmer that the viscera appear soft in texture a **reinjection** of one or more bottles of concentrated cavity fluid is recommended. Under certain circumstances, such as advanced decomposition, the presence of true tissue gas or a death by drowning, reaspiration and reinjection may need to be repeated several times.

Some funeral firms have a rule that **all** bodies must be reaspirated prior to dressing and casketing or the transportation of a body. This is a precaution against the possibility of purge. It is possible for gases to develop in the cavities following embalming if all of the contents of the body cavities were not treated by the first aspiration and injection of cavity fluid. Handling of the body during transportation can cause liquids and gases to relocate and increase the possibility or actually cause a post-embalming purge.

Reaspiration is strongly advised under certain conditions, these would include but are not limited to the following:

1. When prior to dressing the trocar button is removed and a noticeable amount of gas appears to be present in the abdomen
2. When the body is to be transported **to** another funeral establishment (Ship-out)
3. When the body is received **from** another funeral establishment (ship-in)
4. When decomposition is present
5. In the case of recent abdominal surgery
6. When the embalmer is dealing with an obese body
7. When the body shows evidence of gas—distension of the veins of the neck or backs of the hands
8. When purge is present
9. When death involved blood infection or infection of the abdominal cavity (e.g., sepsis, peritonitis, or pneumonia)
10. When death occurred from drowning
11. In the case of bodies with ascites

Reaspiration is also used when the facial tissues have been distended with edema or gases. The neck can be channeled with the trocar during cavity embalming. Repeated aspiration can assist in the removal of liquids and gases out of the tissues of the face and neck.

▶ CONCEPTS FOR STUDY AND DISCUSSION

1. Distinguish between **antemortem subcutaneous emphysema** and "true" tissue gas.
2. Give several reasons for aspiration.
3. Distinguish between stomach purge and lung purge.
4. Describe how the abdomen is divided into nine regions; name each region.
5. Describe how the abdomen is divided into quadrants.
6. List the major visceral contents of the nine abdominal regions.

7. Give the trocar guides for the following organs:
   a. right side of the heart
   b. stomach
   c. cecum, and
   d. urinary bladder.
8. Describe four means of creating a vacuum for aspiration.
9. Discuss the various means of closing the trocar opening in the abdominal wall.
10. Give the standard point of trocar entry into the abdomen and explain why this location is used.
11. List conditions that necessitate reaspiration of the body.
12. Explain why partial aspiration may be necessary prior to or during arterial injection.
13. Explain why cavity embalming is performed.
14. List the advantages and disadvantages of immediate cavity treatment and delayed cavity treatment.

▶ BIBLIOGRAPHY

Burke PA, Sheffner AL. The antimicrobial activity of embalming chemicals and topical disinfectants on the microbial flora of human remains. *Health Lab Sci* 1976;13(4):267–270.

Cavity fluids. In: *Champion Encyclopedia*, No. 454. Springfield, OH: Champion Chemical Co., 1975:1833–1836.

Dorn JM, Hopkins BM. *Thanatochemistry*. Upper Saddle River, NJ: Prentice-Hall, 1998.

Grant ME. Cavity embalming. In: *Champion Encyclopedia*. Springfield, OH: Champion Chemical Co., 1987:2338–2341.

Proper cavity treatment. In: *Champion Encyclopedia*, No. 449. Springfield, OH: Champion Chemical Co., 1974:1813–1816.

Rose GW, Hockett RN. The microbiological evaluation and enumeration of postmortem specimens from human remains. *Health Lab Sci* 1971;8(2):75–78.

Tortora GJ. *Principles of Human Anatomy*, 3rd ed. New York: Harper & Row, 1983.

Trocar and its proper use. In: *Champion Encyclopedia*, No. 422. Springfield, OH: Champion Chemical Co., 1971:1705–1708.

Weed LA, Baggenstoss AH. The isolation of pathogens from tissues of embalmed human bodies. *Am J Clin Pathol* 1951;21:1114.

Weed LA, Baggenstoss AH. The isolation of pathogens from embalmed tissues. *Proc Soc Mayo Clin* 1952;27:124.

CHAPTER 15

TREATMENTS AFTER ARTERIAL INJECTION

CHAPTER OBJECTIVES

▶ Treatments for areas receiving insufficient preservation
▶ Sutures; removal of invasive devices
▶ Treatments for purge, swelling, and discolorations
▶ Terminal disinfection
▶ Surveillance until final disposition

▶ POSTEMBALMING TASKS

The following treatments are generally carried out after the arterial and cavity embalming. Several of the tasks may be performed before or during arterial injection depending on the preference of the embalmer. Examples include the washing of the body, treatment of ulcerations or gangrenous tissues, and removal and closure of a colostomy. Urinary catheter removal and packing of the throat are usually performed before arterial injection. **The following is a list of treatments – they are NOT listed in an order of performance**.

1. Preservative treatments for areas that did not receive arterial solution or did not receive **sufficient** arterial solution.
2. Closure of embalming incisions.
3. Removal (and closure of the opening) of invasive devices, for example, pacemaker, intravenous needles, surgical drains, colostomy apparatus.
4. Washing of the body, turning of the body to dry, and inspect for posterior lesions.
5. Final treatments for ulcerations and discolorations.
6. Corrective treatments for purge and packing of all orifices.
7. Removal of gases or edema from viewable facial areas.
8. Inspection of mouth for purge or moisture; resetting of features if necessary, and insertion of false teeth if these were not available before embalming.
9. Application of adhesives to eyes and mouth.
10. Dressing with plastic garments.
11. Terminal disinfection of instruments and preparation room and personal hygiene.
12. Preparation of documentation, shipping instructions, etc.

▶ TREATMENTS OF AREAS LACKING ARTERIAL SOLUTION

If areas of the body have not received fluid or have not received sufficient arterial solution, the embalmer should inject the area through a secondary injection point.

Appearance of Areas not Receiving or Receiving Insufficient Arterial Solution. Areas that have received insufficient or no arterial solution show little or no evidence of fluid dye. Intravascular blood discolorations may still be present. The tissues exhibit little or no preservative fixation.

When doubt exists as to whether an area has received any or sufficient solution, the simplest corrective treatment is to inject the area arterially.

▶ SUPPLEMENTAL EMBALMING TREATMENTS

There are two supplemental methods of embalming—**surface embalming** and **hypodermic embalming**. These methods are used to embalm either small areas, such as the eyelids, mouth, and fingers, or to treat large body areas such as lower legs obstructed from arterial solution by arteriosclerosis or the trunk walls of autopsied bodies that did not receive arterial solution.

Surface Embalming*

Surface embalming can be used to treat intact skin that has not received sufficient arterial fluid as well as broken skin areas such as abrasions, skin-slip, burned tissues, and surface lesions. Surface embalming may be applied to both **external** and **internal** body surfaces. Examples of internal application of surface packs would include the buccal cavity of the mouth, underneath the eyelids, within the nasal cavity, underneath the scalp in autopsied bodies, and the inner trunk walls in autopsied bodies.

The chemicals used for surface embalming may be liquids, gels, or powders. The liquids most frequently used include accessory surface embalming chemicals and cavity fluid. Cotton compresses saturated with an accessory chemical specifically formulated for surface treatments are designed to preserve, cauterize, dry, deodorize and bleach tissue. Many of these formulations contain phenol. Depending on the condition, these compresses may need to be applied for several hours. When phenol is used after the compresses have been removed, the area can be "washed" with alcohol to stop the action of the phenol. The compresses when used externally should be covered with plastic to prevent evaporation of the chemical and reduce exposure of the embalmer to irritating fumes.

Gels constitute a second surface embalming chemical. Years ago, formalin creams were used for surface embalming. In the early 1960s, surface preservative gels were introduced. These can be applied directly to the skin with a large brush or they can be poured onto cotton and applied as a pack. The gels are available in an almost-liquid form of very low viscosity or in a very heavy "jelly" of very high viscosity. When used on external surfaces, gels should also be covered with plastic to reduce fumes and to prevent evaporation. These chemicals are designed to penetrate the tissues. They can remain affixed to non-viewed body areas. In areas that will be cosmetically treated and viewed, the chemicals should be left on the skin for several hours.

Arterial fluid is not recommended as a surface embalming chemical, for the dyes present in the fluid stain the skin surface. Their penetrating strength and preservative strength may be less than those of cavity fluid, accessory surface chemicals, or gels. When a surface compress (gel or liquid) is removed from an area to which cosmetics will be applied, the area should be cleaned with a solvent and dried before cosmetic treatment begins.

Specific Internal Treatments for Facial Areas

If tissues need the preservative, they will not dehydrate. Underembalmed tissue can dehydrate faster than well-embalmed tissue. Gluing the eyes and mouth further reduces any dehydration problems. Visible areas treated by internal surface compresses or hypodermic preservative treatments can be cosmetized using a cream-based cosmetic to further retard dehydration. These methods allow cosmetic work to be done immediately.

> If time permits, surface compresses and gels can be used over these areas — after several hours removed — surfaces dried and cosmetics applied.

Mouth, Lips. Cotton can be placed over the dentures and saturated with cavity fluid, using a hypodermic needle and syringe to moisten the cotton. The lips can then be glued; the preservative works from the inside of the mouth to preserve the tissues. Cosmetic treatment can be immediately implemented using this method of preservation.

Eyelids. Cotton can be used for eye closure or a small piece of cotton can be inserted over the top of an eye cap. The cotton can be moistened with a few drops of cavity fluid and the eyelids sealed with an adhesive. Cosmetic treatment can begin immediately (Fig. 15–1).

Nose. Cotton saturated with preservative fluid can be inserted into the nostrils. It can later be pushed back far enough that it will not be noticeable. A small gage hypodermic needle can be used to inject a preservative solution from inside the nostrils into various areas of the nose. If hypodermic treatment is used, expect some leakage from the injection sites. Cotton can be placed within the nostrils to absorb the leaking preservative and later removed. The columna nasi and possibly the tip of the nose can also be reached by injecting from within the mouth.

General Treatments for Nonvisible Body Areas

For areas that will **not be seen**, such as the leg or foot, hypodermic treatment, surface gels and preservative compresses can all be used to achieve preservation.

---

*When any surface chemicals are used, the compress or gel should be covered with plastic so as to reduce fumes and to prevent the surface chemical from evaporating.

Figure 15–1. Placing cotton moistened with several drops of concentrated cavity fluid under the eyelids ensures good preservation of the lids. Seal eyelids with superglue. Cosmetic treatment can then begin.

Surface embalming powders have been used for many years.* Diapers can be used to contain the powder or the powder can be placed in plastic garments such as stockings, coveralls, or pants after the garments are in position. Powders can also be used to treat the interior walls of the abdomen and thorax in the autopsied body. Powders are not as effective as gels or liquids. Read the label to be certain the powder is a preservative and not just a deodorant or absorbent.

Hypodermic Embalming

The second and the most effective supplemental method of embalming is hypodermic embalming. This method is used to treat small localized body areas or large areas, such as the trunk walls of the autopsied body or a limb that did not receive sufficient arterial fluid and cannot be injected arterially.

Hypodermic injection involves the use of a hypodermic syringe and needles ranging from 6 to 19 gauges and of varying lengths. The larger needles (6 gauge) are useful for large areas. An infant trocar or specially designed hypovalve trocar can be connected to the centrifugal embalming machine for the injection of large body areas.

The arterial solution used for arterial injection can be used for hypodermic injection. It is recommended that it be strengthened with cavity fluid or a high-index

arterial fluid. **This type of solution should be used only on body areas that will not be viewed, as the dye in the fluid can blotch the skin.** Cavity fluid as well as specially designed accessory embalming chemicals may be used for hypodermic embalming. Phenol solutions should be reserved for localized treatments of discolored areas or tissues when bleaching of tissues is necessary. The phenol solutions would not be used for routine supplemental hypodermic embalming.

In non-viewable areas where the infant trocar or hypovalve trocar has been used, the punctures can be sealed with a trocar button. When machine injection and a trocar is used, phenol products should be avoided. Phenol can be damaging to injection machines. When injection is completed, the embalming machine must be thoroughly flushed and cleaned; clear ammonia run thru the machine will help to eliminate formaldehyde residue.

In facial areas, where hypodermic needles would be used, most of the injections can be made from inside the mouth. In this manner, leakage will not exit onto the face. Unlike tissue builder, these chemicals have a tendency to seep from the point of puncture. In the autopsied body, large portions of the face can be reached through scalp incisions.

The hands and fingers can be injected from the palmar surface of the hand or from between the fingers. Super adhesive (superglue) can be applied to prevent leakage.

The nose can be treated hypodermically by inserting the needle inside the mouth. The ear can be reached by hypodermic injection from behind the ear.

For larger areas, such as the arm and leg, the infant trocar can be inserted into the area of the cubital fossa of the arm to reach the arm and forearm. If the elbow area contains edema, the trocar can also be entered from the upper pectoral region to reach the distended area. The leg can be treated by inserting the infant trocar on the medial side of the leg just inferior or superior to the knee. From this point, both the thigh and lower leg can be reached. Trunk walls, hip, and buttock can be reached by inserting a trocar into the center of the lateral trunk wall.

Combination Treatments for Large Areas

Certain conditions, such as arteriosclerosis, gangrene, and edema, require additional injection of the legs. A combination of supplemental embalming methods (hypodermic and surface) can be used. If arterial treatment has been unsuccessful, the legs can be injected hypodermically. The solution injected can be undiluted arterial or cavity chemical. The legs can also be painted with autopsy gels and embalming powder can be placed into the plastic stockings.

In the trunk area, hypodermic injection can be used when the tissues have received insufficient arterial fluid.

---

*When embalming powders are being used, the embalmer must wear a protective particulate mask and the room should be properly ventilated to remove powder particulate and fumes.

Coveralls, pants, or a Capri garment can be used and embalming powder or autopsy gel painted over the areas being treated. When edema is a problem in the elbow area, hypodermic treatment can be used (inject from the upper arm), paint with autopsy gel and wrap with gauze. A plastic sleeve can then be placed over the treated area.

▶ CLOSURE OF INCISIONS

Today, two methods are used to close incisions—sutures and super adhesive. Regardless of the method of closure, the embalmer must follow several steps to prepare all incisions for closure:

1. Do not suture until after cavity aspiration; aspiration relieves pressure on the vascular system and helps to prevent leakage.
2. Be certain all vessels are securely tied. This prevents any further leakage.
3. If there is edema in the surrounding tissues, force as much liquid out of the incision as possible.
4. Dry the incision.
5. Cotton saturated with a cautery solution can be packed into the incision. This compress can remain within the incision. It, along with incision seal powder, will also help to prevent leakage.
6. Make several sutures before applying the incision seal powder to the incision. In this manner, a "pocket" is created and the powder is retained within the incision and not spread on the surface of the body (Fig. 15–2B–F).
7. After suturing, apply a surface glue over the area to prevent leakage.

Suturing

Cotton or Linen Thread. Linen thread is stronger than cotton thread and is recommended for autopsy, long bone donors and vessel incision sutures. For restorative sutures, which are located on visible areas, dental floss is an excellent material to use.

A ⅜-inch Circle Needle. The ⅜-inch circle needle is used for restorative sutures and to suture incisions made to raise vessels.

Double-Curved Autopsy Needle. The double-curved autopsy needle is easy to grip with the gloved hand. It is used to close autopsy incisions, long-bone donor incisions, surgical incisions, and incisions made to raise vessels.

Needles come in a variety of sizes and shapes, for example, single-curved autopsy needles, loopy needles, and circle needles. Some have a "patented eye." These eyes are threaded by merely pushing the thread against the eye portion of the needle, which eliminates the need to pass thread through the eye of the needle. Regardless of the size or the shape of the needle, it is most important to keep it sharp. Suturing can be very dangerous if the needles are dull, as extra pressure must be applied. In doing so, the embalmer increases the chance of the needle breaking or piercing her or his skin. A sharp needle makes suturing much easier, safer, and faster.

When suturing, one should pull on the thread and not on the needle to tighten the suture. Pulling on the needle weakens the suture cord where it passes through the needle's eye. In closing long sutures, as in autopsies, this may cause the cord to break.

The embalmer can suture using single- or double-stranded thread. This depends on the strength of the suture cord or on the type of suture. It is wise to double the cord when cotton thread or three- or four-twist linen thread is used. Single-stranded suture cord works best with five- and six-twist linen thread (dental floss).

Direction of Suturing

To make suturing more efficient, follow these directions for the various sutures.

- *Common Carotid Artery.* If using the parallel incision, suture from the inferior portion of the incision superiorly. Suture from the medial portion of the incision laterally if using a supraclavicular incision.
- *Axillary Artery.* Suture from the medial area of the incision laterally (with the arm abducted).
- *Brachial Artery.* Suture from the medial portion of the incision laterally with the arm abducted).
- *Radial and Ulnar Arteries.* Suture from the distal portion of the incision medially.
- *Femoral Artery.* Suture from the inferior portion of the incision superiorly.
- *Autopsies (Trunk Standard "Y" Incision).* Use bridge sutures to align the skin into position. Begin the trunk suturing at the pubic symphysis and suture superiorly.
- *Popliteal Artery.* Begin the suture at the inferior (or distal) portion of the incision and suture superiorly.
- *Anterior and Posterior Tibial Arteries.* Begin the sutures distally and suture superiorly.

Sutures

Individual (Bridge) Sutures. Individual sutures are used to align tissues into position prior to, during, or after embalming (Fig. 15–2A). They are temporary and are later replaced by more permanent sutures.

Baseball Sutures. Considered the most secure and commonly used, the baseball suture can be airtight. In

Figure 15–2. A. Individual (bridge) sutures. **B.** Baseball stitch. The ligature is tied in place. Knots should be avoided. **C.** Sutures are made from inside the incision. **D.** A pocket is made before the suture ends and incision seal powder is inserted. **E.** When properly sewn, no string should be visible. **F.** The completed suture. The ligature cord should not be visible. These sutures are airtight.

addition to the injection site incisions, it is used for autopsy, long surgical, and long-bone donor incisions. To make this stitch, pass a suture needle and thread from beneath the incision up through the integument, and cross the needle from side to side with each stitch (Fig. 15–2B). This creates a strong tight closure. In the process, however, the tissues adjacent to the incision are pulled up into a ridge.

When the baseball suture is being used for the closure of long incisions such as an autopsied body or closing the incisions of the legs when the long bones have been removed for donation—about every 5 inches pass the needle through both sides of the incision and tie the suture closed—as if the suture were to be ended. **Do not** cut the ligature but again start the baseball stitch. This "locks down" the suture every 5 inches and takes tension off the suture thread. Also should the thread break it will not be necessary to start the entire suture again—simply, start where the last "lock-down" was made.

Single Intradermal (Hidden) Suture. The single subcutaneous or intradermal suture is made with one needle and a single thread (Fig. 15–3). It is referred to as the "hidden stitch," because it is used on exposed areas of the body and is directed through the subcutaneous tissue only. To begin the closure, insert the needle deep into the tissues at one end of the incision. Make a knot

Figure 15–3. Single intradermal (hidden) suture.

in the thread a short distance from the end and pull the knot to the position of the needle puncture in the integument. Keeping the needle directed through the dermal tissues only, develop a back-and-forth pattern from one side of the incision to the other. Take care to line up the margins as the thread is drawn so that there are no gaps between stitches. To complete the closure, direct the needle through the integument as far as possible from the end of the incision. Once this is completed, draw the margins of the incision together by pulling the free end of the thread. Puckering may result if the thread is pulled too tight. The excess thread is cut off close to the incision as slight pressure is applied, concealing the ends of the thread.

Double Intradermal Suture. The double intradermal suture is made with two needles threaded with opposite ends of the same thread (Fig. 15–4A). Because this suture is permanently fixed at each end, it has greater holding ability than the single intradermal suture. Pass each needle through the dermis at opposite margins so that both stitches are parallel, similar to the lacing on a shoe. Continue the process until the incision is completely sutured. After drawing the margins tight, knot the two ends together within the incision. Correct puckering by light massage or smoothing with the finger. To end the suture, insert both threads onto one needle and insert it under the skin from the end of the incision to a point $1/2$ inch away. The excess threads are then cut as pressure is applied, resulting in the ends of the threads being hidden.

Inversion (Worm) Suture. The inversion suture is used to gather in and turn under excess tissues (Fig. 15–4B). The pattern of this suture is the same as that of the single intradermal suture, except that the stitches are made parallel to the incision edges and do not pierce the margins of the incision. The stitches are generally made as close to the margins as possible. The best results are obtained by making the stitches uniform in length. The stitches do not enter the incision except to start the suture. Each stitch should be drawn taut as sewn. The worm suture is not visible and may be waxed as needed. It is an excellent suture for closing a carotid incision or closing the scalp on the cranial autopsy (Fig. 15–5).

Interlocking (Lock) Suture. The interlocking suture creates a tight, leak proof closure. It has a disadvantage in that an unsightly ridge appears on the surface of the incision. Begin the suture at one end of the incision and direct the needle through the tissue so that it passes through both sides of the incision from the outside. Keep the thread tight with the hand not holding the suture needle. Then, lock the stitch by looping the needle

A

B

Figure 15–4. A. Double intradermal suture. **B.** Inversion (worm) suture.

through the thread. When completing the loop, pull the thread tight. Repeat this process until the incision is closed. The needle insertion should be made consistently from the same side of the incision.

Continuous (Whip) Suture. The continuous suture is generally used to close long incisions (Fig. 15–6). Frequently it is used by the autopsy technician to close the long incisions from the autopsy. This suture prevents leakage of fluids from the body cavities during transfer from the hospital to the funeral home. The suture is also seen in people who have died during surgery; the incision has been drawn closed to prevent leakage of fluids. Organ transplant retrieval teams use the stitch to close long incisions after the removal of visceral organs. To make this stitch, anchor the suture thread. Pass the needle through both sides of the incision, starting on the outside of the tissue on one side of the incision and passing directly through and out the tissues of the opposite side of the incision. Pass the thread over the top of the incision and begin the next stitch ½ to 1 inch beyond the previous stitch. The process is completed when the incision is closed.

Adhesives

The other method of closing incisions involves the use of a super adhesive. Many brands are available today. Most super glues can work in the presence of slightly moist tissues. These adhesives are excellent for closing jagged tears in the skin.

Many embalmers use the glues to close the incisions made to raise vessels. Some use the glues to close the scalp in cranial autopsies. Long autopsy incisions, however, are closed with sutures. As there are many uses for these glues in the embalming room, superglues should be kept in stock.

▶ REMOVAL OF BODY-INVASIVE DEVICES

Several of the following tasks can be performed either before or after arterial injection. It is the position of this text that these tasks, when possible, be performed following arterial injection of the body.

Intravenous Invasive Devices. Often, hospitals do not remove intravenous needles or venous catheters from the body after death. When possible, leave these needles and catheters in place until **after** arterial injection. Considerable swelling and discoloration of the area can occur if the needle or catheter is removed prior to

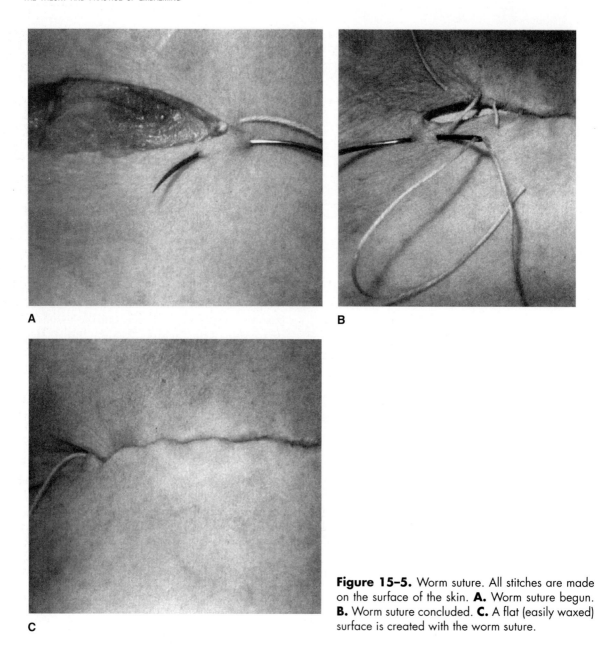

Figure 15–5. Worm suture. All stitches are made on the surface of the skin. **A.** Worm suture begun. **B.** Worm suture concluded. **C.** A flat (easily waxed) surface is created with the worm suture.

arterial injection. **Following arterial embalming, the invasive probe can easily be removed.** These punctures can be sealed with a drop of super glue. Tissue builder or a phenol solution injected beneath the skin also helps to seal these punctures on visible skin areas. When the needle or tube has been placed into the subclavian or jugular vein, a small incision can be made, and the area filled with incision seal powder, then sutured with a small tight baseball suture. If the area will not be seen, a trocar button may be used to seal the puncture.

Pacemakers and Defibrillators. These devices must be removed if the body is to be cremated. Certain radioac-

tive powered units must be returned to the manufacturer. A small incision can be made over the device, which is usually located in the upper pectoral region. The wire leads to the heart are cut. Incision seal powder is placed in the pocket and the incision sutured.

Colostomy. A colostomy is the opening of the colon through the abdominal wall to the skin surface. The **stoma** is the exposed portion of the bowel. Remove the colostomy collecting bag. Pour some cavity fluid into the bag for disinfection before placing it in a hazardous waste container. Disinfect the body area and colostomy stoma with cavity fluid or a phenol solution on cotton.

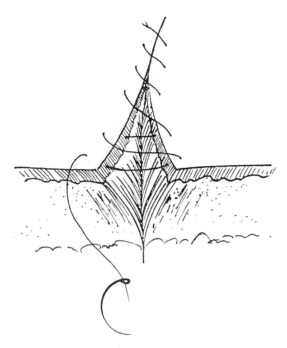

Figure 15-6. Continuous (whip) stitch.

Figure 15-8. Cosmetized hands protected by plastic during dressing and casketing.

By placing pressure on the stoma and slightly twisting, force the piece of bowel back into the abdominal cavity. A pursestring or "N" suture can be used to close the colostomy (Fig. 15–7). Surface glue may be applied to the closure after the body is washed and dried. Dispose of the attaching sleeve and collection bag in a biohazard waste container. The colostomy maybe closed before or after arterial injection.

Surgical Drains. Remove surgical drains and close the openings using a pursestring suture. Surface glue may be applied after the body is washed and dried to prevent leakage.

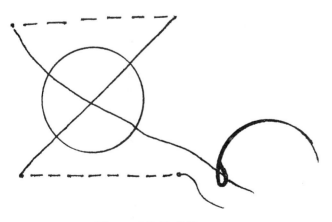

Figure 15-7. "N" suture.

▶ FINAL WASHING AND DRYING OF THE BODY*

After all sutures are completed and points of leakage sealed, the body should be washed and thoroughly dried. Particular attention should be given to the removal of blood from the surface of the body. Adding a small amount of household-bleach to the cleaning solution can assist with removal of any blood. Care should be given to the washing of the hair, especially if the jugular vein has been used for drainage. A conditioner rinse can be massaged into the hair during washing to help eliminate tangles and deodorize the hair. If the scalp exhibits a lot of dander or flaking, wash the hair several times and thoroughly dry with a hair dryer. (This pertains to men as well as women.) Attached hairpieces, naturally curly hair, and permed hair should be dried with cool air so the hair does not straighten. If braids are present, especially in an African-American, it may be wise to consult with the family prior to combing them out when the hair is washed (see Selected Readings, **Professional Hair Care for Human Remains**)

The body should be carefully dried. Good drying eliminates the potential for mold growth on the skin surface, especially in warm climates. **Turning the body on its side gives the embalmer opportunity to examine the posterior area and to thoroughly dry the back and buttocks** (Fig. 15–8).

---

*Proper preparation room attire—gown, gloves, and, if necessary, mask and eye protection—should be worn during these postembalming procedures.

▶ TREATMENT OF ULCERATIONS, LESIONS, AND DISCOLORATIONS

After the body has been washed and dried, incisions closed, invasive devices removed, and their punctures sealed, the embalmer should continue the treatment of lesions (e.g., decubitus ulcers) and discolorations (e.g., an ecchymosis on the back of the hand) on visible areas. Of course, decubitus ulcers should have been treated (preservative surface compresses) at the beginning of the embalming. After embalming, these ulcerations are redressed with compresses of phenol solution, accessory surface embalming chemicals, cavity fluid, or autopsy gels. This redressing helps to ensure preservation and sanitization.

Dry the tissues and deodorize the ulceration. Plastic clothing (coveralls, pants, stockings, etc.) can be placed on the body to help control odors. The buttocks may be diapered. The embalmer can inject the area around the decubitus ulcer with cavity fluid or accessory chemicals designed to combat the gas bacillus that forms tissue gas. The solution may be injected with a large-diameter hypodermic needle (6 gauge) or an infant trocar. Chemicals containing phenol should not be injected by using an embalming machine.

Surface compresses containing phenol solution, an accessory bleaching solution, or cavity fluid can be applied to discolorations (e.g., an ecchymosis on the back of a hand). These discolorations can also be treated internally by hypodermic injection of the same chemical into the discolored areas. With this method, cosmetics may be applied without the delay needed for surface chemicals to work.

▶ TREATMENT OF PURGE

After arterial and cavity embalming, there always exists the possibility of purge from the anus, mouth, or nose. Tightly packing the throat prior to mouth closure and arterial injection should decrease any purge from the mouth. Many embalmers pack the nose and anal orifice after embalming is completed. Packing the nose prior to arterial injection can create a blood and or fluid purge from the nostrils during arterial injection.

Some embalmers prefer to pack the anal orifice prior to embalming. Other embalmers would rather do so at the conclusion of the embalming. After embalming allows the possible escape of fecal matter and or blood from the rectum during the embalming and the cavity treatment.

When anal purge is present after embalming, force as much purge as possible from the rectum by firmly pressing on the lower abdominal area. Pack the rectum using cotton saturated with cavity fluid, autopsy gel, or a phenol solution. Dry packing should be inserted into the anal orifice after the moistened cotton. Leave a portion of the dry cotton so it can be seen. This will help to fully block the anal orifice.

When purge is present from the mouth or nose immediately following arterial injection and cavity treatment, it may be necessary to reaspirate and reinject cavity fluid. Clean out the orifices and be certain they are tightly packed with plenty of dry cotton or cotton webbing. If possible, re-pack the throat area.

▶ TREATMENT OF DISTENSION

Visible areas—face, neck, and hands—that are distended may need to be reduced for viewing of the body. These treatments can be carried out during the postembalming period. Some swellings, such as edema, can be treated by specific arterial solutions during arterial injection. It is necessary to know the cause of the distension to perform a corrective treatment. Swellings present before arterial injection should be noted on the **embalming report**. Examples of such conditions include edema, tumors, swellings caused by trauma, distension from gases of decomposition in the tissues or cavities, tissue gas produced by **Clostridium perfringens**, distension caused by allergic reactions, distension brought about by use of steroid drugs, and gases in the tissues from subcutaneous emphysema.

Distension of facial tissues, the neck, or glandular tissues of the face or the tissues surrounding the eye orbit **during** embalming of the body can be caused by an excessive amount of arterial solution in these tissues. Some of the causes of this swelling are very rapid injection of solution, use of too much injection pressure, poor drainage from these areas, breakdown of the capillaries (e.g. trauma or decomposition), excessive massage, and use of arterial solutions that are too weak. It is essential during embalming of the body that the embalmer is alert to any tissue distension. Injection should be immediately stopped and the situation evaluated.

In pitting edema, excess moisture is present in the tissue spaces. In solid edema, the excess moisture is within the cells. Pitting edema can be moved by mechanical aids such as gravitation, massage, channeling of the area, and application of pressure (e.g., pneumatic collar, weights, elastic bandage, water collar, digital pressure) to move the moisture to another area. Elevation of the head and firm digital pressure slowly drain pitting edema from the facial tissues. During cavity aspiration, the trocar can be used to channel the neck, which may allow some of the edema to drain from the facial tissues into the thorax.

Edema of the eyelids can be treated in several ways: (1) weighted surface compresses; (2) cavity fluid on cotton under the eyelids, during and after injection;

(3) hypodermic injection of phenol compound or cavity fluid after embalming; and (4) by use of a heated electric spatula after embalming.

After preservation of the lids is accomplished, channels can be made under the skin (e.g., from within the mouth, temple area): Carefully apply external pressure to the distended tissues, and "massage" as much of the edema from the tissues as possible. A problem that arises in removing edema from the facial tissues or hands is that the skin may become very wrinkled. Tissue preservation must always be the first concern. The use of an electric spatula may also be used to remove wrinkled eyelids.

Subcutaneous emphysema is air in the subcutaneous tissues. Cardiopulmonary resuscitation, a traumatic event, or surgical procedure can puncture the lung. Gas escapes into the subcutaneous tissues. As the individual struggles to breathe, more air is forced into the body tissues. Gases can easily be detected after death by palpating the tissues. The term **crepitation** is used to describe the spongy feel of the gas as it moves through the tissues when they are pushed on. Arterial injection and blood drainage may remove a small portion of the gas, but gas that is trapped in the facial tissues must be removed by channeling. This channeling can be done **after** the body is embalmed. The lips can be opened and a scalpel, bistoury knife, or large hypodermic needle used to channel the tissues of the face from inside the mouth (Fig. 15–9). Once the channels are made, the gas can be pushed out of the tissues. If the eyes are affected, the lids can be everted and the underside of the lids incised with a suture or hypodermic needle. Cotton can be used to close the eyes; it will also absorb any leakage.

Figure 15–9. After embalming, the lips are lanced to release gases in the tissues.

Subcutaneous emphysema can be differentiated from true tissue gas. True tissue gas has a very distinct foul odor that worsens progressively and is caused by an anaerobic bacterium. Blebbing and skin-slip develop with true tissue gas. (See Chapter 24 for treatments of true tissue gas.)

► RESETTING AND GLUING THE FEATURES

The features can be corrected after embalming. Additional cotton or feature posing compound can be inserted to fill out sunken and emaciated cheeks. If the cotton that was originally used to set the features becomes moist during the embalming, as a result of contact with purge or blood and fluid from the suture or needle injector used for mouth closure, it should be replaced with dry cotton.

The dentures are not always available at the beginning of the embalming. The mouth can be reopened and the dentures inserted afterward. These procedures are, of course, more difficult when the tissues are firm. Eyes, too, can be closed or reset after arterial injection. (Refer to Chapter 18 for a discussion of the postembalming procedures employed when eye enucleation has been performed.)

After the features have been properly aligned, the features can be glued. Adhesive applied to the lips and eyelids helps to avoid the separation caused by dehydration. The area where the adhesive is to be applied should first be cleaned with a solvent. Rubber-based adhesive, which is often used for the mouth and eyes, does not work well on a moist or oily surface. The skin of the lips and margins of the eyelids should be clean, dry, and free of moisture or oils. Super adhesive works very well for securing the eyelids. It ensures good closure of the inner canthus.

When glue is applied to the mucous membranes, it is advised that it should be kept behind the "weather line." This is not always possible. In some elderly persons or in individuals in whom blisters are removed from the mucous membranes after the gluing, the mucous membranes are not even visible. New mucous membranes can be drawn with cosmetics. Gluing helps to place tension on the mucous membranes, and this tension often "pulls" wrinkles from the membranes. Wrinkled lips can be corrected by gluing, waxing, or injecting the mucous membrane with tissue builder.

If the body was shipped from another funeral establishment, the lips may separate as a result of flight vibrations. Because of the delay, the tissues have time to become very firm. In such cases, the lips can be stretched or exercised with the blunt handle of an aneurysm needle or a pair of forceps (Fig. 15–10A). If the eyelids separate, they may also have to be "exercised" or stretched to obtain closure. Super adhesive is more effective in

A

B

Figure 15–10. A. The lips are exercised with the blunt handle of a pair of forceps. **B.** A rubber-based adhesive or a super adhesive is used to seal the lips.

securing the mouth and eyes when the tissues are very firm (Fig. 15–10B).

▶ PLASTIC GARMENTS

Prior to dressing, protective plastic garments can be placed on the body. Be certain the body is thoroughly dried before using a plastic garment. Pants or coveralls can be placed on the trunk. These would protect from

any anal purge or leakage from the genital organs. Pants or coveralls would also be used if a ulcerations or traumatic injuries were present and had been treated by the embalmer. Plastic stockings are used when surface treatments of the legs were necessary. These garments help to prevent soiling of the clothing and to control odors. A Capri pants is a single unit that combines pants and stockings. Embalming powder should be sprinkled into these plastic goods. The powder deodorizes the body and helps to control mold growth. Plastic sleeves may be applied over broken skin at the elbows or on the arms.

If general edema, tissue decomposition or extensive burns are present, a unionall may be necessary to protect the clothing once the body is dressed. The unionall is a plastic garment which covers the arms, trunk (including the shoulders), and legs. The unionall is available up to triple-X size. It is always advised to use a garment slightly larger than necessary.

Terminal Disinfection

Terminal disinfection comprises the disinfection practices carried out after the embalming process to protect the environment and includes personal hygiene for the embalmer as well as disinfection of the instruments, equipment, and preparation room.

Disinfectant Checklist In selecting a disinfectant for instruments and other preparation room paraphernalia, keep in mind the characteristics of a good disinfectant:

- Has a wide range of activity (works against viruses, bacteria, and fungi)
- Is of sufficient strength (active against spore-forming organisms of bacilli and fungi)
- Acts in the presence of water
- Is stable and has a reasonably long shelf life
- Is non-corrosive to metal instruments
- Acts fast
- Is not highly toxic to living tissues or injurious to the respiratory system

Care of the Embalming Machine

After use, the embalming machine should be flushed with warm water. Fluids that contain a humectant such as lanolin or silicon often leave a thick residue in the tank. Ammonia and lukewarm water should be flushed through the machine to remove the residue. Many embalmers prefer to flush the machines with a water softener or the powder used in electric dishwashers. Additives for machine cleaning can be purchased through fluid manufacturers. A final flush with warm water is necessary. It is recommended that the machine be filled with water at this time for the next preparation. This keeps the gaskets moist and allows the water time to release any dissolved gases such as chlorine. Adding embalming fluid (later) to an already-filled machine decreases the release of formaldehyde fumes. A lid must be placed on the water tank of the machine.

Surfaces

All surfaces should first be cleaned with cool water and a small amount of antiseptic soap to remove organic debris. Torn-up sheets make good washcloths and can be disposed of after use. A preliminary wash removes organic debris and also any formaldehyde present. Remember that a number of good disinfectants contain chlorine, and this chemical should not come into contact with formaldehyde. Bleach and warm water make a very good cleaning solution. The table, countertops, and drains can be wiped clean and disinfected with this solution. Lysol products are good disinfectants and are easily available. Be certain to clean the area **under** the table surrounding the drainage outlet. Tops of overhead lighting should also be given attention. Tubing used for aspiration should be soaked in a disinfectant solution. Pay attention to handles on cabinets and drawers. Commercial products used for cleaning the preparation room contain dilution instructions. (Refer to Chapter 3 for a review of disinfection practices.)

Instruments

Clean Instruments Prior to Disinfection. Removing organic material from the instrument makes disinfection more effective. Immerse all instruments including trocars in a solution of Bard-Parker disinfectant (8% by volume formaldehyde in 70% ethanol or isopropanol) or in 200 to 300 ppm of an iodophor for 45 minutes or longer. If possible, destroy cutting blades in a biohazards sharps container. Take special care with cutting instruments when gas gangrene or "tissue gas" has been encountered. The causative agent of this condition, *C. perfringens*, is a spore-forming bacillus and can easily be passed via contaminated cutting instruments. They should remain in this solution several hours. After disinfection, instruments should be rinsed, dried, and properly stored (Fig. 15–11).

Personal Hygiene

Terminal disinfection also applies to the embalmer. **Destroy** gloves after use; gloves are made to be used **once.** Thoroughly wash hands after removing gloves. Keep fingernails short and trimmed to prevent tears in the gloves. Numerous antiseptic preparations are available for washing or applying to the skin after the hands are dried. Consult a hospital-supply catalog. Treat all cuts and punctures immediately: disinfect the area, induce bleeding, and consult a physician. (Review Chapter 3 for preembalming and postembalming sanitation techniques.)

Figure 15–11. Containers of sufficient size must be provided so all instruments can be completely immersed for disinfection.

▶ DOCUMENTATION AND SHIPPING PREPARATION

An **embalming care report** needs to be completed for each deceased embalmed by a funeral facility. The report should contain information pertaining to the preembalming conditions of the deceased and to all personal properties received with the body. Particular attention should be made to the list of jewelry and clothing. The report needs to contain all treatments performed at the funeral facility.

A report needs to accompany all bodies being prepared and shipped to another funeral facility. When the body has been autopsied and is being shipped, the report should contain information indicating if viscera were returned from the hospital or morgue. Organs and tissues removed at autopsy or for donation must be noted, especially if the eyes have been removed. If the viscera were returned from the hospital and replaced in the body cavities, note how the organs were preserved and note that they have been placed in the cavities. Bodies should never be shipped without some partial dressing. Place plastic coveralls or pants and undergarments on the body. If undergarments are not provided, clothe the body in pajamas or a hospital gown.

When positioning instructions have **not** been given by the receiving funeral home, make certain one of the hands is **not** placed over the other. Hands should be placed on the abdomen. Resting one on top of another (which is a custom in many communities) can mark the covered hand.

A very light coating of massage cream can be placed on the face and hands when the body is to be shipped. Large amounts are not necessary and may be difficult to remove even with a solvent.

If instructions have not been given by the receiving funeral home, many embalmers do **not** seal the mouth when the body is being shipped. The lips are coated with massage cream. This allows the receiving funeral home an opportunity to be certain the mouth is dry, allows any gases created by the movement of the shipping of the body to escape from the mouth, and permits tissue building to be done from inside the mouth. The body will be reaspirated by the receiving funeral home; any reconstruction work will be performed by them.

▶ MONITORING: SURVEILLANCE OF THE CASKETED REMAINS UNTIL DISPOSITION

It is the duty of the funeral establishment having custody of the remains (either casketed or waiting to be casketed or to be shipped uncasketed) during the postembalming period to observe the appearance of the body and to correct any problems that might arise.

Detailed examinations should be made before and after each visitation period. Likewise, uncasketed remains should be daily inspected for any changes.

Postembalming problems include, but are not limited to, dehydration of tissues, purge, leakage from incisions (embalming or antemortem surgical), leakage from any antemortem invasive treatments, softening and discoloring of tissues, gas formation, separation of lips or eyelids, leakage from areas where edema is present, odors, maggots, and needed cosmetic changes. If any of these conditions are noted, immediate steps should be taken to make a correction.

Cosmetic Corrections
Areas of the face, neck, hands, or arms may reveal color changes in the skin. The causes include greening of tissues affected by jaundice, darkening of the skin due to dehydration, darkening of the skin due to insufficient preservation of the area, and darkening from minor trauma. Where softening of the skin or darkening from trauma or ecchymosis has occurred, the area should first be treated by hypodermic injection of undiluted cavity fluid or application of a surface compress. (It needs to remain in contact with the skin for several hours.) These areas and dehydrated areas can be covered with a variety of opaque cosmetic "undercoats"; an adjustment can easily be made with cream cosmetics.

Separated Tissues
Tissues such as the lips and eyelids may separate due to dehydration, improper gluing, or motion and handling if the body has been shipped. These tissues should be "exercised" to establish good contact. The contact surfaces should be cleaned with a good solvent and a super adhesive applied. Lips may also be "filled out" with tissue builder to establish contact of the surfaces or they may be waxed.

Leakage
Potential areas of leakage could include some of the following:

- Any area of trauma to the face or hands where the skin was broken or torn
- Cranial autopsy incisions
- Autopsy sutures
- Surgical sutures
- Sutures at sites where vessels were raised for arterial injection
- Areas where edema is present
- Intravenous punctures
- Punctures used for drawing postmortem blood samples
- Any point where the skin has been broken

Minor seepage (e.g., intravenous puncture) maybe corrected by wiping away the accumulated liquid, injecting a phenol compound to cauterize the area, and sealing the puncture with a super adhesive. Where the skin has been torn, a phenol compound surface compress (or a cavity fluid compress) can be applied; later the area can be cleaned with a solvent, dried with a hair dryer, and sealed with a super adhesive or surface glue.

Clothing can be protected by sheets of plastic. The casket interior, pillow, and clothing should be inspected for any signs of leakage. If leakage is judged severe, the body should be removed from the casket and carefully undressed. Incisions can be opened, dried, checked to be certain vessels are ligated, and resutured using large amounts of incision seal powder within the incisions. Plastic garments can be placed on the body and, if necessary, edges sealed with duct tape. Interior damage may be severe enough to require replacement. Casket pillows can be reversed for minor leakage. Blankets and clothing may need to be replaced.

Purge
If purge has occurred, it will be necessary to reaspirate the body. No doubt the body will have to be taken back to the preparation room for this procedure. Not only should the body be thoroughly reaspirated, but the cavities should also be reinjected with undiluted cavity fluid. If gases were noted when the trocar button was removed, leave the body in the preparation room, if possible, for several hours and repeat the treatments again before redressing the body. The mouth and nasal cavities should be checked for dryness and tightly repacked with cotton or cotton webbing. The lips can then be resealed and recosmetized. Distended eyelids may indicate the presence of gases in the tissues. It may be necessary with this condition to aspirate the cranial cavity and inject some

cavity fluid into the anterior cranial cavity. The presence of true tissue gas may necessitate reembalming of the body.

Maggots

Infestation of the body with maggots is a nightmare experienced by few embalmers today. In the summer months, bodies should be carefully examined for fly eggs, in particular the corners of the eyes, within the mouth, and the nostrils. If maggots are present, they can be picked from the surface of the body with cotton saturated with a hydrocarbon solvent. To stimulate maggots to emerge to the surface from areas beneath the skin or from the mouth or nostrils, the areas can be swabbed with a petroleum product. (Kerosene has been used by many embalmers, but its use is not recommended.) As the maggots emerge on the skin surface, they can be removed with cotton saturated with a hydrocarbon solvent. They should be placed in plastic bags before being discarded. The problem with maggots is not known if all have been found. If they persist, it may become necessary to close the casket. Maggots in the clothing and hair can be vacuumed with a suction vacuum. The dust bag then can be destroyed.

Mold

In warm climates, mold can be a problem when bodies are being held for long periods. Bodies should be thoroughly dried to discourage mold growth. Mold needs to be carefully removed with a scalpel or spatula. The area is then swabbed with a phenol compound chemical and later thoroughly dried before cosmetics are applied. Placing embalming powder inside plastic coveralls, pants, and/or stockings helps to control mold growth.

▶ CONCEPTS FOR STUDY AND DISCUSSION

1. You own your own funeral home—make a list of the various plastic garments you need to stock.
2. Describe a body area that is well embalmed.
3. Describe a body area that has not received any arterial solution.
4. Describe a postembalming treatment for a large decubitus ulcer of the buttocks.
5. Give a detailed description of your treatment for a leg that is gangrenous from the knee down and including the foot.

▶ BIBLIOGRAPHY

Grant ME. Chronological order of events in embalming. In: *Champion Expanding Encyclopedia*, No. 571. Springfield, OH: Champion Chemical Co., October 1986.

Venes D. Taber's Cyclopedic Medical Dictionary, 19th ed. Philadelphia: F.A. Davis, 2001.

CHAPTER 16

GENERAL BODY CONSIDERATIONS

CHAPTER OBJECTIVES

▶ Embalming analysis—age of deceased
▶ Preparation of the stillborn, infant and child
▶ Preparation of persons of advanced age
▶ Disease considerations with advanced age

This chapter addresses some of the problems encountered in the preparation of bodies of different age groups. Many factors other than **age** influence preparation techniques. Size and weight of the body, cause of death, moisture conditions in the body, postmortem changes, and discolorations are a few of these other factors which must be considered in the preembalming analysis.

A factor that must always be considered in the preembalming analysis of a body is **age**. Embalmers often think only of the extremes—the techniques that will be used in the preparation of children as compared with those used for adults. If age is taken into careful consideration as a factor influencing embalming technique, four categories become evident.

Infant to child	Birth to approximately age 4
Child to young adult	Approximately age 4 to 12
Young adult to adult	Approximately age 12 to mid-seventies
Old age	Mid-seventies to late nineties

Not only does age influence the techniques used in the embalming process but age also leads the embalmer to expect certain difficulties and conditions with respect to positioning, setting of features, sites for injection and drainage, strength and volume of embalming solution, and injection pressure and rate of flow.

FACTORS DETERMINED IN THE EMBALMING ANALYSIS

1. Vessels for injection and drainage
2. Method of mouth closure
3. Strength of the embalming solution
4. Volume of the embalming solution
5. Injection pressure
6. Injection rate of flow

Note: These factors will vary by the individual body. Several of these factors can also vary in different areas of the same body.

The hands and the head of an infant are positioned differently than those of the adult. Elderly persons may present positioning problems if arthritic conditions are present. Methods of mouth closure in adults and infants differ because the bones of the infant have not yet ossified. In old age the mandible and maxillae may have undergone degenerative changes to the point where a needle injector cannot be used and the mouth must be sutured closed.

The embalmer should not stereotype bodies by age. For example, not all elderly persons are thin-skinned, emaciated, and toothless. Many very elderly persons were in excellent health. Their blood vessels are free of sclerosis and they may have a normal or above-normal weight, good musculature, and excellent teeth. Likewise, not every middle-aged adult will have vessels free of sclerosis, good teeth, good muscular build, and normal weight.

Even in children, it is not always the rule that small quantities of a mild-strength arterial fluid should be used. Many children die from diseases that produced edema or show evidence of advanced postmortem changes. In these cases, seemingly large volumes of strong arterial solutions are needed.

Everybody must be individually judged in making a pre-embalming analysis.

▶ INFANTS AND CHILDREN—GENERAL CONSIDERATIONS

Infants and children require the use of several definite techniques that vary from those used in an adult or very elderly person. As defined in pediatric medicine, the infant period ranges from birth to 18 months and the toddler period from 18 to 48 months. Obviously there are considerable variations in both total weight and development between individuals in these classifications.

In embalming infants, it is important to realize the relationship of body water to body fat. Both contribute to total body weight. At birth, body water is approximately 75% of total body weight. At 1 year of age the body water declines to approximately the normal adult level of 60% of total body weight. It is therefore easy to understand the need for special embalming care for infants.

Similarly, body fat in the new born is approximately 12% of total body weight and normally doubles to 25% at 6 months of age and then increases to approximately 30% at age 1.

Infant skin is much more delicate than adult skin and can easily distend and wrinkle on injection of the arterial solution. The vessels in the infant are extremely small but should be free of sclerosis. Most infants are autopsied, but infants dead from birth defects and systemic disease may not be autopsied. **The embalmer needs to be familiar with the preparation of both autopsied and unautopsied infants.**

The embalmer must have arterial tubes available for embalming infants. These tubes should be cleaned thoroughly after each use because they clog easily. They should always be tested prior to use to be certain they are in working order.

The infant body normally contains a large amount of moisture. In addition to this moisture, disease processes and medications can further increase moisture in the body. Renal and liver failure can bring about the accumulation of toxic wastes in the blood and the tissues. This moisture and the toxic wastes can greatly increase the preservative demand of the body. It is suggested that the embalmer **not** uses preinjection as the preservative solution for embalming infants. Many of these small bodies do not demand as much volume of preservative solution as an adolescent or adult, but they can require an arterial solution strength similar to that used for an adult body. **Use standard arterial and supplemental fluids.**

Certain factors characterize the different cases encountered in the embalming of infants and children:

1. Autopsied bodies; refrigerated and un-refrigerated:
   a. Complete autopsy: cranial, thoracic, and abdominal cavities, spinal autopsy, limbs examined.
   b. Partial autopsy: examination of only cranial, thoracic, or abdominal cavity, spine, or limbs.
   c. Organ examination only: removal of only one organ.
2. Unautopsied bodies; refrigerated and un-refrigerated.
3. Organ donors: removal of eyes and/or any of the visceral organs or skin that may be used for transplantation.
4. Infants whose embalming has been delayed but who have been neither refrigerated nor frozen.
5. Infants that require restorative treatments (these bodies may or may not be autopsied).
6. Fetuses:
   a. Premature infants: referred to as "preterm" in pediatric medicine today, any infant weighing less than five-and-half pounds at birth or born prior to the end of the 37th week of gestation.
   b. Stillborn: fetus that dies prior to delivery from the uterus. (In many states the definition of a stillborn includes a specified number of weeks of gestation, and if that specified time has passed, a death certificate and burial permit are required.)

▶ EMBALMING THE INFANT

All treatment should begin with topical disinfection followed by a washing of the body with good soap and water, cleaning of the nasal, oral, and orbital areas, and gentle extension and manipulation of the head and the extremities to relieve any rigor mortis. Intravenous tubes or any other invasive connections to the arterial or venous systems should be left in place and removed **after** arterial injection. Tracheotomy tubes or any tubing placed into the mouth or nose should be removed **prior to** arterial injection.

After washing and drying of the infant, the body is placed on a towel. The towel will help to position the infant. It can be gathered to hold the head in a proper position. It remains in place during the embalming–after embalming it can be replaced with a clean dry towel.

Eye Closure

Eye caps may be "cut down" and inserted under the lids, or cotton pads can be placed under the lids to effect closure. After embalming, the lids may be glued with rubber-based glue or affixed with superglue. Most embalmers close the eyes prior to arterial embalming, but it should be pointed out that closure can also be done after arterial preparation. In addition, some embalmers prefer to cover eye caps or the cotton with a thin film of massage cream. Care should be taken when using massage cream that the free margins of the eyelids are cleaned with a solvent if the lids are to be glued.

Mouth Closure

In the infant, the needle injector method of closure is may not be possible; however, in an older child this method can easily be used. In the infant, a muscular suture can be used (passing the needle for the suture just in front of the mandible). The suture is completed by passing the needle through the septum of the nose. As the mandible and maxillae are very soft in the infant, closure can also be made by passing a sharp three-eighths–inch circle needle directly through the mandible. The needle can then be passed either through the septum of the nose or directly through the maxillae.

In some small infants the embalmer may wish to use a rubber-based adhesive prior to embalming as a method of closure rather than suturing. After embalming, the mouth can again be cleaned and reglued with a rubber-based glue or super adhesive. Depending on the customs of the community, some embalmers leave the mouth of an infant open. When this is done, massage cream should be placed on the tongue and the walls of the mouth. The corners of the mouth can be glued.

It may be difficult to create a good line of mouth closure in an infant. Use of a thick adhesive emollient cream may help to hold the lips in position. The mouth is generally glued **after** arterial and cavity embalming because air from the lungs can become trapped in the mouth. If gluing is necessary before embalming, use of a rubber-based glue is advised, as the mouth can easily be reopened by the use of a solvent or by reapplication of glue. (The glue acts as its own solvent.) After embalming, a surface coating of mortuary wax may need to be applied to one or both lips to obtain a natural looking line of closure.

Positioning

The position of the arms and head can vary considerably. Generally, the funeral home will have a policy. In some cases the arms are arranged along the sides of the trunk, and forearms and hands are placed on the body, barely touching, so as to encircle or clasp a toy, or stuffed animal.

The head may be so placed that it rests on its side (the right cheek area) or, like an adult, is slightly turned to the right. As it may be impossible to use a head block, pads of cotton or towels can be used. The infant body can firm as strongly as that of the adult. Changes in position can be difficult in the casket. Attention should also be given to the positioning of the legs. Often, the legs are visible during viewing of the infant. If the legs are flexed, they may be straightened by wrapping them with strips of sheeting during the injection of arterial solution.

Blood Vessel Selection: Unautopsied Infants

Common Carotid Artery. All arteries should be usable; size is the varying factor. The common carotid is the largest. It is easily accessible and very shallow. This artery is accompanied by a large vein—internal jugular vein—and affords excellent drainage. Placing support under the shoulders helps to elevate this neck area. Dropping the head backward brings the vessels closer to the surface. Keep in mind that the thymus gland can be quite large in the infant. Turn the head in the direction **opposite** that of the vessel being raised (i.e., to raise the right common carotid turn the head to the left). Place a horizontal incision in one of the horizontal neck wrinkles present in most infants. Later, a super adhesive, a subcutaneous suture, or an inversion (worm) suture can be employed to close the incision. If, because of damage, it is not possible to drain from the right jugular vein, raise and attempt to take drainage from the left internal jugular vein (Fig. 16–1).

Femoral (External Iliac) Artery. The second largest nonaortic vessel that can be used is either the external iliac artery or the femoral artery. The external iliac is slightly larger than the femoral. The same incisions can be used to raise these vessels as are used to raise the vessels of an adult. The accompanying veins are relatively large and may be used as points of drainage. If a small drain tube is not available, these veins can be expanded by inserting a small pair of forceps into the vessels. **Always inject the distal leg first.** This allows the embalmer to observe the effects of the fluid solution on the skin of the leg and to determine if too much or too little fluid dye has been used. If drainage is difficult to establish from the femoral location, the right internal jugular vein can be raised and used as a drainage point.

Use of the axillary vessels is **not** advised in the preparation of the unautopsied infant. The vessel is too small for efficient use, and establishing drainage may be very difficult. In the autopsied infant, however, it may be necessary to inject this vessel. If possible, the embalmer

A

B

Figure 16–1. Unautopsied infant, arterial embalming using restricted cervical injection. **A.** Restricted cervical injection using the right and left common carotid arteries and the right internal jugular vein for drainage. **B.** Completed arterial injection of infant. Note the sutured parallel incision injection sites. **C.** Arms held in temporary position, with soft cloth ties, prior to dressing and casketing.

C

should try to use the larger subclavian artery for arterial injection of the arm.

Abdominal Aorta. The abdominal aorta is a large artery and is accompanied by the largest vein that could be used for drainage. The artery and the vein are deep seated, resting on the anterior surface of the spine. A 2- to 3-in incision can be made just to the left of the midline in the middle of the abdomen, and inferior enough to avoid the liver, which is very large in the infant. The greater omentum must be opened and some of the small and large intestines either held away from the spine or removed from the cavity during arterial injection. The aorta is held in position by its parietal branches (the four pairs of lumbar arteries in particular). Once located, the aorta can be opened and a tube is placed in the direction of the legs and another tube in the direction of the upper portions of the body. The vein can be opened and the blood is allowed to drain into the cavity. It is not necessary to place a drainage instrument into the vein. The lower portion of the body should be injected first, then the upper portion. During injection the viscera can

greatly expand. The viscera can be clipped and drained prior to return to the cavity (Fig. 16–2).

Ascending Aorta. In a variant technique involving the aorta as a primary injection point, the ascending aorta is used. Drainage can be taken from the right auricle of the heart (the small ear-like appendage (right auricle) of the right atrium of the heart). Simply, clip the auricle open.

An incision can be made directly down the midline of the sternum. Because this bone is not ossified but is actually cartilage, a sharp scalpel or strong surgical shears can be used to make this incision. The difficulty is that the incision must be held open with some form of retraction. A 2-in block can be placed in the spread incision to hold it open and to allow the embalmer to work. A second incision, a U-shaped one, is made straight down from the mid-clavicle to the bottom of the rib cage, where it makes a right angle across the inferior margin of the sternum to a point identical to the original mid-clavicle incision. From this point, the cut is directed upward to the mid-clavicle position. The skin is then dissected upward, thus disclosing the sternum,

Figure 16–2. Preparation of an infant using the abdominal aorta. **A.** The incision is made to the left of the midline to raise the abdominal aorta. **B.** The abdominal aorta is exposed. Note that the small intestine has been carefully pulled out and set to the right. The small intestine is lifted out during the injection. These should not be severed. **C.** Viscera are treated after injection. **D.** Plastic is placed over the incision after preparation.

which is then opened by severing the sternal cartilage at its junction with the ribs.

When the sternum is severed free of its lateral attachments it can be bent upward toward the head. With this incision, the internal thoracic arteries may need to be clamped during arterial injection. Once the incision has been made and the pericardium has been exposed, the embalmer must cut open the pericardium and expose the heart and the great vessels (Fig. 16–3). The ascending aorta is observed as it rises from the left ven-

tricle of the heart. It can be opened, or an opening can be made in the arch of the aorta and an arterial tube is inserted. The entire body can be embalmed from this one point.

Be certain permission for embalming should be obtained— especially when using any portion of the aorta artery of the unautopsied infant. The use of any portion of the aorta for injection is very invasive. It may be wise to outline the process for the arranging party, simply because an autopsy was not authorized by the family.

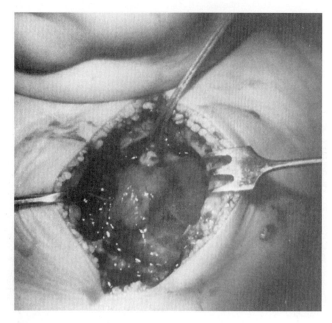

Figure 16–3. The pericardium is opened. Note the string around the ascending aorta. The right auricle is in the center; it will be incised and used for drainage.

Infant Cavity Treatment

For aspirating and injecting the unautopsied infant, use an infant trocar. These trocars are generally approximately 12 in in length with an inside diameter of at least one-fourth inch. The standard trocar point of entry or a lower point, such as the right or the left inguinal abdominal area, may be used.

Cavity embalming may either immediately follow arterial injection or be delayed for several hours. Injection of an undiluted cavity chemical follows aspiration. The amount of cavity chemical depends on the size of the infant. The trocar point of entry can be closed by suture or the trocar button. Reaspiration several hours later is recommended.

Preparation of the Autopsied Infant

The embalmer should prepare autopsied infants by arterial injection, which produces very satisfactory results. Although this process maybe very time consuming, every attempt should be made to effect complete arterial distribution of embalming fluid. Those areas not reached by arterial injection can be treated by hypodermic or surface embalming.

The proportion of infants autopsied in some large hospitals in major cities approaches 70% or more. In these communities, autopsies of infants by coroners or medical examiners may approach 100%.

Four types of autopsies are performed on infants:

- *Complete autopsy:* Cranial and trunk cavities are opened and viscera removed.

- *Partial autopsy:* Only one cavity is opened (cranial, thoracic, abdominal, or spine).
- *Special or local autopsy:* Only one organ is removed or a special examination is made of the route of blood vessels or nerves.
- *Organ donor:* The heart, heart/lungs, liver, kidneys, may be removed as in the adult, and these donations can be treated as partial autopsies.
- *Tissue donor:* Cornea, whole eye, skin, and bones constitute tissues that may be removed for transplant purposes.

When viscera are removed in the autopsy, they may or may not be returned with the body. Generally, any viscera removed by a coroner or a medical examiner are returned with the body. With hospital autopsies, the viscera are not always returned.*

Blood Vessel Selection: Autopsied Infants

Neither the common carotid, common iliac, or external iliac arteries nor their accompanying veins, the iliac and internal jugular, of the adult and infant vary greatly except in **size**. If the autopsy pathologist has left vessels of reasonable length, the difficulty encountered is no greater than when working with an adult. If the vessels are severed excessively short (iliacs at the inguinal ligament, carotids at thyroid cartilage), considerable extensive dissection will be required to locate the vessels and to ligate arterial tubes within them. In lieu of string for ligation, an arterial tube hemostat may be helpful. Do not attempt to locate veins. Drainage can be taken without the use of any instruments. Arteries remain open when cut, this can often help in locating the tiny arteries.

If the iliac arteries cannot be located or if they are too small for the arterial tubes, supplemental methods of embalming can be used to preserve the legs. Hypodermic treatment with long large-gauge needles can be employed. Painting the surface of the legs with an autopsy gel and wrapping the painted limbs in plastic could serve to embalm the limbs. When the carotid arteries are missing the embalmer can place cotton saturated with cavity fluid in the mouth and under the eyelids. With a diluted cavity fluid, deep hypodermic treatment can be made from inside the mouth, from the scalp incisions of the autopsy, and from the opened neck areas of the autopsy. If arterial fluid is going to be injected hypodermically, one with little dye should be used. The dye can create blotches of color as the fluid spreads through the facial tissues. Likewise, the face can be painted with autopsy gel and covered with plastic for several hours. This treatment often bleaches the skin, and corrective cosmetics will be needed. The inside of the scalp and

---

*Refer to Chapter 17 for treatment of viscera.

the base of the cranial cavity can also be painted with autopsy gel.

Subclavian arteries can be located at the usual adult site. If they have been cut short, the axillary artery can be raised at its largest point, as the artery passes into the axilla just at the lateral border of the first rib. To reach the axillary at this point it may be necessary to dissect the pectoralis major and minor muscles. Some embalmers prefer to raise the subclavian artery by elevating the clavicle bones. This exposes the subclavian arteries where they have been severed. An arterial hemostat may be more useful than string ties in securing the arterial tube.

Autopsied Infant: Instruments and Chemicals

Very small arterial tubes are necessary for the preparation of the infant. Infant tubes are approximately $\frac{1}{16}$ to 3.32 in in diameter. These tubes need to be cleaned after each use and should be tested to be certain they are clean and working before being inserted into an artery. **A small arterial-venous catheter may serve as an arterial injection tube.**

There are many suggested chemical combinations, strengths, and dilutions for infant arterial embalming. A false theory is that infants must always be embalmed with very dilute low-index arterial fluids. Infant body tissue contains a higher percentage of water than adult body tissue. In addition, disease processes and drugs may have increased tissue moisture and toxic wastes. It may be necessary to use solution strengths similar to those used for adult bodies. Harsh tissue reactions may be reduced by the addition of supplemental fluids such as humectants and coinjection chemicals or the use of arterial fluids, which contain large amounts of humectants. Some fluid companies even have arterial fluids designed for infants and children. Guidelines for fluid use are provided by the manufacturers. A small amount of fluid dye to add color to the tissues is recommended.

In the autopsied body, the legs are embalmed before the head or the arms. This allows the embalmer to adjust the fluid strengths and the dyes.

The volume to be injected is best determined per case based on the embalming analysis. Intravascular blood discolorations should be cleared and the fluid dyes must appear uniform throughout the tissues. Generally, the tissues may plump slightly. Massage is usually necessary to assist the distribution of the fluid. Pinching the fingertips and the lips helps to clear these areas of blood discolorations. If the eyelids wrinkle after discolorations have cleared, it is recommended that injection be stopped. If any swelling occurs, the arterial solution can be strengthened and only a minimum amount should be injected. (**Weak** arterial solutions easily distend tissues, another reason to use arterial solution at a strength close to that used in the adult.) Conditions of the autopsied infant will dictate strength and quantity of the arterial solution. In general, where no abnormal conditions exist, an infant can be embalmed using one-half to three-fourths gallon of arterial solution made by mixing 6 to 10 oz of an arterial fluid ranging in strength from 18 to 25 index to make a gallon of solution.

Autopsied Infant: Treatment of Areas Not Reached by Arterial Injection

Hypodermic Injection. The head may be injected hypodermically from within an incised neck area or natural openings (mouth and nostrils) or an incised scalp area; arms and legs may be injected from within the open trunk cavity.

In larger children this may entail injection of the arm from the point of insertion of the hypodermic needle or trocar from the antecubital fossa upward toward the shoulder, and then utilizing the same point of insertion, down toward the fingers. The puncture incision is closed with a drop of super glue.

The legs may similarly be injected by inserting the hypodermic needle or infant-trocar from a point: (1) within the abdominal cavity or (2) on the inner aspect of the knee area. All areas of the lower extremities need to be reached with preservative. The point of insertion, if made at the knee, may be sutured closed or closed with superglue. Diluted cavity fluid can be used for injection. Cosmetic arterial fluid should not be used.

Internal Compresses. Internal compresses, referred to as inlays, are cotton or sheeting (well dampened with cavity fluid) inserted into such areas as the interior of the neck, the cranium, and the trunk cavity, when devoid of viscera. Internal packs can also be inserted under the pectoral chest flaps (over the sternum) before trunk incision closure. Autopsy gel can be used in lieu of cavity fluid. Some embalmers will dissect the sidewalls free of the rib cage as deep as the spinal column; into this space they will either paint the exposed tissues with a gel preservative or place inlays of cotton saturated with cavity fluid.

Preservative Gels. Preservative gels are semisolid chemicals that are painted over the calvarium as well as under the anterior chest and abdominal skin flaps before skin suturing. They may also be painted on the skin surface where preservation is needed. The painted areas need to be covered with cotton or plastic to prevent evaporation and release of fumes.

External Compresses. Cotton saturated with undiluted cavity fluid or a topical preservative may be used to preserve areas as small as the ears or, in other cases, the entire body. Compresses should be left in place long enough to accomplish complete preservation. These compresses need to be covered with a thin plastic covering to prevent their evaporation and release of fumes into the air.

Autopsied Infant: Treatment of the Trunk Walls

The back, the shoulders, the trunk walls, and the buttocks, and the scrotum and the penis of the male may require additional chemical treatments for preservation. An infant trocar, a large-diameter hypodermic needle, or a straight long arterial tube can be used to inject these areas with a strong chemical solution. This solution is injected either through the embalming machine or with a large hypodermic syringe. In addition, the inside walls may be treated with autopsy gel or embalming powder. If the viscera are not returned, cavities can be filled with sheeting saturated with cavity fluid.

Autopsied Infant: Viscera Treatments

The viscera of the autopsied body may be immersed in undiluted cavity fluid. Some prefer to place the viscera and the cavity fluid together within a plastic bag and then, later, place the plastic-encased viscera in the abdominal and thoracic cavities. The organs should be clipped and freed of gases after the addition of cavity fluid. It is also recommended that the cavity fluid not be added until the bag of viscera has been positioned within the body cavity. Some embalmers also prefer to make a cut in the thick solid organs (e.g., lungs and liver) to ensure contact with the cavity fluid.

Autopsied Infant: Closure of Cavities

In small infants the scalp has been opened by the usual transverse incision from ear to ear. Access to the floor of the cranial cavity would have been necessary to control leakage from the internal carotids and, possibly, the vertebral or basilar arteries during arterial injection. The scalp should be reflected and the floor of the cavity should be dried. The walls of the cranial vault can be liberally coated with autopsy gel, and the inside surface of the reflected scalp can likewise be coated with a preservative gel. To repair the area, a quantity of cotton may be used to fill the cranial cavity and to reproduce the normal contours as well as act as an absorbent for seepage. The scalp is drawn back to its normal position, and then carefully sutured.

When the fontanelles are still present, it may be helpful to fill the cranial cavity with cotton. With dental floss and a three-eighth–inch circle needle, the soft cranial bones are sutured together. The fontanelle areas can be filled with "mortuary putty." If this is not available, the cranial cavity must be tightly filled with cotton. If the cavity is not tightly filled, sunken areas may be noticed at the locations of the fontanelles. Many embalmers do not want the scalp to rest on the cotton at the fontanelles, so they coat the cotton with massage cream. This prevents the dehydration of the scalp around the fontanelles.

For the scalp, suturing begins on the right side of the cranium and ends on the left side. The inversion (worm) suture is excellent for infants. It helps to tighten the scalp. When the autopsy incision has been made high on the head and the hair is very thin, funeral director recommends that a bonnet be used. Most hospitals make these incisions low enough that the sutured incisions can be hidden by the pillow. Super adhesive can provide a closure that is not easily detected. If the embalmer prefers, a small baseball or intradermal suture using dental floss or thin suture may also be used for closure.

In infants in whom the bones of the cranium are well calcified and the calvarium has been removed as in an adult case, the same procedure used for such repair in the adult is recommended.

If the temporalis muscles have been cut from the cranium or calvarium, the area can easily be filled in with "mortuary putty" to prevent a sunken appearance. Tissue building of the temple is not possible if the muscular tissue has been removed. When the calvarium has not been "notched" it may be very difficult to maintain the calvarium in correct position during and after suturing. Calvarium clamps can be used to hold the calvarium in place. As the bones are not completely ossified, small holes can easily be made on either side of the calvarium and the calvarium is wired into proper position.

The abdominal, thoracic, and pelvic cavities should be coated with autopsy gel or a preservative absorbent powder, following aspiration and drying of the cavities. If neck organs have been removed the neck area should be filled with cotton and saturated with a preservative such as cavity fluid. The trunk cavities should be filled with an absorbent material and also saturated with a preservative chemical. The breast plate should be laid into proper position (and if necessary anchored with sutures); paper toweling can be laid over the plate and saturated with preservative chemical. The skin flaps are tacked together to ensure proper alignment. Suturing is begun at the pubic symphysis and directed upward; a small baseball suture provides a good closure. The body is bathed and the skin surfaces are thoroughly dried. The sutures may be coated with a surface sealer glue. The trunk area can be covered with a thin sheet of plastic to ensure protection of the clothing.

Premature Infants

Although many premature infants are autopsied and may be extremely small (less than 1 lb), there may exist a need to preserve them temporarily for funeral, burial, or cremation services.

If the premature infant has not been autopsied, arterial injection may be attempted by injection of the carotid artery followed by cavity aspiration and injection of a small amount of cavity fluid. Injection of the arterial umbilical vessel has occasionally been advocated, but the difficulty in identifying the artery from the other two veins as well as the poor results obtained when the proper vessel is injected make this procedure unattractive. Other large vessels that could be injection sites are the abdominal aorta, the ascending aorta, and the arch of the aorta.

External compresses may constitute the easiest treatment. The premature infant is wrapped in cotton saturated with cavity fluid or painted with autopsy gel.

The limbs, the trunk cavity and walls, and the head can be injected hypodermically with a strong concentration of preservative chemicals. Cavity treatment and external compresses may be applied as necessary.

▶ EMBALMING THE 4- TO 12 YEAR OLD

The second age group relative to embalming ranges from approximately 4 to 12 years. Although the special techniques used for the infant or the aged are not required, some difficulties may be encountered because of the body size.

Vessel Selection

The vessels in this age group should be healthy and much larger than those of the infant, but still smaller than those of the adult. The two major injection sites used in embalming the adult are also used for embalming the child: (1) the common carotid artery and the internal jugular vein and (2) the femoral artery and femoral vein. There is no need to consider use of the abdominal aorta or the arch of the aorta in this age group. Likewise, the many disadvantages of the axillary artery and vein do not make this a good primary injection site. Many in this age group are autopsied, so most of the embalming is done from the primary autopsy sites—right and left common carotid, right and left external and internal iliac, and right and left subclavian arteries.

In the unautopsied body, the right internal jugular vein is the largest vein that can be used for drainage. It also affords direct access to the right atrium of the heart. Whenever facial blood discolorations are present, this vein affords the best possible clearing of the facial tissues.

Some embalmers prefer the femoral vessels for this age group strictly because their location permits the use of clothing that can be opened at the neck. The possibility of leakage or visibility of the carotid incision should be of little concern if properly prepared, sutured, and sealed.

In this age group (4–12 years), if there has been any trauma to the face or head or if there has been a long delay between death and preparation, the facial tissues may swell during injection. The best control over fluid flow into the head and the face is obtained by the use of restricted cervical injection.

The arteries of children in this age group should all be in excellent condition with no evidence of arteriosclerosis.

FACTORS DETERMINED IN THE EMBALMING ANALYSIS

1. Vessels for injection and drainage
2. Method of mouth closure
3. Strength of the embalming solution
4. Volume of the embalming solution
5. Injection pressure
6. Injection rate of flow

Note: These factors will vary from body to body; or vary within different areas of the same body.

Fluid Strengths and Volume

Fluid strength is determined by the condition of the body. As 4- to 12 year olds have more delicate skin than adults, for routine embalming, a medium-index fluid in the range 18 to 25 is most satisfactory. Dilutions should follow those recommended by the manufacturer. Two schools of thought exist as to embalming solution strengths: the first is to use one mixture strength throughout the entire operation; the second is to begin the injection with a mild solution but following the clearing of intravascular blood discolorations to gradually strengthen the solution. Supplemental chemicals may be used to control harsh reactions of the embalming chemicals. Dye can always be used for its cosmetic effect and to indicate the distribution of arterial solution. In these bodies, however, dyes should be kept to a minimum for, no doubt, cosmetic application will be minimized to produce the most natural appearance.

In cases of trauma and the effects of diseases, such as edema and renal failure, appropriate fluid strengths should be used and, if necessary, special-purpose high-index fluids.

Four- to 12 year olds require a smaller volume of fluid than adults, but a greater volume than that used for infants. Intravascular blood discolorations should have cleared, some firming of the tissues should be present, and there should be evidence of good distribution as indicated by the presence of dye. All of these indicators help to establish the volume of the fluid to be injected.

In this age group, the causes of death include infectious and contagious diseases (e.g., meningitis and pneumonia), childhood viral diseases, and systemic diseases (e.g., leukemia and cystic fibrosis). When contagious or infectious disease is the cause of the death, the arterial solution strength should be of sufficient strength to sanitize the body tissues without any noticeable effect on the appearance of the body. A thorough aspiration of the cavities is necessary, followed by injection of sufficient concentrated cavity fluid to reach all areas of the cavities. Reaspiration and reinjection of the cavities may be necessary.

Pressure and Rate of Flow of Injection

The rate of flow should be a greater concern than pressure to the embalmer, especially in embalming a child. If arterial solution is injected too quickly into the body, the tissues may distend. Injection must be slow enough that the drainage can be restricted at times during the injection. This helps to prevent a loss of the solution through low-resistance paths, especially those vessel connections located near the injection site.

Sufficient force is necessary to establish good distribution, especially in distal body areas such as the hands and the feet. By the use of intermittent drainage, short-circuiting of solution is reduced and retention of solution is increased. Rapid injection with continuous drainage often has the tendency to remove moisture from a child's tissues. This could lead to wrinkling of the skin. A sufficient pressure and rate of flow should be used to achieve a uniform distribution of the solution.

Setting of Features and Positioning

Positioning of the child is similar to that of the adult. The arms can be a little more "relaxed" than those of the adult and, generally, are placed straighter (Fig. 16–4). The head should be slightly tilted to the right.

Facial hair must be removed for good cosmetic treatment. Some drugs stimulate the growth of facial

Figure 16–4. Positioning of the child. Note that the arms are placed at the sides.

hair, and this hair can easily be removed with shaving lather and a sharp razor. It is best not to attempt to shave the forehead.

Mouth closure may pose some difficulty if the child has buck teeth or is wearing braces. For buck teeth, place a small layer of cotton over the **lower** teeth and gum. This helps to push the lower lip forward. The lips can now be glued together with a rubber-based glue prior to arterial injection (Fig. 16–5). Some embalmers prefer to inject the body with the lips slightly parted. This allows the tissues of the lips to "round out." The super adhesives can assist, after injection, with difficult closures.

► EMBALMING THE ADOLESCENT AND THE ADULT

For embalming purposes, the adolescent/adult group comprises persons from 13 to approximately 75 years of age. As in all age categories, individual variations and exceptions exist. Because this age group is characterized by average body conditions for which average embalming treatments are practiced, embalming of the "routine" or "normal" body is outlined. For the beginning practitioner, this overview is suggested in an outline of the step-by-step preparation of the unautopsied or autopsied body (see Chapter 1).

Causes of death in this group include heart disease, malignancies, and accidents. It is important that the embalmer should remember that age is only one factor in the embalming analysis. Other factors are time between death and preparation, progress of decomposition, moisture content, discolorations, condition of the blood vascular system, protein and nutritional condition, traumatic or surgical considerations, time between preparation and disposition, weight, autopsy and organ donation considerations, and pathologic changes.

Chapter 1 provides a recommended sequence for complete embalming of the body. Here, certain points of the chronology are discussed in greater detail.

Vessel Selection

In the embalming of the "normal" adult body, the injection sites could be: (1) **restricted cervical** injection, (2) one-point injection using the common carotid artery, or (3) femoral artery. This order is based on the fact that should there be any arterial coagula in the aorta, it would be best that this material be pushed toward the legs rather than toward the head. The internal jugular vein is the largest vein that can be used for drainage, and any coagula present in the right atrium of the heart can easily be removed with angular spring forceps. Rarely does the common carotid artery show arteriosclerosis, whereas the femoral frequently exhibits sclerosis. Use of restricted cervical injection gives the embalmer control

A

B

C

Figure 16–5. A. Note the large separation of the lips with this child. **B.** The lips are glued prior to arterial injection with a rubber-based glue. **C.** A glued closure is made prior to arterial injection.

of the strength and volume of arterial solutions entering the head and the trunk areas of the body.

Supplemental Fluids

Supplemental chemicals can be used in the embalming of all bodies. These chemicals are designed to enhance the preservative and disinfecting qualities of the preservative fluids, control moisture, add color to the tissues, and adjust pH of the tissues as well as the arterial solution. Supplemental chemicals include preinjection and coinjection fluids, humectants, dyes, and water conditions. In addition, there are specialized supplemental fluids to control tissue gas, bleach internal discolorations, and remove excessive moisture from the tissues. The conditions present within the body to be embalmed will determine the need for the use of specific supplemental fluids.

Preinjection is a supplemental embalming fluid as well as an embalming procedure. As a fluid it is a chemical containing very little or no preservative. As a process it is the injection of this chemical—diluted as recommended by the manufacturer—into the vascular system (via an artery) for the purposes of preparing the vascular system and the body tissues for the injection of the preservative solution. This solution is injected **before** the preservative solution is injected. It is also used to clear intravascular blood discolorations, remove blood in the vascular system, and adjust the pH of the tissues.

Preinjection is done with the unautopsied body; it is rarely done with the autopsied case. There seem to be two schools of thought—those embalmers who frequently practice preinjection and those who never use this process.

Coinjection is a supplemental embalming fluid used to enhance the action of the preservative solution. It is added to the embalming solution to build up almost all of the embalming chemicals with the exception of the preservatives. A purpose of coinjection fluid is to better control the harsh reactions of the preservatives without simply adding more water to the solution. Some embalmers will use coinjection chemicals as a substitute for water, thus producing a **waterless solution** for injection. Coinjection fluids can be used with almost all arterial solutions. Both preinjection and coinjection treatments can be used in the preparation of an unautopsied body.

Some embalmers do not preinject or coinject any bodies. Many embalmers feel that preinjection should be used only when good distribution is anticipated. When circulatory problems are expected (e.g., bodies dead for long periods of time, bodies that evidence early signs of decomposition, arteriosclerotic vessels), the filling of the vascular system and the tissues with a very weak preinjection solution will only bring about tissue distension when the preservative solution is injected. Bodies that have the greatest need for preservative chemicals, such as the previous examples, generally have the least capacity to accept the preservative solution without tissue distension. Preinjection treatment is used by some embalmers as a method for clearing jaundiced bodies.

FACTORS DETERMINED IN THE EMBALMING ANALYSIS

1. Vessels for injection and drainage
2. Method of mouth closure
3. Strength of the embalming solution
4. Volume of the embalming solution
5. Injection pressure
6. Injection rate of flow

Note: These factors will vary from body to body; or vary within different areas of the same body.

Solution Strength and Volume

Age alone cannot be the **single factor** in determining the strength and the volume of the preservative solution to be injected. Conditions within the body such as weight, body build; moisture in the tissues; effects of disease, surgery, or trauma; blood discolorations; and effects of long use of medications all assist in determining arterial solution strength and volume. Several time elements are equally important—the time lapse between the death and the embalming and the time that will lapse between the embalming and the disposition of the body. Sufficient strength and volume of the embalming chemical must be used to assure thorough sanitizing and preservation of all body areas. With respect to the factor of age, in general, it can be stated that infants, children, and the very elderly may display a delicate skin texture, easily subject to the dehydrating and possible wrinkling effects of preservative chemicals.

Several simple rules can be established in determining strength and volume of the embalming solution:

1. *Selection of a particular fluid.* Most fluid companies make a variety of arterial fluids; consider the recommendations of the manufacturer. In producing fluids, some are formulated for infants and children or older individuals where dehydration and wrinkling of the skin might be a concern. Other formulations are produced for bodies with problems such as edema, or bodies with refrigerated, frozen, or decomposition conditions. If formaldehyde is used as a primary preservative, various indexes and buffers in the fluids will produce varying degrees of firmness.

2. *Follow the recommendations of the manufacturer* for the dilution of the concentrated chemical. This is usually measured in ounces per gallon or ounces per half-gallon. These dilutions are often based on the moisture content of the body (e.g., dehydrated, normal, or edema).

3. *For the "average body,"* a milder solution can be used at the start of the embalming. After good distribution of the solution has been established and the intravascular blood discolorations have been cleared, if necessary, the solution can be strengthened. This can be accomplished by: (a) adding more of the same concentrated arterial fluid or (b) adding a stronger arterial fluid to the original dilution. Here are two examples of this process. It may even be necessary to make a gallon or more using not only more of the original fluid but adding to that mixture a number of ounces of a concentrated stronger arterial fluid. It is possible to find body conditions that will call for the use of the injecting pure concentrated fluid without the use of a water dilutant.

Pressure and Rate of Flow of Injection

With most embalming machines the pressure and the rate of flow are related. The important factor is the rate of flow—how fast or in what volume the fluid enters the body.

Figure 16–6. Rate-of-flow meter can be installed on any centrifugal embalming machine.

An "ideal" rate of flow of 10 to 15 minutes per gallon has been recommended for the first gallon of solution. Sufficient pressure and rate of flow should be used to overcome the resistances of the body and to distribute the arterial solution without causing tissue distension. The greater the resistance in a body, the greater the pressure required. A pressure setting of 5 to 20 lb, using the centrifugal machine, should be sufficient to overcome most body resistances. This range is very wide; many embalmers prefer a low pressure, others prefer a higher setting some using a minimum of 140 psi as standard pressure. The rate of flow can be varied with either setting (Fig. 16–6).

The first injection, while the vascular system is filling, should be slow to prevent any arterial coagula from loosening and moving. The arterial solution can then "ride over top" of the coagula. After the first gallon, the speed of injection is increased. Many embalmers inject a gallon of solution at a rate of 10 to 15 minutes per gallon. Healthy body tissues can accept fluid at this rate of speed without distension.

The skin of adolescents should be much firmer and dryer than that of adults, indicating a good protein level. Adolescent tissues are able to assimilate injected arterial solution much better than those of the elderly, in whom skin support is often weak and swelling occurs easily. For this reason, a wide range of pressures and rates of flow can be used to embalm bodies in this category.

Some embalmers prefer to inject at a rapid rate of flow from the very beginning (5–10 min/gal). The theory is that this places greater pressure on the arterial side of the capillaries and increases filtration of the embalming solution through the capillaries. With this method, continuous drainage is used throughout the preparation. The body must be observed carefully to detect any facial or neck distension. This method can also loosen coagula in the arteries creating arterial emboli which will block smaller arterial branches. Multipoint injection and hypodermic embalming may then be required to overcome the problems thus produced.

Pressure and rate of flow must be sufficient to evenly distribute the preservative solution to all body areas without distension of any tissues. Injection speed should be such that restricted drainage can be employed to assist with the solution distribution, penetration, and retention.

▶ EMBALMING THE ELDERLY

Modern medicine has provided health care and control of disease with the result that the average life expectancy has increased to 75.2 years for men and 80.4 years for women. The number of persons living in their eighties and nineties is expected to double within several years. Embalmers are, as a consequence, required to prepare greater numbers of those dying in these upper age groups. Of course, certain afflictions and pathologic conditions are more frequently encountered in the elderly than among the other previously described three age groups. It is useful to identify some of the more common conditions associated with advanced age and to give some general comments on them. As in all age groups, drug therapy can greatly alter the classic conditions of certain diseases, so the medications in and of themselves will play an important role in determining what postmortem conditions exist in the body.

Arthritic Conditions
Many elderly persons are afflicted with arthritis. This condition, which may be longstanding, may be accompanied by atrophy of many muscles. These conditions are manifested many times in a patient restricted to bed rest. Legs are drawn up and the curvature of the spine is evident. Frequently the arms are drawn up onto the chest and the fingers are clenched (Fig. 16–7).

These conditions create a number of positioning problems for the embalmer. Placing head blocks helps to position the body on the embalming table. It may also be necessary to tie the body in position. Generally, blocks under the thighs and head blocks under a shoulder provide adequate support. Turkish towels placed under the shoulders also help to achieve temporary position. After casketing, the bedding of the casket along with pillow supports places the body into a comfortable-looking position. The neck may be difficult to position. Application of firm pressure to arthritic limbs and arms

Figure 16–7. Arthritic arm and hand.

may change their position. It is possible to tear tendons and atrophied muscles. Since the person has had this arthritic condition for many months or years, leaving the arms and legs in these positions may be acceptable to the family. It is not recommended that tendons or skin be cut to achieve good positioning. It is almost impossible to open and expand arthritic fingers. These can be left in their clenched position and partially hidden by the blanket in the casket. When the legs are drawn to one side or into the fetal position, use of the femoral vessels is limited.

The common carotid would be the best site for injection. If it becomes necessary to inject the legs, an attempt can be made to raise the femoral or external iliac artery. The popliteal artery may also be a choice. If these vessels are found to be sclerotic, an attempt should be made to inject using a small arterial tube; if this is not possible the legs should then be hypodermically injected using a small trocar and a dilute solution of cavity fluid injected through the embalming machine. In addition to hypodermic injection, the legs can be painted with a preservative surface gel and placed in plastic stockings.

Mouth Closure Problems

Frequently a loss of weight is manifested in the facial tissues of the elderly. After mouth closure, it is necessary to place either cotton or "mortuary putty" over the teeth or the dentures. This helps to fill out the sunken cheek areas. These areas should not be overfilled, especially if it is known that the deceased did not wear dentures. In this age group, there are natural depressions of the facial tissues. The biggest problem with mouth closure is atrophy of the maxillae and mandible. The mandible in particular has a tendency to atrophy, and for this reason, it is more difficult many times to use the needle injector method of mouth closure. It is necessary to suture using either a muscular or a mandibular suture. The

mandibular suture holds the dentures forward and in a tight position in the mouth.

Arteriosclerosis

Although not a problem exclusively of the elderly, arteriosclerotic arteries are frequently encountered in this age group. The vessel that most frequently exhibits sclerosis that would be used for embalming is the femoral artery. Many times in a very thin individual, the sclerotic condition of the femoral can be palpated. The common carotid artery is thus the best choice in embalming the elderly. Rarely is the carotid found to be sclerotic, and if there is sclerosis, it is generally not sufficient to occlude the carotid (see Chapter 22).

In addition to bringing about occlusion of the arteries, arteriosclerosis can also bring about poor peripheral circulation. As a result of poor circulation, bedfast individuals tend to form bedsores (decubitus ulcers). These sores develop where there is pressure contact. Bacteria invade these areas. Odor control, from the ulcerations, is a concern. It is important to properly disinfect these areas. Undiluted cavity fluid can be applied on cotton compresses to the ulcerated areas. If bandages cover these areas, it may be useful to saturate the bandages with undiluted cavity fluid or a phenol cautery—disinfectant during the embalming procedure. It is also wise to hypodermically treat the areas around these ulcerations using a small trocar and undiluted cavity fluid. This prevents continued bacterial activity and decreases the possibility of tissue gas (Fig. 16–8A).

At the time of dressing, fresh cotton saturated with undiluted cavity chemical, a phenol solution, or autopsy gel is applied to the ulcerations; then the area is wrapped or, if possible, plastic garments should be used to cover these areas. Embalming powder should be placed in the garments to control odors. Some of these ulcerations are quite small, as frequently seen on the shoulders. Others are very large, often involving the entire buttocks or hip area.

Arteriosclerosis can also result in loss of a limb. If the limb was amputated recently, the stump should be treated by hypodermic injection with undiluted cavity chemical (Fig. 16–8B). If stitching is still present, a plastic stocking is placed over the stump to control any leakage.

Gangrene may be seen in the lower leg and the foot. It is very important that these limbs be hypodermically injected with undiluted cavity chemical. They can also be wrapped in cotton saturated with undiluted cavity chemical, phenol solution, or autopsy gel. A plastic garment containing embalming powder can be placed over the leg. Hypodermically inject the tissues immediately superior to the gangrene area.

Arteriosclerosis can also lead to a ruptured aneurysm. This rupture is a site for leakage of embalming

Figure 16–8. A. Diagram of medial sclerosis. **B.** The lower leg had been removed because of arteriosclerosis. This illustrates treatment of upper leg. Arterial fluid did not enter this area of the body.

fluid during arterial injection. On injection there is little or no drainage. The abdomen distends during injection and there are no signs of arterial fluid distribution such as the presence of dye in the tissues. A six-point injection becomes necessary. The trunk walls will have to be hypodermically injected with a small trocar as in an autopsied body for preservation.

Senile Purpura

Senile purpura (or ecchymosis) is an extravascular irregularly shaped blood discoloration that often appears on the arms and the backs of the hands. The condition is brought about by fragility of the capillaries. In the elderly, excessive medications, blood thinning drugs, vitamin deficiencies, uremia, hypertension, thin skin, and slight bruising can easily bring about senile purpura. These discolorations vary greatly in size and do **not** clear during arterial injection. Often, these areas become en-

gorged with fluid and swell during arterial injection. Purpural areas often darken after embalming and are prone to separate from underlying tissue, causing the tissues to tear open. Care should be taken in handling these areas. (Quite often the persons removing the body place a tight strap across the hands, and when the embalmer receives the body, skin areas on the backs of the hands are torn.)

If senile purpura is evidenced over the hands and the arms (and often the base of the neck), the arterial solution should be strengthened. A fast rate of flow is **not** recommended. A slower rate of flow helps to limit further rupture of capillaries. It may be necessary to use multiple injection points. If the arms are separately injected, a special-purpose high-index fluid can be used in an attempt to dry these areas. Surface compresses of cavity fluid, phenol, or autopsy gel can be used. **If the skin over the purpural areas has been torn or break open, all loose skin should be removed. This should be done at the beginning of embalming.** After surface compresses have had time to cauterize or bleach these discolored areas, the surface of the skin can be dried with a hair dryer and restorative and cosmetic treatment is performed. Unseen hemorrhaged areas can be packed with cotton saturated with a proper preservative solution (a phenol solution is preferred) and then covered with plastic. Leakage is always possible with this condition. Care should be taken to protect the clothing of the deceased.

Care should be taken when massage is used to assist in fluid distribution and senile purpura is present. Rough handling of the tissues can bring about postmortem bruising. This bruising is frequently seen when the eyes of the elderly or of individuals on blood thinners have been enucleated.

Malignancy

Improved medical procedures have done much to lengthen the life expectancy. With the extension of life, there is also an increased probability of a malignant tumor. Cancers or neoplasms that begin as localized tumors can easily invade healthy tissues, spread via the blood vascular system, and invade organs. This can interrupt vital functions to the point where death ensues. The embalmer is concerned with the following systemic effects of a malignancy:

- Disseminated intravascular coagulation.
- Disruption of metabolism by uncontrolled secretion of hormones. (This can greatly affect weight control, cell membrane activity, and metabolism of sugars, fats, and proteins.)
- Secretion of both peptide and steroid hormones by many tumors. (Some of these hormones can bring about sustained hypercalcemia.)
- Anemia.

■ Cachexia (caused by the tumor's competition with the body for metabolites and resulting in a wasting away of tissues).

The local effects of a malignant tumor include invasion and destruction of normal tissues; obstruction of intestines, airways, urinary tract, and biliary tract; pathologic fractures; perforation of the hollow viscera; erosion of blood vessel walls, creating acute and chronic hemorrhage; and establishment of portals of entry for infections.

Both local and systemic effects of a malignancy have an effect on the embalming. There can be a loss of weight and emaciation; often, the skin is loose and flabby and has no support. The skin can be dry because of the body's inability to take in proper amounts of water. Localized edema can result when local tumors exert pressure on veins and lymphatics. If the hormone balance has been interrupted and a condition such as sustained hypercalcemia exists, the calcium can easily create a barrier at the cell wall, making it very difficult for embalming solutions to enter the cell and preserve the protoplasm. Because the fluid cannot penetrate the cells, tissue firmness is difficult to establish. When there is loose, flabby tissue, what appears to be firming is only a plumping of the tissues with embalming solution (actually, distension of the tissues). After the solution gravitates away, the tissues become soft along with being underembalmed.

The malignancy in and of itself may not be the cause of death. Most often the actual cause of death is pneumonia leading to respiratory arrest. In embalming these bodies, fluid solutions should be of moderate strength (at least 2% or above) and should be well coordinated. Use of a coinjection fluid is advised. The coinjection helps to increase the distribution and diffusion of the arterial solution. It is especially helpful in the passage of the arterial solution through the cell membranes.

Metabolic disturbances and renal and respiratory failure, which often accompany a malignancy, result in the buildup of metabolic wastes in the tissues. These wastes increase the demand for preservative. Use of a strong arterial solution helps to ensure satisfactory preservation. The rate of flow should be adequate to distribute the fluid throughout the entire body, but if the skin appears flabby and loose, a slower rate of injection may be helpful. Senile, flabby tissue does not assimilate fluid as well as healthy tissue and swelling can result.

If the facial tissues are emaciated, restricted cervical injection is recommended. This allows for separate embalming of the head, at which time a slightly milder solution can be used or a solution containing humectant can be used to moisturize and restore the facial tissues.

If local edema is present as in the arms or the legs, it may be necessary to use multiple sites for injection.

In the elderly, the femoral arteries are often sclerotic. If it is not possible to inject the femoral, the legs can receive supplemental preservation by hypodermic treatment with undiluted cavity chemical. In addition, autopsy gel can be painted on the legs and plastic stockings can be placed over the gel.

A colostomy may be present if there has been a malignancy in the intestinal tract. The collecting bag can remain in place during arterial injection and cavity treatment. After cavity treatment, the bag should be removed and its contents should be disinfected with cavity fluid. The collecting bag and contents should be disposed of in a biohazard waste container. Cotton saturated with cavity fluid or a phenol solution can be inserted into the colostomy opening in the abdominal wall. Closure of the opening is easily achieved with a purse-string suture.

Cardiac Disease

In some diseases of the heart, the medical treatment may include surgical procedures. If the patient died shortly after surgery and if no autopsy was performed, the embalmer may be confronted with extensive incisions of one or both legs and of the anterior chest wall and possibly the abdominal wall. In addition, very pronounced amounts of edema may be present in the facial tissues, especially if death occurred within a day or so of the operation. Generally, the surgery involves bypass repair or valve repair.

The common carotid artery and the internal jugular vein would be the best primary points for injection and drainage on these cardiac patients. A moderate to strong arterial solution should be used. Addition of dye to the solution from the start helps to indicate the distribution of arterial fluid.

If local obstructions exist, sectional embalming is necessary. If there is extensive edema of the facial tissues, restricted cervical injection should be used and strong solutions for the treatment of the edematous face should be employed. If the sutures are recent and leak during injection, the metal staples used to hold them closed should be removed with a hemostat. Dry the incisions and inject a phenol cautery agent by hypodermic needle within the open incisions. Tightly suture them closed with a baseball stitch using incision seal powder to prevent leakage. After washing and drying the body, paint the incisions with a surface glue.

A pacemaker (see chapter 2 Fig. 2-3D) may be present. This device is generally placed in the upper lateral portion of the chest. The contacts for the pacemaker run from the device into the internal jugular vein and then into the heart. Drainage may be difficult to secure from the internal jugular vein. The angular spring forceps is the easiest drainage device to use. A drainage tube may be very difficult to insert. The opposite internal jugular vein or the femoral vein may be a necessary second choice for a point of drainage. If the body is to be cremated, the pacemaker should be removed. Some hospitals also require removal and return of the pacemaker.

Diabetes Mellitus

Diabetes mellitus may be defined as both an acute and a chronic metabolic disorder characterized principally by hyperglycemia (an excess of sugar in the blood) resulting from a deficiency of insulin.

Medical authorities estimate that up to 5% of the population are afflicted with diabetes mellitus and that older than 40 years, women outnumber men so afflicted by approximately 3 to 2. Individuals who are obese are more frequently diabetic than those who are not. The disease usually manifests itself during adult life at the age of 50 to 60. The exception is an acute juvenile type that has a far younger age of onset. Even though the onset of the disease can be in middle age, its effects continue into old age and may contribute to a middle-age death. The affliction affords some merit to the congenital theory of the origin of the disease as researchers have observed that when both parents are diabetic, offspring have a 90% (estimated) chance of acquiring diabetes mellitus.

The principal manifestations of diabetes mellitus include **hyperglycemia**, excess sugar in the blood; **glycosuria**, sugar in the urine; and **ketosis**, acidosis characterized by the presence of ketones in the blood and the body tissues.

Pathologic changes resulting from the disease include poor peripheral circulation brought about by accelerated arteriosclerosis and degenerative changes in small blood vessels that result in poor circulation, particularly in the lower extremities. This often results in gangrene (Fig. 16–9). Kidney failure and enlargement of the liver (very often resulting in infestation of the liver because of the high sugar content of the tissues) and fungal infestations of the lung can also be prevalent. The skin often exhibits scratch marks and infections brought about by pruritus and itching. A strong odor of acetone may be noted, as it is present in the urine and the perspiration.

In embalming these bodies, a strong arterial solution is needed. Peripheral circulation is often poor; therefore, dyes should be added so the embalmer can detect where fluid is present. Areas of the face such as the ears, the tip of the nose, and the cheeks often do not receive an adequate amount of fluid. Likewise, the hands and the legs should be carefully evaluated. The common carotid artery (restricted cervical) would be the best injection point. This artery is the least likely to exhibit arteriosclerosis.

The **restricted cervical injection** is recommended so that higher pressures and two arterial solutions can

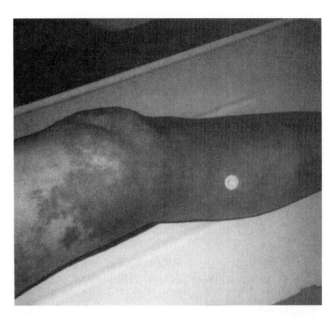

Figure 16–9. Gangrene of the left leg in an individual with diabetes. Treatments included hypodermic injection of cavity fluid and application of surface preservative gel with a plastic stocking.

be employed. Restricted cervical injection also allows the embalmer to inject both sides of the head. This helps to ensure good circulation to all facial tissues. If the lower extremities or the stump of an amputated leg do not receive sufficient fluid by arterial injection, then hypodermic and surface treatment may be needed. Plastic garments, containing surface preservatives or gels, may also be placed on the lower extremities.

If the hands or fingers do not receive sufficient fluid, a small-gauge hypodermic needle can be inserted between the fingers and arterial or cavity fluid can be injected to secure preservation. The hands can also be wrapped with cotton saturated with a surface preservative such as a cavity fluid compress or autopsy gel. Manufacturer's directions may inform how long compresses should be left in place. One must be certain that the preservative is applied to the palm side of the hand in addition to the back of the hand.

The following list summarizes the recommended treatment for diabetics:

1. Use the carotid vessels for primary injection.
2. Use strong arterial solutions.
3. Use fluid dyes for tracers.
4. During injection massage limbs to stimulate fluid distribution.
5. Carefully disinfect the respiratory tract, as fungal infections may be present.
6. Institute hypodermic treatment and surface treatment for areas receiving insufficient arterial fluid.

Cavity embalming should immediately follow arterial injection. The embalmer should be certain that a liberal amount of cavity fluid is injected into the liver and the lungs.

Arteriosclerosis
Arthritis
Atrophy of the mandible and maxillae
Senile diabetes

▶ CONCEPTS FOR STUDY AND DISCUSSION

1. Explain the following:
   Ideal fluid strength for embalming the "normal" adult body.
   Ideal pressure for embalming the "normal" adult body.
   Ideal rate of flow for embalming the "normal" adult body.
2. Explain why it may be necessary to use the same strength arterial solution for embalming an infant or a child and an adult.
3. Discuss the following complications in embalming of the elderly:

▶ BIBLIOGRAPHY

Bickley HC. *Practical Concepts in Human Disease.* Baltimore: Williams & Wilkins, 1974:92–95.

Slocum RE. Type six classification. In: *Pre-embalming Considerations.* Boston: Dodge Chemical Co., 1969:79.

Smith AL. *Microbiology and Pathology,* 12th ed. St. Louis, MO: C.V. Mosby, 1980:513–514.

Spriggs AO. Preparation of children's bodies. In: *The Art and Science of Embalming Springfield,* OH: Champion Chemical Co., 1963:127–128.

The elderly cases. In: *Champion Expanding Encyclopedia,* Nos. 413–415. Springfield, OH: Champion Chemical Co., 1971.

CHAPTER 17

PREPARATION OF AUTOPSIED BODIES

CHAPTER OBJECTIVES

▶ Autopsy types—hospital, medico-legal
▶ Autopsy—purposes
▶ Autopsy work practice controls
▶ Preparation—complete autopsy
▶ Preparation—partial autopsy

An autopsy—necropsy or postmortem—is an examination of the dead human body. There are two types of autopsy: the medical (hospital) autopsy and the medico-legal (forensic) autopsy. In some communities, the pathologist prefers that the arterial embalming of the body be done prior to the autopsy. In contrast, most coroners and medical examiner offices **do not** want the body embalmed prior to the autopsy.

In certain autopsies, particularly hospital autopsies, the family not only must give permission for the autopsy, but they also have the right to limit the extent of the autopsy. Where special instructions have been given, it is important that the pathologist follow the limitations established by the family. The partial autopsy may consist of external examination and/or removal of only one or two organs.

With respect to liability, the embalmer should also note in the funeral home records the type of autopsy performed. In addition, a memorandum should be made as to the disposition of the visceral organs: Were they returned with the body? *This is very important. In a number of instances a second autopsy has been ordered to support insurance claims or to confirm a cause of death. This is especially true in communities where black lung and industrial deaths are linked to claims for insurance compensation. In addition, the next of kin are entitled to the "whole body". Some coroner and medical examiner offices will return tissue samples to the family after the cause and manner of death has been determined and all judicial matters are complete.*

▶ TYPES OF AUTOPSIES

Medical or Hospital Autopsy

Permission for the medical or hospital autopsy is obtained from the person with the proper authority to take charge of the body after death. Several reasons are given by the College of American Pathologists for the performance of the hospital autopsy*:

- When doctors have not made a firm diagnosis.
- When death follows unexpected medical complications.
- When death follows the use of an experimental drug or device, a new procedure, or unusual therapy.
- When death follows a dental or surgical procedure done for diagnostic purposes and the case does not come under the jurisdiction of medical examiner or coroner.
- When death occurs suddenly, unexpectedly, or in mysterious circumstances from apparently natural causes and the case does not come under the jurisdiction of medical examiner or coroner.
- When environmental or workplace hazards are suspected.
- When death occurs during or after childbirth.

---

*Adapted from recommendations of the College of American Pathologists headed by Dr. Hans J. Peters, *New York Times*, July 21, 1988.

- When there are concerns about a hereditary disease that might affect other members of the family.
- When there are concerns about the possible spread of a contagious disease.
- When the cause of death could affect insurance settlements (e.g., policies that cover cancer or that grant double indemnity for accidental death).
- When death occurs in a hospital and the patient comes from a nursing home and the quality of care is questioned.

In addition to the preceding reasons, hospital autopsies are requested to confirm or to verify a diagnosis. Also, many of these institutions are teaching hospitals, and the autopsy serves as a tool in explaining a diagnostic technique or disease process.

Coroner or Medical Examiner Autopsy

Reasons for a medico-legal autopsy ordered by a coroner or medical examiner include: (1) determination of the cause of death; (2) determination of the manner of death; (3) establishment of the time of death; (4) recovering, identifying, and preserving evidence;(5) provide factual objective information for legal authorities; and (6) separate deaths due to disease from deaths due to external causes. The cases that come under the jurisdiction of a coroner or medical examiner vary from state to state and from county to county **within** a state. The following general list represents typical cases that would be reported to a coroner or a medical examiner (see Chapter 1 for additional medico-legal referrals):

- All sudden deaths not caused by readily recognizable disease or wherein the cause of death cannot be properly certified by a physician on the basis of prior (recent) medical attendance.
- All deaths occurring in suspicious circumstances, including those where alcohol, drugs, or other toxic substances may have had a direct bearing on the outcome.
- All deaths occurring as a result of violence or trauma, whether apparently homicidal, suicidal, or accidental (including those caused by mechanical, thermal, chemical, electrical, or radiation injury, drowning, cave-ins, and subsidences), regardless of the time elapsed between injury and death
- Any fetal death, stillbirth, or death of a baby within 24 hours of birth, where the mother has not been under the care of a physician.
- All therapeutic and criminal abortions, regardless of the length of pregnancy, and spontaneous abortions beyond 16 weeks' gestation.
- All operative and perioperative deaths in which the death is not readily explainable on the basis of prior disease.

- Any death wherein the body is unidentified or unclaimed.
- Any death where there is uncertainty as to whether or not it should be reported to the coroner's office.

Death within 24 hours of admission to a hospital is not considered a reportable death unless it falls into one of the specific categories defined.

► GUIDELINES TO DETERMINE WHEN AUTOPSIES ARE TO BE PERFORMED

The following list includes not only the cases that fall under the jurisdiction of a coroner or a medical examiner, but **specific cases on which an autopsy must be performed.** (This list is only representative.) This list will vary from state to state and within counties of a particular state:

- Victims of homicide.
- Victims of deaths in the workplace.
- Motor vehicle drivers who have been involved in accidents.
- Pedestrians who have been involved in accidents.
- Passengers who have been involved in accidents but who lack clear evidence of trauma.
- Victims of intra- and perioperative accidental deaths.
- Epileptics.
- Possible victims of sudden infant death syndrome.
- Infants or children with evidence of bodily injury.
- Inmate fatalities in correctional facilities, nursing homes, or medical institutions.
- Victims of trauma.
- Victims of nontraumatic, sudden, unexpected deaths.
- Victims of anorexia nervosa.
- Multiple victims of coincidental, unexplained death at one location.
- Victims of possible poisoning or overdose deaths.
- Any other case in which the pathologist holds a bona fide belief that the death is unexplained and/or an autopsy is in the best interest of the public or that it is necessary for the proper administration of the statutory duties of the office of the coroner.

► GENERAL CONSIDERATIONS IN AUTOPSY TREATMENT

Order in Working

When the embalmer is working alone, do one item at a time in preparation of the autopsied body. In injection of the legs, that must be the only concern—that is, check for distribution, use intermittent drainage by clamping off the external iliac vein, massage the leg to assist distribution, and so on. Do not try to set features or raise other vessels while injecting the legs. Do one procedure at a time. Time is not saved by trying to do several things at the same time.

Work Practice Controls

1. Be aware where cutting and sharp instruments are laid during preparation.
2. Cover broken or cut bones (e.g., ribs) prior to placement of embalmer's hands into a body cavity.
3. Wash gloved hands or change gloves often during the embalming procedure.
4. Avoid use of high water pressure when water is used to flush blood and fluids from the embalming table.
5. Practice continuous aspiration of the cavities during arterial injection to remove drainage and excess arterial fluid.
6. Clamp leaking arteries and small veins to avoid excessive embalming solution loss and improve solution distribution during arterial injection.
7. Run table water continuously to dilute and carry away any blood or chemicals on the table surface.
8. Pack external orifices: rectum, esophagus, trachea, ears, and vagina.
9. During embalming, the calvarium and the removed portions of the sternum can be soaked in a preservative solution in a closed container or sealed plastic bag.

FACTORS DETERMINED IN THE EMBALMING ANALYSIS

1. Vessels for injection and drainage
2. Method of mouth closure
3. Strength of the embalming solution
4. Volume of the embalming solution
5. Injection pressure
6. Injection rate of flow

Note: These factors will vary by the individual body; or vary in different areas of the same body.

Fluid Strength

Preparation of the autopsied body is usually **delayed**. The delay may occur between death and autopsy or between autopsy and release of the body. The autopsy for a drowning victim is usually delayed for 24 hours and

if a body is frozen the autopsy can be delayed for 48 hours. Most institutions **refrigerate** bodies during these time delays. These factors combined with the pathologic conditions of the body generally require that somewhat **stronger-than-average arterial solutions** be used; however, improper and delayed refrigeration could also produce dehydrated tissues, which will demand a different type of arterial solution. Delays increase the possibility of **distension** during arterial injection and also increase the preservative demand of the tissues.

Refrigerated bodies, bodies dead 12 to 24 hours, and bodies that evidence early decomposition—all increase the preservative demand.

Use of Fluid Dyes

Delay also brings about rigor mortis and, if long enough, the passing of rigor. Rigor can cause poor arterial solution distribution and may also be a false sign of fluid firming. Fluid reactions with body proteins do not proceed normally when a body is in rigor mortis. Refrigeration can bring about hemolysis of the blood trapped in the superficial tissues. This hemolysis can create an appearance similar to that of the dye present in arterial solutions. The tissue thus appears "embalmed." In addition, refrigerated tissues feel "embalmed" because the fats in the subcutaneous tissues have hardened. Use dye in the arterial solution; it serves as the best sign of arterial solution distribution. Keep in mind that dyes show only **surface** distribution of arterial solutions. Massage deep tissues, such as the muscles of the legs (especially in rigor). Employ intermittent drainage to "force" fluids into the deep tissues.

▶ PRESSURES AND RATES OF FLOW

Tissues can assimilate only a certain amount of fluid in a given time period. Often, arterial solution is injected too fast into the body and swelling results. In preparation of the autopsied body, inject each section separately. During injection into a specific body region, such as an arm or a leg, higher pressures and faster rates of flow can be safely used to help establish good circulation. The embalmer can vary the rate of flow for each area and, if necessary, vary the pressure to overcome the resistances of a particular body part. In addition, intermittent drainage and pulsation can be used for each area to establish good distribution and diffusion.

▶ DRAINAGE

With the autopsied body it is **not** necessary to insert drainage devices (drain tubes or angular spring forceps) into the veins. Drainage can be taken directly from the cut vein and the drainage material can flow directly into the body cavities. Once in the cavities, an autopsy aspirator is used to keep accumulated drainage at a minimum. These instruments are useful because they are designed not to clog. These accumulated fluids can be aspirated into a sanitary sewer system. Clamping the vein with a hemostat or applying digital pressure with a piece of cotton temporarily stops the drainage. Intermittent and alternate drainage greatly assists in fluid distribution, diffusion, and retention of the arterial solution.

▶ COMPLETE AUTOPSY/PARTIAL AUTOPSY

In this chapter, autopsies are divided into two categories (based on the extent of the autopsy): the **complete autopsy** and the **partial autopsy**. The hospital or forensic autopsy can be either type. The coroner or the medical examiner autopsy is generally a complete autopsy (Fig. 17–1).

The **complete autopsy** involves opening of the following body cavities and removal of the following organs:

1. Cranial cavity and its contents:
   a. Possibly removal of the inner ear.
   b. Brain.
   c. Removal of the pituitary gland.
2. Eye enucleation or vitreous humors of the eye:
   a. Electrolytes can indicate if dehydration is present.
   b. Glucose levels can indicate diabetes.

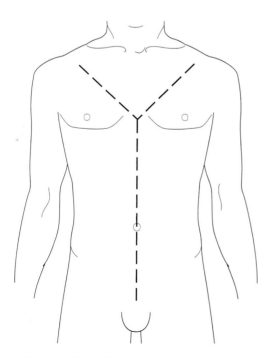

Figure 17–1. Standard Y autopsy incision.

Figure 17–2. Spinal cord removed for examination by the dorsal approach.

   c. Vitreous ethanol can indicate alcohol increasing or decreasing when compared to the blood alcohol.
3. Removal of the neck organs:
   a. Thyroid gland.
   b. Larynx.
   c. Cervical portion of the esophagus and the trachea.
   d. Possibly removal of the common carotid arteries.
   e. Removal of the tongue (especially if a "cafe coronary" is suspected). Removal is also necessary to completely examine the contents of the throat.
4. Thoracic cavity and its contents.
5. Abdominal cavity and its contents.
6. Pelvic cavity contents.
7. Removal of spinal cord:
   a. *Dorsal* approach: body is turned over and vertebral column is opened (Fig. 17–2).
   b. *Ventral* approach: vertebral column is opened from within the body cavities and cervical area.
   c. Removal from the foramen magnum.
   OR
   d. *Sample* removal of the spinal cord, usually through the ventral approach (a "wedge" cut from the vertebral column).
8. Removal of testes from the scrotum.
9. Tissue samples may be taken from any region of the body.

In the **partial autopsy**, generally only one body cavity (cranial, thoracic, or abdominopelvic cavity) is opened to examine one specific item. This type of autopsy is most frequently performed as the medical (or hospital) autopsy.

Some institutions remove and examine only one organ, usually because they are limited by the person granting permission for the autopsy. If only one organ is removed and all vessels ligated, the embalmer should have little difficulty. Many pathologists, however, remove the one organ but do not ligate the vessels. Failure to tie off vessels can cause a loss of arterial solution during arterial injection.

▶ SUGGESTED ORDER FOR PREPARATION OF THE AUTOPSIED BODY

1. Unwrap the body. Apply a topical droplet spray to the surface of the body and the orifices. Wash the body with germicidal soap and dry it. Relieve (as much as possible) any rigor mortis present. Position the head and the shoulders.
2. Shave the body and set the features.
3. Open the cavities. Remove the viscera if they have been returned. Disinfect the internal surfaces of the body cavities with droplet spray.
4. Locate and place ligatures around the six vessels needed for sectional arterial injection:
   a. Right and left external iliac arteries.*
   b. Right and left axillary or subclavian arteries.
   c. Right and left common carotid arteries.
5. Prepare the arterial solution. Consider a variety of factors in determining the strength of the solution:
   a. Cause of death.
   b. Size and weight of body.
   c. Time between death and preparation.
   d. Presence of decomposition changes.
   e. Moisture content of tissues.
   f. Protein content of body.
   g. Refrigeration.
      (Different solutions may have to be prepared for different sections of the body, e.g., if edema is present in the legs but not in the arms or the head.)
6. Inject at rates of flow and pressures that meet the demands of the various body areas. Drainage may be concurrent or intermittent:
   a. Inject the legs first, one at a time.
   b. Inject the arms second, one at a time.
   c. Inject the head.
      (1) Inject the left side **first**.
      (2) Inject the right side.
7. Institute supplemental treatments: hypodermic injection of **the trunk walls, the shoulders, the neck,** and **the buttocks**.
8. Drain all liquids from body cavities and treat internal surfaces with hardening compound or autopsy gel.
9. Prepare abdominal and thoracic cavities and neck area:
   a. Return the bag of viscera and add preservative chemical **OR** replace viscera (after treatment) directly into the body cavities using liberal amounts of hardening compound on the viscera.
   b. If viscera are not returned, fill cavities with absorbent material such as sheeting or cotton and saturate material with preservative chemical.
   c. Fill out neck area with cotton saturated with preservative chemical or autopsy gel.
10. Suture thoracic and abdominal cavities.
11. Dry cranial cavity. Treat walls with preservative powder or gel and attach calvarium.
12. Suture scalp.
13. Wash and dry body.
14. Apply glue to incisions of the thoracic and abdominal cavity.
15. If necessary place appropriate plastic protective garments on the body: embalming powders should be placed inside the garment.
16. Prepare the embalming report.

▶ PREPARATION OF THE AUTOPSIED BODY*

Carefully open the zippered pouch or the plastic or cotton sheeting enveloping the autopsied remains. Liberally, using a droplet spray, disinfect the exposed surfaces and inner wrappings. Several minutes later, roll up the covering material, and gently roll the body from side to side to remove all of the wrappings. Place these immediately in a biohazard container. Next, wash the body with a disinfectant solution. Let this topical solution remain on the body for at least 10 minutes. The body can then be rinsed and dried. Relieve any rigor mortis present and proceed to position the body:

1. Remove the pathologist's stitches and lay back the flaps of skin, exposing the thoracic and abdominal and cranial cavities. Spray these cavities with a broad-spectrum disinfectant droplet spray. Remove the stitches from the scalp and

---

*Common iliacs can be injected when present. Internal iliacs may be injected if they are present.

*See also selected readings armed services specifications for mortuary services.

remove the calvarium. Disinfect the cranial cavity or better yet, swab it with autopsy gel, especially in cases of systemic infection (meningitis, hepatitis, acquired immunodeficiency syndrome (AIDS)). Support the scalp in the forehead area, especially during arterial injection, to avoid a "creased" area across the forehead and to assist distribution of fluid through the scalp.

2. Inspect the arteries needed for injection.

3. *Option:* Some embalmers prefer to shave and set the features at this time; others prefer to inject the legs and arms prior to setting the features.

4. *Mix arterial solution.* If there has been a delay between death and preparation or if the body has been refrigerated, or both, a slightly stronger arterial solution is needed: *either a higher-index fluid or a standard arterial solution to which 4 to 6 oz of a high-index fluid has been added.* Add some tracer dye to indicate the distribution of arterial solution in the body. Fluid selection and solution strength will also be determined by the conditions present in the area of the body being injected. (*Example: the legs may have edema, but the arms and the hands have no edema.*)

5. Inject the lower extremities:

    a. The ideal vessels to use for injection of the legs are the right and the left common iliac. Any leakage from the internal iliac branch can be clamped (vessels were severed when the pelvic organs were removed). Arterial solution will reach the legs by the external iliac and the internal iliac artery will supply solution to the buttocks, the anal area, and the perineal tissues. Injection of the common iliac would also supply solution to the trunk walls through branches off the external iliac artery. In some autopsies, the common iliac and the internal iliac arteries have been excised. In this situation, the embalmer will use the external iliac artery to inject each leg. Injecting each common iliac artery or external iliac artery separately permits more control over the flow of the solution into the extremity being injected. The embalmer can control massage, pressure, rate of flow, and strength of the solution being used for each leg. Separate direct injection of the internal iliac artery accompanied by massage to the buttocks and the upper thighs can bring about a noticeable amount of arterial solution distribution to these areas. It should always be attempted; leakage may need to be controlled with hemostats.

    b. Some autopsy technicians and/or pathologists sever the external iliac artery directly beneath the inguinal ligament. It is important to remember that arteries remain open when severed. In the nose of a hemostat, grasp the cut end of the artery and gently expose it sufficiently to insert an arterial tube. If possible place a tight ligature around the artery to secure the tube; if this is not possible, use an arterial hemostat to secure the tube in the artery. Always attempt to place strings around arteries to hold arterial tubes in place rather than holding them in position using hemostats.

    c. If necessary, raise the femoral artery to inject the lower extremities.

    d. Allow drainage to enter the abdominopelvic cavity. If intermittent drainage is desired, use a hemostat to stop drainage for intervals.

    e. If fluid does not reach the foot, institute the following procedures:

        (1) Very firmly massage the leg, pushing strongly along the arterial route (femoral, popliteal, and anterior and posterior tibial arteries). Rotate the foot medially. This squeezes all the muscles of the lower leg.

        (2) Use a higher injection pressure and pulsation.

        (3) Limit drainage by using intermittent drainage.

        Many times, the vessels of the leg are sclerotic. If injection of the lower arteries is impossible, inject the legs hypodermically (using an infant trocar) with a preservative. Then paint the legs with autopsy gel and clothe them in plastic stockings.

        The volume and the strength of the solution depend on pathologic conditions, leakage, and postmortem conditions. Sometimes, one-half gallon is sufficient. With edema, two or more gallons might be needed per leg. **There is no set** volume or strength.

6. Inject the upper extremities:

    a. If the arch of the aorta or its branches are present, use the subclavian arteries for injection. In this way, fluid is distributed to the shoulders, to the back of the neck, and to the upper back regions. In the complete autopsy, however, the following vessels must be clamped if the subclavian artery is injected:

        (1) Vertebral artery (if a cranial autopsy has been done).

        (2) Internal thoracic artery.

        (3) Inferior thyroid artery (when neck organs have been removed).

        The right subclavian is a branch of the brachiocephalic artery. It can be distinguished from the right common carotid artery, because the subclavian is usually larger in diameter. Follow the direction

A

B

C

Figure 17–3. Autopsy injection of arms using the axillary artery. **A.** Note the pectoralis muscle. **B.** The axillary artery is shown; inject from this location. **C.** The arm may be positioned during injection.

of the insertion of an arterial tube to determine if the right subclavian artery has been entered; it heads laterally toward the arm. The left subclavian branches off the arch of the aorta. If, after clamping off the leakage from the severed branches of the subclavian, leakage still continues, it may be necessary to raise and inject the axillary artery. The problem with using the axillary is that the shoulder, the upper portions of the back, and the deep muscles of the neck do not receive arterial solution distribution.

b. The axillary artery can be raised by cutting the pectoralis major and minor muscles (Fig. 17–3). It is easy to raise this artery just as it leaves the cervicoaxillary canal. This canal is bounded by the scapula, the first rib, and the clavicle. If the axillary artery is raised at this point, all its branches can be used to distribute fluid to the trunk walls and the shoulder areas. In addition, the arm can be placed in a natural position. Use of the axillary artery avoids many of the leakage problems seen with the subclavian artery, and the axillary can be raised from the incision the pathologist has already made (if that incision rises to the shoulder area). *If fluid does not flow easily down the arm, pull the arterial tube out a little. This usually frees the tube of any blockage.*

c. Drainage can be taken from the subclavian vein. If intermittent drainage is desired, place a hemostat on either the subclavian or the axillary vein.

d. Fluid strength and volume vary from body to body or even from right side to left side. Continue injection until the hand has cleared and distribution is evident. Manipulate the arm, flexing at the elbow and the wrist, to assist distribution along with intermittent drainage. It may also be necessary to place digital pressure on the cephalic vein to increase distribution by blocking the loss of fluid from the superficial drainage route.

If fluid is not flowing into the hand, try the following: lower the hand while injecting, massage by pushing very firmly along the arterial route (axillary, brachial, radial, and ulnar arteries), increase injection pressure (using pulsation if available), and use intermittent drainage. Finally, the radial and the ulnar arteries can be raised and injected. If fluid still does not enter the fingers, treat by hypodermic injection of a preservative fluid.

7. Inject the head:

a. Place arterial tubes in the right and the left common carotid arteries. If the common carotid has been cut by the pathologist, try to find the external carotid. The common carotid bifurcates at the level of the superior border of the thyroid cartilage. This point is quite high in the neck. If the artery can be located, insert a small arterial tube. Clamp it in place with a hemostat.

Option 1. Inject the left side of the head first. Certain arteries must be clamped for leakage if the **left common carotid** artery is injected. The **left internal carotid** is located inside the cranial cavity just lateral to the sella turcica of the sphenoid bone. Clamp this vessel after arterial injection has begun. In this way, filling of the vascular system supplied by the common carotid artery can be observed. This will not be necessary if the cranial cavity was not autopsied. The **superior thyroid artery** is located in the neck; this branch of external carotid artery leaks if the neck organs have been removed.

Inject the right side of the head. Arteries to be clamped are the **right internal carotid**, found lateral to the sella turcica in the cranial cavity when the cranial cavity has been autopsied, and the **right superior thyroid**, found in the neck if the neck organs have been removed.

The left is injected first so that a certain amount of fluid flows to the right side via anastomosis. It also gives the embalmer a chance to observe the effects of the fluid and the dyes on the left side. If there is any problem, the arterial solution can be changed before the right side is injected. This method also prevents overinjection of the right side of the face.

Option 2. Once tubes are in place in the right and the left common carotid arteries, attach them to a Y tube. Inject both right and left sides at the same time. Clamp all arteries, such as internal carotids and superior thyroids or any other major leaking arteries, with hemostats.

Option 3. When no cranial autopsy has been performed but the major cavities have been autopsied, inject the left and the right sides of the head. If each side of the head is being separately injected, the carotid artery not being injected should be clamped, tied or if a tube has been placed in the artery, the stop-cock should be closed. This will assist in distribution and prevent a loss of arterial solution. Because the cranial autopsy was not performed collateral circulation will occur through the circle of Willis. Where there is an anastomosis of vessels (such as the lips) arterial solution will pass from one side of the face to the opposite. An alternative injection technique is to inject right and left sides of the head simultaneously. This is done by using a "Y" tube for the injection.

b. *Enucleation.* If the eyes have been enucleated, loosely pack the eye orbits with cotton saturated with autopsy gel. Close and pose the lids. A light coating of massage cream can be placed on the surrounding facial tissues. Slightly increase the strength of the arterial solution. Inject using a low rate of flow and low pressure. If leakage occurs from the corner of the closed eyelid allow the fluid to escape. If the leakage is stopped by tightly packing the base of the orbit, it increases the possibility of the eyelids swelling during injection. After arterial injection, the cotton will be removed and the eyes will be restored.

c. If the inner ear has been removed, tightly pack the area of the temporal bone from which the tissues were removed with cotton saturated with autopsy gel. If this area leaks profusely during injection, if possible apply a hemostat to the leaking vessels.

d. *Tongue removed.* Many medico-legal autopsies remove the neck organs, the floor of the mouth, and the tongue (glossectomy). Distribution of the embalming solution to the facial tissues will be interrupted due to the severance of a sufficient number of small arteries. It is difficult to clamp these leaking vessels during arterial injection with hemostats. First close the mouth and pose the lips. A light coating of massage cream can be placed on the tissues of the buccal cavity and lips. Insert a large piece of cotton saturated with cavity fluid or covered with autopsy gel through the neck. Tightly pack the cotton into the floor of the mouth. This puts pressure on the severed arteries and limits leakage of the arterial solution. The arterial solution can be slightly increased in strength when this condition exists. Dye should be added to the arterial mixture so evidence of arterial fluid in the facial tissues can be easily observed. The packed cotton can remain in place and need not be removed after arterial injection.

e. Observe the parotid, sublingual, and submaxillary glands for swelling. Use of a stronger solution and pulsation, a slower rate flow, and a reduced pressure during the injection helps to limit swelling of these glands. If swelling occurs, apply digital pressure against the glands. These glands can also be pierced from under the skin with a scalpel, which, together with digital pressure, helps to reduce swelling. If the swelling is too pronounced, the glands may have to be excised from under the skin by going up through the neck.

▶ SUPPLEMENTAL HYPODERMIC INJECTION

Depending on the incisions made by the pathologist and the extent of vessel removal, only a small portion of the trunk may receive arterial fluid. It now becomes necessary for the embalmer to preserve those areas lacking fluid, as best as possible, by hypodermic embalming (Fig. 17–4). Preservative solution is injected via a trocar attached to the embalming machine. Some embalmers prefer arterial solution for this work; others use a mixture of cavity fluid and water.

It is important that all tissues be channeled: the trunk walls (anterior, lateral, and posterior), with special emphasis on injection of the buttocks, the breasts in the female, and the shoulder and the neck regions. Channel these regions first; then turn on the machine or allow the fluid to pass through the trocar into the channels. Avoid accidents that expose the embalmer to excessive amounts of embalming solution. Universal precautions require eye protection during all embalming procedures; hypodermic treatments certainly demand this protection. In addition to the hypodermic treatment of the trunk walls, surface embalming can be used in the following ways:

A   B

Figure 17–4. A. Hypodermic treatment of the walls after autopsy. **B.** After the intercostal muscles are incised, the cavity walls are painted with autopsy gel.

1. A scalpel can be used to cut the intercostal muscles in the thoracic area. Later, this area can be painted with autopsy gel, which, over time, penetrates the tissues of the back (Fig. 17–4B).

2. The trunk walls on the outside of the rib cage can be cut further back (some embalmers do this as far back as the vertebral column) and then painted with autopsy gel. In lieu of autopsy gel, cotton, paper towels, or strips of sheeting can be placed between the trunk wall and the rib cage and saturated with cavity fluid.

3. All inside surfaces of the cavities can be painted with autopsy gel.

4. If viscera are not returned, sheeting can be placed in the cavities and saturated with cavity fluid. This provides an "inside compress" for surface embalming.

5. Even if viscera are returned, the cavity can be lined with cotton, paper towels, or sheeting and saturated with cavity fluid before the plastic bag of viscera is placed back in the cavity. This material can be saturated with preservative or cavity fluid, in lieu of autopsy gel.

Autopsy gels are made to cling to the lateral walls. In addition, they are formulated to penetrate the tissues, so their use may be preferred to that of inlays of cavity fluid. The autopsy gels are a little easier to work with from the standpoint of formaldehyde irritation.

Care should be taken to pack the pelvic cavity so there is no leakage from the rectum. If the pathologist has removed the entire rectum, it may be necessary to turn the body over and suture the area closed. The rectum, the esophagus, and the trachea can be tightly ligated from within the cavities.

Attention should also be given to the neck area if the neck organs have been removed. Cotton is used to replace the missing organs, and once it is in place, the cotton is saturated with preservative fluid. This is necessary, because circulation to the skin of the neck is interrupted when the neck organs are removed. Again, all inside areas of the neck can be painted with autopsy gel before cotton is inserted.

▶ TREATMENT OF THE VISCERA

The embalming report should indicate if the viscera were or were not returned with the remains. If the viscera were returned, the report should state whether they were: (1) placed within the body or (2) prepared and placed in a separate container with the body in the casket or shipping case. If returned, the viscera are usually enclosed in a plastic bag. Several methods can be used to treat the viscera.

If the viscera are to be returned to the abdominal and the thoracic cavities, a minimum of two bottles of cavity fluid should be mixed and poured over the viscera before the bag is returned to the cavities. It is much easier to position and "find room" for the viscera in the cavities if the preservative fluids are not poured over the viscera until the bag is in position. After being covered with cavity chemical, the hollow organs can be incised using shears to release any gases.

Some embalmers return the viscera to the cavities but **not** in plastic bags. The viscera should be soaked in cavity fluid several hours, returned to the abdominal and thoracic cavities, and covered well with absorbent autopsy hardening compound. Then, the cavities are tightly sutured closed.

▶ CLOSURE OF THE CAVITIES

Abdominal and Thoracic

After **walls of the cavities** have been treated **hypodermically** and by **surface embalming** and the viscera returned (preferably in a plastic bag) to the abdominal and thoracic cavities: if not returned the cavities filled with an absorbent material, the next step is closure of the cavities.

Position the breastplate, being certain that it is coated on both sides with autopsy gel or preservative powder.

Begin to suture using a double-curved needle and linen suture cord. Linen suture cord is much stronger than cotton suture cord. A minimum of a five-twist (strand) linen suture cord should be used. When pulling the cord to tighten the stitches, **pull on the thread, not on the needle.** Otherwise, the thread may break as it rubs against the eye of the needle.

If cotton is used as filler for the cavities, be certain that paper toweling or sheeting is placed over the cotton. Cotton has a tendency to get caught in the suturing and can be quite troublesome to work with.

Bring all the three flaps of the incision together and tie them together with one suture. From this point, if desired, sew to the shoulder area along one of the branches of the incision extending from the xiphoid process of the sternum to the shoulder (Fig. 17–5).

Start the suture for the abdominal cavity at the level of the pubic symphysis. Begin the suture by **tying the suture in place** rather than tying a knot on the end of the suture. Knots have a tendency to pull through the skin. Use a baseball suture for closure. This suture is very tight. String from the suture pattern should not be seen. If the suture looks like the lacing pattern of a baseball, it is **too loose.** Pull the sutures **very tight.** Single- or double-cord suture thread may be used. If linen is used, single-strand thread should be sufficient and should not cause any breakage. (If the hole made by the suture needle

Figure 17–5. Align autopsy incisions before suturing the abdominal incisions.

appears large, double-stranded thread may be preferred to close (fill) the hole.)

Approximately every 4 or 5 inch pass the needle through both sides of the incision as if the suture were being ended. This will "lock down" the completed sutures; it will also take the tension off the suture thread. This is repeated throughout the suturing process.

If the suture thread should break, assess the situation. Rather than tearing out all the suturing and starting over, it may be more convenient to begin sewing from another direction and tie the two sutures together.

When the tie at the location of the xiphoid process is reached, continue the suture up the branch of the Y incision that was not previously closed to the shoulder. It is important, especially in the shoulder areas, to use **incision seal powder** to prevent any leakage. This is the one area of the Y incision that is most likely to leak.

The skin of bodies with certain wasting diseases may be difficult to suture because it tears easily. Try using a large inversion (worm) suture to close these incisions. In the female, suturing is easier if the pathologist made a Y incision over rather than under the breasts. This might be suggested to the pathologist.

Cranial Cavity

During the embalming of the body, a phenol cautery chemical can be placed on cotton compresses and laid along the autopsy incision where the scalp has been opened. This will assist in drying the marginal tissues and reduce the possibility of leakage from this incision when the scalp is closed by suturing.

Arterial solution or blood that has accumulated in the posterior portion of the cranial cavity should be re-

moved by aspirating or sponging. The walls of the cavity can be painted with autopsy gel or dusted with a preservative powder. An absorbent material should be placed in the cavity to absorb the liquids that may accumulate. In addition, some embalmers place incision seal powder in the foramen magnum and the posterior areas of the cranium to absorb the liquids that might leak.

Some embalmers force a long wood dowel into the foramen magnum. This holds the head steady if the vertebral column has been opened for examination.

The calvarium, at the start of preparing the body, can be removed and placed into a plastic bag. Some cavity fluid or a phenol cautery can be poured into the bag. This is allowed to sit until it is time to attach the calvarium. This treatment will preserve and help to dry any tissues which are still attached to the calvarium.

Next, the calvarium should be replaced. If the autopsy has been properly performed, there should be one **notch** in the area of the **frontal bone** and other **notches** laterally in the **area of the temporal bone**. If notches are present, the calvarium will not be able to move forward, backward, or laterally (from side to side). If notches are not present, several methods of attachment can be used to prevent the calvarium from moving:

1. Suture through the temporalis muscles and up across the calvarium. Suture through the cut portion of the temporalis muscle still attached to the temporal bone and through that portion of the muscle still attached to the calvarium.
2. Separately suture the cut temporalis muscles on either side of the head.
3. Use calvarium "clamps." Several varieties are available.
4. Drill opposing holes in the calvarium and the temporal bone and wire the calvarium into position.
5. Use superglue to help hold the calvarium in position.
6. Use plaster of Paris. This older method of attachment may have advantages if the skull was fractured. The base of the skull would be aligned and plastered into position (prior to arterial injection). Later, the cranial cavity can be filled with cotton and this can be covered with plaster, and the calvarium (or its pieces) can be placed into position.
7. Use needle injector wires. Use four wires on each side: two attached to the calvarium and two attached to the temporal bone. Then crisscross the wires.

After the calvarium is attached, place a small amount of "mortuary putty" along the cut line of the calvarium in the region of the **forehead**. Mortuary putty can also be used to fill in the area of the temple where some of the muscle may have been cut away.

Figure 17–6. Treatment of the autopsied skull. **A.** The base of the skull is prepared using absorbent powders and cotton. Cavity walls are painted with gel preservatives. **B.** The temporalis muscle is sutured to the calvarium. The scalp is painted with a preservative gel. **C.** Begin on the right side when suturing the scalp. **D.** Use a "worm" suture for scalp closure. Spread incision seal powder along the incision. **E–F.** Completed suture.

338

Mortuary putty is a useful substitute for incision seal powder along the scalp incision. The putty helps to prevent leakage, especially if some of the material is pulled through the punctures made by the suture needle. If "mortuary putty" is not available and the temple muscles have been cut away, mortuary wax or cotton and glue can substitute as a filler. "Tissue builder" cannot be used if the muscles are missing.

Next, coat the calvarium with autopsy gel or preservative powder (Fig. 17–6). Reflect the scalp over the calvarium. While attaching the calvarium, pull the scalp down over the face. Doing so prevents wrinkles in the area of the forehead. After reflecting the scalp, spread some incision seal powder or mortuary putty along the posterior portion of the area where the scalp meets the occipital and temporal bones to help prevent leakage through the sutures.

Begin sutures on the right side of the head and end them on the left side.

There are several ways in which the hair can be kept out of the suture line:

1. Comb the hair out of the way with water.
2. Use hair clamps to "clamp" the hair away from the sutures.
3. Moisten the hair with liquid soap and comb the hair away from the incision line.

Using a double-curved needle, tie the first suture into place behind the right ear. **Do not use knots;** they have a tendency to pull through the scalp. Single- or double-linen suture cord can be used. Single is preferred and the cord should be a minimum of five-twist (strand) linen suture cord. Two sutures can be used to close the scalp incision. The **inversion (worm) suture** is made entirely on the surface of the scalp. The area between the edge on the scalp and the needle "rolls under" if each stitch is tightly pulled when the sutures are completed. Only a straight line should be seen. On a bald head, the line can easily be waxed or covered with glue, and cosmetics placed over the dried glue. If a **baseball suture** is used, be sure each suture is tightly placed. No thread should be seen.

Some embalmers use **super adhesive** in place of sutures on the scalp. In the preparation of infants and in difficult circumstances (such as when surgery has been performed on the cranium), super adhesive may be advantageous.

▶ FINAL PROCEDURES

After suturing, the hair and the body should be washed and thoroughly dried. The sutures can be sealed with a surface glue. Some embalmers cover the glue (while still wet) with cotton or cotton webbing. If air appears to be trapped in the thoracic area, insert a trocar through the abdominal wall just under the skin surface to draw out the air. Dress the body in coveralls (or cover the sutures with plastic); embalming powder should be placed in the coveralls to control moisture, mold, and odor.

▶ ADDITIONAL EXAMINATIONS

Cervical Vertebrae

In some autopsies, the posterior of the cervical vertebrae is opened externally and examined (Fig. 17–7). Cervical vertebrae are usually examined when a broken neck is suspected or when bleeding may have occurred along the vertebrae (as might occur in falls or automobile accidents).

For the pathologist to examine the vertebrae, an incision is made along the back of the neck, above the line where the shirt collar would pass to as high as the hair-line.

Roll the body on its side or, if necessary, completely over prior to arterial injection and remove any sutures. Pack the area with a phenol cautery chemical. Hold the edges together with bridge sutures or several strips of duct tape. After the body is embalmed again, roll the body on its side or completely over. Remove the cautery packing, dry the deep tissues, fill the incision with incision seal powder or "mortuary putty," and tightly suture closed using a baseball stitch. The sutures can be coated with a thick layer of surface glue.

Tissues are sometimes taken from the knee areas. These incisions can be opened prior to arterial embalming. They should be dried with cotton and packed with a cautery agent on cotton swabs. After injection, dry out

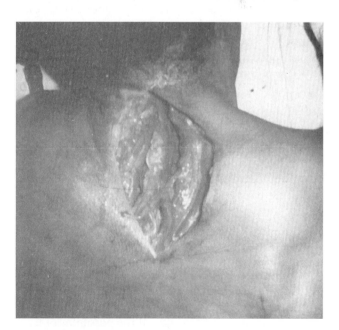

Figure 17–7. Examination of cervical vertebrae.

the area, fill with incision seal powder, and suture tightly closed with a baseball stitch. The incisions can then be glued. If leakage might be a problem, place plastic stockings on the body.

▶ BATTERED CHILD SYNDROME

An extensive medico-legal autopsy will follow a detailed external and x-ray examination of all body areas. The visceral organs will be examined for traumatic as well as any pathological changes. Inner walls of the body cavities will be examined for evidence of blunt force trauma and fractures. The battered child syndrome autopsy can be very extensive and invasive. Any external body surface suspect of blunt force injuries may be incised. This incising of subcutaneous fatty areas can reveal evidence of bruising and contusions caused by of blunt force injuries that may not be visible on the skin surface. Tissue samples for microscopic examination my be taken from these incised areas as well as from any lacerations, contusions or bone fractures.

All external incisions and lacerations will need to be dried and closed by suture or a strong bonding super glue. Facial areas may be involved which would require wax reconstruction.

Death from Pulmonary Embolism

If the autopsy reveals a pulmonary embolism, the pathologist may trace its origins. Incisions are often made along the medial and the posterior areas of the lower legs. The pathologist is looking for the source of the clot that moved into the lungs. These incisions can be filled with cotton packs dipped in a phenol cautery solution or cavity fluid while the rest of the body is embalmed. After the other incisions have been closed, the cotton packs can be removed and the incisions can be packed with dry, absorbent cotton. Use sufficient amounts of incision seal powder or mortuary putty when suturing these long incisions. A baseball suture is the tightest stitch and the easiest to use. The stitching can be coated with a surface glue. Plastic stockings may be used if any leakage is anticipated.

Death from Drug Overdoses

In the autopsy of persons dead from suspected drug overdoses, the pathologist is likely to excise tissue where old keloid scars (fibrous tissue) have formed from the use of needles. Generally, a square of tissue is cut out, quite often in the bend of the elbow. **The excision cannot be closed by suturing.** It is best to cover these open areas with cotton saturated with phenol chemical prior to embalming. After arterial injection, remove the cotton, dry with a hair dryer, and paint the area with glue. Apply fresh cotton and wrap the area. If the possibility of leakage exists, place a plastic "sleeve" on the arm or self-clinging food wrap around the arm. Some embalmers

cut out a portion of plastic stocking to make a sleeve, slip it onto the arm, and tape it in place with duct tape.

▶ PARTIAL AUTOPSIES

Cranial Autopsy Only

In this partial autopsy, the cranial cavity is opened and the brain is removed. The body can be embalmed by one of the three procedures.

Method 1. Raise the right and the left common carotid arteries. Insert tubes in both, directed upward toward the head. Insert one tube directed downward toward the trunk in the right common carotid. Tie off (ligate) the lower portion of the left common carotid.

Use the right internal jugular vein for drainage.

Inject downward **first** to embalm the extremities and the trunk. Clamp off leakage in the cranium from the right and the left vertebral arteries (which are branches of the subclavian arteries). Inject the left and the right sides of the head, clamping off the left and the right internal carotid arteries.

Method 2. Raise the right common carotid artery and the right internal jugular vein. Insert two tubes directed upward toward the head and one tube directed downward toward the trunk.

Inject downward, clamping off the right and the left vertebral arteries and the left internal carotid artery. These are found in the base of the cranial cavity.

Inject up the right side of the head. Clamp off the right internal carotid artery in the base of the skull.

Method 3. Raise the right femoral artery and vein. Insert into the artery one tube directed upward and one tube directed to the foot.

Inject the right leg.

Inject upward toward the trunk and the head. Clamp off the right and the left internal carotid arteries and the right and the left vertebral arteries. After arterial injection, dry the cranial cavity, paint it with autopsy gel, and fill it with cotton.

Attach the calvarium and suture the scalp back into position using the inversion or baseball suture. Spread plenty of incision seal powder or mortuary putty within the incision as the suturing progresses. Begin suturing on the right side of the head and end on the left side.

▶ THORACIC AUTOPSY ONLY

In a thoracic partial autopsy, one or more organs of the cavity have been removed (assuming that the neck organs have not been removed). Drainage taken for the lower extremities and the abdomen are drained through

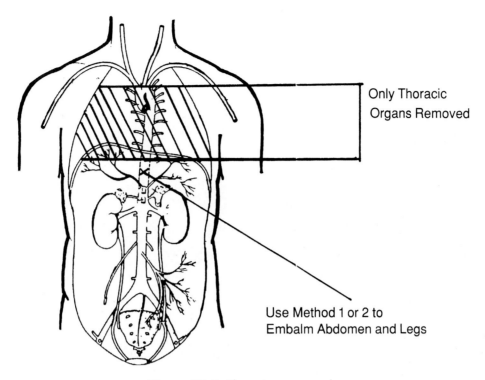

Only Thoracic
Organs Removed

Use Method 1 or 2 to
Embalm Abdomen and Legs

Figure 17–8. Thoracic autopsy only.

the inferior vena cava, which is located at the lower right area of the diaphragm (Fig. 17–8).

There is only one way to prepare the head and the arms. It is similar to the technique used after a complete autopsy, when the head and the arms are separately injected. Inject the left arm using the left subclavian or the left axillary artery. Inject the right arm using the right subclavian or the right axillary artery. Inject the left side of the head using the left common carotid artery. Inject the right side of the head using the right common carotid artery. Two methods can be used to inject the abdomen and the lower extremities:

Method 1. Locate the terminal portion of the thoracic aorta on the vertebral column at the central posterior portion of the diaphragm. Insert a large arterial tube into the aorta. Either clamp the tube in place with an arterial hemostat or, if possible, tie the tube in place. Inject downward through the arterial tube. This embalms the abdominal walls, abdominal contents, and lower extremities. Leakage may occur from the right and the left inferior or superior epigastric arteries, depending on how the pathologist made incisions.

Method 2. Raise the right femoral artery and insert a tube directed upward toward the abdomen. Also, insert a tube downward to inject the right leg. Inject the right leg first. Next, inject upward. This embalms the left leg, the abdominal contents, and the trunk. Ligate by tying or clamping the thoracic aorta when fluid is observed flowing from this artery into the thoracic cavity.

After arterial injection, check for preservation of the thoracic walls and the back and the shoulders. If the preservation is inadequate, the walls should be treated by hypodermic injection. The thoracic cavity can be painted with autopsy gel and filled with sheeting or an appropriate absorbent material. This material, in turn, can be saturated with cavity fluid or some other preservative, the breastplate can be put into position, and the incisions can be closed with a baseball suture. Aspirate the abdominal cavity and inject cavity fluid over the abdominal viscera (Fig. 17–9).

▶ ABDOMINAL AUTOPSY ONLY

In an abdominal partial autopsy, the contents of the abdominal cavity are removed (Fig. 17–10). If only the abdominal cavity is opened and the organs are removed, two methods can be employed for arterial embalming of the thorax, the upper extremities, and the head. The legs can be injected from the external iliac arteries. Drainage from the arterial injection of the upper trunk, the arms, and the head can be taken from the **inferior vena cava**, found in the lower right area of the diaphragm, where it would be attached to the liver:

Method 1. To inject the thorax, the upper extremities, and the head, locate the abdominal aorta as it passes through the diaphragm. The aorta can be located at the level of the vertebral column in the central posterior position of the diaphragm. Tie or clamp an arterial tube into the aorta. Upward injection should embalm the thorax and its contents, the arms, and the head.

Method 2. Raise the right common carotid artery. Insert a tube upward for the right side of the head. Insert a tube downward. Inject downward toward the trunk; the arms, the thorax, and the left side of the head should receive arterial solution. When leakage is noted from the aorta, clamp or tie the aorta in the abdominal cavity. After the

downward injection, inject the right side of the head. (The restricted cervical method of injection could also be used.)

Check the abdominal walls, the buttocks, and the back for fluid distribution. Depending on the pathologist's incision there may be leakage from the superior epigastric arteries during injection. (**Hypodermic injection can be used to preserve the abdominal walls and buttocks.**) Injection of the male genitalia may also be

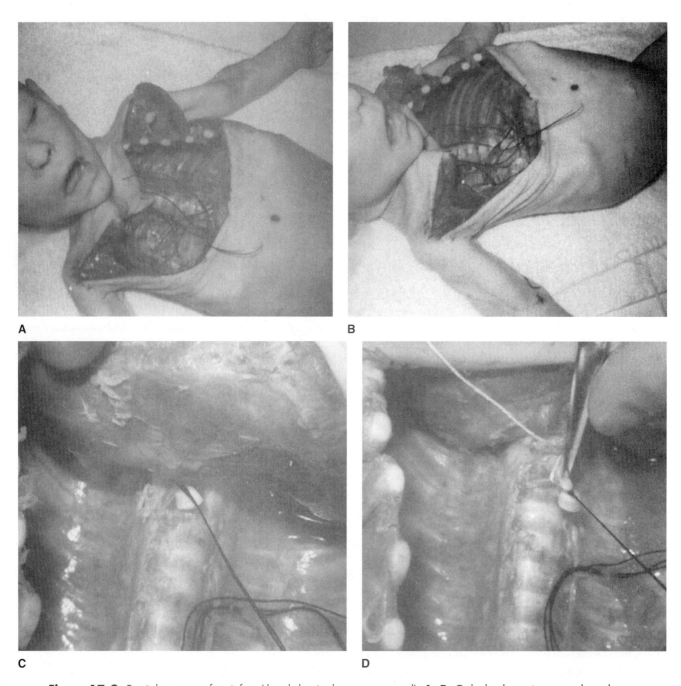

Figure 17–9. Partial autopsy of an infant (the abdominal aorta was used). **A, B.** Only the thoracic organs have been removed. **C.** The thoracic aorta is located on the spinal column. The diaphragm is at the top of the picture. **D.** The aorta being opened. Drainage is taken from the inferior vena cava located at the diaphragm. No drainage instruments are needed.

E   F

Figure 17–9. (*Continued*) **E.** The arterial tube is inserted into the aorta. **F.** Treatment of the abdominal viscera.

necessary. Direct injection of both internal iliac arteries will provide good distribution of arterial solution to the buttocks, the genitalia, and the upper thighs. The walls of the cavity can be painted with autopsy gel and the abdominal cavity can be filled with sheeting or other absorbent material. This filler can then be saturated with cavity chemical or other preservative.

Suture the abdominal incisions using a baseball suture. After washing and drying the body, cover the incisions with surface glue.

Aspiration and cavity fluid injection of the thorax can be done either through the diaphragm or by inserting the trocar through the rib cage. If aspiration and injection are to be done through the external rib cage

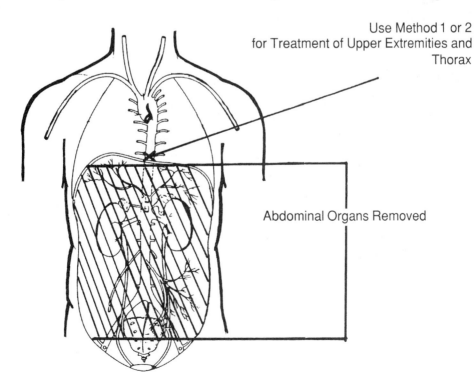

Use Method 1 or 2
for Treatment of Upper Extremities and
Thorax

Abdominal Organs Removed

Figure 17–10. Abdominal autopsy only.

wall, this treatment can be done **before or after** the autopsied cavity has been closed by suturing.

► PROTOCOL FOR THE TREATMENT OF AUTOPSIED BODIES WHEN RESTORATIVE TREATMENTS ARE NECESSARY

Restoration of the deceased to natural **form** and **color** is directly related to **embalming**. Many restorative treatments begin in the preembalming period and some are carried out during embalming. The majority of restorative work, however, is accomplished in the postembalming period. Accidental deaths may involve **trauma**, to the face and/or the hands. Because these deaths are accidental, the certification of death is under the jurisdiction of the coroner or the medical examiner. In most instances, the official will have the body autopsied to determine the exact cause and manner of death.

The outline that follows suggests the order of preparation of bodies that have sustained traumatic injuries to the face and have also been autopsied. Restorative art is a subject unto itself, and this protocol involves only some of those restorative treatments that should be carried out before and during arterial embalming. Two important criteria must be achieved for good restorative work. Tissues of the body must be **firm** and completely **dry**. It is the goal of the embalmer to adequately preserve and, thus, firm the tissue. By the use of embalming chemicals, solvents, and manual aids, the embalmer can dry the tissue.

In addition to trauma—be it lacerations, abrasions, bruising, or fractures—pathologic conditions may exist in the body prior to accidental death. Consideration must also be given to postmortem changes. Preparation of the body with facial trauma and a complete autopsy allows the embalmer to use a different strength of arterial solution for each area of the body injected. If trauma is in the facial tissues, a stronger solution can be injected to control swelling, and dry and firm these tissues; a milder solution may be desired for the arms and/or the legs. These factors, taken together, constitute the basis for the embalming analysis:

1. Disinfect and position the body:
   a. Be cautious of shards of glass that may be embedded in the skin if glass was involved in the accident. Sometimes these shards can be flushed out with water or picked out with forceps.
   b. Use cool water and plenty of liquid soap to remove blood, grease, and oils.
2. Assess the damage to all body areas.
3. Begin with injection of the legs; then inject the arms.
4. Prepare the head and face:

   a. Open the cranial cavity and check for fractured bones. Inspect for scalp lacerations or abrasions.
   b. Shave the body. Observe punctures, lacerations, abrasions, and hematomas. Remove all loose skin and dehydrated edges of lacerated tissues using a sharp razor or scalpel.
   c. By application of digital pressure to face, inspect for fractures of the mandible, maxillae, and nasal bones and for the presence of air (subcutaneous emphysema).
   d. Close the mouth using a method that keeps the lips in contact and align the jaw bones if they are fractured. Suturing may be required. Temporarily gluing lips may help.
   e. Close the eyes using cotton support or eye caps. Depending on the damage to the eyelids, it may be necessary to glue the lids prior to injection.
   f. Attempt to realign fractured bones and support depressed fractures.
   g. Align lacerated tissues. Temporary individual sutures of dental floss or superglue can be used. After embalming, remove the temporary sutures or glue anchors and place permanent sutures or glue.
   h. Prepare a very strong arterial solution using a high-index fluid (25-index and above). Dye should be added to the arterial solution.
   i. Inject the left side of the face first. Pulse the fluid into the head and observe the dye to check fluid distribution.

In many of these bodies there will be a great amount of fluid leakage. This leakage helps to control some of the swelling. What is important is that the tissues receive fluid; this will be indicated by the presence of the dye.

► CONCEPTS FOR STUDY AND DISCUSSION

1. Consult your local coroner or medical examiner and prepare a list of all bodies which must be referred to their office. Make an additional list of bodies which they require to be autopsied.
2. Describe the general order for embalming the autopsied body.
3. Describe several methods for securing the calvarium.
4. List the branches of the external carotid artery.
5. Give the location where the common carotid artery divides.
6. In the complete autopsy (neck organs removed), name the major arteries that must be clamped if the **left subclavian artery** is injected.

7. In the complete autopsy (neck organs removed), name the major arteries that must be clamped.
8. List the branches of the internal iliac artery and the area each supplies.
9. Describe several methods for preserving autopsy viscera.
10. Discuss several treatments for embalming the trunk walls in the autopsied body.
11. Describe two methods of injection to embalm the abdomen and the legs when a partial autopsy has been performed and the contents of the thoracic cavity have been removed.

▶ BIBLIOGRAPHY

Altman LK. Sharp drop in autopsies stirs fears that quality of care may also fall. *New York Times*, July 21, 1988.

Altman LK. Diagnosis and the autopsies are found to differ greatly. *New York Times*, October 14, 1998.

DiMaio V, DiMaio D. *Forensic Pathology*, 2nd ed. Boca Raton, FL: CRC Press, 2001.

Ninker R. Ethics goes beyond self interest. *The Director* 1997;7:18.

Slocum RE. *Pre-embalming Considerations*. Boston, MA: Dodge Chemical Co.

CHAPTER 18

PREPARATION OF ORGAN AND TISSUE DONORS

CHAPTER OBJECTIVES

► Organ vs. tissue donation
► Uniform Anatomical Gift Act
► Procurement agency and funeral home communication
► Organ donor preparation
► Tissue donor preparations

Although **tissue donation** and **organ donation** share many similar goals and objectives, they are not exclusively the same. The differences are better understood by comparing the definition of **tissue** with the definition of **organ**. **Tissue** is defined as a collection of similar cells and the intercellular substances surrounding them. Tissue donation involves, skin, eye tissue, ligaments, and bones.* An **organ** is defined as any part of the body exercising a specific function, such as respiration, secretion, and digestion.† Organ donation refers to the procurement and transplantation of a body part that fulfills such a specific function. Organ transplantation would include procedures to transplant a kidney, heart, liver, and so on.

There are common issues and objectives that arise from the procurement and transplantation of organs and tissues. The nature of transplanting organs versus transplanting tissues also gives rise to different conditions and circumstances, which must be carefully controlled. Organ recovery and transplantation is very time sensitive. The patient must still be on a ventilator and remain in the Intensive Care Unit until taken to the operating room. Tissue recovery must be completed within 24 hours of death when the deceased has been refrigerated and 15 hours when there has been no refrigeration. Tissue can be preserved for a longer period of time allowing for a longer time until it can be transplanted.

---

*Stedman's Medical Dictionary**, 26th ed. Baltimore, MD: Williams & Wilkins, 1995:1816.
†*Stedman's Medical Dictionary*, p. 1257.

► FEDERAL REGULATIONS REQUIRING REFERRAL

In 1998, the United States Department of Health and Human Services through the Centers for Medicare and Medicaid Services enacted new regulations that require the referral of all "imminent deaths and actual deaths" by hospitals receiving Medicaid and Medicare funds. If the hospital does not comply with the referral process, it can lose that federal funding. This regulation was meant to insure that all families are offered the opportunity to donate and thus decrease the organ transplant waiting list. Today, that list has more than 100,000 men, women, and children listed on it. It also looks to help nearly one million people who need a tissue transplant during any given year.

► CONSENT FOR ORGAN AND TISSUE DONATION

The **Uniform Anatomical Gift Act** has been enacted in all states and the District of Columbia to provide statutory regulations regarding postmortem organ and tissue donation. The Act allows any person 18 years or older to donate all organs and tissues of his or her body for transplantation, research, or educational purposes after his or her death. Many states (43 as of this writing) have adopted what is called "First Person Consent or Donors Designation" that allows an individual to make a legally binding decision to become and organ/tissue donor. At

Figure 18–1. Incisions frequently used for organ transplantation.

the time of death, no further consent is needed from the family or next of kin. The Uniform Anatomical Gift Act provides the order of priority for consenting persons and specifically protects physicians who act in good faith from civil liabilities and criminal prosecution. It is responsibility of the hospitals and the organ procurement organizations to insure they have consent when needed from the correct person entitled to make that decision.

▶ ORGAN DONORS

Every effort is made to recover as many organs from a donor as possible. Currently, the following organs are being recovered for transplantation: heart, lung(s), heart and lungs en bloc, liver, kidney(s), pancreas, and small bowel. The number of organs that are actually recovered may depend on consent or on the viability of each individual organ. For example, the next of kin may only give consent for the procurement of a certain organ, or the cause and circumstances of death may affect the viability and transplantability of organs. Because of the variations that can occur in organ recovery, the embalmer must be prepared to deal with a variety of embalming issues that arise from organ donation. Dealing with embalming complications of organ donation will require the embalmer to (1) assess the situation, (2) analyze the embalming complications, (3) develop a plan for the application of embalming treatments, (4) implement the embalming plan, and then (5) engage in concurrent evaluation of the effectiveness of the embalming treatments, making any changes in procedure that might be indicated.

Embalming an organ donor is almost like embalming an autopsy case. The embalmer has two options for the arterial injection of an organ donor. First, there is the option of **external access**, in which embalming is accomplished by raising vessels at one of the commonly used injection and drainage sites. Second, there is the option of **internal access**, in which the embalmer opens the procurement incision(s) and attempts to inject the body utilizing the arterial structures that remain intact in the area(s) where organ recovery has taken place.

Embalming an organ donor using the external access option requires the embalmer to raise arteries and veins at one of the commonly used injection and drainage sites. Realistically, the embalmer can anticipate having to use two or more injection sites, depending on the extent of vascular disruption. In addition to the considerations for the organ procurement, the procedure would involve many of the same case analysis considerations that embalmers routinely apply. As the embalming proceeds, the embalmer needs to carefully monitor the body for signs that arterial solution is being adequately distributed in the body, and for indicators that the ligatures on vessels affected by the procurement are preventing leakage. If procurement ligatures are absent, or if they fail, the embalmer can anticipate excess leakage from the procurement incision or distension caused by an accumulation of liquids in body cavities. If the leakage and/or distension are too severe, the procurement incision will likely have to be opened to deal with the complication.

If the internal access option is selected for embalming an organ donor, the embalmer can anticipate finding one of the following four procurement incisions* (Fig. 18–1).

1. A midline incision that runs from the base of the neck to a point superior to the umbilicus for a heart, lung, or heart and lung procurement.
2. A midline incision that runs from the base of the sternum to the pubic bone for liver, kidney, pancreas, and/or small bowel recovery.

---

*From Toledo-Pereya LH. *Organ Procurement and Preservation for Transplantation*, 2nd ed. Austin, TX: Landes Bioscience, 1997.

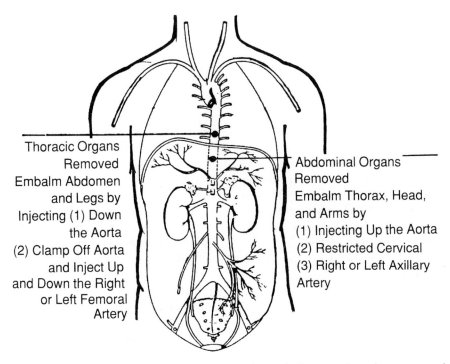

Figure 18–2. Embalming sites in bodies from which organs have been removed.

3. A "T" incision that transverses the abdomen along the inferior margin of the ribcage, and a midline incision from the base of the sternum to the pubic bone for liver, kidney, pancreas, and/or small bowel recovery.

4. A midline incision that runs from the base of the neck to the pubic bone if a full recovery was done.

Today, most embalmers have become experienced with the preparation of the autopsy case. The knowledge, skill, and experience of autopsy embalming can be applied when the embalmer is called upon to embalm an organ donor. In cases where the procurement has been limited, embalming can be approached in a manner similar to embalming a partial autopsy. In cases where a full organ procurement has taken place (heart, lungs, liver, kidney, pancreas, and small bowel), the embalming can be approached in a manner very similar to a full autopsy (Fig. 18–2). Keys to successful autopsy and organ donor embalming include (1) knowing anatomical structures and relationships and (2) anticipating which vessels have been cut. Because of time delay, a stronger arterial solution may be necessary. In addition, hypodermic injection of some areas will be necessary. As the body cavity may be empty, the embalmer will need to provide a filling to the chest and abdominal cavities to restore the natural form and also act as an absorbent. A drying or hardening compound is also recommended.

Other Issues

The embalmer will have to take into consideration the nature of the death when preparing the body. Frequently, organ donors have died as a result of trauma or some other sudden illness requiring time in the intensive care unit for life-sustaining measures. These issues must also be analyzed and approached in manner that leaves the entire body preserved.

▶ TISSUE DONORS

Eye Enucleation

One of the tissues most commonly transplanted today is the human cornea. Every year, thousands of individuals undergo corneal transplantation. Although the cornea itself can be removed from the organ donor, most frequently the entire eyeball is removed or **enucleated**.

The most common problem in the aftermath of an enucleation is swelling or distension in and around the orbital cavity. In addition, ecchymosis may be present, and there is always the possibility of small lacerations.

To help control swelling of the eyelids during embalming, the following procedures are recommended: (1) use restricted cervical injection to control arterial solution entering the head; (2) avoid preinjection procedures; (3) **do not** use weak arterial solutions—it is recommended that the solution be slightly stronger than average; (4) avoid excessive manipulation of the eyelids prior to and during embalming; (5) let embalming solution drain from the eye during arterial injection; (6) avoid rapid rates of flow and high injection pressure during arterial injection.

The following treatments have produced very satisfactory results:

1. **Before arterial injection**, apply massage cream around the eye to protect facial skin areas.
2. Remove packing from the eye.
3. Saturate pieces of cotton with autopsy gel and **loosely** fill the orbital cavity. Autopsy gel on the outside of the eyelids will not create additional problems. **Do not** pack the material tightly into the orbit—this will allow some leakage but will help to prevent swelling of the eyelids.
4. Fill the eye with sufficient cotton to recreate the normal appearance of the closed eye.
5. **Embalm the body**; use the procedures previously suggested to avoid swelling. If swelling does begin, strengthen the arterial solution so only a minimum amount can be injected. Stop injection if swelling becomes excessive and, if necessary, use surface embalming.
6. **After arterial injection**, remove the autopsy gel saturated cotton and dry the orbit.
7. Carefully place a small amount of incision seal powder or mortuary putty in the base of the orbit. Many incision seal powders swell in contact with moisture. Use only a minimum amount.
8. Pack the orbital cavity with cotton, kapok, or mortuary putty.
9. Exercise the eyelids and insert an eyecap over the filler.
10. Glue the eyelids closed.

With this method, major treatment of the eye occurs after the arterial injection (Fig. 18–3).

Cornea Removal

When only the cornea has been removed, the preparation work is greatly reduced. The body can be embalmed using whatever injection technique and arterial solution strength that the embalmer feels necessary. The eyes can be set after the arterial injection.

As the front of the eye is opened when the cornea is removed, the embalmer may find it necessary to aspirate the fluids from the eye to prevent leakage. During embalming, the hollow eye globe can be filled with cotton saturated with autopsy gel or undiluted cavity fluid. After embalming, the eye orbit is then filled with mortuary putty or incision sealer. An eyecap can be placed over the eyeball to support the eyelids, and create a natural contour and form. The eyelids can be secured with superglue (Fig. 18–4).

Vertebral Body Donor

Recovery of vertebral bodies involves removing sections of the spinal column. Once removed, the tissue is processed into biomedical products that are used in a number of orthopedic surgical procedures. As a rule, tissue procurement specialists will attempt to recover as large a section of the spinal column as possible but the size of the section removed may vary depending on the use to which the tissue will be put, the accessibility of the spine, and other factors. The embalmer can anticipate that varying lengths of spine may be removed from the donor depending on circumstances.

Access to the vertebral bodies can be gained in a number of ways. Vertebral bodies may be harvested following organ recovery or autopsy where an incision already exists, and the spine is partially or completely exposed. Vertebral bodies may be harvested from an anterior incision where no organ recovery or autopsy has been performed. Vertebral bodies may be harvested through a posterior incision. This usually occurs when no previous postmortem invasive procedures have occurred, but can also be used in cases where autopsy or organ recovery has taken place.

Recovery Following Autopsy or Organ Recovery. As embalmers know well, an autopsy will include the removal of thoracic, abdominal, and pelvic organs, exposing the spinal column. In this instance, removal of vertebral bodies will not significantly alter injection and drainage techniques for the embalmer, because recovery of the vertebral bodies requires no additional disruption to the cardiovascular system beyond what has already taken place at autopsy. One major concern will be the possibility that the tissue specialist has punctured skin on the donor's back during vertebral body recovery. The embalmer must carefully inspect the donor's back for leakage. Another major concern will be the loss of rigidity that results from having a section of the spinal column removed. Many tissue banks are reconstructing vertebral body donors with prosthetic devices intended to recreate the support previously provided by the tissues that have been removed, thus making the spine and back area rigid. One of the most effective of these devices is a Limbz product, which is made of adjustable lengths of polyvinyl chloride piping and end caps containing surgical screws. The device's adjustability allows it to be fitted to the size of the opening in the spinal column. Turning the surgical screws into the remaining bony structures allows the device to be securely attached at the top and the bottom of the opening. The secure, custom-fitted device assures stability during dressing and casketing.

In those cases where vertebral bodies have been removed following organ donation, the embalmer will encounter circumstances quite different from autopsy. In

Figure 18-3. Procedure for eye enucleation restoration.

Figure 18–4. A. Aspiration of the eye globe after the cornea is removed. **B.** Packing inserted into aspirated eye globe. The packing is saturated with autopsy gel or cavity fluid. **C.** After embalming, the eye globe is dried and incision seal powder is placed in the globe to prevent any leakage. **D.** Cotton is placed over the incision seal powder to fill the eye globe. An eyecap is placed over the filled globe. **E.** The lids are sealed with glue. **F.** Completed restoration. Only the cornea was removed from each eye.

such cases, a majority of viscera will be left in the body, with the notable exception of the organ or organs that have been harvested.

The embalming procedures required for this type of case would include locating the transected vascular structures, watching for leakage from skin punctures that may have been made in the back during vertebral body recovery, and the loss of rigidity in the spinal column.

For example, in a case where the heart has been removed for transplant, the embalmer deals with the vascular disruptions of the organ donation during the arterial injection and the structural disruptions of the vertebral body recovery during reconstruction. The transected ends of the subclavian arteries and common carotid arteries are located and injected to embalm the head, neck, and arms, in much the same manner as an autopsied case. The lower portion of the body can be embalmed by injecting interiorly from the thoracic or abdominal aorta.

Recovery via an Anterior Incision. Some tissue banks recover vertebral bodies using an anterior midline incision that runs from the xiphoid process to the pubic bone. The primary consideration in this method is to avoid making an incision on the back of the donor, which creates obvious complications for the embalmer. When the anterior incision is utilized, however, the embalmer can anticipate that the aorta will be cut in both the thoracic and abdominal cavities, and that a renal vein(s) will be cut. Once the incision has been made, the tissue specialist mobilizes and retracts the necessary organs to allow the spinal column to be visualized. It is at this time that the aorta will be cut. Once the vertebral tissue has been recovered, a prosthesis may be put in position. The tissue procurement specialist will then place the viscera back into position. Although it is necessary for some vascular structures to be sacrificed, procurement procedures caution the tissue specialist to avoid cutting or damaging vascular structures needlessly. Procurement procedures also instruct tissue procurement specialists to ligate any vessel that is damaged or cut. The embalmer would be wise to anticipate the possibility that accidental damage or disruptions will occur from time to time. As such, it is prudent for the embalmer to open the incision to determine whether vascular disruptions exist, and take the appropriate steps to deal with them. The embalmer may be able to arterially inject such a case using the ends of the transected vessels, carefully watching for signs that solution is being lost in the abdominal or thoracic cavities.

Recovery via a Posterior Incision. This method requires that a posterior midline incision be made: beginning at the level of the scapula, ending at about the level of the sacrum. Once the incision is made, the surrounding tissues are dissected to expose the spine. The section of spine to be removed is transected and rotated in such a manner that leaves the spinal cord in the body. If proper skill and care are utilized, this procedure will not cut or damage the vascular structures that are necessary for embalming. Once the section of spine is taken from the body, the tissue procurement specialist will install a prosthetic device as described previously, and suture the incision closed.

Because the vascular system should not be disrupted by this procedure, the embalmer can approach arterial injection and venous drainage in a manner that is determined by evaluating factors common to case analysis. The embalmer must consider leakage from the procurement incision as a major postembalming problem, and take appropriate steps to stop leakage and seal the incision.

The embalmer must be aware of several factors that will affect embalming results in the aftermath of vertebral body recovery. First and foremost, vertebral body recovery seldom takes place without other tissues also being taken. If the patient is a full tissue donor, the embalmer will be dealing with a multitude of conditions that will require special attention. Second, depending on the procedure utilized by the tissue bank, the embalmer will most certainly have to deal with the possibility of leakage from the body following vertebral body recovery. Third, again depending on the procedure utilized by the tissue bank and the length of spine taken, the embalmer will need to take steps to reconstruct the body in such a way as to provide rigidity previously provided by the tissue that has been removed. This type of recovery generally requires the use of plastic coveralls or unionalls to insure there is no leakage following the preparation.

Long Bone Donor (Femur, Tibia, Fibula, Hemipelvis)

The recovery of long bone tissue from a donor involves making an incision along the anterior surface of each leg from the tip of the hip to the mid-foot. Long bone procurement is the most dramatic of all tissue recovery. In some cases, no type of internal tissue will be found in the lower extremities from mid-thigh to the mid-foot area, only skin will remain. It involves a great amount of time, not only for the removal of the tissue, but also for the treatments that will be applied by the embalmer. Because of the delays that are involved in this process, and the large-scale disruptions of the circulatory system, it is recommended that arterial injection be accomplished with a stronger arterial solution than normal. These bodies should not be preinjected. The increased strength of the arterial solution accomplishes two things: (1) if a smaller volume of solution is distributed to the tissues and the muscles, the higher concentration of preservative will,

Figure 18-5. Removal of long bones from the legs. The procedure was performed under sterile conditions.

to a certain extent, offset the lack of volume; (2) there is some possibility that arterial solution which pools in the tissue spaces will penetrate the tissues and provide some preservation (Fig. 18–5).

Two methods of preparation for the legs are discussed. In the first technique, the incisions are opened; in the second, if the sutures are tight, they are not opened.

Method 1. Supports, such as head blocks, can be placed along the medial and lateral sides of the legs in preparation of removing the sutures. This work practice helps to create a "channel" to drain blood and embalming chemicals flow to the foot of the table, thus allowing the embalmer to maintain a cleaner work area.

In those cases where the donor's legs have been sutured, **all** suture lines are removed from the extremities. The prosthetic device should not be removed as it may not be able to be put back in the same manner it was inserted by the tissue recovery staff. The embalmer then locates and identifies any ligatures that have been put in place by the tissue procurement team. The practice of ligating vessels during procurement varies widely, and it will not be uncommon for the embalmer to find no ligatures.

The embalmer will then dissect and ligate the left and right femoral arteries to isolate each extremity for injection separately from the rest of the body.

The trunk, hips, head, neck, and upper extremities of the body can be injected by using cervical and/or femoral vessels as injection and drainage sites. If necessary, the embalmer can choose other injection sites as needed to complete this portion of the preparation.

Care is taken to ensure that embalming solution does not freely flow into either the lower extremities during injection of the trunk, hips, head, and neck, or the upper extremities.

The thigh and leg areas are injected by using the left and right femoral arteries. Care is taken to clamp off other vessels as loss of embalming solution becomes apparent. Particular attention is paid to the multiple branches of the genicular arteries found just above the knee, because they will likely have been cut during sharp dissection. A large number of hemostats may be required.

The leg and foot are injected by using the left and right popliteal arteries. In some instances, the popliteal may not be accessible and the embalmer may use the superior aspects of either the anterior or posterior tibial artery for injection. Care is again taken to clamp off other vessels as loss of embalming solution becomes apparent. Here, also, the multiple branches of the genicular arteries found just below the knee will likely have been cut during sharp dissection. A large number of hemostats may be required.

Hypodermic injection may be required to supplement arterial injection. The embalmer must carefully assess the success of arterial injection to determine where hypodermic supplement might be required.

At the conclusion of the arterial and hypodermic injections, the embalmer dries the tissue bed with absorbent cotton.

A light coating of preservative/drying compound is applied to the tissue beds. It is to the embalmer's advantage to use a substance that has both preservative and absorptive qualities.

If no internal structures are found from mid-thigh to mid-ankle, the embalmer must still preserve the skin tissue left behind. This can be accomplished by use of undiluted cavity packs or mortuary gels placed prior to arterial injection of the rest of the body. The musculature of the mid-thigh can be hypodermically injected following arterial injection.

The incisions are then sutured closed. Care is taken to make the sutures tight. Additional preservative/drying compound may be added during the suturing process. Following suturing, the body is thoroughly bathed. Cotton and liquid sealer are then applied to the incision to provide an additional barrier to leakage. Finally, plastic stockings and pants are placed on the body as a further barrier to leakage. The body is now ready for dressing and casketing.

Method 2. Free-flow method. There is a second method for preparing the lower extremities when the long bones (femur, tibia, and fibula) have been removed. This method leaves the procurement sutures in place. Some embalmers prefer to open the procurement sutures and pack the entire leg with an absorbent material and then resuture the leg. If tight baseball stitches have been used to close the incisions, leakage from these sutures should be minimal. Raise the right and left external iliac arteries (or right and left femoral arteries) and insert arterial tubes directed down the legs in each vessel. Prepare an arterial solution of very strong concentration: a high-index arterial fluid with equal parts of water or 100% arterial fluid. Inject each leg using at least a half-gallon of solution. The tissues of the leg will distend slightly (Fig. 18–6). Be certain that the solution has reached portions of the leg below the knee. Stop the injection and let the arterial solution saturate the tissues while the arms, and the head and trunk areas of the body are embalmed. After the solution has had time to thoroughly saturate the tissues of the leg with a scalpel, place a puncture in the area of the lower leg. Insert a drain tube or trocar and force as much of the solution as possible from the leg. The tissue procurement specialists will have placed prosthetic devices into the legs and heavily padded them with gauze sponges. These will now act as internal compresses. The procurement team's suturing can then be coated with a surface glue and the leg placed in a plastic stocking containing preservative powder or autopsy gel.

Method 3. Saturated packing. The embalmer opens all of the procurement sutures. The legs are packed with an absorbent material and the leg is resutured. The resuturing should begin at the foot. As the packing and suturing proceeds, the packing material is saturated with an undiluted cavity fluid or a strong arterial fluid. This creates an internal preservative compress. The larger muscles of the thigh area can be injected with a strong preser-

A

B

Figure 18–6. Injection of the leg using the femoral artery. The recovery team has sutured the leg using a tight baseball suture. **B.** Drainage of excess fluids, 1 hour after injection, from the lower leg.

vative solution using an infant trocar. Both the baseball and the worm suture work well for this procedure. The sutures should be "locked-down" about every 5 in. as the suturing proceeds. If necessary, a preservative gel can be applied to the skin areas of the leg and a Capri garment or stocking placed on the legs.

Proximal Humerus and Scapula Donors

In spite of the steady increase in the number of bone donors encountered by embalmers, tissue banks still operate in an environment where demand for tissue products far exceeds the supply. As a result of this shortage, tissue banks are constantly evaluating the possibility of procuring bones in addition to the pelvis and long bones from which suitable tissue products can be processed.

The proximal humerus and scapula have been identified as additional sources of bone, and embalmers can anticipate seeing cases where these structures have been

Figure 18–7. Anterior incision for removal of the proximal humerus.

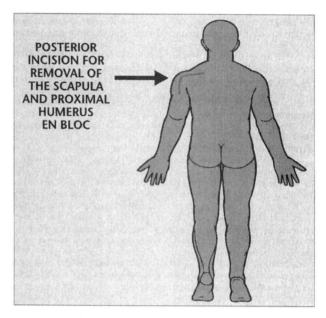

Figure 18–9. Incision for scapula recovery. (*Drawing used with permission from NFDA.*)

taken, procurement technicians will usually take them en bloc. In those cases where the scapula will not be recovered, only the proximal humerus will be taken from the donor (Figures 18-7 to 18-10).

Restoration by the Procurement Technician. It is the responsibility of the procurement technician to restore the body to a condition and appearance as similar to the preprocurement condition and appearance as possible.

In those cases where the tissue has been harvested in a funeral home preparation room, the funeral home staff may request that the procurement technician **not**

procured. The term "proximal humerus" is used by tissue banks to indicate that only the humeral head and upper portion of the humerus are recovered. The scapula is commonly known as the shoulder blade. In those cases where both the proximal humerus and the scapula are

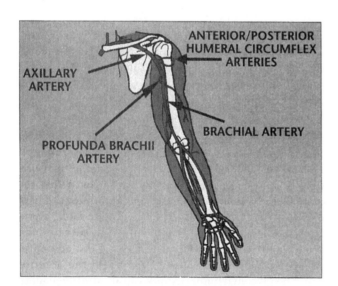

Figure 18–8. Arteries of the upper arm. [*Courtesy of National Funeral Directors Association (NFDA).*]

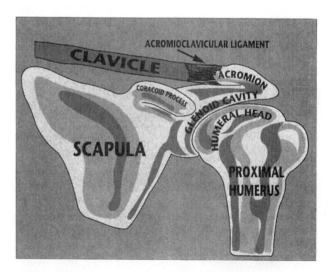

Figure 18–10. The acromioclavicular ligament attaches the scapula to the clavicle. (*Used with permission from NFDA.*)

do the restoration at the conclusion of the procurement. It makes little sense for the procurement technician to do restorative work on a donor, only to have the embalmer come in and remove the sutures and prosthesis in order to prepare the body. The funeral home can request that the prosthesis and any other materials needed for the restoration be left for use at the time of postembalming restoration. Communication between the tissue bank and the funeral home is important in these cases, so that both know the other's capabilities, needs, and preferences.

In those cases where the restoration is completed by the procurement technician, it will be necessary to utilize a prosthetic device to recreate the shape and support that was once provided by the harvested bone. Some tissue banks employ devices made of plastic tubing that can be secured by means of surgical screws to the glenoid cavity and to the distal end of the humerus. Once the prosthesis is in place, the incision is closed with a tight suture.

Any leakage that might occur after a proximal humerus recovery would generally be easier to manage because the procurement incision occurs on the anterior surface of the shoulder. The anterior location of the incision causes blood and other fluids to gravitate away from the opening of the incision. Greater difficulty could be anticipated for a proximal humerus and scapula en bloc procurement where the incision is made on the posterior surface of the shoulder. The posterior location of the incision would cause blood and other fluids to gravitate toward the opening of the incision.

Embalming. Unlike many other types of tissue procurement, proximal humerus and scapula removal can be done with little disruption to the blood vascular system. If the procurement technician exercises the necessary skill and care, major blood vessels in the arm and shoulder will be intact for arterial embalming. This circumstance has obvious implications for the embalmer. The major vessels most likely to be severed would be the axillary or brachial arteries.

EMBALMING WITHOUT OPENING THE PROCUREMENT INCISION. If proper technique has been employed in procurement and restoration, it may be possible to embalm the body without opening the procurement incisions. Selecting this option requires that the embalmer know, or trust, that the technician has done the procurement without disrupting major blood vessels. In this situation, the embalmer employs standard procedures, using either a cervical or a femoral injection and drainage site. As the arterial injection proceeds, the embalmer must carefully monitor the procurement site for distension and/or leakage. If neither occurs, the embalming can be completed with a normal application of embalming

Figure 18–11. Injection of the arm using the brachial artery.

procedures. If distension occurs, it is likely that either blood or embalming solution is causing the problem. The embalmer must assess the problem, and make a determination as to whether the procurement incision should be opened, and alternative embalming procedures be applied.

OPENING THE PROCUREMENT INCISION. In cases where the procurement incision is opened before or during arterial injection, the embalmer first examines the procurement site for cut or broken blood vessels. If no disruption is found in either the axillary or brachial arteries, the embalmer looks for cuts or breaks in the anterior and/or posterior humeral circumflex arteries, or in the profunda brachii artery (Fig. 18–11). Cuts or breaks in smaller branch arteries may not represent a significant enough disruption to prevent the perfusion of arterial solution into the arm and hand. If either the axillary or brachial artery is cut or broken, the embalmer ligates the proximal (close to the midline) and distal (away from the midline) end of the vessel. Ligation of the proximal end helps to control leakage as the rest of the body was embalmed. Ligation of the distal end would serve as an anatomical marker for locating the vessel as an injection site when the arm and hand are embalmed. If either the axillary or basilic vein has been cut or broken, the embalmer will clamp the proximal and distal ends of the vessel so that they are marked. The embalmer may choose to allow drainage to flow from cut or broken veins as arterial injection takes place. If controlled drainage is desired, the open ends of the axillary or basilic vein can be clamped.

Other Embalming Considerations. Opening the incision and examining the procurement site may not always reveal cut or broken vessels. As the arterial injection is proceeding, the embalmer will monitor the site for signs of leakage. Blood leaking into the procurement site during arterial injection should prompt the embalmer to look for a cut or a break in the axillary vein, basilic vein, or one of their tributaries. In this case, it is possible to continue embalming from the primary injection site. Leakage from the veins is not a significant problem during arterial injection, but it is necessary for the embalmer to make certain that any cut or broken veins are properly ligated, if possible, at the conclusion of the arterial injection to prevent postembalming leakage.

Arterial solution leaking into the procurement site indicates that vessels providing circulation to the arm and hand have been disrupted. The embalmer can thus conclude that the arm and hand are likely to have to be injected separately from the rest of the body. The embalmer examines the procurement site for a cut or break in the axillary artery or the brachial artery. If either has been cut or broken, the embalmer must locate the distal and proximal ends of the vessel. The proximal end is clamped, and the distal end used as a secondary injection site to embalm the arm and hand separately from the rest of the body. If examination reveals the artery has only been punctured, the embalmer may attempt to clamp the puncture and continue with the injection. It may also be possible for the embalmer to utilize the puncture as a secondary injection site. For those cases where the axillary or brachial arteries have been cut or broken, the axillary and basilic veins may also have been cut. Leakage or drainage from these vessels can be controlled with hemostats.

At the conclusion of arterial injection, the embalmer should assess embalming results to determine if supplemental embalming techniques are necessary. The embalmer must securely ligate all vessels that have been cut or broken. Once the embalmer has determined that leakage has been stopped, the procurement site should then be thoroughly dried. The incision can be packed with cotton saturated with a chemical cautery. This can remain in place or removed in several hours. Once removed, pack the cavity with absorbent material, and treated with powdered incision sealer. A tight suture will then be used to hold the incision closed. The sutures should be treated with a coating of liquid sealer, and a layer of absorbent material. The embalmer should take effective steps to stop or contain any postembalming leakage that might occur.

Embalming proximal humerus and scapula donors does not present great difficulty, providing the procure-

Figure 18–12. Areas from which skin is most often removed.

ment has been done with reasonable skill and care. Many of the procedures are not significantly different from procedures frequently applied in autopsied cases or in sectional embalming.

Skin Donors

Donor skin is recovered by two different methods: **partial thickness and full thickness.** Skin can be removed from the back, buttocks, thighs, and lower legs, and in some instances the chest. The partial thickness method employs an instrument called a **dermatome**, and it is used to peel or shave very thin layers of the skin (Fig. 18–12). The full thickness or the free-hand method removes skin and connective tissue structures down to the muscle layer using a scalpel. This method removes the vascular layer of the skin. Generally, less leakage will be seen during the embalming when the free hand method is used.

The recovery of skin from the dead human body presents three major problems for the embalmer. First, during the process of the skin removal, the body has been turned and has rested on its abdomen, this may create a blood discoloration of the facial tissues. Second, drying of the affected areas from which skin has been taken. Third, control of the (1) seepage or leakage from the area where skin has been taken and (2) leakage from the borders surrounding the areas where skin was removed.

Discolored Facial Tissues. When the body is received at the funeral facility and it is noted that the facial tissues exhibit a blood discoloration, the following steps can be taken:

1. Position the body with elevation to the shoulders and elevation to the head.
2. Disinfect the facial tissues, eyes, nasal, and oral cavities. Wash and dry the face and hair. Apply a thin coating of massage cream to the facial tissues.
3. Pack the throat and set the features.
4. Using the **restricted cervical technique**. For the unautopsied body, inject the head draining from the right internal jugular vein (possibly draining from both jugular veins).
5. Because of time delays, use an arterial solution of moderate strength and inject slowly; during injection massage, the discolored tissues encouraging a flow of arterial solution into these tissues and a displacement of the blood and resultant discoloration. The arterial solution should contain added dye.

A similar technique can be followed for the embalming of the autopsied body when blood discolorations are present in the facial tissues.

Treatment of Areas from which Skin has been Removed (see color plate section of text)

PARTIAL THICKNESS DONOR. After removing the body from the body bag, with assistance, turn the body on its side and inspect the areas from which the skin has been removed. These areas can be sprayed with a disinfectant and patted dry:

1. Position the body on the embalming table where the feet are secured at the bottom of the table. This will prevent slippage of the body.
2. Elevate the body on **body bridges**.

EMBALM THE BODY. During the embalming, with the partial thickness method, it is possible for a great amount of blood and fluid drainage to occur through the areas where skin has been removed. If time permits, let the body sit to allow leakage and drying of the areas where the skin has been removed. Time permitting air drying will help to seal the affected areas. Treatment can next include:

1. Turn the body on its side. Dry and inspect the raw areas.
2. The nude skin areas can be painted with a cautery agent or preservative gel.
3. Cover the painted areas with an absorbent material.
4. Lay the body down onto an absorbent sheet, if skin has been removed from the legs cut the sheet so each leg can be wrapped. Excess sheeting can be cut away. The sheet will also allow better maneuvering of the body.
5. Place the body in an appropriate plastic garment – a unionall may be necessary. A dusting of hardening or autopsy compound can be placed inside the plastic garment.

FULL THICKNESS DONOR. The full thickness or the free hand method of skin removal is gradually replacing the partial thickness method of removal. Treatment can follow similar steps as that outlined for the partial thickness recovery. The full thickness recovery removes the vascular layer of the tissues so usually very little leakage during arterial injection will be noted. If possible, allow the tissues to dry as much as possible following the arterial embalming. Keeping the body elevated on body bridges will permit air to come into contact with the affected areas and promote drying of the tissues.

BONE AND SKIN DONOR. Often, with skin recovery, there is also a recovery of long bones. These same methods of treatment can be followed.

1. First, embalm the body.
2. Prepare the limbs from which the bones have been removed. Complete this task by tightly suturing the extremities from which the bones have been removed.
3. Finally, prepare the areas of the body from which the skin has been removed.

Plastic garments are very helpful in containing any leakage that may occur. Many of the procurement agencies will supply these garments.

Mandible Donors

Mandible recovery does not occur as frequently as other types of tissue donation. In most cases, mandibles are recovered from bodies that will not be viewed. There are two methods by which mandibles are removed from the body. Both methods have significant embalming and restorative consequences.

Method 1. An incision is made on the undersurface of the jaw starting at the angle of the jaw on one side, following the jawline under and around the chin to the angle of the jaw on the other side. The skin, muscle, and fascia are then dissected away, exposing the bone. Once the bone has been freed from soft tissue, it is manually disarticulated from the temporomandibular joint, and removed.

Method 2. An incision is made between the lip and gum on the inside of the mouth, following the jawline from approximately the angle of the jaw on one side of the face, passing over the chin to the angle of the jaw on the other side of the face. The soft tissues are then dissected away so that the mandible can be freed, disarticulated, and removed.

In both cases, the arterial system supplying the facial surface will be disrupted. In particular, the facial artery will be cut and/or broken in the process. The external incision method will leave obvious restorative problems, although the internal incision method, if not done carefully, can result in tears or cuts in the surface tissue along the jawline as well.

Rib Donors

Ribs are usually recovered through the same incision used for vascular organ recovery. After organ recovery, a scalpel is used to peel back the skin, and every other rib is removed. The embalmer will have to contend with disruptions to the intercostal arteries as a result of this procedure. This may not present a problem that would cause the embalmer to make any significant changes in procedure, but will definitely contribute to leakage during embalming. The embalmer must ensure that the leakage is stopped so that it does not create problems after embalming.

Temporal Bone Donors

Two techniques are employed to recover the temporal bone: (1) exterior approach and (2) interior approach.

Generally, leakage can be controlled with hemostats or by tightly packing cotton into the area where the temporal bone has been removed and applying hand pressure. After embalming, mortuary putty or incision seal powder can be placed in the area from which the bone was removed. Some embalmers prefer plaster of Paris as a filler for this cavity. These measures ensure against further leakage from the external ear as well as from the scalp. Plenty of absorbent cotton filler can be placed in the cranial cavity prior to suturing the scalp. It is wise to pack the external auditory meatus with cotton and some incision seal powder to prevent leakage from the external ear.

If the bone was removed by the external approach and the ear has been partially excised after embalming, the temporal area should be packed with a phenol cautery agent. This material should be left in place for a time, and then replaced with dry cotton and incision seal powder. Mortuary putty can also be used as a filler. The ear can be reattached with intradermal sutures or superglue.

▶ CONCLUSIONS

In an environment where the demand for organs and tissue exceeds supply, organ and tissue procurement organizations will continue to work very hard to perpetuate the growth in donations that has already been realized. Embalmers can anticipate an ever-increasing number of cases where the deceased has been a donor. Knowing what steps to take in the preparation of donors is a professional requirement for the embalmer.

There is a great need for embalmers and organ and tissue procurement organizations to become professional colleagues because the work done by each group is vital to fulfilling the wishes of the deceased and/or the deceased's next of kin. Unfortunately, the lack of regard that sometimes exists between the two groups has created a number of adversarial situations. *It is important to remember that both the funeral home and these organizations are involved in postdeath activities at the invitation of, and with the permission of, the donor and/or the donor family.*

The funeral service community, however, has every right to insist that procurements be done in a manner that preserves options for open-casket viewing. Procurement organizations go to great lengths to ensure donor families that consent to recovering organs and tissues will not significantly disrupt funeral plans. Donor families, therefore, have a right to expect that these organizations are true to that claim. Funeral directors are in a unique position, because they know when procurement agencies have failed to keep their word. Funeral directors, therefore, can serve families by communicating with procurement organizations regarding any issues and problems that arise from procurement. That does not mean the funeral director becomes a watchdog. Rather, the funeral director and the procurement organizations are colleagues who must deal in a professional manner with each other, and the families they serve.

▶ CONCEPTS FOR STUDY

1. Contact your local organ/tissue procurement agency and make a list of the types of bodies or conditions which would prohibit the decedent from becoming a donor.
2. Discuss the difference in the preparation of a body from which the whole eye has been removed vs. the donor from which only the cornea has been removed.

3. Discuss under what conditions can a decedent may not be an organ donor but can be a tissue donor.

▶ BIBLIOGRAPHY

Koosmann S. Bone transplantation. In *Champion Expanding Encyclopedia.* Springfield, OH: Champion Chemical Co., 1984:2210–2217.

Kroshus TJ, Stroud D, Klitzke K, et al. Embalming techniques in long bone donor cases. *American Funeral Director* 1995;118(30):26–27.

Kroshus TJ. Embalming the vertebral body donor. *The Director.* 1997;69(30):32–34.

Kroshus TJ, Stroud D, Klitzke K, et al. Heart transplantation. In Hakim NS, ed. *Introduction to Organ Transplantation.* London: Imperial College Press, 1997:121–132.

Kroshus TJ. Embalming proximal humerus and scapula donors. *The Director.* 1998;70:44–48.

Mayer RG. Enucleation restoration. In *Champion Expanding Encyclopedia.* Springfield, OH: Champion Chemical Co., 1987:2322–2325.

Toledo-Pereya, LH. *Organ Procurement and Preservation for Transplantation,* 2nd ed. Austin, TX: Landes Bioscience, 1997.

CHAPTER 19

DELAYED EMBALMING

CHAPTER OBJECTIVES

▶ Preparation of the body in the state of rigor mortis
▶ Preparation of the refrigerated body
▶ Preparation of the body showing signs of decomposition

This chapter discusses the preparation of bodies where there has been a time delay between death and embalming. Over the years, the broad rule has been, the sooner the embalming is performed, following the death, the better the results that can be obtained and the fewest complications encountered. It seems as the time between death and preparation increases so to do the difficulties. In addition to time, internal and external temperatures, cause and manner of death, medications, activity prior to death, and others—all speed and/or slow postmortem changes. Thus, it is easy to see the ideal time for preparation will vary from body to body.

Preparations discussed in this chapter include the following:

■ Bodies embalmed in a state of rigor mortis.
■ Bodies that have been refrigerated.
■ Bodies displaying early signs of decomposition after the passage of rigor mortis.

The common external factor with all these bodies is an extended period of time between death and embalming.

Six factors enter into the embalming analysis of a body:

1. The body itself—for example, age, weight, musculature.
2. Immediate cause and manner of death.
3. Disease(s) within the body.
4. Effects of medications.
5. Postmortem physical and chemical changes.
6. Postembalming conditions, for example, firmness desired, time between preparation and disposition, shipping.

Postmortem changes begin at the time of death. Embalming of the body retards or stops most of these changes. A detailed discussion of these 11 physical and chemical changes can be found in Chapter 5. These changes do not occur simultaneously throughout the body. Bodies in which there has been a time delay between death and preparation exhibit three common problems. These problems are common with both the autopsied body and the unautopsied body. The unautopsied body will be the subject of discussion unless otherwise noted.

First, the embalmer can anticipate problems in achieving an **even distribution** of the injected arterial solution. This can be caused by any of the following: the presence of rigor mortis, increased postmortem coagula, increased viscosity of both arterial and venous blood, or the breakdown of portions of the capillary system. This results in some areas receiving too much solution and other body areas receiving too little or no arterial solution.

Second, these bodies can easily **swell**, especially unsupported tissues such as the neck and eyelids. Noticeable too will be the easy distension of the facial glands (parotids) and the submandibular and submaxillary glands. Bodies dead for long periods of time do not assimilate the arterial solution well.

Third, these bodies all exhibit an increased preservative demand. A time delay between death and embalming allows for the breakdown of body proteins (Fig. 19–1). Even with refrigerated bodies, there has been a slowing of decomposition but not a stoppage of decomposition. A breakdown of body proteins increases the sites for attachment of preservative.

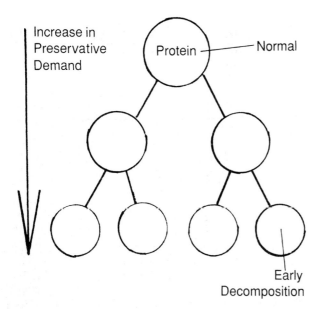

Figure 19–1. Demand for preservative is increased in bodies as protein breaks down.

Preservative absorption by tissue proteins is usually greatest immediately after injection. Most bodies exhibit some degree of firming during the injection process. One reason for this early fixation is that the concentration of preservative (fixative) is greatest when the arterial solution is first introduced into the tissues. If a sufficient amount of preservative has been injected, complete firming of the body will occur several hours to a day later. Degree of decomposition, tissue pH, and temperature and concentration of arterial solution all play a role in determining the speed and degree of fixation. Cool temperature slows these reactions; alkaline pH above 7.4 slows fixation; and decomposed protein demands more concentrated preservative.

This increased fluid need is brought about by the breakdown of tissues. As circulation is impaired in most of these bodies, distribution problems can be anticipated. As these bodies are all subject to distension, use **of a minimum amount** of **a stronger** arterial solution best establishes good preservation and minimizes tissue distension. Stronger (hypertonic) arterial solutions help to minimize swelling of the tissues.

▶ MECHANICAL, MANUAL, AND OPERATIVE AIDS

Achieving adequate distribution of the preservative solution with a minimum amount of tissue swelling is of great concern in the preparation of bodies where there has been an extended time delay between death and embalming. Manual aids—**during arterial injection**—such as lowering the arms; firm massage; squeezing the sides

of the fingers and the nailbeds; bending, rotating, and flexing of limbs; and massaging the areas of the buttocks and shoulders where there is contact with the embalming table surface or positioning devices, will help to distribute the arterial solution. Mechanical aids in the form of drainage tubes, controlled pressure and rate of flow, use of pulsation, and size of the arterial tube will all help to control the speed and the amount of embalming solution entering the body or a body area.

When localized swelling of unsupported tissues such as the eyelids or neck occurs, operative aids that involve invasive treatments such as channeling, incising, and if necessary excising can be used to correct the swollen condition. Manual aids such as elevation, weights, compresses, and pneumatic collars can be used to correct minor swellings.

▶ GENERAL EMBALMING TREATMENTS INJECTION PROTOCOL

Embalming of a body involves four steps: (1) observation of the body, (2) evaluation of the conditions present, (3) implementation of an injection and drainage plan, and (4) observation of the results achieved.

During the injection of the arterial solution, the embalmer needs to ask the following questions:

1. Which body areas are receiving arterial solution and which are not?
2. What can be done to stimulate arterial solution into body areas where the arterial solution is not being distributed?
3. Is there sufficient arterial solution in all body areas?

For underembalmed areas, the embalmer has three choices: (1) arterial injection, (2) hypodermic embalming, and (3) surface embalming.

Restricted cervical injection or a six-point injection plan is the best injection choices when embalming unautopsied bodies dead for long periods of time. With restricted cervical injection, drainage can be taken from the right internal jugular vein with the six-point injection from each injection site, or from one drainage point such as the right internal jugular vein. A one-point injection is not recommended for these bodies since it is difficult to control the amount of fluid entering the head.

Restricted Cervical Injection
Restricted cervical injection, using the two carotid arteries, works well in the preparation of these bodies. First, inject the trunk and limb areas. **Be certain that the tubes directed toward the head remain open during injection of the trunk**. Arterial solution that has reached the face and head by collateral routes will exit from the body and

Color Plate 1. Ecchymosis of eyes (a).

Color Plate 3. Discoloration covered with opaque cosmetic (c).

Color Plate 2. Cavity fluid on cotton under eyelids (b).

Color Plate 4. Ecchymosis and IV Puncture, back of hand.

Color Plate 5. Bleach injected after embalming.

Color Plate 7. Ecchymosis and post-mortem Stain, and Tardieu spots (a).

Color Plate 6. Swelling of IV puncture during embalming.

Color Plate 8. Eyes set after embalming (b).

Color Plate 9. Opaque cosmetic application (c).

Color Plate 11. Hands lowered before and during injection, to stimulate fluid distribution (b).

Color Plate 10. Livor mortis in fingers—diabetic (a).

Color Plate 12. Hands and fingers cleared (c).

Color Plate 13. Excessive facial dehydration post-embalming.

Color Plate 15. Body in river 3 months—post-mortem stain.

Color Plate 14. Carbon monoxide death. Note intense discoloration in the dependent areas.

Color Plate 16. CO death. Hematoma of eye, purge (a).

Color Plate 17. Post embalming—note bleaching (b).

Color Plate 19. Chicken pox (a).

Color Plate 18. Cosmetic application (c).

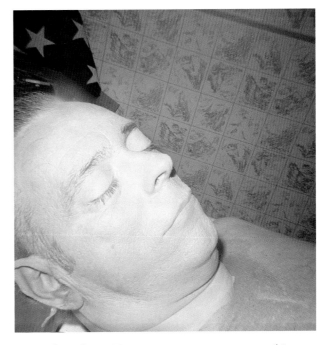

Color Plate 20. Opaque cosmetic treatment (b).

Color Plate 21. Vitamin B. deficiency—note lesions (a).

Color Plate 23. Cosmetic treatment. Hair restoration (c).

Color Plate 22. Lesions dried (b).

Color Plate 24. Burns of arm and hand.

Color Plate 25. Facial abrasions—dried.

Color Plate 27. Auto victim—cosmetic treatment (b).

Color Plate 26. Auto victim—moist lacerations (a).

Color Plate 28. Gunshot within mouth—fractures (a).

Color Plate 29. Gunshot—pre-cosmetic treatment (b).

Color Plate 31. Body prepared with non-formaldehyde fluid.

Color Plate 30. Hand treated with non-form aldehyde fluid, note pebbling, which will dissipate.

Color Plate 32. Obese—PVC shoulder elevation to clear livor mortis from face and neck.

thus prevent the head from receiving fluid. The head should be injected last. If purge develops during the downward injection, this method allows the features to be set and the body to be aspirated **before** the head is injected.

Six-Point Injection

If this method is used first, raise all six arteries; common carotids, axillaries, and femorals. First inject the legs, then the arms, then the trunk, and finally the head. If purge develops, the body can be aspirated and the features set before the head is injected. Drainage can be taken from each site or from the right internal jugular vein.

Autopsied Remains

If the body has been autopsied, a six-point or a multi-point injection is necessary. Drainage will be taken from each injection site.

FACTORS DETERMINED BY THE EMBALMING ANALYSIS

1. Vessels for injection and drainage
2. Method of mouth closure
3. Strength of the embalming solution
4. Volume of the embalming solution
5. Injection pressure
6. Injection rate of flow

Note: These factors will vary by the individual body and can vary in different areas of the same body.

Arterial Solution Strength and Volume

As previously stated, a stronger-than-average arterial solution is needed for the bodies discussed in this chapter, especially when signs of decomposition are evident. Arterial fluids of 25 index or higher are recommended. When decomposition is present, a *high-index special-purpose fluid* is advised.

In preparing the arterial solution, the first recommendation is to follow the suggestions of the manufacturer. Many labels carry dilution instructions for delayed, refrigerated, or decomposed bodies. Preinjection fluids should be avoided. Use of a coinjection would be a better choice.

The first half-gallon may be made milder in an attempt to clear blood discolorations in the unautopsied body, but should be followed by stronger fluid solutions, 2.0% strength or higher. In the treatment of bodies that show evidence of decomposition, 100% arterial fluid with a coinjection fluid (waterless) may be required. Fluid dye can be added to the embalming solutions because it will serve as an indicator of arterial solution dis-

tribution. The dye will also help to prevent graying of the embalmed tissues.

For extreme situations, the **instant tissue fixation** method may be helpful. It can be used to inject each section of the autopsied or the unautopsied body. With respect to the face, it can minimize swelling while establishing maximum fluid distribution throughout the facial tissues.

The amount of solution injected depends on the size of the body and the success in distributing the arterial solution. The tissues of these bodies can easily distend, necessitating the use of a concentrated, well-coordinated embalming solution. Such a solution should require less amount (volume) to establish maximum preservation and a minimum amount of tissue distension.

Pressure and Rate of Flow. When there has been a long delay between death and embalming, the unautopsied body should be *very slowly injected.* Slower injection helps to prevent coagula in the arterial system from moving (solution flows over the coagula) into the smaller distal arteries. Rapid injection can easily cause intestinal distension, which puts pressure on the stomach and can create purge. Even in embalming the "normal" body, the first gallon of arterial fluid is slowly injected; then the process may be speeded to facilitate distribution of the arterial solution.

In the injection of arms or legs of the autopsied body, higher pressures and faster rates of flow may be needed to establish distribution. Pulsation may be helpful in distributing fluid to the extremities, and higher pressures can be used with pulsation.

A pulsed flow can be created in several ways: use an embalming machine with a pulse setting; manually turn the rate of flow valve on and off; turn the stopcock valve on and off; bend the delivery hose, starting and stopping the flow of fluid.

▶ PREPARATION OF BODIES IN RIGOR MORTIS

One of the most difficult preparations is that of the body in the intense state of **rigor mortis**, in particular, the body that is well nourished and has a well-developed musculature. These bodies with well-developed musculature develop a very intense rigor mortis. It may be impossible for the embalmer to remove this rigor by manipulating the body prior to injection of the arterial solution. Thin bodies, bodies that demonstrate the effects of wasting disease, and bodies in which the musculature is not well developed undergo the complete rigor mortis cycle; however, the rigor can be more easily relieved prior to injection.

Rigor mortis, which affects all body muscles begins as soon as the body cannot replenish adenosine triphosphate (ATP). Any activity that reduces ATP prior to death will speed the onset of rigor. It rapidly occurs in bodies with high temperatures and where exertion or exercise have preceded death. Rigor can even occur instantaneously (cadaveric spasm) in situations such as automobile crashes. It can be recognized in the "average" body within the first 2 to 4 hours following death. Within 6 to 12 hours, it will generally be fully established. It passes generally in approximately 36 hours following death. An old rule states, "the sooner the onset, the sooner the passage." Depending on cause of death, environmental temperature, and activity prior to death, the rigor can occur sooner or be delayed. It is easy to see how easily this postmortem change varies from body to body. (See Chapter 5 for further details concerning the rigor mortis cycle in the dead human body.) The passage of rigor is actually brought about by the start of decomposition.

Rigor comprises three general stages: (1) primary flaccidity, the period in which the rigor develops and is hardly noticeable; (2) the period of rigor; (3) secondary flaccidity, in which the rigor has passed from the body. The most problems are encountered when the body is to be embalmed while in intense rigor.

Table 19–1 summarizes the preservative demand of the muscle tissues during the stages of rigor.

As noted in Table 19–1, a body in rigor absorbs a very small amount of preservative. The problem, however, arises in that once the rigor passes the demand for preservative increases greatly. **It is imperative that the embalmer saturate the tissues with a well-coordinated solution of sufficient strength to meet the preservative demands of the body when the rigor has passed.** Otherwise, the body will soften not only from the passage of rigor, but from the decomposition processes that break down body proteins. Therefore, the bodies embalmed prior to the onset of rigor should be injected with a sufficient strength of arterial solution to meet the preservation needs as determined from body weight and effects of disease or drugs; bodies embalmed during and after rigor mortis have a higher preservative demand.

Problems Associated with Embalming Bodies in Rigor

Rigor may be relieved by physical manipulation of the muscle tissues. Firmly massaging, rotating, flexing, and bending the joints help to relieve the rigor condition. **Once broken, the condition does not recur.** In persons with a well-developed musculature, it may be very difficult to attempt to relieve rigor in areas such as the thighs or arms. The following problems may be encountered in the preparation of the body in intense rigor:

- Positioning may be difficult.
- The features may be difficult to set if the jaw is firmly fixed. Packing of the throat may be difficult if not impossible.
- Distribution of fluid may be poor because of the pressure on arteries and the narrowed arterial lumens resulting from contraction of muscle cells in the arterial walls.
- Drainage may be poor because of the pressure exerted by contracted muscles on the small veins.
- Tissues tend to swell, because fluid does not penetrate muscles during rigor but flows to surface areas where there is little resistance.
- The pH of the tissues is not ideal for fluid reactions.
- Tissues may not firm well after the passage of rigor, because it may not have been possible to inject sufficient quantities of the arterial solution.
- Firmness of rigor can be a false sign of tissue fixation.

Other Considerations for Bodies in Rigor Mortis. During the period in which rigor occurs, the pH of the tissues is slightly acid. It has been found that the preservative-protein reaction occurs most readily at slightly basic pH, about the same as that of normal, healthy tissues (7.38 to 7.4). Also, pH will not be the same in the various muscles. Where rigor has passed from the muscles, autolysis and hydrolysis have proceeded to a point where protein has decomposed and the pH has become increasingly alkaline (basic).

Increase of tissue pH into the alkaline pH range after rigor mortis indicates that the muscle proteins have

TABLE 19–1. PRESERVATIVE DEMAND OF THE MUSCLE TISSUES DURING RIGOR

Prerigor	Great absorption of preservative	The protein centers to which preservative attaches and cross-links the proteins are readily available. Tissue pH is slightly alkaline and fluids work best in this pH range.
Rigor	Little absorption of preservative	The protein centers to which preservative attaches are engaged in maintaining the state of rigor mortis; vessel lumens are reduced so distribution is decreased. Muscle protein is contracted so fluid does not penetrate the muscle fibers well. The acid pH retards the absorption of preservative.
After rigor	Great preservative demand	Proteins have disorganized (or broken) and many centers are available for preservative attachment. The alkaline pH increases preservative absorption; nitrogenous wastes increase the need for preservative.

begun to break down or decompose. There are now additional sites for reaction with preservative. During rigor, there are few sites for the reaction of preservative and proteins. A body being embalmed while in rigor should be saturated with sufficient preservative, so that it will be available later as the state of rigor passes.

Rigor and varying pH combine to make it very difficult for the embalmer to obtain uniform preservation of the body. Some of the factors that contribute to this lack of uniform embalming are outlined in the following chart:

BODIES IN RIGOR MORTIS

▶ Degree of rigor varies in the different muscle groups.
▶ Tissue pH varies throughout the body.
▶ There is a lack of uniform distribution of fluid as a result of rigor mortis.
▶ Depending on the degree of rigor, tissues vary in their preservative demand.

As the absorption of preservative results in firming, there is a relationship between the rate of preservative absorption by tissues and the rate of firming. This is why bodies embalmed prior to the onset of rigor rapidly firm; preservative is rapidly absorbed and rapidly attaches to the proteins. During rigor, the proteins are "locked" together, and it is difficult for the preservative to attach to the proteins. As a result, there is little absorption of preservative by muscles in the state of rigor mortis. Most of the firming that occurs during the injection of a body in rigor is caused by the swelling of the tissues. If a mild or a weak arterial solution is used, these tissues soften later. After the passage of rigor, demand for preservative increases greatly.

As well as a need to use strong solutions in the preparation of bodies in rigor, there is a need for a coinjection chemical. This chemical helps to adjust tissue pH as the various areas of the body are at different pH. The buffers in arterial fluids help to achieve the uniform pH necessary for the action of the preservative. It is easily seen that distribution is not uniform in these bodies, dyes are not evenly distributed, firming is not uniform, and the preservative needs of the tissues vary throughout the body.

PRESERVATIVE ABSORPTION AND FIRMING

Prerigor	Good absorption	Firming is good
Rigor	Little absorption	Firming is due to the rigor present and swelling
Postrigor	Great need for preservative	Firming is difficult to achieve

Firmness cannot be relied on as a test of preservation, for the firmness may be a result of the rigor present in the muscles. Firmness can also result from the distension of tissues during injection of arterial solution. In addition, if the embalmer attempted to relieve the rigor by manipulating the muscles, many capillary beds may have been torn, which would also account for the swelling of muscles and tissues during arterial injection. Tissues also swell because fluid follows the path(s) of least resistance. These paths lead to surface areas because the rigor present in the deep muscles resists the flow of fluid.

Features
In setting the features of a body in intense rigor, use a towel to firmly manipulate the jaw. Begin by raising the jaw, even if the lips are firmly pressed together. Massaging the temporalis muscles may also be helpful. Firmly push the chin, covering the chin with a towel and pressing firmly with the palm of the hand. Cotton may also be forced into the mouth to help open it. As soon as the lips can be properly aligned, suture or use a needle injector to ensure that the lower jaw remains in the proper position.

Positioning
Firmly rotate, bend, flex, and massage the joints and muscles of the neck, arms, and, if possible, legs. This may be necessary to position the body properly. Relieve the rigor in the arms by first rotating the shoulder joint. Next, flex the elbow and wrist areas. Grasp all the fingers and gently pull them into a straightened position if the hand is firmly closed. To relieve rigor in the legs, exercise the hip joint first. Next, flex the knee joint. Finally, rotate the foot inward very firmly. These manipulations help to relieve some of the rigor present.

Injection
Restricted cervical or a six-point injection may be needed to thoroughly embalm these bodies. The right internal jugular vein is the best drainage site. If a six-point injection is used in addition to the right internal jugular, drainage can be taken at each injection site. A medium to strong arterial solution should be used. Follow the manufacturer's recommendations for dilutions. Dye and coinjection fluid can be added to the solution. The extra dye not only serves as a fluid tracer, but helps to prevent the tissues from graying. In the embalming of these bodies, blood drainage is often minimal and formaldehyde gray can easily develop hours after embalming. The coinjection fluid assists in fluid penetration and adjustment of tissue pH. The dye merely indicates that surface tissues have received fluid; there is no indicator for the deeper tissues.

Some embalmers prefer to begin the injection of most bodies with a mild arterial solution (1.25–1.50%)

until surface blood discolorations are cleared. Subsequent injections are then made using stronger arterial solutions. Avoid the use of preinjection fluids with the body in intense rigor condition. Whenever distribution difficulties are expected, preinjection should not be used.

As soon as the body is undressed and treated with a surface disinfectant, attempt to reduce the intensity of the rigor mortis by flexing, bending, and manipulating the limbs. Hands can be lowered to encourage the flow of the arterial solution into the hands. Inject slowly. During arterial injection, continue massage and manipulation of the limbs to encourage distribution. When drainage is established, the injection speed can be slightly increased to encourage better distribution. If a six-point injection is used, higher pressure and rate of flow can be used for direct injection of the body limbs. Injection pulsation may assist in distribution of the solution. This technique may prove useful in the injection of the autopsied body in intense rigor mortis.

Use of a minimum amount of a strong solution helps to control swelling and achieve good preservation and tissue fixation.

▶ PREPARATION OF REFRIGERATED BODIES

Almost all bodies removed from medical or forensic institutions have been refrigerated for some period of time. It is difficult to set an exact length of time after which refrigeration would pose special problems for the embalmer. Some advantages of short-term refrigeration include (1) slows the progress of rigor mortis, (2) slows decomposition, and (3) maintains blood in a liquid state. Because the blood remains liquid, livor mortis can be expected to be more intense. Long-term refrigeration, however, can cause a number of problems for the embalmer.

For years, one effect of refrigeration has been a major subject of discussion—**dehydration**; however, this situation has changed. When bodies were wrapped in cotton sheets and refrigerated, surface dehydration occurred easily. Lips, eyes, and fingertips seem to be the first tissues noticeably affected.

Internally, the blood gradually thickened as the moisture was removed from the surface tissues. Movement of water out of the surface tissues forced the liquid portion of the blood into the dry tissues, causing a mild postmortem edema. This especially occurs in the dependent tissues. Gradually, this moisture also worked itself to the skin surface. If the body were exposed to the cool, dry air for a sufficient period, the tissues could even mummify as a result of dehydration. Today, however, most bodies are wrapped in plastic or placed into large zippered plastic pouches. Dehydration is no longer as great a problem. The plastic wrapping or pouch can

help to bring about other problems for the embalmer. Frequently bodies refrigerated over a period of a day or more will evidence decomposition (discolorations, abdominal gases, skin slip) encouraged by the trapped heat within the body and moisture in the pouch.

There is usually a slight elevation of body temperature after death (postmortem caloricity) because metabolism continues until the oxygen trapped in the body is exhausted. As the blood no longer circulates, the heat produced by the catabolic phase of metabolism is trapped in the body. Therefore, the body temperature increases slightly. Heat speeds the cycles of rigor mortis and decomposition. Because of this trapped heat, it is not unusual to find green discolorations on abdominal areas when the bodies are removed from refrigeration. Autolysis and bacterial activity continue while the body is in refrigeration, faster at first while the body is still warm and then slower as the tissues gradually cool.

Figure 19–2 illustrates some of the problems associated with refrigeration.

When bodies have been refrigerated for long periods and wrapped in plastic or placed in a plastic pouch, the embalmer can expect some of the following problems:

- Increased capillary permeability.
- Easy rupture of the capillaries during arterial injection.
- Tissue structure breakdown as a result of the slow, continuous processes of autolysis and bacterial enzymes.
- Increased coagula in the vascular system; increased blood viscosity.
- Gravitation of blood and body liquids into the dependent body tissues, resulting in an increase in moisture in these tissues.
- Intense livor mortis.
- Rapid hemolysis resulting in postmortem extravascular stain.
- Moist clammy tissues caused by the plastic wrapping of the surface tissues; possibly skin-slip.
- Decomposition signs (e.g., abdominal discoloration, purge, and skin-slip).
- Rapid distension of abdominal organs during injection, resulting in stomach and/or lung purge.
- Cold solidified subcutaneous fatty tissues can give a **false sign** of firm tissues similar to firmness brought about by embalming.

Blood gravitates to dependent areas. Blood thinners and cooling of the body both contribute to the hypostasis of the blood. In refrigerated bodies, livor mortis can be intense. Postmortem stain can rapidly occur and often postmortem petechiae and purpura (Tardieu spots) will be seen as capillaries rupture in the dependent tissues. As the body cools, hemolysis easily occurs, causing the

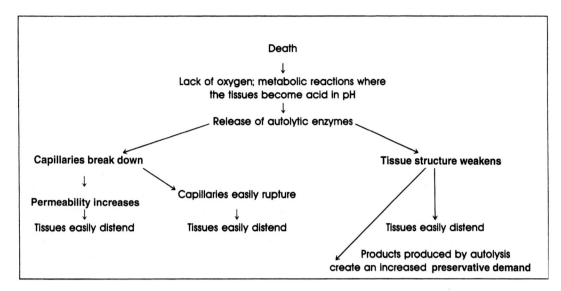

Figure 19–2. Problems associated with refrigeration: time–temperature effects.

blood cells to rupture and release **heme** into the tissues. This results in **postmortem staining**. This type of blood discoloration cannot be removed by arterial injection and blood drainage. If the head has not been raised, these discolorations may be present in the facial tissues. Some bleaching is possible with the use of a strong arterial solution, a bleaching coinjection fluid, and surface bleaches. Postmortem stain and the Tardieu spots can be lightened but **not** removed. Opaque cosmetics are needed to hide the discoloration.

If the body has been refrigerated for a long period and wrapped in cloth sheeting, dehydration will be a problem. The amount of moisture in the dependent tissues increases because of hypostasis of the blood and tissue fluids into these areas. The upper areas of the body may be browned from dehydration. Of particular interest to the embalmer are the drying and browning of the lips, eyelids, fingers, and base of the nose. The cheeks and forehead may also exhibit dehydration. The dehydrated tissues can range in color from yellow to brown

to black in both Caucasians and African-Americans. This discoloration cannot be removed by arterial injection. Opaque cosmetics are used to hide the discolorations. Surface dehydration water also creates a loss of moisture from the blood vascular system. There will be increased amount of coagula in the vascular system, making distribution of the arterial solution very difficult.

During refrigeration, the progress of rigor mortis slows, but still occurs. Rigor usually passes in 36+ hours after death. Because it is slowed by cooling, it may still be present in some muscles at the time of embalming. Decomposition is what breaks rigor, and it too is slowed in a body that is cooled.

Arterial Preparation

Swelling is always a concern when embalming has been delayed, this includes. Distension of visible body areas as well as the swelling of the hollow abdominal viscera (Fig. 19–3). Visceral swelling can create sufficient pressure

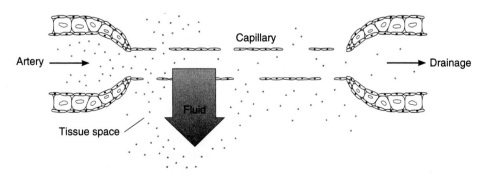

Figure 19–3. Refrigerated bodies and bodies in which decomposition has begun easily swell because of capillary breakdown and increased capillary permeability.

on the stomach and create purge. There is an increased demand for preservative, as the processes of autolysis and decomposition slowly continue. The presence of rigor mortis and the increased moisture content of the dependent tissues increase the preservative demand. Arterial injection of the trunk areas should be **slow** using a strong, well-coordinated arterial solution with tracer dye added. Distribution may be difficult to achieve and drainage may be limited. The amount of fluid and volume of solution, of course, is determined by the size of the body and the embalmer's satisfaction that the tissues have received sufficient preservative solution.

Extra amounts of fluid dye should be used to trace the distribution of arterial fluid. When postmortem stain is present, the tissues can easily gray several hours after embalming. The dye helps to cover the gray discoloration produced when formaldehyde and hemoglobin combine. The skin of refrigerated bodies can have a slight pinkness. This is caused by the hemolysis of red blood cells trapped in surface tissues. The tissues appear to be embalmed. In addition, the cold has a tendency to solidify the fatty tissues of the body, so the tissues may also feel embalmed. False signs of embalming include firmness from swollen tissues, pink from hemolysis which resembles fluid dye, and firmness from solidified subcutaneous body fats.

If the head has been excessively elevated during extended refrigeration, the tissues of the face can be dehydrated. This is caused by the gravitation of interstitial fluids in addition to any moisture loss created by the refrigeration environment. A good application of massage cream on the outside and inside of the buccal cavity can help to moisturize the lips, eyelids can be also be treated with a light application of massage cream. The entire face can be lightly coated with massage cream. Eyes may be sunken. This is due to a loss of moisture from the eyeball. Setting the eyes with cotton can help to elevate the lids. Some embalmers inject tissue builder into the eyeball or behind the eyeball to elevate the eyes—this is best done after arterial injection. (Eyes can be set before or after arterial embalming.) A milder arterial solution may be best for injection of the head. A coinjection and/or humectant can be added to the arterial solution in an attempt to moisturize the tissues.

As strong arterial solutions are necessary for the body trunk and limbs and a milder arterial solution for the face and head, use of **restricted cervical** injection is recommended. Drainage may be difficult to establish because of increased blood viscosity and coagula; therefore, the right internal jugular vein would be the best choice for the primary drainage site. Multipoint injection should be used for arms and legs not receiving sufficient arterial solution. Injection should be slow to prevent abdominal distension and to keep arterial coagula from moving and blocking smaller arteries.

Dependent areas of the trunk, buttocks, and shoulders that do not receive sufficient fluid can be treated by thorough hypodermic injection. Cavity fluid can be injected (by infant trocar) into these areas through use of the embalming machine. These dependent areas are very moist and, thus, may be sites of bacterial activity. Surface treatment is of little or no value in these high-moisture areas.

Cavity Embalming

If restricted cervical injection is used, the cavities can be aspirated before the features are set and the head and the facial tissues are embalmed. If purge develops during embalming of trunk areas, aspirating **before** setting of the features eliminates the need to reopen the mouth and remove **purge**. Cavity embalming should be thorough. A minimum of one bottle of concentrated cavity fluid should be injected into each major body cavity. Reaspiration is always advised. If any gases escape when the trocar button is removed for reaspiration, if the abdomen appears distended or if the large surface veins of the neck appear distended, the cavities should also be reinjected with concentrated cavity fluid after reaspiration.

Final Treatments

The hair and the body should be washed at the completion of the preparation. As little water as possible should be run over the body during embalming and with the final washing. The body should be thoroughly dried—often a hair dryer will help with this process. Drying of the body will help to bring the cold tissues to room temperature. Having the skin at room temperature will stop moisture condensation on the face and the hands. Surface moisture can interfere with cosmetic application. Cosmetic application should be delayed until the tissues have had time to warm and condensation has stopped. Face and hands can be lightly coated with massage cream and tissue builder if necessary can be used to plump out dehydrated fingers and facial areas.

Frozen Tissues

Some refrigeration units may freeze body tissues. Ice crystals form when body tissues freeze and ice crystals tear tissues. The body should **not** be warmed by pouring warm water over it. Allow the body to warm gradually by letting it sit in the preparation room for several hours. Manipulation of the tissues while ice crystals are still present will cause more tearing. Try to manipulate the body as little as possible.

For the unautopsied body, restricted cervical or a six-point injection is vital. Some embalmers prefer to inject these bodies as soon as it is possible to raise an artery and a vein. When raising vessels, it will be noted most of the structures within the incision will have a similar pink color. There will be little or no blood drainage. A strong arterial solution should be used and injected very slowly. The blood acts as a vehicle for the arterial solution as it does in bodies from which blood is not drained. Some embalmers prefer to use a strong arterial solution prepared with warm to hot water. There are fluid manufacturers that make arterial fluids specifically for refrigerated and frozen bodies. **Follow recommendations of the fluid manufacturer.**

The facial tissues will, no doubt, be thawed so a stronger-than-average solution can be used to inject the head. If the embalmer feels that distension of the face will be a problem, a waterless solution should be considered.

Additional fluid dyes as a fluid tracer should be used in embalming these bodies.

▶ PREPARATION OF BODIES THAT SHOW SIGNS OF DECOMPOSITION

In the period between death and embalming, the cycles of rigor mortis and decomposition play out their roles in the dead human body. These cycles are both part of the postmortem chemical changes, and are speeded by elevated environmental and body temperature. While the cycle of rigor mortis affects directly the muscle cells of the body, decomposition in time will affect all body cells through the destructive action of autolytic and bacterial enzymes. The rigor and decomposition are integrated but rigor mortis is the first to be recognized. After the passage of rigor mortis, noticeable signs of decomposition can begin to be observed (Fig. 19–4). Some of the factors that speed the onset of decomposition include elevated environmental heat, elevated and retained body heat, high moisture content within the body, and translocation of intestinal bacteria.

Color Changes

Trunk Areas. One of the first external signs of decomposition is a green discoloration in the lower right quadrant of the abdomen. Gradually, the outline of the large intestine can be identified by the green discoloration over the abdominal wall. Hydrogen sulfide produced in the colon after death reacts with hemoglobin breakdown products to produce the greenish discoloration seen in the bowel and the structures that contact the bowel. The color change in time proceeds up the anterior abdominal and thoracic walls as far as the neck and chin.

Vascular Changes. Early decomposition color changes can affect the small veins in almost any area of the body. The blood in these superficial vessels breaks down and the hemoglobin combines with hydrogen sulfide to pro-

Figure 19–4. Early signs of decomposition (color changes, purge). Note ecchymosis of the right eyelid.

duce a green–black discoloration. The vessels take on a spider web appearance. This extravascular decomposition discoloration is called "marbling."

Livor Mortis and Stain. Livor mortis is completely established in the dependent tissues of these bodies. Some of these purple discolorations clear during injection of the arterial solution. The majority, however, have become postmortem stains. Stain develops as the hemoglobin breaks down (hemolysis) and allows the heme portion of the molecule to pass from the capillaries into the tissue spaces. This light red discoloration cannot be removed by arterial injection. At best, it may be bleached. This is of particular concern when the body is found face down. Some of the small capillaries will have broken down causing petechia and purpura called Tardieu spots. Postmortem stain and Tardieu are extravascular discolorations and will not clear by arterial injection.

Dehydration. Most bodies exposed to air will in addition to decomposition changes also exhibit dehydration of areas such as the lips, eyelids, and fingertips. If the body is unclothed, the male scrotum often exhibits dehydration.

Odors

As autolysis and putrefaction occur, some products of protein breakdown emit very foul odors. Foul amines and mercaptans combine with ammonia and hydrogen sulfide to produce the odors of decomposition. Embalming converts the amines, mercaptans, and hydrogen sulfide to odorless methylol compounds. Formaldehyde converts ammonia to odorless hexamethylene. Odors can be reduced by bathing the surface of the body with a solution prepared by mixing 2 pints of hydrogen peroxide with one-half cup of baking soda and adding a tablespoon of liquid soap. This solution is left on the skin surface for several minutes before rinsing and drying.

Clostridium perfringens is an anaerobic bacterium. In some bodies, its postmortem activity can create intense gas accompanied by a very foul odor.

Purges

If gases have developed in the abdominal cavity and products of partial digestion were present in the stomach at the time of death, purge can be expected (Fig. 19–5). Ruptured capillaries and congested lung passageways may also create a "lung" purge. Abdominal pressures may also cause purging from the rectum through the anal orifice.

Gases

In some bodies, especially those in which bacterial activity increased after death, the tissues and cavities may contain gases. Conditions favoring gas formation are heat and humidity; those hindering formation are cold and dry environments. Gas can cause bloating and swelling of the body, protrusion of the tongue and eyes, and distension of the male genitalia. The pressure resulting from distension of the abdominal cavity creates lung, stomach, and anal purges.

Desquamation

The autolytic changes that begin immediately after death weaken the superficial layer of the skin. Gas can easily move into the weakened superficial tissues, resulting in blisters and separation of the skin layers. Frequently, the embalmer encounters skin-slip when there are no gases in the tissues. Then, mere handling of the body causes the epidermis to loosen and separate.

Chemical Changes

Although not visible, important postmortem chemical changes occur in the tissues that the embalmer must be concerned about. Autolytic and proteolytic decomposition of the body proteins result in numerous nitrogenous products. These products greatly increase the preservative demand of the body. Their presence also shifts the body pH to alkaline (basic). Embalming solutions react best with proteins under slightly (not strong) alkaline pH conditions.

Embalming Protocol

The following factors concerning the body enter into a **preembalming analysis**: (1) general conditions of the body, (2) immediate cause and manner of the death, (3) disease processes, (4) effects of drugs and medications, (5) postmortem changes, and (6) postmortem conditions such as time between death and disposition. The postmortem changes may be the most important factor in determining the embalming techniques to be used.

The protocols for embalming the bodies discussed in this chapter are similar, because all of these bodies have undergone a delay between death and preparation and all have a high preservative demand. Some of the complications encountered during embalming of the body with early signs of decomposition follow:

- Fluid distribution is poor, because coagula are present in the arterial system.
- Drainage is poor because blood elements have decomposed.
- Tissues easily swell, because capillaries have broken down or are easily torn by the pressure of the fluid; tissue structure has been weakened by autolytic and putrefactive changes.
- Ammonia and nitrogenous products in the tissues greatly increase the preservative demand.
- Little or no firming is exhibited because of protein breakdown.

Figure 19–5. Early decomposition. Purge, discolorations, and distension from gases are evident.

Maximum-strength fluid can be used to prepare these bodies—25 to 30 index or higher. For this type of body, maximum-strength arterial solutions are necessary. Supplemental chemicals can be used to increase the working ability of these arterial solutions. Again, follow the instructions of the manufacturer. The goal here is to use a minimum amount of a very strong arterial solution. **Do not preinject these bodies**. Only a strong arterial solution should be injected into the vascular system. Use additional fluid dye, because firming cannot be used to judge distribution or preservation. The dye only indicates the presence of fluid in the surface tissues.

Two protocols are recommended for injection, **six-point injection** and **restricted cervical injection**. Drainage can be taken from each injection site or from the right internal jugular vein. Little or no drainage can be expected from these bodies. With both protocols, the head should be injected last.

The purpose in using a **six-point injection** is to minimize the number of arterial coagula that may move into the smaller arteries. Keep in mind that the aorta may contain a number of large coagula. If these coagula move, they will block small arteries.

1. Raise the right and left common carotid, right and left axillary (brachial), and right and left femoral (external iliac) arteries.
2. Inject the right and left femoral artery.
3. Inject the right and left axillary artery.
4. Inject the body trunk and limbs using the right common carotid artery. (Both the left and right common carotid arteries should have been raised and an arterial tube inserted in both toward the head—the stopcocks on these tubes should remain open. The lower portion of the left carotid should be tied closed.)
5. Aspirate the body after the trunk is injected.
6. Set the features.
7. Inject the left side of the head.
8. Inject the right side of the head.
9. Aspirate the cavities again and inject them with a suitable undiluted cavity chemical.
10. Evaluate the distribution of fluid and use hypodermic and surface embalming treatments where fluid has not been distributed.

Restricted Cervical Injection

1. Raise the right and left common carotid arteries; drain from the right internal jugular vein.
2. Inject down the right common carotid to embalm the arms, legs, and trunk. The left common carotid should be tied off and a tube directed toward the head inserted; this tube should remain open.

3. Evaluate the distribution of arterial solution. Inject the arms and legs separately if these areas lack fluid.
4. Aspirate the body cavities.
5. Set the features.
6. Inject the left side of the head.
7. Inject the right side of the head.
8. Reaspirate the cavities and inject a suitable undiluted cavity chemical.
9. Evaluate the distribution of arterial solution and treat area needing fluid with hypodermic and surface embalming.

If the abdomen is distended tightly with gas prior to arterial injection, introduce a trocar into the abdominal cavity to relieve this pressure. The trocar should be kept just beneath the anterior wall. An attempt can be made to puncture the transverse colon and the distended stomach.

The trunk should be injected at a very slow rate of flow to prevent swelling of the abdominal viscera and purge. Limbs can be injected slowly at first, and then at a higher pressure and faster rate of flow to secure distribution. Pulsation is recommended. If desired, each extremity can also be injected by the instant tissue fixation method (100% arterial fluid injected in pulses under high pressure) or by using waterless embalming.

If sectional arterial embalming has produced unsatisfactory results, sectional hypodermic injection will be necessary. Undiluted arterial or cavity fluid may be injected by machine through a hypo-valve or infant trocar. To inject the arms, insert the trocar into the area of the bend of the elbow; from this point, the upper as well as the distal portion of the arm can be reached, possibly as far as the palm of the hand. An alternative point of entry can be at the upper anterior portion of the arm—from this point, the upper portion of the arm can be reached, shoulder, back of the neck, and upper pectoral regions of the chest. To inject the legs, insert the trocar on the medial side of the leg either above or below the knee; from this point, fluid can be injected as far as the buttocks and as far as the foot. An alternative point of entry is the base of the foot. From this point of entry, fluid could be injected as far as the knee. The trunk walls can be injected from points of entry on the lateral walls of the trunk at approximately the level of the midaxillary line. It may be necessary to insert the infant trocar into the upper shoulder area to inject the posterior portions of the back, shoulder, and neck. All of these points of entry can be closed with trocar buttons or, if necessary, sutured closed with a pursestring suture. Glue can be applied over the trocar button or suture to ensure against leakage. Fingers and the foot can be separately injected with a hypodermic syringe and a small-gauge needle.

The use of super adhesive helps to ensure against leakage from each point where the needle is inserted.

These bodies need to be reaspirated several hours after embalming. Reinjection is strongly advised, especially if any gases are evident during the reaspiration. If desquamation is present, the loose skin should be removed at the beginning of embalming. Surface compresses can be applied to help dry these areas. Air drying also helps to dry the raw skin after the compresses have been removed.

Plastic garments can be used and embalming powder or moisture-absorbent kitty litter should be placed inside these garments. This powder produces some surface preservation but, more importantly, helps to control odors.

Treatment of the Features

In preparing a body in which decomposition is evident, the embalmer may wish to vary the technique used to set features.

The mouth can be closed after arterial injection. As the lips and areas around the mouth may swell, it may be easier to obtain a proper closure after injection. Firming is not a problem in these bodies, because it is delayed. Difficulty in closing will be a result of the swelling.

The embalmer should evaluate the preservation of tissues surrounding the mouth. It may be necessary to place cotton in the mouth and saturate it with concentrated cavity fluid to help ensure preservation. Dehydration should not be a concern. The lips can be secured with a super adhesive.

Eyes can also be closed after arterial injection. In this way, the embalmer has an opportunity to observe if the eyelids have received sufficient fluid. If the lids appear under-embalmed, cotton can be used for closure. This cotton can be saturated with some concentrated cavity fluid to help ensure preservation of the lids. Several hours later, the cotton packs can be removed from under the eyelids and the eyes reset or they may remain in place. Eyelids, especially if underembalmed, should be handled very gently to avoid skin-slip. A super adhesive can be used to secure eye closure. Dehydration is not a concern in the preparation of these bodies.

Areas of the face that appear not to have received sufficient arterial solution can be reached by hypodermic injection from inside the mouth. Cavity fluid should be used to treat these areas. Do not dilute the cavity fluid; use the concentrated fluid. Make all injections from inside the mouth, because cavity fluid, unlike tissue builder, has a tendency to leak from the tissues. This leakage occurs on the inside of the closed mouth. The sides of the nose can be reached as well as the cheeks and the lower eyelids from inside the mouth. A 17- to 19-gauge needle is excellent for this work.

In bodies dead for a long period, the submaxillary, sublingual, and parotid glands tend to swell during injection. If this happens, apply very firm digital pressure to these areas immediately after arterial injection. If the swelling is not reduced, make a flap incision at the base of the neck. Using an infant trocar as an operative aid, lance the glandular tissue several times and apply digital pressure again. If this treatment is unsuccessful, another operative correction—excision of the swollen tissues—may be necessary.

In bodies exhibiting decomposition, the tongue often protrudes and is swollen. Attempt to force the tongue back into the mouth by using firm digital pressure prior to arterial injection. The protruding tongue can be covered with a piece of cloth and firm pressure applied to the cloth. When teeth or dentures are present, try to force the tongue behind them and then secure the jaw shut. This helps to contain the tongue. Excision of the tongue should be a last resort.

Advanced Decomposition

There should be some preparation of the body in advanced stages of decomposition.

If the embalmer thinks it is possible, raise and inject the right common carotid artery with about 1 gallon of undiluted high-index fluid, there are fluids made for such cases (decomposition, burns, etc.). Some cavity fluids (undiluted) can be injected arterially in special situations. Be certain to follow manufacturer's instructions. Drainage would not be indicated.

The abdominal and thoracic cavities should be aspirated and filled with three or more bottles of undiluted cavity fluid. The extremities and trunk walls can be treated by hypodermic injection of undiluted cavity fluid by use of an infant trocar and the embalming machine. The primary purpose here is to diminish some of the odor and slow the progress of decomposition.

The body can be wrapped in one or more sheets and placed in a clean, zippered pouch. Before wrapping the blankets around the body, sprinkle embalming powder over the surface of the body. The entire body surface may also be painted with autopsy gel. Place the wrapped body in the pouch. If desired, saturate the sheets surrounding the body with cavity fluid or an external preservative solution. Any chemical used to saturate the sheeting should be concentrated and not diluted.

Before zippering the pouch, sprinkle additional embalming powder over the sheeting and the inside of the pouch. Placing moisture-absorbent kitty litter inside the pouch will assist in the control of odors. Some embalmers prefer to place a surface glue along the zipper of the pouch to help control the escape of any odors. A double pouch may be necessary to ensure that the odors are contained and the pouch does not rip when it is lifted. To prevent the pouch from tearing, place a sheet under it; the pouch can be lifted and moved with the sheet.

▶ CONCEPTS FOR STUDY AND DISCUSSION

1. Discuss the concepts of restricted cervical injection; instant tissue fixation; waterless embalming.
2. List the postmortem chemical and physical changes.
3. Explain why restricted cervical injection should be used when strong arterial solutions are to be injected.
4. Describe the effects of rigor mortis on the embalming process.
5. Describe the postmortem pH changes in the unembalmed body.
6. Describe the effects of postmortem cooling of the body. What are its advantages and its disadvantages.
7. List the classic signs of decomposition.
8. How does formaldehyde work to slow or stop decomposition?
9. Describe how you would prepare a body in advanced decomposition.
10. What primary factors within the body are responsible for decomposition? Make a list of intrinsic and extrinsic factors that speed decomposition. In intrinsic and extrinsic factors which slow decomposition.

▶ BIBLIOGRAPHY

Boehringer PR. *Controlled Embalming of the Head.* Westport, CT: ESCO Tech Notes, February–March, 1969: No. 57.

DiMaio VJ, DiMaio D. *Forensic Pathology,* 2nd ed. Boca Raton, FL: CRC Press, 2001.

Dorn JM, Hopkins BM. *Thanatochemistry,* 3rd ed. Upper Saddle River, NJ: Prentice Hall, 2010.

Jones H. A chemist looks at embalming problems. *Casket and Sunnyside* May 1968.

Pervier NC. *A Textbook of Chemistry for Embalming.* Minneapolis, MN: University of Minnesota, 1961.

Sanders CR. Refrigeration (Parts 1-2-3). *Dodge Magazine* March/April/May 1987.

Sawyer D. Treatment of refrigerated bodies. *Dodge Magazine* June/July/August 1989.

Slocum RE. *Pre-embalming Considerations.* Boston, MA: Dodge Chemical Co., 1945.

Strub CG. Why bodies decay. *Casket and Sunnyside* February–March 1959.

Weber DL. *Autopsy Pathology Procedure and Protocol.* Springfield, IL: Charles C. Thomas, 1973:69–70.

DISCOLORATIONS

In this chapter, the acceptable appearance of the embalmed body is explored. In this context, one would refer to what the family and friends of the decedent actually see. This chapter will concentrate on the appearance of the face, neck, hands, and arms of the deceased. In some instances, the legs and feet of an infant or a young child may also be viewed. **Embalming** is defined as a process that chemically treats the dead human body to reduce the presence and growth of microorganisms, to retard organic decomposition, and to restore an acceptable appearance of the body. Achieving an acceptable appearance of the body depends on successful sanitation and preservation. However, sanitizing and preserving the body can be accomplished without creating an acceptable appearance. This is the type of embalming used for the preparation of the anatomical bodies used for dissection in medical schools. They are well preserved and sanitized but generally badly discolored and often facial features are grossly swollen.

The term **discoloration** has two important meanings for the embalmer. First, to discolor means "color is removed or lost." An objective of embalming is to restore lost skin color either internally by the use of arterial fluid dyes or externally by the application of a cosmetic medium to the skin surface. A second meaning is "to change color." These discolorations are further defined for the embalmer as "any abnormal color appearing in or on the dead human body." Discolorations can be **localized**, for example, "black-eye" or razor "burn,"

others, **generalized**, for example, livor mortis, dehydration, and jaundice. Arterial injection and subsequent drainage can remove discolorations such as livor mortis. The bleaching agents of some arterially injected fluids and supplemental surface and hypodermic treatments can lighten and/or alter such discolorations as ecchymosis and purpura.

► GENERAL SKIN COLOR

Skin has been defined as the organ that forms the outer surface of the human body. It consists of two major divisions, the superficial **epidermis** and a deeper **dermis**. It is classified as thin and hairy—which covers most of our bodies; and, thick and hairless—which covers the palms of the hands, soles of the feet, and the flexor surface of the digits. For all races, the color of skin has been defined as, "straw color with pink overtone." Three pigments create skin color, melanin (browns to black), carotene (yellow), and hemoglobin (oxyhemoglobin) (red). While all the three are common to all individuals and races, the amount and distribution of **melanin** plays the most influential role. Melanin and carotene are cellular elements, which remain in the skin after death. Hemoglobin and oxyhemoglobin are blood elements, which undergo changes after death. First, the red blood cells, which contain the hemoglobin, no longer receive a fresh supply of oxygen so their bright red color is diminished; second, those red blood cells that are oxygenated rapidly give up their oxygen as the dying cells of the body undergo for the last time the metabolic stages of anabolism and catabolism. Blood also begins to drain from upper areas of the body into the dependent vessels, a process called postmortem hypostasis. Hypostasis can begin even before the death in what is described as the agonal phase of dying.

The deceased body is often described as having a **death pallor** or a paleness to the skin. In effect, the pinkness or redness of the skin is lost. This may not be as noticeable in the African American, who belongs to a racial culture where environmental factors have darkened the skin, and in the suntanned Caucasian—in these persons the large amounts of melanin and carotene pigmentation remain in the skin cells after death. They have a greater influence on the color of the skin than the lost postmortem blood elements.

Restoration of the visible skin areas to a natural color and acceptable appearance involves the internal use of (1) fluid dyes and (2) arterial injection and drainage. It also may require the external application of mortuary cosmetics. The dyes and the base (or foundation) cosmetics help to reinstate the lost red to the skin. Special emphasis is placed on the reinstatement of the red or **warm** areas of the face and the hands. These are areas where the red pigment is most noticed, they include the lips, the cheeks, the base of the chin and nose, the ears, and the joints of the backs of the hand as well as any palmer surfaces that may be seen, for example, the fingertips and the sides of the thumb. This creates a **natural** appearance to the skin. With respect to women often an **ornamental** cosmetic effect is desired. Here special emphasis is placed on the color of the lips, the eyelids, and the cheeks.

▶ DISCOLORED AREAS

Nearly every body to be embalmed today has some localized or generalized discolorations. These deviations from normal skin coloration may require a change in the embalming technique, the chemicals employed, and the cosmetic and restorative techniques. The embalmer should be able to identify any and all discolorations present on the body. Quite often, a family member asks questions concerning the antemortem discolorations and if they will be visible after the preparation. The embalmer should understand the **cause** of a discoloration, to know which discolorations **can** and **cannot** be reduced by arterial injection, to know which discolorations can be altered or bleached by proper chemicals, and to know which discolorations will have to be treated by opaque cosmetics to hide them.

FACTORS DETERMINED IN THE EMBALMING ANALYSIS

1. Vessels for injection and drainage
2. Method of mouth closure
3. Strength of the embalming solution
4. Volume of the embalming solution
5. Injection pressure
6. Injection rate of flow

Note: These factors will vary by the individual body and can vary in different areas of the same body.

Classification of Discolorations According to Cause

There are six classifications of discolorations that the embalmer can identify.

The following charts summarize the classifications of the various discolorations. Examples are given for each category. Some brief explanation should be made regarding discolorations labeled as blood, pathological, and drug discolorations. Keep in mind the classification is by the cause of the discoloration. Thus, "ecchymosis" is a blood discoloration if caused by trauma, is a pathological discoloration if it occurs during a disease, and is a drug discoloration when brought about by a drug. Jaundice can be classified as a drug or a pathological discoloration depending on its **cause**:

1. Blood discolorations.
2. Drug and therapeutic discolorations (pharmaceutical agents).
3. Pathological discolorations.
4. Surface discoloring agent discolorations.
5. Reactions to embalming chemicals on the body.
6. Decomposition changes.

Classification of Discolorations According to Time of Occurrence

Antemortem discolorations appear on the human body during life. The fact that they remain after life is extinct will not change their classification. Postmortem discolorations appear on the human body only after the death of the body.

1. Antemortem
   a. Blood discolorations
   b. Drug and therapeutic discolorations
   c. Pathological discolorations
   d. Surface discoloring agent discolorations
2. Postmortem
   a. Blood discolorations
   b. Surface discoloring agent discolorations

c. Reactions to embalming chemicals on the body
d. Decomposition discolorations

Classification by Location

Blood discolorations are also classified as intravascular (within the circulatory system) or extravascular (outside of the circulatory system). Intravascular blood discolorations either antemortem or postmortem are easily removed by arterial injection and drainage. Some extravascular discolorations may be slightly altered but most **are not** substantially reduced.

Blood Discolorations

Blood discolorations (see Table 20-1) are discolorations resulting from changes in blood composition, content, and location.

1. Antemortem blood discolorations
   a. Intravascular
      (1) Hypostasis of blood (blue–black discoloration).
      (2) Result of carbon monoxide (CO) poisoning (cherry red coloring).
      (3) Capillary congestion (hypostatic, active, or passive).
   b. Extravascular
      (1) Ecchymosis: a large bruise caused by escape of the blood into the tissues.
      (2) Purpura: flat medium-sized hemorrhage beneath the skin surface.
      (3) Petechia: small pinpoint skin hemorrhage.
      (4) Hematoma: swollen blood-filled area within the skin.

2. Postmortem blood discolorations
   a. Intravascular
      (1) Livor mortis.
   b. Extravascular
      (1) Postmortem stain.
      (2) Tardieu spots.

Intravascular Blood Discolorations

Intravascular blood discolorations respond best to arterial injection and blood drainage. These discolorations include antemortem hypostasis of blood into dependent tissues, cyanosis, results of CO poisoning, capillary congestion, and livor mortis.

Livor mortis (a postmortem **physical** change) is a postmortem intravascular blood discoloration. It is brought about by the gravitation of blood into the dependent capillaries (Fig. 20–1). It is first observed approximately 20 to 30 minutes after death and is well established by the sixth hour after death. Refrigeration and drugs such as blood thinners speed the onset and increase in intensity of livor mortis. If the darkened area is pushed on and the area clears, this is an indication that the discoloration is intravascular. Livor mortis can be gravitated. If a body is laid on a flat surface, the heart is slightly higher than the head. Blood thus has a tendency to gravitate into the facial and neck tissues.

The head and the shoulders should always be elevated to help drain blood from these upper tissues. While the body is shaved, the face and the hair are washed, and the features are set, most of the blood gravitates from facial and neck tissues if the shoulders and the head have been elevated. If the discoloration does not clear, this may be an indication that there is blockage (e.g., a coagulum) in the right atrium of the heart or in the right or left internal jugular veins. The best vessels for injection and drainage of this body would be the right and left common carotid arteries and the right internal jugular vein. The internal jugular allows access to the right atrium of the heart. Coagula present can be removed with an angular spring forceps.

Preinjection fluids were developed to help clear blood discolorations such as livor mortis. If the body has not been dead very long, the embalmer may wish to inject a preinjection fluid solution. A large enough volume of solution should be injected to clear the livor mortis. If a preinjection fluid is not used, a mild arterial solution may be used to clear the blood discolorations. Subsequent injections can be stronger. This method helps to prevent setting of the livor mortis as a stain. Most of the fluids manufactured today are of such a nature that strong solutions can be injected and the fluid will clear the blood discolorations without setting the livor mortis as a stain. Many of these fluids are labeled "reaction-controlled fluids," meaning that they are able to be distributed throughout the body and diffuse into the tissue spaces before the chemical reaction with the proteins of the body. **Note:** In attempting to clear livor mortis, the drainage used should be continuous until the livor has cleared. Then, intermittent or alternate methods of drainage can be employed. Manual massage and mechanical raising and flexing of a body limb may assist the flow of the injection solution into a discolored body region and the blood drainage from the region.

Livor mortis can also be an advantage for the embalmer. The breaking and clearing of the livor mortis indicates that fluid has been distributed into those tissues. Most bodies exhibit some degree of livor mortis. Some, however, are quite dramatic and the face may be almost blue–black. Elevation, continuous drainage, use of the internal jugular veins for drainage, and a mild arterial solution all help to clear the discoloration of livor mortis.

TABLE 20–1. EMBALMING CONSIDERATIONS AND BLOOD DISCOLORATIONS

Antemortem Hypostasis	Postmortem Hypostasis	Time	Livor Mortis	Time	Postmortem Stain	Time	Formaldehyde Gray
Occurs prior to death or during the agonal period	Begins at death		Seen as soon as blood fills superficial vessels; begins approximately 20 min after death; depends on postmortem/antemortem hypostasis		Normally occurs approximately 6 h after death; rate varies with the cause of death and the blood chemistry		Occurs after embalming
Intravascular Movement of blood to dependent tissues	*Intravascular* Movement of blood to dependent tissues		*Intravascular* Postmortem blood discoloration as a result of postmortem/antemortem hypostasis		*Extravascular* Postmortem blood discoloration as a result of hemolysis		*Intravascular or Extravascular* Embalming discoloration
Antemortem physical change	Postmortem physical change		Postmortem physical change		Postmortem chemical change		–
–	Speed depends on blood viscosity		Color varies with blood volume and viscosity and the amount of O_2 in blood		May occur prior to, during, or after arterial injection		Seen after arterial injection
Antemortem	Postmortem		Postmortem		Postmortem		Postmortem
–	–		Clears when pressed on. Removed by blood drainage		Does not clear when pressed on. Not removed by blood drainage		Seen as a gray stain Methemoglobin (HCHO and blood)
–	Arterial injection stops progress		Arterial injection (mild) clears with drainage		Strong solutions bleach and "set" livor as stain		–
–	Speeded by cooling of body, low blood viscosity		Speeded by cooling, blood "thinners," low blood viscosity, CO deaths		Speeded by cooling, rapid red blood cell hemolysis, CO deaths		Speeded by poor drainage, small amount of arterial fluid
							Vascular system not well cleared of blood

Figure 20–1. Livor mortis of the facial tissues, the ear, and the neck.

In making an embalming analysis, the nail beds should be observed for livor. This is especially important in the embalming of African Americans in whom the livor in the skin tissues is not always evident. Clearing of the nail beds indicates the distribution of the fluid.

Antemortem as well as postmortem intravascular blood discolorations should respond to arterial injection and subsequent blood drainage.

To summarize, the embalmer must consider several factors in embalming the body with livor mortis:

1. It is a postmortem physical change.
2. It appears in dependent tissues.
3. It is speeded by refrigeration and blood thinners, CO deaths, low blood viscosity, and large blood volume.
4. It is an intravascular condition.
5. It may be cleared by arterial injection and blood drainage.
6. It may be gravitated and massaged from a body region.
7. Color varies from light pink to almost black depending on blood volume and viscosity.
8. When pushed on (or palpated), tissues clear.
9. It is cleared best by the use of mild arterial solutions or preinjection solutions.

The discolorations caused by CO poisoning are antemortem blood discolorations classified as intravascular and thus should be cleared by arterial injection. Often there is a delay between death and preparation. The body might not be found for a period of time or the death must be investigated by the coroner or the medi-

cal examiner. Generally the **intra**vascular condition becomes an **extra**vascular condition because of the delay. Hemolysis also occurs creating a postmortem stain. This bright red discoloration does not clear. Care should be taken to use a dye with the arterial solution to be certain of the distribution of the arterial fluid and to prevent the condition of formaldehyde gray.

Extravascular Blood Discolorations

Extravascular blood discolorations do not respond well to arterial treatment. Examples of these discolorations are ecchymosis, purpura, petechia, hematoma, and postmortem stain and Tardieu spots. Injection of a stronger arterial solution assists in bleaching some of these discolorations. Both livor mortis and postmortem stain can be present in the same dependent area. The livor might be "washed out" but the stain remains. Preinjection, coinjection, or "special arterial" fluids cannot completely remove these extravascular discolorations. When formaldehyde reacts with these discolorations they usually turn gray in color.

Ecchymosis, purpura, and petechia are all extravascular. They are classified as blood discolorations but can also be classified as pathological and drug discolorations, for they can be **caused** by diseases as well as by extended use of many pharmaceutical and chemotherapeutic agents. The treatment of these extravascular conditions can involve all three types of embalming: arterial, hypodermic, and surface.

Tardieu spots are pinpoint hemorrhages seen in the areas of advanced livor mortis. The skin capillaries have burst, thus causing the pinpoint hemorrhages into the skin. This is an extravascular condition and the dark spots cannot be removed by arterial injection and blood drainage.

Ecchymoses are very large discolorations. Purpura and petechiae are smaller discolorations, and very frequently, simple arterial embalming satisfactorily bleaches and preserves these discolorations. Ecchymoses are of concern when they occur in a visible area such as on the face, the neck, the arms, and the back of the hands. If the ecchymosis was caused by a needle puncture, the area may distend during arterial injection (Fig. 20–2A).

Let us assume that a large ecchymosis on the back of the hand was caused by a intravenous puncture (Fig. 20–2B). Three conditions can occur during arterial injection of this body: (1) Arterial solution will perfuse the area, there will be little distension, and the area will be well preserved and may even bleach a little. (2) The area will distend, often very dramatically. (3) Nothing will happen. The area will not receive arterial solution. It will be neither preserved nor bleached. The ecchymosis must now be treated by hypodermic or surface embalming, or both.

A

B

Figure 20–2. A. Swelling of an ecchymotic area during arterial injection. **B.** Large ecchymosis caused by intravenous needles. Application of superglue after embalming can easily prevent leakage.

Hypodermic Treatment (After Arterial Injection). Two chemicals can be used: a phenol cautery solution or formaldehyde (a cavity fluid). The phenol solution is a better bleaching agent. It also works much faster and cauterizes as well as preserves and disinfects the area.

1. If the ecchymosis is on the back of the hand, insert a hypodermic needle between the fingers.
2. Repeatedly push the needle through the discolored tissues prior to injecting any of the solution.

3. Inject the solution and massage the area to uniformly distribute the chemical beneath the skin.
4. Some of the chemical will leak out of the points of entry between fingers. Some may also exit from the needle puncture on the back of the hand, if an IV had caused the discoloration.
5. Let the chemical remain for 15 to 20 minutes. Then, massage as much of the chemical as possible through the punctures in item 4.
6. Seal the needle punctures with a drop of super adhesive.

Surface Embalming. In addition to formaldehyde and phenol solutions, a variety of surface preservatives are available. The autopsy gels are quite popular for surface embalming. Surface treatments can be done before, during, or after arterial injection.

1. Coat the surface of the ecchymosis with autopsy gel. Or, saturate cotton compresses with the preservative chemical (undiluted cavity fluid or a bleaching chemical) and apply the cotton packs to the ecchymosis.
2. Cover the cotton compresses with plastic. This helps to decrease odors and prevent dehydration of the chemical.
3. Allow sufficient time for these chemicals to penetrate and preserve the ecchymotic tissues. Several hours will be required. Phenol solutions work very fast. Autopsy gels have a good penetrating ability.
4. Later, remove the surface compresses. Clean the area with a solvent and dry the tissues.
5. If there is any puncture to the skin (i.e., from an intravenous line), the puncture can be sealed with a drop of super adhesive.

Ecchymosis or Hematoma of the Eye. In treating an ecchymosis or hematoma of the eye (Fig. 20–3), commonly known as a "black eye," raise and separately inject the left and the right common carotid arteries. A stronger solution can be employed and the embalmer can control the amount of solution entering the head. Using the stronger solution, a smaller volume can be used in the event that the eye (or eyes) begins to distend. Do not inject the head of these bodies with a preinjection fluid.

Use cotton to close the eyes. Place a few drops of cavity fluid on the cotton. This acts as a compress under the eyelids and assists in preserving the tissues and bleaching some of the discoloration. This method is also good for routine embalming when the embalmer feels the eyelids have not received sufficient preservative. The eyelids can be glued and dehydration need not be a concern. The important factor is preservation. Cavity fluid does not contain dye; over time, arterial fluids with dyes could stain the tissues.

Figure 20–3. Ecchymosis or hematoma of the right eye.

Another approach can be taken to the treatment of swollen black eyes. Inject the tissues around the eyes and the lids with a phenol cautery chemical prior to arterial injection. Wait approximately 20 minutes for the chemical to cauterize the tissues; then proceed with the arterial injection. This method cauterizes the tissues and does not permit arterial solution to flow into the area. Many phenol chemicals are accompanied by **specific directions** for their use. Follow the time periods set by the manufacturer. A postembalming operative correction may be needed to directly incise or puncture and channel the swollen discolored eyelids. This can be done under the eyelids. It will allow a direct outflow of the extravasated blood and the accumulated serum.

Postmortem Stain. Postmortem stain (a postmortem **chemical** change) is an extravascular blood discoloration. It occurs in tissues where livor mortis was present or in surface tissues from which blood could not be drained. Stain usually indicates a period of time has elapsed between death and embalming. It is the result of the decomposition or breakdown of the red blood cells. The coloring matter (heme) has moved through the capillaries and into the tissue spaces. Postmortem stain can occur along with livor mortis in the same tissue regions. When pressed upon (or palpated), the skin does not clear. During arterial injection the discolored area will lighten but not entirely clear.

A stronger arterial solution needs to be used in the embalming of bodies with this condition. Circulation may be difficult to establish. There is also a tendency for these bodies to easily swell. The embalming solution used should be of sufficient strength so that a minimum volume effects preservation but at the same time minimizes distension.

Some dye should be added to this solution, because when the formaldehyde and the coloring portion of the blood mix to produce a gray hue, the extra dye not only indicates surface distribution of the fluid but also acts to counterstain the adverse discoloration.

Avoid using preinjection solutions in the preparation of these bodies. Bodies dead for long periods require strong, well-coordinated solutions. A preinjection treatment would only fill the vascular system with a weak and often non-preservative solution and possibly cause distension. If a supplemental fluid is to be used a coinjection fluid is recommended.

Factors to consider with respect to embalming the body with postmortem stain:

1. A number of hours (approximately 6 or more) have elapsed since death.
2. Pressed on skin does not clear.
3. It is extravascular.
4. It cannot be removed by arterial injection and blood drainage.
5. It is caused by hemolysis and is not by blood in the tissues.

Pharmaceutical (Drug) Discolorations

Pharmaceutical, drug, or chemotherapeutic discolorations occur from the administration of these agents. These discolorations are all antemortem. There are many discolorations under this classification. Some are specific to a particular drug. Large amounts of drugs, in time, affect the vascular, renal, and hepatic systems as well as the skin. Frequently, drug discolorations such as ecchymosis and purpura result from the breakdown of capillaries by the drugs. Often, the capillaries are fragile and bruising occurs easily. A second frequently encountered drug discoloration is jaundice, a result of the toxic effect of drugs on the liver or the red blood cells. These discolorations are very common. Usually, the arms are affected by hemorrhagic discolorations, and the entire body is affected by jaundice. The extravascular pathological discolorations such as ecchymosis and purpura should be treated using those embalming treatments for extravascular blood discolorations. Renal failure can also be a result of extensive drug therapy. Renal failure can produce a yellow discoloration to the skin. A build-up of nitrogenous wastes will require the injection of strong arterial solutions.

Pathological Discolorations

Pathological discolorations are antemortem discolorations that occur during the course of certain diseases. Some examples include:

1. Gangrene
    a. Wet: caused by venous obstruction; infected tissues red to black in color
    b. Dry: caused by arterial insufficiency; a dark red-brown to black color
    When gangrene occurs in a facial area or affects the fingers, it becomes cosmetic concern to the embalmer. Frostbite and diabetes can be responsible for this condition in the facial areas and the hands. Arterial preservation is difficult to establish, and surface and hypodermic preservation are necessary.
2. Jaundice: caused by many disease processes, for example, diseases of the liver, a bile problem, or a blood problem
3. Specific diseases
    a. Addison's disease: a bronze discoloration produced in the skin
    b. Leukemia: petechiae
    c. Meningitis: discolorations can include cyanosis; a blotchy erythematous rash (reddening) of the skin; petechia and purpura
    d. Tumors: discolorations in and around the tumor itself may be caused by pathological changes
    e. Lupus erythematosus: a chronic skin disease characterized by scaling, red, macular rash

Jaundice. There are three general types of jaundice: toxic jaundice, hemolytic jaundice, and obstructive jaundice. Within each category are a large number of diseases that bring about the antemortem discoloration.

Healthy human blood serum contains approximately 1.0 to 1.5 mg of the bile pigment bilirubin (which is yellow in color) per 100 mL as a result of the breakdown of red blood cells. Most red blood cells live approximately for 120 days. Because of a variety of diseases that result in **hepatic failure, excessive blood hemolysis, or obstruction of the contents of the gallbladder**, the level of bilirubin reaches above 1.5 mg per 100 mL of blood serum and the tissues of the body begin to take on the yellow jaundiced condition (Fig. 20–4).

In embalming, it was once widely believed that a strong arterial solution was the cause of a conversion of the bilirubin (yellow discoloration) to biliverdin (green discoloration). This chemical reaction is not caused by formaldehyde; it is however, caused by the presence of a strong acidic environment. A purely strong formaldehyde solution may form such an environment since formaldehyde is a **reducing agent**. However, most jaundice fluids today contain the proper amounts of buffers to balance the pH level within the tissues to prevent a strongly acidic environment. The use of an acidic fluid (usually classified as "fast acting" fluid) is not recommended when jaundice is present. The following state-

Figure 20–4. Yellow or mild jaundice is often first detected in the sclera (white) of the eye.

ment by Lee Rendon for Champion Chemical Company points out what is thought to be the actual cause of this conversion. Remember that formaldehyde is a chemical **reducing agent** and the conversion from a yellow discoloration to a green discoloration is an **oxidation** chemical reaction.

When aldehydes react with proteins, one of the chemical reactions that occur is said to be that of release of hydrogen ions which, of course, results in a low pH (acid) that is acid in nature. A given amount of formaldehyde or aldehyde can unite with a given amount of protein to form a given aldehyde condensation resin (fixed protein). Once the proteins have received the necessary amount of aldehyde to form these condensation resins, any excess aldehyde tends to become more acid in character and, therefore, causes oxidation changes. From another point of view, aldehydes, in combining with protein or amino acid, increase the local acidity in the tissues by the release of proton. The hydrogen (H[1]) ions which produce the acid condition result from the chemical reaction between aldehyde and protein. This acid medium, in turn, results in oxidation changes. The yellow (bilirubin) is converted to green (biliverdin). **It is not the formaldehyde** which causes the oxidation (formaldehyde is a reducing agent). It is the chemical reaction (oxidation) as a result of the presence of the acid.

Six methods for the treatment of the jaundiced body are discussed in this chapter with the explanations of the benefits and the risks with each method. Note that no one solution will ever treat every jaundiced body. Careful preembalming analysis and monitoring of distribution will ensure the best results. Each method will employ a different type of chemicals and while most funeral homes will not stock all of the chemicals mentioned here, it is the responsibility of the embalmer to have the proper chemicals to clear the mild to moderate jaundiced condition.

Those methods based on the assumption that the embalmer uses a small amount of formaldehyde to prevent the conversion of a yellow discoloration to a green discoloration are acting adversely to the goal of proper preservation and may lead to a poorly embalmed body. In addition to discolorations an embalmer must consider many other conditions when making a preembalming analysis. A common mistake when embalming the jaundiced body is for the embalmer to focus strictly on the discoloration and give little or no consideration to other conditions present such as edema, tissue gas, emaciation, or decomposition. These other conditions cannot be ignored.

As the primary concern of the embalmer in the preparation of the jaundiced body is the clearing of the discoloration present in the face and the hands, only the face and the hands need to be treated with a jaundice clearing or counterstaining solution. Generally it is found that the hands are minimally affected by the jaundice so the head and the face become the primary concern for the embalmer. **Restricted cervical** injection is recommended for embalming the jaundiced body. This allows the use of two embalming solutions: first, a jaundice clearing solution which will be directly injected into the head and, second, a preservative solution of sufficient strength and volume is injected into the trunk and the limbs.

The following methods give an overview of what a majority of embalmers have used to address the jaundice condition. These methods are not clearly defined "rules" or prescriptions for the treatment of jaundice. Each embalming is different for each dead human body. Medications administered during a last illness alone may alter chemical reactions with an embalming solution. Some discolorations cannot be overcome by embalming techniques so these bodies need to be corrected by opaque cosmetic application.

In the embalming of all jaundiced bodies, preservation takes precedence over clearing of the discoloration.

METHOD 1: USE OF A JAUNDICE FLUID. Almost every chemical manufacturer produces a jaundice fluid. Most of these fluids are very low in formaldehyde. Some even substitute other preservatives for formaldehyde. For the most part, these fluids are not strong preservatives. Use the recommended dilutions and solution volume as a minimum. Never use less arterial fluid than recommended by the manufacturer; use of a slightly stronger solution may be necessary.

At the completion of the arterial embalming if preservation is a concern, reinject the body with a stronger preservative solution of standard embalming fluid. Most jaundice fluids contain a large amount of dye but additional dye can always be added. The dyes not only indicate to the embalmer where the fluid has distributed, but even more important, they serve to counterstain the jaundice and, thus, cover the discoloration. Counterstaining is explained in greater detail in Method 6, below.

METHOD 2: USE OF A PREINJECTION SOLUTION. In the treatment of mild jaundice a preinjection fluid can be injected prior to the arterial preservative. The theory here is to wash out as much of the discoloration as possible. Sufficient volume of preinjection solution should be used to thoroughly rid the body of as much blood as possible. After the preinjection solution has remained in the body for a short period, inject a normal (1.25%–2%) arterial solution containing dye. Again, sufficient volume should be injected to satisfy the preservative demands of the body. Dye can be added to the preinjection solution. This method is of little help in clearing jaundice since jaundice causes a true stain. The dye in the solutions will counterstain the discoloration. This method is not recommended when difficult distribution is anticipated and when edema or decomposition is present.

METHOD 3: USE OF MILD ARTERIAL SOLUTION. If preinjection fluids are not used and jaundice fluids are not purchased, it was once thought that injecting the body with a mild arterial solution with additional dyes added would correct the jaundice condition. This method can easily result in underembalmed bodies with the jaundice still a problem and soft tissues making cosmetic application difficult. Injecting large volumes of mild fluid can also contribute to swelling of the face and the neck. Sufficient volume needs to be injected to satisfy the preservative demands of the body.

> The new non-fomaldehyde fluids are proving to be beneficial in the clearing of jaundice. Using restricted cervical injection these fluids could be used for injection of the head and face. Standard preservatives could be used for the remainder of the body. Strictly follow the instructions when using the non-formaldehyde fluids.

METHOD 4: USE OF CAVITY FLUIDS AS ARTERIAL FLUIDS. Certain **specific** cavity fluids may also be used as arterial fluids for specific treatments. One of these treatments is the embalming of jaundiced bodies. Be positive the manufacturer states the fluid can be used as a jaundice treatment. It is the bleaching chemicals in the cavity chemical that clears or lightens the jaundice. Not all cavity fluids are of high index, so their formaldehyde content is not high. Again, dye should be added to these arterial solutions.

METHOD 5: USE OF BLEACHING COINJECTION SOLUTIONS. Instructions for several coinjection fluids state that they may be used for the treatment of bodies with extravascular discolorations such as postmortem stain, ecchymosis, gangrene, and jaundice. It is the bleaching property of this fluid which acts on these discolorations. The fluid is injected along with a preservative arterial solution. Dilutions are indicated on the labels of these coinjection fluids. They tend to work best on **mild jaundice**. They lighten the dark jaundice but the remaining discoloration must be covered with opaque cosmetics.

METHOD 6: USE OF THE RELATIVE COUNTERSTAINING METHOD. The theory of the Relative Counterstaining Method combines several properties of other methods currently used for the embalming of jaundiced bodies. This method is based on the practice that a true jaundice stain is indeed a stain. The only proper solution is to counterstain the discoloration. With many cases of jaundice, especially those more moderate to severe cases, the jaundice can never be completely covered or bleached. A counterstain will add a solid base color that will aid in the application of cosmetics. The counterstain is created by the extensive use of fluid dyes in the arterial solutions.

As always with any embalming a constant analysis is very important and alterations in the embalming solution must be made to maintain a desirable balance between preservation and restoration. Proper control of the rate of flow of any embalming machine is crucial to the prevention of swelling of any kind during the embalming process.

If, and in many cases they do, another consideration is present (edema, emaciation, decomposition) treat this condition along with the jaundice. Adding an edema-reducing chemical in increments or a humectant may be indicated.

Preservation is most important in the preparation of a jaundiced body. These bodies can always be treated with opaque cosmetics to successfully hide the discoloration. A good foundation even for cosmetic treatment is good preservation.

Nephritis. One of the signs of chronic renal failure is a "sallow yellow color" or bronzing to the skin resulting from the presence of urochrome in the tissues. This antemortem pathological discoloration takes on the appearance of mild jaundice. In cases with chronic renal failure, urea in the blood system is converted to ammonia. Ammonia in the tissues and the blood acts to neutralize formaldehyde. The discoloration is generally

treated easily by mixing additional dye into the arterial solution. Treatment of bodies with renal failure requires strong arterial solutions to establish firming and good preservation.

Chronic renal failure often accompanies diabetes mellitus. One of the major problems for the embalmer in the preparation of bodies with diabetes mellitus is poor peripheral circulation. This calls for strong arterial solutions. A coinjection fluid can be added to help increase distribution and diffusion of the chemical. In many of these bodies gangrene has already been established in the lower limbs. A good dye is recommended to indicate fluid distribution.

Should a preinjection solution be used to rid the blood vascular system of the nitrogenous wastes prior to injection of the preservative arterial solution? Here, the embalmer needs to use extreme caution. When it is felt that the circulation and the drainage will be good, this preinjection treatment can be used. If, however, there is evidence of poor circulation and drainage may be difficult to establish (if the body has been dead for a long period, gangrene is present, or there is heavy clotting and ischemic necrosis is present), avoid the preinjection treatment and employ a good strong arterial solution, possibly using a coinjection fluid to assist in distribution and diffusion of the preservative. Waterless embalming treatment may be necessary in establishing good preservation in these bodies.

Surface Discoloring Agents

Surface discoloring agents are antemortem or postmortem discolorations that occur prior to (or during) embalming as the result of the deposit of matter on the body surface. Examples include blood, betadine, adhesive tape marks, gentian violet, paint, mercurochrome, and tobacco tars. Most of these can easily be removed with soap and water or with a solvent such as the dry hair washes.

Surface discolorations should be cleaned away prior to arterial injection. The pores of the skin are easier to clean at this time. After arterial injection the pores close and it is more difficult to completely clean off the discoloration. A second reason is that the embalmer must see the skin to evaluate if arterial solution is present in a particular location. For example, cleaning blood, dirt, and grease from the fingers, if present, prior to embalming allows the embalmer to observe the presence of livor mortis in the nail beds. During arterial injection the embalmer can then observe the clearing of the nail beds and the replacement of the livor by the dye of the arterial solution.

Mechanical and chemical methods can be used to remove surface discoloring matter. Mechanical means include the use of abraded scrubbing pads, soft cloths, gauze, and brushes. Warm water and antiseptic soap can be used along with these mechanical aids. Chemical solvents can be used to remove specific discolorations that do not respond well to mechanical scrubbing.

Blood is one of the most common discolorations and it can be removed very simply by washing the skin surface with cold water. A mild liquid soap is also of help, and an abrasive cloth such as cheesecloth or a gauze pad assists in the removal of dried blood.

Most of the discolorations described above (gentian violet, adhesive tape, surface antiseptics, etc.) respond well to a cleaning with the "dry" hair wash solvents or a hydrocarbon solvent.

Discolorations Related to Embalming Chemicals

Reactions to embalming chemicals are postmortem discolorations that may be present before embalming that becomes more intense, changed in color, or evolved as a result of the embalming. They occur either during or following the embalming of the body. Examples include razor burns, dehydration of tissues, formaldehyde burn, formaldehyde gray, flushing and conversion of yellow to green jaundice, eye enucleation discoloration, and postmortem (bruising) contusions.

Dehydration. Dehydration is a drying of the skin. The classic colors of this discoloration are yellow, brown, and black. Dehydration can be caused internally by (1) injection of too much arterial solution, (2) use of an arterial solution that is too strong, and (3) continuous or concurrent drainage. It can also be caused externally by the passage of air over the body. Dehydration can also be the result of loss of the superficial layer of skin (e.g.,

abrasion) or the drying of cut edges of skin (e.g., laceration). Dehydrated tissues cannot be bleached and usually progressively darkens. The application of opaque cosmetics is the best treatment for this discoloration. The embalmer must be able to distinguish this darkening of the tissues from a similar darkening caused by decomposition. Dehydrated skin areas are generally very hard to touch, whereas a skin area that has decomposed is generally very soft and on touching, skin-slip may be evidenced (Fig. 20–5).

Dehydration of the fingers should be mentioned. If strong chemicals were employed (or an edema-reducing chemical), the ends of the fingers may have wrinkled and darkened because of dehydration. An application of massage cream or mineral oil over the fingers and the hands will help to reduce further dehydration. To correct this condition, tissue builder can be injected into each finger after embalming. Another area of the hand that frequently darkens as a result of dehydration brought about by the embalming is the tissue between the thumb and the index finger. Again, filling out this area with some tissue builder after arterial injection will hide the discoloration. The arterial solution may also bring about a loss of moisture from the lips. Wrinkling and, possibly, separation can occur. Tissue builder (after arterial injection) can be injected, from the end of each mucous membrane, to round out the lips and restore their natural fullness.

Many embalmers add a humectant coinjection fluid to the arterial solution for the purpose of adding and/or retaining moisture in the tissues of the body. When using a humectant the embalmer should carefully follow

Figure 20–5. Abraded tissues and small lacerations of the left side of the face.

the instructions of the manufacturer, so a proper osmotic balance can be achieved. Overuse of some humectants can actually create more dehydration. Restricted drainage (intermittent, alternate) should also be used to help retain tissue moisture.

Every fluid company today produces humectant-based arterial fluids. These fluids help to maintain a good moisture balance in the embalmed tissues.

Yellow to Green Jaundice. This conversion of bilirubin (yellow) to biliverdin (green) is an oxidation reaction. One theory is that formaldehyde, being a strong reducing agent, is only indirect to the cause of this reaction. Strong formaldehyde solutions can create an excess of formaldehyde in the tissues. The excess formaldehyde gradually converts to acid. The acid condition in the tissues, it is thought, converts the yellow jaundice to green jaundice. Oxygen from the air no doubt also may play a role in this conversion. Coating the face and the hands with massage cream can possibly help to prevent the oxygen contact with the tissues. The most important point is the **preservation** of the body. This is more important than clearing the discoloration. Counterstaining with an arterial fluid dye is one of the better treatments. The dye helps to cover the jaundice. If this fails to cover the jaundice condition, an opaque cosmetic treatment will be necessary.

Embalmer's (Formaldehyde) Gray. Embalmer's gray, a graying of the tissues, is due to failure of the embalmer to remove as much of the blood out of the body as possible. The remaining blood mixes with the preservation fluids in the tissues, and the resulting color is a dark gray. This condition can be avoided by the injection of a large volume of arterial solution accompanied by thorough drainage and thorough aspiration of the heart. It is also important the head and the shoulders of the embalmed body are kept elevated. This elevation prevents blood present in the heart after embalming from moving into the facial and neck tissues, and, thus, prevents embalmer's gray. The discoloration can create a cosmetic problem which can be corrected by the use of opaque cosmetics.

Flushing. Flushing is seen in those body areas into which the embalmer has been able to distribute arterial solution but has been unable to obtain good drainage of blood. Take as an example the body in which the femoral artery is used for injection and the accompanying femoral vein for drainage. If drainage is poor because of clotting in the right atrium of the heart or in one of the internal jugular veins or because of abdominal pressures, arterial solution will quite often flow into the facial tissues. Blood, however, will not be able to rapidly drain from these tissues. The facial tissues and the neck take on a cyanotic appearance. Establishing drainage

from another point such as the right internal jugular vein will clear this problem. If there is edema of the pleural sacs, often seen with pneumonia, drainage from the jugular will help to remove blood from the facial tissues and the neck. Flushing can result from leaving the drainage closed too long when using intermittent or alternate drainage. The establishment of drainage should clear the problem.

Razor Abrasion (Razor Burn). A razor "burn" abrasion is a cut of the skin during the shaving of the dead human body. Air drying alone turns these areas dark brown. With razor burn, application of a light layer of massage cream during embalming helps to prevent the nicked area from dehydrating and browning. If cream cosmetics are to be used and a small layer of wax is placed over the area, the discoloration should not darken or be noticed. The darkening may also be considered an advantage, because it indicates that the areas have dried, and an opaque cosmetic can be used to cover the discoloration. Dried tissues accept cosmetics and, when necessary, wax very well. The embalmer can promote the drying of these areas by using a hair dryer for few minutes. This ensures that there will be no further leakage and establishes a good surface for cosmetics.

Postmortem Bruising. Postmortem bruising is rare; it occurs if sufficient pressure is applied to tissues to damage the capillaries. This condition is particularly noted in persons who have been on blood thinners and in elderly people whose skin is thin. When an eye enucleation has been incorrectly performed—if the eye speculum used to keep the lids open has crushed capillaries in the lids, blood will escape into the eyelids. The discoloration resembles an ecchymosis or "black eye." It will possibly further discolor and swell during the injection of the head. When present, restricted cervical injection is advised. Use a preservative solution that is a little stronger than that normally used so only a minimum of solution need be injected to ensure preservation. Avoid preinjection treatment of the head and facial tissues in these bodies. Injection using a lower pressure and slower rate of flow will help to control swelling. Postembalming treatments include: hypodermic injection of a phenol solution may help preserve and reduce the distension or surface compresses of a phenol solution or other preservatives such as cavity fluid or the autopsy gels may also be used to reduce any distension, bleach the discoloration, and ensure preservation.

Confluent hemorrhage into the eyelids is also seen when death occurs due to head trauma. This is caused by fracturing of the orbital plates. Almost all gunshot wounds to the head will exhibit some amount of hemorrhage into the eyelids. Restricted cervical injection is recommended to control swelling along with those recommendations suggested in the previous paragraph.

Formaldehyde Burn. In bodies dead for long periods of time some of the capillaries in the skin may have broken. When a large volume of a strong formaldehyde solution circulates through such localized skin areas—fluid can escape directly into the tissues. This can create a raised rash-like appearance. Often this is seen near the injection site and is possibly caused by excessive collateral circulation through the tissues. In a few hours the raised skin areas will decrease. The tissues generally feel very firm to the touch and depending on dyes in the fluid the area can remain discolored.

Decomposition Discolorations

Decomposition color changes are postmortem discolorations brought about by the action of bacterial and/or autolytic enzymes on the body tissues as a result of decomposition. These colors may be yellow, green, or blue-black to black. Examples are progressive skin color changes and "marbling" of the veins on the skin surface.

Decomposition is evidenced by five signs: odor, desquamation, gas, purge, and color changes. The first external sign of decomposition is a color change, usually a green discoloration of the right inguinal or iliac area of the abdomen. This green discoloration enlarges over a period and outlines on the abdominal wall, the ascending, transverse, and descending colon. The green then proceeds upward over the chest area into the tissues of the neck and the face. A color change is also evidenced throughout the skeletal tissues. Generally the color changes from yellow to green to blue-black to black. In addition, the blood in the veins begins to break down. This discoloration progresses from the red of the postmortem stain to a black, and follows the course of the particular vein. The pattern thus forms a "spider web" and the veins are described as being marbled.

Both the general progression of color changes resulting from decomposition and the marbling of the veins are discolorations that can be bleached with external compresses such as phenol solutions, cavity fluid, or autopsy gel. These discolorations can be lightened but not to normal skin color. Postembalming hypodermic treatment can also be used to lessen the discolorations and to help ensure preservation.

▶ CONDITIONS RELATED TO DISCOLORATIONS*

A discoloration is simply any abnormal color appearing in and on the dead human body. The discolorations already described involved color changes and possibly some swellings. There were no breaks or tears in the skin surface with the exception of the razor abrasion. In the following conditions, a discoloration is present but, in addition, there is some form of disruption of the skin surface (Fig. 20–6). The emphasis is not so much on the pathological origins of these conditions, but rather on the treatment of these conditions from an embalming standpoint.

A **skin lesion** is any **traumatic** or **pathological** change in the structure of the skin. The objective of the embalmer is to properly sanitize skin lesions, clean them of debris, remove skin that cannot be used in the restorative treatment, and secure adequate preservation and drying of the tissues. There are four categories of skin lesions: (1) unbroken skin but discolored, (2) skin scaling as in exanthematous diseases, (3) skin that is broken or separated from the body, and (4) pustular or ulcerative lesions.

All eruptive and scaling skin conditions should be treated as if they were infectious and/or contagious. Thoroughly disinfect these areas prior to any treatments.

Unbroken but Discolored Skin

Skin may remain unbroken but discolored for a variety of pathological and traumatic cases, for example, allergic reaction, inflammation, trauma, and tumors. Generally, a discoloration will result from an increase in blood flow into the tissues of the affected area and some swelling. If this area is to be viewed (face, neck, or hands), a strong arterial solution can be used to help decrease further swelling or surface compresses can be used to help bleach the area and possibly reduce some of the distension. A phenol solution can be injected beneath the skin after arterial injection to preserve, bleach, and reduce the swelling.

Scaling Skin

Exanthematous diseases such as measles and chickenpox can result in small discolored skin eruptions. Dry skin and large amounts of medications can result in extensive scaling of the skin on the face and the hands. Some of the skin breaks away, as in the healing of sunburn. The embalmer must make certain that as much of the loose skin as possible is removed. This is necessary for a good cosmetic treatment on the affected area. Methods of removal include: shaving off the loose skin with a razor; firmly wiping with a solvent (e.g., hydrocarbon solvent and the dry hair washes); and cleaning the area using an abrasive gauze pad and massage cream. This helps to remove skin debris.

If there is any question as to preservation, brush autopsy gel over the affected area for several hours or apply compresses of a surface preservative. The gels work well because they can be evenly applied and are not harsh bleaching agents. Surface compresses or gels should always be covered with plastic to reduce fumes.

---

*Conditions discussed relating to discolorations and lesions pertain to those conditions located on the face and/or the hands of the deceased or other areas of the body that will possibly be viewed.

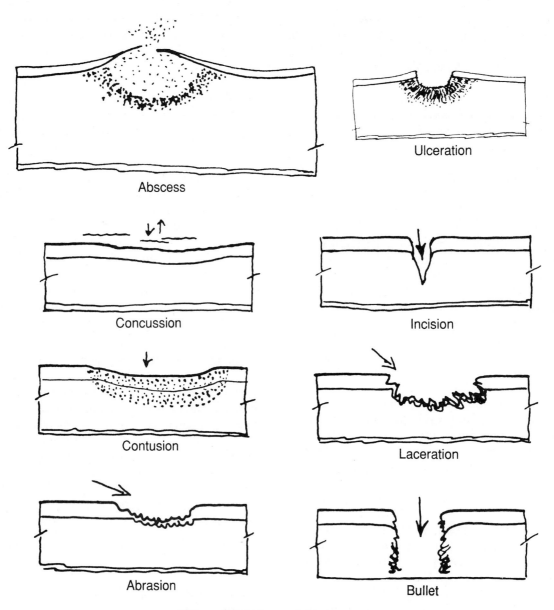

Figure 20–6. Types of skin trauma.

Broken Skin

Three types of broken skin are discussed: abrasions, blisters, and skin-slip.

An **abrasion** is defined as an antemortem injury resulting from friction of the skin against a firm object resulting in the removal of the epidermis. When the raw skin is exposed to the air and dries, it discolors to a brown color or as deep as a black color (Fig. 20–7). An abrasion must be dried before restorative treatment commences. During embalming, the surrounding tissues can be protected with massage cream. **Do not apply massage cream to the abrasion.** Let the fluid flow through the broken skin. After embalming use a hair dryer to dry the tissues. The tissues will darken and will be firm and dry and ready for restorative treatment. If there is a preservation prob-

lem and fluid did not reach the abraded tissue, a surface compress of phenol cautery or cavity fluid will help promote preservation and drying of the tissues. Abraded tissue cannot be bleached with surface packs because it is dehydrated.

Blisters are elevations of the epidermis containing a watery liquid. The embalmer must make some decisions here. When blisters are present on an area of the face and preservation has been adequate, they could be coated with a preservative gel for a period, then merely treated with cosmetics. On the lip, however, where glue must be applied, blisters can be "glued under," and no treatment is needed except the creation of a new lip line with cosmetics. If the embalmer feels that blisters should be opened and drained, this can be done prior to arterial

Figure 20–7. Minute lacerations and abrasions, once dried, turn dark brown.

treatment. Be certain to remove all loose skin. A phenol cautery solution compress can be used to help cauterize the raw tissue (Fig. 20–8), and after embalming, a hair dryer can be used to force-dry the tissue.

Tissues must be dry before they are treated with cosmetics, waxes, or surface glues.

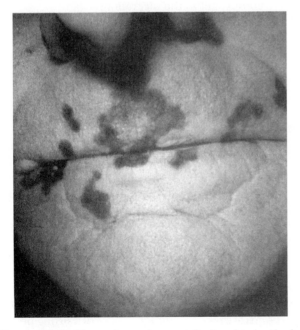

Figure 20–8. Blisters from a herpes infection dried with phenol. Note the dark brown color.

Blisters are characteristic of second-degree burns. In most second-degree burns, the individual lives for a time during which the blisters are opened and drained as part of the treatment. When present on the face, these lesions should be cleaned of loose skin with a sharp razor. A stronger than average solution should be used to embalm the affected area. Then the lesions could be force-dried with a hair dryer, or phenol solution.

▶ TREATMENT

1. Lance and drain.
2. Remove all damaged skin.
3. Cauterize.
4. Dry.

Desquamation (Skin-Slip)

Desquamation, separation of the upper layer of skin (the epidermis) from the deeper dermal layer, can be a sign of decomposition. The embalmer's goal is to achieve good preservation and make sure the areas are dried. Remove all loose skin prior to arterial injection. Peel all loose skin away then use a scalpel to cut at the point where freed skin joins attached skin. For exposed areas with desquamation the following protocol is recommended:

1. Apply a topical disinfectant.
2. Open and drain vesicles if present.
3. Remove all loose skin.
4. Apply surface compresses of cavity fluid or phenol solution to the "raw" tissue or coat the "raw" tissue with autopsy gel.
5. Sectional embalming may be necessary. Use a strong arterial solution.
6. Check preservation. Compresses can be continued or hypodermic treatment instituted with cavity fluid or phenol solution.
7. Allow time for these chemicals to take effect.
8. Clean away all preservative chemicals with a solvent (e.g., dry hair washes or hydrocarbon solvents).
9. Dry the area with a hair dryer to ensure no further leakage.

If desquamation is present on the eyelids or in the vicinity of the eye orbit, cotton can be used to close the eye. Saturate the cotton with a few drops of cavity fluid. This will serve as an additional internal compress to help establish good preservation. Leave it in place and use cosmetics over the affected skin areas when dried.

Desquamation in unexposed body areas can be treated in the following manner:

1. Apply a topical disinfectant.
2. Open and drain any vesicles that are present.

Figure 20–9. Chickenpox lesions on the forehead.

3. Remove all loose skin.
4. Embalm the body with a strong, well-coordinated arterial solution.
5. If possible apply a cavity or phenol compress to the raw tissue or paint it with an autopsy gel.
6. Check for preservation. If not complete, hypodermically treat the area with cavity fluid.
7. Paint again with autopsy gel, cover with embalming powder, or do both.
8. Cover the area with absorbent cotton.
9. Use plastic garments over the affected area.

Pustular and Ulcerative Lesions

Examples of pustular or ulcerative lesions are ulcerations, pustules, herpes fever blisters (Fig. 20–9), boils, carbuncles, and furuncles. These lesions are pustular and contain dead tissue. Treat these lesions in the following manner:

1. Disinfect the surface of the lesion.
2. Open and drain or remove any material in the lesion; clean the lesion and coat with autopsy gel or compress with cotton saturated with cavity fluid or a phenol cautery solution.
3. Embalm the body.
4. Check for preservation. Hypodermic treatment with a preservative or surface compress may be necessary.
5. Dry the area with a solvent and force-dry with a hair dryer.

Decubitus Ulcers (Bedsores)

Because of their size and the fact that most occur on body areas that are not visible, decubitus ulcers bear special mention. These lesions are the result of a constant inadequate blood supply to the tissues overlying a bony part of the body against which prolonged pressure has been applied. These ulcerations can be very large and are most frequently seen over the sacrum, heels, ankles, and buttocks. In addition, bacterial infections occur at these locations. Not only does the skin break and drain, but an odor is emitted because of the infection, usually staph infections.

Routine treatment of these ulcerations (when present on body areas that are not visible) can be summarized:

1. Disinfect the surface. Remove all bandages and apply a droplet spray.
2. Temporarily pack the area to reduce odors and to promote surface preservation.
   a. Autopsy gel can be painted over the ulceration.
   b. A cavity or phenol solution compress can be placed over the ulcer. When the lesions are located on the sides of the body, it may be helpful to leave taped bandages in place and soak them with cavity fluid.
3. Embalm the body.
4. Hypodermically inject cavity fluid (via infant trocar) into all the areas surrounding the ulceration.
5. Apply new surface compresses of cavity fluid or autopsy gel to the ulceration.
6. Clothe the body in plastic garments (stockings, pants, coveralls, etc.). If plastic garments are not available for the buttocks, make a larger diaper.
7. Spread embalming powder in the plastic garments to control odors.

Conditions Related to Discolorations—Unnatural

Almost all deaths from unnatural causes are investigated by legal authority, either the coroner or a medical examiner. Some of these deaths may be work related and the subject of workmen's compensation and insurance claims. Investigation by the coroner or the medical examiner, in most states, leads to autopsy. The autopsy presents its own set of problems for the embalmer. Many of these deaths occur in the absence of other individuals, and there may be a considerable delay between death and finding of the body (Table 20–2). With time delays, circulation and preservative problems can be expected. Two points are recommended: the use of a strong preservative arterial solution and the use of restricted cervical injection if the body is not autopsied.

TABLE 20–2. UNNATURAL CONDITIONS RELATED TO DISCOLORATIONS

Burns	First degree—redness of the skin Second degree—blistering and redness Third degree—charred tissue
CO poisoning	Bright red color to the blood Low blood viscosity, intense livor Rapid postmortem staining
Drowning	Low blood viscosity, intense livor Head faced downward, livor and stain Possible abrasions and bruising
Electrocution	Point of contact, burn marks can be present
Exsanguination	Little livor mortis, paleness to skin surfaces
Gunshot wounds	Eyelids can show ecchymosis, swelling of eye area when injury is to face or head
Hanging	Intensive livor in facial tissues; some capillary rupture showing petechial discolorations; no blood present in facial tissues
Mutilation	Loss of blood—little livor mortis Ecchymosis and bruising at affected areas
Poisons	Variable—from generalized conditions such as jaundice and cyanosis to localized discolorations such as caustic burns and petechiae
Refrigeration	Low blood viscosity, intense livor Postmortem stain speeded Dehydration of mucous membranes and skin surface after long exposure to cold air

Preservation must be the most important goal in embalming these bodies. Discolorations can always be masked with opaque cosmetics.

Two postmortem conditions, which are not causes of death, but have a relationship to discolorations, are also included here: bodies refrigerated prior to embalming and mold.

Hangings and Strangulation. Hanging and strangulation is death due to closure of the blood vessels and possible blockage of the air passages of the neck as a result of external pressure. Hanging can result in two very different situations. First, extensive blood discoloration and petechia can occur due to local blood congestion. The discoloration appears on the face as a result of the pressure placed on the jugular veins in the last moments of life, when blood was able to enter the facial tissues via the common carotids and vertebral routes, but was unable to drain from these tissues. The eyes and tongue may also protrude. The discoloration can be intense enough that the face appears almost black. If there is delay in finding the body, postmortem stain can be expected.

Second, no blood or discoloration is present in the face because the veins are able to drain and there was obstruction of the arterial system and blood could not enter the face.

Many cyanotic and blood discolorations in the facial tissues clear after the pressure has been relieved from the neck. Additionally, almost all of these bodies come under the jurisdiction of the coroner or the medical examiner and most would be examined by autopsy. During autopsy a great amount of blood is drained from the facial tissues. Restricted cervical injection and no preinjection treatment are recommended in the preparation of unautopsied bodies dead from hanging. The strength of the solution depends on the time between death and preparation, pathological conditions, and so on. As in most cases of delay, a medium to strong 2.0% to 2.5% well-coordinated arterial solution should be used.

Markings from rope (etc.) on the neck may be abraded. They will dry and turn brown when exposed to air. Some grooves may be deep, others will make only a shallow furrow. A very thin ligature such as wire may cut deeply into neck tissue.

Burned Bodies. Burns may be caused by heat (thermal burns), electrical shock, radioactive agents, or chemical agents. It is not always the local effect of the burn that should concern the embalmer, but rather the systemic effects brought about by major burns: bacterial infections, lack of blood flow to peripheral areas of the body, and kidney failure and the resulting buildup of wastes in blood and tissue fluids.

Burns are classified into three categories:

- **First degree:** The skin surface is red (erythema); only the surface epithelium is involved.
- **Second degree:** The skin blisters and edema is present. Blisters beneath or within the epidermis are called **bullae.** There is destruction of the deep layers of the epidermis and the upper layers of the dermis (Fig. 20–10).
- **Third degree:** The tissues are charred. The epidermis, the dermis, and epidermal derivatives such as hair follicles and glandular inclusions are destroyed.

Many victims of second-degree burns will have lived for a period between the injury and their death. The blistering of second-degree burns is rarely seen. These blisters are opened, drained, and treated long before the death. It is the systemic effects of kidney failure and generalized edema that must concern the embalmer. These bodies have a very high preservative demand. Circulation may be very difficult to establish. Very strong or waterless arterial solutions are needed to prepare these

Figure 20–10. Second-degree burns. Burned bodies often have a very high preservative demand because of kidney failure.

bodies. Dye is added to trace the distribution of solution. Multipoint injection, if the body has not been autopsied, is often needed. A major objective is creating dry clean skin for cosmetic work which includes:

1. Remove all loose skin before arterial injection using a good sharp razor (on visible areas).
2. Apply surface cavity (or phenol) compresses or paint the visible areas with autopsy gel. These gels can be painted over damaged skin areas that will not be viewed. (It is not necessary to clean these areas as they will be covered with plastic and clothing.)
3. Clean the skin surface with a good solvent.
4. Air-dry or force-dry with a hair dryer.

Often burns (and scalds) affect large regions of the body. The affected areas may emit an odor. Painting these areas with an autopsy preservative gel helps to ensure preservation and reduce odors. Edema and swelling are often present with second-degree burns. To prevent leakage and again to control odors, use of a **unionall** garment is recommended. This plastic garment covers all of the body except the face and the hands. Ample embalming powder should be spread in the unionall, especially over the burned areas. The autopsy gel may be left in place. The sprinkled powder adheres to the gel surface. Moisture-absorbent kitty litter can be liberally sprinkled over the burnt tissues to help control odor.

The need to achieve preservation cannot be overemphasized in the preparation of burned bodies. Many of these bodies should be embalmed with a waterless solution using a high-index arterial fluid.

Many bodies cannot be viewed because the facial tissues are severely swollen. All the embalmer can obtain some preservation and control leakage and odors.

Since suturing of incisions may be difficult, a worm suture may be more successful than use of the baseball suture.

Electrocution. Electrocution is related to discoloration because of the burn that results from contact with the electrical source. Often the palms of the hands are burned. Low-voltage burns appear either as an erythematous area of blistering or as chalky white lesions. High-voltage burns can char body tissue where contact is made. Rigor mortis often occurs very rapidly in these deaths.

The cause of death, the electrical contact, should present no problem to the embalmer. Restoration of the burn area is a restorative art problem only if the burn exists in a viewable area. Often, these bodies are autopsied, as the death must be investigated by a coroner or a medical examiner. For the preparation, the routine autopsy protocol is followed. In some instances the coroner or the medical examiner may have excised the area of tissue where the electrical burn occurred. If so, a strong cautery phenol solution should be applied to the raw tissue to dry and firm the area.

CO Poisoning. The primary concern in discolorations associated with deaths from CO poisoning is the classic "cherry-red" color. The bright color of the blood is due to carboxyhemoglobin, a component of blood. These bodies generally have a very low blood viscosity and few clots. These conditions assist distribution of the embalming solution and blood drainage. Of course, as time progresses so do the problems of distribution and drainage.

The bright reddish color is found in the dependent areas of the body to which the blood gravitates after death—the areas where livor mortis is present (Fig. 20–11). If the facial tissues and the neck are dependent, however, intense livor and staining can be expected. When some discoloration exists after embalming, a semiopaque or opaque cream cosmetic is advised, as the tissues tend to gray over time. Again, counterstaining with extra dye in the arterial solution helps to overcome this graying.

Most areas of the body where livor mortis is not present appear normal, although some blood is usually trapped in the anterior surface tissues and appears as pink in color. It looks as if the tissue was well embalmed and fluid dye was employed.

This discoloration is classified as an antemortem, intravascular blood discoloration. It should clear during arterial injection and subsequent blood drainage; however, there are usually some time delays between the death and the preparation of the body. Because most

Figure 20–11. Dependent areas are bright red in this unembalmed autopsied body. The cause of death was CO poisoning.

of these deaths must be investigated by a coroner or a medical examiner, preparation is delayed and the blood rapidly undergoes hemolysis and staining results. Therefore, in the majority of these bodies, some, but not complete, clearing of the discoloration occurs.

Solution strength should be based on the embalming analysis. Delay and refrigeration necessitate use of a stronger-than-average solution. Extra dye should be used to indicate solution distribution and diffusion. Once circulation is established, the solution strength can be increased further.

With regard to the selection of vessels, if there are no major problems or delays, any vessel is appropriate. Where there has been a delay, pathological problems, and so on, the best vessels are the common carotid artery and the internal jugular vein. If the embalmer feels that large volumes of solution are needed, restricted cervical injection is recommended.

CO poisoning in and of itself should not be a big problem for the embalmer. In many cases, the blood is quite thin and there is minimal clotting. Most of these bodies are autopsied for medicolegal purposes. In these situations, follow the normal autopsy preparation protocol.

Drownings. All asphyxia deaths exhibit cyanosis due to a change in the hemoglobin; petechia in the facial tissues is common and generally the blood has a low viscosity due to the rapid death. In a victim of drowning, the most noticeable discolorations are intense livor mortis, petechia, and possibly cyanosis. The livor mortis is due to the low temperature of the water, similar to refrigeration; the blood remains liquid and rapidly settles to the dependent tissues. If enough gas is generated to bring the body to the surface, the body floats **face downward**. Therefore, the livor and the resulting postmortem stain are intense in the facial areas. The cyanosis would be the result of the asphyxia (from the water in the respiratory system).

Each case must be handled on an individual basis. Preparation of some bodies has been delayed for months because the drowning occurred in winter but the body was not recovered until spring. These bodies were viewable. Other drowned bodies that have been in the water for a matter of hours have been so decomposed that they could not be prepared for viewing.

In addition to livor, postmortem stain, and cyanosis, some bodies may be dragged by water currents and bruised (lacerations). Large abrasions are frequently seen. Cool water preserves the body. Warm water speeds decomposition. In addition, fish and marine animals may desecrate the body.

A constant problem in the preparation of a drowned person who has not been autopsied is the possibility of **purge**, either lung or stomach purge. Be certain an adequate amount of cotton or cotton webbing is packed into the throat and respiratory passageways. Selection of vessels should be based on the condition of the body. If the embalmer has any doubts, use of the common carotid artery and the internal jugular vein is recommended. The ideal is restricted cervical injection. The strength of the fluid again depends on the extent of decomposition, the size of the body, pathological complications, and other factors in the case analysis. Aspiration should be thorough, with a minimum of two to three bottles of cavity fluid used on adult bodies. These bodies should be reaspirated, and if gases are evident or the viscera do not appear firm, reinject cavity fluid.

Gunshot Wounds

FACE AND HEAD. Each body where death involved trauma in the form of gunshot to the face or the head must be considered on an individual basis. Some of these wounds will appear quite simple with the points of entry and exit being difficult to locate. Other firearm deaths cause extensive damage to bones and tissues—entire portions of the skull or face may be removed.

Several common factors can be cited with most trauma to head or face:

- Eyelids and surrounding eye tissues discolored (ecchymosis)
- Eyelids and surrounding tissues swollen
- Torn or bruised tissues easily swell during arterial injection
- A majority of these bodies will be autopsied
- Fractures of the facial and cranial bones

A

B

Figure 20–12. Bullet wound. **A.** The bullet entry wound is used to aspirate the cranial cavity. **B.** Wound is closed with a trocar button.

If the missile passed into the cranial vault, and the body is not autopsied, leakage of arterial fluid into the cranium is a possibility (Fig. 20–12). If sufficient arterial fluid fills the cranial cavity, sufficient pressure can be created to create brain or fluid purge. Frequently these purges are seen from the nose or the ear if surrounding bones are fractured. Purge may also exit at the site of the missile entry or exit. The embalmer needs to make a thorough examination of the face and the skull to determine where there is bone and tissue damage. Preembalming local treatments include:

- Clean and disinfect the face, cranium, and cranial hair.
- Pack entry and exit points with cotton saturated with a phenol-cautery chemical to dry and firm surrounding tissues.
- Protect good skin by a light application of massage cream.
- Align fractured bones to achieve a normal contour to the head or the face.
- Temporary bridge sutures or superglue may be needed to align torn tissues.
- Apply compresses of bleaching or cavity chemical over discolored and/or swollen facial areas, e.g., eyelids, skin of the forehead, etc.

Injecting the head with a strong, well-coordinated, arterial solution or a **waterless** arterial solution accomplishes the following:

- Good preservation.
- Firm and dry tissues for restorative treatments.
- Control and reduction of swollen tissues.
- Bleaching of discolored tissues.

Sectional embalming is used for injection of the autopsied body. **Restricted cervical** injection is recommended for the unautopsied body. Restricted cervical injection will give the embalmer greatest control over fluid entering the face and the head—not only can solution strength be controlled but also pressure and rate of flow of the solution.

Some embalmers use **instant tissue fixation** for this type of body. Restricted cervical injection is used for the unautopsied body and sectional embalming for the autopsied body. A very strong arterial solution or a waterless solution is prepared. Additional fluid dye should be added to the solution. The solution is injected in "spurts" or "pulses" into the head using a high-pressure setting. Twenty pounds pressure with the centrifugal pump machine is sufficient (some embalmers use as much as 140 psi). The pressure is set with the rate of flow **closed**. Optional is to inject each side of the head separately or to inject both sides at the same time using a "Y" tube. If injecting each side of the body separately, the left side should be injected first and the right side second. Once the injection hose is attached to the arterial tube and the machine pressure set (rate of flow off) the embalmer **OPENS the rate of flow valve**—then immediately **CLOSES the rate of flow valve.** This spurts the solution into the head. This is repeated several times until the dye in the fluid becomes evident. Only a very small amount of arterial solution is usually required. **This technique allows the embalmer to inject a minimum amount of fluid the furthest distance and achieve the maximum preservation.**

After arterial embalming is completed, a phenol cautery chemical (or cavity fluid) can be injected using a hypodermic syringe and needle into the discolored or distended tissues. This solution should be injected from a "hidden point" of entry for these chemicals can leak. It may be necessary to aspirate the cranial cavity of the unautopsied body. Undiluted cavity fluid should be injected into the cranial cavity. Aspiration and injection can be performed through the point of entry or exit of the bullet or through the nose, passing the instruments through the ethmoid foramen of the cribriform plate of the ethmoid bone.

Postembalming if the eyelids are distended, a phenol-reducing and bleaching agent can be hypodermically injected using "hidden points of entry." It is possible for this solution to leak out of the hypodermic needle punctures; the hidden points provide a location where leakage is least likely to be seen. The following points of entry are suggested:

1. Lower eyelid and surrounding tissues
   a. Inside the mouth
   b. Inside the nostril
   c. Behind the ear or in the hairline
2. Upper eyelid and surrounding tissues
   a. Eyebrow
   b. Hairline

Let the phenol solution remain undisturbed for 20 to 30 minutes; then apply pressure to decrease swelling. Remove excess liquids through the needle punctures.

Surface compresses (of cavity fluid or a surface bleaching compound) may be applied to add weight to help reduce the distension as well as to preserve and bleach tissues. These compresses take more time to work and are much less effective than injection of a phenol solution into the tissues. If there is doubt about preservation, cotton may be used to close the eyelids; it can be saturated with cavity fluid and then the lids glued.

If eyelids are grossly distended, surgical reduction may be necessary. First achieve good preservation of the eyelids. The eyeball can be collapsed by aspiration. The eyelids should be reflected and the tissue excised from beneath the eyelids.

When eye problems have existed, always encourage the use of glasses on the deceased. The lights over the casket or on either end of the casket reflect off the lenses and hide some of the problem areas.

See Selected Readings, "Management Techniques for the Eyes" by V. Fountain later in this book.

Poisoning. A variety of discolorations are associated with poisoning deaths. Some poisons act in a very short time. Others have a cumulative effect on the body. The latter poisons may affect the liver, which, in turn, leads to jaundice. Some poisons induce shock; the blood is drawn into the large veins and the body exhibits very little livor mortis.

A large number of poisons act on the nervous and muscular systems. Respiration becomes difficult and the body becomes cyanotic. Other poisons are corrosive and burn areas such as the mouth and the hands with which they come into contact. In addition, the corrosive agent destroys tissues of the gastrointestinal tract, causing the rupture of veins and arteries in these organs. Some poisons cause petechiae on the skin surface. Others bring about anaphylactic shock, causing the skin to redden and swell. Cyanide produces a bright pink to the blood similar to CO poisoning. It is oxyhemoglobin that gives the blood the bright color.

Most of these bodies are autopsied. Dyes can be used to counterstain discolorations. Preservation should be the first concern. Areas burned by corrosive poisons need to be cleaned and dried before restorative treatment begins.

Mutilations and Blunt Force Trauma. The conditions caused by the various types of mutilation and blunt force trauma could fill an entire book. Tissues can be crushed, lacerated, punctured, and abraded. If injuries are to the face, the area affected can easily swell during arterial injection.

These bodies should not be embalmed by the "one-point" method of arterial embalming. Most require multipoint arterial embalming. In addition, some amount of hypodermic and surface embalming is necessary to achieve adequate preservation of the body (Fig. 20–13).

Figure 20–13. Corner of mouth deformed from use of a gastric tube.

In these bodies discolorations usually manifest as ecchymoses and antemortem and postmortem bruises. As with most unnatural causes of death, an autopsy is likely, but even with the autopsy, additional sectional and regional arterial injection may be necessary.

In mutilated areas severed arteries remain open making them somewhat easy to locate. An embalmer familiar with the arterial pathways can easily dissect to find the arteries. These vessels can be used for the injection of embalming solution. Drainage need not be a concern as many of these bodies have sustained a major blood loss and drainage will be minimal. Strong arterial solutions should be used. Such cases constitute an excellent example of the type of body for which special-purpose high-index fluids can be used. Use dyes to trace arterial solution distribution.

Exsanguination. Exsanguination is excessive blood loss to the point of death. The blood loss is not always external, as in massive hemorrhage. It can be internal, for example, rupture of a blood vessel caused by ulceration of an area or rupture of an aneurysm in one of the large body cavities. Blood loss can also occur without a break in the blood vascular system, as seen in shock. Here, the blood flows to the large, deep veins of the body, draining the capillaries of needed blood.

Exsanguination deaths are characterized not so much by discoloration as by a lack of color. Whether blood is lost externally, internally, or into the deep veins, very little livor mortis is evident. In cases of shock, the blood tends to congeal in the large veins and drainage may be difficult to establish. The largest vein possible should be employed in the preparation of these bodies. That would be the right internal jugular vein, which leads directly into the right atrium of the heart.

In injecting the bodies that have sustained a large blood loss, a slightly stronger arterial solution should be used, for there is likely to be a loss of arterial solution depending on the cause of blood loss. Additional dye should be added to the arterial solution to trace the distribution of arterial solution.

When necessary, sectional arterial embalming should be employed. The most difficult area to embalm, when there has been a "break" in the circulatory system, is the trunk. The legs, the arms, and the head pose no difficulty as these can be directly injected. The trunk may absorb some solution, but if an artery such as the aorta has ruptured, the trunk walls will have to be embalmed hypodermically, using a small trocar attached to the embalming machine.

A strong solution should be used for the hypodermic injection. This work must be thorough, as areas not reached by the hypodermic treatment stand little chance of contact with fluid by gravitation or diffusion from other areas. Several points will have to be used to introduce the trocar into the trunk. Special emphasis should be placed on the buttocks and the shoulder areas.

Refrigerated Bodies. From a discoloration standpoint, intense livor mortis can be expected in bodies that are refrigerated shortly after death. The cooling process helps to keep the blood liquid. When the body has been stored 6 to 12 hours prior to preparation, the dependent tissues can turn a variety of dark hues from red to blue-black. It is important to elevate the head and the shoulders of refrigerated bodies to avoid intense livor mortis in the tissues of the neck and the face.

Postmortem stain and Tardieu spots are also prevalent in these bodies. Hemolysis is speeded by cooling. In addition, the capillaries are more porous. Thus, stain can be expected in the areas where livor is present if the body has been refrigerated more than 12 hours. Blood trapped in any of the tissues can take on a light pink hue. This needs to be noted so it will not be mistaken for a sign of embalming fluid dye.

If the body has been refrigerated several days, expect surface dehydration of the body. The lips and the fingertips darken because of dehydration, as does the remaining skin, after a long period of refrigeration. This is not as much a problem today for most bodies are in body bags that do not permit the flow of air across the body.

Mold. The surface growth of mold, which may occur when the body has been stored for a time, should be scraped away and the area swabbed with a 1% phenol, 1% creosote solution, or a mixture of half methyl alcohol and half acetic acid. Cosmetic treatment will be necessary.

When the embalmed body is to be stored for several weeks, air should be allowed to circulate around the body. The exposed tissues (face and hands) can be sprayed with a surface mold preventative or carbolated Vaseline.

Darkness and moisture encourage mold growth. Molds will grow on both the unembalmed and the embalmed body. Cold molds will also grow on the body surface in refrigeration.

▶ CONCEPTS FOR STUDY AND DISCUSSION

1. Describe in detail how you would embalm an autopsied body, dead from traumatic head injuries, the eyelids and the surrounding orbital tissues of both eyes are "black" and swollen. How would you prepare an unautopsied body exhibiting the same condition of the eyes?
2. Discuss the embalming treatments for a body with "mild" jaundice.

3. Discuss the arterial solutions that can be used to help clear livor mortis in embalming a body that still retains heat.

4. Discuss the problems that can be encountered, with respect to discolorations, in the preparation of a drowned body, a body dead from hanging, and a body dead from CO poisoning.

5. Discuss the differences between postmortem hypostasis, livor mortis, and postmortem stain.

▶ BIBLIOGRAPHY

Adams J. Embalming the jaundice case—Part IV. *Dodge Magazine,* January-February 1995.

American Board of Funeral Service Education, *Course Content Syllabus,* St. Joseph, MO: American Board of Funeral Service, 2008.

Bedino JH. Waterless embalming—an investigation. *Champion Expanding Encyclopedia no. 656* 1993:619–620.

DiMaio VJ, DiMaio D. *Forensic Pathology,* 2nd ed. Boca Raton, FL: CRC Press, 2001.

Dorn JM, Hopkins BM. *Thanatochemistry,* 3rd ed. Upper Saddle River, NJ: Prentice-Hall, 2010.

Embalming Course Content Syllabus. Portland, ME: American Board of Funeral Service Education, 2001.

Kazmier H. *Essentials of Systemic Pathology.* Dubuque, IA: Kendell-Hunt Publishing Co., 1976.

Knight B. *Simpson's Forensic Medicine,* 11th ed. London: Arnold, Hodder Headline Group, 1997.

Mayer JS. *Color and Cosmetics,* 3rd ed. Dallas: Professional Training Schools, Inc., 1986.

Mayer JS. *Restorative Art,* 6th ed. Bergenfield, NJ: Paula Publishing Co., 1974.

New Jersey State Funeral Directors Assn. "Putting Alternative Preservations to the Test." In *The Forum,* Vol. 76, No. 3, Wall, NJ: New Jersey State Funeral Directors Assn., January 2010.

CHAPTER **21**

MOISTURE CONSIDERATIONS

CHAPTER OBJECTIVES

▸ Dehydration
▸ Body fluid accumulation—edema—tissues
▸ Body fluid accumulation by location—cavities
▸ Embalming treatments with edema
▸ Burned bodies—renal failure

There are three objectives in the embalming process: temporary preservation, sanitizing, and restoration to an acceptable appearance of the dead human body. Water plays an important role in achieving each of these objectives. The viewed areas of the body: face, neck, arms, and hands should appear "normal" to the family and the public—not shrunken and discolored by dehydration or swollen by edema. In unseen areas of the body, these moisture extremes should be controlled by the arterial embalming and by the supplemental embalming treatments along with proper postembalming care. The control of moisture is a primary concern for the embalmer. **A major objective of the embalming process should be to establish or to maintain a proper moisture balance in the dead human body.**

Three conditions characterize the various tissues of the dead human body with regard to moisture: normal body moisture, dehydration, and body fluid accumulation. Dehydration and fluid accumulation (edema) are generally the results of either disease processes, drug therapy, surgical procedure, or improper postmortem sheltering (refrigeration). These moisture extremes can be local or generalized within a body. It is possible that all the three conditions can be found within the same body! An excellent example is the patient who dies following open heart surgery or aortic repair. The face can be grossly swollen with edema, while the rest of the body is perfectly normal with regard to moisture.

In this chapter, bodies with generalized normal water balance are considered first. It is important that this normal water balance be maintained during the funeral. It is the job of the embalmer to prevent bodies with normal tissue moisture from dehydration. Dehydration is discussed next, as are the methods the embalmer can employ to moisturize tissues. Finally, localized and generalized edema is discussed together with the methods that can be employed to reduce moisture.

Embalming analysis determines what embalming chemicals are to be used and in what manner these chemicals should be injected. Body moisture plays a significant role in these decisions. Some examples of chemicals and injection techniques the use of which is determined by the moisture condition of the body follow:

- Arterial fluid (index, firming action, etc.).
- Dilution of the arterial fluid.
- Volume of arterial solution to inject.
- Use of coinjection or humectant fluid and its dilution.
- Vessel or vessels for injection and drainage.
- Injection and drainage techniques to add, maintain, or remove moisture.
- Speed of arterial injection.
- Use of the special techniques and fluids that add or remove moisture.

FACTORS DETERMINED IN THE EMBALMING ANALYSIS

1. Vessels for injection and drainage
2. Method of mouth closure
3. Strength of the embalming solution
4. Volume of the embalming solution
5. Injection pressure
6. Injection rate of flow

Note: These factors will vary by the individual body and can vary in different areas of the same body.

▶ NORMAL BODY MOISTURE

For the healthy, average, 160-lb male adult, **total body water** constitutes 55% to 60% (for normal to obese bodies) and approximately 65% (for thin bodies) of **total body weight.** For the female adult, the proportions are, on average, 10% less than those for the corresponding male body types. **Edema is said to be established when there is a 10% increase in total body water.**

After death, several factors bring about dehydration. Storage of the body in a refrigerator is one of the leading causes of a postmortem loss of moisture. Dry, cool, or warm air moving across the body promotes dehydration. Between death and embalming, the blood and the tissue fluids begin to gravitate into dependent body regions, increasing the moisture levels in the dependent tissues but reducing the moisture in the elevated body areas.

The embalming process itself can either add or greatly reduce moisture. The primary ingredient in almost all embalming fluids is formaldehyde, and formaldehyde dries tissues. During arterial injection, the skin becomes dry to the touch. The lips, the fingers, and the area between the thumb and the index have a tendency to rapidly dehydrate; wrinkling of these body areas is easily evidenced if the arterial embalming produces dehydration. This dehydrating effect can often be seen even before arterial injection is completed.

The embalmer must see that a good moisture balance is established or maintained. The well-embalmed body should not show signs of wrinkled, dark dehydrated tissue during the funeral. **Thoroughly embalmed tissues dehydrate LESS than under embalmed tissues.** Today, many bodies are shipped to other locations for funeral services and disposition, which results in delays. It is more important that there should be a little change in the appearance of the body during these delays.

An article published many years ago by Philip Boehringer in **Esco Review** cited some interesting re-

lationships dealing with the loss of moisture from the dead human body:

> If a pint of water weighs approximately 1 lb, consider the following: If the embalmer injects 3 gal of arterial solution, 24 lb of liquid is injected.
> The following liquid losses were estimated: $1\frac{1}{2}$ gal of drainage = 12 lb of moisture lost; 1 qt of liquid aspirated = 2 lb of moisture lost. Up to 3 pt can be lost per day by dehydration; funerals average 3 days = 9 lb of moisture lost.

One pound of moisture remains (or was added) by the preceding example. This body should not have evidenced any dehydration during viewing. These are conservative figures, but they do present an interesting challenge for the embalmer.

A simple way to maintain the proper moisture level during the embalming process is simply to follow the dilution recommendations on the label of the arterial fluid. Almost all fluid manufacturers recommend dilutions based on the moisture conditions of the body. Many times, they recommend the volume to be injected, the type of drainage, and the rate of flow at which to inject the arterial solution. The temperature of the water is also often stated on the label. For example, a typical fluid label might state the dilution for "normal" bodies, the dilution for "dehydrated" bodies, and the dilution for "edematous" bodies.

The dilution rule also applies to the use of coinjection and humectant fluids. Improperly used, these fluids can act in an opposite manner. Some humectants can act as a dehydrating chemical as well as a moisturizing chemical.

The following techniques can help to maintain a good balance of moisture in the body:

1. Avoid the use of astringent or hypertonic arterial solutions. Follow dilutions recommended by the manufacturer. Hypotonic solutions penetrate better, and their diffusion and retention will be increased. Strengths of 0.75% to 1.5% help to add moisture to the tissues. Most manufacturers recommend dilutions for dry, moist, and normal bodies.

2. Avoid the use of concurrent or continuous drainage after surface discolorations have cleared. Intermittent or alternate drainage helps to distribute and diffuse the arterial solution. These methods also help the body to retain arterial solution.

3. Avoid rapid arterial injection and drainage. A slower injection helps fluid to penetrate the tissues and reduces "short-circuiting" of fluids, so the solution is better distributed. Less tissue fluid is withdrawn from the tissues.

4. The delay of aspiration, if just for a short time, assists in diffusing arterial solution into the tissues. For best results, the final portion of arterial solution should be injected with the drainage closed. If aspiration is then delayed for a short time, the solution will have ample time to properly diffuse into the tissues.

5. If refrigerated prior to embalming, the body should be covered with plastic sheet during refrigeration to prevent the surrounding air from dehydrating the surface tissues.

6. Strong alkaline or acid fluids can alter the reaction between protein and preservative. Formaldehyde has a drying effect on the tissues. Acid or rapid-acting arterial fluids often produce very firm and dry tissues. Old (outdated) fluids should be avoided. These fluids cause the tissues to dehydrate rapidly.

7. Disinfectants should not dry and bleach the surface tissues.

8. Use of cotton to set features can cause tissues to dry. Massage cream and cream cosmetics help to slow the dehydrating effect of cotton. Nonabsorbent cotton can be used as a substitute.

9. Fumes from the injection of cavity fluids into the neck area can dehydrate the mouth and the nose. These areas can be packed tightly so fumes cannot enter.

10. Short-circuiting of arterial solution causes dehydration of the areas in which the solution is circulating. Distribution is uneven and the short-circuiting regions are very firm and dry.

11. Warm water solutions increase fluid reaction. Follow the manufacturer's recommendations for water dilution temperatures. Cool solutions slow the formaldehyde reaction, thus allowing better distribution and diffusion of the arterial solution throughout the entire body.

12. After embalming, the body should be covered to prevent circulating air from dehydrating the surface. Application of cream cosmetics and massage cream to the surface tissues helps to reduce moisture loss to the atmosphere (Fig. 21–1).

13. If there is to be a long delay between embalming and viewing of the body **do not** excessively elevate the head during storage of the body— elevation will cause gravitation of liquids from the facial tissues.

14. Tissue building the cheeks, the temples and the finger tips, after embalming, will help to prevent dehydration of these areas.

15. A light coating of massage cream applied to face, neck and hands, during and following embalming, will help to prevent dehydration of these tissues.

Normal

Dehydrated

Figure 21–1. Dehydration causes horizontal wrinkles to form on the lips. With the disease processes seen today it is necessary that the body be properly sanitized. A moderate arterial solution by today's standards is 1.5% to 2.0%. Many fluids are reaction controlled and do not release the preservative ingredients until they come into contact with body cells.

It is important that the embalmer should maintain the moisture present in the "normal" body. Because of drainage and the arterial fluid itself (formaldehyde dries tissues), the embalmer must actually **add** moisture to the normal body. This is why so much of water is used to dilute arterial fluid. Almost 15 oz of water is added for each ounce of arterial fluid!

▶ PREPARATION OF THE DEHYDRATED BODY

Antemortem Dehydration

A number of disease processes can result in a loss of fluid from the body cells and tissues: hemorrhage, febrile diseases, kidney diseases, diabetes, some cancers and localized neoplasms, and some first-degree burns. For many years, tuberculosis was a classic example of a disease whose symptoms produced severe emaciation and dehydration. More recently, emaciation and dehydration were seen in the early years of AIDS. However, most patients today under medical care are given hydrating therapies, so the "classic" dehydrated body is rarely seen. Those bodies that do exhibit severe dehydration are of persons who either did not seek medical treatment or withdrawn treatment under physician care as in some hospice situations.

Postmortem Dehydration—Preembalming

Dehydration following death is classified as a postmortem physical change. Following death and before embalming of the body, refrigeration and gravitation can remove moisture from the upper areas of the body such as the face and the neck. If the body is refrigerated, the dry, cool air moves around the body and gradually draws the moisture in the tissues to the surface of the body and into the surrounding air. (Refrigerated bodies are discussed in Chapter 19.) Even the unrefrigerated bodies exposed to environmental forced air heating and air conditioning can rapidly dehydrate.

Refrigeration also helps to keep the blood in a fluid state. Thus, the blood and the tissue fluids slowly gravitate (hypostasis) to the dependent tissues of the body. The upper areas of the body lose moisture because of the surface evaporation and the gravitation of fluids. Gradually the viscosity of the blood will thicken due to loss of moisture. This will increase postmortem coagula in the vascular system. Postmortem emboli in the arteries prevent a good distribution of the arterial embalming solution and coagula in the veins can make drainage difficult to establish.

Embalming Treatments to Control Dehydration

The skin on a dehydrated body is very dry. Often, the skin is quite "flaky." These small scaly flakes of skin must be removed from the facial areas or they will create a problem when cosmetics are applied. A liberal application of massage cream helps to control the flaking. The massage cream can be firmly wiped off with a gauze pad saturated with solvent, completely removing the loose skin cells. Several applications of cream and cleaning may be necessary.

The skin of the dehydrated bodies is often very dark. A condition similar to a suntan may exist. It may be difficult to trace the distribution of arterial solution through these areas of the skin. Dehydrated skin is very firm to the touch. The skin feels as if it has already been embalmed. Additional fluid dye is needed to be certain of arterial solution distribution.

Desiccation

Regardless of the antemortem or postmortem conditions that have brought about the condition of dehydration, there is only one positive benefit to the embalmer. Dehydrated bodies tend to decompose more slowly, as water is necessary for decomposition. Extreme dehydration is called **desiccation.** Desiccation is a form of preservation; however, desiccated bodies are not viewable.

Often, certain areas are desiccated in bodies that have been frozen or refrigerated for a long period. For example, desiccated lips appear black, very wrinkled, and shrunken. The lips are drawn back and the teeth are exposed. When the tips of the fingers are desiccated, the skin becomes parchment like and turns a yellow brown. Other body areas easily desiccated are the thin skin areas such as the ears, the nose, and the eyelids. Arterial injection or hypodermic injection is very ineffective in correcting this problem.

▶ LOCAL DEHYDRATION PROBLEMS

Dehydration is associated with several situations where the epidermis layer of the skin has been removed. When the epidermis is removed and the area is allowed to dry or force dried, the affected area will turn dark brown in color and appear quite firm to the touch. Examples frequently encountered: **abrasion**, which dries, **razor burn** (**abrasion**), nicking of the face during shaving of the body, **skin-slip**, where the dermis has dried, **epidermis removed** for transplant. This type of discoloration does not respond to bleaching by preservative surface compresses. Opaque cosmetic treatment is necessary when this occurs in a visible body area.

The drying of the tissues in the preceding examples is actually desired by the embalmer, for the skin surface is now sealed and there is no leakage from these areas. Opaque cosmetics (or waxes) can be applied over these dried areas. To speed the drying of abraded tissues, following arterial injection, a hair dryer can be used. Massage cream should not be applied to these areas, because it slows the drying of tissues.

▶ ARTERIAL EMBALMING PROBLEMS

Dehydration occurring during the antemortem, agonal, and postmortem periods prior to arterial embalming can result in a thickening of the blood. Satisfactory blood removal is essential to establish uniform distribution and even diffusion of arterial solution. Drainage may be difficult to establish in these bodies. A more important problem, however, may be congealing and clumping of this thick blood in the arterial system. On arterial injection, the heavy arterial blood and any clots may be forced into small arteries, thus cutting the flow of arterial solution, supplied by these small arteries, into the tissues.

Blood should be drained from the best location possible, the right internal jugular vein. Likewise, arterial injection from the right common carotid artery or restricted cervical injection pushes arterial coagula toward the legs. A secondary injection point (e.g., femoral vessels) may be necessary, and if this is not successful, hypodermic and surface treatment of the legs can be used to establish preservation.

It is unwise to inject from the femoral or external iliac arteries if clots are present. The arterial clots can be pushed into the carotid arteries, making embalming

TABLE 21–1. PROBLEMS ASSOCIATED WITH DEHYDRATION

Darkened skin	Corrected by cosmetic application; use fluid dyes to ensure fluid distribution to all body areas
"Flaking" or peeling of skin, especially in facial areas	Apply massage cream and then clean with a solvent to remove all loose skin; mortuary cream cosmetics further reduce skin drying
Firm feel to the skin	Skin feels embalmed; additional dye helps to trace the distribution of fluid
Desiccated lips, eyelids, or fingertips	May need correction with restorative waxes; tissue building; opaque cosmetics needed to hide discolorations
Thickened blood	May be diluted with a preinjection fluid; use right internal jugular as drainage point; inject from the carotids to push arterial coagula toward the lower extremities
Dehydration created by the embalmer; wrinkled lips, fingertips; facial areas	Use correct dilutions for arterial and humectant fluids; areas may be filled out with tissue builder after embalming
Dehydration of large facial area from embalming and passage of air over body	Use massage cream on exposed areas prior to cosmetic application; if skin is discolored, opaque cosmetics will be needed; cream cosmetics further reduce dehydration; fingertips and facial areas may also be treated with tissue builder to reduce dehydration

of the face a most difficult task. Slow injection will minimize arterial coagula from being dislodged and moved to block smaller arteries.

From an arterial chemical standpoint, preinjection fluids, coinjection fluids, and dilute arterial solutions can be used to prepare the dehydrated body (Table 21–1).

▶ TREATMENTS THAT MINIMIZE OR PREVENT POSTEMBALMING DEHYDRATION

Everybody that is embalmed dehydrates to a certain extent. Formaldehyde solutions not only firm tissues but also **dry** them. Drainage removes a large amount of moisture from the body tissues. These factors account for a great amount of dehydration during and after embalming. Some treatments can be used to maintain the level of moisture in or add moisture to these dehydrated bodies:

1. Use a moderate arterial solution. A moderate arterial solution by today's standards is 1.5% to 2.0%. Many fluids are reaction controlled and do not release the preservative ingredients until they come into contact with body cells. Many arterial fluids contain antidehydrants in their formulations. Large volumes of a mild solution can be used to moisturize and secure preservation. Follow the recommendations of the manufacturers of the arterial fluid. They generally recommend dilutions for dehydrated bodies.
2. Very slow injection of the arterial solution will help to fill the vascular system without creating arterial emboli which will block small arterial branches.

3. Use a coinjection fluid with the arterial solution. The coinjection fluid helps to reduce the astringent dehydrating action of the arterial solution and also adds moisture to the tissues. It is recommended that equal amounts of coinjection and preservative arterial fluids be used.
4. Use a humectant coinjection fluid along with the arterial solution. These fluids are designed to maintain or add body moisture. It is very important that the dilution recommended by the manufacturer be used. If improperly used, humectants can dehydrate the body.
5. Run large amounts of fluid through these bodies to replenish the lost moisture.
6. Intermittent or alternate drainage can be used to help the tissues retain the arterial solution and also to reduce short-circuiting of fluids and, thus, achieve more uniform embalming. This type of drainage also helps the arterial solution to penetrate the deeper body tissues (Fig. 21–2).
7. Apply massage cream, petroleum jelly, lanolin, or silicone to the exposed skin surfaces of the face and the hands during and immediately after arterial injection to retard water loss to the surrounding atmosphere. In the preparation of infants, the arms and the legs should also receive treatment. It is not necessary to use a large amount of lubricant. A light layer is sufficient. Cream cosmetics also retard surface dehydration.
8. Avoid excessive massage of the hands, the neck, and the face. Massage is often necessary to distribute fluid through these regions, but excessive massage not only draws additional fluid into these areas but also removes tissue and arterial solution from these areas.

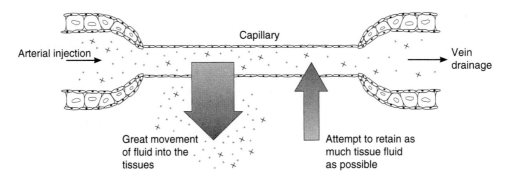

Figure 21–2. Hypotonic arterial solutions help the tissues to retain moisture.

9. Do not expose reposing or stored bodies to air currents. Forced air heating and air conditioning currents quickly dehydrate the exposed areas of the body.

► EDEMA

Edema, whether localized or generalized, creates many problems for the embalmer. This condition is one of the most frequently encountered problems in embalming today. **Edema is defined as the abnormal collection of fluid in tissue spaces, serous cavities, or both.**

Interstitial or tissue fluids enter and leave the bloodstream (in a similar manner to embalming fluids) through the walls and the pores of the capillaries, the small vessels connecting the smallest arteries (arterioles), and the smallest veins (venules). If more fluid leaves the blood vascular system and enters the tissues than is absorbed from the tissues into the blood, the tissues become filled with moisture; this condition is called **edema.**

Abnormal amounts of fluid (edema) can be found in three body sites:

1. *Intracellular*—within the individual cells.
2. *Intercellular*—within the spaces between the cells.
3. Within the body cavities.

Edema can be **local,** for example, when surgery has involved the heart or repair of the aorta. Following these surgeries, the head and the face can be grossly swollen with fluid, while the body trunk and the limbs display no trace of edema. It may be **generalized** (anasarca) and present in all the dependent tissues. A number of diseases and conditions can cause generalized edema: diseases that affect cardiac function and result in increased venous pressures, diseases that affect the renal system, increased permeability of the capillary walls, inflammation, and allergic reactions. In addition, long-term use of drugs can damage such vital organs as the liver and kidneys and the circulatory system. Failure of these organs or systems can lead to edema. Some drugs also act on cell membranes, causing cells to retain or take up moisture, thus creating a condition of edema within the cell. This is often seen in individuals who have used corticosteroids over long periods of time.

Often the embalmer encounters edema of one or more body cavities but no edema in the skeletal tissues. Likewise edema can be demonstrated in the skeletal tissues but with no edema in the body cavities.

It is not the purpose of this discussion to explain the disease processes that bring about edema. The embalmer should have an understanding of pathology and microbiology to recognize the relationship between certain conditions and edema. The following diseases/conditions are often associated with edema. The embalmer should be able to relate the cause of the edema with the condition:

■ Alcoholism.
■ Burns.
■ Cirrhosis of the liver.
■ Carbon monoxide poisoning.
■ Congestive heart failure.
■ Allergic reactions.
■ Inflammatory reactions.
■ Extended drug therapy.
■ Renal failure.
■ Trauma.
■ Lymphatic obstruction.
■ Steroid therapy.
■ Venous obstruction.
■ Phlebitis.
■ Malnutrition.
■ Hepatic failure and/or obstruction.
■ Surgical and transplant procedures.

► CLASSIFICATION OF EDEMA BY LOCATION

Cellular (Solid) Edema

When moisture is retained by the cell, or abnormal amounts of moisture are allowed to pass into the cell, a condition called solid edema results. The tissues appear

Figure 21–3. Pitting edema of the leg.

swollen and, when pushed on by the embalmer, feel very firm. Indentations are not made by pushing on these tissues. Frequently, this condition arises when large doses of corticosteroids have been administered over a long period. This form of edema, often seen in the facial tissues, does **not** respond to embalming treatments. The swelling and the distortion remain. The only possible, although not practical, method of reducing the swelling is excision of the deep tissues after arterial treatment is completed.

Intercellular (Pitting) Edema

In intercellular edema, fluids accumulate between the cells of the body. When these swollen areas are pushed on by the embalmer, the imprint of the fingers remains for a short period after the fingers are withdrawn. This form of edema, also known as **pitting edema** (Fig. 21–3), responds well to embalming treatments and can be gravitated to the dependent body areas. It can be drained from the tissues into the circulatory system and removed with the blood drainage. This edema may be localized as is frequently seen in bodies dead from cardiac diseases where only the legs are distended, and pulmonary edema (edema of the alveolar spaces in the lung tissue). Or, it may be generalized as is frequently encountered after death from liver or renal failure. Generalized edema is referred to as anasarca.

Edema of the Body Cavities

Ascites is edema of the abdominal (or peritoneal) cavity; the edema is found within the cavity and surrounds the abdominal viscera. **Hydrothorax** is edema of the pleural cavity; it may involve one or both pleural cavities. **Hydro-**

cephalus is edema of the cranial cavity, and **hydropericardium** is edema of the pericardial sac surrounding the heart. **Hydrocele** is an accumulation of serous fluid in the saclike cavity in the tunica vaginalis testis of the male scrotum.

> Edema of the cavities does not dilute the arterial solution. If the body being prepared has ascites, it is not necessary to increase the strength of the arterial solution because of the edema in the abdominal cavity. Edema of the cavities does not mix with the arterial solution. The embalmer's concern is that the edema in the abdominal cavity might dilute the cavity fluid when it is injected.

▶ EMBALMING PROBLEMS CREATED BY EDEMA

Generalized edema presents a number of problems for the embalmer. The tissues in which edema is present are swollen. When this involves the face and the hands, measures must be taken to reduce the distortion. Edema of the skeletal tissues has a tendency to gravitate into the dependent body areas, during life as well as after death.

In the bedridden patient, the edema is found largely in the dependent areas such as the back, the buttocks, the shoulders, and the backs of the legs. After death, this edema in the dependent tissues can in time lead to the passage of this fluid through the skin. This exit of fluid from the body can dampen the clothing of the deceased and the casket bedding, unless precautions are taken (e.g., use plastic garments and absorbent powders to trap and hold the fluids).

Bodies with large amounts of edema also exhibit leakage from intravenous punctures and small openings such as those made with hypodermic needles. Any surgical or embalming incisions are possible sites of leakage. Another major concern with edema is that the excess moisture in the tissues will hasten the decomposition cycle. A good, moist environment for bacterial growth is provided. Autolytic and hydrolytic enzymes will have an ample source of water for their role in decomposition. A secondary dilution of the embalming fluid is created by this excess fluid.

▶ EMBALMING PROBLEMS CREATED BY ANASARCA

1. Affected tissues are swollen with fluid.
2. When edema gravitates or moves from a region, the skin can wrinkle and appear distorted.

3. Fluid can leak from intravenous or invasive punctures through the skin surface by gravitation, through hypodermic needle punctures, through surgical incisions, and through incisions made for embalming purposes.
4. Arterial fluid is diluted (secondary dilution).
5. Decomposition is speeded.
6. The possibility of separation of the skin layers (skin-slip) is increased.

When the face is affected by edema, the embalmer must first determine whether **solid** or **pitting** edema is involved. This can be done by gently applying digital pressure to the swollen tissues. Solid edema **cannot** be indented by pressure from the fingers. With solid edema, the extra fluids are located within the individual cells of the tissues. This type of edema is seen in allergic reactions and as the result of certain drug therapies, such as the extended use of corticosteroid drugs. Solid edema cannot be removed by arterial or mechanical means. It would not be wise to attempt to reduce the swelling by surgical removal of subcutaneous tissues after arterial embalming. Uniformity of the tissue reduction and leakage would be major concerns. Solid edema, especially of the facial tissues, is not as frequently encountered as pitting edema.

In pitting edema, the fluid is in the interstitial spaces (between the cells). **Pitting edema can be gravitated**. Merely elevating the head helps to drain some of the fluid from the tissue spaces. Elevation of the head and the shoulders, during and following arterial injection, can drain a considerable amount of edematous fluids from the facial tissues. Passing the trocar through the tissues of the neck, while aspirating, will provide channels through which these fluids can pass from the face into the thorax. A sufficient amount must be given for this drainage to occur.

▶ ARTERIAL TREATMENT FOR GENERALIZED EDEMA

Generalized edema presents a number of problems for the embalmer. First and foremost is the increased rate of decomposition resulting from the presence of a large amount of body moisture. Water is necessary for decomposition. In generalized edema, vast quantities of water can be found in almost all the dependent skeletal tissues. In addition, the excess moisture causes a great secondary dilution of the arterial fluid, reducing the ability of the embalming solution to dry, sanitize, and preserve. The edema will, in time, seep through the skin, soiling the clothing and the casket interior. The large blebs that can form at edematous sites can break open and release fluids.

The objectives of the embalmer are to: (1) inject an arterial solution of sufficient strength and volume to counteract the secondary dilution that occurs in the tissues and (2) remove as much of the edema from the tissues as possible. **It is very important that the embalmer should know what condition caused the edema.**

For example, generalized edema can be the result of heart disease or renal failure. With renal failure, in addition to the edema, there is a buildup of nitrogenous wastes in the tissues. The nitrogenous wastes have the ability to neutralize the preservative solution. Therefore, very astringent solutions should be used.

Edema also coexists with nitrogenous wastes in the bodies dead from second-degree burns, especially when the patient lived several days or weeks after being burned. These bodies demand large amounts of preservation solution.

Edema can be present in all body types. Edema can and does quite often exist in emaciated bodies. The first concern, even in an emaciated body, is to achieve preservation and dry the tissues. Overdehydration of the face and the features is best avoided by raising both common carotid arteries at the beginning of the embalming and injecting the head separately.

Frequently in cases such as cancer of the liver, the body with generalized edema may also be jaundiced. Again, of primary importance are the preservation and the drying of the tissues. The discoloration is secondary. Only the face and the hands will be viewed. The restricted cervical method of injection allows the head to be embalmed separately. A jaundice fluid could be employed for embalming the head and a strong arterial solution in large amounts for the preparation of the trunk.

When arterial methods have not been completely successful, hypodermic injection of cavity fluid (or concentrated arterial solution) via the embalming machine can be used to inject local body areas. A small trocar can be used for the injection. The puncture is easily closed with a trocar button. Application of super adhesive around the trocar button helps to prevent leakage. The body is clothed in plastic garments. This technique works well with edematous legs.

Methods of Treatment

In treating the body with generalized edema, the embalmer should realize that large amounts of arterial solution must often be injected. Generally, the facial tissues are not affected by the edema (because in life the head is kept elevated), so to control the amount of the arterial fluid entering the facial tissues it is wise to use restricted cervical injection. In this method, both right and left common carotid arteries are raised at the start of the embalming. The left artery is opened and a large tube is inserted toward the head; the lower portion of the artery is ligated. A tube directed toward the head is

Figure 21–4. Restricted cervical injection allows large volumes of very strong arterial solution to be injected without over embalming the head.

placed in the right artery, as is a tube directed toward the trunk. Both tubes directed toward the head remain open during the injection of the trunk.

In some of these treatments, several gallons of arterial solution are injected or waterless solutions are employed. The fluid that enters the head and the facial areas exits through the open tubes while the lower portion of the body is being injected (Fig. 21–4). After satisfactory injection of the lower portion, the head can then be injected using a strength and quantity of arterial solution desired by the embalmer.

In bodies in which the head and the facial tissues are affected by edema, the restricted cervical injection is still recommended. The embalmer can inject the head separately with arterial solution of sufficient strength and quantity to ensure proper preservation of the facial tissues. The embalmer may wish to employ a specially prepared arterial solution with the osmotic qualities that assist in removing the excess fluids from the facial tissues.

When edema affects the head and the facial tissues, the tongue and the eyes may be grossly distended. Digital pressure on the scalp (especially the dependent portions) can also reveal the presence of pitting edema. Elevation of the head and the shoulders is necessary. In addition to employing a strong arterial solution for the injection of the head, the embalmer may wish to channel neck tissues during cavity embalming to provide a route for fluids to drain from the face, the scalp, and the neck into the thoracic cavities. Downward massage of the fa-

cial tissues also assists in draining the excess fluids from these regions.

Following arterial injection and cavity treatment, some embalmers place the body onto the removal cot and secure the body to the cot. The head end of the cot is then fully elevated, thus placing the body in a standing position. The body remains in this position for several hours to encourage as much edema as possible to gravitate from the head, the face, and the neck. Thorough aspiration and re-aspiration are recommended.

Local areas such as the eyes can be treated by a variety of techniques to restore swollen tissues. The first concern for the embalmer should be the complete preservation of these tissues. By injecting the left and right sides of the face separately, the embalmer can control the quantity of arterial solution entering the facial tissues. If the eyelids exhibit large amounts of edema and do not seem to be adequately embalmed, cotton can be placed under the eyelids and saturated with undiluted cavity fluid to ensure their preservation.

If areas of the face appear to lack adequate arterial solution, surface compresses of undiluted cavity fluid or preservative gels can be applied and left in place several hours. Facial areas can also be preserved hypodermically, but the points of entry must be carefully considered, as the edema may leak through the entry points. Most of this work should be done from within the mouth. When the head has been autopsied, a long hypodermic needle can be introduced from within the margins of the cut scalp areas.

In summary, arterial treatment for facial edema consists of injection of both common carotid arteries with a solution of sufficient strength and quantity to ensure complete preservation. Keep the shoulders and the head elevated. Use fluid dyes to locate areas of the face not receiving adequate arterial solution. These areas can then be treated by hypodermic or surface embalming methods. To drain fluid from the face and the neck, channel the neck with the trocar during aspiration of the body cavities. Reaspiration and cavity fluid reinjection of bodies with edema are always recommended. Excessive elevation of the head and the shoulders is essential.

Several types of arterial solutions can be used to treat bodies with generalized edema (Fig. 21–5): a very large volume of an average-strength solution; a sufficient volume of a very strong "hypertonic" solution; a special "high-index" dehydrating arterial solution; an average to strong arterial solution accompanied by a salt coinjection (Epsom salts); and an average to strong arterial solution accompanied by a vegetable humectant to help draw moisture out of the tissues into the capillaries.

Most bodies with generalized edema exhibit very good circulation. Few clots are found in the drainage from these bodies. There should be good distribution of the arterial solution, probably because the blood was

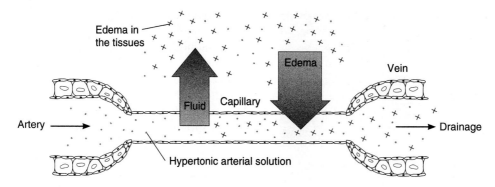

Figure 21–5. Hypertonic arterial solutions and arterial solutions containing large colloid molecules help to draw the edema from the tissues into the circulatory system.

diluted and thinned by the edema during life and after death. Therefore, formation of coagula in the blood vascular system postmortem is minimal.

In the majority of bodies with generalized edema, the embalmer can expect copious drainage and good fluid distribution and, thus, can inject large volumes of arterial solution. There are two means by which the preservative demand (or formaldehyde demand) of the body is met: by injection of strong arterial solution and by injection of a large volume of mild (average) arterial solution.

Injection Site. In the body with generalized edema, it is recommended that restricted cervical injection be employed. This allows saturation of the trunk without over injection of the head and separate injection of the head after the trunk has been embalmed (the body can be aspirated prior to injection of the head; features may be set after the trunk has been embalmed and after aspiration).

Drainage Site. The center of blood drainage is the right atrium of the heart. If the right internal jugular vein is used for drainage, instruments can be inserted directly into the right atrium and the head and neck drained from this site. Some embalmers prefer to drain from both the right and the left internal jugular veins when preparing a body with severe facial edema. Continuous drainage encourages removal of edematous fluids from the body.

Rate of Flow. All embalming should begin at a slow rate of flow. Once distribution has been established, the embalmer can increase the rate of flow to ensure good distribution to distal body areas.

Interrupted Injection. It is very important in removing edematous fluids from the tissue spaces to allow the embalming fluid, once injected, time to bring about osmotic exchange wherein the edematous fluids move into the capillaries and the preservatives move from the capillaries into the tissue spaces. After injecting $1\frac{1}{2}$ to 2 gal,

stop injection for one-and-half hour to allow these physical exchanges to occur. Then inject about $\frac{1}{2}$ to 1 gal and again stop and allow the physical exchange. Massage and squeeze the limbs from their distal portion toward the heart to encourage drainage of the edematous fluids from the veins into the blood drainage. Elevation of the arms and the legs also encourages the edematous fluids to move into the large veins. The injection of additional arterial solution after a rest period helps to force edematous fluid out of the vascular system into the drainage.

Arterial Solutions

Arterial Solution 1. A very large volume of a mild or average (standard) arterial solution is used. By today's standards, the strength of this solution would be 1.5% to 2.0% formaldehyde (approximately 8 oz of a 25-index arterial fluid is used to make a gallon of arterial solution). Continuous drainage is established with the injection of the solution. It is recommended that fluid dye be added to the last gallon to trace the distribution of the arterial solution. It is not uncommon to inject at least 2 to 3 gal of arterial solution into each leg of the autopsied body with generalized edema. The theory is that injection of large volumes of mild solution ensures good distribution of the solution and instills into the body a large volume of preservative, but at the same time washes as much of the edema as possible out of the tissues. To accomplish the fluid removal, a steady to fast rate of flow is recommended along with continuous or concurrent drainage. If the embalmer feels that preservation is inadequate, it is recommended that he or she should add several ounces of a high-index special-purpose arterial fluid to the embalming solution and make use of intermittent drainage to ensure that a sufficient amount of preservative solution remains in the tissues.

Arterial Solution 2. A very strong (or astringent) arterial solution is used. Some of the high-index fluids are accompanied by instructions on their use for embalming bodies with edema. The solutions for edema are generally quite strong, and dilution occurs when the arterial solution mixes with the edema in the tissue spaces. Arterial solution 2 should be used when the embalmer feels that circulation will not be good. As previously stated, circulation is generally good in bodies with generalized edema. There may be long delays, however, between death and embalming, and signs of decomposition may already be noticed. Use of large volumes of mild solution is not advised for these bodies. It is important to establish preservation first, then to dry the tissues. These strong solutions help both to preserve the tissues and to remove the edema. As these solutions are hypertonic relative to the moist tissues, the edematous fluids in the tissues are drawn back into the capillaries and, thus, removed with the drainage. It has been stated that use of these strong or astringent solutions is advised when the body with edema has been dead for a long period. Many of the capillaries are broken, so it is very difficult to inject arterial solution without causing even more swelling than already exists. Therefore, the strongest fluids possible should reach the tissues to establish preservation; injection of a large fluid volume would result in distortion from the swelling caused by the broken circulatory system. The embalmer's goal is to deliver the least amount necessary of the strongest arterial fluid. Knowledge of the cause of the edema is also important (e.g., renal failure or burns). Kidney wastes in the tissues neutralize preservative and necessitate use of strong solution. Concurrent drainage can be instituted with this solution. The embalmer, however, may wish to use some form of restricted drainage during injection of the last gallon to ensure solution retention. Cavity embalming can be delayed a short time to ensure fluid diffusion and saturation of the tissues. Again, fluid dye is recommended so the embalmer can see where the arterial solution has distributed. Firming may be minimal in these preparations. Firming of the tissues and drying of the skin are not dependable signs of arterial distribution. Areas that do not receive adequate solution should be arterially embalmed separately or treated by surface or hypodermic embalming techniques.

Arterial Solution 3. Some fluid companies manufacture special-purpose high-index fluids designed specifically to preserve and dry tissues with edema. Some companies further describe these arterial fluids as either dehydrating or nondehydrating. For treatment of the body with generalized edema, the dehydrating fluid is preferred. These high-index fluids are especially useful in the embalming of the bodies dead from second-degree burns or liver or renal failure. Directions on the bottle should be followed to ensure proper dilution of the arterial solutions. The quantity of the fluid injected depends on the size and the weight of the body, the dilution effected within the body by the edema present, the amount of edema present, and the distribution of embalming solution. Fluid dyes can be used to trace the distribution of arterial fluid. Use of coinjection fluid depends on the recommendations of the fluid manufacturer. Because these special fluids are strong, have a dehydrating effect, and must be injected in a large volume, it is strongly urged that the restricted cervical injection be implemented (raising both right and left common carotid arteries). If the head and the facial tissues have not been affected by the edema, the embalmer will, no doubt, want to use a standard arterial solution to embalm the head. Keep in mind that renal failure also affects the facial tissues; these tissues will contain nitrogenous waste, which neutralizes formaldehyde. Be certain that an adequate amount of sufficient-strength arterial solution is injected into the head.

Arterial Solution 4. Arterial solution 4 works to reduce the presence of edema by the use of dehydrating coinjection chemicals. Almost every embalming fluid manufacturer has such a coinjection product available. These coinjection products are designed to be injected with a preservative arterial solution. Follow manufacturers' instructions as to the amount of chemical to use and the time at which the chemical should be added to the preservative solution. These coinjection chemicals increase the osmotic qualities of the arterial solution either through the addition of salts or through large colloidal molecules. They are especially effective for facial edema. Facial edema responds well for not only there is a chemical drying of the tissues by the coinjection chemical, but also elevation of the head allows for gravitation of the edematous fluids from the facial tissues. Firm massage and pressure should also be applied to the facial tissues especially after the chemical has been injected. Aspiration of the cavities can help to relieve additional pressure caused by edema in the thoracic and the abdominal cavities. This also helps edema to drain from the facial tissues. Restricted cervical injection is advised when using this method of treatment for facial edema.

The hands respond well to the use of a dehydrating coinjection fluid. They should be well massaged during and after arterial injection. Elevation will assist in the movement of the edematous fluids from the hands to the upper arms. Sectional injection using the coinjection fluid solution may be necessary.

Manufacturers' instructions as to the quantity and methods of use of these fluids should be followed. Overdehydration of the face and the hands is always a possibility. Post embalming tissue building can be used to correct this problem.

Arterial Solution 5. Arterial solution 5 works to reduce the swollen condition brought about by the edema. It is made using Epsom salts, which create a hypertonic solution. This hypertonic solution sets up an osmotic gradient that draws the edema from the tissue spaces toward this concentrated salt solution in the capillaries. The embalmer may wish to begin the embalming and clear the blood vascular system with either strong or average arterial solution. Injection continues until the blood drainage clears and the distribution appears uniform. When strong dehydrating solutions such as this arterial mixture are used, it is very important that both common carotid arteries be raised as the primary injection site. In this manner, the head can be separately injected. If the head is grossly distended by the edema, arterial solution 5 should help to remove it. The following arterial solution is suggested.

Fill a container with half a gallon of cool water; add as much Epsom salts as can be dissolved. Thoroughly stir this solution. Next, add 4 to 6 oz of a high-index (25 to 35) arterial fluid. Pour this solution into the embalming machine but do not pour any of the undissolved salt that may have settled to the bottom of the container.

Inject this solution into the area affected by the edema. Massage the tissues (after they are injected). Assume that the head and the face are grossly distended with edema (often seen after cardiac surgery or aortic repair). First inject the left side of the head; then inject the right side. Massage the swollen tissues downward to encourage the edema to drain through the veins. (Some embalmers allow this solution to remain in place approximately one-and-half hour and then reinject with a strong arterial solution. Thus the Epsom salt solution remains in the capillaries long enough to draw the edematous fluid from the tissue spaces. This edematous fluid is then flushed away by the reinjection.) Massage plays a very large role in the success of this process. This is an excellent technique to use on an arm or a leg grossly distended with edema. Care should be taken to keep the solution thoroughly stirred, for it is easy to clog the delivery lines of the embalming machine. If this should occur, flush the machine with warm water to dissolve the Epsom salt crystals. An aspirator hose can be attached to the delivery line to pull the crystallized materials out of the machine. After using a solution containing Epsom salts, always flush the machine with warm water. This very old technique can be quite effective (Fig. 21–6). The Epsom salt solution works best on the facial tissues, especially when the edema is recent (e.g., recent surgical patients, heart or aortic surgery). This process does not work well when the edema has been present for a long period (e.g., trauma cases, drug therapy cases).

Arterial Solution 6. Use of waterless arterial solutions containing, in addition to standard co-injection and water-corrective chemicals, the addition of an edema reducing co-injection chemical.

▶ LOCAL TREATMENT FOR EDEMA

General Techniques
1. Sectional injection
2. Direct hypodermic injections
3. Elevation and gravitation
4. Channeling and wicking
5. Lancing and draining
6. Plastic protective garments and absorbent powders

Legs
When only the legs are affected by edema, it is best to embalm the body with a standard-strength arterial solution. This, of course, depends on the general condition of the body. The important point is not to prepare a strong arterial solution for the entire body based on the fact that edema is present only in the legs (Fig. 21–7).

After embalming the body, raise the femoral or iliac vessels and separately inject the legs using one of the arterial solutions just discussed. If the edema is severe, after arterial injection use the trocar to pierce the upper thighs beneath the inguinal ligaments while embalming the cavities. Elevate the legs and, if desired, wrap them with an elastic bandage beginning at the foot and moving up the leg. This pushes some of the edema into the pelvic cavity from which it can later be aspirated. The legs should be elevated several hours to make this treatment effective.

The legs can also be injected with cavity fluid or a high-index arterial fluid using a trocar. This is done **after** the arterial injection of the legs. The fluid is placed in the injection machine, and the delivery tube is attached to an infant trocar. The inside of the calf is a good point of entry. From this point, the lower leg and thigh can be reached. Saturate the leg with the fluid and close the entry point with a trocar button. The leg can also be painted with autopsy gel and accompanied with the use of a plastic stocking. Embalming powder can also be placed inside the stocking. The powder and the gel assist in the preservation of the leg. When edema is more extensive and affects the hips and the buttocks, plastic coveralls or pants should also be used. When shoulders and trunk walls are affected along with legs and arms, use of a unionall is advised, for it covers all these areas.

"Wicking" is a post-embalming process used to remove edema from body regions. One or more small holes are placed into the dependent area of the edematous tissue. A portion of about a 12-inch cotton, webbed cotton or cloth wick is inserted into the tissue. The longer portion of the wick is placed into the side drain of the embalming table. The capillary action of the wick will draw the edema from the tissues over a period of time. Manual pressure placed on the edematous area can increase the drainage of the edema. This process does take time. After drainage, the wick is removed; the opening can be closed with a trocar button (see Fig. 21–8).

A

B

C

Figure 21–6. Facial edema after repair of an aortic aneurysm. The swelling was reduced by the addition of Epsom salts to the arterial solution. **A.** Facial edema prior to injection. **B** and **C.** Reduction of the facial edema at completion of the embalming.

Arms

When only the arms and the hands are affected with edema, the arm can be separately injected after the body has been embalmed. The hand and the arm can be elevated to gravitate some of the edema into the upper arm. Wrinkling of the back of the hand now becomes a problem.

If distal areas such as the fingers become badly wrinkled, a small amount of tissue builder can be injected into each finger. Some wrinkling may be removed by

Figure 21-7. Extreme edema of lower extremities.

the injection of tissue builder; good points of needle entry would be between the fingers. If there are intravenous or needle punctures on the back of the hand, the embalmer can remove a considerable amount of edema through these openings by squeezing and then sealing the openings with a drop or two of super adhesive.

If only the elbow area is swollen with edema, it may be unwise to lance and drain the edema after embalming, UNLESS a sufficient amount of time is available for the fluids to drain and the tissues would be strong enough to be sewn closed. Wicking the edema is possible—time permitting. Cavity fluid can be injected into the elbow area by use of an infant trocar. The trocar can be inserted through a high point in the upper arm. The opening can be securely closed with a trocar button.

Figure 21-8. Wicking of the forearm to remove edema.

Edema of the Trunk

After death, edematous fluid gravitates to the dependent areas. Sectional arterial injection of the trunk is not possible. When edema is present in the dependent trunk areas (e.g., shoulders, buttocks, lateral walls), direct hypodermic injection will serve best to increase the preservation of these regions. An infant trocar can be inserted into the lateral walls on each side of the body. The point of entry can be along the midaxillary line in the soft tissues inferior to the rib cage. From this point of entry, the trocar should be able to reach as far up as the axilla and also as far down as the buttocks. Cavity fluid or very concentrated arterial solution can be injected through the embalming machine. This added embalming measure, of course, is done after arterial injection of the body. Coveralls or a unionall can be placed on the body, and a liberal amount of preservative powder can be sprinkled into the plastic garment. Eventually this edema will pass through the skin of the back and the dependent trunk walls. This exit of fluid can occur even before the disposition of the body. It is essential to protect the clothing and the interior of the casket by use of the plastic garments.

Ascites (Edema of the Abdominal Cavity)

Ascites can exist almost unnoticed until the embalmer begins to aspirate the cavity or it can severely distend the abdominal cavity, because the edematous fluid is located within the cavity and around the visceral organs. **It is unaffected by arterial fluid treatment or blood drainage. Ascites will not dilute arterial fluid, because the arterial solution and the edema in the abdominal cavity do not come into contact.**

When ascites is present and noticeable, do not mix arterial solutions in the belief that ascites will be a secondary dilution for arterial fluid. Ascites **will** be a diluting factor for cavity fluid. When ascites is present and the abdomen is very tense prior to arterial embalming, the pressure in the abdominal cavity may be sufficient to interfere with arterial distribution. More importantly, the pressure can interfere with blood drainage. This pressure is created not only by the enormous amount of fluid in the abdominal cavity (often several gallons) but also by possible gases in the intestinal tract. The pressure should be removed prior to arterial injection. Several techniques can be used:

1. Using a scalpel, make a small opening in the abdominal cavity and insert a drain tube or a trocar from which the point has been removed. Many embalmers prefer to make this incision in the inguinal or the hypogastric area of the abdominal wall. At this lower point more liquid can be removed from the cavity. Attach the aspirating hose to the drainage tube or trocar for delivery of the edematous fluids directly into the drainage or collection system.
2. Insert a trocar keeping the point just under the anterior abdominal wall. Pierce the transverse colon to release gases. Attach the aspirating hose to the trocar.
3. Make a small incision over the area of the transverse colon, exposing the colon (which can be opened). The incision is an outlet for the edema. This technique is most unsanitary and, if possible, should be avoided.

When the distension of the abdomen is not severe enough to restrict the flow of arterial solution or interfere with blood drainage, the ascites can be removed during the normal period for aspiration of the abdominal cavity. These bodies should be reaspirated.

Hydrothorax

In hydrothorax, edema is present in the space between the wall of the thoracic cavity and the lung. This condition is not easy to recognize because the rib cage cannot expand like the abdomen does when edema is present. This condition can be expected in the bodies dead from heart disease or pneumonia. Often, there is some distension of the neck, and, very frequently, both the face and the neck exhibit a great amount of livor mortis after death. Aspiration of the thoracic cavity removes the fluid. Aspiration is done after arterial embalming. The trocar should be directed to the posterior portions of the thorax, where the fluid will have gravitated. It is possible to remove one or more gallons of fluid from the thorax when this condition is present.

If it is necessary to relieve some of this pressure prior to or during arterial injection, a trocar can be introduced from the standard point of trocar entry and guided along the lateral wall of the abdomen into the thoracic cavity. This provides a drainage outlet for the fluid, but does not rupture any large arteries or veins. When hydrothorax is suspected, use the common carotid artery for injection and drain from the right internal jugular vein. This is the best location from which to drain the head and the arms. Aspiration should immediately follow arterial injection. Very often distension of the neck will diminish and any swelling that may have occurred in the facial tissues will be reduced.

Hydrocele

In the male, the scrotum can become distended with edematous fluid. Quite frequently, insufficient arterial solution reaches the tissues of the scrotum, which can be a site for decomposition. This condition is treated during aspiration and injection of the body cavities, after arterial injection. During aspiration pass the trocar over the pubic symphysis and pubic bone and enter both sides of the scrotum. Place a towel around the scrotum and apply pressure. This forces the edematous fluid through the channels that have been made with the trocar and into the pelvic cavity. Both sides of the scrotum can then be filled with undiluted cavity fluid to ensure preservation. Care should be taken not to puncture the scrotum with the trocar. If the scrotum is punctured, superglue or a trocar button can be used for closure. If the leakage cannot be stopped, drain the edematous fluids and the cavity fluids that were injected. Let the drainage continue several hours.

Hydrocephalus

When edematous fluid fills the cranial cavity during fetal development, the head is grossly distended. Some individuals survive after birth and live many years with this condition. In the unautopsied infant, it is necessary to drain some of this fluid, or very rapid decomposition of the brain and fluids of the cranial cavity may occur. Drainage can be established by passing a large hypodermic needle through the nostril and directing it through the anterior portion of the cribriform plate of the ethmoid bone. This process should be done after arterial embalming.

Several ounces of undiluted cavity fluid or phenol solution can be injected in the same manner as the fluid was aspirated. The nostrils should be tightly packed with cotton to protect against leakage. When there has been ossification of the bones of the cranial cavity, it is not always necessary to aspirate and inject the cavity. Leakage must always be considered when the cranial cavity is aspirated.

► SPECIAL CONDITIONS

Burned Bodies

Edema accompanies burns, especially second-degree burns. Generally, these victims live for days or weeks after the burns. Blistering of the skin is characteristic of second-degree burns. The embalmer, however, very rarely sees the blistering condition. The blisters have been opened and drained and preparations are placed on the denuded skin area to encourage cellular growth and skin replacement. Death usually results from renal failure. Because of the skin damage, many waste products that normally leave the body via the skin are retained in the blood. As a result, the kidneys cannot handle the wastes that rapidly build up in the body. These bodies are often so grossly distended with edema that the face is not recognizable.

The first concern of the embalmer is preservation. These bodies have a very high preservative demand. Restricted cervical injection with drainage from the right internal jugular vein is recommended for these bodies when they are not autopsied. Waterless or very strong arterial solutions should be injected. Fluid dye can be added to the arterial solution to identify those body areas receiving arterial solution. Areas not reached by the arterial solution are best treated by hypodermic injection of cavity fluid or a very strong arterial solution. These bodies are very difficult to handle as they are often covered with various ointments. Washing the skin surface with a good disinfectant soap removes surface medications and debris.

Long open incisions are the result of one method used to treat the patients with burns. The embalmer cannot suture these long incisions. The surface can be thoroughly dried after it has been bathed with a soapy solution. Exposure to air also helps to dry the skin surface. These bodies can be placed in a unionall; this plastic garment covers all body areas except the hands, the neck, and the face. The body surface can be liberally covered with embalming powder. In addition, the skin surface can be painted with autopsy gel, or cavity compresses can be applied before the body is clothed in the unionall. Strips of sheeting or gauze can be used to wrap extremities when long incisions are present.

Leakage can be a major problem with these bodies. Allowing the body to drain as much as possible and to air-dry prior to placing plastic garments on the body diminishes the amount of leakage into the plastic garments after the body is casketed. Frequently, these persons have had a tracheotomy. It may be very difficult to close the tracheotomy opening if the neck area was affected by the burns. In these cases, after aspiration of the unautopsied body, fill the opening with cotton and incision seal powder and liberally apply surface glue over the opening.

Renal Failure

Chronic renal failure brings about an increase in toxic wastes (urea, uric acid, ammonia, and creatine) in the blood and the tissues of the body. Retention of these wastes results in acidosis (the tissues become acidic). Over time, there is a decrease in cardiac function leading to congestive heart failure and pulmonary edema. Gastric ulcerations occur and gastrointestinal bleeding can be expected. The patient becomes anemic and the skin turns sallow as a result of the retention of urochrome.

This condition is very important to the embalmer. Bodies with renal failure rapidly decompose. The edema present dilutes the arterial solution. The waste products in the bloodstream and the tissues neutralize the formaldehyde. The color can deepen after embalming and become more pronounced, creating a cosmetic problem. Tissues do not firm normally, for the proteins of the body have been altered. Such bodies have a very high preservative demand. It is important that the embalmer should use strong arterial solutions. Special-purpose high-index fluids are recommended. Preinjection should be avoided if there has been a delay between death and embalming or if the embalmer feels circulation may be difficult to establish. Restricted cervical injection, for the unautopsied body, with drainage from the right internal jugular vein is recommended.

A very strong arterial solution should be used. Dye can be added to the arterial solution not only to trace the distribution of fluid, but also to counterstain the sallow color produced by the urochrome in the tissues. In many bodies that have been in chronic renal failure, other visceral organ damage has taken place. The body may be very jaundiced, and ecchymoses from disease and medications may be seen on the skin surface. Emaciation and protein damage may have occurred in the tissues. The embalmer will have problems with discolorations, firming, and preservation.

The most important objective in embalming these bodies is good preservation. Firming is not always necessary. Tissue can be preserved without being intensely firmed. Discolorations are secondary and can always be treated with cosmetics.

Cavity embalming is very important. Frequently, bleeding has occurred in the gastrointestinal tract, providing an excellent medium for bacterial proliferation and a good site for the formation of gas. Thorough aspiration of the cavities is necessary. The embalmer may note arterial solution in the cavities or hollow viscera where bleeding occurred in life. A minimum of two to three bottles of undiluted cavity fluid should be injected. Several hours later, the body should be reaspirated and reinjected with cavity fluid. Renal failure is a condition that the embalmer must learn to recognize. **Check the death certificate carefully if available for references to renal involvement.** Areas not receiving adequate

TABLE 21–2. SUMMARY OF EDEMA

Edema	Definition	Problems	Treatment
Solid	Edema within body cells	Swollen tissues; difficult preservation	Must be excised for reduction Strong arterial solutions; coinjection fluids
Pitting	Edema in tissue spaces, between the cells	Distension; fluid dilution; leakage; difficult preservation	May be gravitated; use strong arterial solutions; may be punctured and drained; use plastic garments to protect from leakage
Anasarca	Generalized edema in all body tissues	Leakage; distension; arterial fluid dilution	Strong arterial solutions; hypodermic and surface embalming; plastic garments; gravitation; puncture and drain
Edema of face	Edema in facial tissues	Swollen tissues, eyelids, and tongue	Restricted cervical injection; strong coordinated arterial solutions; possible use of salt solutions or high-index solutions to reduce swelling; elevate head; channel with trocar neck area for drainage into thorax; surface weights for eyes and lips; surface and hypodermic embalming to ensure preservation with cavity fluid
Edema of hands	Edema in tissues of the backs of the hands	Swollen tissues; possible leakage from intravenous punctures; wrinkles after removal	Sectional injection from axillary artery; surface packs with cavity fluid to ensure preservation; bleach any discolorations; elevate to gravitate edema into arm
Edema of legs	Edema in thighs and lower legs	Dilution of arterial fluid; leakage	Sectional injection of legs from femoral or external iliac artery; use of strong arterial solutions; use of salt solutions or dehydrating solutions to remove edema; hypodermic injection with undiluted cavity fluid; surface treatment using autopsy gel; plastic stockings containing embalming powder and autopsy gel; elevate to gravitate edema into abdominal cavity; puncture and drain
Pulmonary edema	Edema in the alveoli of the lungs	Purge	Aspiration and injection of lungs
Hydrothorax	Edema in the thoracic cavity	Purge; dilution of cavity fluid; pressure can cause venous congestion of neck and face; facial distension	Aspiration; injection of cavity fluid; careful draining prior to arterial injection
Ascites	Edema of abdominal cavity	Pressure can cause purge of stomach contents; anal purge; dilution of cavity fluid	Aspiration and injection of undiluted cavity fluid; preembalming draining via trocar or drainage tube; reaspiration and reinjection
Hydropericardium	Edema of pericardial cavity	Dilution of cavity fluid pressure could cause drainage problems	Aspiration and injection of undiluted cavity fluid
Hydrocele	Edema of scrotum	Leakage; dilution of arterial fluid; distension; problems in dressing	Channel with trocar to drain into abdominal cavity; inject via trocar undiluted cavity fluid; surface coating with autopsy gel; use of plastic garments and embalming powder
Hydrocephalus	Edema of cranial cavity	Purge in infant	Drain in infant via ethmoid foramen; inject cavity fluid via ethmoid foramen

arterial solution should be sectionally injected. If necessary, undiluted cavity fluid can be injected hypodermically, or compresses of undiluted cavity fluid or autopsy gel can be applied to the surface to ensure preservation.

The embalming complications associated with chronic renal failure can be summarized:

1. Decomposition occurs rapidly.
2. Acidosis alters the reaction between proteins and the preservative.
3. The body appears sallow because urochrome is present in the tissues.
4. Sites of gastrointestinal bleeding may be sites of arterial fluid loss and sources of purge.
5. Edema dilutes the arterial fluid.
6. Uremic wastes in the blood and tissues neutralize preservatives.
7. Skin infections may be caused by uremic pruritis.

See Table 21–2 for a summary of edema.

▶ CONCEPTS FOR STUDY AND DISCUSSION

1. Explain how a supplemental edema reducing chemical works.
2. Discuss what treatments can be employed to help restore moisture to a body that is badly dehydrated during embalming.
3. List some of the conditions, both antemortem and postmortem, that cause dehydration.
4. Discuss some of the complications created by the presence of skeletal edema.

5. Discuss the arterial solutions and embalming techniques that can be used to remove edema from the skeletal tissues.
6. Discuss the complications that arise in the preparation of a body dead from renal failure.

▶ BIBLIOGRAPHY

American Board of Funeral Service Education, *Course Content Syllabus*, St. Joseph, MO: American Board of Funeral Service, 2008.

Elkins J. Major body elevation as a technique for the reduction of swelling in the face and hands of embalmed bodies. In: *Champion Expanding Encyclopedia*, No. 554. Springfield, OH: Champion Chemical Co., 1985.

Henson RW. Controlling the moisture content of the tissues. *Professional Embalmer*, November 1940.

Henson RW. Controlling the moisture content of the tissues. *Professional Embalmer*, October 1940.

Regulating the Moisture Content of Tissues. Wilmette, IL: Hizone Supplements; 1938:11.

Sheldon H. *Boyd's Introduction to the Study of Disease*, 10th ed. Philadelphia: Lea & Febiger, 1988.

Shor MM. Can magnesium sulfate be safely used to rid body of fluid in lower extremities? *Casket and Sunnyside*, July 1965.

Sturb CG. Distribution and diffusion. *Funeral Directors Journal*, May 1939.

Venes D. *Taber's Cyclopedic Medical Dictionary*, 19th ed. Philadelphia: F.A. Davis, 2001.

CHAPTER 22

VASCULAR CONSIDERATIONS

CHAPTER OBJECTIVES

▶ Intravascular conditions
▶ Extravascular conditions
▶ Vascular coagula
▶ Diabetes

The blood vascular system is the distribution route for the embalming solution. Any pathological or traumatic change that obstructs or breaks open this delivery system either completely blocks or reduces flow of arterial solution to a body region.

As people age, many degenerative changes can occur in the circulatory system. Although heart or blood vessel disease may not be the immediate cause of death, such a condition can greatly influence the embalming procedure. Likewise, drugs given for the treatment of heart or vascular diseases may have more influence on the embalming procedure than the condition of the diseased vessels. Intravascular conditions, diseases, or tissue changes in the walls of or within the blood vessels is of concern to the embalmer. The arteries are the vessels that carry the embalming solution to the capillaries. At the capillaries, some of the arterial solution will leave the vascular system to enter the interstitial spaces, where it will come into contact with the body cells and cellular proteins. The solution remaining in the vascular system travels into the veins and helps push the blood from the body in the form of drainage. Arteries have three layers:

- *Intima.* The inner lining of endothelial cells, which continue to form the walls of the capillaries and then the inner walls of the veins and arteries (this endothelial layer of cells lines the entire blood vascular system).
- *Media.* The middle layer, composed of muscle cells and elastic tissue.
- *Adventitia.* The outer layer, composed mostly of connective tissue.

The cavity of the vessel is called the **lumen.** Narrowing or obstruction of the lumen can decrease or stop flow of arterial solution to a body area. Intravascular problems can also result in breaks or tears in vessels. These can be very small ruptures such as petechiae or major ruptures such as aortic aneurysms.

Table 22–1 lists intravascular arterial conditions that can limit the distribution of arterial solution to various body areas. Arteriosclerosis and arterial coagula are the problems most frequently encountered by the embalmer.

Preinjection fluid should not be used when it is thought it will be difficult to establish arterial solution distribution. If the system is filled with the preinjection solution, swelling could result when the preservative solution is injected. Preinjection fluid should be used only if circulation is thought to be good; in such cases it maintains the good distribution and drainage. Many persons who had vascular diseases were given blood thinners and anticoagulants. These bodies generally exhibit good arterial solution distribution and few or no clots in the drainage.

▶ ARTERIOSCLEROSIS

Almost anyone older than 30 years may exhibit arteriosclerosis. Most people think of this degenerative condition as occurring in old age. Many persons who die from heart disease in their mid-fifties exhibit more

TABLE 22–1. CONDITIONS RESULTING FROM INTRAVASCULAR DISEASE PROCESSES

Vascular Condition or Injury	Description	Embalming Concern
Advanced decomposition	Breakdown of the body tissues	Arteries are one of the last "organs" to decompose. Some circulation may be possible. Expect a large number of intravascular clots. Distribution is very poor. Capillary decomposition causes rapid swelling of the tissues.
Aneurysm	Localized dilation of an artery	If aneurysm ruptures, fluid cannot distribute.
Arteriosclerosis	Hardening of the arteries	Vessel may not be suitable as an injection site. Narrowed arteries may easily trap arterial coagula.
Arteritis	Inflammation of an artery	Artery may narrow, resulting in poor distribution of arterial solution. Artery may also weaken and rupture from pressure of injection.
Asphyxiation	Insufficient oxygen supply	Right side of heart is congested (poor drainage). Purging can result as blood flows back into lungs instead of draining. Tissue is cyanotic. Intense livor mortis is present in neck and facial tissues. Blood may remain liquid. Capillary permeability is increased. Swelling could easily occur.
Atheroma, atherosclerosis	Patchy or nodular thickening of the intima of an artery	Flow of arterial solution may be restricted or occluded. Arterial coagula may be easily trapped during injection. Vessel is poor injection site.
Burns	Local or general damage to tissue from heat	Capillaries constrict resulting in extensive coagulation. Distribution of arterial solution may be reduced. Large burns can result in kidney failure, with retention of nitrogenous wastes, thus increasing the preservative demand of the tissues.
Cerebrovascular accident	"Stroke" caused by a clot or the rupture of a small artery in the brain.	Vasoconstriction may occur on one side of the body, reducing the distribution of arterial solution.
Clots or coagula	Antemortem or postmortem clumping of blood elements	Arterial clots can block or reduce fluid flow to a body region, and may not be removed through drainage. Venous clots may often be removed; if clots are unmovable, swelling and discoloration can result.
Congestive heart failure	Decreased heart function	Venous congestion and clotting and cyanosis occur. Legs and feet are edematous. Capillary permeability increases. Tissues can easily swell.
Corrosive poisons	Toxic and corrosive chemicals	If poisons are swallowed, purge can usually be expected. Corrosive action may destroy blood vessels causing loss of solution or blood into the gastrointestinal tract.
Diabetes	An endocrine disease affecting the control of blood glucose levels	Poor peripheral circulation can reduce solution distribution. Gangrenous areas require surface and/or hypodermic embalming treatments. Dehydration frequently occurs. Breakdown of protein results in poor firming of tissues.
Emboli	Detached blood clot	Blockage of a small artery interrupts solution distribution. Venous emboli can block drainage.
Esophageal varices	Swollen, tortuous veins caused by a stagnation of blood and generally seen in the superficial veins	Drainage may be difficult to establish. Rupture and massive purge may occur.
Extracerebral clot (stroke)	A clot, usually in the carotid artery, that stops blood supply to the brain	The clot can occlude the artery, making it impossible for arterial solution to flow to one side of the face. Blockage may occlude the carotid so it cannot be used as an injection site. Resulting stroke may cause vasoconstriction on one side of the body, reducing arterial solution distribution.
Febrile disease	A disease or condition accompanied by an elevation of body temperature	Decomposition may be speeded. Dehydration is possible. Blood coagulates and causes congestion. Distribution and drainage may be hard to establish.

Condition	Description	Embalming Considerations
Freezing (postmortem)	Cooling of the body to the point where ice crystals form in body tissues	Small vessels and tissues easily swell on injection of solution.
Gangrene (dry)	Poor arterial circulation into an area of the body, causing death of body cells	Distribution of arterial solution into the affected area is impossible to establish. Surface and hypodermic treatment is needed.
Gangrene (moist)	Occlusion of veins draining a body area that becomes the site of bacterial infection	Very strong fluid must be injected into the general area arterially. The affected necrotic tissues require hypodermic and surface treatments.
Gunshot wounds	Entry of a foreign missile into the body	Arterial system may rupture. Multisite injection may be needed. Conditions vary depending on location of wound. Blood loss may result in very little drainage. Bodies are usually autopsied.
Hanging	Asphyxiation resulting from exertion of pressure against the large vessels of the neck	Livor mortis is intense or absent in facial tissues. Vessels may be damaged or severed. Restricted cervical injection and jugular drainage are recommended.
Hemorrhage	Loss of blood caused by a break in the vascular system	Blood volume may be quite low so there is little drainage. Livor mortis may be minimal. If hemorrhage is the result of a ruptured artery, arterial solution may be lost to body cavities. Multisite injection may be necessary. If a vein has ruptured, much of the drainage may collect in the body cavity where the hemorrhage occurred. If the stomach or esophageal veins are affected, stomach purge can be expected.
Ischemia	Lack of blood supply to an area, frequently resulting in tissue necrosis	Arterial solution cannot reach the affected tissues. Hypodermic and surface embalming treatments are needed.
Leukemia	Cancer of the tissues that form white blood cells	Purpura are observed over the thorax, arms, and abdomen. Edema may be present. Circulation of arterial solution and drainage may be difficult to establish.
Mutilation	Traumatic tissue injuries	Several arteries may result in difficulty in establishing distribution. Multipoint injections may be needed.
Phlebitis	Inflammation of a vein	Edema may be present in the area. Blood does not easily drain from the area and discolorations may result.
Pneumonia	Acute inflammation of the lung	Broken lung capillaries can result in lung purge. Fever speeds the onset of rigor and decomposition. Congestion may lead to hydrothorax. Distension of the neck can easily occur. Body should be aspirated immediately after arterial injection.
Shock	Sudden vital depression, reduced blood return to the heart	Vasodilation may be present, which can cause swelling. In other types of shock, capillaries constrict and blood congestion occurs in the large veins, making drainage difficult to establish. Capillary congestion may interfere with the distribution and diffusion of arterial solution.
Syphilis	Venereal disease caused by the spirochete Treponema pallidum	Aneurysms may occur in arteries. Rupture can make distribution of arterial solution impossible.
Thrombosis	Blood clots attached to the inner wall of a blood vessel	Arterial solution distribution may be difficult. If occurring in a vein, drainage may be hard to establish from the affected tissues.
Tuberculosis	Infection of the lungs by Mycobacterium tuberculosis that may spread to other organs (e.g., bone, brain, kidney)	When the lungs are affected, cavitation may result; this causes small vessels and capillaries to rupture. There may be a great loss of arterial solution through purging. Purge can be expected. Untreated dehydration and emaciation may be observed.
Tumor	Benign or malignant growth of cells	Pressure may be exerted on the outside of an artery or a vein. Distribution to and drainage from an area may be difficult to establish.
Vasoconstriction	Narrowing of a blood vessel	When arteries are affected, as in a "stroke," it may be difficult to supply sufficient arterial solution to the affected side of the body. Multipoint injection may be necessary.

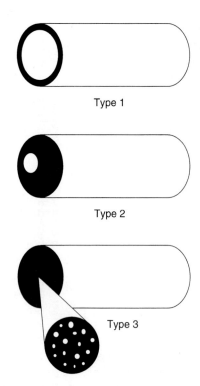

Figure 22–1. Types of arteriosclerosis seen in arteries used for arterial injection.

sclerosis than a 90-year-old person. Of the vessels used for embalming, the femoral artery is the most likely to be affected by arteriosclerosis. Thus, use of the common carotid artery as the primary site for injection is recommended.

The embalmer encounters three types of arteriosclerosis (Fig. 22–1):

- *Type 1*. The inner wall of the artery is hardened and thickened but the lumen is well defined and large. These vessels can usually be used for arterial injection. This condition is frequently observed in the autopsied body when the common iliac arteries are exposed.
- *Type 2*. The lumen is quite reduced in size and pushed to one side of the artery. The lumen can usually be identified and a small arterial tube can be used for injection.
- *Type 3*. The artery is completely occluded. If ischemia or gangrene is **not** present in the area supplied (e.g., the leg), the collateral circulation may have increased to supply blood to the limb **or** there may be minute paths in the occluded artery through which the blood can pass. The formation of these paths or canals is called **canalization**. These arteries **cannot** be used for injection.

In the presence of sclerosis, the strength of the arterial solution can be increased if distribution is poor or slow. Use of a stronger solution ensures that sufficient preservative reaches the tissues even if a large amount of solution cannot be injected. Coinjection chemicals may be used to help distribute the preservative solution. Dye can be added to the solution; it will help to indicate what tissues are receiving the arterial solution.

Lowering the hands over the sides of the table and gently but firmly massaging the limbs helps to distribute fluid in sclerotic bodies. Begin injection using a very slow rate of flow. After the vascular system is filled, rate of flow can be increased. When multisite injection is used, higher pressures and pulsation can be used to establish local distribution. Once circulation is established, the pressure and the rate of flow can be reduced.

When vascular problems are anticipated, the use of the common carotid artery is advised for injection. This vessel rarely exhibits arteriosclerosis. In those instances, when sclerosis is present, the size of the lumen of the carotid generally allows for easy insertion of arterial tubes. The accompanying internal jugular vein is large; the superior portion directly drains the head. The inferior portion of this vein leads directly into the right atrium of the heart. This chamber serves as the center of blood drainage during embalming. The use of angular spring forceps as an aid to drainage will help to remove venous coagula.

If a femoral vessel must be used, avoid cutting into the artery where an atheroma can be felt. Make the incision a little larger at a point where the vessel is softest. Avoid raising these sclerotic arteries to the surface. Work with them from within the incision. Ligate the arterial tubes in place with an arterial hemostat or a thick cotton ligature. Thin linen ligatures may separate and tear the vessel. Use an arterial tube small enough that it easily slips into the lumen.

A large arterial tube can damage the lumen of the artery and possibly make it unusable as an injection point (Fig. 22–2).

▶ AORTIC ANEURYSM

A ruptured aortic aneurysm can seriously affect fluid distribution in the unautopsied body. If surgical repair of the vessel was performed, extreme facial edema can often accompany this surgical repair. In the unautopsied body, determine whether fluid can be distributed from a single-site injection. Inject from the right common carotid artery or use restricted cervical injection. Usually, the femoral vessels in these bodies are sclerotic.

Use a strong arterial solution with additional fluid dye as a tracer. Inject slowly. If **drainage** is established, continue to inject. **If there is no drainage and the abdomen begins to swell, stop the injection** and institute a multipoint injection to embalm the various body areas. No drainage indicates a loss of the embalming solution into the thoracic or abdominal cavity. The trunk walls may have to be injected by use of an infant trocar with

Figure 22–2. Common sites of arteriosclerosis. (*Courtesy of HE Kazmier*.)

cavity fluid. Often, when the death certificate cites the immediate cause of death as a ruptured aortic aneurysm, it may be possible to embalm the entire body from one injection site.

▶ VALVULAR HEART DISEASES

The following extract from the article, "Damage to aorta may bring embalming problems," written by Murray M. Shor, describes how disease or malformation may prevent the aorta from being the center of arterial solution circulation.

> Because of the position of the aortic semilunar valve, embalmers generally consider the aorta as the center of arterial fluid circulation. In most cases, this seems to be true. In the absence of damage to the circulatory system or the heart, it is only after the aorta is filled with fluid that its branches can be expected to receive fluid under any appreciable pressure.

> Were it not for the position and construction of the aortic valve, fluid would pass from the ascending portion of the aorta into the left ventricle. Under those conditions, the aorta would not be considered the center of embalming fluid circulation. If because of disease or malformation of the aortic semilunar valve fluid did pass into the left ventricle and was confined there by the proper functioning of the mitral valve, the problem would be merely academic. It is when other heart valves are impaired concurrently that embalming problems are created.

Anatomy of the Heart

Let us pause here for a brief review of the anatomy of the heart. The functioning valves are the left atrioventricular or mitral, which allows blood to pass from the left atrium to the left ventricle; the right atrioventricular or tricuspid, which opens from the right atrium into the right ventricle; the pulmonary semilunar, a tricuspid valve which opens to allow blood to flow from the right ventricle into the lungs via the pulmonary artery; and the aforementioned aortic semilunar, a tricuspid valve that opens into the aorta from the left ventricle.

During life, any one or any combination of these valves can be affected by the same degenerative diseases that affect the arteries. They can also be attacked by bacteria and damaged irreparably or suffer a congenital malformation. In all of these conditions, the circulation of blood during life and of the preservative during embalming is substantially altered.

The great strides made by the medical profession in the fields of infant mortality and infectious diseases leave an older population; one more likely to die of degenerative diseases. Also, because of better medical care, some of the infectious diseases that damage the heart, such as diphtheria and rheumatic fever, have been controlled to such an extent that victims of these diseases survive the infectious stage and live many years afterward, often with a damaged heart valve or valves.

In the United States, we have reached a point where one in every two deaths is attributable to cardiovascular disease. Therefore, it behooves the embalmer to become thoroughly familiar with embalming problems associated with these diseases.

In situations where the mitral and the aortic semilunar valves are damaged, embalming fluid under pressure will pass from the aorta into the left ventricle and from there into the left atrium. The left atrium receives the pulmonary veins from the lungs. These veins have no valves. Therefore, a fluid in the atrium, under pressure, would pass back into the capillaries of the lung.

Lung Purge

During most embalming procedures, the pulmonary capillaries also receive fluid from the bronchial arteries, coming from the descending thoracic aorta. When the two fluid masses, one from the bronchial arteries and the other from the pulmonary veins, meet, their collective volume and pressure create a lung purge by virtually squeezing the contents of the hollow portions of the lung out through the trachea.

This event should not cause too much apprehension. The matter thus emanating from the mouth or the nostrils is the material the embalmer seeks to remove during routine cavity work.

▶ CONGESTIVE HEART FAILURE

Frequently, death certificates cite congestive heart failure as the primary cause of death. Some complications of the end stage of congestive heart failure are of particular interest to the embalmer:

1. Blood is congested in the right side of the heart.
2. The neck veins are engorged with blood; the facial tissues are dark because of the congestion of blood in the right side of the heart and the veins of the neck.
3. Lips, ears, and fingers are cyanotic.
4. Generalized pitting edema may be present. Edema of the legs and feet is pronounced in most bodies. Ascites may be present.
5. Blood may be more viscous because of an increase in red blood cells (polycythemia).
6. Salt is retained in the body fluids.

The carotid artery is used for injection and the right internal jugular vein for drainage, or restricted cervical injection is employed. This helps to ensure good drainage from the head and the right atrium of the heart. The first gallon of arterial solution is made mild to clear the blood congestion and discolorations. If edema is present, the subsequent gallons should be stronger to meet the preservative demand of the body. If the ascites (and intestinal gases) is severe, enough pressure can be placed on the inferior vena cava to diminish drainage from the lower areas of the body. Some of the fluid can be drained with a trocar or drain tube inserted into the abdominal cavity. Keep the trocar or drain tube in the ventral portion of the abdominal cavity so as not to puncture any of the major vessels.

Lowering the arms over the table at the start of arterial injection helps to establish good distribution so the discolorations of the hands and fingers can be cleared. The facial tissues may need to be massaged to clear the blood discolorations. It may be necessary to inject both common carotid arteries. When there is extensive discoloration of the face, some embalmers prefer to drain from both the right and left internal jugular veins.

Begin injection at a high enough pressure and rapid enough rate of flow to establish good distribution. Continuous drainage should be used to clear the congested blood. Pressure and rate of flow may be increased as the embalming progresses; the pressure and the rate of flow should be sufficient to move arterial solution through the entire body. In the presence of generalized edema, distribution and drainage can be expected to be good.

The liver may be enlarged and its functions decreased. This should improve drainage, as the level of clotting factor in the blood will be low.

Pulmonary edema, often observed in cases of congestive heart failure, may cause lung purge. The purge should be allowed to continue during the embalming process. Cavity treatment and repacking of the nasal cavity with cotton after embalming should correct this condition.

Thorough aspiration is necessary to remove distension in the neck tissues resulting from the engorgement with blood. Remove (as much as possible) the edema that led to the ascites. This edema dilutes cavity fluid. It is best to reaspirate and, if necessary, reinject the cavities several hours after the first treatment. Bodies dead from congestive heart failure should be aspirated immediately after arterial injection to help reduce distension in the neck and the facial tissues.

▶ VASODILATION AND VASOCONSTRICTION

Sometimes, the dye used to trace the distribution of arterial solution indicates that one side of the body has received a large amount of solution and the other side a small amount. This difference is often evident down the midline of the body. This unequal distribution of arterial solution frequently occurs after death from cerebrovascular accident. The vessels on one side of the body have undergone vasoconstriction. In an effort to supply more oxygen to the tissues in life, the vessels on the opposite side of the body have undergone vasodilation. Multisite injection may be necessary, but in most bodies injection of a sufficient quantity of solution should overcome the problem. This condition may be seen when the deceased has suffered a stroke.

▶ ARTERIAL COAGULA

At death, some blood remains in the arteries, especially in the large aorta. During the postmortem period, this blood can congeal (Fig. 22–3). Injection of the arterial solution may loosen and push coagula into the smaller arteries. By injecting the common carotid arteries, these coagula would be moved toward the legs.

If the femoral artery is used as the primary injection point, coagula can be moved into the common carotid arteries and stop the flow of arterial solution into the facial tissues. When the femoral artery is injected upward arterial coagula, most frequently, flow into the left subclavian artery, and it becomes necessary to raise and

Figure 22–3. Dark areas are large dots in this sclerotic segment of the aorta.

inject the axillary or brachial artery of the left arm. When the common carotid is used as the primary injection site, arterial coagula are moved into the iliac and femoral arteries. The femoral arteries can be raised to embalm the legs; should this prove unsuccessful, the legs can be treated by hypodermic or surface embalming, or both.

If embalming is begun at a slower rate of flow and the use of preinjection fluids (which may loosen arterial coagula) is avoided, the arterial solution can pass **over** but not loosen coagula.

▶ VENOUS COAGULA

As veins enlarge toward the drainage site, venous coagula do not pose as serious a problem as arterial coagula. Failure to move the coagula, however, can block a vein, and this blockage can lead to tissue distension and discoloration. Massage from distal points toward the heart. Use the right internal jugular vein for drainage, as coagula in the right atrium can be easily reached with angular spring forceps and removed. Intermittent drainage helps to increase venous pressure and loosen coagula from the veins. Multisite injection and drainage may be warranted. When this condition is encountered in a localized area, use a stronger arterial solution to ensure that a minimum amount of arterial fluid delivers the maximum preservative.

▶ DIABETES

Various problems arise in the embalming of a person with diabetes. Of primary concern to the embalmer is

Figure 22–4. Discolored fingertips of an individual with diabetes. Poor peripheral circulation is often seen in the person with diabetes.

the establishment of good fluid distribution. Individuals with diabetes tend to develop arteriosclerosis, especially in the smaller vessels, and poor peripheral circulation can be anticipated (Fig. 22–4). These persons are also subject to increased bacterial and mycotic infections; all these conditions require use of a strong arterial solution. The first gallon can be slightly milder than subsequent gallons. To assist in establishing distribution and clearing of blood discolorations, the first gallon of arterial solution can be milder than subsequent injections. Some embalmers prefer to use a coinjection fluid to assist in the clearing of discolorations. Restricted cervical injection is suggested, and the embalmer should use moderate to high pressure to help distribute the solution. Massaging the extremities and using intermittent drainage also facilitate fluid distribution. High pressure and pulsation promote flow to the peripheral tissues (fingers, toes, ears, nose, and lips). Fluid dye can be used to trace the distribution of solution in the tissues.

The tissues of the diabetic may exhibit abnormal pH values. This may result in difficult tissue firming. Use of a moderate to a strong solution accompanied by a coinjection fluid and dye should meet the preservative demands.

Many individuals with obesity are diabetic. Restricted cervical injection and drainage from the right internal jugular vein ensure tissue saturation. A large volume of solution can be injected without concern that the face may be overembalmed. The large volume of solution also promotes better fluid distribution.

Cavity embalming should be thorough. Mycotic infections are often found in the lungs of persons with diabetes. A minimum of 16 oz of cavity fluid should be used for each major body cavity. Abscesses, necrosis, and gangrene may be present in the pancreas and the liver. Arterial solution may not have reached these tissues. The cavity fluid is the only preservative that will be available to halt the decomposition that occurs in the tissues of these diseased organs.

Gangrene may also be present in distal tissues such as the fingers and the toes. These areas will **not** receive arterial solution when the body is injected. Cavity fluid should be injected into these areas by hypodermic injection or injection with an infant trocar. The surface of feet affected by gangrene should be painted with autopsy gel or cavity fluid compresses should be applied and the leg clothed in a plastic stocking.

Persons with diabetes are also subject to decubitus ulcers. These lesions should be disinfected topically and the tissue around them injected hypodermically with cavity fluid or a phenol cautery solution. Surface compresses of autopsy gel, cavity fluid, or phenol cautery solution should be applied to the necrotic surface tissues.

Restricted cervical injection allows the injection of a milder arterial solution into emaciated and dehydrated facial tissues. Coinjection chemicals and humectants may be used to help restore some moisture. After arterial preparation, tissue builder can be used to restore emaciated and sunken facial tissues.

▶ EXTRAVASCULAR RESISTANCE

Pressure on the outside of an artery or a vein is referred to as **extravascular resistance**, and may restrict the flow of arterial solution into a body region or may restrict drainage through a vein.

A slightly stronger, well-coordinated arterial solution should be used as distribution may be limited. Multisite injection may be necessary if extravascular resistance is present. Use of higher embalming pressures may promote distribution. Stopping the injection and allowing time for drainage may help to prevent blood discolorations: inject—drain without injecting—inject. Use concurrent drainage throughout the entire operation. Massage and manipulate the tissues to promote both fluid distribution and blood drainage.

Sources of extravascular resistance and suggestions on how to overcome the resulting problems are listed here:

- *Rigor mortis.* Relieve as much rigor as possible by manipulation prior to arterial injection.

- *Ascites.* Relieve the abdominal pressure by draining prior to or during arterial injection.
- *Gas in cavities.* Puncture the abdomen and relieve gases prior to or during arterial injection.
- *Bandages.* Remove tight bandages prior to injection.
- *Contact pressure.* Massage these areas.
- *Tumors.* Excise, with permission, if absolutely necessary. Sectional injection may be necessary.
- *Swollen lymph nodes.* Sectional injection may be necessary.
- *Hydrothorax.* Drainage may be possible prior to injection but can be difficult.
- *Visceral weight.* Above- and below-heart injection and drainage points can be employed.

▶ CONCEPTS FOR STUDY AND DISCUSSION

1. Discuss, from an embalming standpoint, the differences between postmortem venous coagula and postmortem arterial coagula.
2. Describe the vascular problems created by diabetes.
3. Discuss the problems created by congestive heart failure.
4. The embalmer has raised the right common carotid artery, as a point for arterial injection, an arterial tube is inserted toward the heart but it is a long tube and it passes through the aortic semi-lunar valve. Trace the various routes that the arterial fluid might take because of the location of the arterial tube.
5. The embalmer is injecting and draining from the right common carotid artery and the right internal jugular vein. All areas of the body are receiving arterial solution with the exception of the buttocks, the genital area, and the legs. Explain the problem and what can be done to solve it.

▶ BIBLIOGRAPHY

American Board of Funeral Service, *Course Content Syllabus,* St. Joseph, MO: American Board of Funeral Service, 2008.

Day DD, Poston G. Embalming the diabetic case. In: *Champion Expanding Encyclopedia,* No. 560. Springfield, OH: Champion Chemical Co., 1985:2254–2257.

Mulvihill ML. *Human Diseases: A Systemic Approach,* 2nd ed. Norwalk, CT: Appleton & Lange, 1987.

Sheldon H. Boyd's Introduction to the Study of Disease, 9th ed. Philadelphia, PA: Lea & Febiger, 1984.

Shor MM. Damage to aorta may bring embalming problems. *Casket and Sunnyside* June 1960.

CHAPTER 23

EFFECT OF DRUGS ON THE EMBALMING PROCESS

CHAPTER OBJECTIVES

▶ Preservative demand
▶ Effects of various drug types
▶ Chemotherapy effects
▶ Radiation effects

The contemporary professional embalmer practices this art and science in an age that has often been referred to as the **Chemotherapy era**. (**Chemotherapy is the treatment of disease with chemical agents and drugs**.) The aims of modern medicine are to cure disease and alleviate pain via the long-sought-for "magic bullet" of Dr. Paul Ehrlich. Today, there is not a single case on which the embalmer works that has not been injected or made to ingest some type of chemical substance or substances (pharmaceuticals) prior to death. In many cases, particularly those received from medical facilities and institutions, many different types of drugs were used prior to the patient's death. Although the chemotherapy era began with Ehrlich's "magic bullet" for the treatment of syphilis, today we live in an age of **multiple-agent** chemotherapy.

The way antibiotics are used today exemplifies the multiple-drug approach common to the medical profession. It is very unlikely nowadays that a single antibiotic is prescribed for the treatment of an infection. Usually, two or more antibiotics are administered. In cancer chemotherapy, the multiple-drug approach is also common. It is not unusual for an oncologist to administer both a **cytotoxic** drug (one that kills the cancer cell directly) and an **antimetabolite** (one that slowly "starves" the cancer cell by depriving it of a needed nutrient). One result of this multiple-agent approach has been an increase in the number and types of embalming problems.

Before the embalming problems caused by chemotherapeutic agents are discussed, "normal" embalming must be defined. There is **no** "ideal case." It is probably impossible to find a person who has not

been treated by one or more doctors with one or more drugs prior to death. So, in addition to the problems caused by the pathological processes resulting in death, the chemotherapeutic agent or agents administered for various intervals prior to death have physiological effects. The longer the drug was taken before death, often the more intense are the embalming problems likely to be encountered.

Another problem may arise from the chemical reaction between the administered drugs and the components of the embalming fluid. For example, are there any components of arterial embalming fluid that form insoluble precipitates when they react with antibiotics? If so, the circulatory path may become blocked, thus preventing the preservative components of the arterial fluid from reaching the tissues for preservation.

▶ THE CHEMISTRY OF PROTEINS

To discuss the chemistry of embalming, it is essential to understand the chemistry of proteins. These materials form the physical structures of the body. They give the body form. **The professional embalmer must achieve the absolute preservation of these structures.** This means that the proteinaceous materials forming portions of the various tissues and organs of the human body must be rendered chemically inert. Essentially, these structures must be frozen in time and space!

Proteins are labile substances. The molecules break down quite rapidly even without bacterial action. There exist proteins that break down other proteins. These specialized proteins, called **enzymes,** are endowed with a physicochemical structure that allows catalytic activity. These enzymes can speed up decomposition reactions. It must be realized that even if a cadaver were completely sterile, the proteolytic enzymes in the cells and tissues of that body would still be fully active and capable of causing the breakdown of tissue proteins.

One goal of embalming must be to render the proteins resistant to attack by catalytic enzymes. There are two ways to do this: (1) The proteins themselves can be treated so that they are no longer susceptible to the action of proteolytic enzymes. (2) The enzymes themselves can be so changed or inactivated that they cannot exert catalytic action on other proteins. Modern embalming chemicals are formulated to do both.

To determine how both of these goals can be achieved in a so-called "ideal" case, a brief mathematical formula is helpful.

What this means in terms of actual chemicals used to embalm a case should be discussed from a practical standpoint.

AVERAGE BODY PROTEIN

The average body = 150 lb = 65.3 kg
A 65.3-kg body contains 10.7 kg of protein = 10,700 g of protein

FORMALDEHYDE DEMAND

100 g of soluble protein requires 4.4 g of formaldehyde for preservation
The average body contains 10,700 g of protein
Therefore,

$$\frac{10,700}{100} \times 4.4 = 470.8 \text{ grams of formaldehyde needed}$$

SOLUTION NEEDED

Given: Standard 30-index arterial fluid contains 16 oz of 30% formaldehyde = 142.08 g of formaldehyde
Need: 470.80 g of formaldehyde

$$\frac{470,80}{142.08} = 3.31 \text{ sixteen-ounce bottles of a 30-index}$$
fluid needed, or approximately 53 ounces of arterial fluid

For a nonideal case (as practically all cases today are), the conclusion that some of the formaldehyde will be lost in embalming seems obvious. For example, many chemotherapeutic agents are nephrotoxic and, therefore, cause a breakdown of kidney function. As the kidneys are the main organs responsible for elimination of nitrogenous wastes, these waste materials (ammonia, urea, uric acid, etc.) are retained by the body. There is no better way to neutralize formaldehyde than to react it with ammonia, and this is exactly what happens in the body. If there has been a buildup of nitrogenous waste materials as a result of chemotherapy-induced kidney dysfunction, a standard dilution of arterial embalming fluid will not be sufficient. A large proportion of the formaldehyde in the embalming fluid will be neutralized when it encounters the nitrogenous wastes in the body. The remainder is insufficient to preserve the tissues, and the body starts to decay.

Normally, arterial embalming fluids are supplied as 16-oz concentrates. These are diluted with water and additives prior to injection into the body. An embalming fluid containing 30% formaldehyde supplies 142 g of formaldehyde per bottle. To embalm the "average" or "ideal" body containing 10.7 kg of protein, 470 g of formaldehyde is needed, that is, a minimum of three bottles of arterial embalming fluid. (If the body has been on a drug regimen, more than double this amount of formaldehyde may be necessary!)

(See Selected Readings. Mathematics of Embalming Chemistry: Part I. A Critical Evaluation of "One Bottle" Embalming Claims.)

▶ THE CHEMOTHERAPY CASE

All chemotherapeutic agents are toxic. This is the one axiom universally applicable to all drugs. Cellular and tissue changes occur when drugs are used. It does not matter what drug is administered; even the seemingly innocuous aspirin tablet has its effects (aspirin acts as a blood thinner). Drug-induced changes may be relatively minor, perhaps limited to slight skin discolorations, which, in the deceased, readily respond to cosmetic treatment. When drugs cause major problems, such as acute jaundice, or saturate the body tissues with uremic wastes, the fixative action of the preservative chemicals in the arterial embalming fluid is seriously impaired.

The chemotherapeutic agents common to modern medicine exert their effects in many ways. They may impair function of the liver, the circulatory system (heart and blood vessels), the kidneys, the lungs, and the skin. These drugs can inactivate the embalming fluid by causing the buildup of nitrogenous wastes or decreasing the permeability of the cell membrane (Fig. 23–1).

Because the **liver** is the main detoxification center, every drug eventually enters the hepatic circulation.

Figure 23–1. Chemotherapy patient showing weight loss and hair loss.

While in the liver, the drug may be changed to an innocuous form by hepatic enzymes or the drug may cause profound changes in the liver itself. When the liver is damaged, the embalmer may have to cope with a jaundiced body.

All drugs ultimately pass through the kidneys. Even those that accumulate in other body areas must pass at least once (and often more) through the kidneys. If the drugs cause extensive changes in this organ, renal insufficiency follows, resulting in the buildup of nitrogenous wastes in body tissues. Saturated with urea, uric acid, ammonia, creatinine, and other wastes, the tissues become spongy and difficult to preserve. In such cases, preservation is almost impossible to achieve unless the treatment is modified.

Drugs also change the biochemical constituents of the blood. Some drugs damage even the connecting blood vessels themselves extensively. The circulatory system may become impaired as a result of extensive clot formation, lysis of the blood cells, or extensive damage to the walls of the arteries and veins.

The effects on **skin** are closely associated with the changes in the circulatory system and may include the formation of widespread areas of discoloration stemming from lysis and release of blood pigments from red blood cells. Ecchymosis and purpural hemorrhages are frequent discolorations seen on the surface of the skin.

Pharmacologically, the dividing line between the beneficial effects and toxic effects of drugs is very slen-

der. The professional embalmer must learn to cope with these effects.

▶ INACTIVATION OF PRESERVATIVE AGENTS BY DRUGS

The problems likely to be confronted while embalming a body that has been administered chemotherapy do **not** result from the reactions of formaldehyde or other preservative aldehydes with the drug or the drugs. Much too little drug is present, even after aggressive therapy. **It is the physiological effect of the drug that is culpable.** A drug that causes nephrotoxic changes enhances the accumulation of nitrogenous waste products in the body. These waste products, which result indirectly from the physiological effect of the drug, are responsible for the inactivation or, more specifically, the neutralization of the formaldehyde:

$$4NH_3 + 6CH_2O \rightarrow (CH_2)_6N_4 + 6H_2O$$

This neutralization reaction, whereby formaldehyde is converted to hexamethylene, is probably at the root of at least 90% of the contemporary embalmer's problems.

A change in permeability of the cell membrane is another effect of most systemically administered drugs. It is through this membrane that everything must pass, either to enter or to leave the cell. Preservative chemicals such as formaldehyde must pass through this membrane if they are going to inactivate the intracellular enzymes that decompose the proteins there.

If a chemotherapeutic agent reduces or destroys membrane permeability, preservative solutions may not be able to enter the cell. The antibiotic tetracycline is a case in point. Although most antibiotics exert their effects on bacteria, they also have an effect on the human cell. They are chelating agents and tend to lodge in the cell membrane, causing calcium to form an impenetrable layer around the cell. "Chelating" means they have an affinity for metallic ions, particularly calcium and magnesium. Antibiotics appear to act selectively on cell membranes. After they are entrenched in the membrane, they start chelating or sequestering calcium and magnesium ions. [There is generally no shortage of calcium in the body; it is present in all biological fluids (secretions, excretions, etc.).]

Eventually, as more calcium and magnesium ions become lodged in the chelate in the cell membrane, the permeability of the membrane changes; the membrane becomes less permeable. It becomes increasingly more difficult for some chemicals to enter such a cell. Because the goal of embalming is to inactive the intracellular enzymes present, it is essential that the preservative enter the cell. If it does not, the proteolytic enzymes inside the cell can proceed to break down the proteinaceous materials in the cell, and the tissue is subject to decomposition and lysis of its structural features.

▶ COMBINATION ANTIBIOTIC CHEMOTHERAPY

Today, it is routine procedure for physicians to prescribe two or more antibiotics at the same time. This, of course, intensifies the embalming problems. The embalming problems resulting from synergistic combination chemotherapy are not new, only more intense. Use of a combination such as gentamicin and a synthetic penicillin (e.g., methicillin) makes preservation and firming difficult to achieve. These bodies are usually saturated with ammoniacal and other nitrogenous wastes. The arterial fluid in such cases must be very concentrated if any embalming is to be accomplished.

▶ CORTICOSTEROIDS AND ANTI-INFLAMMATORY DRUGS

If antibiotics are the most widely used drugs, then cortisone and its derivatives constitute a close second. The anti-inflammatory drugs have many uses (e.g., itching caused by allergies) and are the drugs of choice for arthritic and rheumatic conditions. Corticosteroids are also widely used in the chemotherapy of cancer.

With regard to specific embalming problems caused by these drugs, the chief effect is blockade of the cell membrane. **Corticosteroids decrease the permeability of this membrane** and thereby block passage of liquids into the cell. On a gross macroscopic level, liquids are retained by the cells and tissues, resulting in an increase in cell turgor and waterlogging of tissues.

The use of cortisone for the treatment of chronic diseases (over long periods) may result in **gastrointestinal ulcerations with possible perforations of the gut.** Prolonged use in the treatment of ulcerative colitis has also resulted in dehydration of the body.

Corticosteroids have been shown to exert a "protective" effect on proteolytic enzymes. This is demonstrated by the difficult task one has in trying to denature these enzymes in cortisone-treated bodies. Even if these enzymes are extracted from such cortisone-treated tissues and are obtained in an almost pure form, they are still difficult to inactivate. They retain the "protective" effect originally conferred by the corticosteroids. This means that more undenatured proteolytic enzymes remain in the body after embalming. Such bodies tend to "go bad" (decompose) very rapidly after an apparently trouble-free embalming.

What has so far been described with respect to corticosteroids can also occur as the result of the use of oral contraceptives by women. Progesterone and its derivatives have chemical structures similar to that of cortisone. It has long been known in pharmacology that similar chemical structures elicit similar biological reactions. Many of the embalming problems observed after the use of corticosteroids are identical to those encountered in bodies of young women who died while taking oral contraceptives.

Another problem encountered when corticosteroids have been administered for some time prior to death is of a more insidious nature. These persons have been shown to have disseminated tuberculosis. The anti-inflammatory action of the corticosteroids results from their suppression of immunity. In cases of "arrested" (or so-called "cured") tuberculosis in which large doses of cortisone were administered before death, it is not uncommon to find that because immunity was suppressed the mycobacterium was reactivated and spread throughout the body. Such cases offer hidden hazards to the embalmer's health and sanitation precautions should be observed.

To secure preservation in these bodies, some permeability should be restored to the cell membranes so that preservatives can enter the cells. This can be done through the use of adjunct fluids. Preinjecting such a body restores some of the permeability; and the surface-active chemicals in such preparations facilitate entry of the preservative components of the arterials into cells. At the same time, a stronger-than-normal arterial injection should be used together with a coinjection fluid. (It is also possible to use some coinjection fluids as a preinjection.)

▶ CANCER CHEMOTHERAPEUTIC AGENTS AND THEIR EFFECTS

Various drugs are used to treat malignancies, but generally they fall into two main classes. **Cytotoxic** drugs act directly on the tumor cells to bring about their death. **Antimetabolite** drugs substitute for an essential metabolite required by the cancer cell for growth. It is not unusual for both types to be given to the cancer patient. This multiple-agent chemotherapy creates tremendous problems for the professional embalmer.

Cytotoxic drugs (e.g., nitrogen mustards, alkylating agents) kill both malignant and normal cells. (A "magic bullet" for cancer has not yet been found.) When cells die, proteins break down and large amounts of nitrogenous wastes are released. Therefore, the tissues in these bodies, besides containing a small amount of protein as a result of the extreme cachexia associated with cancer, are saturated with nitrogenous waste products.

Achievement of preservation under these conditions is a Herculean task in itself, but the embalming problems that arise from the coadministration of antimetabolites must be added. These are sure to cause symptoms of extensive vitamin deficiency. Such bodies may exhibit everything from scurvy to brittle rickets-like bone disease. If radiation therapy has been administered, there may be extensive skin and circulatory problems (e.g., purpura and body clots).

▶ RADIOACTIVE ISOTOPES AND THEIR EFFECTS

Because radioactive materials are used for cancer therapy, it is not amiss to discuss the radiation-treated body. An embalmer should not attempt to embalm a radiation-treated body unless a radiation safety officer has certified the body as safe because of the possibility of gamma radiation. The main radioisotopes used to diagnose and treat malignancies are cobalt-60, iodine-131, phosphorus-32, radium-226, gold-198, and strontium-89. Beta rays are stopped much more readily than gamma rays, which are similar to X-rays and require lead shielding. In addition, tiny needles or "seeds" of gold-198, as well as radon needles, are implanted in tissues to treat metastatic tumors in the abdomen and lungs. These bodies, if declared safe, may be embalmed as would any cancer case.

A second source of radiation exposure is an occupational accident. Radioactive materials are measured in **millicuries.** A **millicurie** (mCi) is defined as that amount of radioactive material in which 37 million atoms disintegrate each second. Medical institutions must "tag" bodies, warning that radioactive isotopes are present in the body or that the body has had a high exposure to radiation by accident. The medical institution is not permitted to release the body until the level of radioactivity has dropped below 30 mCi, for unautopsied bodies. Autopsied remains are not to be released until the radiation level drops to 5 mCi or below. It is necessary for the embalmer to follow any instructions issued by the radiation protection officer. If embalming is permitted when radiation levels are above the figures cited, the preparation should occur at the hospital under the strict supervision of the radiation officer.

When radiation levels are below 30 mCi for unautopsied remains and 5 mCi or below for autopsied remains, standard embalming procedures can be used that would be determined by the conditions present in the dead human body. There are certain recommended precautions the embalmer should exercise. These precautions can be summarized in the words **protection**, **time of exposure**, and **distance.** During the preparation of bodies that have been exposed to high doses of radioactivity, the embalmer should wear rubber gloves, if possible two pairs, and a heavy rubber apron. In addition, of course, standard Universal Precautions attire should also be worn. The shortest time of exposure should be employed. Time of exposure can be shortened, when possible, by working in pairs; two embalmers can work together performing different tasks (e.g., one embalmer raises vessels and a second sets features). This helps to reduce the exposure time. Having instruments ready and fluids mixed, as soon as the body is observed, again reduces the time spent in preparation. It would be most wise to avoid raising vessels in a body region where tissues have been seeded with the radioactive isotope; for example, if seeds are present in tissues of the neck, use of the femoral vessels would reduce contact with the seeds.

Distance also plays a large role in reducing exposure to radiation. For every 3 feet of distance from the body, exposure is reduced by a substantial amount. When not actually performing a procedure, the embalmer should stand at a distance from the body (e.g., during injection of the arterial solution when massage may not be necessary). There should be a constant flow of water under the body. New tables allow the body to be positioned on body bridges, which allow water to flow beneath the body without coming into contact with the body. The constant flow of water is necessary to dilute and flush away all drainage matter as it exits the body. Care should be taken to cover the area around the preparation table with sheeting, which can be destroyed by incineration or placed in a biohazard container after the embalming; this ensures that all waste matter is removed from the areas surrounding the preparation table. Gloves should be frequently flushed with soap and water during the embalming procedure. Any spillage should be removed immediately with the use of forceps or tongs and new sheeting or a portion of the sheeting draped onto the floor.

Final cleanup should include the following:

- Instruments should be thoroughly flushed with running water, then soaked in a good soap or a detergent and rinsed well with running water.
- Disposable waste matter and gloves should be collected in a suitable biohazard container and disposed of (if permitted) by incineration.
- Gowns, towels, clothing, and so on should be monitored and stored for suitable decay before being sent to the laundry (consult the radiation officer of the medical facility for assistance in this matter).
- If the embalmer suffers any introduction of material from the body into lesions on his or her hands, the injured area should be washed with copious amounts of running water and a physician or a radiation safety officer consulted.

The embalmer should follow any instructions that have been made by the radiation safety officer with regard to preparation of the body. An example would be if the officer stated that aspiration and injection of the cavities should not be carried out until a certain time. Strengths of arterial solutions, volume of fluid injected, and so on do not directly affect radiation exposure. Some examples of radioactive isotopes employed in disease diagnosis and treatment are cobalt-60, iodine-131, radium-226, gold-198, and strontium-89. A more detailed discussion of radioactive isotopes can be found in the text **Thanatochemistry,** 2nd ed., by James M. Dorn and Barbara Hopkins, published by Prentice-Hall, Upper Saddle River, NJ 07458, 1998.

▶ TRANQUILIZERS AND MOOD-ALTERING DRUGS

It is not easy to discuss prescribed legal drugs without venturing into the field of drug abuse. No matter what the drug is, if it is taken beyond the period prescribed or if more than the dose prescribed is taken, it becomes "abused." For example, if amphetamines are prescribed for dietary or psychiatric reasons and are taken longer than necessary to alleviate the condition, they become illegal or abused drugs. It should be realized that such components of the drug culture as benzedrine, dexedrine, and methedrine were all at one time (and some still are) rigorously and ethically prescribed by physicians to treat specific ills. The same holds true for such tranquilizers as phenothiazine and its derivatives.

There are roughly five classes of tranquilizers and mood-altering drugs. In general, they have one common characteristic: they result in a loss of weight of the abuser. Embalming these bodies is very frustrating because of the lack of protein (most of the protein stores have been depleted). A person on a "trip" does not care about nutrition.

- *Sedatives:* barbiturates [amobarbital (Amytal), secobarbital (Seconal), etc.]; meprobamate (Quanil, Miltown, etc.).
- *Stimulants:* amphetamines (Benzedrine, Dexedrine, etc.); cocaine; phenmetrazine (Preludin).
- *Tranquilizers:* phenothiazines [chlorpromazine (Thorazine), prochlorperazine (Compazine), etc.]; reserpine (Serpalan, Serpasil); chlordiazepoxide (Librium); diazepam (Valium)].
- *Narcotics:* opiates (opium, heroin, morphine, etc.).
- *Antidepressants:* methylphenidate (Ritalin); imipramine (Tofranil).

The continued use (or abuse) of tranquilizers can also result in such embalming problems as jaundice because of the destructive effect of these drugs on liver cells. In addition, tranquilizers may cause hemolysis of the red blood cells and thereby add to the jaundice problem because pigments are released from these red blood cells. Also common to abusers of all five classes of drugs is the depletion of protein stores resulting from their neglect of nutrition. Protein depletion results in the release of large amounts of nitrogenous waste products. If kidney function is impaired (particularly in heroin addicts in whom both constipation and anuresis occur), these waste materials cannot exit the body. They are retained in the tissues and rapidly neutralize formaldehyde (or any aldehyde).

▶ PROBLEMS CAUSED BY ORAL DRUGS THAT CONTROL DIABETES

A group of chemotherapeutic agents with broad-spectrum effects comprises those drugs used to control diabetes, the oral diabetic agents. Use of such drugs as tolbutamide (Orinase) and chlorpropamide (Diabinese) to control adult (type II) diabetes is increasing. These drugs certainly are more convenient (for those who can use them) than the daily (or more frequent) self-injections of insulin.

Tolbutamide was used widely until recently, when it was replaced with another second-generation sulfonylurea called **chlorpropamide**. Both may cause jaundice. Most of the sulfonylureas can induce changes in the voluntary muscles (site of glycogen storage and breakdown) and the liver (main glycogen storage organ of the body). Continuous use of oral diabetic agents has been linked with circulatory problems, which can result in poor distribution of the arterial chemicals. (This has been observed to be the result of extensive clot formation in the cadaver.) Acidosis sometimes occurs as a result of the altered carbohydrate metabolism and leads to the formation of high concentrations of lactic acid in muscle tissue. Such bodies firm very rapidly unless an alkaline coinjection is used with the arterial embalming fluid.

In general, although oral diabetic agents may cause a large variety of embalming problems, they do not cause as severe embalming problems as do other drugs.

▶ NEUTRALIZING CHEMOTHERAPEUTIC AGENTS

It must be understood that chemotherapeutic agents cause embalming problems not through their reactions with embalming chemicals but through their physiological effects on the body prior to death (Table 23–1). No drug, no matter how often, how long, or in what concentration it is used, could ever be administered long enough during life to react significantly with the components of an arterial chemical injected after death. As

TABLE 23–1. PROBLEMS CAUSED BY CHEMOTHERAPEUTIC AGENTS[a]

Drug	Problem
Antibiotics (penicillins, synthetic penicillins, aminoglycosides, tetracyclines)	Cotton-like circulatory blockages (fungal overgrowth); jaundice; bleeding into skin; poor penetration
Corticosteroids (cortisone)	Cell membranes less permeable; retention of fluids; mild to severe waterlogging of tissues; "protects" proteolysis enzymes, resulting in more rapid breakdown of body proteins
Cancer chemotherapy (antimetabolites, cytotoxic agents, radioisotopes)	Emaciation and dehydration; extensive purpura; jaundice; low protein (because of anorexia and vomiting); perforation of gut; brittleness of bone; nitrogenous waste retention
Tranquilizers (phenothiazines)	Dehydration; weight loss and emaciation; low protein; kidney dysfunction and retention of nitrogenous waste products
Stimulants (amphetamines, cocaine)	Weight loss; emaciation; low protein; mucous membranes bleed easily; other problems as for tranquilizers
Sedatives (barbiturates, meprobamate)	Emaciation; dehydration; low protein; difficult to firm
Oral antidiabetic agents (tolbutamide)	Muscle atrophy; mild to severe jaundice; some emaciation and edema
Circulatory drugs (antihypertensives, anticlotting agents)	Blood clots; impairment of circulation; poor distribution of fluids; purpura; urine retention and spongy nitrogenous waste-filled tissues

[a]Table has been adapted and summarized from many published works. It is neither complete nor exhaustive. It is designed to point out categories of chemotherapeutic agents in use now. It is hoped that this table will stimulate both the student of embalming and the licensed professional to read about the latest developments in journals and trade magazines. As new chemical agents are introduced so frequently by the medical profession, it is impossible to publish up-to-the-minute tables. Keeping up with the literature is of the utmost importance.

has previously been stressed, **it is the physiological reaction the drug induces that causes the problem**. For example, the embalming problem created by the aminoglycoside antibiotics is produced not by the reaction between formaldehyde and kanamycin (even if a few grams of the antibiotic were present), but rather by the reaction between formaldehyde and the nitrogenous waste products released into the tissues through the action of the antibiotic.

Once absorbed into the bloodstream, a drug is rapidly diluted. An average body contains about 6 L (1 L is equivalent to 2.1 pints) of blood. This volume of blood circulates once per minute. It comes into contact with additional 35 L of liquid. (58% of the body weight of an average 150-lb male is water.) **Therefore, there is a total of 41 L of liquid (including blood volume) in the average body.** Any drug, usually given in milligram doses, would be so diluted as to have no significant effect in a direct chemical reaction with formaldehyde or any component of embalming fluid. Refer to the section on renal failure for embalming treatments for bodies with high levels of nitrogenous wastes in the tissues and bloodstream.

▶ POSSIBLE SOLUTIONS TO CHEMOTHERAPY PROBLEMS

The problems arising from chemotherapy vary in severity, but can be divided into a few broad categories. Several preventive and ameliorative treatments are available that have been shown to work in the majority of cases. **The professional embalmer must consider each case as unique**. Just as a physician does not prescribe the same dosage of a medication for all patients, the embalmer must vary procedures (and preservative fluids) to meet the requirements of the particular case.

FACTORS DETERMINED IN THE EMBALMING ANALYSIS

1. Vessels for injection and drainage
2. Method of mouth closure
3. Strength of the embalming solution
4. Volume of the embalming solution
5. Injection pressure
6. Injection rate of flow

Note: These factors will vary by the individual body and can vary in different areas of the same body.

In Table 23–1, five different embalming treatments are recommended to combat most chemotherapy-derived problems. Obviously, these cannot solve all the problems that the professional embalmer will face. They do, however, serve as a springboard for further research and, therefore, offer the embalmer an opportunity for experimentation and learning—both the marks of professionalism.

► CONCLUSION

Mistaken ideas about the specificity of a particular chemotherapeutic agent are quite common. For example, one may believe that a drug known to have a pronounced effect on a particular organ will be found only in that organ. This is not so. That a drug shows a more dramatic effect on a particular tissue does not mean that the effect is limited only to that tissue.

In general, no matter what chemotherapeutic agent is used, it is concentrated, metabolized, and detoxified in the liver and excreted via the kidneys (and, sometimes, the lungs and skin). But before it reaches these organs, it passes through other tissues of the body, which is contrary to the "magic bullet" concept. Actually, there is no magic bullet! It is impossible for a drug to bring about a single reaction in a single organ or in a tissue. It should not be surprising then that a single drug can cause a plethora of embalming problems. Simultaneous use of two or more drugs, as is common in medical practice today, intensifies the problems.

In the body, a drug is subject to great dilution. The problems it causes do not result from its direct reaction with components of the embalming fluid, but from the chronic physiological effects it produces.

On the basis of both laboratory studies and field work, five embalming treatments for the problems encountered in bodies that have undergone chemotherapy have been recommended. It is the responsibility of the embalmer to modify the treatment to suit the particular case.

► CONCEPTS FOR STUDY AND DISCUSSION

1. It is known that elderly persons present chemotherapy-derived embalming problems because the ability of the body to circulate, detoxify, and excrete drugs decreases with age. Discuss, on this basis, the possible effects of an aminoglycoside antibiotic such as gentamicin when the "usual" dilution is used.
2. If approximately 58% of the human body is composed of water, is it defeating the purpose to embalm the body that has undergone chemotherapy, particularly if there is little protein (as in the drug addict) in that body, by further diluting the embalming fluid with water before it is injected? Discuss how this intracellular water can be used as a diluent for concentrated arterial fluid. As this "tissue" water is known to be high in calcium, should it be conditioned with a water softener or conditioner?
3. It is a fact that a body treated with antibiotics usually contains all types of fungi. Certain fungi may pose a hazard to the embalmer. Discuss the possibility of contracting **Candida**, **Cryptococcus**, and **Histoplasma** infections from cadavers. What can be done to protect the embalmer?
4. It has been shown that to embalm an "average" body, at least three to four 16-oz bottles of a 30% formaldehyde arterial solution are necessary. Discuss whether enough preservative is contained in this amount of arterial fluid to embalm a body treated with corticosteroids. What adjunct embalming chemicals should be added to the arterial injection?
5. A young housewife is killed in an automobile accident. The embalmer is told that she has been taking a fertility drug (progesterone) because she was childless and wanted a family. What types of embalming problems might be expected?
6. A chronic diabetic is brought to the preparation room. The embalmer discovers that instead of insulin, the man had taken tolbutamide (Orinase) two times daily for the past 3 years. What embalming fluids should be used on this case, taking into consideration dilution of arterial chemicals, rapidity of firming, and use of preinjection fluid, water conditioners, and other fluids?
7. After arterial injection, the drainage is observed to contain small wads of greenish "cotton." The patient had been taking massive doses of penicillin prior to death. What could these "cotton wads" be?
8. A radiation safety officer has certified the release and permission to embalm a body that contains implanted seeds containing a radioisotope. Discuss the personal protective hygiene practices that the embalmer should use during the preparation of this body.
9. Discuss why an embalmer cannot use one type and one concentration of arterial embalming fluid in all cases.
10. A particular drug exerts its effect on only one specific organ. Therefore, after a patient treated with cortisone for an arthritic condition dies, high concentrations of cortisone will be found only in the joints. Discuss the fallacy of this type of thinking.

► BIBLIOGRAPHY

American Board of Funeral Service, *Course Syllabus*, St. Joseph, MO: American Board of Funeral Service, 2008.

Brozek J. *Body Composition*. New York, NY: New York Academy of Sciences, 1963.

Dorn J, Hopkins B. *Thanatochemistry*, 3rd ed. Upper Saddle River, NJ: Prentice-Hall, 2010.

Fredrick JF. An alpha-glucan phosphorylase which requires adenosine-5-phosphate as coenzyme. *Phytochemistry* 1963,2:413–415.

Fredrick JF. *Embalming Problems Caused by Chemotherapeutic Agents*. Boston, MA: Dodge Institute for Advanced Studies, 1968.

Gomori G. Microtechnical demonstration of phosphatase enzymes in tissue sections. *Proceedings of Society for Experimental Biology and Medicine* 1939,42:23–26.

Goodman L, Gilman A, eds. *The Pharmacological Basis of Therapeutics*, 4th ed. New York, NY: Macmillan, 1970.

Goth A. *Medical Pharmacology*, 6th ed. St. Louis, MO: C.V. Mosby, 1972.

Julian RM. *A Primer of Drug Action*. San Francisco, CA: Freeman, 1975.

Long YG. *Neuropharmacology and Behavior*. San Francisco, CA: Freeman, 1972.

Merck, Sharpe, & Dohme. *Merck Index*, 10th ed. Rahway, NJ: Merck & Co., 1983.

Physician's Desk Reference (PDR). Oradale, NJ: Medical Economics, 1984, No. 38.

Windholz M, Budavari S. In: *Merck Index*, 10th ed. Rahway, NJ: Merck & Co., 1983.

Yessell ES, Braude MC. *Interaction of Drugs of Abuse*. New York, NY: New York Academy of Sciences, 1976.

SELECTED CONDITIONS

▶ PURGE

Purge is defined as the postmortem evacuation of any substance from any external orifice of the body as a result of pressure. This condition can occur **prior to**, **during**, and **after embalming**. Purge is generally described by its source—stomach, lung, brain, and anal. The pressure responsible for the purge can develop in several ways:

1. **Gas**—Gas in the abdominal cavity or in the hollow intestinal tract can create sufficient pressure on the stomach to force the contents of the stomach through the mouth or the nose. This abdominal pressure can also push on the diaphragm with sufficient force to cause the contents of the lungs to purge through the mouth or the nose. Gas can originate from early decomposition or from partial digestion of foods or may be true tissue gas formed by **Clostridium perfringens.**
2. **Visceral Expansion**—When bodies have been dead for several hours and arterial solution is injected too fast, the hollow visceral organs (intestinal tract) tend to expand. Because the abdomen is a closed cavity, this expansion creates sufficient pressure to push on the stomach walls and create a stomach purge. The expansion also pushes on the diaphragm and squeezes on the lungs, possibly resulting in lung purge.
3. **Arterial Solution**

   a. Injection of arterial solution at a faster rate of flow, especially in bodies dead for long periods, causes expansion of the viscera (see item 2).
   b. If an area of the stomach, the upper bowel, or the lung is ulcerated, the arterial solution can leak through the ulcerated vessels, fill the stomach, the esophagus, or the lung tissue, and the trachea, and develop into a purge.
   c. If esophageal varices break, sufficient blood and arterial solution can exit to create purge.
   d. Gastrointestinal bleeding accompanies a variety of diseases and the long-term use of many drugs. If a sufficient amount of arterial solution and blood leak from these tissues during injection, anal purge results.
   c. Purge can occur when leakage of arterial solution from an aneurysm in the thoracic or abdominal cavity develops sufficient pressure to push on the lungs or the stomach.
   f. Sufficient injection pressure can cause leakage from recent surgical incisions. The arterial solution lost to the stomach or the abdominal cavity builds up enough pressure to create purge.
4. **Ascites and Hydrothorax**—When edema fills the thoracic or abdominal cavity prior to death, a great amount of pressure builds up and, on injection of arterial solution forces purge.

CONDITIONS PREDISPOSING TO PURGE

▶ Decomposition
▶ Long delay between death and embalming
▶ Drowning or asphyxia
▶ Recent abdominal, thoracic, or cranial surgery
▶ Tissue gas
▶ Hydrothorax or ascites
▶ Peritonitis or bloodstream infections
▶ Esophageal varices, ulcerations of the gastrointestinal tract, or internal hemorrhages
▶ Warm environment which speeds decomposition

Protecting Skin Areas from Purge

When purge occurs prior to or during arterial injection from the nose or the mouth, the surrounding tissues of the face should be protected by an application of massage cream. Stomach purge contains hydrochloric acid and can desiccate and discolor the skin. If arterial fluid is contained in the purge material, the dye from the fluid can stain the skin. Cover the facial tissues and the neck area with the massage cream. Only a light coating is needed. Be certain that the inside of the lips is covered as well as the base of the nose. Tightly packing with cotton or webbed cotton the throat, the nostrils, the ears, and the anus prior to embalming should greatly reduce the possibility of a purge during or after embalming.

General Preembalming and Embalming Treatments

When the abdomen is tightly distended from gas or edema (ascites) prior to embalming, a trocar should be introduced into the upper (ventral) area of the cavity. Piercing the transverse colon can help to relieve gas pressure. The stomach can also be punctured, as it can contain a large quantity of liquid. If ascites is present, removing some of the edema from the abdominal cavity will relieve the pressure. To drain ascites, insert a trocar or make a puncture in the lower left inguinal area of the abdomen (just above the inguinal ligament). Insert either a trocar or a drain tube to which a drainage hose is attached. From this location a portion of the liquid should gravitate from the cavity. By keeping the trocar (or drain tube) just under the abdominal wall (ventral), there should be no piercing of any large blood vessels.

Time Period Treatments

Two factors are necessary for purge to occur. First, there must be a substance to purge, such as stomach contents, blood, arterial fluid, and respiratory tract contents. Second, there must be pressure on an organ such as the stomach, the rectum, or the lung to evacuate the material.

Preembalming Purge

Stomach or Lung Purge. Preembalming purge generally consists of the stomach contents (Table 24–1). If esophageal varices have ruptured or if a stomach ulcer has eroded a blood vessel, blood can also be expected in the purge. As the stomach contains acid, this purge usually is brown. Stomach purge is often described as "coffee grounds" in appearance. Removal of this material at the beginning of embalming decreases the possibility of a postembalming purge. A nasal tube aspirator can be used to remove purge from the throat and the nasal passages. Some embalmers prefer to disinfect the oral cavity and the nose and tightly pack the passage with cotton. Others prefer to let the purge continue during embalming and make a final setting of the features after embalming. When restricted cervical injection is used, the body can purge during injection. After arterial injection, the body can be aspirated, nasal and throat passages can be tightly packed, the features can be set, and the head can be separately embalmed. Any purge on the face before or during embalming can create cosmetic problems. To protect the facial tissues, a massage cream should be applied to the skin surface and the neck. Be certain that the lips are coated on the inside as well as the outside.

Anal Purge. Preembalming anal purge material should be forced from the body by applying firm pressure to the lower abdomen and flushed away with running water. Use a very controlled water pressure so no fecal material is splattered. It is recommended that this purge be allowed to continue during embalming. Quite often, fecal matter is difficult to aspirate from the body. The anal orifice can be tightly packed with cotton saturated with cavity fluid or a phenol cauterant solution **after** cavity treatment. When it is time to finally wash the body, turn the body on its side so the buttocks, the back of the legs, and the embalming table can be cleaned and disinfected. A solution of fresh laundry bleach can be used for this postembalming cleaning. To protect the clothing of the deceased from any further soilage dress the deceased first in plastic garments—pants or Capri garment. Always sprinkle an embalming powder into these garments to control any odors.

Brain Purge. Preembalming brain purge results from a fracture of the skull, a surgical procedure in the cranial cavity, or a trauma such as a bullet penetrating the bone of the skull. It is possible for gas (a type of purge) to build up in the cranium and travel along the nerve routes to distend such tissues as the eyelids. Numerous foramina in the eye orbit communicate with the cranial cavity. Brain purge from the nose is rare and is usually the result of a fracture of the cribriform plate in the

TABLE 24–1. POSTMORTEM PURGE

Source	Orifice	Description	Contents	Time
Stomach	Mouth/nose	Liquid/semisolid "Coffee grounds" appearance Foul odor Acids pH	Stomach contents Blood Arterial solution	Preembalming Embalming Postembalming
Lung	Mouth/nose	Frothy Blood remains red Little odor	Respiratory tract liquids Residual air from lungs Blood Arterial solution	Preembalming Embalming Postembalming
Esophageal varices	Mouth/nose	Bloody liquid	Blood Arterial solution	Preembalming Embalming Postembalming
Brain	Fracture in skull Nose Fractured ethmoid Fractured ear Temporal bone Surgical opening	White semisolid	Brain tissue Blood Arterial solution	Preembalming Embalming Postembalming
Anus	Anal orifice	Semisolid/liquid	Fecal matter Blood Arterial solution	Preembalming Embalming Postembalming
Embalming solution	Mouth/nose Anus/ear	Color of arterial solution injected	Arterial solution	Embalming
Cavity fluid	Mouth/nose Anal orifice	Color of cavity fluid Blood present is brown in color	Cavity fluid	Postembalming

floor of the anterior cranial cavity. The ear can also be the site of brain purge, usually as a result of a fracture of the temporal bone. It is best to let these purges continue during the embalming procedure.

Embalming Purge

During arterial injection, the injected solution can expand the viscera. Pressure on the stomach or diaphragm can result in expulsion of the contents of the stomach and/or the respiratory tract. Also during arterial injection, arterial solution can be lost to the respiratory tract, the stomach, or the esophagus as a result of ruptured capillaries, small arteries, or veins. Ulcerated or cancerous tissues easily rupture because of the pressure of the solution being injected.

Tuberculosis of the lungs, cancer, pneumonia, and bacterial infections of the lung can cause fluid loss through weakened capillaries. A second cause of lung purge during embalming is congestion in the right atrium of the heart, which easily occurs if disease has involved the valves of the heart. Assume that drainage is being taken from the right femoral vein but has been very difficult to establish. Blood continues to push into the right atrium but cannot be drained away. The pressure builds to the point where the blood flows into the right ventricle and into the pulmonary arteries, squeez-ing the lung tissues and forcing a purge. Rupture of small veins can also produce a bloody lung purge.

During embalming purge may simply be composed of the contents of the stomach, lung, or rectum or, as already explained, arterial solution. As a large amount of arterial solution is lost in the drainage and possibly as purge, be certain that a sufficient volume of arterial solution is injected to replace these losses. It is not always necessary to turn off the machine and begin a multipoint injection when purge contains arterial solution. When arterial solution is present in purge during arterial injection and **drainage is occurring**, inject a sufficient volume to satisfy the preservative demands of the body. When arterial solution is present in purge during arterial injection and **drainage has stopped,** a major fluid loss is occurring and distribution is not taking place. Evaluate the body and use sectional arterial injection where needed.

Rarely does anal purge contain arterial solution; however, long-term use of some drugs can cause gastrointestinal bleeding; rectal and colon cancers can erode tissues; and ulcerative colitis can destroy vessels. These conditions make possible a loss of arterial solution as well as blood drainage into the colon and the rectum. If a sufficient amount of blood or arterial solution accumulates in the lower bowel, purge containing arterial solution can exit from the anal orifice.

It is usually during arterial injection that brain purge occurs. As already stated, for brain purge to occur, an opening must be present in the skull as a result of fracture, surgery, or trauma. Arterial solution escapes through small leaking arteries within the cranium, building up pressure that forces blood, arterial solution, and tissues of the brain through the openings.

Postembalming Purge

Purge that occurs prior to or during arterial injection can easily be controlled by the embalmer. It is the postembalming purge that should be of utmost concern to the embalmer. After cavity embalming, possibility of purge should be minimal. Many times, purge from the mouth, the nose, or the anal orifice after cavity embalming is simply cavity fluid that has been injected into passages of these orifices. Tightly repack the nostrils with cotton and replace moist cotton in the mouth with dry cotton.

Reaspirate prior to dressing whenever possible. If there appears to be a buildup of gas in the abdominal cavity, consider reinjection. Treat postembalming anal purge by forcing as much of the purge material from the body as possible. Then pack the rectum with the cotton saturated with a phenol solution, autopsy gel, or cavity fluid. Clothe the body in plastic pants or coveralls as added protection.

A purge that occurs from the mouth or the nose after the body has been dressed and casketed may be temporarily stopped by removing the trocar button and passing a trocar through the viscera to relieve the pressure that has accumulated. The body should be reaspirated and reinjected.

Prevention of Postembalming Purge

1. Thoroughly aspirate the body cavities. Inject (in the adult body) at least 16 oz (one bottle) of cavity fluid into the abdominal cavity, 16 oz into the thoracic cavity, and, if possible, 16 oz into the pelvic cavity.
2. Inject additional cavity fluid into obese bodies, bodies with ascites, bodies that have recently undergone abdominal surgery, and bodies which evidence decomposition.
3. If the abdominal trunk or buttock walls do not appear to have received sufficient fluid, hypodermically inject these areas with cavity fluids. Gases can form in unembalmed tissues and gradually move into the body cavities.
4. Reaspirate, especially those bodies that exhibit abdominal gas. This gas is easily detected when the trocar button is removed.
5. Reaspirate all the bodies that have been shipped from another funeral home.
6. Pack the throat and the nose with cotton. Nonabsorbent cotton should be used, because absorbent cotton may act as a "wick" to draw cavity fluid into the throat or the upper nasal passages. Apply massage cream or autopsy gel to the nonabsorbent cotton before it is inserted into the nostrils or the throat.
7. Remove moist cotton if purge has occurred during embalming. Be certain that the mouth is completely dried.
8. When purge has been expelled from the skull as a result of fracture, decomposition, or surgical procedure (brain purge), the cranial cavity can be aspirated by passing an infant trocar or large hypodermic needle through the surgical opening, the body fracture, or the cribriform plate. To aspirate through the cribriform plate, insert the needle through the nostril. Direct the needle toward the anterior portion of the cranial cavity. The brain can be injected with a small amount of cavity fluid. This is best done with a large hypodermic needle and a syringe.
9. A body that has had "tissue gas" in an extremity or a cavity may need to be reaspirated and reinjected several times before dressing.
10. Inject a cavity fluid supplement (phenol solutions used for external bleaches) along with the cavity fluid into "problem" body cavities. (Labels of these products will indicate cavity injection.)
11. Tie off or sever the trachea and the esophagus. This can be done through the incision used to raise the carotid artery.

▶ GASES

Five types of gases may be found in the tissues of the dead human body: (1) subcutaneous emphysema, (2) air from the embalming apparatus, (3) gas gangrene, (4) tissue gas, and (5) decomposition gas (Table 24–2).

In the dead human body, gases move over time to the higher body areas. When the body is in the supine position with the head elevated, the gas will move into the unsupported tissues of the neck and the face. The **source** of the gas can be in the **dependent** body areas. Gas can be detected in three ways in the body. It distends weak unsupported tissues such as the eyelids and the tissues surrounding the eye orbit, the temples, the neck, and the backs of the hands. In a firmly embalmed body, distension of veins is a possible sign that gas has formed. Pushing on the tissues where the gas is present may elicit a crackling sound that is both heard and felt. This is called **crepitation.** The area under the skin feels as if it is filled with cellophane.

TABLE 24–2. GASES THAT CAUSE DISTENSION

Type	Source	Characteristics	Treatment
Subcutaneous emphysema	Puncture of lung or pleural sac; seen after CPR; puncture wounds to thorax; rib fractures; tracheotomy	No odor; no skin-slip; no blebs; gas can reach distal points, even toes; can create intense swelling; rises to highest body areas	Gas escape through incisions; establishment of good arterial preservation; channeling of tissues after arterial injection to release gases
"True" tissue gas	Anaerobic bacteria (gas gangrene), C. perfringens	Very strong odor of decomposition; skin-slip; skin blebs; increase in intensity and amount of gas; possible transfer of spore-forming bacterium via cutting instruments to other bodies	Special "tissue gas" arterial solutions; localized hypodermic injection of cavity fluid; channeling of tissues to release gases
Gas gangrene	Anaerobic bacteria, C. perfringens	Foul odor, infection	Strong arterial solutions; local hypodermic injection of cavity chemical
Decomposition	Bacterial breakdown of body tissues; autolytic breakdown of body tissues	Possible odor; skin-slip in time; color changes; purging	Arterial injection of sufficient amount of the appropriate strong chemical; hypodermic and surface treatments; channeling to release gases
Air from embalming apparatus	Air injected by embalming machine (air pressure machines and hand pumps are in limited use today)	First evidence in eyelids; no odors; no skin-slip; amount depends on injection time	If distension is present, channeling after arterial injection to release gases

Types of Gases Found in Tissues

Subcutaneous Emphysema. The most frequently encountered gas condition is caused by antemortem subcutaneous emphysema, brought about by a puncture or a tear in the pleural sac or the lung tissue. As the living individual gasps for air, more and more air is drawn into the tissues. Subcutaneous emphysema frequently follows compound fracture of a rib, tracheotomy, lung surgery, or projection of an object (such as a bullet) into the pleural sac. A rib can be broken and the pleural sac or the lung itself torn if cardiopulmonary resuscitation (CPR) is not administered with care, permitting a large amount of air to escape into the tissues.

This condition is **not** caused by a microbe and does not continue to intensify after death. The gas, however, moves from the dependent areas to the upper body areas such as the neck and the face. No odor accompanies this condition; skin-slip or blebs do not form on the skin surface. In the male, the scrotum can distend to several times its normal size. It is best to remove the gas from the tissues **after** the body is embalmed.

COMMON CONDITIONS CAUSING ANTEMORTEM SUBCUTANEOUS EMPHYSEMA.

- Rib fractures that puncture the pleura or a lung
- Puncture wounds of the thorax
- Thoracic surgical procedures
- CPR compression causing a fractured rib or sternum to puncture a lung or pleura
- Tracheotomy surgery

Air from the Embalming Apparatus. The injection of air from the embalming machine is NOT a frequent problem today. Most machines automatically shut off when the tank has been emptied. This condition is most likely to occur when an air pressure machine or hand pump is used for injection. Air is forced into the closed container that contains the embalming solution. The pressure from the air forces the fluid into the body. The problem is of most concern if the face is being injected. The eyelids are one of the first areas to distend, even if a very small amount of air is accidentally injected.

Gas Gangrene. Gas gangrene is a fatal disease caused by contamination of a wound infection by a toxin-producing, spore-forming, anaerobic bacterium. This bacterium can be found in soil and the intestinal tract of humans and animals. *C. perfringens* is the most common of the Clostridium bacteria responsible for this condition. The organisms grow in the tissue of the wound, especially muscle, releasing exotoxins and fermenting muscle sugars with such vigor that the pressure build up by the accumulated gas tears the tissues apart.

The gas causes swelling and death of tissues locally. The exotoxins break down red blood cells in the bloodstream and, thereby, damage various organs throughout the body. The bacteria enter the blood just before death (the incubation period is 1 to 5 days). Because of the destructive action of the exotoxins and the enzymes produced, tissue involvement and spread are very rapid. Gas gangrene usually occurs after severe trauma, especially farm or automobile accidents and close-range shotgun discharges, where the wound may be contaminated with filth, manure, or surface soil. Gas gangrene is particularly likely after compound fractures; the bone splinters provide foreign bodies that enhance the infection as well as permit entrance of embedded debris or dirt.

The gangrenous process begins at the margins of the wound. The skin, dark red at first, turns green and then black, and there is considerable swelling that extends rapidly over the body. The tissues are filled with gas, sometimes to the point of bursting. The affected tissue decomposes, blisters and skin-slip form on the surface, and there is no line of demarcation. A very foul odor permeates the surroundings.

Gas causes the tissue to crackle when touched. The danger involved, as an embalming complication, lies in the fact that if death occurs shortly after injury, the gas gangrene may not be visible; it may be totally internal. If embalming treatment is not sufficient to control the spread of the organisms or their by-products, the symptoms of gas gangrene may show up several hours after embalming. In addition, if the postmortem examination is delayed, internal spread will be extensive and could create disastrous postembalming complications.

Tissue Gas. Tissue gas is caused primarily by *C. perfringens*. It may begin prior to death as gas gangrene. After death, the condition may result from the contamination of tissues by the gas bacillus, which has translocated from the intestinal tract. Contaminated hypodermic needles have also been known to transfer *C. perfringens* to the tissues of the extremities. Contaminated autopsy instruments have spread this condition from one body to another. This condition may also be spread when embalming instruments (cutting instruments, i.e., scalpels, scissors, trocar, suture needles) are not thoroughly disinfected. These organisms are very resistant to most disinfectants. Thus, the condition can occur after the body has been embalmed if all the tissues of the body and the visceral organs have not been adequately sanitized and preserved (Fig. 24–1).

The gas is ordinarily formed more rapidly and with greater intensity in the dependent tissues and the organs. These areas are frequently congested with blood and later poorly saturated with arterial solution and, therefore, provide an ideal medium for bacterial growth. Being lighter than the liquids it displaces, the gas rises to the highest receptive parts of the body. In addition,

Figure 24–1. Body distended within 2 hours of death by tissue gas.

the gas is larger in volume than the liquid it displaces, and thus tears and distends the tissues.

Distension is usually greatest in soft tissue areas such as the eyelids, the neck, and the scrotum of the male. The gas spreads rather rapidly through the tissue, causing blebs to form on the surface. As the condition progresses, the blebs grow and burst, releasing the gas and putrefactive fluids and causing skin-slip.

CONDITIONS PREDISPOSING TO TISSUE GAS..

- Recent abdominal surgery
- Presence of gangrene at the time of death
- Intestinal ulcerations or perforations
- Contaminated skin wounds or punctures
- Intestinal obstruction or hemorrhage
- Unsatisfactory embalming
- Contact with contaminated instruments

Decomposition. In the dead human body two factors are responsible for decomposition: bacterial enzymes and autolytic enzymes. Gases are formed that accumulate in the visceral organs, body cavities, and the skeletal tissues. These gases are responsible for the odor of decomposition. As the gases accumulate in the body cavities, sufficient pressure is produced to cause purge. The gases produced by decomposition are not often as intense as tissue gas or gas gangrene. Likewise, decomposition cannot be spread from body to body by contaminated instruments. The generation of gas ceases when the tissues are properly embalmed. Gases can be removed by cavity aspiration and postembalming channeling of the tissues.

Embalming Protocol

Subcutaneous Emphysema. Because subcutaneous emphysema does not involve microbes, treatment involves merely removal of the gas from the tissues. There are no foul odors, blebbing, or skin-slip with this condition. During arterial injection, some of the gas in the tissues may relocate, especially into higher body regions such as the neck and the facial tissues.

Restricted cervical injection should be used for the arterial injection. Fluid strength should be based on the postmortem and pathological conditions. A slightly stronger solution should be used to embalm the head, because if gas should relocate into the head after embalming (if the tissues are firm), sufficient resistance will be exerted to prevent distension. In restricted cervical injection, two incisions are made at the base of the neck. These incisions provide an exit for the gas in the tissues. The incisions can also be used as points from which to channel the neck so air can be pushed from the facial tissues.

Decomposition Gas, Gas Gangrene, and True Tissue Gas. Decomposition gas, gas gangrene, and true tissue gas all have a bacterial origin. It is very important to saturate the tissues of the body with a very strong arterial solution. Restricted cervical injection should be used so large quantities of sufficient-strength arterial solution can be injected into the trunk. Chemicals specifically made for the treatment of decomposing bodies and tissue gas should be used, for example, special-purpose arterial fluids, coinjection chemicals, and cavity fluids that can be injected arterially.

If the gas appears to have originated in an extremity, sectional arterial embalming should be done. If the condition is well advanced, 100% chemical should be injected into the localized area. A coinjection chemical can be added for each ounce of the arterial chemical. High pressure may be needed to inject the solution into the affected area. Often tissue gas is not noticeable at the time of death. As the organism responsible is anaerobic, after death the human body becomes an ideal medium.

Gases can form very rapidly after death. These postmortem changes can be devastating enough that a viewing of the body would be impossible. It is imperative that the preparation be started as soon after death as possible. If the gas source is an extremity or an area such as the buttocks, a **barrier** can be made by hypodermic injection of undiluted cavity fluid in addition to sectional embalming.

Clinical Example

The source of the tissue gas appears to be a gangrenous condition of the left foot. The lower portion of the leg has turned a deep purple-black. The leg is swollen and gas can be felt beneath the tissues. Injection is begun using a high-index special-purpose arterial fluid and employing restricted cervical injection as the primary injection point. Drainage is taken from the right internal jugular vein. After injection of the body, attention is turned to the left leg. The left femoral artery is then raised and the left leg arterially injected. Pulsation and high pressure are used to distribute the solution. After arterial injection, the femoral incision can remain open for a period of time to allow gas to escape. A trocar is introduced from the medial side of the middle of the thigh. Cavity fluid is injected through the embalming machine throughout the area above the knee. In addition, the trocar is thrust into the deep tissues of the lower leg. Undiluted cavity fluid is injected. A barrier has now been formed with cavity fluid in an attempt to contain the *C. perfringens* and prevent it from migrating to other body areas.

In treatment of a body with true tissue gas, six-point injection can be employed with a strong arterial solution to ensure good preservation. The incisions for the arterial injection can remain open several hours, providing an exit for the gas.

Cavity treatment should be very thorough. Gas rises to the anterior portions of the viscera and the cavity. Carefully aspirate the cavity, including the walls, to provide exits for the gas if it can be felt in the trunk walls. Inject a minimum of 16 oz (or more) into each cavity. The trocar puncture can remain open to allow the escape of gases, later to be closed after reaspiration and reinjection.

Such bodies can be reaspirated and reinjected several times to ensure that bacterial activity has ceased. The treatments so far suggested are radical, but tissue gas is a very serious problem.

Tissue gas can form in bodies that have not been thoroughly embalmed. *C. perfringens* is a normal inhabitant of the gastrointestinal tract, which after death rapidly moves to other body areas.

Removal of Gas from Tissues

Regardless of the source of the gas, the method of removing it is the same. There is only one effective way to remove gas from the distended tissues and that is to lance and channel the tissues and release the gas. Arterial injection and subsequent blood drainage may remove gases in the circulatory system, but do little to remove gas trapped in the subcutaneous tissue. The incision made to raise any vessels is an escape route for gas from the body.

Remember that in bodies with true tissue gas, release of the gas from the tissues does not stop its generation. The microbe causing the gas must be killed. Although gas accumulates in the superficial body tissues, the source of the gas may be located in a distal extremity or in the dependent tissues.

Trunk Tissues. Gases in trunk tissues can be removed by trocar after arterial injection. During aspiration of the cavity, the trocar is channeled through the thoracic and the abdominal walls. If the scrotum is affected, it too can be channeled by passing the trocar over the pubic bone.

Neck and Face. After arterial embalming, the trocar can be used to channel the neck to remove gas. Insert the trocar into the abdominal wall, after making certain that the trocar can reach the neck tissues. Pass the trocar beneath the rib cage and under the clavicle to reach the neck. The trocar can also be inserted into the neck by passing under the clavicle. Make a large half-moon incision at the base of the neck lateral from the center of the right clavicle to a point lateral from the center of the left clavicle. Reflect this flap and, with an infant trocar or scalpel, channel the neck tissue. Squeeze the neck tissues. Force the gas toward the openings. The half-moon incision can also be used for restricted cervical injection. If restricted cervical injection is used, this incision prevents more gases from entering the neck and the facial tissues. If possible, leave these incisions open several hours or until the body is to be dressed and casketed.

Eyelids and Orbital Areas. The eyelids are loose unsupported tissues, gas easily distends the lids. After embalming, the eyelids can be opened and slightly everted. Using a large suture needle, make punctures along the undersurface of the lids. Deep channels can also be made from this location to the surrounding orbital areas. By digital pressure move the gases from the most distal areas toward the punctures. A bistoury knife or large hypodermic needle can also be inserted from within the hairline of the temple area to remove gases in the orbital area and the temple. Cotton should be used for eye closure. It absorbs the small amount of liquid that may seep from the punctures. It may be best not to seal these punctures, for they are an escape route for any further gas that may accumulate in the orbital area. In the autopsied body, after arterial injection, the orbital area can be channeled by carefully reflecting the scalp. A bistoury blade can be used to dissect into the orbital areas. All this can be done from beneath the skin surface through the tissues exposed by the cranial autopsy.

Facial Tissues. Gases present in the cheeks and the facial tissues can easily be removed after arterial injection and cavity embalming (Fig. 24–2). Aspiration of the tho-

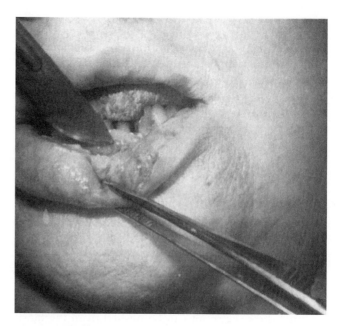

Figure 24–2. Lips are lanced to allow gas to escape (a postembalming treatment).

racic cavity and channeling of the neck tissues may help to remove some of the gas in the facial tissues. Open the mouth and insert a bistoury knife into the tissues of the face; run it deep to the facial bones to make channels for the gas to escape. This channeling provides escape routes for the gas. Digital pressure is needed to force the gas from the tissues to the exits. Begin at the distal points of the face and work the gas to the points where the bistoury knife or large hypodermic needle has been inserted. Any liquid leakage will drain into the mouth and the throat areas. The lips can be glued. This is a radical treatment, but is the only way to provide an escape route for the gas. In the autopsied body, reflect the scalp with a bistoury knife or large hypodermic needle and make channels into the facial tissues from the temple areas (Fig. 24–3). This may be sufficient to release the accumulated facial gases.

Instrument Disinfection

Tissue gas and gas gangrene involve a spore-forming bacillus, *C. perfringens,* which can easily be passed from one body to another via contaminated instruments. Great care should be taken in the disinfection of cutting instruments and suture needles. Wash instruments in cool running water using a good disinfectant soap. Then, soak them in a very strong disinfectant solution for several hours. Be certain that the disinfectants used in the preparation room are active (most disinfectants have a specific shelf life). Place disposable scalpel blades in a sharps container. Care should be given to the

Figure 24–3. A scalpel is used to cut channels through which gas in the tissues can escape (postembalming treatment).

disinfection of the trocar and the suture needles. See Chapter 3 for specific disinfectant recommendations.

▶ BODIES WITH FACIAL TRAUMA

In the preparation of bodies with facial trauma, the embalmer's goal is maximum tissue preservation with a minimum amount of swelling. If good preservation can be established, the restorative and cosmetic procedures will be easier to perform and will provide satisfactory results.

Traumatic injuries vary greatly; however, blunt force facial trauma can be classified into two categories: injuries in which the skin is broken (abrasion, laceration) and injuries in which the skin is not broken (contusion, hematoma).

Skin	Broken Skin
Depressed fractures	Abrasion
Swollen tissues (hematoma)	Laceration
Ecchymosis	Incision
Simple fracture	Compound fracture
Contusion	

Traumatic injuries also vary with respect to their location on the head. A laceration of the cheek may be simple to restore; however, a lacerated upper eyelid may involve swelling and discoloration, as well as torn skin, resulting in a much more serious problem for the embalmer to restore.

It is not within the scope of this text to detail the restorative treatments for each type of facial trauma and describe how treatment varies with location. It is the intent of this text to give a general outline of embalming protocol for traumatic facial injuries. Most of these injuries involve delay, for there usually is an inquiry by the coroner or the medical examiner. Quite frequently, when an autopsy is performed, refrigeration may precede or follow the postmortem examination. This discussion is concerned only with preparation of the head. If the body has been autopsied, the head is separately embalmed by injecting first the left common carotid artery and then the right common carotid. In the unautopsied body, restricted cervical injection can be used (right and left common carotid arteries are raised at the beginning of the embalming). Insert two arterial tubes into the right common carotid, one directed toward the trunk of the body and the other directed toward the right side of the head. Open the left common carotid artery, tie off the lower portion of the artery, and insert one tube into the artery directed toward the left side of the head. Leave both arterial tubes directed toward the head **open**. Inject the trunk first, then the left side of the head, and, finally, the right side. Drainage can be taken from the right internal jugular vein. Some embalmers prefer to drain from both the right and the left internal jugular veins when they inject the head.

General Considerations

Begin the preparation of these bodies by spraying the body with an effective topical disinfectant. Next, run cool water over the facial areas and hair to remove debris and blood. If glass was involved in the trauma, watch for small shards of glass that can easily rip gloves and cut the embalmer's fingers. Some glass can be flushed from the wounds with water, and forceps may be needed to pick glass pieces from broken tissues.

Align fractures. Incisions may have to be made prior to embalming to prop or align simple and depressed fractures. Next, align lacerated or incised skin areas. This is accomplished with a drop or two of super adhesive, or single (bridge) sutures of dental floss can be sewn with a small curved needle. Remove loose skin that cannot be embalmed by arterial means (this includes loose scabs). Apply surface preservative and bleaching compresses at this point or, if preferred, wait until the arterial injection is completed. Compresses of cavity fluid or phenol help to bleach, preserve, and dry the tissues. Phenol solutions work much faster than formaldehyde. Good tissue may be protected with a very small amount of massage cream.

Instant Tissue Fixation

Prepare a strong arterial solution. These solutions can vary depending on the arterial fluid chosen. Two examples are given here:

Solution 1	One bottle (16 oz) of 25- to 35-index arterial fluid
	One bottle (16 oz) of coinjection chemical
	Several drops of arterial fluid dye
Solution 2	One bottle (16 oz) of 25- to 35-index arterial fluid
	One-fourth gallon water
	Several drops of arterial fluid dye

These solutions are very strong because the index of the fluid is high and there is little dilution.

Set the pressure gauge on the centrifugal injection machine at 20 psi (or higher) with the rate-of-flow valve closed.

After running some of the arterial solution through the machine to evacuate all air from the delivery hose, attach the delivery hose to the left common carotid artery. Now, open the rate-of-flow valve and allow the fluid to surge into the left side of the face. As soon as the fluid starts to flow, shut the valve off. Pause a few moments and repeat the process. The dye rises to the skin surface immediately so the embalmer is able to see what tissues are receiving fluid. In the autopsied body, the internal carotid artery may have to be clamped.

This method allows the embalmer maximum distribution, using a minimum amount of arterial solution. Keep in mind the strength of this solution. The dye helps to prevent postmortem graying of the tissues and also serves as a tracer for the fluid. Drainage is minimal and is not a concern. This method can also be used to inject the legs and the arms when problems exist in the extremities.

In the unautopsied body, the trunk would generally be embalmed first and the facial area last. A suitable solution for preservation of the trunk and the limbs can be used for injection. In the autopsied body, the legs and the arms are embalmed first, and the instant tissue fixation method is used to embalm the head.

▶ RENAL FAILURE

A more common complication associated with embalming today is due to kidney failure. Improvements in medicine and long-term drug therapy have increased the life span of persons with terminal diseases. The embalmer must check the death certificate carefully for references to renal failure or dysfunction. If the death certificate is not available, the embalmer should look for the signs of renal failure when making the preembalming analysis. Also, during and after embalming, if tissues fail to respond (by firming), the embalmer may suspect renal failure.

It has been estimated that six times more preservative chemical is needed to preserve tissues of bodies dead from the complications of renal failure. The embalmer can use some of the following signs to determine whether renal failure has affected a body:

- Sallow color to the skin as a result of urochrome buildup.
- Uremic pruritus (scratch marks on the extremities).
- Increase in the amount of urea, uric acid, ammonia, and creatine (urea and ammonia can be detected by their odor).
- Acidosis.
- Edema (retention of sodium by the kidneys leads to increased retention of water).
- Anemia.
- Gastrointestinal bleeding (blood in the gastrointestinal tract and purging).

As can be seen, a variety of signs indicate renal failure. The embalmer should realize that renal failure may be only a contributory cause of death, as it often accompanies other life-threatening diseases. Thus, the cancer or heart patient will display the bodily changes associated with these diseases, as well as the signs associated with kidney failure.

The importance of this disease to the embalmer lies in the fact that these bodies rapidly decompose. The acidity of the tissues leads to rupture of lysosomes, which contain the autolytic hydroenzymes that begin the decomposition cycle. The edema present provides the moisture needed for the hydrolytic enzymes to act, the blood in the intestinal tract provides an excellent medium for the growth of putrefactive microorganisms, and the abundant ammonia in the tissues readily neutralizes formaldehyde.

Embalming Protocol

Preparation of the body affected by renal failure calls for the use of strong arterial solutions. Preinjection fluid should be avoided, because if circulation is impaired, tissues can easily swell. Begin with at least a 2.0% formaldehyde-based arterial solution. The use of a 30- to 35-index fluid is advised. Many fluid manufacturers make high-index arterial fluid specifically for the bodies dead from uremia. Follow the dilution instructions of the manufacturer. After surface blood discolorations have cleared and circulation is established, arterial solution in subsequent injections can be increased in strength. Use dye to indicate the distribution of arterial solution. If edema is extensive, inject a sufficient amount of fluid to dry some of the edema.

Some embalmers prefer to use an "average-strength arterial solution" made from a 20- to 30-index fluid. After surface blood discolorations are cleared and circulation is established, they add several ounces of a high-index formaldehyde-based arterial fluid to the arterial solution. This increases the strength of the solution being injected.

Two theories are held with respect to arterial solutions: (1) solution of one strength is used throughout the embalming procedure; (2) average solution is used at the beginning, and then strength is increased gradually until the desired tissue firmness is obtained.

When both edema and renal failure are present (in addition to side effects of drug therapy, effects of the immediate cause of death, and postmortem changes that have occurred if embalming was delayed), it is easy to understand why these bodies are so difficult to prepare and why fixation of the protein can be so difficult. It is most important to saturate these tissues with a strong preservative arterial solution. If this is not done the body will soften in a few hours, blebs can form, desquamation can develop, and the body can discolor and show signs of decomposition within a day or so.

To inject these strong solutions without over embalming the facial tissues, restricted cervical injection is advised. A large volume of very strong arterial solution can be injected into the trunk, and later a milder solution can be used to embalm the facial tissues.

The cavities should be thoroughly aspirated. Inject a minimum of one bottle of concentrated cavity fluid into each cavity. During arterial injection purge is possible from gastrointestinal ulcerations, so a large amount of blood and arterial solution may be present in the contents aspirated from the abdominal cavity. These bodies should be aspirated immediately after arterial injection. It is also advised that these bodies be reaspirated and reinjected.

Some of the dependent areas press against the embalming table. These pressure point areas often do not receive sufficient arterial solution. These dependent areas are high in moisture, and so hydrolytic changes occur and the putrefactive bacteria flourish. Coveralls and possibly a union all may be needed to prevent leakage if pitting edema is present. Preservative-deodorant powder should always be sprinkled inside the plastic goods.

▶ ALCOHOLISM

The preparation of the body that has suffered from chronic alcoholism can present a number of problems for the embalmer.

Many of these bodies exhibit jaundice as a result of liver failure. The primary goal is good preservation. Liver failure can also cause edema in the skeletal tissues or the cavities (ascites, hydrothorax). In addition, hepatic failure depletes the blood of clotting factors; therefore, good drainage can be expected if the body is prepared a reasonable time after death. Both the common carotid artery and the femoral artery are good primary injection sites; however, if skeletal edema is extensive and a large volume of strong arterial solution must be injected, restricted cervical injection is recommended. Injection should proceed at a moderate rate of flow so the tissues can assimilate the arterial solution without swelling. A moderate rate of flow also helps to prevent purging and rupture of weakened esophageal veins.

Purge is often seen in these bodies. Bloody purge may exit the mouth or the nose during arterial injection. Later, it turns into a fluid purge. A good sign that fluid is being distributed to the tissues is blood drainage. Inject a large volume of arterial solution to compensate for the fluid lost through purge. Arterial fluid dye is used to trace fluid distribution and to counter stain jaundice.

Because of the effect of long-term alcohol abuse on tissues, firming may be difficult to establish. These bodies should be injected with a moderate to strong preservative arterial solution. Do not use weak solutions even when the tissues may be emaciated or jaundiced. Add sufficient arterial fluid to firm the tissues.

Ecchymoses on the back of the hands can be treated by hypodermic injection of cavity fluid or phenol cautery solution after arterial injection. Before, during, and after arterial injection, compresses of cavity fluid, autopsy gel, or phenol solution may be applied to the skin surfaces to bleach and firm the ecchymotic areas.

Most of these bodies require tissue building after arterial injection. Tissues may be built up by injection of a restorative humectant in the last gallon of arterial solution.

At the beginning of the embalming, if ascites is present and the abdomen is much distended, puncture and drain the abdomen of this serous fluid prior to or during arterial injection. By keeping the point of the trocar just beneath the surface of the anterior abdominal wall, no large vessels will be punctured. Cavity embalming should be thorough, and, of course, reaspiration is recommended.

▶ OBESITY

Preparation of the obese body has been discussed elsewhere in this book. Some of the items discussed are reviewed here. The first concern is positioning. The shoulders of an obese body should be raised high off the table. The body should occupy three levels: the head is highest, then the chest, and, finally, the abdomen. Keeping the head high facilitates raising of the vessels and helps to prevent purge. Keep the elbows as close to the body wall as possible. It may be necessary to tie the arms into position with cloth straps after embalming to keep the elbows high and as close as possible to the body. Just moving the heavy body on the preparation table can be difficult. Movement of a body is easier if it rests on a sheet or is clothed. Unclothed bodies are easier to move on a wet table.

Position the elbows close to the body. Because the neck is usually quite short, keep the head straight and tie the feet together. Later, when the body is placed in the casket, tilt the shoulders and the head slightly to the right. The preceding scheme illustrates some of the complications associated with obesity.

Restricted cervical injection affords the use of the largest arteries, which should be free of arteriosclerosis. These vessels are not as deep as the femoral arteries. The right internal jugular vein can be used for drainage. It is the largest vein the embalmer can use in the un autopsied body.

Because of the short neck, drainage forceps are easier to use than a drain tube. The forceps can be inserted directly into the right atrium of the heart through the right internal jugular vein. If varicose veins are present, large clots may be observed in the drainage. The internal jugular vein allows passage of these clots out of the body.

If the obese person was also a diabetic, begin the embalming with the arms lowered over the sides of the table. Leave them in this position until the arterial solution reaches the tissues of the hands. Massaging the hands and radial and ulnar arteries promotes the flow of fluid into these peripheral areas.

This body will demand large volumes of solution. The solution can be an average dilution unless edema or other complications are present that call for stronger arterial solution mixtures. If restricted cervical injection is used, large volumes of solution can easily be injected without over embalming the facial tissues. Some embalmers prefer to increase the strength of the solution toward the conclusion of the embalming, before the head and the face are injected. This increased solution strength helps to dry and firm tissues. A well-firmed body is much easier to dress and lift. Sufficient pressure should be used to overcome the resistance, particularly the resistance exerted against the large vessels by the weight of the viscera. Massage, manipulation, and intermittent drainage assist in fluid distribution.

If the legs do not receive sufficient arterial solution, try raising the external iliac artery at the level of the inguinal ligament. The vessels here are more superficial than the femoral artery. It is often observed that the arteries in obese bodies are quite small in size.

Purge is always a problem with obese bodies. Weight of the viscera pushing against the stomach can easily create sufficient pressure to cause a stomach purge. These bodies also retain heat for extended periods after death and gases easily form in the gastrointestinal tract. Again, restricted cervical injection allows the trunk to be embalmed first; then the cavities can be aspirated, the features set, and the head embalmed. Purge is thus easily dealt with. This order of embalming also eliminates the need to set features twice if the mouth becomes filled with purge material.

▶ MYCOTIC INFECTIONS

Mycotic infections are fungal infections that may have been present as an antemortem condition or occurred as the result of a postmortem invasion. Fungi may be saprophytic or parasitic; that is, they obtain their nourishment from a dead organic material or from a living organism. Fungal infections are not rare in humans and frequently are serious. Often, skin and mucous membranes are affected by the fungal infection, as in athlete's foot and thrush. The more destructive parasitic fungi produce widespread chronic lesions.

In some fungal infections, the inflammatory response and tissue damage are the result of hypersensitivity to the fungal antigens. Fungi that are ordinarily saprophytic, such as Aspergillus, Mucor, and Candida, proliferate in patients receiving prolonged antibiotic, immunosuppressive, or steroid therapy and in those with predisposing diseases such as diabetes mellitus, leukemia, and acquired immunodeficiency syndrome (AIDS). Although there are many types of fungal infections, discussion is limited to those specific to embalming.

Candidiasis (Moniliasis)

Candida species are commonly found in the mouth, intestinal tract, and vagina of healthy individuals. **Candida albicans** is the most common cause of candidiasis. A common form of the disease known as thrush affects the oral mucosa (tongue, gums, lips, and cheeks) and the pharynx and is seen most often in debilitated infants (especially premature) and children. The lesions, white patches on the mucosa, comprise an overgrowth of yeast cells and hyphae and a nonspecific acute or subacute inflammation of the underlying tissue. Similar lesions occur on the vulvovaginal mucosa, particularly in diabetic and pregnant women and women on birth control pills. The skin, especially moist skin (e.g., perineum, inframammary folds, and between the fingers), may be affected.

Candida may produce lesions of the nails (onychia) and around the nails (paronychia), particularly in people whose hands are always in water (e.g., cooks). Occasionally, esophageal, bronchopulmonary, and widely disseminated forms of candidiasis are observed. Invasiveness is promoted by the lowered resistance of the host, as may occur in various debilitating illnesses and with intensive antibiotic, immunosuppressive, or steroid therapy. Candidal endocarditis has been reported in drug addicts, as a result of the intravenous injection of narcotics, and in patients who have undergone cardiac surgery.

Oral candidiasis can occur at any age during the course of a debilitating disease. It can also occur under dentures and orthodontic appliances and can complicate other erosive mucosal diseases (e.g., pemphigus vulgaris). The moist folds at the corners of the mouth provide a friendly environment for a troublesome candidal infection.

Oropharyngeal candidiasis is a specific complication of AIDS, because individuals with AIDS are immunosuppressed. Mouth lesions can spread down the trachea and the esophagus and produce extensive gastrointestinal infections.

Aspergillosis
Most species of the genus Aspergillus are saprophytic and nonpathogenic. Some are found as harmless invaders of the external auditory canal, nasal sinuses, and external genitalia and as secondary invaders in lung abscesses.

In involvement of the ear, the external auditory canal may be partially filled with foul moist material spotted with black granules. The lung appears to be the most common site of serious infection. Pulmonary lesions manifest as bronchopneumonia, abscesses, small infarcts (resulting from thrombosis caused by vascular invasion), or masses of Aspergillus mycelia ("fungus balls") in a newly formed cavity or a preexisting inflammatory (e.g., tuberculosis) or carcinomatous cavity. Chronic granulomatous reactions to the organisms in the lungs are also possible.

A primary fatal disseminated infection is relatively uncommon. Generalized aspergillosis is more frequent as a secondary complication and tends to occur in patients with debilitating diseases and in those who have received steroid, antibiotic, or immunosuppressive therapy. Aspergillosis occurs in various tissues and organs and is characterized by abscesses, necrotic and necrotizing lesions, and sometimes chronic granulomatous inflammation.

Phycomycosis
Phycomycosis is an infection of the lungs, the ears, the nervous system, and the intestinal tract caused by a fungus commonly encountered as a saprophyte or a contaminant. The lesions may display an intense necrotizing and suppurative inflammation process. Although this infection is commonly called mucormycosis, it may be caused by several members of the group Phycomycetes, including Mucor, Rhizopus, and Absidia. These fungi invade vessels and cause thrombosis and infarction. Phycomycosis is especially seen in patients with uncontrolled diabetes mellitus, leukemia, AIDS, and other debilitating diseases and in those receiving antibiotics, corticosteroids, chemotherapeutic agents, and irradiation. The resulting lesions are similar to those mentioned earlier.

Histoplasmosis (Reticuloendothelial Cytomycosis)
Histoplasmosis is caused by the oval, yeast-like organism **Histoplasma capsulatum**. Histoplasmosis occurs worldwide, although infection is particularly common in the Mississippi Valley of the United States. Positive diagnosis depends on the identification of the organisms in cultures of sputum, blood, or bone marrow or in biopsied tissue from the lymph nodes. This infection may spread throughout the body.

Histoplasmosis is not generally spread between individuals. It appears to be contracted from soil contaminated with fecal material of chickens, pigeons, starlings, other birds, and bats. In South Africa, most of the recognized benign pulmonary infections seem to have been acquired from contaminated caves (cave disease). Histoplasmosis is endemic in many parts of the world, particularly near large rivers and in high-humidity warm-temperature regions. The lungs are believed to be the usual portal of entry of the organisms. Histoplasmosis can be classified into four forms: acute pulmonary, chronic pulmonary, acute disseminated, and chronic disseminated.

The acute pulmonary form may be asymptomatic or symptomatic. The basic reaction in the lungs and the lymph nodes consists of foci of tuberculoid granulomas that tend to heal. Most cases of histoplasmosis are benign, asymptomatic pulmonary infections, with positive histoplasmin skin tests and healed calcified nodules in the lung and the peribronchial lymph nodes, often resembling the healed primary complex of tuberculosis. The symptomatic pulmonary infections may be either mild and "flu-like" or more severe, resembling atypical pneumonia. Usually the prognosis is good. Multiple pulmonary infiltrations, with or without hilar lymphadenopathy (involvement with the entrance to the glands), may be indicated in x-rays of the chest and, in the more prolonged cases, tend to calcify and simulate healed miliary tuberculosis. In some cases, a localized pulmonary tuberculoid granulomatous lesion with caseation necrosis, calcification, and fibrotic border (histoplasmoma) may occur, appearing in an x-ray of the chest as a "coin" lesion. This lesion is sometimes removed surgically because of the clinical suspicion of lung cancer.

The **chronic pulmonary** form is progressive, forming granulomatous inflammation with caseation necrosis and cavitation, and frequently is misdiagnosed as pulmonary tuberculosis, or it may occur as a secondary complication of tuberculosis. It is seen most commonly in otherwise healthy males older than 40 years. The prognosis is poor. Occasionally, either the acute primary complex or the chronic pulmonary type is disseminated, spreading through the blood to involve many organs. Involvement of the lymph system, the liver, the spleen, and the bone marrow dominates the clinical picture. The organs involved are packed with macrophages stuffed with organisms, so the histologic picture resembles that of visceral leishmaniasis. Jaundice, fever, leukopenia, and anemia lead to a condition that mimics acute miliary tuberculosis.

The **acute disseminated** form may be either benign or progressive. The acute progressive form is rapidly fatal and is usually encountered in young children or immunosuppressed (AIDS) adults. The spleen, the lymph nodes, and the liver are enlarged. There is a septic type fever with anemia and leukopenia. Bone marrow smears may reveal the organisms or granulomas. Occasionally, the organisms may be found in mononuclear cells in blood smears.

The **chronic disseminated** form may occur in the elderly and otherwise healthy individuals and may be fatal. In the more protracted form, which occurs in otherwise healthy individuals, the clinical features vary according to the organ most severely involved. For instance, involvement of the heart valves leads to endocarditis, and involvement of the adrenal glands leads to Addison's disease. Other organs that can be affected are the gastrointestinal tract, the spleen, the liver, the lymph nodes, the lungs, the bone marrow, and the meninges. In some cases, infection and ulceration of the colon, the tongue, the larynx, the pharynx, the mouth, the nose, and the lips are initial manifestations.

Other Mycotic Infections

Several other mycotic infections may be encountered but are rare. These include dermatomycosis, cryptococcosis, North American blastomycosis, and protothecosis. More than 100,000 species of fungi are known, of which approximately 100 are human pathogens. For the most part, they occur as secondary complications of other diseases.

Significance of Mycotic Infections to Embalming

Mycotic infections are frequently encountered, especially in those with debilitating or immunosuppressive diseases and diabetes mellitus. The widespread use of immunosuppressive drugs, combined with modern medical advances that keep patients alive but debilitated, has led to a considerable increase in the incidence of fungal infections. In the modern hospital, they are one of the most important and lethal examples of opportunistic infection.

The greatest danger presented is to the embalmer and to others who work directly with the dead human bodies. Many fungal infections produce superficial lesions on the skin and the mucous membranes. As many of the fungi involved are saprophytic, they continue to multiply until they are effectively arrested. Other fungal infections involve the oral/nasal cavity, the larynx, the pharynx, the esophagus, and the lungs. These may also be saprophytic and continue to multiply in untreated or poorly embalmed dead human bodies.

In all fungal infections or unidentified lesions, careful handling of the remains is essential. When moving the remains, do not compress the abdominal or thoracic cavity. Such compression causes air and fungal organisms (including spores) to be expelled into the environment. The spores may lay dormant in the environment until the conditions conducive to fungal growth arise. The spores and fungal organisms may also be inhaled by embalming personnel, establish colonies in the lungs and the throat, and cause further infections.

Bodies with superficial lesions should never be handled with bare hands. A cut or break in the skin of the hands of embalming personnel represents a portal of entry for fungal and other organisms. Should the organisms enter the bloodstream, they can spread throughout the body and cause serious infections. In addition, the embalmer's clothing may harbor fungal organisms and spores, as well as other infectious organisms, which could be spread to other persons with whom the embalmer comes into contact.

Most, if not all, fungal organisms form spores. These spores may be resistant to weak disinfecting agents. Therefore, the spores may lay dormant in an improperly cleaned and disinfected preparation room and on improperly disinfected instruments. These spores could contaminate subsequent remains embalmed in that preparation room. The greater danger, however, lies in the possibility that unsuspecting embalming personnel might inhale airborne spores or contract them through cuts or breaks in the skin. Spores may enter the ventilation system and be spread to other areas.

Embalming personnel should wear protective garments in the preparation room (gloves, apron and/or impermeable disposable coveralls, oral/nasal mask, goggles, head and shoe coverings). Personal garments or bed clothing should be removed carefully and disposed of properly. The body should be thoroughly bathed with a proper disinfectant solution as soon as it is undressed. All superficial lesions should be treated immediately, and the mouth, the nose, and the eyes should be properly disinfected. All of these procedures must be accomplished before any embalming procedure is initiated (this would be true of all cases).

FACTORS DETERMINED IN THE EMBALMING ANALYSIS

1. Vessels for injection and drainage
2. Method of mouth closure
3. Strength of the embalming solution
4. Volume of the embalming solution
5. Injection pressure
6. Injection rate of flow

Note: These factors will vary by the individual body and can vary in different areas of the same body.

Once the external disinfection has been completed, embalming procedures may be carried out as prescribed by the preembalming analysis. Routine arterial injection of a solution of sufficient strength and thorough cavity treatment should control internal fungal infections. Oral, nasal, vaginal, and anal cavities may be packed with disinfectant-soaked cotton as an added precaution. For autopsied bodies, careful handling of drainage is recommended.

Students of funeral service education are taught that everybody should be treated as though it were infectious, because it very well may be. This has been sound advice for many years and is especially important today in light of the fact that it is not always known what diseases the deceased may have had or may have come into contact with. Whether the body is a seemingly routine case or a victim of a severe infectious disease (e.g., hepatitis or AIDS), the protection of the embalmer rests solely in employing precautionary procedures.

▶ CONCEPTS FOR STUDY AND DISCUSSION

1. You are injecting an unautopsied body—but what you do not know is this individual died from a ruptured aortic aneurysm—what signs will indicate to you that this condition is present? Discuss the thorough embalming of this body.
2. Discuss the measures that can be taken to prevent postembalming purge.
3. Discuss the difference between subcutaneous emphysema and "true" tissue gas.
4. Outline the embalming of a body with tissue gas in the tissues of the right leg.
5. Discuss the problems encountered in embalming a body dead from chronic alcoholism.
6. List some mycotic infections encountered by the embalmer.
7. Discuss the problems encountered in preparation of the obese dead human body.
8. Discuss the complications encountered in embalming bodies dead from renal failure.

▶ BIBLIOGRAPHY

Anderson WAD, Scotti M. *Synopsis of Pathology,* 10th ed. St. Louis, MO: C.V. Mosby, 1980.

Boehringer PR. Uremic poisoning. *ESCO Rev* 1964; Second Quarter.

Boehringer PR. *Controlled Embalming of the Head.* Westport, CT: ESCO Technical Notes, 1967:57.

Grant M. Selected embalming complications and their treatment. In: *Champion Expanding Encyclopedia,* No. 573. Springfield, OH: Champion Chemical Co., 1987.

Mulvihill ML. *Human Diseases,* 2nd ed. Norwalk, CT: Appleton & Lange, 1987.

Robbins SL. *Pathology,* 6th ed. Philadelphia, PA: W.B. Saunders Co., 1999.

Sheldon H. *Boyd's Introduction to the Study of Disease,* 9th ed. Philadelphia, PA: Lea & Febiger, 1984.

Tissue gas cause and treatment. In: *Champion Expanding Encyclopedia,* No. 420. Springfield, OH: Champion Chemical Co., 1971.

Walter JB. *Pathology of Human Disease.* Philadelphia, PA: Lea & Febiger, 1989.

CHAPTER 25

EMBALMING FOR DELAYED VIEWING, RE-EMBALMING OF THE BODY, EMBALMING FOR SHIPPING, AND SHIPPED-IN BODIES

CHAPTER OBJECTIVES

▶ Embalming for delayed viewing
▶ Re-embalming of the body
▶ Preparation of the body for anatomical study
▶ Preparation for shipping human remains
▶ Protocol for receiving shipped human remains

In 1989, the American Board of Funeral Service Education curriculum committee on embalming clarified the definition of **embalming** from "the preservation of the dead human body" to "the **temporary preservation** of the dead human body." Standard embalming practices never guaranteed a **permanent** or **indefinite** preservation of remains. Embalming for funeralization is not the same as preparations for museum or laboratory study. Objectives of embalming for funeralization not only involve preservation of the body but also the creation of an acceptable appearance of the body. This acceptable appearance would not be possible using preservation methods such as mummification, desiccation, freeze drying, vulcanization, or even embalming for dissection. In time, all organic matter will be reduced; we even see this with the desiccated mummies of ancient Egypt. Embalming slows this reduction process. In time—perhaps many years—a gradual breakdown of the embalmed body will take place, rather than a putrefactive process involving liquefaction and odors.

A standard for each preparation should be that the preservation of the body last more than several days or "until the burial." Standard embalming and preservation practices should conceivably keep the remains intact for months or possibly years with no special treatments. Three major factors affect the degree and length of preservation:

1. Condition of the body at the time of the preparation
2. Embalming thoroughness and chemical formulations
3. Aftercare

A unique and interesting opportunity to study many hundreds of embalmed and entombed bodies was afforded, Professor John Pludeman, a Funeral Service Instructor at the Milwaukee Area Technical College in Milwaukee, Wisconsin, in 1996. His discussion is included here because it pertains to the past and present of long-term embalming.

In recent years, funeral service professionals have begun to question the need for long-term preservation of human remains. Funeral directors, mortuary college professors, and other funeral service professionals have engaged in serious discussions on the subject. Because of the ethical, moral, and legal issues related to preservation of human remains, the issue raises important questions worthy of consideration. Frequently debated questions include:

■ How long should modern embalming preserve human remains?
■ What are the purposes and benefits of long-term preservation?

- What does the consumer have a right to expect in terms of long-term preservation?

The answers to these important questions of today may be partially answered by looking to the past. In the United States, it was not so many years ago that nearly all human remains were embalmed as a matter of standard practice. The society, the surviving relatives, and the funeral director correctly assumed that preservation was a customary and proper part of the traditional funeral.

More recently, diverse societal attitudes and cultural changes have raised questions about the value of the funeral altogether, not to mention the value of embalming and long-term preservation. As a result, the funeral director can no longer assume that embalming and preservation will be authorized by the relatives of the deceased. Further, certain federal regulations forbid the funeral director from making statements guaranteeing long-term preservation.

Several years ago, I managed a very unique project involving the demolition of an 85-year-old mausoleum that was in ruins. The massive project first required the disinterment of all human remains entombed within. Once completed, more than 650 casketed human remains and about 350 cremated remains were reinterred in another, well-maintained cemetery. Because the mausoleum entombment records were vandalized and incomplete, every casket was opened to confirm occupancy and reestablish identities. By observing large numbers of embalmed human remains that had been preserved and entombed over an 85-year period, the following anecdotal information was derived about the subjects of this study.

- Between 1900 and 1960, nearly 99% of human remains were embalmed.
- In most cases, there was strong evidence of successful long-term preservation, lasting many decades.
- There was much evidence of thorough preservation through the use of adequate embalming chemicals and implementation of proper embalming methods of the day.
- In numerous cases, the deceased were very well preserved and distinctly recognizable. Facial features, hands, jewelry, and clothing remained intact.
- Some remains were completely desiccated but still recognizable while others were only skeletons. In either case, there was no odor present.
- Less than 15% (approximately 35) of all 650 disinterments were in a state of active decomposition. The majority of these cases were in sealer caskets and it appears that moisture was trapped inside the casket and could not escape, or the crypt accumulated water and it seeped into the casket.
- There was consistent evidence of extreme care given to the deceased in respectful final preparation (dressing, positioning, cosmetizing, hair dressing, etc.).
- Funeral directors achieved these admirable accomplishments without the assistance of modern embalming machines, advanced embalming chemicals, eye caps, needle wire injectors, hydroaspirators, and so on.

If the previous observation and examples are an indication of successful long-term preservation from the past, does this not set a certain professional standard for the present?

Most ancient and modern funeral customs around the world include the remains of the deceased as a ceremonial focal point. Some societies believe in expedient disposition of the remains, usually through cremation, while other societies have recognized the benefits of long-term preservation to accomplish their funeral objectives.

Should the professional embalmer of today strive to achieve short-term or long-term preservation? What are the purposes and the benefits of long-term embalming? Are the family and the public concerned about preservation beyond the funeral and final disposition? Are they entitled to a certain degree of preservation because they requested and paid for embalming by a professionally licensed funeral director?

Today, consumers are better informed, better educated, and demand value in exchange for the money they spend. So when faced with the decision of paying for the cost of embalming, some may question just how long embalming will preserve their loved one. If the funeral director is asked this question directly, his response may be influenced by a Federal Trade Commission (FTC) requirement that prevents the funeral director from representing that preservation will delay the natural decomposition of human remains.

There exists yet another consumer-related argument for long-term preservation, which involves the offering of protective funeral merchandise. Considering the many well-constructed, durable, highly protective caskets, burial vaults, crypts, and mausoleums offered to the consumer, what is it these products are protecting if long-term preservation is not possible? And will the consumer be willing to select these products if they perceive long-term preservation as an unlikely possibility?

The mausoleum disinterment project mentioned earlier demonstrates another important principle of protection for the deceased: A thoroughly embalmed, well-preserved body is fundamental to long-term protection of that body. Without initial preservation, no casket, crypt, or other product will retard decomposition and protect the body in the efficient manner that embalming can accomplish. Consequently, caskets, burial vaults, crypts, and other protective devices offer added protection of the deceased and then provide good value.

Long-term preservation accomplishes a number of objectives. Families have the assurance of a professionally prepared loved one and the peace of mind that it affords. Also, there will be greater value, function, and purpose of the protective products surrounding the deceased.

How long will quality embalming preserve the deceased? Because the extent of preservation and the rate of decomposition is subject to many intrinsic and extrinsic factors, the degree of the length of preservation cannot be accurately predicted. However, a generally accepted consensus states that preservation should far surpass the period of the funeral.

▶ GENERAL CONCEPTS

All three groups of embalming chemicals may be necessary to use in the preparation of bodies for extended preservation and delayed viewing: (1) preservative embalming chemicals, (2) supplemental embalming chemicals (injectable chemicals such as humectants, co- or pre-injection chemicals, dyes, and other preservative chemicals), and (3) accessory embalming chemicals (noninjectable chemicals such as mold retardants, embalming powders and gels, and autopsy compounds). In addition, many funeral homes have the luxury of a refrigeration unit. This is particularly helpful when the decision about embalming is delayed several days. It is also helpful to have a refrigeration unit for the remains that will have a delayed viewing. However, refrigeration is not necessary for a delayed viewing of the body.

Some considerations for the preparation of a remains for delayed viewing include the following:

- Restricted cervical injection allows the injection of large volumes of arterial solution without over-injecting the facial tissues; one solution strength can be used for the face and another for the trunk and limbs.
- Intermittent or restricted drainage.
- Delay aspiration and cavity treatment. This helps the arterial solution to thoroughly saturate the body tissues and organs.
- Place the remains on "body bridges" or "blocks" so that as little body surface as possible makes contact with the surface it is laying on. This is

important during embalming and storage of the body.

- Avoid excessive elevation of the head. This can cause fluids to drain from the face and neck, bringing about a sunken appearance.
- Because some tissue and embalming fluids can be removed from facial tissues by dehydration and gravitation, it is recommended to do some feature tissue building prior to storage of the embalmed body. Restore by filling out the areas of the cheeks, temples, lips, and fingertips.
- Hypodermically treat all areas of ecchymosis; left untreated over time they will turn black. Use a phenol cautery solution or cavity fluid; this will bleach the tissues and ensure good preservation.
- Apply liberal amounts of massage cream to the face, neck, hands, and wrist areas. These areas can also be covered with cotton to prevent further evaporation of the massage cream.
- Spray the remains with a mold retardant (there are some specific mold retardants available, but any topical embalming spray should prevent the growth of mold) initially, and at regular intervals, during storage.
- Do not place the remains in a closed, sealed environment; it encourages mold growth.
- The remains must be inspected on a regular basis once in storage. If problems develop, they can be corrected immediately (Fig. 25–1A to 25–1H).

Embalming for delayed viewing can adversely affect the remains:

- Overdrying or desiccation of tissue
- Development of mold on the surface of the remains
- Insufficient preservation, requiring re-embalming

Desiccation (an over drying of tissue that causes dehydration or a leathery appearance to the remains) can also make it difficult to keep the eyes and mouth properly closed (Fig. 25–2). Closure should be done preferably with a superglue; this will help to retain the closure for the duration of storage. Use of liberal amounts of massage cream throughout the storage period will also help to reduce dehydration. Mold formation can be prevented by the topical use of a mold-retardant chemical. The remains should never be placed in a closed, dark environment as this promotes the growth of mold. During the time of storage, if any area exhibits inadequate preservation, it should be treated by hypodermic injection of undiluted preservative chemical or reinjected using undiluted preservative chemical. This should be done as soon as problems are identified.

Figure 25–1. A. Preparation using restricted cervical injection. **B.** After embalming, soft areas such as the lips require treatment using cotton within the mouth saturated with cavity fluid, and lips are sealed with superglue. **C.** Each finger tissue built after embalming. **D.** Massage cream placed on facial tissues; Vaseline used to cover lips and eyelids. **E.** Loose cotton covering face and hands. **F.** Body stored on body bridges. (*Continued*)

G

H

Figure 25–1. (*Continued*) **G.** Face at end of 1 week; no dehydration, eyes and lips closed. **H.** Face at end of 2 weeks; no dehydration, eyes and lips closed.

▶ BODIES THAT REQUIRE RE-EMBALMING

There are occasions when it may be necessary to re-embalm a body or section of a body:

- Fluid was not distributed to all areas
- Too little solution was injected
- The concentration of the fluid was too low to meet the preservative demands of the body
- The injected solution was neutralized by the body chemistry (often seen in bodies dead from renal failure or edema)

Figure 25–2. Extreme desiccation 3 days after embalming.

- Rigor mortis was mistaken for embalming fluid tissue fixation

The embalmer has three methods by which to re-embalm a body or area of a body: arterial injection, hypodermic injection, and surface embalming. Time may play a significant role in selecting a method of treatment. If the body is received from an out-of-town funeral establishment, and problems exist, there is always the possibility the time between receipt of the body and viewing will be minimal. If a problem such as purge or tissue gas develops during a visitation, the time slot **between** the visitation hours or the time period after the visitation may be when the corrections can be made. Visitation in a church or a public building may also mean transport of the body back to the embalming facility for corrections.

In the treatment of the unautopsied body, a multipoint injection may be required depending upon the extent of the problem. This is necessary because cavity embalming will have been completed, so begin by **reaspiration before arterial injection**. In this manner, the drainage can be taken from the heart. It is not necessary to drain from each site of injection. As only a minimum amount of fluid is used in the reinjection process, drainage should not be a big concern. After injection, thoroughly aspirate again, and then inject a minimum of two or three bottles of concentrated cavity fluid into the cavities. It is always suggested that these bodies be reaspirated before dressing.

If time is a serious factor areas such as the trunk walls, buttocks, shoulders, and legs can be directly injected using a trocar directly attached to the embalming machine. Undiluted cavity fluid or high-index fluid should be injected. Points of entry can be sealed using trocar buttons.

Small areas of the face that appear underembalmed can be injected from within the mouth by hypodermic treatment. Undiluted cavity fluid works best for this re-embalming. Arterial fluids may contain dye and in a few hours the dye can actually create a surface stain on the face. Hidden points of entry are recommended for leakage of the injected fluid is a possibility.

Eyelids and mouth. These areas can be easily treated by placing cotton under the eyelids or over the teeth. Saturate the cotton with a few drops of undiluted cavity fluid and seal the lids or mouth with a superglue. This will serve as an **internal** compress which in a few hours should have the surrounding tissues well preserved. This technique will allow the embalmer to proceed with cosmetic treatment.

If time permits, external preservative surface compresses can be placed over an affected area but generally these treatments take several hours to take effect. At the conclusion of the treatment, the areas will have to be force dried if cosmetics are to be applied to the area.

Internal treatments. Arterial, hypodermic, and where possible internal compresses (face) are the most effective.

If an entire side of the face or hand needs to be re-embalmed, arterial injection is recommended. Inject the artery that supplies the area using a waterless embalming solution. One formula is to mix equal parts high-index arterial fluid and coinjection fluid. If coinjection is not available, use two parts high-index arterial fluid and one part water. Dye should be added to help trace the solution.

If the body has developed tissue gas, it is recommended that each section of the body be injected using a waterless solution as described in the preceding paragraph. Some chemical companies manufacture a fluid for tissue gas treatment. If available, this should be used. Trunk walls, buttocks, and shoulders will need to be injected by trocar using undiluted cavity fluid. Following injection treatment, the cavities should be thoroughly reaspirated and reinjected with undiluted cavity chemical. Gasses can be forced from incision sites where arteries are raised.

Embalming for Delayed Viewing

Embalming for delayed viewing or interment can be defined as a preparation of a remains that will allow the initial viewing up to several weeks after death. Initial viewing may be delayed for a number of reasons. Examples include the following:

- The family of the deceased needs to make travel arrangements.
- There is difficulty in locating the family of the deceased.

- The remains are being shipped to a foreign country.
- Family members are waiting for someone to be released from the hospital or awaiting the imminent death of another family member, for example, accident cases.

In embalming any remains, it is important to base choice of arterial fluids and amounts of solution to be injected on the condition of the remains, length of time since death, and refrigeration status. This is done through an analysis of the remains before making any selection of fluids. (During the embalming of the body, a further analysis will be necessary to determine fluid strengths and volume and possible multipoint injections; this analysis is based on the reaction of the body to the solutions being injected.) Some important factors to be considered include the following:

- Edema or emaciation
- Kidney or liver failure
- Trauma
- Infectious diseases
- Obesity
- Signs and/or degree of decomposition present

The United States Army Regulation 638–2 **Care and Disposition of Remains and Personal Effects** in Appendix D—Armed Service Specifications for Mortuary Services (Care of Remains of Deceased Personnel and Regular and Port of Entry Requirements for Casket and Shipping Cases) in Section D-5 (5) under **Treatment of Remains** (see the Selected Readings section) states:

> Frequently, final disposition of processed or reprocessed remains may not be effected for a period of 10 days or more; remains may be transported over long distances or subjected to hot, humid conditions. At all times the remains must be free of putrefaction and infectious agents. This requires the thorough disinfection and uniform preservation of all body tissues. Employment of continuous injection and intermittent drainage will enhance chemical distribution and penetration. Use of humectants (moisture retention chemicals) in the arterial injection solution will help to achieve greater tissue penetration and to restore normal body moisture content.

This description adequately states the desired results of all remains, not just those that will be subject to delayed viewing. The military takes an aggressive methodology toward the preparation of its deceased members as described in section D-6 **Preparation of Remains,** Processing Viewable Remains: "a thorough pre-embalming case analysis shall be made in order to determine the best embalming techniques to be used to obtain optimum results." It goes on to state the specific preferred method of treatment:

> Whenever possible, a six-point arterial injection with multi-site drainage shall be accomplished. The arterial chemical injection solution shall contain a 2 to 3 percent concentration, by volume, of aldehyde or aldehyde derivative preservative agents, with equal parts of a humectant chemical also being added to the injection solution. The thoracic, abdominal, and pelvic cavities shall be thoroughly aspirated and injected with full strength cavity chemicals having a 30-index (percent) or greater, using a minimum of 16 ounces for each cavity.

Embalming for Delayed Viewing for More Than 1 Month

In some rare instances, it may be necessary to keep remains for longer than 1 month. Any of the examples presented earlier on delayed viewing can be applied to a situation that grows into greater than a 1-month period of time. Some suggested formulations for this type of delayed viewing are include in the Selected Reading "The two-year fix: long-term preservation for delayed viewing" by Kerry Don Peterson,

When no signs of decomposition exist in the remains, use the following solution (1 gallon of solution):

- 32 oz arterial humectant fluid
- 32 oz coinjection
- 16 oz water corrective
- 16 oz humectant
- 32 oz tepid water

For remains showing early or intermediate signs of decomposition, use the following solution:

- 32 oz high-index fluid
- 32 oz coinjection fluid
- 32 oz water corrective
- 16 oz humectant
- 0 oz water

Many funeral homes in the United States do not use supplemental chemicals or they might use only one or two such formulations. Excellent results are possible without the use of supplemental chemicals; many preservative arterial fluids contain humectants and high amounts of dye. Restricted cervical injection is the preferred method of injection for treatment of these bodies. The use of intermittent drainage and delaying aspiration of the cavities will allow for more thorough distribution, penetration, and diffusion of the preservative chemicals.

The body must be thoroughly analyzed after embalming and if necessary additional steps taken to ensure that all areas are well preserved. This can be thought of as a quality assurance inspection.

Storage for Delayed Viewing

Refrigeration is not necessary for storage of embalmed remains for delayed viewing, but a cool location is preferred. If refrigeration is available, it would be recommended to use as a storage site. Carefully inspect the body before placing it in storage. Some storage suggestions include the following.

- Lay a large sheet of thick plastic down, place body bridges on top of the plastic sheet, and lay remains on top of body bridges.
- Cover the remains with a cotton hospital gown or a sheet, but do not cover the face or feet.
- Prepare a chemical wetting agent by mixing two-thirds of a gallon of humectant, 4-oz mold retardant (thymol or phenol), and 1 gallon of water. Semisaturate the body covering with the wetting agent. Reserve the rest in a spray bottle.
- Loosely cover the remains with the sheeting, trapping a moderate amount of air inside the sheeting.
- Place in a cool area.
- Check the remains every 3 to 4 days; aspirate or sponge out any liquid that has collected on the plastic, spray the gown or the sheet with the wetting agent, and reapply massage cream to facial and hand areas.
- Follow these guidelines until day of final viewing.
- Thoroughly wash and dry (so that no evidence of moisture exists) the remains, dress, and cosmetize.

Alternate preparation and storage methods can be found in the Selected Readings section of this book – see "The two year fix: long-term preservation for delayed viewing" by Kerry Don Peterson.

Anatomical Embalming

Today, medical schools around the country continue the practice of embalming bodies donated for anatomical purposes. Anatomical donation in the past has precluded the traditional funeral for the family. This in some cases has caused families not to proceed with donation. To address this issue, some state anatomical boards have created stipulations that allow funeral homes to initially embalm the bodies so that the families may have a visitation and funeral. In these situations, the anatomical board provides the directions for the embalming of the body. After the funeral, the body is delivered to the medical school and is re-embalmed. The majority of schools use a combination of pressure injection and gravity injection overnight to thoroughly perfuse the embalming fluid. Gravity injection is done through large

A

B

C

Figure 25–3. A. Excessive dehydration 2 years after preparation. **B.** Mold on foot and ankle 2 years after preparation. **C.** Loose epidermis of fingertips 4 years after preparation.

"percolators"; some will hold as much 8 gallons of solution. These are raised to a height of 6 to 9 feet above the body creating the pressure for the perfusion. The use of large arterial tubes helps to increase the rate of perfusion.

Most schools inject between 4.5 and 9 gallons of preservative, depending on the size of the body. Some medical schools use arterial embalming fluids available commercially from embalming fluid companies; other schools use special anatomical formulations. Formulations for anatomical embalming contain some or all of the following ingredients: formaldehyde, phenol, methanol, glycerine, formol, ethylene glycol, and isopropyl alcohol. Depending on how the body will be used, some schools drain the blood while others do not. There is no aspiration of bodies for medical schools (Fig. 25–3).

Many of the bodies used by medical schools are kept for 2 years or more. At the University of Pittsburgh, they currently have an embalmed body for 5 years and have in the past had one for 9 years. Desiccation and mold are two major concerns in keeping bodies for long time periods at medical schools. Some schools feel it is not necessary to submerge and soak the bodies after embalming; rather, they can be maintained indefinitely by using body bags with an antimold agent and humectant. Some schools refrigerate the bodies—not so much for preservation but for mold growth prevention.

Depending upon the use of the body, some bodies or body parts may indeed be frozen.

Preservation in this manner would be of value for either teaching or developing new surgical techniques.

▶ SHIPPING OF HUMAN REMAINS

Terminology

■ **Air tray:** used for casketed remains, only the bottom is made of wood, top sides and ends are made of heavy grade cardboard
■ **Burial-transit permit:** a disposition permit which is a legal document issued by a governmental agency, authorizing transportation and/or disposition of a dead human body

- **Combination case:** a transfer container consisting of a particleboard box with a cardboard cover used to ship a remains in place of a casket or air-tray
- **Common carrier:** any carrier required by law to convey passengers or freight without refusal if the approved fare of charge is paid; travels according to a set schedule (e.g., airlines, railroads)
- **Death certificate:** a legal document containing vital statistics, disposition, and final medical cause of death pertaining to a deceased human body
- **Hermetically sealed:** airtight, impervious to external influence; completely sealed by fusion or soldering
- **Human remains:** a dead human body or cremains
- **International:** between countries
- **Interstate:** between two or more states
- **Intrastate:** within one state
- **Private carrier:** an individual or a company that transports only in particular instances and only for those it chooses to contract with, for example, livery companies, private aircraft
- **Removal:** (first call or transfer of remains) transfer of remains from the place of death to a funeral establishment
- **TSA:** Transportation Security Administration
- **Ziegler case:** (liner) a gasket-sealed container that can be used as an insert into a casket or a separate shipping container

Shipping is the transportation of human remains away from the place of death to another location for final disposition. Human remains can be defined as a dead human body or cremains. The shipping (transportation) may be via a private carrier (e.g., hearse, van, airplane) operated by a funeral home, livery company, or family of the deceased; or a common carrier (e.g., commercial airline, train, bus). There are no definitive data on the number of human remains transported in a given year, but a conservative estimate might be 20,000 by common carrier within the United States. Shipping can be divided into three categories based on the destination of the remains: (1) intrastate, between cities within a state; (2) interstate, between cities located in two different states; and (3) international, between countries. Intrastate shipping or transporting of a body is the least complicated of the three. Each of these divisions can have its own rules and regulations for the transportation of human remains. A general rule is that all remains transported by common carrier **must** be accompanied by a burial-transit permit (or similar document). Some states issue a provisional transit permit when a death certificate has not been signed by a physician or a coroner; other states require that the medical examiner or the coroner be notified and provided with the cause of

death prior to consent being given for the transportation of the deceased. In some states, the local jurisdiction at the place of death may impose additional requirements, such as that the death certificate must be signed by a doctor before removing the deceased from a hospital or a place of death. From a legal standpoint, all the same criteria for release of the remains from the location of death must be met. This may include written authorization from the decedent's immediate next of kin or legal representative, an executor of the estate, or if no next of kin exists, the public administrator's office at the place of death can authorize release of the remains. Several states (e.g., California) require written authorization for embalming beyond what is required by the FTC. The FTC regulations do not change when the death takes place away from the area where the purchaser of the goods and services resides. If a funeral home embalms remains and it was not authorized by the person in charge of disposition, no charge can be made for the embalming. A funeral home serving an out-of-town funeral director must also release the remains, without receiving payment for its services, to another funeral home should there be a request to do so. A funeral home may not hold remains for payment.

Regardless of the type of shipment or carrier, certain rules apply for the preparation of the body.

- Thoroughly cleanse and embalm the remains; thoroughly dry the body.
- Pack all external orifices.
- Place the remains in a plastic garment (pants, coveralls, or unionalls).
- Partially dress the remains using underclothing, pajamas, or a hospital gown, and envelop in a clean sheet.
- When shipping by common carrier place the shrouded body on a sheet of plastic that can envelop the body.
- Do **not** place one hand over another, as this might not be the desired position.
- When shipping casketed remains, place a very heavy layer of cotton around the head and face to protect the casket and clothing from any purge; be certain to turn the pillow over for shipping to prevent soilage from purge or cosmetics.
- Secure the body on a cot if shipping within the container; if casketed, place the bed of the casket in the lowest position and move the feet to the furthest end; secure the head end so the body will not slide.
- Document the condition of the body before, during, and after embalming. Send a copy of the embalming report with the remains.
- Notify the receiving funeral director of any unusual conditions (e.g., trauma, obesity, edema).

Intrastate and interstate shipping regulations will usually be set by a governmental agency in the state where the death occurs (certification of the death would be filed in the state or county of the state where the death occurred). One or more agencies may formulate the rules relative to the removal of a dead human remains from the place of death to another location within or outside of the state. Shipping regulatory agencies may include a local or a state board of health, local or state bureau of vital statistics, state board of embalmers and funeral directors, local or state coroner or medical examiner's office, and transportation agencies (airline regulations, livery regulatory unions, etc.). There is no uniform, universal death certificate and vital statistics registry shared by all states and likewise there are no uniform regulations governing the transportation of dead human remains between states. For example, some states allow the transportation of dead human remains between cities within the state and outside of the state by private carrier without a burial transit permit; other states allow the transport of a body by private carrier with a temporary transit permit or no permit at all. Some local municipalities may make requirements such as the need for a signed death certificate before a body can be removed from an institution such as a nursing home, hospice, or hospital. Intrastate transportation is the least complicated of the three types of shipping.

For all human remains that will be shipped by common carrier (airline is the most utilized) new federal regulations were put into place after September 11, 2001. A new agency was formed called the TSA. They put into place the "Known Shipper Program" to identify all shippers of cargo (including funeral homes/services) and freight. Each individual airline is responsible to approve cargo shippers including funeral homes as a "known" shipper through their inspection and approval process. As of August 1, 2010, all human remains must be screened just as all carry on items are prior to placement on an aircraft. This may result in an earlier drop off time at the airport for the screening process prior to flight.

The type of screening that is being done includes X-ray of cargo and odor identifier that is used to detect explosives. The odor identifier however has been found to be triggered by formaldehyde. Any human remains that sets off alerts from a screening procedure must be quarantined and cannot be released back to the shipper. An approved Certified Cargo Screening Facility (CCSF) can then inspect the shipment and resolve the alarm issue. A funeral home can be certified as a CCSF. If a human remains shipment triggers an alarm, it will not be placed aboard any flight until it can be cleared. This can cause delays in the arrival of the deceased to their destination.

For intrastate and interstate shipping of cremated remains, the United States Post Office is the only method available. Federal Express, United Parcel Service (UPS), and other carrier services will not accept cremated remains for shipment. The majority of airlines will accept cremated remains for shipment within their small package cargo systems.

Regardless of the final destination—within the state, between states, or to a foreign country—there are responsibilities for both the shipping and the receiving funeral establishments. The shipping facility must

- Remove the remains from the place of death.
- Embalm and thoroughly preserve the remains, the exception being if shipping is to Israel.
- Prepare the Embalming Case Report—one copy to accompany the body and a second copy to remain in the shipping funeral home case file. If the deceased exhibits, facial disfigurement photos before and after preparation may be taken (with permission) to document the disfigurement.
- Secure the necessary documents for shipping and disposition.
- Arrange for private or common carrier transportation and, if necessary, the required container.
- Communicate to the receiving funeral establishment the condition of the remains and the time schedules of the carrier and provide the service as expediently as possible to relieve any anxiety on the part of the family and the receiving funeral establishment.

The receiving funeral establishment must

- Avoid making promises to the family about the time and the date of the funeral services.
- Cooperate with the shipping funeral establishment in providing statistical information for the filing of the death certificate and disposition information.
- Be prepared for unexpected delays due to weather, flight cancellations, and problems with a local coroner, medical examiner, or organ retrieval teams.

There are two types of containers used when shipping a body by common carrier. The "combination air tray," which is a wood-based container that has sides, ends, and inside top all made of wood (plywood or fiber board) with an exterior covering of cardboard. The shrouded remains are placed directly in the wood bottom and the sides, ends, and top are closed around the body. The second container is referred to as an "air tray." This container is for casketed remains with only the bottom being made of wood and the sides, ends, and top being of heavy-grade cardboard. These two containers are used throughout the United States and some foreign countries such as Great Britain. They come in infant, child, adult, and oversized units and are meant to be used **once,** with most airlines stringently enforcing this rule. Because of cargo door size limitations, the airline should always be consulted when using an oversized container. When booking the flight, advise the airline of the outside dimensions of the container. Many foreign countries still require an all-wooden box (previously known as a railroad box). The airline needs to be advised of the dimensions of the wooden box because some cargo holds for international flights will only accommodate one all-wooden box. Information on international shipping containers can be obtained from the consulate or shipping directory publications (e.g., **American Blue Book of Funeral Directors).**

International shipping is by far the most complicated type. The country where the body is to be buried has rules and regulations that must be followed before the transportation can take place. The funeral director at the place of death must notify the local consulate of the foreign country and obtain the regulations. In almost all countries today, permission must be granted for the deceased to enter the country. The foreign government where the remains are being shipped has an embassy in Washington, D.C. The embassy then has smaller branch offices in various locations within the United States called "consulates." Smaller countries may offer only an embassy to deal with; other countries may have consulates in most major cities. The consulate of jurisdiction may handle the affairs for a specific geographic region of the United States. The local funeral director who is shipping the remains will generally deal with this office in obtaining the necessary requirements and documentation. It should be noted that there are countries that have no diplomatic relations with the United States (e.g., Cuba), and shipping remains to these countries may not be possible or may need to be done through another foreign government. Remains cannot be shipped to countries where war has been declared between that country and the United States.

The consulate of jurisdiction will request documentation to be presented and will in turn provide documents that will allow entry of the remains into the country. Some consulates will accept faxing of the documents as originals. It is advised to check with the consulate to obtain its policy. Documents generally required can include the following:

- Certified copy of the death certificate
- Noncontagious disease letter issued by the local health department where the death occurred stating there are no contagious diseases or epidemics in the city or county of death

- Embalmer's affidavit saying the remains were embalmed in accordance with the laws of the state where the death occurred
- Noncontraband letter stating the casket contains only the body and clothing necessary for burial

A fee is usually paid to the foreign consulate for processing of the documents

When shipping overseas, some unusual requirements can be made by the foreign country. Examples include the following:

- Need for a sealing casket or a wood casket with a sealing Ziegler case inside
- An all-wood shipping container possibly lined with zinc and soldered closed
- Exact dimensions for the outer shipping box and the material of composition
- Bottom of the casket be filled with sawdust (Egypt)
- Israel does not require embalming, but if embalmed, the remains must be embalmed by the gravity method and no drainage taken
- Require embalming using chemicals illegal in the United States such as bichloride of mercury (Italy)

Individual airlines may also impose regulations on foreign shipments. Puerto Rico airlines, for example, requires a noncertified copy of the death certificate to be presented to the airline officials when the body is delivered to the airport. Some airlines require that they have written permission from the foreign country to allow them to bring the remains into the country. There are also significant security precautions taken. Examples include a security endorsement stating the container has no explosive devices, requiring the person dropping off the shipment to have two picture IDs, and a letter of certification that the shipment meets all Federal Aviation Administration rules and regulations. The shipment may need to be x-rayed, must arrive in the cargo area at a certain time, and no additional items are allowed to be placed inside the container. Shipments sent **unembalmed** can either be packaged in dry ice or in freezer packs similar to the kind used for food. Many airlines charge a premium for the shipment of dry ice because it is considered a hazardous material. The freezer packs come in much larger sizes and do not carry the tariff that dry ice does. The cost of shipment is per pound (or kilogram) weight and the airlines all require that the shipment be paid for at the time it is dropped off at their cargo area. It cannot be charged to an airline account. The length of time involved to process an international shipment can take anywhere from 5 to 14 business days. Most foreign consulates observe American holidays and do not work on weekends. Additionally, some foreign consulates require that one of their officers inspect the casket and container, and seal the outer box with wax and the seal of their government. This may require that the shipment first go to another larger city (e.g., Chicago, New York, Los Angeles) to fulfill this obligation.

Preparation of the Body for Shipping

Once the remains have arrived in the funeral home, the embalmer should inspect the body noting any problem conditions. The embalming process for shipping is based on the condition of the remains as they enter the preparation room from the place of death. The decision on arterial embalming solution should be based on these factors. All areas of the body need to be treated to guard against decomposition during the transportation, viewing, and the funeral. To achieve this, arterial injection supplemented by hypodermic injection and/or surface treatments may be necessary. If additional treatments are required, it may be necessary to communicate this to the receiving funeral home. This information should be contained on the embalming case report form but it is also advisable to relay the information over the phone. The communication of "a condition report" should be done by the embalmer to, at least, a funeral director at the receiving funeral home, **not** to secretarial help or an answering service. Both parties should clearly know the names of the person they spoke to in the event that questions come up later.

After embalming, the remains should be thoroughly bathed and dried so that no moisture is evident on the body. The nails, nose, and mouth should be cleaned. The nose and ears should have any hair removed. For women, facial hair should also be removed before embalming. Pack **all** external body orifices. Minimally, plastic pants or coveralls should be placed on all remains that are to be shipped—use additional plastic garments should any leakage be anticipated. An embalming powder should be placed inside the plastic garments to absorb any moisture and prevent mold or mildew.

Unless requested, restorative and cosmetic treatments are the responsibility of the receiving funeral home. Many embalmers who provide embalming for shipping **do not** glue the mouth and eyes shut. It would be advisable to check with the receiving funeral home to determine what they want done before shipping the remains. A light layer of massage cream can be applied to the face and hands.

Today, it is very important to prepare an embalming case report for all embalming cases regardless of the shipping status. This document can help protect all parties involved in case of a legal dispute. It is of particular importance when shipping because the receiving funeral home has no firsthand knowledge of the condi-

tion of the remains before embalming, what was done during the course of embalming, and what follow-up treatment might be needed upon arrival.

The body should be placed in underclothing, hospital gown, or pajamas and wrapped in a clean sheet prior to placement in the shipping container. The inside of the container should have a large sheet of plastic laid down and the body placed inside of it. This will prevent the wooden bottom of the combination unit from becoming soaked with body fluids in the event that the body develops leakage during transportation. The body should then be securely tied in place. The head should be placed on a Styrofoam head block or other elevation device. When the lid of the container is in place, it should not touch the nose or forehead. **The lid of the container must be nailed or screwed in place**. This prevents it from collapsing inside the container and causing damage to the remains. The "head" end should be clearly marked on the outside of the container along with the name of the deceased, the consignee (receiving funeral home and phone number), and the transportation arrangements. The necessary legal documents and embalming case report should be placed in a sealed envelope and placed on top of the container in the document envelope.

When the body is to be shipped in a casket, the remains should be secured in place with padding along the elbows and at the feet to prevent sliding during transit before shipping. Plastic should be placed around the head and neck to prevent any soilage should purge occur. The pillow should be turned over or have a piece of plastic covering it. Cover the face and hands to prevent any make-up from damaging the interior of the casket. If the casket has a moveable bed, it should be lowered to its lowest position. If the casket is a sealing type, it should **not** be cranked all the way shut to allow for any air pressure changes inside the cargo hold of the plane. The crank for the casket should be wrapped and placed on the outside of the casket so that it can be used by the receiving funeral home to open the casket. This is important as there are many different casket companies and some have a crank that is unique to a particular casket. The casket will be placed in an air tray and the information placed on the outside as suggested above.

▶ PREPARATION OF HUMAN REMAINS BY THE RECEIVING FUNERAL HOME

Under the best of circumstances, a funeral home that receives a human remains shipment will have to do only a small amount of preparation for viewing. This might be dressing and cosmetics or adjustments of cosmetics or clothing from flight air disturbances. In some situations, there might need to be extensive work and the paragraphs on re-embalming in this chapter should be reviewed.

Some general suggestions the funeral home may want to consider are as follows:

1. Inspect the remains and the external areas of the casket upon arrival at the funeral home for any problems or issues needing resolution. (Ideally, this should be within hours of the arrival.)
2. Use an **"embalming care report"** to document the condition of the remains and to identify any action that was taken to further prepare the remains. (This would include cosmetics, dressing, or any "embalming" that might need to be done.)
3. If extensive problems are present, a decision about family notification needs to be made. More documentation of the condition (i.e. photographs) may be required:
   a. Minor adjustments such as cosmetics or clothing generally do not require family notification unless the funeral home will be making a charge for the work done.
   b. For extensive problems, the funeral home will have to decide about charges for the care of the remains and whether a replacement casket is needed. The shipping funeral home may also need to be contacted if there are extensive problems.

Suggested protocol for inspection of the shipped-in body not casketed:

- Undress the remains and inspect all body areas for adequate preservation.
- Reinjection of localized areas may be necessary. Small areas can best be treated by hypodermic embalming.
- Reaspirate the body and if necessary reinject the cavities.
- Remove excess massage cream from face and hands.
- Be certain the mouth is dry and free of any purge material; reset and glue the mouth.
- Dry eyes and re-set and glue eyes (**often bodies shipped the mouth and eyes are not glued**).
- Tissue build hands and face where necessary.
- Apply cosmetics.
- Dress and casket the remains.
- Prepare **two copies** of the Embalming-Care Report – noting the condition of the body at the time of arrival and any necessary corrections and treatments. Retain one copy and send the other to the shipping funeral director or embalming facility.

▶ BIBLIOGRAPHY

American Board of Funeral Service Education, *Course Content Syllabus,* St. Joseph, MO: American Board of Funeral Service, 2008.

Army Regulation 638–2. Care and Disposition of Remains and Disposition of Personal Effects. Headquarters, Department of the Army, Washington, D.C., February 9 1996 (unclassified).

Basic factors relating to the embalming process. In: *Champion Expanding Encyclopedia,* Springfield, OH: Champion Chemical Co., September 1981.

Hirst T. Diagnose your cases before you start embalming. *American Funeral Director* March 1930.

Mayer R. The secret is in its strength. *The Director* April 1992.

Peterson KD. The two year fix: Long-term preservation for delayed viewing. *The Director* April 1992.

Sanders CR. Preventing restorative problems caused by delayed interment. *The Dodge Magazine* March/ November, 1997; January, 1998.

Shor M. Condition of the body dictates the proper embalming treatment, not cause of death. *Casket and Sunnyside* November 1972.

Strub CG. Embalmed body may become "disembalmed." *Casket and Sunnyside* 1966.

SECTION II
THE ORIGIN AND HISTORY OF EMBALMING

Edward C. Johnson, Gail R. Johnson, and Melissa Johnson

A statement in 1875 by the New York State Supreme Court is still relevant, concise, and conceptually complete:

> The decent burial of the dead is a matter in which the public have concern. It is against the Public Health if it does not take place at all and against a proper public sentiment should it not take place with decency.

Winston Churchill stated in his gifted style:

> Without a sense of history, no man can understand the problems of our time, the longer you can look back, the further you can look forward—the wider the span, the longer the continuity, the greater is the sense of duty in individual men and women, each contributing their brief life's work to the preservation and progress of the land in which they live, the society of which they are the servants.

Esmond R. Long, M.D., a medical historian, wrote:

> Nothing gives a better perspective of the subject than an appreciation of the steps by which it has reached its present state.

So it is with the subject of embalming. The authors of this chapter trust that this brief exposition of the origin and history of embalming will impart to the reader a sense of the tradition and technical advances achieved over nearly 5000 years that the art and science of embalming have been practiced. There is a clear indication that both tradition and new technical advances will continue to be maintained in the future.

Embalming, one of humankind's longest practiced arts, is a means of artificially preserving the dead human body.

1. **Natural means of preservation:** obtained without the deliberate intervention of humans
   a. *Freezing:* By this method, bodies are preserved for centuries in the ice and snow of glaciers or snow-capped mountains.
   b. *Dry cold:* A morgue located on the top of St. Bernard Mountain in Switzerland was so constructed to permit free admission of the elements. True mummies were produced as a result of the passage of the cold, dry air currents over the corpses.
   c. *Dry heat:* Natural mummies are produced in the extremely dry, warm areas of Egypt, south western America, and Peru.
   d. *Nature of the soil at the place of interment:* There are recorded instances of the discovery of bodies in a good state of preservation after long-term burial in a peat bog that had a high tannin content or in soils strongly impregnated with salts of aluminum or copper.

2. **Artificial means of preservation:** secured by the deliberate action of humans
   a. *Simple heat:* Simple heat is the means employed to preserve bodies in the Capuchin Monastery near Palermo, on the island of Sicily. The monastery is connected to a catacomb or underground burial vault composed of four separate chambers. Treatment of the bodies consists of slow drying in an oven that is heated by a mixture of slaked lime. The desiccated bodies, quite shrunken and light in weight, are placed in upright positions along the walls of the catacombs.
   b. *Powders:* In powder methods, the body is placed on a bed of sawdust mixed with zinc sulfate or other preserving powder.
   c. *Evisceration and immersion* (used by the Egyptians and others)
   d. *Evisceration and drying* (the Guanche method)
   e. *Evisceration, local incision, and immersion* (employed in Europe, particularly in France, during the period AD 650–1830)
   f. *Simple immersion* (in alcohol, brine, or other liquid preservatives)
   g. *Arterial injection and evisceration* (used by the Hunter brothers and others)
   h. *Cavity injection and immersion* (method of Gabriel Clauderus)
   i. *Arterial injection* (mode of treatment of Gannal, Sucquet, and many others)
   j. *Arterial injection and cavity treatment* (method in daily use by all present-day embalmers; generally taught in schools and colleges of embalming today)
   k. *Artificial cold* (by a system of refrigeration to reduce the body temperature to inhibit bacterial activity; in use in most hospitals and morgues today)

▶ PERIODS OF EMBALMING HISTORY

Embalming originated in Egypt during the period of the first dynasty. It is estimated to have begun around 3200 BC and continued until AD 650. The motive of Egyptian embalming was religious in that preservation of the human body (intact) was a necessary requirement for resurrection, which is their religious goal. During this nearly 4000-year period of embalming practice, there obviously existed a number of variations in this technique. Egyptian embalming began to decline with the advent of Christianity, as the early Christians rejected the practice, associating embalming with various "pagan religious rites." When the Arabs conquered Egypt, they too rejected the practice of embalming.

The second period of embalming history extends from AD 650 to 1861, and its principal geographical area of practice and growth was Europe. This era is termed the *Period of the Anatomists*, as the motive was to advance the development of embalming techniques for the preservation of the dead to permit detailed anatomical dissection and study.

The third or modern period of embalming history extends from 1861 to the present day. It is during this period that embalming knowledge, which had been transferred from Europe to America during the previous period, finally reverted to its original use, principally for funeral purposes. Embalming again became available to all who requested it. Motives in this period are diverse, with sentiment probably predominant, as the average person desires to view the decedent free of evidence of the ravages of disease or injury. Public transportation is another reason to embalm, as the procedure prevents a dead body from becoming offensive during a protracted period of travel and is required by many public transport agencies.

Although the value of embalming is disputed and debated to the public health, it is most apparent that a decaying, unembalmed body is surely a health menace to those exposed to its effluvia. From earliest Egyptian times, embalmers have been closely associated with the medical profession. In fact, most embalmers in the United States were doctors of medicine until the later portion of the nineteenth century.

▶ EGYPTIAN PERIOD

During the early predynastic period, well before 3200 BC, the Egyptians had a very simple culture. When death occurred, the unembalmed body was placed in the fetal position (arms and legs folded), wrapped in cloth or straw mats, and placed in a shallow grave scooped out of the desert sand west of the Nile River. A few pieces of pottery and other artifacts were placed in the grave with the body, which were positioned on its side. The body was preserved by drying, and from contact with the arid, porous sand and the total absence of rainfall, or other moisture. From time to time, desert winds uncovered the bodies in their shallow graves, and cemetery guards or relatives saw that the bodies were indeed preserved (Fig. 1).

Then, as now, there existed members of the society who were criminals, and some devoted themselves to grave robbing. When the cemetery custodians or family survivors of such elaborate burials noted the opening and desecration of burials, they also noted and were appalled that the corpse was no longer preserved, but had begun to decay. One attempt to forestall decomposition was the enclosure of the body within a solid stone coffin cut from a single mass of stone. The body of the coffin was without seams and the cover fit tightly. These burials were subsequently plundered, and again, the custodians or relatives contemplated the remains, which, to their horror, had on many occasions completely decomposed to a skeletal status. Without a scientific knowledge of the process of putrefaction, they expressed the belief that the stone coffin ate the soft tissues. To this day, massive bronze and copper caskets are termed *sarcophagi* from the Greek *sarco* for "flesh" and *phagus* for "eater." The Egyptians, not wishing to revert to their simple method of burial in the sands, found it necessary to devise some system of preserving the human body—embalming.

It is not too difficult to understand how Egyptian embalming was first developed when it is kept in mind that Egypt has a basically warm climate. The culture was such that hunting and fishing provided some of

Figure 1. Predynastic (3200 BC) Egyptian burial site, west of the Nile. The unembalmed corpse is in the fetal position, wrapped in straw matting. (*Courtesy of the Royal Ontario Museum.*)

the food requirements. Thus, a hunter or a fisherman might have a successful catch and secure more birds, fish, or game than he or his family could consume immediately. Such animals, fish, or birds could, like the human body, quickly decay and become worthless for food. The hunter, however, knew how to prepare his catch and to preserve it. He eviscerated and bled his catch and then, by one or another method such as salting, sun drying, smoking, or cooking, preserved it for future consumption. *(This procedure for the preservation of food was common knowledge and it requires little imagination to recognize the ease with which the basic food preservation process could be adapted with refinements to the preservation of the dead human body.)*

Variation in Embalming Methods

The actual methods of embalming employed by the Egyptians varied from dynasty to dynasty according to the custom and the technique of the individual embalmer. History provides views of four contemporary writers on the subject who have frequently been quoted.

The earliest account is that of the Greek historian Herodotus, who lived around 484 BC:

There are certain individuals appointed for the purpose [the embalming], and who profess the art; these persons, when any body is brought to them, show the bearers some wooden models of corpses; the most perfect they assert to be the representation of him whose name I take it impious to mention in this matter; they show a second, which is inferior to the first and cheaper; and a third which is cheapest of all. They then ask according to which of the models they will have the deceased prepared; having settled upon the price, the relations immediately depart, and the embalmers, remaining at home, thus proceed to perform the embalming in the most costly manner.

In the first place, with a crooked piece of iron, they pull out the brain by the nostrils; a part of it they extract in this manner, the rest by means of pouring in certain drugs; in the next place, after making an incision in the flank with a sharp Ethiopian stone, they empty the whole of the inside; and after cleansing the cavity, and rinsing it with palm wine, scour it out with pounded aromatics. Then, having filled the belly with pure myrrh pounded, and cinnamon, and all other perfumes, frankincense excepted, they sew it up again; having so done, they "steep" the body in natrum, keeping it covered for 70 days, for it is not lawful to leave the body any longer.

When the 70 days are gone by, they first wash the corpse, and then wrap up the whole body in bandages cut out of cotton cloth, which they smear with gum, a substance the Egyptians use instead of paste. The relations, having then received back the body, get a wooden case in the shape of a man to be made; and when completed, they place the body in the inside and then, shutting it up, keep it in a sepulchral repository, where they stand it upright against the wall. The above is the most costly manner in which they prepare the dead.

For such who choose the middle mode, from a desire of avoiding expense, they prepare the body as follows: They first fill syringes with oil of cedar to inject into the belly of the deceased, without making any incision, or emptying the inside, but by sending it in by the anus. This they then cork, to hinder the injection from flowing backwards, and lay the body in salt for the specified number of days, on the last of which they release what they had previously injected, and such is the strength it possesses that it brings away with it the bowels and insides in a state of dissolution; on the other hand, the natrum dissolves the flesh so that, in fact, there remains nothing but the skin and bones. When they have done this they give the body back without any further operation upon it.

The third mode of embalming, which is used for such as have but scanty means, is as follows: after washing the insides with syrmaea, they salt the body for the 70 days and return it to be taken back.

The second writer is Diodorus Siculus, who lived around 45 BC:

When anyone among the Egyptians dies, all his relations and friends, putting dirt upon their heads, go lamenting about the city, till such time as the body shall be buried. In the mean time they abstain from baths and wine, and all kinds of delicate meats, neither do they during that time wear any costly apparel. The manner of their burials is three-fold: one very costly, a second sort less chargeable, and a third very mean. In the first, they say, there is spent a talent of silver [$1,200]; in the second, 20 minae [$300]; but in the last there is very little expense [$75]. Those who have the care of ordering the body are such as have been taught that art by their ancestors. These, showing to the kindred of the deceased a bill of each kind of burial, ask them after which manner they will have the body prepared. When they have agreed upon the matter, they deliver the body to such as are usually appointed for this office. First, he who has the name scribe marks about the flank of the left side how much is to be cut away. Then he who is called the cutter or dissector, with an Ethiopian stone, cuts away as much of the flesh as the law commands, and presently runs away as fast as he can. Those who are present pursue him, cast stones at him, curse him, thereby turning all the execrations which they imagine due to his office upon him.

For whosoever offers violence, wounds, or does any kind of injury to a body of the same nature with himself, they think him worthy of hatred; but those who are called embalmers are worthy of honor and respect; for they are familiar with their priests and go into the temples as holy men without any prohibition. So soon as they come to embalm the dissected body, one of them thrusts his hand through the wound into the abdomen and draws out all the viscera but the heart and kidneys, which another washes and cleanses with wine made of palms and aromatic odors.

Lastly having washed the body, they anoint it with oil of cedar and other things for 30 days, and afterwards with myrrh, cinnamon, and other such like matters, which have not only a power to preserve it for a long time, but also give it a sweet smell; afterwards they deliver it to the kindred in such manner that every member remains whole and entire, and no part of it changed. The beauty and shape of the face seems just as it was before, and may be known, even the hairs of the eyebrows and eyelids remaining as they were at first. By this method many of the Egyptians, keeping the dead bodies of their ancestors in magnificent houses, so perfectly see the true visage and countenance of those that died many ages before they themselves were born that in viewing the proportions of every one of them, and the lineaments of their faces, they take as much delight as if they were still living among them.

The third account is given by Plutarch, who lived between AD 50 and 100:

The belly being opened, the bowels were removed and cast into the River Nile and the body exposed to the sun. The cavities of the chest and belly were then filled with the unguents and odorous substances.

The fourth description is by Perphry, who lived around AD 230 to 300:

When those who have care of the dead proceed to embalm the body of any person of respectable rank, they first take out the contents of the belly and place them in a separate vessel, addressing the sun, and utter on behalf of the deceased the following prayer, which Euphantus has translated from the original language into Greek: "O thou sun, our lord, and all ye gods who are the givers of life to men, accept me, and receive me into the mansions of the eternal gods; for I have worshiped piously, while I have lived in this world, those divinities whom my parents taught me to adore. I have ever honored those parents who gave origin to my body; and of other men I have neither killed any, nor robbed them of their treasure, nor inflicted upon them any grievous evil; but if I have done anything injurious to my soul, either by eating or drinking anything unlawfully, this offense has not been committed by me, but by what is contained in this chest." This refers to the intestines in the vessel, which is then cast into the River Nile. The body is afterwards regarded as pure, the apology having been made for its offenses, and the embalmer prepares it according to the appointed rites.

Differences in Translations

As may be observed, there were differences in embalming methods as described by the foregoing writers. This may be, in part, due to inaccuracies in copying and translating of the original manuscripts.

Present-day translations of the *Book of the Dead*, a textbook guide for the Egyptian embalmer, do not agree on the 70-day period for the covering with natron. One of the chronologies of the most costly method states that the 1st to the 16th days were occupied with evisceration, washing, and cleansing of the body; from the 16th to the 36th days, the body was kept under natron; from the 36th to the 68th days, the spicing and bandaging took place; and from the 68th to the 70th days, the body was coffined.

Steps in Egyptian Preparation

Step 1: Removal of the Brain. The brain was generally removed by introducing a metal hook or spoon into the nostril and by forcing it through the ethmoid bone to the brain. As much as possible was scooped out in this way. In some mummies, the brain was not removed. A few craniums had the brain removed through the eye socket. There is one case on record in which the evacuation of the cranium was accomplished through the foramen magnum, after excision of the atlas vertebra. After the body was removed from under natron, the cranium was usually repacked with linen bandages soaked in resin or bitumen. One writer tells of removing 27 feet of 3-inch linen bandage from the cranium of a mummy. Sometimes the cranium was filled with resin believed to have been introduced while molten with the aid of a funnel.

Step 2: Evisceration. Many bodies were not eviscerated. The earliest incision was made vertically in the left side, extending from the lower margin of the ribs to the anterior superior spine (crest) of the ilium. This incision would measure between 5 and 6 inches in length. At a later period, the incision became oblique, extending from a point near the left anterior spine (crest) of the ilium toward the pubis. A variant incision extended vertically from the symphysis pubis toward the umbilicus. In the very late 26th dynasty (665–527 BC), some bodies were eviscerated through the anus. The incision was usually made with a flint knife called Ethiopian stone because of its black color. All the viscera, with the exception of the kidneys and usually the heart, were removed, washed, and immersed in palm wine or packed in natron. (*Their disposition will be referred to later.*)

Step 3: Covering with Natron. Natron is a salt obtained from the dry lakes of the desert and is composed of chloride, carbonate, and sulfate of sodium and nitrate of potassium and sodium. Because of its corrosive action on the body, the embalmers had to affix the toes and fingernails to the body during the macerating period. This was accomplished by tying the nails on with thread or copper or gold wire. Alternatively, metal thimbles were fit over the ends of the fingers and toes for the same purpose. The body was then ready for the natron treatment. Early Egyptologists believed that the bodies were placed in a solution composed of natron dissolved in water, as described by Herodotus. Present-day authorities, in studying the original writing of Herodotus and other prime sources, detect a flaw in the translation of the text that is responsible for the misrepresentation. Present-day research, where the embalming process was recreated, indicates conclusively that only application of the concentrated dry salt over the body to some depth could dehydrate and preserve it. Experiments with different concentrations of the natron solution and immersion of specimens therein were largely unsuccessful in preventing decay.

Step 4: Removal from Natron. At the end of the 20th day of immersion in natron, the body was washed with water and dried in the sun.

Step 5: Wrapping and Spicing. The body was coated within and without by resin or a mixture of resin and fat. The skull was treated as in Step 1. The viscera, when removed from the body and not returned to the body, were placed in four canopic jars, the tops of which were surmounted by the images of the four children of Horus. Each jar held a specific portion of the viscera. The jar topped with the human head represented Imset and contained the liver. The jar covered with the jackal's head represented Duamutef and contained the stomach. The jar topped with the ape's head represented Hapy and held the lungs. The fourth jar, surmounted by a hawk's head, represented Qebeh-Snewef and contained the intestines. No mention is made of the disposition of the spleen, pancreas, or pelvic organs (Fig. 2).

Figure 2. Canopic urns—containers of the viscera removed during embalming preparation and not returned to trunk of body. From left to right are the jackal's head, Duamutef (contained stomach); the human head, Imset (contained liver); the ape's head, Hapy (contained lungs); and the hawk's head, Qebeh-Snewef (contained intestines). (*Courtesy of Paula Johnson De Smet.*)

The canopic jars varied in size and material. They were from about 9 to 18 inches in height and 4 inches in diameter and were made of alabaster, limestone, basalt, clay, and other materials. The canopic jars were usually placed in a wooden box and kept near the body. When the viscera were placed in these jars, images in miniature of the jars were returned to the cavity, which was padded in straw, resin-soaked linen bandages, or lichen moss. On return to the body cavity, the viscera were usually wrapped in four separate parcels to which specific images were attached, as mentioned earlier. Originally, the incision was not sewn but merely had the edges drawn together. Sometimes the edges were stuck together by resin or wax; however, there are recorded instances in the 18th, 20th, and 21st dynasties (respectively, 1700, 1250, and 1000 BC) of closure effected by sewing, which closely resembles the familiar embalmer's stitch of today. The incision was covered, whether sewn or not, by a plate of wax or metal on which the eye of Osiris (Egyptian god of the dead) was engraved.

Ancient Restorative Art

It was during this part of the preparation in the 20th dynasty (1288–1110 BC) that a little-known process was performed. Most present-day embalmers feel that the restoration to normal of emaciated facial features of a corpse is of comparatively recent origin. On the contrary, the Egyptian embalmers performed this operation, but on a much more extensive scale. Not only were the facial features restored, but the entire bodily contours were subcutaneously padded to regain their normal shape. The methods and materials used varied.

The mouth was usually internally packed with sawdust to pad out the cheeks, while the eyelids were stuffed with linen pads. Then, working from the original abdominal incision by burrowing under the skin of the trunk in all directions, the packing material was forced into these channels. In places such as the back and arms that could not be reached from the original incision, additional local incisions were made through which to pass the padding material. In later periods, the cheeks and temples were padded with resin introduced through openings in front of the ears. This material, introduced while warm, could be molded to conform to the desired contour. The packing materials most commonly used were resin, linen bandages, mud, sand, sawdust, and butter mixed with soda. It was also during this stage of preparation that repair of bodily injuries took place. Broken limbs were splinted, and bed sores were packed with resin-soaked linen bandages and covered with thin strips of antelope hide.

There is a case of a crooked spine having been straightened. Eyes were sometimes replaced with ones of stone or, as in one instance, with small onions. The bodies that were to be gilded (covered with golden leaf) were then treated. Some were completely covered with a gold leaf; on others, only the face, fingernails, and toenails, or genitals were gilded, as there was much variation on this matter. After the complete covering of the body with a paste of resin and fat, the bandagers set to work. It is believed that there were individuals who specialized in wrapping certain parts of the body such as the fingers, arms, legs, and head. Each finger or toe was first separately swathed; then each limb. The body was first covered with a kind of tunic and the face covered with a large square bandage followed by the regular spiral bandages. Pads were placed between the bandages to aid in restoration and maintenance of the bodily contour. Lotus blossoms have been found between the layers of linen bandages. Some authorities claim that the living saved cloth all their lives to provide bandages for use as mummy wrappings. The bandages varied from 3 to 9 inches in width and up to 1200 yards in length and were inscribed at intervals with hieroglyphics indicating the identity of the enswathed person. Authorities believed that only 1 of 10 mummies was prepared by the first method. The others were prepared by the cheaper methods, as described by the earlier writers. Another means of embalming used then was simple covering of the entire body with natron or molten resin. This latter process, while preserving the body, destroyed the hair and most of the facial features, fingers, and toes.

During the last 1000 years of Egyptian embalming practice, the emphasis gradually changed from producing a well-preserved body capable of withstanding decay for all eternity to creating an increasingly elaborate external appearance of the wrapped body. Wrapping patterns became quite elaborate and cartonage and plaster were employed to present a sometimes fanciful external recreation of the deceased. During the terminal centuries of Egyptian embalming, portraits on a flat surface were painted and placed over the head area, which more faithfully resembled the dead.

The Receptacles

The wrapped mummies were usually additionally encased and placed in boxes or coffins. An additional encasement, termed *cartonage*, was made of 20 or 30 sheets of linen cloth or papyrus saturated in resin, plaster of Paris, or gum acacia and placed over the wrapped body while wet. To ensure a tight fit, the material was drawn together in the back of the body by a kind of lacing not unlike present-day shoelacing. The cartonage, when dry, was as hard as wood and was covered with a thin coating of plaster, then painted with a representation of a human head and other designs. Two or more wood cases of cedar or sycamore might encase the cartonage and each other. These coffins or mummy cases were of different shape, depending on the period when they were

Figure 3. Wooden coffin. The body, placed inside, lies on its left side with the head at the end where eyes are drawn thus looking outward. (*Courtesy of Paula Johnson De Smet.*)

made. The outer wooden case was, at times, rectangular in shape with a cover resembling the roof of a house. Early coffined embalmed bodies were placed within the coffins lying on their side. The exterior of the coffin contained the representation of a pair of eyes on one side near the head of the coffin (Fig. 3). This indicated the position of the body facing outward at this point. Coffins shaped like the human form were termed anthropoid or mummiform (Fig. 4). If the deceased was a member

Figure 4. Wooden anthropoid or mummiform coffin. (*Courtesy of Paula Johnson De Smet.*)

of a great family, he might be enclosed within a stone sarcophagus, which was a stone coffin or vault fashioned of marble, limestone, granite, or slate.

Even in Egyptian times, the tombs of the dead were plundered for their valuables. Many mummy cases were broken open and the mummies themselves were damaged. The embalmers were called on to repair the damaged mummies and to rewrap and recoffin them. This may explain, in part, the so-called faking of mummies. In the Field Museum of Natural History in Chicago there are numerous x-ray pictures of unopened mummy cases and unwrapped mummies. Some of these pictures show damage that may have occurred prior to or during the course of embalming. One x-ray photo of a young child displays the complete absence of the arms and bilateral fractures of the femurs at about their midpoint, with the lower broken portion entirely missing. Museum authorities advance the theory that this was done to fit the child into a smaller mummy case. Another x-ray photo reveals a wrapped mummy lacking arms and the trunk of the body. The head was connected to the legs by a board and the body has been represented by padding of straw or lichen moss.

Additional faking may be the result of a curious custom of the early middle ages of using bits of mummies as good luck pieces and as a drug for internal consumption. This demand created a brisk business for the Arabs of North Africa, and as the supply of natural mummies was difficult to maintain, the Arabs began to produce their own from the bodies of lepers and criminal dead.

Animals were also embalmed, wrapped, and coffined in a manner similar to humans. The variety of animals so treated was large and included baboons, monkeys, full-grown bulls, gazelles, goats, sheep, antelopes, crocodiles, cats, dogs, mice, rats, shrews, hawks, geese, ibis, snakes, and lizards. X-ray examination of these wrapped packages discloses an occasional falsity. Some of these false mummies are composed of straw or rags wrapped in the form of the animal they were to represent. G. Elliot Smith, in his article on "The significance of geographical distribution of practice of mummification," states that knowledge of the Egyptian method of embalming was carried westward as far as the Canary Islands. He bases his decision on the similarity of the embalming procedures carried on in these areas of the world and the knowledge that the Egyptian method preceded those in all other known parts of the world.

Recreation of the Ancient Mummification Process
The Greek historian Herodotus wrote of the ancient mummification practice while visiting Egypt in approximately 450 BC. It was a fascinating description of the nearly 70-day process and the tools, processes, and ceremony that surrounded the preservation process.

Although this account has existed for centuries and we have seen the mummies that have been preserved through this process, there has never been a modern understanding of what takes place. In 1994, Robert Brier, an Egyptologist with the C.W. Post Campus of Long Island University, and Ronald Wade, the Director of Anatomical Services at the University of Maryland Medical School in Baltimore, Maryland, embarked on an amazing research study. They set out to recreate an authentic Egyptian mummy using the process and tools described by Herodotus. To be true to the process, they had replicas of the original tools made by a silversmith, they had a wood artisan construct an embalming table, and they visited Egypt to obtain the oils, spices, amulets, and Nile natron salt. Additionally, they had the ceramics department at C.W. Post make canopic jars to hold the internal organs.

The modern day mummy was an elderly gentleman who donated his body to science. The body was placed on the embalming table and the process of making the mummy began with the removal of the subject's brain through the nose. Brier and Wade used the replicated "hook" to break through the ethmoid bone. The ethmoid bone is a thin bone that is located at the back of the nose and leads directly into the brain. Although the description by Herodotus suggests that the hook was used to actually remove the brain, Brier and Wade found that this was not the case. They used the hook to pulverize the brain and then turned the body over on its stomach and allowed it to drain out of the nose.

The procedure then calls for the removal of the thoracic and abdominal organs. This was done using a sharpened black stone according to Herodotus. The recreated bronze tools initially did not work because they dulled too quickly. Brier and Wade then used a stone called obsidian that was sharpened, and they made an incision in the left side of the abdomen to remove all the organs except the heart. The heart was considered to be the essence of the individual. The body cavities were then washed with a combination of palm wine and myrrh, whereas the brain cavity was washed with palm wine and frankincense. The body cavities were then filled with bags filled with natron. The body was then completely covered with 600 pounds of natron and placed in a room to recreate the climatic conditions that would have been found in ancient Egypt 3000 years before. The body was left for 35 days and then rubbed with oils of frankincense, myrrh, palm, lotus, and cedar. The body itself had lost over 100 pounds of water from its original weight of 160 pounds. Brier and Wade then removed tissue samples for bacterial sampling and the results were all negative for any growth. Using linen bandages and shrouds purchased in Egypt, they wrapped the body over a 6-day time period. The body was wrapped in six layers and the traditional amulet was placed directly above the heart. The mummy currently resides at the University of Maryland Anatomical Services Laboratory.

► THE PRACTICE OF BODY PRESERVATION OF VARIOUS ETHNIC GROUPS AND PLACES

Jews. The Jews did not embalm but simply washed and shaved the body and swathed it in sheets, between the folds of which were placed spices such as myrrh and aloes. The purpose of herbs and spices was to disguise the odor of decay of the body, not to preserve it.

Ancient Persians, Syrians, and Babylonians. Sometimes the ancient Persians, Syrians, and Babylonians immersed their human dead in jars of honey or wax. Alexander the Great was said to have been so treated to preserve his body during the long journey from his place of death in Babylon in 323 BC (during a military campaign) to Egypt.

Ancient Ethiopians. The ancient Ethiopians eviscerated and desiccated their dead in a manner similar to the Egyptian method. The bodily contours were restored by applying plaster over the shrunken skin. The plaster-covered corpse was then painted with lifelike colors and given a coating of clear resinlike substance believed by some authorities to be a fossil salt and by others to be a type of amber, somehow rendered fluid at the time of application.

Canary Islands. (from at least 900 BC). In the Atlantic Ocean, about 4 degrees south of the Madeira Islands, on the northwest coast of Africa, there is a cluster of 13 islands known as the Canary Islands. These islands were not subdued by any European nation until the Spaniards overran them in the late fifteenth century. The original inhabitants, known as Guanches, are thought to have been descendants of the lost continent of Atlantis. It is believed that only prominent and influential families had the dead embalmed. The Guanches' method of embalming their dead is very similar to the Egyptian method.

The Guanche embalmers were both men and women who performed the services for their own sex. These embalmers were well paid, although their touch was considered contaminating and they lived in seclusion in remote parts of the islands. On the death of a person, the family bore the body to the embalmers and then retired. The embalmers placed the body on a stone table and an opening was made in the lower abdomen with a flint knife called a *tabona*. The intestines were withdrawn, washed, cleaned, and later returned to the body. The entire body, inside and outside, was very thoroughly saturated with salt and the intestines were returned to the body along with numerous aromatic plants and herbs.

The body, anointed with butter, powdered resin, brushwood, and pumice, was exposed to the sun, or, if the sun was not hot enough, the body was placed in a stove to dry. During the drying period, the body was maintained in an extended position; the arms of men were placed along the sides of the body, whereas women's arms were placed across the abdomen.

The embalmers maintained a constant vigil over the body during this period to prevent it from being devoured by vultures. On the 15th or 16th day, the drying process should have been complete and the relatives would claim the body and sew it in goatskins. Kings and nobles were, in addition, placed in coffins of hollowed juniper logs. All bodies were deposited in caves in the hilly regions of the islands.

In another method of preparation described, a corrosive liquid believed to be juice of the spurge or euphorbia plant was either introduced through the belly wall or poured down the throat; this was followed by the drying process described earlier. The mummies produced by these processes were called *xaxos* and the method of embalming was believed to have been introduced from Egypt about 900 BC. In T. J. Pettigrew's *History of Egyptian Mummies*, there is a description of a *xaxos* as found by a sea captain in 1764. The author points out the "flesh of the body is perfectly preserved, but it is dry, inflexible and hard as wood . . . nor is any part decayed. The body is no more shrunk than if the person had been dead only two or three days. Only the skin appears a little shriveled and of a deeply tanned, copper color." The *xaxos* were extremely light in weight, averaging about 6 to 9 pounds for bodies up to 5 1/2 feet in length.

Peru. Preservation of the body in Peru was practiced for at least a 1000 years before the Spanish conquest in the early sixteenth century. It had for its motive a religious belief in the resurrection of the body. Most authorities agree that the Peruvians had no process of embalming, but that their mummies were a product of the extremely dry climate of the region. There are reports that the Incas or ruling classes were embalmed, and because only mummies of the common people have been discovered, this report may be true. The manner in which the Inca rulers are believed to have been prepared was by evisceration. The intestines were placed in gold vases, the cavity filled with an unspecified resin, and the body coated with bitumen. The bodies were said to have been seated on their thrones, clothed in their regal robes, hands clasped on the breast, and head inclined downward. There is mention of the use of gold to plate or replace the eyes.

The usual Peruvian mummy, of which there are many specimens in the Field Museum at Chicago, was often found buried with the face toward the west, together with provisions of corn and coca contained in earthen jars. The mummies themselves were wrapped in cloth and tied with a coarse rope. The outer covering was of matting and followed a roll of cotton that, in turn, enveloped a red or varied-color wool cloth wrapped about the body. The innermost wrapping was a white cotton sheet. The corpse was found in a squatting position, knees under chin, arm over breast, with the fists touching the jaws. The hands were usually fastened together, and on most mummies, there was a rope passed three or four times around the neck. In the mouth, there was usually a small copper, silver, or gold disk. The greater part of the mummies was well preserved, but the flesh was shriveled and the features were disfigured. The hair was preserved, with the women's hair braided. Nearly all types of animals and birds have been found mummified, including parrots, dogs, cats, doves, hawks, heron, ducks, llamas, vicunas, and alpacas wrapped in the manner of human mummies.

Ecuador. The Jivaro Indians of the Marano River region of South America had a method of preserving heads by shrinking them. Technically, this process does not come under the heading of embalming, but a brief general description of the process is of interest.

The bones of the skull were first removed through long slits in the scalp. The skin of the head, with the hair attached, was boiled in water containing astringent herbs. On completion of this process, hot stones of gradually diminishing size were inserted into the space formerly occupied by the skull bones. When the shrinking process was completed, the stones were removed and the incisions were sutured as were the mouth and eyes. The finished shrunken head is about the size of a man's fist, with the features rather clear and retaining their proper proportions. It has been stated that this same process has been applied to an entire human body with equal success, although no such specimens have been found.

Mexico and Central America—Aztecs, Toltecs, and Mayans. On the basis of information received from Alfonso Caso, Mexico's outstanding anthropologist, there is no evidence of the employment of any artificial means of preservation of the body in the pre-Spanish era in these regions. There are accounts of finding mummies wrapped in matting and buried in the earth or in caves, but it is the opinion of Caso and others that such mummification was the result of the natural climate of the region.

North American Indians. Although no proof exists to substantiate claims that some of the Indian tribes embalmed their dead, there are quotes from two accounts of embalming means as recounted by H. C. Yarrow in his *Study of Mortuary Customs of North American Indians* from 1880, collected from earlier publications. On page 185 of the *History of Virginia* (Beverly, 1722), this statement is found:

> The Indians are religious in preserving the corpses of their kings and rulers after death. First they neatly flay off the skin as entire as they can, slitting only the back; then they pick all the flesh off the bones as clean as possible, leaving the sinews fastened to the bones, that they may preserve the joints together. Then they dry the bones in the sun and put them into the skin again, which in the meantime has been kept from shrinking. When the bones are placed right in the skin, the attendants nicely fill up the vacuities with a very fine white sand. After this they sew up the skin again, and the body looks as if the flesh had not been removed. They take care to keep the skin from shrinking by the help of a little oil or grease, which saves it from corruption. The skin being thus prepared, they lay it in an apartment for that purpose, upon a large shelf raised above the floor. This shelf is spread with mats for the corpse to rest easy on, and screened with the same to keep it from the dust. The flesh they lay upon hurdles in the sun to dry, and when it is thoroughly dried, it is sewed up in a basket and set at the feet of the corpse, to which it belongs.

Another account appeared in Volume XIII, page 39, of *Collection of Voyages* (Pinkerton, 1812), concerning the Werowance Indians:

> Their bodies are first bowelled, then dried upon hurdles till they be very dry, and so about most of their joints and neck they hang bracelets or chains of copper, pearl and such like, as they are used to wear. Their innards they stuff with copper beads, hatchets and such trash. Then they lap them very carefully in white skins and so roll them in mats for their winding-sheets.

The Indians are known to have wrapped their dead in cloth or leather and to have suspended the bodies in a horizontal manner in trees or buried them in the earth, in caves, or in the ground covered by rocks. This may have had a religious significance, but more likely it was done to prevent vultures or animals from devouring the dead.

Aleutian Islands and Kodiak Archipelago. It is believed that the inhabitants of the Aleutian Islands and Kodiak Archipelago practiced preservation of their dead from at least AD 1000, although the custom did not prevail on the mainland. The internal organs were removed through an incision in the pelvic region and the cavity was refilled with dry grass. The body was placed in a stream of cold running water, which was said to have removed the fatty tissues in a short time. The corpse was removed from the water and wrapped in the fetal posture, knees under the chin and arms compressed about the legs. This position was accomplished by use of force, breaking bones if necessary. In this posture, the body was sun-dried and, as a final gesture, was wrapped in animal skins and matting.

▶ PERIOD OF THE ANATOMISTS (AD 650–1861)

With the Arabic conquest of Egypt and the fall of the Roman Empire, European and Mediterranean civilizations declined virtually to the vanishing point. The old world of law and order as the Romans and others knew it was replaced by anarchy. Geographical areas were ruled by bands of armed men with little stability of control. The Dark Ages were to continue until the year 1000 when a gradual elimination of unstable leaders left a few more wise and capable individuals in charge of substantial geographical divisions of Europe. With a return to a more normal civilized existence came the establishment of schools and colleges in what is today Sicily, Italy, France, and England and later in Germany, Holland, Belgium, and Switzerland. The schools were, in part, the product of the Catholic Church, which throughout the Dark Ages had maintained and served as a sanctuary for work in the fields of medicine, nursing, teaching, copying of manuscripts, and establishment of orphanages and poorhouses.

The medical schools that were established used some texts originally written during the glory era of Egypt. In Alexandria, on the Mediterranean at the mouth of the Nile, there existed the greatest center for teaching that history had known. The library, before its destruction, was said to have contained more than half a million manuscripts on subjects varying from astronomy to mathematics to engineering to medicine. It was here that a famous teacher and practitioner of medicine, Claudius Galen (130–200 AD), born in Pergamum, Asia Minor, taught and wrote on the subject of anatomy. His textbook on anatomy described human anatomy principally from dissections of animals such as the pig or monkey. It must be obvious today that there are substantial differences or variations between the anatomical structure of the pig or monkey and those of the human being. Galen and others were not encouraged to dissect the human body as it was considered a mutilation and a crime under Egyptian law. Nevertheless, Galen's teachings and writings on human anatomy were to be considered as the unchallengeable authority for the next 1000 to 1200 years.

With the emergence of Europe from the Dark Ages came a craving for learning that had to that time been suppressed. The medical schools lacked the authority to legally acquire dead human bodies for dissection and anatomical study until the thirteenth and early fourteenth centuries. Such authority was granted in 1242 by Frederick II, King of the Two Sicilies, and again in 1302 for the delivery of two executed criminals to the medical school at Bologna, Italy, each year for dissection. Such dissections were public affairs, often conducted in open areas or amphitheaters always during the cold months of the year because the dissection subjects were not preserved. The dissection itself was rapid, frequently confined to a 4-day period. In the actual procedure, the anatomy professor, who was seated, read from Galen's text on anatomy while pointing out (with a wand) the body structures mentioned by Galen. An assistant, a barber-surgeon, did the actual dissection as the lecture progressed. Obviously, there were frequent contradictions between Galen's description of a body part and its actual appearance as disclosed by the dissection. These most evident discrepancies encouraged the more intelligent student and medical practitioner to steal bodies from cemeteries and gallows for personal study and research. Every part of such a purloined cadaver was probed speedily for knowledge of its structure or function until it became too loathsome to conceal and had to be disposed of. In many cases, the soft tissues were thrown away and the bones boiled to secure the skeleton.

Military Religious Campaigns

During the period from 1095 to 1291, a series of military religious campaigns mounted by the Christian nations of Europe, termed the *crusades*, were conducted to recapture the Holy Land from the Moslems. The campaigns were successful early on, but with the passing of time, the Christian occupation forces in the Holy Land became complacent and less martial and eventually were expelled from the entire conquered territory. Many prominent members of the nobility, including King Louis XIX of France, died far from home during the crusades. To allow the return to their homeland of their remains, it was necessary to develop what became a gruesome procedure, as no certain means of embalming was available during the campaigns. The procedure consisted of disemboweling and disarticulating the body, cutting off all soft tissues, and then boiling the bones until they were free of all soft tissues. The bones were then dried and wrapped within bull hides and returned to their homeland by the couriers who maintained the communication lines.

In 1300, Pope Boniface VIII issued a papal bull (a directive) that prohibited the cutting up of the dead for the purpose of transport and burial under penalty of excommunication. For a brief period, this papal bull was interpreted by some members of the medical profession as a directive to ban anatomical dissection. For example, in 1345, Vigevano stated that dissection was prohibited, and Mondino (1270–1326) said sin was involved in boiling bones. In any case, such interpretations were rare and were seldom given any regard by the majority of anatomists.

As the years passed, it became obvious that some system of preservation, even temporary, had to be contrived to permit a more careful and intensive study of body structure. Early efforts of preservation followed the ancient regimen of drying the parts, for moisture was and is the enemy of preservation. Preservation by drying of cadavers or their components was first sought by exposure to the natural heat of the sun. Later, use of controlled heat in ovens was employed to accomplish desiccation. Eventually, while probing the nature and extent of the hollow blood vessels, it was noted that warm air forced through the blood vessels removed blood and eventually dried out the tissue.

Reports of preservation attempts from the fifteenth century did not include injections of the blood vascular system. Such early injections into hollow structures of the body were made to trace the direction and continuity of blood vessels or to inflate hollow organs so as to reveal their size and shape or to make internal castings of areas under study. As early as 1326, Alessandra Giliani of Italy injected blood vessels with colored solutions that hardened; Jacobus Berengarius (1470–1550) employed a syringe and injected veins with warm water; Bartolomeo Eustaschio (1520–1574) used warm ink; Regnier De Graaf (1641–1673) invented a syringe and injected mercury; Jan Swammerdam (1637–1680) injected a waxlike material that later hardened. The great artist Leonardo Da Vinci (1452–1519), who is said to have dissected more than 30 corpses to produce hundreds of accurate anatomical illustrations, injected wax to secure castings of the ventricles of the brain and other internal areas.

Early Instruments for Injection

Early instruments for injection were crude and usually made in two parts: a container for the injection material and some form of cannula. The cannula was often contrived from a hollow straw, feather quill, hollow metal, or glass tube that was attached by ligature to an animal bladder (stomach or intestine). The cannula was inserted into the hollow opening being studied and the bladder tied onto its free end. The bladder, in turn, was filled with a liquid and then tied to retain the bladder full. Entrance of the liquid material into the hollow area was secured by squeezing the bladder until it emptied.

As early as 1521, Berengarius wrote of using a forerunner of the modern syringe. Early syringes similar to the hypodermic syringes employed today were constructed. They were filled and then attached to a cannula in position within the opening to be injected. To refill the syringe, the operator had to detach the syringe from the cannula, refill it, and then reattach it.

Bartholin (1585–1629) developed the first continuous-flow syringe. It could be recharged during use without halting the injection process.

One of the best accounts of nonanatomical embalming for burial purposes is related by the Dutch physician Peter Forestus (1522–1597), who wrote about embalming. His account, in German, is contained as an appendix in the 1605 edition of Peter Offenbach's treatise on *Wound Surgery*. Forestus specifically described the embalming process and the materials used in five named cases between 1410 and 1548, two of which he personally performed:

1410	Pope Alexander V of Bologna, Italy
1511	Lady Johanna of Burgundy, Holland
1537	Bishop Magoluetus of Bologna, Italy
1582	Countess of Hautekerken of The Hague, Holland
1584	Princess Auracius of Holland

As these cases are essentially similar, only one embalming report is cited in its entirety.

Most of the above-mentioned embalmings were performed in the room of the residence where the death occurred, a practice rather commonly followed later (well into the twentieth century) in many countries including the United States.

The following is the full description of the Forestus embalming of the Countess of Hautekerken. The others listed are quite similar with some individual variations such as opening the cranium and removing the brain and making long and deep incisions in the extremities to press out the blood, then filling the incisions with the powdered mixture.

I personally was bidden to embalm the Countess of Hautekerken, who was a daughter of a nobleman of Egmont (Holland) and who died of childbirth on January 9, 1582 at The Hague (Holland) before Johannes Heurnius (1543–1604), my good friend, and professor at Leyden in Holland was asked. Preceding all things, before the embalmment was begun, there was made the following preparation . . . I took $2\frac{1}{2}$ lbs. aloes; myrrh, $1\frac{1}{2}$ lbs.; ordinary wermut, seven hands-full; rosemary, four handsfull; pumice, $1\frac{1}{2}$ lbs.; marjoran, 4 lbs.; storacis calamata, 2 loht; the zeltlinalipta muscata, $\frac{1}{2}$ loht. Mix all and reduce to a powder. Lay open the trunk of the body, remove all the viscera, afterwards take such sponges which were previously immersed in cold fresh water, afterwards dipped in aqua vita, and wash out the interior of the body by hand with the sponge. This having been done, fill the cavities (of the body) with a layer of cotton moistened in aqua vita; sprinkle over it a layer of the previously mentioned powders; place another layer of the moistened cotton and a layer of powder one over the other until the abdomen together with the chest is entirely full. Afterwards sew the above (abdominal walls) again together. Wrap around (the body) with waxed cloth and other things. Now having heard this you understand this embalmment was performed by me, the aforementioned Heurnius and Arnold the Surgeon on January 10, 1562, in the dwelling of the wellborn Count and Countess Von Wassenaer in The Hague.

Ambroise Paré (1510–1590)

Born in France, Ambroise Pare was military barber-surgeon and eventually surgeon to French Kings Henri II, Francois II, and Charles IX. He was famous for re-discovery and improvement of use of ligature to control bleeding after amputations, podalic version (changing the position of an unborn infant within the uterus) to facilitate delivery, and designing of artificial limbs. Paré, like many surgeons of the period, embalmed the bodies of prominent military leaders and noblemen killed during military campaigns as well as similarly prominent civilians dying of natural causes.

In one of his books written in 1585 and entitled *Apology and Account of His Journeys into Diverse Places*, Paré described embalming a follower of the Duke of Savoy, a Monsier de Martiques, who died following a gunshot wound through the chest received in battle. The embalming was followed by coffining and transportation to the home of the deceased.

In his book, *The Works of Ambroise Pare*, translated into English and published in London in 1634, he devotes a portion of the 28th chapter, "On the Manner Howe to Embalme the Dead":

> But the body which is to be embalmed with spices for very long continuance must first of all be embowelled, keeping the heart apart, that it may be embalmed and kept as the kinsfolkes shall thinke fit. Also the braine, the scull being divided with a saw, shall be taken out. Then shall you make deepe incisions along the armes, thighes, legges, backe, loynes, and buttockes, especially where the greater veines and arteries runne, first that by this means the blood may be pressed forth, which otherwise would putrifie and give occasion and beginning to putrefaction to the rest of the body; and then that there may be space to put in the aromaticke powders; and then the whole body shall be washed over with a spunge dipped in aqua vita and strong vinegar, wherein shall be boyled wormewood, aloes, coloquintida, common salt and alume. Then these incisions, and all the passages and open places of the body and the three bellyes shall be stuffed with the following spices grossely powdered. Rx pul rosar, chamomile, balsami, menthe, anethi, salvia, lavend, rorismar, marjoran, thymi, absinthi, cyperi, calami aromat, gentiana, ireosflorent, assacederata, caryophyll, nucis moschat, cinamoni, styracis, calamita, benjoini, myrrha, aloes, san-

tel, omnium quod sut ficit. Let the incisions be sowed up and the open spaces that nothing fall out; then forthwith let the whole body be anointed with turpentine, dissolved oyle of roses and chamomile, adding if you shall thinke it fit, some chymicall oyles of spices, and then let it be againe strewed over with the forementioned powder; then wrap it in a linnen cloath, and then in cearecloathes. Lastly, let be put in a coffin of lead, sure soudred and filled up with dry sweete hearbes. But if there be no plenty of the forementioned spices, as it usuall happens in besieged townes, the chirurgion shall be contented with the powder of quenched lime, common ashes made of oake wood.

The procedure described by Paré was the most prevalent in use from the end of the Egyptian system to well past the discovery of arterial injection.

Discovery of a New Technique

Anatomical dissection, nonpreservative injections, and study continued until inevitably the technique of arterial injection of some preservative substance into the blood vascular system to secure an embalmed subject was stumbled upon. Contrary to popular belief, three men, all Dutch and all friends, were involved and must be recognized for their contributions to the technique: Jan Swammerdam (1637–1680), the original inventor or discoverer; Frederick Ruysch (1638–1731), the great practitioner who refined the technique; and Stephen Blanchard (1650–1720), the person who openly published the method.

Swammerdam was educated in medicine but devoted the greatest part of his life to the study of insects and small animals. He perfected a system of injection to preserve even insects through tiny cannulas made of glass and manipulated by the aid of microscopes designed by Leeuwenhoek (the inventor of the microscope). His preservatives were said to have included various forms of alcohol, turpentine, wine, rum, spirits of wine (purer form of alcohol), and colored waxes. This injection technique was transmitted to Ruysch who applied it to human subjects, both entire bodies and portions thereof. His superb collections of anatomical specimens provided great teaching aids. His embalming of complete human remains included individuals such as British Admiral Sir William Berkley, who was killed during a sea battle off Holland in 1666, and whose body was recovered from the sea in a decomposing condition. Ruysch was requested by the Dutch government to embalm the body so that it might be returned to England for funeral and burial. It is said that the body was normal in appearance and color after his treatment.

In another episode, the Russian Czar Peter the Great, during one of his visits to western Europe, visited the medical school of Leiden, Holland, and Ruysch's home, where his museum was situated. During the visit with Ruysch, it is related that some domestic problem required Ruysch's attention and he left Czar Peter alone for a few minutes. Czar Peter began to explore the various rooms and, in opening one door, discovered an infant apparently asleep. Tiptoeing into the room he contemplated the beautiful pink child, then bent down and kissed it, only to discover by its cold exterior that it was one of Ruysch's many preparations. Czar Peter purchased one entire museum collection from Ruysch, which some historians report was lost or destroyed. The truth is that it is still on exhibit in Leningrad today. Ruysch personally never did make a full disclosure of his technique or preservative. There are many who conjecture that his preservative was alcohol, turpentine, or even arsenic.

Blanchard, an anatomist of Leiden, published a book in 1688 entitled *A New Anatomy with Concise Directions for Dissection of the Human Body with a New Method of Embalming*. Pages 281 to 287 and several diagrams of syringes and instruments constitute the appendix describing his method of embalming. He mentions the use of spirits of wine and turpentine. In one of his embalming treatments, he began by flushing out the intestinal tract by first forcing water from the mouth to the anus. Then he repeated the flushing with spirits of wine and retained it in place by corking the rectum. He opened large veins and arteries and flushed out the blood with water, then injected the preservative spirits of wine. **(This technique described in the book appears to be the earliest mention of injection of the blood vessels for the specific purpose of embalming.)**

Gabriel Clauderus (Late Seventeenth Century)

Gabriel Clauderus, a physician from Altenburg, Germany, was a contemporary of De Bils. In 1695, he published a book, *Methodus Balsamundi Corpora Humani, Alique Majora Sine Evisceratione*, in which he described his method of embalming, which omitted evisceration. His fluid was made from 1 pound of ashes of tartar dissolved in 6 pounds of water, to which was added $\frac{1}{2}$ pound of sal ammoniac. After filtration, it was ready for use and was denominated by Clauderus as his "balsamic spirit." He injected this fluid into the cavities of the body and then immersed the cadaver in the fluid for 6 to 8 weeks. The treatment was concluded by drying the corpse either in the sun or in a stove.

England's Customs and Achievements

Although the British Isles are geographically grouped with Europe, they developed different customs and their scientific achievements advanced at a pace different from that in continental Europe.

Some individuals regard the Company of Barber–Surgeons of London to be the first group licensed to embalm. A brief examination of the background of this organization reveals that from about 1300 to 1540, the Company of Barbers and the Guild of Surgeons were separate entities. In 1540, they received a charter from Henry VIII consolidating these two groups under the title of the Company of Barber–Surgeons and granting them the right to anatomize four executed criminals each year. In 1565, Queen Elizabeth I granted the same privilege to the College of Physicians. In 1745, the Surgeons and Barbers ended their joint relationship and again became two separate organizations. During the Barber–Surgeons period, they were permitted to be the sole agency for embalming and for performing anatomical dissections in the city of London, although there is no record of any of the bodies for anatomy being embalmed.

This was never a well-respected or enforced monopoly. In their 200-year existence, there were fewer than 10 complaints, and in several of the cases cited in the College of Barber–Surgeons records, no fines or other punishment is noted. In several cases, no conclusion of the case appears. Most complaints were lodged against members for performing private anatomical dissections not on the premises of the College. The more influential members such as William Cheselden and John Ram simply ignored the rule and even withdrew from the organization as William Hunter did. **(The Barber–Surgeons made no progress in the development of licensing of embalmers as such, and even today in the British Isles, no license or permit is needed from any governmental agency to perform embalming and never has been so required.)**

William Hunter, M.D.

William Hunter (1718–1783) was born in Scotland and studied medicine at the University of Glasgow and at Edinburgh. He finally settled in London where he specialized in the practice of obstetrics and taught anatomy. He became one of the great teachers of anatomy in English medical history and received many awards and appointments to honor societies, climaxed in 1764 by his appointment as Physician-Extraordinary to Queen Charlotte of England. He was the author of many brilliant treatises on medical subjects, perhaps the greatest being his *Anatomy of the Gravid Uterus*. His private collections of anatomical and pathological specimens, together with his lecture and dissecting rooms, occupied a portion of his home. All of this, plus a large sum of money, were donated to the University of Glasgow after his death.

Hunter was in the habit of delivering, at his private school at the close of the anatomical lectures, an account of the preparation of anatomical specimens and embalming of corpses. He injected the femoral artery with a solution composed of oil of turpentine, to which had been added Venice turpentine, oil of chamomile, and oil of lavender, to which had been added a portion of vermillion dye. This mixture was forced into the body until the skin exhibited a red appearance. After a few hours during which the body lay undisturbed, the thoracic and abdominal cavities were opened, the viscera were removed, and the fluid was squeezed out of them. The viscera were separately arterially injected and bathed in camphorated spirits of wine. The body was again injected from the aorta and the cavities were washed with camphorated spirits of wine. The viscera were returned to the body, intermixed with powder composed of camphor, resin, and niter, and placed in the eyes, ears, nostrils, and other cavities. The entire skin surface of the body was then rubbed with the "essential" oils of rosemary and lavender. The body was placed in a box on a bed of plaster of Paris for about 4 years. When the box was reopened, and if desiccation appeared imperfect, a bed of gypsum was added to complete the process.

One of Hunter's admonitions to his students, which is still applicable to attainment of the finest results, was to begin the embalming process within 8 hours of the death in the summer and within 24 hours in the winter.

Until the wartime aerial bombing of the Royal College of Surgeons Museum in 1941, the embalmed body of the wife of eccentric dentist Martin Van Butchell, a pupil of William Hunter, was on exhibition. There was a letter in Van Butchell's handwriting describing the embalming process. It is reproduced here verbatim:

12–Jan.–1775: At one half past two this morning my wife died. At eight this morning the statuary took off her face in plaster. At half past two this afternoon Mr. Cruikshank injected at the crural arteries five pints of oil of turpentine mixed with Venice turpentine and vermillion.

15–Jan.: At nine this morning Dr. Hunter and Mr. Cruikshank began to open and embalm my wife. Her diseases were a large empyema in the left lung (which would not receive any air), accompanied with pleuropneumony and much adhesion. The right lung was also beginning to decay and had some pus in it. The spleen was hard and much contracted; the liver diseased, called rata malphigi. The stomach was very sound. The kidneys, uterus, bladder and intestines were in good order. Injected at the large arteries oil of turpentine mixed with camphored spirits, i.e., ten ounces camphor to a quart of spirits, so as to make the whole vascular system turgid; put into the belly part six pounds of rosin powder, three pounds camphor and three pounds niter powder mixed rec. spirit.

17–Jan.: I opened the abdomen to put in the remainder of the powders and added four pounds of rosin, three pounds niter and one pound camphor.

In all there were ten pounds rosin, six pounds niter and four pounds camphor, twenty pounds of powder mixed with spirits of wine.

18–Jan.: Dr. Hunter and Mr. Cruikshank came at nine this morning and put my wife into the box on and in 130 pounds of Paris plaster at eighteen d. a bag. I put between the thighs three arquebusade bottles, one full of camphored spirits, very rich of the gum, containing eight ounces of oil of rosemary, and in the other two ounces of lavender.

19–Jan.: I closed up the joints of the box lid and glasses with Paris plaster mixed with gum water and spirits wine.

25–Jan.: Dr. Hunter came with Sir Thos. Wynn and his lady.

7–Feb.: Dr. Hunter came with Sir John Pringle, Dr. Heberden, Dr. Watson and about twelve more fellows of The Royal Society.

11–Feb.: Dr. Hunter came with Dr. Solander, Dr.——, Mr. Banks and another gentleman. I unlocked the glasses to clean the face and legs with spirits of wine and oil of lavender.

12–Feb.: Dr. Hunter came to look at the neck and shoulders.

13–Feb.: I put four ounces of camphored spirits into the box and on both sides of neck and six pounds of plaster.

16–Feb.: I put four ounces oil of lavender, an ounce of rosemary and $\frac{1}{2}$ ounce of oil of camomile flowers (the last cost four Sh.) on sides of the face and three ounces of very dry camomile flowers on the breast, neck, and shoulders.

The body was said to resemble a Guanche or Peruvian mummy and was very dry and shrunken.

John Hunter, M.D.

John Hunter (1728–1793) was born in Scotland, the younger brother of William Hunter, in whose anatomy classes he first proved so adept. After studying under the great surgeons of his time, he was appointed to hospital staffs and lectured on anatomy. A region of the body he described was named in his honor: "Hunter's canal." He served as a surgeon in the British army during the campaign in Portugal (1761–1763) and, on his discharge from the service, settled in general practice in London. There he continued the collection and study of anatomical and natural subjects. He was a most brilliant and prolific writer on all phases of medicine and surgery and later founded his own private anatomy classes, which were unexcelled for the number of students who later distinguished themselves in medicine. Among these students were Jenner, Abernathy, Carlisle, Chevalier, Cline, Coleman, Astley Cooper, Home, Lynn, and Macartney.

In 1776, Hunter was honored by appointment as Surgeon-Extraordinary to the King of England. In 1782, he constructed a museum between his two homes in London to house his anatomical and natural history collections. These eventually contained nearly 14,000 items, and at his death, they were purchased by the British government for the Royal College of Surgeons. The main exhibit hall, measuring 52 by 28 feet, was lighted from above and had a gallery for visitors.

Many stories are told of body stealing for dissection and for securing specimens for collections. None would better illustrate this than John Hunter's acquisition of the body of the Irish giant O'Brien in 1783, at a cost to him of about $2500.00. O'Brien, about 7 feet 7 inches in height and dreading dissection by Hunter had, shortly before his death, arranged with several of his friends that his corpse be transported to the sea and sunk in deep water. The undertaker, who it was said had entered into a pecuniary agreement with Hunter, managed that while the escort was drinking at a certain stage of the journey to the sea the coffin should be locked in a barn. Confederates, who the undertaker had concealed in the barn, speedily substituted an equivalent weight of stones for the body. At night, O'Brien's body was forwarded to Hunter who took it immediately to his museum, where it was dissected and boiled to procure the bones. The skeleton was on exhibit until May 1941, when three-fourths of the museum of the Royal College of Surgeons, London, was destroyed by German bombers. Joshua Reynold's portrait of John Hunter displays the huge skeletal feet of O'Brien in the background.

Matthew Baillie

Baillie (1761–1823) was a nephew of William and John Hunter. He was educated by his uncles and became famous as a physician and writer on medical subjects. He modified the Hunterian method of embalming so as to provide as good preservation as ever in a shorter period. Using a solution of oil of turpentine, Venice turpentine, oil of chamomile, and oil of lavender (to which was added vermillion dye) he injected the femoral artery. He allowed several hours of elapse before he opened the body as in a postmortem examination and made a small incision in the bowel below the stomach, into which he inserted a small piece of pipe through which he introduced water to wash out the contents of the bowels. Then, ligating the rectum above the anus and the small bowel below the stomach, he filled the intestinal tract with camphorated spirits of wine. The lungs were filled with camphorated spirits of wine via the trachea. The bladder was opened and emptied of its contents and a powder of camphor, resin, and niter was dusted over the viscera and the incision was closed. The eyeballs were pierced and emptied of their contents and repacked to normal with the powder mixture, as were the mouth and ears. The body was rubbed with oil of rosemary or lavender and placed on a bed of deep plaster.

Europe's Access to Cadavers

Continental European countries such as France, Germany, and Italy did not encounter the problems in supplying medical schools with cadavers as existed in Great Britain. Medical schools had access to bodies unclaimed for burial, a situation not present in the British Isles until after passage of the **Warburton Act** in 1832. The problem in continental Europe was different, consisting of securing a means to preserve cadavers for dissection with nonpoisonous chemicals. In France, for example, medical schools in the north had scheduled anatomical dissection classes during the cold months of the year as the cadavers were unembalmed.

By the late eighteenth and early nineteenth centuries, France and Italy had a number of different techniques and chemicals for embalming proposed by members of the medical or scientific communities.

Giuseppe Tranchina (1797–1837) of Palermo, Italy, openly advocated and successfully used arsenical solutions, arterially injected, to preserve bodies for both funeral and anatomical purposes. An anatomist at the Royal University, he used a method involving an injection into the carotid artery. It is known he used this method as early as 1833 on the body of Prince Corrado Valguarnera of Niscemi and, later, on that of Cardinal Giacinto Placido Zurla (1834). The ingredients he used were revealed during a demonstration in the Naples Military Hospital in 1835 and consisted of a solution of white arsenic diluted in water or alcohol and then colored with either cinnabar or red lead oxide. No evisceration, drainage, or cavity treatment was performed. Tranchina's technique, which would lead to a perfect body exposure for 3 or 4 months, represents the very first documented method that did not involve evisceration but was uniquely relying upon arterial injection.

J. P. Sucquet of France (mid-nineteenth century) was one of the earliest proponents of the use of zinc chloride as a preservative agent. He injected about 5 quarts of a 20% solution of zinc chloride in water through the popliteal artery and also introduced some of this solution into the abdomen. One body prepared in this way was buried for 2 years, then disinterred and found to be in an excellent state of preservation. About 1845, an agent representing Sucquet sold the U.S. rights to his method and chemical to Chas. D. Brown and Joseph Alexander of New York City.

Jean Nicolas Gannal (1791–1852), a chemist in France (Fig. 5), began his life's work as an apothecary's assistant. From 1808 to 1812, he served in the medical department of the French Army, including the Russian campaign under Napoleon. After his discharge from the

Figure 5. Portrait of J. N. Gannal at age 40. (*Courtesy of Ordre National de Pharmacien.*)

army, he reentered the field of chemistry and was appointed assistant to the great French chemistry teacher Thenard. He later became interested in industrial chemistry and did research on methods of refining borax and improving the quality of glues and gelatins. In 1827, he was awarded the Montyon science prize for developing a method of treating catarrh and tuberculosis with chlorine gas. In 1831, he was asked to devote his time to devising an improved method of preserving cadavers for anatomical purposes. Close application to the problem resulted in success, which was recognized in 1836 by the award to Gannal of a second Montyon science prize.

His experiments included the use of solutions of acids (acetic–arsenous–nitric–hydrochloric), alkali salts (copper–mercury–alum), tannin–creosote–alcohol, and various combinations such as alum, sodium chloride, and nitrate of potash, and acetate of alumina and the chloride of alumina, the latter of which obliterated the lumen of blood vessels. His perfected method of embalming cadavers for anatomical purposes comprised the injection of about 6 quarts of a solution of acetate of alumina through the carotid artery without drainage of any blood. No evisceration or other treatment was used,

although occasionally the bodies were immersed in the injecting solution until ready for dissection. Gannal used practically the same solution for embalming bodies for funeral purposes, although he did add a small quantity of arsenic and carmine to the solution. He injected about 2 gallons of this mixture, first upward and then downward in the carotid artery in less than one-half hour. No special treatment was given to the trunk viscera. In his book *History of Embalming*, he cited case histories of bodies he had embalmed and subsequently disinterred from 3 to 13 months after burial. Gannal states that in every such case, the body was found in exactly the same state of preservation and appearance as when buried.

Gannal was involved in several precedent-making events. In mid-April 1840, a Paris newspaper published the following article:

> The young boy found murdered in a field near Villete not having been recognized and the process of decomposition having commenced, the Magistrates ordered it to be embalmed by M. Gannal's simple method of injection through the carotid arteries, so that this evidence of the crime may remain producible. This is the first operation of the kind performed by order of the Justices, and it was completed in a quarter of an hour.

In his translation of Gannal's *History of Embalming* (1840) (Fig. 6), Harlan mentions that the Paris police have access to Gannal's embalming process to preserve bodies in the Paris morgue where murder has been suspected.

Gannal was indirectly responsible for the passage of the first law prohibiting the use of arsenic in embalming solutions in 1846 (to which the use of bichloride of mercury was also prohibited in 1848).

There are several versions of the story. In one, Gannal had omitted stating that a portion of arsenic was added to his alumina salts embalming chemical, and when this solution was analyzed and arsenic was found, the medical community was enraged and compelled the law to be decreed. The other tale, never documented, relates that Gannal was retained to embalm the corpse of a member of the nobility who died suddenly. The members of the nobleman's family accused the decedent's mistress of poisoning him with arsenic. Under French law, she was arrested and tried, the burden of her defense on her shoulders. Gannal followed the progress of the trial in the Paris newspapers and noted that the accused mistress was unable to prove her innocence. Finally, at the last possible moment, Gannal appeared at the trial and requested permission to testify on her behalf. He states that in his opinion the arsenic found in the body tissues of the deceased came there during the embalming with his embalming solution, as it contained arsenic.

HISTORY

OF

EMBALMING,

AND OF

PREPARATIONS IN ANATOMY, PATHOLOGY

AND NATURAL HISTORY;

INCLUDING

An Account Of A New Process

For Embalming.

BY J. N. GANNAL.

Paris, 1838.

Translated From The French, With
Notes And Additions.
By R. Harlan, M.D.

PHILADELPHIA;

PUBLISHED BY JUDAH DOBSON,

NO. 106 CHESNUT STREET.

. . . .

1840

Figure 6. Title page of Harlan's translation of the *History of Embalming.*

She was freed and the legal community petitioned for the abolition of arsenic in embalming solutions.

Gannal had two sons, Adolphe Antoine and Felix, who became physicians and continued the embalming practice after his death. They embalmed many famous people including De Lessups, who constructed the Suez Canal. The sons died in the early 1900s.

Richard Harlan (1796–1843) of Philadelphia, Pennsylvania, graduated from the Pennsylvania Medical College in 1818 and was placed in charge of Joseph Parrish's private anatomical dissection rooms in Philadelphia. After engaging in various projects in company with other Philadelphia physicians, he became a member of the city health council. In 1838, he traveled to Europe and spent a portion of his time in Paris visiting various medical facilities and meeting local savants, among whom was J. N. Gannal. After being presented with a copy of Gannal's *History of Embalming*, he became so fascinated with it that he requested and received permission to publish an American edition translated into English. **The book,**

published in Philadelphia in 1840, became the first book devoted entirely to embalming procedures, which was published in the United States in English (Fig. 6).

Other Physicians and Anatomists

Girolamo Segato. (1792–1836). A naturalist, explorer, and cartographer residing in Florence, Italy, Segato is known to have converted the human body to stone ("petrification"), allegedly by infiltrating the bodily tissues with a solution of silicate of potash and succeeded this treatment by immersion of the body in a weak acid solution. The exact modus operandi is unknown. His technique was emulated by other notable Italian scientists including Bartolommeo Zanon, Giovan Battista Rini, Giambattista Messedaglia, Paolo Gorini, and Efisio Marini.

Thomas Joseph Pettigrew. A London physician and surgeon, graduate of Guys Hospital, and fellow of the Royal College of Surgeons, Pettigrew (1791–1865), was one of the great historians of the science of embalming. His treatise *History of Egyptian Mummies*, published in London in 1834, is a masterpiece revealing Pettigrew's ability to accurately observe and minutely describe objects and processes of interest to students and practitioners of the art of embalming. This volume is to this day considered one of the finest works on Egyptian embalming methods and customs. In 1854, he withdrew from the practice of medicine and devoted his entire energy to the study of archaeology.

Dr. Falconi. A French physician of the mid-nineteenth century, Falconi employed a means of preservation of cadavers for anatomical purposes, which is of interest because of its simplicity. The corpse was placed on a bed of dry saw dust to which about a gallon of powdered zinc sulfate had been added. No injections, incisions, baths, or any additional treatment was used. The bodies so treated were said to have remained flexible for about 40 days, after which time they dried and assumed the appearance of mummies.

Dr. John Morgan (Circa 1863). A professor of anatomy at the University of Dublin, Morgan made use of two principles that are widely recognized as necessary to achieve the best embalming results: (1) the use of the largest possible artery for injection and (2) the use of force or pressure to push the preserving fluid through the blood vessels. Also noted are his use of a preinjection solution (the earliest mention found) and his controlled technique of drainage. Morgan cut the sternum down its center, opened the pericardium to expose the heart, made an incision into the left ventricle or into the aorta, and inserted a piece of pipe about 8 inches long. This injecting pipe was connected by 15 feet of tubing to a

Figure 7. Gravity fluid injector. The jar filled with arterial chemical could be elevated several feet above the corpse, thus creating pressure for injection. (*Courtesy of Paula Johnson De Smet.*)

fluid container that was maintained 12 feet above the corpse, thereby producing about 5 pounds of pressure (Fig. 7).

The tip of the right auricular appendage was clipped off to allow blood drainage. The first injection was composed of $\frac{1}{2}$ gallon of a saturated salt solution to which was added 4 ounces of niter. After this solution was allowed to "rush" through the circulatory system, a clamp was fastened over the auricular appendage when the drainage stopped. Several more gallons of a solution of common salt, niter, alum, and arsenate of potash were injected until the body was thoroughly saturated with the fluid. No special treatment of the internal organs or viscera was mentioned.

At this time, there was virtually no embalming of the dead for funeral purposes available for the largest percentage of deaths. Many books were written regarding the dangers to the living of exposure to the dead buried or entombed (unembalmed) in churches or in city cemeteries. There was also concern for those who handled the dead.

Alfredo Salafia. One of the world's oldest and best known examples of modern day embalming is a 2-year-old child by the name of Rosalia Lombardo. Little Ros-

alia died in December of 1920 in Palermo, Italy. Her father full of grief over the loss of his child called upon a local embalmer with more than 20 years of embalming experience to prepare his daughter. Today, Rosalia is known as "Sleeping Beauty" as she appears to just be sleeping.

It is not known how Salafia became interested in embalming. He worked with Francesco Randacio, a professor of anatomy at Palermo University, where he achieved excellent results after he was granted permission to apply his embalming procedure to unclaimed human bodies. His embalming skills were extraordinary. He was able to restore the remains of Francesco Crispi, the Italian Premier, in 1902, after the original embalming had failed to preserve his body. He worked for months using hypodermic injections, performing restorative art by replacing the eyeballs with glass eyes and reattaching the hair and beard that had fallen out. He injected paraffin into the facial features to "regain the form and lost volume." The local press wrote of his work that allowed the body to be viewed three times from 1902 to 1914 following exhumation.

Salafia manufactured embalming chemicals through his "Salafia Permanent Method Embalming Company." He came to New York City on multiple visits to give demonstrations and sell his fluid. The company provided embalming using Salafia Perfection Fluid. The method he used was a single point injection through the carotid artery using 1.5 gallons of his nonpoisonous chemical.

Along with his nephews Oreste Maggio and Achille Salamone (who went to the Renouard School of Embalming and opened a funeral home), Salafia would demonstrate his chemicals and method on unclaimed bodies on two occasions. The first was in April of 1910. The body was embalmed and then enclosed in a glass case for 6 months. It was examined by a group of leading embalmers including Professor William P. Hohenschuch along with Frank E. Campbell, Charles F. Moadinger, Jr., and Fred Hulberg, Jr. The autopsy revealed well-preserved tissue throughout with no decomposition. It was proclaimed a success. He demonstrated it again in September of 1910 for the New York Embalmers Association. Again, the body was embalmed and examined 6 months. It was also found to be in an excellent state of preservation. Although he sold chemicals throughout the United States from this point through 1911, there was no further evidence of his corporation after December, 1911.

Although he never revealed his chemical formulation before his death, he did keep a beautifully handwritten and illustrated memoir. This memoir contained accounts of his embalming and formula. Through the generosity of his family, the memoir was shared with researchers at EURAC in Bolzano, Italy. His formulation included formaldehyde, possibly the first use in Europe. Professor Salafia understood not only the chemistry of preservation but also the sentiment of what embalmers do. He wrote in the opening of his memoir "A Noble Tradition. The sentiment of the people is innate with human nature and it is not always the real determinant of civil progress. The proof can be found in the most ancient of peoples where we find nobler traditions, much more moving than we do in the people of today, too evolved and too calculating and thus too cold. To hand down to the posterity the intact appearance of dear ones just as they were when they left us at the moment eternal departure, it is among these compassionate customs that antiquity has handed down to us and that time has preserved."

Bernardino Ramazzini. The founder of occupational medicine, Ramazzini (1633–1714) wrote the *Diseases of Workers* in 1700, and an enlarged edition of that text was published in 1713. The latter edition contained a chapter on the disease of corpse bearers.

Numerous publications varying in size from leaflets to bound books were printed inveighing against existing burial practices. A few relevant titles are *Considerations on the Indecent and Dangerous Custom of Burying in Churches and Churchyards etc.*, 1721, London, A. Batesworth; *Blame of Kirk Burial, Tending to Persuade Cemeterial Civility*, 1606 NP, Rev. William Birnie; *Gatherings from Graveyards, Particularly Those of London etc.*, 1830, G. A. Walker, surgeon, London; and *Sepulture, History, Methods and Sanitary Requisites*, 1884, Stephen Wickes, Philadelphia. The astonishing accounts contained in these or similar works should convince even the most skeptical opponent of embalming of the sanitary value of the embalming process.

From Europe to the Colonies

The transfer of embalming knowledge from Europe to the colonies in what today is the United States was accomplished by several means.

Anatomical study in the colonies as early as 1676 in Boston and again in 1750 recorded that "Drs. John Bard and Peter Middleton injected and dissected the body of an executed criminal for the instruction of young men engaged in the study of medicine." In 1752, the *N.Y. Weekly Post-Boy* carried an advertisement offering anatomy instruction by Dr. Thomas Wood. From 1754 to 1756, William Hunter, physician and student of the famed anatomy teacher Alexander Monroe I of Edinburgh, Scotland (and a relative of the Hunter brothers), lectured on anatomy at Newport, Rhode Island. Doctors William Shippen and John Morgan of Philadelphia studied medicine in Europe and anatomy under British anatomists. On their return to the United States between 1762 and 1765, they became engaged in teaching medical subjects, especially anatomy, in Philadelphia.

In 1840, the translation of Gannal's book, *The History of Embalming*, into English was to provide the first text in English printed in the United States devoted to embalming. In the mid-1840s, the acquisition of Sucquet's embalming technique and chemicals as a franchise by Dr. Charles D. Brown and Dr. Joseph Alexander of New York City added to the increasing amount of embalming knowledge transferred to the United States.

▶ MODERN PERIOD

By the year 1861 and the onset of the Civil War, the transfer of embalming knowledge from Europe to the United States was virtually concluded. A small group of medically trained embalmers existed together with printed information such as Harlan's translation of Gannal's textbook and various European embalming formulas and techniques that had been acquired.

Until the Civil War, however, little or no embalming was performed for funeral purposes. Most preservation, such as it was, for brief periods was provided by ice refrigeration when available.

With the outbreak of the Civil War in April 1861, there began the raising of troops by the North and South to prosecute the war. Little, if any, embalming was available to the Southerners during the war. Virtually all embalming was done by Northerners. As Washington, D.C. was the capital city of the north, it became a center for troop concentration both to protect the city and to serve as a marshalling point for the armies moving against the south.

Northern troops composed of individual companies from small geographical areas and regiments from individual states as disparate as Vermont and Maine, Minnesota and Wisconsin, and Ohio, Pennsylvania, and New York crowded into the Washington, D.C. area. Civilian embalmers Dr. Thomas Holmes, William J. Bunnell, Dr. Charles Da Costa Brown, Dr. Joseph B. Alexander, Dr. Richard Burr, Dr. Daniel H. Prunk, Frank A. Hutton, G. W. Scollay, C. B. Chamberlain, Henry P. Cattell, Dr. Benjamin Lyford, Samuel Rodgers, Dr. E. C. Lewis, W. P. Cornelius, and Prince Greer are known to have embalmed during the Civil War. There are others who, to this day, remain anonymous.

None of the embalming surgeons, as they were called, were ever employed in the military as embalmers. Some had been or would become military surgeons but did not perform embalming while in the military service.

Civil War Times

At the beginning of the Civil War, as in all previous wars fought by the United States, there was no provision for return of the dead to their homes. In the Seminole Indian Wars (during the 1830s), the Mexican War

(1846–1848), and the campaigns against the Indians up to the outbreak of the Civil War, the military dead were buried in the field near where they fell in battle. It was possible for the relatives to have the remains returned to their home for local burial under certain conditions:

1. The next of kin was to request the disinterment and return of the body in a written request to the Quartermaster General.
2. On military authority confirmation that the burial place was known and disinterment could be effected, the family was advised to send a coffin capable of being hermetically sealed to a designated Quartermaster Officer nearest the place of burial.
3. Such Quartermaster Officer would provide a force of men to take the coffin to the grave, disinter the remains, and place them in the coffin and seal it. The coffined remains would then be returned to the place of ultimate reinterment.

During the early days of the Civil War and less frequently as the war dragged on, some family members of the deceased personally went to hospitals and battlefields to search for their dead and bring them home for burial. Civil War embalming was carried out with various chemicals and techniques. Arterial embalming was applied when possible. An artery, usually the femoral or carotid, was raised and injected without any venous drainage in most cases. Usually, no cavity treatment was administered. When arterial embalming was believed impossible because of the nature of wounds or decomposition, other means of preparation of the body for transport were resorted to. In some cases, the trunk was eviscerated and the cavity filled with sawdust or powdered charcoal or lime. The body was then placed in a coffin completely imbedded in sawdust or similar material. In other cases, the body was coffined as mentioned without evisceration.

Chemicals employed during the Civil War were totally self-manufactured by the embalmer and included, as basic preservatives, arsenicals, zinc chloride, bichloride of mercury, salts of alumina, sugar of lead, and a host of salts, alkalies, and acids. An example of fluid manufacture of one of the most popular embalming chemicals, zinc chloride, was the immersion of sheets of zinc in hydrochloric acid until a saturated solution was obtained. The resulting zinc chloride solution was injected without further dilution. Many of the injection pumps employed were quite similar to what would be described as greatly enlarged hypodermic syringes. Many required filling of the syringe, attachment of a cannula, emptying of the syringe, unfastening of the syringe, and refilling. It was an extremely slow process! A few pumps were designed to provide continuous flow, aspirating the embalming chemical continuously from a large source into the pump during the injection process. Others, such as the Holmes invention, were designed to fit over a bucket that could hold a gallon or more of liquid.

On May 24, 1861, 24-year-old Colonel Elmer Ellsworth, commander of the 11th N.Y. Volunteer Infantry, was shot to death in Alexandria, Virginia, as he seized a confederate flag displayed atop the Marshall House Hotel. He became the first prominent military figure killed in the war. His body was embalmed by Dr. Thomas Holmes, who had set up an embalming establishment in Washington, D.C. Funeral services for Colonel Ellsworth were performed in the White House, in New York City, and in Albany, New York, and he was buried in his home town of Mechanicsburg, New York. His funeral set a pattern to be followed by prominent members of the military, culminating in President Lincoln's historic funeral services. Colonel Ellsworth's embalming and viewable appearance were widely and favorably commented on in the press and did much to familiarize the previously uninformed public with embalming.

The Army issued only two sets of orders relative to fatal casualties in the early stages of the war. On September 11, 1861, War Department General Order 75 directed the Quartermaster Department to supply all general and post hospitals with blank books and forms for the preservation of accurate death records and to provide material for headboards to be erected over soldiers' graves. On April 3, 1862, Section II of War Department General Order 33 stated:

> In order to secure as far as possible the decent interment of those who have fallen, or may fall in battle, it is made the duty of commanding generals to lay off lots of ground in some suitable spot near every battlefield, as soon as it may be in their power, and to cause the remains of those killed to be interred, with head boards to the graves bearing numbers, and when practicable the names of the persons buried in them. A register for each burial ground will be preserved, in which will be noted the marks corresponding with the headboards.

This was the origin of what was to become the National Cemetery System.

Embalming Surgeons of the Civil War

Dr. Thomas Holmes (1817–1900). Holmes was born in New York City in 1817 and educated in local public schools and New York University Medical College, though the records of the period are incomplete and document only his attendance, not his graduation. He did practice medicine and was a coroner's physician in New York during the 1850s as numerous newspaper stories attest. He apparently moved to Williamsburg (now

DR. THOMAS H. HOLMES.

Figure 8. Portrait of Thomas H. Holmes.

Figure 9. Front page of *The Sunnyside*, June 1886, featuring an article on Holmes's removal bag, citing its all-around utility as a sleeping bag and stretcher, its ability to be inflated as a raft, and, of course, its use as a corpse removal bag or coffin.

Brooklyn) and experimented with various chemicals for embalming and techniques. When the Civil War broke out, he opened an embalming office in Washington, D.C. and Colonel Ellsworth became his first prominent client. Holmes subsequently embalmed Colonel E. D. Baker, a prominent politician and soldier killed in battle. This case brought more publicity both for Holmes and for embalming (Fig. 8).

Holmes ultimately prepared about 4000 bodies (including eight generals) and patented many inventions relating to embalming during his lifetime. One in particular, a rubber-coated canvas removal bag, was far ahead of its time (Fig. 9).

When the war ended, Dr. Holmes returned home to Brooklyn and only occasionally practiced embalming. He operated a drugstore and manufactured various products as diverse as embalming fluid and root beer! He invested heavily in a health resort and lost the investment. He wrote little about embalming, did not teach, and had no children. After a serious fall in his home, he became periodically psychotic and occasionally required confinement. When he died in 1900, it was said that he wanted no embalming.

William J. Bunnell (1823–1891). Bunnell was born in New Jersey, moved to New York City, and in the 1850s became acquainted with Dr. Holmes and married his sister. Dr. Holmes found him employment as an anatomy technician for some New York medical schools while teaching him embalming. When war broke out, Bunnell did not work directly with Dr. Holmes but formed his own Embalming Surgeon's organization with Dr. R. B. Heintzelman from Philadelphia as his active partner. Holmes and Bunnell did occasionally work together during the war at Gettysburg and at City Point, Virginia. After the war, it was reported that Bunnell was practicing medicine briefly in Omaha, Nebraska, and eventually opened an undertaking establishment in Jersey City, New Jersey. He became a marshall at the funeral of General Grant and became prominent in undertakers' associations. His son, George Holmes Bunnell (1855–1932), followed his father in the business and was given assistance by his uncle, Dr. Holmes. George H. Bunnell had twin sons: Milton

Figure 10. Portrait of Henry P. Cattell, an associate of Brown and Alexander, the embalming surgeons who embalmed Willie Lincoln in 1862 and President Lincoln in 1865.

became a funeral director, and Chester became a physician.

Charles Da Costa Brown, Joseph B. Alexander, and Henry P. Cattell. Brown, Alexander, and Cattell were all active in the firm of Brown and Alexander, Embalming Surgeons. It is not known whether Brown and Alexander met in New York City in the late 1850s or in Washington, D.C. in early wartime. Cattell (Fig. 10) is believed to have been the stepson of Dr. Charles Brown's brother, as his mother married a brown in 1860. In any event, he entered the employment of the firm that embalmed Willie Lincoln, son of President Abraham Lincoln, and later embalmed the President Lincoln himself in 1865. After the war, Dr. Brown abandoned embalming, returned to New York City, practiced dentistry, and became very active in the Masonic Lodge. He died in 1896 and is buried in Greenwood Cemetery in Brooklyn.

Alexander died in 1871 in Washington, D.C. H. P. Cattell halted his embalming practice after the war, became a lithographer, and then entered the Washington, D.C. police force. None of his family was ever aware that he had embalmed President Lincoln. He died in 1915 and is buried in Washington, D.C.

Frank A. Hutton. Little is known of Hutton's personal biography. Born in or near Harrisburg, Pennsylvania, about 1835, he was a pharmacist by occupation. He had

military service in the 110th Pennsylvania Volunteer Infantry ending in June 1862, was discharged in Washington, D.C., and became a partner in the firm of Chamberlain and Hutton, Surgeons. This partnership did not last long and Hutton withdrew in February 1863. He formed the firm of Hutton and Company with E. A. Williams, son of a Washington, D.C. undertaker as his partner. Hutton advertised in the Washington City Directory, taking a full-page space to extol his embalming expertise. He was also issued Patent 38,747 for an embalming fluid on June 1, 1863. The formula included alcohol, arsenic, bichloride of mercury, and zinc chloride.

During mid-April 1863, Hutton became embroiled in an argument with a client over charges for shipping his son's body to him. The client complained to Colonel L. C. Baker, provost marshall of the capitol, who, on April 20, 1863, arrested Hutton and seized the contents of his office as evidence. Hutton was confined in the Old Capitol Prison for about 10 days and then released. No details of his release or trial have been found. He subsequently relocated his quarters and continued in business with a much diminished clientele. Hutton is said to have returned to Harrisburg after the war ended and died there within a year.

Daniel H. Prunk (1829–1923). Born in Virginia in 1829, Prunk and his family migrated to Illinois where he attended college. After attending medical school in Cincinnati, he began medical practice in Illinois and in April 1861 moved to Indianapolis where he joined the 19th Indiana Volunteer Infantry as an assistant surgeon in September 1861. He was transferred to the 20th Indiana Volunteer Infantry in June 1862 and was arrested in November of that year and incarcerated in the Old Capitol Prison in Washington, D.C. for about 3 months for conduct unbecoming an officer. He was then dismissed from the service. From July to October 1863, he was acting assistant surgeon at the 2nd Division Army Hospital at Nashville, Tennessee, and subsequently requested permission to provide embalming services in Nashville. The request was initially refused but finally granted late in 1863. He eventually had embalming establishments located not only in Nashville but also in Chattanooga and Knoxville in Tennessee; at East Point, Atlanta, Dalton, and Marietta in Georgia; and at Huntsville in Alabama (Fig. 11).

In 1865, Dr. Prunk was licensed by the Army to practice embalming and undertaking. (He was also engaged in a wholesale grocery business, cotton trading, and money lending.) He made his own embalming fluid by dissolving sheets of zinc in muriatic acid (hydrochloric acid) until a saturated solution of zinc chloride was obtained to which a quantity of arsenious acid was added. The fluid obtained was injected quite warm without dilution or blood drainage.

Figure 11. Injection syringe and cannulas of Daniel H. Prunk, Civil War embalming surgeon. (*Courtesy of the Illinois Funeral Directors' Foundation.*)

Prunk sold all his embalming establishments in 1866 and returned to Indianapolis to practice medicine. It seems that he never engaged in embalming after his return to Indianapolis. He made one of the earliest written statements regarding the necessity of cavity treatment in a letter written in 1872, to Dr. J. P. Buckes to of San Jose, California.

If I were going to ship a corpse from San Jose to New York City, we have advised for sometime the puncturing of the stomach to give vent to gases which accumulate at this time. In a subject with a large abdomen, where the bowels are discolored, the introduction of a couple of quarts into the peritoneal cavity by making a puncture near the umbilicus and throwing a thread of strong silk around it like a drawstring on a button cushion which can be readily closed after you are thru injecting.

Dr. Richard Burr. Although little biographical information other than his rumored origin in Philadelphia is available concerning Burr (who apparently practiced during the period 1862–1865), he has achieved immortality as the embalmer photographed by the Civil War photographer Matthew Brady in front of his embalming tent while injecting a subject (Fig. 12). W. J. Bunnell complained about Burr's unprofessional conduct, alleging that, among other things, he set Bunnell's embalming tent on fire! He was also one of the men against whom complaints had been issued regarding inflated prices and poor services, which resulted in all embalmers being excluded from military areas by order of General U. S. Grant in January 1865. **This resulted in establishment of the first set of rules and regulations for the licensing of embalmers and undertakers in the United States.**

The final Army order for embalmers contained some of the suggestions made by Dr. Barnes, chief of

Figure 12. Richard Burr embalming near a battlefield during the Civil War. (*Courtesy of Library of Congress.*)

the Army Medical Service in December 1863, to the effect that a performance bond should be posted by any embalmer desiring to practice. In addition, the requirement stipulated by the Provost Marshall General ordered the embalmer to furnish a list of his prices as charged for work or merchandise to the Provost Marshall General, the medical director of the department, and the Post Provost Marshall.

U.S. Army General Order 39 concerning embalmers (March 15, 1865) read as follows:

1. Here after no persons will be permitted to embalm or remove the bodies of deceased officers or soldiers unless acting under the special license of the Provost Marshall of the Army, department, or district in which the bodies may be.
2. Provost mar shalls will restrict disinterments to seasons when they can be made without endangering the health of the troops. They will grant licenses only to such persons as furnish proof of skill and ability as embalmers, and will require bonds for the faithful performance of the orders given them. They will also establish a scale of prices by which embalmers are to be governed, with such other regulations as will protect the interest of the friends and relatives of deceased soldiers.
3. Applicants for license will apply directly to the Provost Marshall of the Army or department in which they may desire to pursue their business, submitting in distinct terms the process adopted by them, materials, length of time its preservative effect can be relied on and such other information as may be necessary to establish their proficiency and success. Medical directors will give such assistance in the examination of these applications as may be required by the Provost Marshall.

In the Army of the Cumberland the following additional requirements were stipulated:

1. No disinterments will be permitted within the department between the 15th day of May and the 15th day of October.
2. The following scale of prices will be observed from and after this date: At Nashville and Memphis: for embalming bodies each at $15.00 to disinter, furnish metallic burial cases, well boxed, marked and delivered to the express office each at $75.00, zinc coffins and the above listed services each at $40.00. An additional charge of $5.00 may be made for embalming and also for either of the above styles of coffins at Murfreesboro, Chattanooga, Knoxville, and Huntsville, Alabama, or in the field.
3. No person will be permitted to operate as an embalmer under any license issued to him until he shall have filed a bond in this office in the pe-

nal sum of $1000 conditioned for the faithful observance of this order, and for the skillful performance of such works he shall undertake by virtue of his license. [Such licenses were not transferable from one individual to another.]

By 1864, the Armory Square Military Hospital in Washington, D.C. had all its deceased patients routinely embalmed and the grave recorded so that the body could be disinterred and sent to family or friends when requested.

C. B. Chamberlain. Chamberlain is said to have been born in Philadelphia. Although very little is known of the man, he definitely was an early partner of F. A. Hutton. He and Hutton apparently were not compatible, and he formed a new partnership with Ben Lyford. They both can be documented as practicing embalming surgeons on the scene at Gettysburg after the battle. Chamberlain is listed in the Washington, D.C. City Directory as late as 1865 as a partner in Chamberlain and Waters Embalmers at 431 Pennsylvania Avenue. He is mentioned by F. C. Beinhauer, Pittsburgh undertaker, as being in the Pittsburgh area prior to and during the Civil War. Joseph H. Clarke also mentioned Chamberlain as a teacher of embalming in the post–Civil War period.

Benjamin F. Lyford. Lyford was born in Vermont in 1841 and received public school education there. Lyford attended and graduated from Philadelphia University's 6-month course of medical studies. He first appeared on the Civil War scene as a partner of C. B. Chamberlain, who provided embalming after the Battle of Gettysburg. Later, he had altercations with Provost Marshall General Rudolf Patrick of the Army of the Potomac. This series of disagreements stimulated him to accept appointment on July 13, 1864, as assistant surgeon of the 68th Regiment of Infantry—U.S. Colored Troops. He reported to the unit in Missouri and subsequently served in Memphis. For a time, he served as commanding officer of a small cavalry and artillery contingent in southern Alabama.

He returned to his regiment stationed near New Orleans, Louisiana, and went on leave in New Orleans. He was arrested inside a bordello in full uniform and faced court-martial charges. Apparently found innocent of the charges, he was discharged from the Army on February 5, 1866, traveled to San Francisco, and opened an office for medical practice. One of his early patients was a wealthy widowed landowner who had an attractive daughter whom he fell in love with and married. The mother owned large tracts of land in Marin County across the bay north of San Francisco. Lyford built a health resort and dairy as well as his own home on this property and prospered.

In 1871, Lyford patented "An Improvement in Embalming," which was a very complicated system consisting of the introduction through the blood vessels of specially distilled chemicals (including creosote, zinc chloride, potassium nitrate, and alcohol) while the body was enclosed in a sealed container. The container that had the air within it alternatively evacuated to create a vacuum and reversed to create pressure. Finally, the body was eviscerated and the trunk cavity filled with an arsenical powder. His final recommendation was the use of cosmetics to color the features; he was one of the first to make this recommendation. In 1870, a local newspaper carried a story describing a body he had successfully embalmed. Lyford died in 1906 without issue and had a large, well-attended funeral.

Dr. E. C. Lewis, W. P. Cornelius, and Prince Greer. This most interesting account of the Civil War embalming surgeons relates the method of the transmission of embalming technique from a medically trained practitioner to an undertaker, who, in turn, trained a layman in the skill. Dr. E. C. Lewis was a former U.S. Army surgeon, W. P. Cornelius (1824–1910) was a successful undertaker in Nashville, Tennessee, and Prince Greer was a former orderly, body servant, slave of a Colonel Greer of a Texas cavalry regiment who died in the fighting in Tennessee.

Thomas Holmes wrote:

> In the forepart of the war a young ex-Army doctor named E. C. Lewis called at my headquarters in Washington and wished me to instruct him in the embalming profession and sell him an outfit to go to the western Army and locate at Nashville. He offered as security a property holding in Georgetown, DC for any amount of fluid I would trust him for. I made a bargain with him and he used many barrels of fluid. I was often surprised at his large orders. [*Note:* Dr. Lewis's headquarters were at Mr. Cornelius's undertaking establishment in Nashville.]

Cornelius stated:

> It was during the year 1862 that one Dr. E. C. Lewis came to me from the employ of Dr. Holmes and proposed to embalm bodies. It was new to me but I at once put him to work with the Holmes fluid and Holmes injector. He was quite an expert, but like many men could not stand prosperity and soon wanted to get into some other kind of business, which he did. When Lewis the embalmer quit, I then undertook the embalming myself with a colored assistant named Prince Greer.

Cornelius explained that Prince Greer had earlier brought the body of Colonel Greer of a Texas cavalry regiment to Cornelius for shipment back to Texas. After shipping back the body, Prince Greer remained at Cornelius's premises and was asked what he wanted to do to earn his room and board. Prince Greer indicated he would do anything.

Cornelius continued:

> Prince Greer appeared to enjoy embalming so much that he himself became an expert, kept on at work embalming during the balance of the war, and was very successful at it. It was but a short time before he could raise an artery as quickly as anyone and was always careful, always of course coming to me in a difficult case. He remained with me until I quit the business in 1871.

Prince Greer is the first documented black embalmer in U.S. history.

Establishment of Embalming Schools

The incentive for embalming in the period AD 650 to 1861 was the preservation of anatomical material to further the study of and research in anatomy. Those who made the early strides in embalming were the anatomists, but about the time of J. N. Gannal (early nineteenth-century France) and Thomas H. Holmes (late nineteenth-century United States), general public interest was aroused in the preservation of the dead. This interest and the later demand for preservation for funeral purposes of all human dead grew far beyond the means and desires of the few, trained embalmers in the medical profession. During the late nineteenth century in the United States, schools of embalming instruction were established by experienced embalmers. Many funeral directors and doctors attended the schools to study embalming and to seek employment. By the beginning of the twentieth century in the United States, separation of the fields of embalming and medicine was complete. This brought about the advancement of both professions, particularly that of embalming, because it placed a complex art in the hands of specialists who are still striving to acquire more knowledge and skill in preserving the human dead.

Public and Professional Acceptance

With the ending of the war and the assassination of President Lincoln, the Civil War's last major casualty, the public had been familiarized with the term *embalming* and obtained personal knowledge of the appearance of an embalmed body. This knowledge was acquired by the hundreds of thousands who viewed not only President Lincoln but also other prominent military and civilian figures as well as the ordinary soldiers embalmed and shipped to their homes.

Despite the end of the war and the establishment of peace, there was no wide adoption of embalming by civilian undertakers of the United States. There were many reasons for this apparent reluctance to adopt a worthwhile new practice. Undertakers in the United States at the end of the Civil War were an unorganized, largely rural group of individuals lacking a professional body of knowledge and skills. Specifically, they lacked textbooks of instruction on embalming, instructors and schools of embalming, professional journals, and professional associations. Until these necessities became available, embalming would not flourish.

The first step taken was to attempt the sale of embalming fluid to undertakers. Some Civil War embalming surgeons, such as Dr. Thomas Holmes, engaged in this endeavor on returning home. Holmes had a large local market (metropolitan New York City) for his preservative chemical, which he had named *Innominata*, and he promoted it well. Holmes, like other embalming chemical salesmen, realized quickly that the undertakers were interested in the preservative qualities of such chemicals but the clients were without knowledge of embalming techniques. Holmes therefore promoted the use of his Innominata as an external application, to wash the body and to saturate cloths to place over the face. His fluid was also poured into the mouth and nose to reach the lungs and stomach. Holmes' early practices were duplicated by other purveyors of embalming chemicals.

Examples of chemical embalming fluid patents include one issued to C. H. Crane of Burr Oak, Michigan, in September 1868. It was a powdered mixture of alum salt, ammonium chloride, arsenic, bichloride of mercury, camphor, and zinc chloride. It could be used as a dry powder or dissolved in water or alcohol to form an arterial solution and was named Crane's Electrodynamic Mummifier. In 1876, he sold the patent rights to this or a similar formulation to a Professor George M. Rhodes of Michigan. Another early embalming chemical manufacturer in 1877 was the Mills and Lacey Manufacturing Company of Grand Rapids, Michigan, whose embalming fluid featured arsenic as its preservative.

Instruments and chemicals available in the post–Civil War period included rubber gloves at $2 per pair (1877); anatomical syringes and three cannulas in a case for $20 to $22; surgical instruments in cases for $4 to $5; Rulon's wax eyecaps and mouth closers at $1 each; and Segestor embalming fluid for $4.50 per dozen pint bottles (1873). Professor George M. Rhodes was said to have sold 10,000 bottles of his dynamic Electro Balm in 1876 with more than 3000 undertakers using the product. Egyptian Embalmer Fluid (1877) sold for $6.50 per dozen pint bottles and was also available in 5- and 10-gallon kegs as well as $\frac{1}{2}$- and 1-gallon carboys at $3.00 per gallon.

Until the first quarter of the twentieth century, embalming was most frequently carried out in the home of the deceased or, in some communities, in the hospital where death occurred. There were early attempts in some funeral homes in the 1870s to provide both a preparation room and chapel space for the wake and services. In issues as early as 1876 of both *The Casket* and *The Sunnyside*,* there were accounts of the installation of preparation rooms. For example:

Hubbard and Searles Undertaking establishment at Auburn, New York, could provide seating for 100 persons at a service and had a cooling room with cement floor and marble slabs (2 × 8 feet) and running water connection.
Knowles Undertaking establishment at Providence, Rhode Island, had a preserver room and a corpse room where surgical procedures and postmortems were made.

Dr. Auguste Renouard. In 1876, Dr. Renouard (1839–1912) became a regular contributor to *The Casket* of articles on all phases of embalming knowledge, which greatly implemented interest in embalming. He was born on a plantation in Point Coupee Parish, Louisiana, and received his early schooling locally. He is said to have attended the McDowell Medical School in St. Louis, Missouri, and, at the outbreak of the Civil War, to have returned to Louisiana to enlist in the Confederate Army. Despite his claim to military service in the confederate forces, no documented evidence has been found in some 50 years of searching. In the postwar period, he secured employment as a pharmacist in various cities such as New York, Memphis, and Chicago, where he was married. His son, Charles A. Renouard, was born shortly before the Chicago fire of 1871. Losing everything in the fire, Renouard traveled to Denver, Colorado, and secured employment as a bookkeeper for a combination furniture store and undertaking establishment. Because of its altitude, Denver at this time was regarded as a health resort for treatment of lung diseases.

The undertaking section of the firm returned many bodies to the east and south for hometown burial, and Renouard became interested in the procedures employed at his firm for shipment of the bodies. After studying the existing rudimentary system, he suggested to his employer that he be permitted to prepare the bodies for shipment by arterial embalming. This consent was given and it almost immediately produced a volume of letters from the receiving undertakers inquiring about the procedure used to create such beautiful corpses, which resembled a person asleep. Renouard graciously replied, explaining his chemicals and technique to the extent

---

*The most significant impetus to spreading embalming knowledge was the founding of the professional journals *The Sunnyside* in 1871 and *The Casket* in 1876. Both, from their inception, carried advertisements for various embalming chemicals.

that it assumed the proportions of a correspondence course. Additionally, there were a number of individual undertakers who traveled to Denver to receive personal instruction in embalming from Renouard.

The publisher of *The Casket* urged Dr. Renouard to write a textbook on embalming and undertaking for use by undertakers. In 1878, he published *The Undertaker's Manual*, which contained 230 pages of detailed instruction on anatomy, chemistry, embalming procedures, instruments, and details of undertaking practice (Fig. 13). **This was the first book published specifically as an embalming textbook in the United States and followed by a horde of others.** In 1879, notices appeared in *The Casket* that undertakers in states such as Connecticut and Pennsylvania were agents for the sale of Auguste Renouard's chemical formulas and techniques (Fig. 14).

In 1881, Dr. Renouard was requested to open a school of embalming in Rochester, New York, but, for various reasons, this did not become a reality until early 1883. In 1880, the state of Michigan was the first to form an undertakers' association, which, in 1881, changed its name to Funeral Directors Association. Other states quickly followed the Michigan lead and organized state associations. **The various state associations met in 1882 in Rochester and organized the National Funeral Directors Association (NFDA), another important step toward professionalism.** Renouard provided demonstrations of embalming in Rochester at the first national convention of the Association. This set a pattern for many years of an obligatory embalming demonstration at state and national conventions. During the 1882 gathering, agents of an English firm (Dotridge Brothers, Funeral Supply Firm) offered Renouard a 5-year contract to teach embalming in London at $5000 per year, which he rejected.

The Rochester School of Embalming headed by Dr. Renouard under the auspices of the Egyptian Chemical Company opened in 1883 and he continued his affil-

THE
UNDERTAKERS' MANUAL:

A TREATISE OF
USEFUL AND RELIABLE INFORMATION;
EMBRACING COMPLETE AND DETAILED
INSTRUCTIONS FOR THE PRESERVATION
OF BODIES.

ALSO, THE
MOST APPROVED EMBALMING METHODS;
WITH
HINTS ON THE PROFESSION OF UNDERTAKING.

BY AUGUSTE RENOUARD

Rochester, N. Y.
A. H. Nirdlinger & Co., Publishers.
1878

Figure 13. Title page of Auguste Renouard's first edition of *The Undertaker's Manual.*

iation with this school until December 1884. He then entered into an agreement with Hallett and Company Undertakers in Kansas City, Missouri, to locate his school, the School of Embalming and Organic Chemistry, on the company's premises. By mid-1886, he terminated his school in Kansas City and returned to Denver. He then began to travel to distant points such as Ft. Worth,

Figure 14. Auguste Renouard's advertisement for embalming fluid.

Texas, and Toronto and Montreal, Canada, providing embalming instruction for periods ranging from 3 days to 2 weeks.

In 1894, Dr. Renouard made his final move to New York City and established the U.S. College of Embalming. The school had no fixed-term classes and the student remained until he was able to embalm. In 1889, the doctor's son, Charles A. Renouard, was reported to be a shipping clerk with the firm of Dolge and Huncke—Embalming Chemical Manufacturers. Early in 1899, Charles Renouard opened the Renouard Training School for Embalmers in New York City, and in February, 1900, Auguste Renouard closed the U.S. College of Embalming and joined Charles at his school. Charles provided several months of embalming instruction in London, England, on behalf of the O. K. Buckhout Chemical Company of Grand Rapids, Michigan. In 1906, Auguste traveled to England and continental Europe where he was most graciously received and entertained.

Auguste Renouard died in his home in 1912. A monument paid for by voluntary subscription of his former students was an example of the esteem in which he was held by those he instructed. **He can, without question, be regarded as the first major figure to provide embalming instruction for undertakers in the United States.** His son Charles continued the Renouard Training School for Embalmers until his death in 1950.

Joseph Henry Clarke. Born in Connersville, Indiana, Joseph Henry Clarke (1840–1916) received his early education in pharmacy and enrolled as a student in a medical college in Keokuk, Iowa. His studies, however, were interrupted by the Civil War. He volunteered for service with the Union Army but was rejected because of physical defects. He was permitted to serve as a civilian and later held the position of assistant hospital steward in the Fifth Iowa Infantry. After the death of his father, he returned home before the end of the war to support his family. He married and secured employment as a casket salesman. During the course of his travel, he became acquainted with a fluid manufacturer and became sufficiently interested in embalming to sell embalming fluids as a sideline. His interest in embalming grew as he realized the need to demonstrate the method of use of the fluid he hoped to sell to his patrons. This, in turn, led to his study of and experimentation with embalming chemicals to solve problems relating to preservation of the dead. He enrolled in an anatomy course conducted by Dr. C. M. Lukens of the Pulte Medical College in Cincinnati, Ohio, which broadened into a lifetime friendship and professional partnership in the founding of the Clarke School of Embalming at Cincinnati in 1882 (Fig. 15).

The school lacked permanence because Mr. Clarke traveled most of the year giving courses of instruction,

Figure 15. Portrait of Joseph Henry Clarke, founder of the Cincinnati College of Embalming.

each course varying in length from 2 to 7 days. His second course of instruction away from Cincinnati was presented in New York City. One class member was Felix A. Sullivan, who later became a well-known teacher and writer in the embalming field. Sullivan and Clarke became rivals and bitter enemies. One major clash occurred when General and ex-President Ulysses S. Grant died on July 23, 1885, at Mt. McGregor, New York. Clarke had been advised by the Holmes Undertaking Company (no relation to Thomas Holmes) of Saratoga, New York, that the company would be retained to handle the funeral of General Grant and that they wanted Clarke to do the embalming. Clarke was in Baltimore on the day of Grant's death, but he became ill and went to his Springfield, Ohio, home where he was bedridden for 3 to 4 weeks. The embalming was accordingly performed by one member of the Holmes Undertaking Company family and Dr. McEwen using Clarke's proprietary embalming chemical (Fig. 16).

After the body had been embalmed, Rev. Stephen Merritt, clergyman and undertaker of New York City and also General Grant's religious adviser, arrived together with Felix A. Sullivan and announced that they were to take charge. The Holmes personnel withdrew from the premises and Sullivan proceeded to reembalm the body. He claimed he withdrew all previously injected arterial

Reminiscences of Early Embalming

By Joseph Henry Clarke

Father of American Embalming Schools

The Sunnyside
New York
1917

Figure 16. Title page of an article by Joseph Henry Clarke for *The Sunnyside*.

fluid and replaced it with the chemical made by the company he represented. Clarke rebuffed these claims in the professional journals. A reporter from *The New York Times* wrote that Mr. Holmes (of Saratoga, New York) was too drunk to carry out the necessary preparation of the body. *The New York Times* was subsequently sued for libel and lost the case, and Mr. Holmes was awarded several thousand dollars in damages.

The name of the embalming school was changed to the Cincinnati College of Embalming in 1899 and was established on a permanent basis. Mr. Clarke conducted only occasional lecture tours at that time. He was ably assisted in the management of the school by his son, C. Horace Clarke. In 1907, Charles O. Dhonau became associated with him and later took over operation of the school. Mr. Clarke was a capable teacher, lecturer, and author of several texts on embalming, and he held several patents in the embalming field. He retired in 1909 to San Diego, California, where he died in 1916.

Felix Aloysius Sullivan (1843–1931). Sullivan was born in Toronto, Ontario, Canada, in 1843, the son of a Scottish immigrant undertaker and an Irish mother. He unquestionably had the most interesting, controversial, riotous, and successful career as a practitioner, writer, teacher, and lecturer of embalming and related subjects. His career was so full of incidents that it would be impossible to recount all but a few highlights.

After the Civil War, he followed various occupations and traveled. He eventually drifted to New York City where he secured employment with various casket companies and finally became a funeral director for hire. He studied anatomy and other medical sciences and, by 1881, became an embalmer of some local repute. He was hired to go to Cleveland, Ohio, to reembalm President Garfield, who died from an assassin's bullet, and seems to have been successful in this venture. Sullivan attended Clarke's embalming class in New York City in 1882 to learn how such a class of instruction was conducted. Sullivan, together with W. G. Robinson, opened the New York School of Embalming in 1884 and a year later was again involved in the embalming of a president, this time President Ulysses Grant (see previous information on Clarke's career). He then entered and left along list of employers. In 1887, he was in Chicago when the anarchists who bombed the police in 1886, killing and wounding police and civilians, were condemned to die. One exploded a dynamite cap in his mouth in jail and the others were hung. He prepared all bodies and was praised for his plastic surgery on the "mad bomber."

Sullivan continued his erratic employment or work habits, working for one firm, quitting, and then working for another. By 1891, he was again a lecturer/demonstrator, this time for the Egyptian Chemical Company. By 1892, he reached the height of his career as a lecturer, speaking and teaching in more cities to larger classes than anyone previously had. He was expelled from the State Funeral Directors convention in 1893 in St. Louis, Missouri, and a resolution was passed to forbid ever inviting his return. Sullivan settled in Chicago and opened a school of embalming. Local papers relate his arrest there together with a female companion (not his wife) on charges of adultery and wife and child desertion. When he finally settled the charges, he underwent a cure for alcoholism and resumed teaching in a succession of short-lived appointments at various schools.

In 1900, the O. K. Buckhout Company of Michigan, a manufacturer of embalming chemicals, had Charles A. Renouard under contract to lecture and sent him to London, England, to present a 3-week course of instruction that was very well received. Renouard returned home to attend similar engagements in the United States. The Buckhout Company had to find someone to continue the successful course of instruction in England, and the position was offered to Sullivan, who immediately accepted. Sullivan began teaching in London on October 8, 1900, a career that would extend to 1903. He lectured throughout the British Isles and helped to organize the British Embalmers Society as well as a journal entitled the *British Embalmer.*

He related that when Queen Victoria died in 1901, he was consulted about the possibility of embalming her. He recommended against it because it was impossible to guarantee perfect results. When he returned to the United States, he purchased an embalming school in St. Louis, Missouri, but the venture proved unprofitable. He then moved to Denver and Salt Lake City and eventually back to St. Louis, where he died. Sullivan wrote hundreds of articles plus eight books, taught thousands to embalm, and probably received more gifts from his classes than any other teacher before or since his time.

A. Johnson Dodge (1848–1926). Little did A. Johnson Dodge know in 1889 that he and his family were about to embark on a remarkable history of service to the funeral profession. At that time, he was a Maine legislator and general store owner, while his brother George B. Dodge ran a printing company in Boston. When the owner of the Egyptian Chemical Company was not able to pay a bill to the printing company, George was given the company to pay the indebtedness. A. J. was an avid student of anatomy and chemistry and George knew that he had always dreamed of being physician. By 1890, George had convinced A. J. to close the store and come to Boston to learn embalming. His love of knowledge and learning went hand in hand with his ability to teach. He authored three textbooks of the day: *The Embalmer's Guide, The Essentials of Anatomy,* and *Sanitary Science and Embalming and the Practical Embalmer.*

Embalming instruction in those days was provided by embalming chemical companies through teachers who traveled around the country giving 2-day courses. In 1893, George and A. J. Dodge bought the Oriental School of Embalming, a traveling school based in Boston. By the end of that year, A. J. Dodge had resigned from the Egyptian Chemical Company but continued with the Oriental School. The school was renamed the Massachusetts College of Embalming in 1895 and incorporated under the Massachusetts nonprofit educational act. A. J. Dodge founded a new school in 1907, the New England Institute of Anatomy, Sanitary Science and Embalming, after selling his interest in the Massachusetts College. The New England Institute was chartered by the Commonwealth of Massachusetts as a nonprofit educational institution in 1910 and is still in operation today. In addition to these activities, A. J. Dodge served as a principal lecturer at the Barnes School of Anatomy and had founded his own manufacturing company after leaving the Egyptian Company.

A. J. Dodge's son, Walter Dodge, continued the family business by learning embalming and taking his skills to Detroit where he opened the Dodge Chemical Company. At the same time, his father was also opening the Dodge Chemical Company in Boston. They decided to join forces and the first plant was run out of A. J.'s home. A. J.'s knowledge of chemistry [leads] led him to develop a research arm of the company while still conducting all the lectures on the road. He traveled by train to various cities where he would arrange for demonstrations when bodies were available. By 1913 A. J.'s younger son George B. Dodge II joined the firm as a very successful salesman for the company.

The facilities for manufacturing at the home were becoming inadequate to keep up with the demand for their products. The next four decades saw tremendous growth of the company, leading to the move to its present location in Cambridge, Massachusetts. During this time, not only was the company expanding locally in the Boston area but it was also opening branch offices in other U.S. cities and Canada as well. Branch offices and warehouses were opened in Los Angeles, Fort Worth, Texas, and Chicago to provide its customers all over the country with prompt service. The Dodge Chemical Company (Canada) was formed in Toronto and had complete manufacturing facilities. By 1982, the company had expanded to Europe and now also has distributors in Australia, New Zealand, Mexico, and Japan.

One thing that A. J. Dodge clearly understood from very early on was the importance of research. He was always striving to create better products and techniques for the embalmer. To this end, he hired a full-time graduate chemist from Yale University, William B. O'Brien. O'Brien remained with Dodge until the time of his death. Research was to continue as an important part of the manufacturing process throughout the company's history. Important studies and discoveries were made by the likes of Louis McDonald, Dr. Jerome Frederick, and Margaret Boothe.

Even after A. J. Dodge's death, the family continued to devote significant time and resources to continuing education for embalmers and funeral directors. Today, the Dodge Company is still owned and operated by the Dodge family. They have remained true to A. J.'s vision of service to the funeral profession in everything they do.

Increase in Embalming Schools

Some early "graduates" of embalming courses of instruction gave up regular employment at an undertaking establishment to provide embalming service to a number of undertakers who had no staff member trained to embalm. **This is how the terms *embalmer to the trade* or *trade embalmer originated.***

Many undertakers and/or their assistants were eager to learn to embalm but were unable to absent

Figure 17. Old Indianapolis College of Embalming, Indianapolis, Indiana.

themselves from their business or employment to take advantage of such training. Some, however, managed to attend the 3- to 5-day schools, sponsored by the embalming chemical companies, in their city where they were taught the basic skills by the itinerant instructors. Others augmented their meager knowledge by enrolling in home study courses offered by many of the established schools of embalming.

Schools of instruction in embalming increased in number and activity by the beginning of the twentieth century. Many manufacturers of embalming chemicals entered into the business of teaching embalming to maintain and increase the market for their products. Although the repair of injuries to the dead caused by disease or trauma had been dealt with since Egyptian times, it was not until 1912 that a systematic treatment for such cases was developed by a New York City embalmer, Joel E. Crandall (1878–1942). From this time on, the schools of embalming slowly began to adopt instruction in this special phase of embalming treatment. Today, the subject area is commonly referred to as **restorative art.** It would be impossible to list in this text every personality who became an embalming professor or every school that was established, but a few should be mentioned.

Carl Lewis Barnes. Born into a family that operated an undertaking establishment in Connellsville, Pennsylvania, Barnes (1872–1927) studied medicine in Indiana, opened an embalming school there (Fig. 17), and moved it to Chicago. He manufactured embalming chemicals, wrote many books and articles on the subject, and had the largest chain of fixed-location schools in history in New York, Chicago, Boston, Minneapolis, and Dallas. While serving overseas as a medical colonel in the U.S. Army in World War I, his business failed. He never reopened the schools, continuing the practice of medicine until his death (Fig. 18).

Albert H. Worsham. Worsham (1868–1939) attended Barnes's school and was on the faculty from 1903 to 1911 when he opened his own school in Chicago, with his wife Laura and brother Robert as faculty members. He lectured widely and was noted principally for contributing to the early foundation of postmortem plastic surgery.

Howard S. Eckels. Eckels (1865–1937) was a manufacturer of embalming chemicals and the founder of Eckels College of Embalming in Philadelphia, Pennsylvania. *(The school and chemical plant were in the same building, which*

Figure 18. Advertisement for Barnes's handless injector.

closed after a period of affiliation with Temple University.

William Peter Hohenschuh. Born in Iowa City, Iowa, the son of an undertaker, Hohenschuh (1858–1920) took over the family business on the death of his father and began to teach embalming, which he had learned by correspondence from Auguste Renouard in the mid-1870s. Hohenschuh was active in the Iowa State Association and was elected president to the NFDA. He operated an embalming school in Chicago and, in 1900, in partnership with Dr. William S. Carpenter (1871–1944), opened the Hohenschuh-Carpenter School of Embalming in Des Moines, Iowa. He also operated a funeral home. In 1930, Dr. Carpenter moved the school to St. Louis and merged it with the Moribund American College of Embalming owned by F. A. Sullivan. After Dr. Carpenter's death, his daughter Helene Craig and her son Golden Craig operated the school as well as the American Academy in New York City. This continued well into the post–World War II period.

Clarence G. Strub. Born in Iowa March 1, 1906, Strub attended the University of Iowa in Iowa City, Washington University in St. Louis, Missouri, and the Hohenschuh-Carpenter College of Embalming in Des Moines, Iowa. He became an instructor at the Hohenschuh-Carpenter College in 1929. In 1930, the school was moved to St. Louis where it merged with the American College of Embalming and operated under the name of the St. Louis College of Mortuary Science. In 1934, he became a member of the staff of the Undertaker's Supply Company of Chicago and conducted clinics and demonstrations throughout the United States and Canada. He taught embalming and funeral management at the University of Minnesota and the Wisconsin Institute of Mortuary Science and was the director of research for the Royal Bond Chemical Company for many years (Fig. 19).

His greatest contributions to embalming lie in his ability to write clearly and simply, explaining embalming theory and practices. During his career, he published well over 1000 articles as well as many teaching outlines and quiz compendia. His little text, *The Principles of Restorative Art*, was the true prototype of all present-day texts on the subject. He also authored the monumental textbook *Principles and Practice of Embalming*, published by L. G. "Darko" Fredericks, which became the standard embalming text used by most colleges of mortuary science. Strub also wrote several technical movies such as the *Conquest of Jaundice* and *The Eye Bank Story* as well as many children's stories and movies. He was the architect of the Eye Bank System in Iowa, which set the national pattern, as well as the curator of the state of Iowa's anatomical donation program. He died in Iowa City, Iowa, on August 6, 1974.

was not an uncommon arrangement.) Eckels wrote many articles and books, was successfully sued for plagiarism, and was not adverse to engaging in prolonged debates in the press. After his death, his son John managed the school well into the post–World War II period when it

Figure 19. Photograph of Clarence G. Strub.

Women Embalmers. Women as well as men were trained as embalmers and not only practiced embalming but founded schools of instruction. Among these women were **Mrs. E. G. Bernard** of Newark, New Jersey, who founded the Bernard School of Embalming; **Mme. Linda D. Odou,** who founded the Odou Embalming Institute in New York City (Fig. 20); and **Lena R. Simmons**, who founded and operated the Simmons School of Embalming in Syracuse, New York, until her son Baxter took over the management.

▶ MORTUARY EDUCATION

Each course in a college of mortuary science employs a basic course content. Now overseen by various committees of the American Board of Funeral Service Education, the basic course content in embalming is a foundation for uniform performance standards in the preparation of all bodies embalmed in the United States. This basic course content also allows the Conference of Funeral Service Examining Boards to administer a uniform objective examination to those who are candidates for a license. As an introduction to this chapter, we are going to take an overview of the development of the basic course content in embalming, as it lays the foundation for professional performance standards.

Mortuary colleges, as we know them today, are relatively recent in origin. The development of mortuary education has followed the general pattern common to all professional fields. It emerged slowly from a period in which knowledge was transmitted from preceptor to student by means of observation and informal discussion, to its present academic status.

Following the American Civil War, when funeral homes first came into existence, the pioneers in funeral service experimented with materials, equipment, and methods for their use. There were no channels for wide distribution of the knowledge they gained through trial and error. Training was conducted solely by means of apprenticeship.

As the scope of funeral service expanded and as embalming came into wider use, commercial companies were organized to supply the needs of the embalmer and funeral director. Research was directed to developing

Figure 20. Anatomy class at Odou Institute of Embalming, New York, circa 1900 (Professor Odou at center of group).

better products, and this resulted in a rapid increase in knowledge of what today is termed *mortuary science.* During the latter decades of the nineteenth century, the establishment of trade journals made possible a wider distribution of this knowledge. These same companies employed skilled lecturers and demonstrators to instruct funeral directors in the use of these products and in improved methods of embalming. These early "classes," lasting from a few hours to a few days, provided the first formal vocational instruction.

As the public health and welfare aspects of funeral service became more widely recognized, state licensing laws were established. For the first time, educational requirements were formulated and a definite course of training was legally prescribed. At about this same time, educators established the first schools of embalming to train students in a relatively new art. Over the years, these pioneers in mortuary education expanded and improved the scope of training, often keeping far ahead of requirements prescribed by law and by licensing authorities.

A system for national accreditation of mortuary schools was first introduced in 1927 by the Conference of Funeral Service Examining Boards, a national association of state licensing boards. Higher standards governing qualifications of faculty, the curriculum, and teaching facilities were established and enforced. Details of

the development of mortuary schools can be found in Part II of this textbook.

The National Council on Mortuary Education was established in 1942 by the NFDA and the National Association of Embalming Schools and Colleges. After World War II, with the termination of restrictions on assembly, a formal meeting was held in December of 1945 in Cleveland, Ohio. Officers for the Council were Chairman, Ralph Millard; Vice-Chairman, Jacob Van't Hof; and Secretary Treasurer, R. P. Mac Fate. The Council was attended by 62 school administrators, faculty members, state board authorities, and various funeral service association officers. The program committee comprised John Eckles, Jacob Van't Hof, and Otto Margolis. This meeting gave a fresh impetus to progress toward educational competence and professional status in funeral service. In March of 1947, the First National Teacher's Institute was held in Cincinnati, Ohio. Forty-four representatives from 14 schools met to lay the foundation for the course content in Chemistry and Mortuary Administration. Charles O. Dhonau of the Cincinnati College of Embalming presided over the meeting. In November of 1947, the Second Teacher's Institute was held in Pittsburgh, Pennsylvania (Fig. 21). More than 75 individuals from 23 schools and associations were present. Adopted at this meeting was the first basic course content syllabus for anatomy and embalming and the Mortician's

Figure 21. Educators from across the United States gathered for the Second Teachers Institute held in Pittsburgh, Pennsylvania, November 8 and 9, 1947. At this meeting, the first curriculum in anatomy and embalming was established and the Mortician's Oath was adopted. (*Courtesy of the Pittsburgh Institute of Mortuary Science, Pittsburgh, Pennsylvania.*)

Oath (drafted by R. P. Mac Fate). The Oath has been administered to all graduates of a mortuary college since 1948. Dr. Emory S. James of Pittsburgh was chair of the anatomy course content committee. The committee on the basic course content in embalming consisted of R. H. Hannum (Cleveland), L. G. Frederick (Dallas), R. Victor Landig (Houston), J. E. Shea (Boston), and E. L. Heidenreich (Wisconsin). The formulation and analysis of the embalming basic course content was brought about through the efforts of mortuary colleges, state boards, state associations, and the profession in general. The task was difficult because it meant resolving many individualistic teaching procedures into one common, sound educational basis. Once the basic course content was established, it was immediately recognized there would be an imperative need to review and update the curriculum every few years. Revision of the course content has continued over the years and is currently overseen by the American Board of Funeral Service Education. In their July 1994 meeting in Denver, Colorado, a glossary of terminology was appended to the basic course content in embalming. In a meeting in Denver as late as July of 2000, the basic course content in embalming was again reviewed, amended, and prepared for editing and input by the member schools of the American Board of Funeral Service Education. This basic course content is an example of a professional performance standard in the field of embalming in America.

▶ CONCERN FOR TREATMENT

Early embalming reports concerning arterial injection indicated some concern for special treatment of the trunk viscera. Most such treatments consisted of removal, treatment, and replacement of viscera in the trunk cavity together with some preservative material, either powdered or liquid. Other reports, such as those of the Gannal-Sucquet era, indicate dependence for total preservation solely on the arterial injection unaccompanied by any special treatment for the trunk cavities. Gabriel Clauderus had advocated preservation based on introduction of his preservative chemical into the trunk cavity followed by immersion of the entire body in the preservative.

It was not until the mid-1870s that a "modern" system of treatment for the cavities was designed. The inventor of the trocar, Samuel Rodgers (listing Los Angeles, New York City, and San Francisco as his residences) secured two patents for the trocar, one in 1878 and the second in 1880. The 1878 patent described the trocar much as it exists today. The 1880 patent was issued for a system of embalming that consisted of introduction of his trocar, thrust through a single point in the navel into all the organs of the trunk to distribute a preservative fluid throughout the trunk viscera. The simplicity of this treatment and its modest success made it appealing to those who, for whatever reason, did not adopt arterial embalming, which required greater knowledge of anatomy and surgical skill. The inevitable result was a confrontation between "belly punchers" (cavity treatment advocates) and "throat cutters" (arterial embalmers) concerning the merits of their respective means of preservation.

It slowly became evident that neither system was always completely successful and that combination of the two systems, arterial injection followed by cavity treatment, offered the greatest promise of embalming success. Although Rodgers did not mention aspiration prior to injection of preservative chemicals in his process, Auguste Renouard did specifically recommend this in his *Undertaker's Manual*. Rodgers's method of a single-entrance opening into the trunk cavity was a brilliant concept not followed by all his contemporary "authorities." Espy's and Taylor's books of embalming instruction, for example, advocated multiple (three to four) points of insertion through the trunk wall for the trocar. Rodgers formulated an embalming preservative chemical named *Alekton*, which was believed to have phenol as its principal preservative. He also recommended cavity treatment followed by hypodermic injections using his trocar, inserted into the limbs of the corpse.

Since the introduction of arterial injection of the blood vessels in the late seventeenth century, no other system of corpse preservation explored had ever been seriously used. In 1884, a British physician, Dr. B. W. Richardson, devised what he termed **needle embalming.** The process consisted of inserting a trocar (the needle), such as Rodgers's invention, at the medial corner of the eye socket and forcing it into the brain area, where the injection process was repeated. After removal of the trocar from the brain area, cavity treatment, aspiration, and injection were carried out. This process was most often referred to as the **eye process.** Rodgers in his early patent had proposed insertion of his trocar through the nose to inject preservative chemicals into the brain area, but did not suggest that this process would preserve the entire body as Richardson contended. It eventually was to be called the **nasal process.** Professor Sullivan, ever alert for any new procedure to interest his students, adopted Richardson's eye process and exploited its simplicity to the maximum.

Carl Barnes offered a variation of the procedure by inserting the trocar through the neck and into the brain via the foramen magnum. T. B. Barnes, his brother and school instructor associate, inserted the trocar between dorsal vertebrae into the spinal canal. In this method, Dr. Eliab Meyers drilled a hole through the center of the vertex of the skull, permitting direct access for a small trocar into the superior sagittal sinus. The process, regardless of point of access, is said to have delivered the preservative chemical eventually into blood vessels within the cranium and then to the rest of the body.

A dramatic test demonstration of the process is both described and illustrated in Barnes' textbook, *The Art and Science of Embalming*. A severed head of a dissection room subject had trocars inserted into the brain area through the eye socket route. Rubber tubes connected the carotid arteries and jugular veins with collecting bottles. As fluid was injected through the trocars into the brain area, fluid flowed into the collecting bottles via the carotid arteries and jugular veins. The process achieved moderate popularity until about 1905 when it became extinct. Not all teachers of embalming were advocates of it, and J. H. Clarke was a vigorous critic.

A variation of the process was the short-lived attempt to insert the trocar into the left ventricle of the heart and inject the arterial system. The great difficulty encountered in positively locating the left ventricle quickly discouraged this procedure. The intentional application of an electric current directly to a corpse for the intended purpose of simulating the effect of lightning or accidental electrocution on the blood—destruction of blood coagulation—has been attempted many times without any appreciable success.

One early experimenter was Charles T. Schade of McAlester, Oklahoma, who as early as 1909 conceived the idea of applying an electric current, powered by dry cell batteries, to the body surface, in the belief that this would cause small muscles to contract and hence force blood out of the areas of discoloration. No effect was noted concerning the ability of an electric current applied externally to a corpse to prevent normal postmortem blood coagulation or promote dissolution of any existing intravascular clots. Similar attempts to accomplish this desirable effect have been attempted through the years down to the present both in the United States and in England without success. Those who have experimented have concluded that the dead human body does not conduct an electrical current well enough to accomplish the intended purpose.

Toward the end of the nineteenth century and on into the twentieth century, a number of events were to occur that would accelerate embalming toward the level of professionalism. A convergence of two movements became apparent around 1897, with the appearance of advertisements by embalming fluid companies stating that their fluid contained formalin. For some years, there had been arguments to eliminate arsenic and other poisons from inclusion in embalming fluid formulas for the same medicolegal reason that the French prohibited arsenic in 1846 and bichloride of mercury in 1848. Now that a powerful disinfectant, **formalin**, was available and reasonably priced, the opportunity to eliminate poisonous

chemicals was at hand. The state of Michigan led the way in 1901 and was followed by other states.

The second movement was to require regulations for both licensing and governing those who practiced embalming, and in 1893–1894, the state of Virginia became the first state to do so. Formalin content fluids were not a total blessing and were not as favorably received as might have been expected. Embalmers of the period were unaccustomed to the very different characteristics of the new preservative. For example, bodies embalmed with arsenic were said to have been relatively supple, making dressing and positioning relatively easy. Many of the poisonous chemicals had bleaching qualities and left the body quite white. Only a few left any undesirable coloration, such as those reported to contain copper, which tended to produce a bluish color in the skin. Then too, little or no problem was reportedly encountered to the penetration of all the body tissues, with or without blood drainage. There was also the proven ability of such poisonous chemicals to preserve the body tissues. There were, of course, some negatives such as the possible absorption of poisonous chemicals through the embalmer's unprotected skin, various skin irritations, and thickened and cracked fingernails.

Embalmers beginning to experiment with the formalin-based embalming fluids had to learn that they must remove the blood in all cases and began to use low-formalin-content or nonformalin fluids to wash the blood out before injection of the preservative formalin-based solutions. They also learned that they had to position the body properly before injection and the hardening effected by formalin or they would encounter serious problems later in trying to properly position hands together. To their astonishment, embalmers also discovered that formalin reacted with the bile pigments present in the skin of jaundiced bodies to produce an unsightly green-colored skin.

The opponents of formalin fluids were highly critical of the formaldehyde fumes, which irritated mucous membranes, claiming these effects were more dangerous to health than the poisonous chemicals. Reason and science prevailed, and the embalming fluid formulas were improved to overcome most of the early problems. With the eventual transfer of the site of embalming from the family home bedroom to the funeral home preparation room, proper ventilation tended to eliminate most of the irritation problem. Chemicals became more diverse. For example, different formulas were developed for specific uses, such as arterial and cavity, preinjection, coinjection, and for special purposes as in decomposing cases. The delivery of embalming fluids in concentrated form, to be added to water to create the desired dilution strength, was a distinct contrast to the former embalming chemical packaging, which was delivered in containers already combined with water ready to inject. Thus, embalmers had to become more experienced and intelligent in the mixing of the formalin embalming solution than they had formerly been.

▶ UTILIZATION OF NEW DEVICES

Over the years of embalming in bedrooms of the home of the deceased, little in the way of improvements was instituted in injection pumps or aspirating devices. With the transfer of the majority of embalming preparations to the funeral home, however, new devices could be used. In the last quarter of the nineteenth century, most embalming pumps or injectors were based on the gravity bowl, the hand pump, or the rubber bulb syringe. The gravity bowl was simply a container suspended above the body and connected to the arterial tube by a length of rubber tubing. The height of the bowl above the body determined the pressure. Its main advantage was that it did not require the constant pumping by the embalmer and, therefore, left hands free to perform other tasks. The hand pump could produce either pressure or vacuum for injection or aspiration into or from a glass container.

When the preparation of the body was moved to the funeral home, water pressure was used to create suction to aspirate. Special aspirators, such as the Penberthy, Worsham, and Slaughter models, generated suction by water pressure and were made to attach to preparation room sink faucets, connected by rubber tubing to the trocar. Later in the 1950s, special electric motor-driven aspirators were devised and were found to overcome the aggravation encountered by low water pressure during high-water-use periods. *Most communities today have requirements relating to the need for preventing suction of aspirated material into the water system.*

At a New York state convention in 1914, a battery-powered electric pump, the Falcon Electric Embalmer for injecting embalming chemicals, was demonstrated but was not widely adopted. Some new instruments devised to simplify or improve certain embalming procedures were developed in the 1920s and 1930s. A new method of jaw closure was devised involving "barbed tacks" driven into the mandible and maxillae by a spring-propelled hammer. Wires attached to the "tacks" were then twisted together to secure the desired degree of jaw closure. A plastic, threaded, screwlike device called the **trocar button** became the most useful waterproof seal for trocar punctures, bullet wounds, and even for intravenous needle punctures (when surgically enlarged). A metal dispensing device that was attached directly to any standard 16-ounce bottle of cavity fluid (by screwing it into the bottle opening in place of the cap) simplified cavity fluid injection. The dispenser was connected to the trocar by a length of rubber hose and injection was

accomplished by gravity after the cavity fluid bottle was elevated and inverted.

It was not until the mid-1930s that electric-powered injection machines were available and in use. Some were simply electric motors with fittings to produce pressure or vacuum-connected to suitable containers by rubber tubing. One of the first "self-contained" embalming fluid injection machines put on the market in the 1930s was the Snyder–Westberg device. It was originally designed to hold one half gallon of embalming fluid. The machine was compact, durable, and trouble free, and was originally designed with motor and the fluid container side by side. Model II of the Snyder–Westberg device was designed so that the fluid container was placed above the injection motor; thus, the fluid was "gravity fed" to the pump. This arrangement has become standard on all self-contained units. In 1937, the Slaughter Company developed an all-metal fluid injection tank equipped with a pressure gauge; in 1938, the Flow master electric-powered injection machine was announced; in 1939, the Frigid Fluid Company developed a pressure injector consisting of a metal container for holding embalming fluid complete with exit connection with shut-off and a carbon dioxide gas cylinder to create the necessary pressure to inject the fluid. **In mid-1939, the Turner Company announced the availability of the Porti Boy, which was to become the all-time most popular injection machine.** Several improvements over the years included a pulsator device, a larger fluid tank, and the ability to produce extreme high-pressure injections. By the 1960s, extreme high-pressure injection machines such as the Sawyer were available and in use.

▶ AVAILABILITY OF MODERN MATERIALS

With the end of World War II, metal and other materials became available to produce various new embalming devices. The concept of using externally generated agitation to assist in blood removal became popular. Some embalming tables had such pulsating devices built in as an integral part of the structure. Other pulsating devices were devised to be attached to existing operating tables or were handheld devices to be applied to the body over the course of the major blood vessels. Disillusionment with this development came after a short period of use. The vibrations produced by such devices made it impossible to keep instruments, and even the body itself, from sliding downward toward the foot of the table.

Another innovation was the development of a conventional embalming fluid by the Switzer Corporation of Cleveland that contained a large quantity of fluorescent dye. The dye was to act as a tracer or indicator of the degree of circulation or penetration of the embalming fluid when viewed under an ultraviolet light illuminator furnished with the embalming fluid. Although the system did indeed disclose the extent of the distribution of the embalming chemical and its fluorescent dye, it never was proof positive that areas of the body beneath the skin were thoroughly embalmed.

In the wake of Hiroshima and Nagasaki and other major disasters such as airline crashes, earthquakes, mudslides, and building collapses, a search was instituted for some new means of quickly processing (preserving) huge numbers of dead. Over the years, different means of processing (preserving) the victims of such tragedies were devised, tested, and found unsuitable for various reasons. Experiments were conducted with processes using ultrasound, radiation, atomic bombardment, and ultracold. No process tried seemed to be capable of preserving a tremendous number of bodies in a brief period. The search continues!

Indisputably, the greatest change in embalming procedures began in the 1980s by the intervention of federal government agencies. The Federal Trade Commission (FTC) adopted rules concerning the necessity for embalming and the securing of consent for same. The Occupational Safety and Health Administration (OSHA) adopted rules relating to embalming procedures, funeral home personnel protection, and similar public health and hygienic measures. The Environmental Protection Agency (EPA) issued rules concerning the use and control of formaldehyde and chemicals used by embalmers.

Although it has been generally conceded that formaldehyde-based fluids performed well as preserving and fixing agents for the embalming process, chemical research for an improvement in embalming chemicals has always been active.

During the 1930s, Hilton Ira Jones of the Hizone Company performed extensive research on glyoxal, a chemical that seemed to display much promise for use in an embalming formula. World War II, however, reduced the available supply and thus the research in this direction.

Another chemical, glutaraldehyde, was thoroughly researched and developed into an embalming formula by the Champion Company.

At the time of publication of this textbook edition, several embalming fluid companies have formulations that replace formaldehyde in embalming solutions. We also have the development of the first computerized embalming machine by Trinity Fluids, LLC. This machine allows for a closed system of delivery of a chosen chemical solution through the use of a computer-based system. The Embalmatron machine may well assist with the problems some firms see with OSHA compliance for the formaldehyde rule.

Since the intervention of OSHA in embalming procedures, the search has intensified to find a substitute for formaldehyde and thus eliminate the vexatious problems of monitoring formaldehyde fume levels and wearing filter masks as required by OSHA regulations.

It is astonishing what has been achieved in the embalming field in nearly 5000 years of growth of knowledge, skill, and experience. Naturally, what the future holds is unknown, but those working in the field feel it will be as exciting and rewarding as the past millennia.

▶ PROFESSIONALISM IN EMBALMING

In many states, a single license to practice as a funeral director and embalmer is issued. The remaining states issue a separate license for embalming and a separate license for funeral directing. As a result, members of large funeral directors state associations and trade associations such as the NFDA, International Order of the Golden Rule (OGR), International Cemetery, Cremation and Funeral Association (ICCFA), or Selected Funeral Directors Association include individuals who are both embalmers and funeral directors. Their educational and convention programs attempt to include both groups. However, in more recent years, programming emphasis has been placed on the subjects related to funeral directing.

Trade associations devoted solely to embalmers are very few in number. The oldest international association (and by far the largest with over 1300 members in Britain alone) is the British Institute of Embalmers (BIE) founded in 1927. It has 14 divisions; 9 divisions within England and Scotland, while other divisions include Ireland, Belgium, Australia, Overseas, and the latest the North American division established in 1994. In the United States, the Ohio Embalmers Association founded in 1931 is the oldest and one of the largest. The second oldest is the Academy of Graduate Embalmers in Georgia founded in 1955. A recent but very active association is the Michigan Embalmers Association. In 2004, The American Society of Embalmers was established. These organizations provide educational programs for their members along with publications and Web sites with resources for the embalmer.

With many states beginning to require continuing education for licensees and with the increasing difficulty of the types of embalming cases being seen in preparation rooms around the country, there became the need for embalming seminars for mortuary school graduates.

The Dodge Seminars have been providing funeral directors and embalmers with educational seminars since the 1950s. With lectures and demonstrations by men like Ray Slocum, Louis Fitzpatrick, and other Dodge staff members, they have kept education as an important part of their mission. In 1921, the company began producing a house journal that published articles on various subjects on both embalming and funeral directing and continues today as *The Dodge Magazine*.

Vernie Fountain's Fountain National Academy in Springfield, Missouri, focuses on those difficult case embalmings. He brings in attendees from around the world for extended day preparation room sessions. In 2010, he organized the first international embalmers conference. *See the History of Restorative Art chapter for more detailed information.*

Since the Civil War period, the transportation of the deceased from the place of death back to their home has been on the increase. From the days when train transportation was the most common method of transportation within the United States to today when we transport remains around the world, embalming is the best way to preserve the deceased for this purpose. Traveling to foreign countries can take more than 14 days to accomplish due to individual foreign country laws. Many of these laws are outdated but still must be followed or risk having the deceased returned to the funeral director of shipping origin. One of the concerns that were observed here in the United States during the late 1940s and early 1950s was that a family that had a death away from home would be paying for services and merchandise they did not need or necessarily want. To transfer the deceased to their home, they would be purchasing caskets as a means to enclose the deceased during the transport period. The invention of the combination shipping air tray benefited both funeral service and families. This allowed protection of the deceased and the ability of the family to purchase the casket of their choice with the local funeral home. During this time frame, we begin to see the "shipping specialist" emerge. Either local funeral homes that would help to minimize the cost for the family and local funeral home or a company that would have a network of funeral homes that they worked with to effect the speedy and competent preparation of the deceased. The first of these was Inman Nationwide Shipping founded by Robert J. Inman of Cleveland, Ohio. Other companies had been formed but not to the extent that Mr. Inman had successfully created. He eventually expanded services into the international shipping arena as this need arose. Today, the shipping of human remains is done approximately 25 to 30,000 times per year. There are no firm statistics, but this is based on information from the major airlines that handle the majority of human remains shipments.

Unfortunately today, in the modern period of embalming, the evolution of malpractice lawsuits developed against funeral homes for poor preparation of the remains. On a regular basis, we hear horror stories recounted in the media. How these two situations have impacted the public's perception of the need for embalming is unknown. Although there is very little research on the value of viewing the deceased, there are medical journal publications that suggest that there *is a value to the grieving family to see the properly embalmed and presented remains of their loved one.* This remains one of the foremost purposes for embalming.

▶ BIBLIOGRAPHY

Beverly R. *History of Virginia*. 1922:185.

McClelland EH. *Bibliography on Embalming*. New York: National Association of Mortuary Science, 1949. [Mimeographed copy, limited to 100 copies]

McCurdy CW. *Embalming and Embalming Fluids—With Bibliography of Embalming*. Wooster, OH: Herald Printing, 1896.

Oatfield H. *Literature of the Chemical Periphery—Embalming*. Advances in Chemistry Series, No. 16. Washington, DC: American Chemical Society. [A key to pharmaceutical and medicinal chemistry literature]

Pinkerton J. *Collection of Voyages*, Vol. 13. 1812.

Surgeon General's Catalogue. Washington, DC: U.S. Army, 1883–1884.

Townshend J. *Grave Literature*. New York (private collection), 1887. [A catalogue of some books relating to the disposal of bodies and perpetuating the memories of the dead]

Egypt

Aliki. *Mummies Made in Egypt*. New York: Thomas J. Crowell, 1979.

Arcieri GP. *Note E Ricordi—Sulla Preservatione Del Corppo Umano*, No. 1. Florence, Italy: Rivista Di Storia Delle Scienze Medicine E Naturoli, 1956.

Bardeen CR. Anatomy in America. *Bulletin of University of Wisconsin* September 1905, No. 115.

Brier B, Wade RS. The use of natron in human mummification: A modern experiment. *ZAS*, No. 124, 1997.

Brier B, Wade RS, Zimmerman MR. Brief communication: Twentieth-century replication of an Egyptian mummy: Implications of paleopathology. *American Journal of Physical Anthropology* 1998;107.

Budge EAW. *The Mummy*. Cambridge, UK: Cambridge University Press, 1893.

Choulant L. *History and Bibliography of Anatomical Illustration*. New York; 1962. [Reprint]

David AR, ed. *Manchester Museum Mummy Project*. Manchester, UK: Maney and Sons, 1979.

Harris JE, Weeks KR. *X-Raying the Pharaohs*. New York: Charles Scribner's Sons, 1973.

Hemneter E. *Embalming in Ancient Egypt. Ciba Symposia*; Vol. 1, No. 10. Summit, NJ: Ciba Pharmaceuticals, January 1940.

Herodotus. *History*. Rawlinson G, trans. New York: Dial and Tudor Presses, 1928.

Liebling R, et al. *Time Line of Culture in the Nile Valley and Its Relationship to Other Countries*. New York: Metropolitan Museum of Art, 1978.

Martin RA. *Mummies*. Anthropology Leaflet No. 36. Chicago: Chicago Natural History Museum Press, 1945.

Mendelsohn S. *Embalming*. Ciba Symposia, Vol. 6, No. 2. Summit, NJ: Ciba Pharmaceuticals, May 1944.

Moodie RL. *Anthropology Memoir, Vol. III: Roentgenologic Studies of Egyptian and Peruvian Mummies*. Chicago: Field Museum Press, 1931.

Pettigrew TJ. *History of Egyptian Mummies*. London: Longman, Rees, 1834.

Piombino-Mascali D. *Il Maestro del Sonno Eterno*. La Zisa, Palermo, 2009.

Piombino-Mascali D, Williams, MJ. Rosalia Lombardo and her Master Embalmer. *The Director* July 2009.

Pons A. *Les Origines de L'Embaumement et L'Egypte Predynastique*. Montpelier, France: Imprimerie Grollier, 1910.

Smith GE, Dawson WR. *Egyptian Mummies*. New York: Dial Press, 1924.

Steuer RO, Saunders JB de CM. *Ancient Egyptian and Indian Medicine*. Berkeley–Los Angeles: University of California Press, 1959.

Touchette N. MUMAB, The Making of a Modern Mummy. *ChemMatters* February 1996.

Wade RS. Medical mummies: The history of the Burns Collection. *The Anatomical Record*, 1998.

Peru*

Garcillaso de la Vega. *Royal Commentaries of Peru*. Rycant P, trans. London, 1688.

Prescott WH. *History of the Conquest of Peru*, 2 vols. Philadelphia: J.B. Lippincott, 1882.

Rivero ME, Von Tschudi JJ. *Peruvian Antiquities*. Hawks FL, trans. New York: George Putnam, 1853.

Von Hagen VW. *Realm of the Incas*. New York: New American Library of World Literature, 1957.

Alaska and Aleutian Islands

Quimby GI. *Aleutian Islanders*. Anthropology Leaflet, No. 35. Chicago: Natural History Museum, 1944.

North American Indians

Yarrow HC. *Study of Mortuary Customs among the North American Indians*. Washington, DC: U.S. Government Printing Office, 1880.

Ecuador—Jivaro Indians

Cottlow LN. *Amazon Head Hunters*. New York: Signet. Book/Henry Holt, 1953.

Flornoy B. *Jivaro*. New York: Library Publishers, 1954.

*Also see Moodie in list under Egypt.

Canary Islands

De Espinosa A. *The Guanches of Tenerife*. London: Hakluyt Society, 1907.

Hooton EA. *The Ancient Inhabitants of the Canary Islands*. Harvard African Studies, Vol. II. Cambridge, MA: Harvard University Press, 1925.

Europe (Early Period)

Bradford CA. *Heart Burial*. London: Allen & Unwin, 1933.

Castiglioni A, Robinson V. *The Anatomical Theater*. Ciba Symposia, Vol. 3, No. 4. Summit, NJ: Ciba Pharmaceuticals, May 1941.

Clauderus G. *Methodus Balsamundi Corpora Humane Aliaque Majora sine Evisceratione et Sectione Hucusque Solita*. Altenberg, Germany: G. Richterum, 1679.

De Villihardouin G, DeJoinville J. *Memoirs of the Crusades*. New York: E. P. Dutton, 1938.

Dionis M. *Cours D'Operations de Chirurqie*. Paris: d'Houry, 1746.

Dobson J. Some eighteenth century experiments in embalming. *Journal of the History of Medicine* 1953.

Garrison FH. *Introduction to the History of Medicine*. Philadelphia, 1929.

Greenhill T. *Nekrokadeia—Or the Art of Embalming*. London: printed for the author; 1705.

Guichard C. *Des Funerailles et diverses Manieres*. Lyon, France: D'ensevelir, 1582.

Guichard C. *Funerailles*. Lyon, France: Jean de Tovrnes, 1581.

Guybert P. The charitable physitian showing the manner to embalm a dead corpse. In *The Charitable Physitian*. London: Thomas Harper Printer, 1639.

Paré A. *How to Make Reports and to Embalm the Dead* (translated). London: Cotes & Young, 1634.

Pilcher LS. The Mondino myth (reprint). *Medical Library and History Journal* 1906;4(4, December).

The art and science of embalming dead bodies. In Offenbach P, M.D. *A New Medical Treatise*. Frankfort: Zacharian Palthenium, 1605. [Taken from the 29th book of Peter Forestus and translated from the Latin into German]

Treece H. *The Crusades*. New York: Random House, 1962.

Walsh JJ. *The Popes and Science*. New York: Fordham University Press, 1908.

Walsh JJ. *The 13th—Greatest of Centuries*. New York: Catholic Summer School Press, 1907.

Wellcome HS. *The Evolution of Antiseptic Surgery*. London: Burroughs Wellcome, 1910.

Young S. *The Annals of the Barber Surgeons of London*. London: Blades East & Blades, 1890.

Europe (Late Period)

Bailey JB. *The Diary of a Resurrectionist 1811–1812*. London: Swan-Sonnenschein, 1896.

Ball JM. *The Sack em Up Men.* London: Oliver & Boyd, 1928.

Bayle DC. *L'Embaumement.* Paris: Adrien Delahaye, 1873.

Blanchard S. *Anatomia Reformata—Balsamatione, Novus Methodus.* Leiden: Boutesteyn & Lughtmans, 1687.

Cole FJ. *A History of Comparative Anatomy.* London: MacMillan, 1944.

Coliez A. *Conservation Artificielle des Corps.* Paris: Amedee Legrand, 1927.

Cope Z. *The History of the Royal College of Surgeons.* Springfield, IL: Charles C. Thomas, 1959.

Dawson WR. Life and times of Thomas J. Pettigrew. *Med Life* (3 issues) 1931;38(1–3, January–February–March).

DeLint JG. *Atlas of the History of Medicine,* Vol. I. London: H. K. Lewis, 1926.

Eriksson R, ed., trans. *Andreas Vesalius 1st Public Anatomy at Bologna—1540.* Uppsala, Sweden: Almquist & Wikselle, 1959.

Gannal JN. *Histoire des Embaumements.* Paris: Ferra Librairie, 1838.

Gannal JN. Harlan R, trans. *History of Embalming.* Philadelphia: Judah Dobson, 1840.

Gerlt-Wernich-Hirsch. *Biographisches Lexikon Der Herrvorragenden Arzte Aller Zeiten und Volker.* Berlin: Urban & Schwarzenberg, 1932.

Laskowski S. *L'Embaumement, la conservatione des Sujets et les Preparations Anatomiques.* Geneva: H. Georg, 1886.

Mann G. The anatomical collections of Fredrick Ruysch at Leningrad. *Bull Cleve Med Library* 1964;11 (1, January).

Nordenskiold E. *The History of Biology.* New York: Tudor, 1928.

Paget S. *John Hunter.* London: T. Fisher University, 1898.

Peachy GC. *The Homes of Hunter in London.* London: Bailliere, Tindall & Cox, 1928.

Pettigrew JT. Fredrick Ruysch. In *Pettigrew's Medical Portrait Gallery.* London: Whitaker, 1840.

Ramazzini B. *De Morbio Artificum* (2nd ed., 1713). *Diseases of Workers.* Wright WC, trans. New York: Hafner, 1964.

Richardson BW. The art of embalming. In *Wood's Medical and Surgical Monographs,* Vol. III. New York: 1889.

Sigerist HE. *The Great Doctors.* Garden City, NY: Doubleday; 1958.

Singer C. *Studies in the History and Method of Science,* Vol I.—1917, Vol II.—1921. Oxford, England: Clarendon Press.

Sucquet JP. *De L'embaumement et des conservation pour l'etude de l'anatomie.* Paris: Adrien Delahaye, 1872.

Sucquet JP. *Traits du visage dans l'embaumement.* Paris: Adrien Delahaye, 1862.

United States

Barnes CL. *The Art and Science of Embalming.* Chicago: Trade Periodical, 1905.

Clarke CH. *Practical Embalming.* Cincinnati, OH: C. H. Clarke, 1917.

Clarke JH. Reminiscences of Early Embalming. *The Sunnyside,* 1917.

Crane EH. *Manual of Instructions to Undertakers,* 8th ed. Kalamazoo, MI: Kalamazoo, 1888.

Dodge AJ. *The Practical Embalmer.* Boston: A. Johnson Dodge, 1908.

Eckels HS. *Practical Embalmer.* Philadelphia: H. S. Eckels Co., 1903.

Espy JB. *Espy's Embalmer.* Springfield, OH: Espy Fluid Co., 1895.

Gallagher T. The body snatchers. *American Heritage* June 1967.

Johnson EC. Civil war embalming. *Funeral Directors Rev* June–July–August 1965.

Johnson EC, Johnson GR. A Civil War Embalming Surgeon—the story of Dr. Daniel H. Prunk. *The Director* (NFDA publication) January 1970.

Johnson EC, Johnson GR. *Alone in His Glory.* Unpublished manuscript, Civil War Mortuary Practices.

Johnson EC, Johnson GR. *Prince Greer—America's First Negro Embalmer.* Liaison Bulletin, International Federation of Thanatopractic Association, Paris, April 1973.

Johnson EC, Johnson GR. The undertakers manual. *Canadian Funeral News* July 1980.

Johnson EC, Johnson GR, Johnson M. Dr. Thomas Holmes—pioneer embalmer. *American Funeral Director* July–August 1984.

Johnson EC, Johnson GR, Johnson WM. Dr. Renouard's role in embalming history. *American Funeral Director* August 1987.

Johnson EC, Johnson GR, Johnson WM. History of modern restorative art. *American Funeral Director* January–April 1988.

Johnson EC, Johnson GR, Johnson WM. The trial, execution and embalming of two Civil War soldiers. *American Funeral Director* December 1986.

Johnson EC, Johnson M. H. Rhodes—conscientious caretaker of Arlington National Cemetery. *American Funeral Director* January 1984.

Johnson M. A historic precedent to the FTC rules of 1977 (Civil War licensing for embalmer requirements). *NFDA Bulletin* 1979.

Johnson M, Lena R. Simmons—The grand dame of early embalmers. *American Funeral Director* January 1977.

Johnson M, Lina D. Odou—Embalmer. July 1977.

Keen WW. *Addresses and Other Papers.* Philadelphia: Saunders, 1905.

Mendelsohn S. *Embalming Fluids.* New York: Chemical Publishing, 1940.

Mills and Lacey Mfg. Co. *Practical Directions for Embalming the Dead.* Grand Rapids, MI: Stevens, Cornell and Dean, 1881. [No author stated]

Myers E. *Champion Textbook on Embalming.* Springfield, OH: Champion Chemical Co., 1908.

Renouard A. *Undertakers Manual.* Rochester, NY: A. Nirdlinger, 1878.

Renouard CA, ed. *Taylor's Art of Embalming.* New York: H. E. Taylor, 1903.

Samson H, Crane ON, Perrigo AB, et al. *Pharmaceutical, Anatomical and Chemical Lexicon.* Chicago: Donohue & Henneberry, 1886. (The NFDA official textbook)

Strub CA, Frederick LG. *The Principles and Practice of Embalming,* 4th ed. Dallas, TX: L. G. Frederick, 1986.

Sullivan FA. *Practical Embalming.* Boston: Egyptian Chemical Co., 1887.

The faculty of the Cincinnati School for Embalming. In Lukens CM, Clarke JH. *Textbook on Embalming.* Springfield, OH: Limbocker, 1883.

War Department. General Order 75, September 11, 1861.

War Department. General Order 33, April 3, 1862.

War Department. General Order 39, March 15, 1865.

Wightman SK. In search of my son (Civil War). *American Heritage* February 1963.

PART

II

RESTORATIVE ART AND MORTUARY
COSMETOLOGY

SECTION I
RESTORATIVE ART

RESTORATIVE ART—PART 1

Restorative art is defined as "care of the deceased to recreate natural form and color." Two divisions are seen in this definition. The first is the establishment of natural contour or form to the visible surfaces. Examples include reduction of swollen tissue; elevation of sunken tissue; closure of broken tissue; replacement of missing skin; and alignment, elevation, or depression of fractured bones. Second is establishment of normal skin color. Examples include bleaching and/or covering a discoloration, replacement of natural skin color lost through the embalming process, and application of ornamental cosmetics for women. This phase of restorative art is often referred to as mortuary cosmetology.

A practical approach to restorative work is taken in this text. For detailed study of the bones, muscles, tissues, and vascular systems of the head and hands and an in-depth study of physiognomy of the face refer to anatomical publications or texts devoted entirely to restorative art. Throughout this portion of the text, the term *embalmer* will be used rather than *restorative artist* or *cosmetologist*.

Since the mid-1930s, funeral service professionals and the public expect the body to be prepared so that viewing is possible by family and friends. Damage from traumatic injuries, tissue and organ donations, the effects of disease, therapeutic drug and surgical treatments, or early postmortem changes should not be evident when proper restorative treatments have been performed. The goal here is to bring about a change from an appearance which is unacceptable to one which family and friends will find acceptable.

► CONSERVATIVE APPROACH

The funeral director and the embalmer should always take a conservative approach to restorative work and its end results. Statements of assured physical improvement should be limited, and no guarantees should be made. No more restorative work should be performed than is necessary. Discuss with the family about changes that

may have occurred through extended illness, traumatic injury, autopsy examination, organ and tissue donation, or postmortem changes. If there has been a long illness, the family should be aware of facial and body appearance. This may not be so if death was traumatic or if changes occurred during the postmortem interval prior to embalming. Assure the persons making arrangements that everything possible will be done to improve the appearance of the deceased. A final decision as to public, private, or no viewing should be decided by those making the arrangements.

The funeral director must make every effort to **see the body before** meeting with the persons making funeral arrangements. If this is not possible (e.g., the body is at a medical examiner's office or at a central embalming facility), a verbal description of the body should be given to the funeral director. Unusual conditions should be discussed with the arranging party for instructions, for example, discolorations such as jaundice, facial tumor, or crippling arthritic deformities. Distinguishing markings and characteristics should also be discussed to inquire if they should be altered or removed. Examples include moles, facial scars, facial hair, visible birthmarks, goiter, or visible tattoos.

► PERMISSION

Permission for embalming and restorative work should be obtained by the funeral director. These permissions, if first obtained by oral agreement, need to be later confirmed and signed in writing. Embalming and restorative treatments are interdependent and interrelated—many restorative treatments are actually performed during the embalming of the body. The closure of the mouth and eyes accomplishes a restorative function; embalming injection techniques can swell sunken tissues of the face or reduce swollen tissues, and fluid dyes can restore the skin to natural color. If excisions or similar extensive restorative procedures are to be performed, specific restorative permission should be obtained (see Part I, Chapter 1).

▶ PHOTOGRAPHS

A recent photograph of the deceased should be obtained. Recent photos provide information about facial characteristics, hairstyle, and with men valuable information about facial hair, for example, moustache, beard, or sideburns.

Desirable Characteristics of the Photos.

1. The photo should be recent.
2. The individual should appear in normal good health in the photo.
3. Shadows should not appear on the face.
4. Snapshots are preferred over professional portraits, which may have been retouched.
5. Hairstyle of the deceased should be visible.
6. Symmetry and asymmetry of the facial features can be observed.
7. Shape of the attached mucous membranes (lips) can be observed.
8. A photo in three-quarter profile shows the fullness of the cheeks and the jaw line.
9. Projection of the mouth and lips can be noted in a three-quarter profile photo.
10. A frontal view photo will depict length and width relationships and distances can easily be measured.
11. A profile view photo will show projections and recessions of the face.

Study the photo by holding the picture upside down. In this manner, the embalmer is not distracted by the features; it allows a better comparison of facial features and characteristics. Digital photos (before and after) of the decedent can be part of the embalming care report. This can be very important when a body is to be embalmed and shipped to another funeral home. Photos taken by a funeral home, as part of the embalming report, must be kept confidential—NEVER should they be sent over the Internet. **Permission for funeral home photos can be included in the embalming permission form.**

▶ VIEWING

The presentation of the prepared body is very important. Viewing of the deceased may be in a casket, on a dressing table, or placed on a bed. Local customs, church affiliation, and ethnic background are all factors that can contribute to how the deceased is to be viewed. When restorative work has been performed or there is concern about facial swelling or extreme weight loss, some

Figure 1. Local and ethnic custom can dictate body casket position.

of the following suggestions may be of value in posing the decedent:

1. The body is generally viewed with the head tilted about 15 degrees to the right; the head is elevated on a pillow to decrease the angle between the chin and the chest. Local and ethnic customs may dictate that the head be kept perfectly straight so that the deceased appears to be looking directly upward (see Fig. 1).
2. For obese bodies, keep the head in a straight position and elevate the left shoulder to tilt the deceased slightly to the right. By keeping the head straight and the chin high, there will be less bulging of the neck, making it appear smaller.
3. If there is a problem on the right side of the head, reversing the body in the casket (or having the body viewed from the opposite side) may solve the problem. When this is done, keep the head perfectly straight and do not tilt the head toward the viewer (see Fig. 2A–C).
4. When there are extensive facial problems, the casket can be covered with a "casket veil." The veil prevents persons from touching restored areas and hides imperfections if wax work was performed. The veil may also provide complexion coloring.
5. Profiles change the least; if a kneeler is to be used, place it toward the head of the casket. The person kneeling sees the profile of the deceased rather than the bilateral view.
6. When facial problems exist, especially problems with the eyes, encourage the use of glasses (if worn by the deceased). Glasses actually reflect

A

B

C

Figure 2. A. Early decomposition; note ecchymosis of right eye. **B.** Opaque undercoat cosmetic applied; normal cream cosmetics applied over the opaque undercoat. **C.** Body reversed in full couch casket; kneeler at head so profile is seen by the person kneeling.

light and may help to hide problems; they also help to distract from problem facial areas.

7. Stanchions with roping can be used to keep persons a short distance from the decedent. These are often used when the body is viewed in a public place such as a church or public building.

Clothing

It is generally unnecessary to recommend any specific clothing color. For women, it is recommended, if the family is using their own clothing, that the garment has sleeves of sufficient length to cover the arms. For men, proper measurements should be taken so that clothing fits properly. Care should be taken when dressing men that the collar of a shirt be properly seen when dressed

with a tie and coat. A small portion of the shirt cuff should be seen when the deceased is dressed in a suit or sportcoat.

When the deceased has jaundice, it is helpful if clothing of cold colors is avoided, such as blue, green, or violet. Yellow is also not recommended. In addition, black and white should be avoided for they provide too much contrast with the skin tone. All warm colors from peach through pink, even to maroon, are recommended. Gray is also excellent for this type of body. Casket interior color can also enhance the cosmetic appearance of the deceased. A white casket interior provides the most difficult background for a cosmetized body because it provides too much contrast. For bodies with a normal skin color, after they have been cosmetized, grays and other dark tones provide the best background for display of the body.

Lighting

Illumination of the casketed body not only provides light to view the deceased, but it also contributes to the cosmetic color effect on the deceased. It is ideal to apply the cosmetics to the deceased using the same lighting that will be used to display the casketed remains. When colored lights (pink or red lights) are used to illuminate the cosmetized body, they have the effect of decreasing the red tones that are present in the skin cosmetic, because there is a general increase in the overall reddish or pink appearance. It becomes necessary, using this lighting, to increase the amount of red color used in the warm (red) areas of the face, such as the cheeks, lips, and ears.

Bodies viewed under normal lighting (no tinting) appear overcosmetized and theatrical, but when viewed under slightly tinted pink lighting, they will appear quite normal. Colored lights do have value, particularly when you want to create the illusion of the presence of reddish tones in the face. This is of particular value with jaundiced bodies.

Use of a standard incandescent bulb with shaded lamps, which have eggshell or ivory glass globes or shades, will compliment the cosmetized body. The combination of the incandescent bulb with the eggshell shade adds yellow color to the face. A great deal of yellow is found in the natural skin complexion, especially in the elderly. Many funeral homes also use point lighting over the casket to add color to the cosmetized body. The color magenta (magenta adds a small amount of blue to the cosmetic, and this helps to emphasize facial reds) works well for point lighting. The body and casket should be lighted evenly. Lighting that is too strong and uneven will have a tendency to create unnatural shadows on the face.

▶ CLASSIFICATION OF CONDITIONS AND TREATMENTS

Some degree of restorative treatment is necessary in the preparation of every body. Proper support and closure of the eyelids and mouth could be considered a restorative treatment. Application of some cosmetic treatment, if only to reinstate the warm areas of the cheeks and lips, is a form of restoration. More than one restorative treatment may be performed in the preparation of a body for viewing. For example, a typical preparation of an elderly female may involve some of the following restorative treatments:

- If there has been a loss of weight, cotton or a mortuary mastic will be needed to fill out sunken areas of the mouth, even if teeth or dentures are present. If there are no dentures, the entire reshaping of the mouth contour will be necessary. Cotton and/or eyecaps will be necessary to help shape, support, close, and raise sunken eyes.
- Eyelids and lips need to be closed and sealed.
- Dyes may be added to the arterial solution to help restore a natural coloring to the skin.
- Restorative fluids can be added to the arterial solution to assist in swelling sunken areas of the face and hands.
- After arterial injection, tissue building can be done to hands and face to restore emaciated or dehydrated areas.
- Ecchymosis or purpural hemorrhage may be present on the back of a hand as a result of use of medication, and these areas need to be bleached and covered with an opaque cosmetic.
- A small fever blister on the lips may need to be removed, and the area dried and waxed.
- Facial hair needs to be removed prior to embalming.
- Cosmetics need to be applied to face and hands to restore their natural coloring.
- The hair needs to be washed and properly styled.

Here, we see with just a "normal" preparation, a variety of minor restorations are needed. Facial trauma and tissue changes from disease or decomposition can result in the need for major restorative work (see Fig. 3A–B).

Classification of tissue conditions and restorative treatments may seem like an academic exercise for the classroom. By recognizing the various problems present and treatments available, guidelines for treatment can be established.

Conditions Requiring Restorative Treatment.

1. Pathological (disease)—tumor, ecchymosis discoloration, and edema
2. Trauma (injury)—abrasions, contusions, torn tissue, and fractures
3. Postmortem changes—skin slip, gases in the tissues, and discolorations
4. Embalming—swollen tissue and dehydrated (wrinkled) areas (e.g., lips)

Changes can occur in the antemortem and postmortem time periods, which will necessitate restorative treatments. In the antemortem time period, two groups can be listed.

Antemortem Time Period.

1. *Pathological conditions:* Disease processes that result in visible manifestations.

A

B

Figure 3. A. Emaciation of the face, an antemortem condition. **B.** Facial trauma; note facial abrasions and lacerations. The body has also been autopsied.

- loss of weight in the facial tissues
- loss of hair; increased growth of hair in areas such as the forehead
- discolorations
- skin eruptions
- tumors
- swelling of face and/or hands

Drug and surgical treatments can result in visible body changes, for example, scars, incisions, discolorations, swelling, and loss of hair (alopecia). The effects of some drugs or surgical procedures create greater restorative problems than the disease processes.

2. *Injury:* Trauma restoration is the procedure most associated by the public with the embalming process. Degree of trauma is widely variable. **It is absolutely necessary for the funeral director to see the extent of the injury before assuring a family that the deceased can be viewed.** Most often, a traumatic death will require an autopsy or examination by a coroner or medical examiner. There can be a considerable time delay until the embalmer knows the extent of damage from injuries or autopsy. Trauma does not always result in immediate death. It may be days, weeks, or even years until the death finally occurs. Medical treatments, as in the disease category above, may create more need for restorative work than the traumatic injury itself.

Postmortem Time Period.

1. Preembalming changes:
   a. Discoloration resulting from the movement of blood to dependent parts of the body (e.g., if the body dies with the head in a dependent position, the resulting discoloration may require treatment with opaque cosmetics to conceal the discoloration).
   b. Compression from surface contact. If the face or hands were pressed against a solid object such as a floor or wall, the soft tissues could be flattened; thus, the contour of the skin surface would need to be corrected.
   c. *Gases.* If cardiopulmonary resuscitation (CPR) was attempted, the rupture of the plural sac could result in air entering the subcutaneous tissues. These gases will frequently move into elevated areas such as the neck and face.
   d. *Decomposition changes.* These changes are the most obvious postmortem tissue changes requiring restorative treatment. Discolorations, gases in the tissues, and separation of the epidermis from the dermis (desquamation) can all create major problems.
   e. *Dehydration of the face and hands.* This postmortem loss of body moisture can result in fingers and features such as the lips, eyelids, and ears discoloring to deep brown or black and shrinking in size to a point where they cannot be rehydrated.
   f. *Organ and tissue donation.* Donation of the whole eye, inner ear, pituitary gland, and mandible would all require restorative treatments to the head and/or facial tissues.

g. Autopsy procedures and/or postmortem examinations.
2. Embalming changes:
   a. *Swelling.* As a result of injecting embalming solution under pressure, there is the possibility of distension of unsupported tissues and glands, particularly in the face or neck area (e.g., eye, neck, submaxillary and parotid glands, and cheeks). Bodies where decomposition has begun or where the tissues have been frozen distend easily during arterial injection.
   b. *Discolorations.* Livor mortis, if present in the face, can often be converted to a stain if too strong an arterial solution is employed. Yellow jaundice can be converted to a green discoloration. Harsh formaldehyde solutions and inadequate aspiration of the heart can create a graying of the face. The shoulder and head area of the embalmed body should always be elevated to help prevent "formaldehyde gray"—a graying of the tissues resulting from a mixing of blood not removed during the embalming process with formaldehyde. The use of fluid dye can help to prevent graying of the tissues.
   c. *Dehydration.* Excessive dehydration of the facial tissues can result if these areas are overembalmed using solutions that are too strong or if an excess of solution is run through these areas. Improper storage of the body following embalming can also cause dehydration necessitating restorative treatments.
   d. *Overembalmed tissues.* Too strong an arterial solution or too much arterial solution injected into the face can result in a number of conditions that may make restorative treatment quite difficult to perform, including separation of lips and eyelids, inability to tissue build the face or features, and wrinkling of the face and features.
   e. *Poorly preserved* local and general body areas.

► CLASSIFICATION OF RESTORATIVE TREATMENTS

Wax and Nonwax Treatment

Classification of a restoration as a wax or nonwax restoration simply means that wax will or will not be employed in the restoration. Wax plays a major role in replacing missing skin or covering skin areas where the skin has been broken. Typical wax restorations include correction of abrasions; second- and third-degree burns; repair where fever blisters have been removed; a treatment for skin slip; replacing torn skin; use of wax as a filler for deep wound restoration; and repair to close separated lips and eyelids.

Today, there are some excellent surface glues and opaque paints that can be used as wax substitutes for some restorations (e.g., replacement of missing or abraded skin). Mortuary mastics (mortuary putty) can be used as a deep filler as well as a surface filler for deep wound restorations.

Moist or Dry Tissue Condition

Tissue conditions can be classified as either dry or moist. Examples of **dry conditions** might be treatments for swollen or emaciated tissues, simple fractures, hair that needs to be replaced, discolorations, and separated lips or eyelids. These nonbroken skin conditions would almost always be considered dry tissue conditions. When the skin is dry, cosmetics, waxes, and glues can be applied to the surface.

Examples of **moist conditions** might include skin slip, lacerated tissues, compound fractures, second- and third-degree burns, blisters, scabs, pustules, and abrasions. Broken skin conditions may be moist or dry, depending on the amount of dehydration that has occurred. Frequently embalming solution will be seen exiting from moist skin areas (e.g., abrasions and lacerations) during arterial injection. This indicates the area is receiving good preservation treatment. Massage cream should be placed on the surrounding "good tissues," **not** over the moist tissues. This will protect the "good" tissues and allow faster drying of the problem area. Moist tissue must be dried. Following arterial injection, treatments with an electric spatula or hairdryer, or chemical compresses of phenol solutions or concentrated formaldehyde, can be used to dry moist tissue. When chemical compresses have been used, after their removal, the tissues need to be cleaned with a solvent and then air-dried with a hair dryer. Dry tissue is necessary for opaque cosmetics, waxes, and surface glues to adhere.

Condensation can occur on the surface of bodies that have been refrigerated. This can make cosmetic application difficult, especially cream cosmetics. A dry surface is necessary for cosmetic application.

Time Periods for Restorative Treatments

Restorative treatments can be divided into three time periods: (1) before the arterial injection of the body (preembalming), (2) during the arterial injection, and (3) a postembalming period, during which most restorative and cosmetic treatments are performed. Before the final time period, the body should be left undisturbed so that the tissues dry and become firm.

Knowing in which time period a particular procedure should be performed results in more orderly and satisfactory work. Body conditions and personal preference guidelines of the embalmer can and will vary. **The treatment periods outlined below serve only as guidelines**.

Guidelines for Restorative Treatments Made in the Pre-embalming Period. Objectives: It is in this time period that a restoration analysis, along with the embalming analysis, is made. Conditions of the body are evaluated and a plan is designed for restorative treatments. General treatments performed in this time period will include the following:

- alignment of fractured bones
- posing of the mouth and eyelids
- drainage of skin eruptions and blisters
- cleaning all skin surfaces, hair, and nails
- alignment of torn tissues and deep cuts
- removal of loose or torn epidermis
- removal of surface discolorations
- shaving of the face.

Treatments Performed During This Time Period.

1. Surface sanitizing of the body and external orifices
2. Removal of tubes or devices that in any way mark the face; removal of any facial bandages
3. Washing of the skin surface and hair with warm water and soap (borax can be used to assist in cleansing); cleaning of the fingernails and removal of any old nail polish
4. Removal of surface stains caused by adhesive tape, gentian violet, and so on; solvents such as dry hair washes or hydrocarbon solvent remove most stains; blood can be removed by using cool water with laundry bleach added
5. Shaving of facial hair
6. Positioning of head and hands; alignment of features
   a. Place cotton in the nostrils to expand them if they have become depressed.
   b. Cotton is placed behind the ear to expose the lobe, important when earrings are to be worn by the deceased.
   c. Hands can be laid at the sides or hang off the table until fluid distribution is established. Later a towel can be placed on the abdomen to position the hands and cup the fingers.
7. Mouth and lip closure
   a. Lips may be held together with thick petroleum jelly or mortuary compound. Later, this can be removed and the mucous membranes sealed with lip adhesive or superglue.
   b. Prognathism of the upper teeth may require gluing of the lips to hold the membranes together during embalming. Cotton can be placed over the lower teeth or dentures when the upper teeth protrude. This will bring the lower lip into alignment with the protruding upper lip. (Rubber-based glue is recommended for temporary gluing; superglue is recommended for permanent sealing.)
   c. Sunken facial areas may be raised by inserting cotton or mortuary mastic in the buccal cavity.
   d. Scabs, oozing scabs, and fever blisters should be removed from the lips or face and a cotton compress of phenol or formaldehyde can be placed over the raw tissue to sanitize, preserve, and eventually dry the exposed tissues.
   e. *Correct misalignment of the mandible.* If the lower jaw has separated from the mandibular fossa of the temporal bone, the mandible should be massaged back into position at this time. Lip closure cannot be made if the mandible is not in proper alignment.
8. Closure of the eyelids
   a. Sunken eyes can be elevated by closure with cotton, or a combination of cotton and an eyecap.
   b. When a glass eye is present, the lids may need to be glued or the artificial eye removed and a closure made with cotton or eyecaps.
   c. Eyelashes should be cleaned and properly aligned. A brush moistened with water or a solvent such as dry hair wash can be used to clean the lashes.
   d. Enucleated eyes
      (1) Remove any packing from the orbit.
      (2) Gently clean the orbit with cotton.
      (3) Very loosely place a cotton pack saturated with autopsy gel in the orbit using enough cotton to establish the contour of the closed eyelid.
      (4) Gently abut the lids to give a natural closure to the eye.
9. Glass shards should be removed with the embalmer wearing heavy gloves. Some shards can be flushed loose with water, and others will need to be removed with spring forceps.
10. Align lacerated and cut tissue edges.
    a. Small bridge sutures of dental floss can be used.
    b. A drop or two of superglue along the laceration can be used to align surface skin edges.
    c. Deep lacerations can be pulled into alignment with deep sutures using dental floss.

11. Remove torn epidermal tissue and visible desquamation.

12. Open and drain blisters, pustules, boils, or similar skin eruptions.

13. Remove loose skin from opened blisters and skin eruptions. Remove loose scabs.

14. If a tumor of the face is pushing a feature out of alignment, it may be necessary to excise the tumor at this time. Some embalmers prefer to do all excisions in this time period.

15. Apply surface compresses over blood discolorations to begin bleaching the affected areas.

16. Apply surface compresses of phenol or concentrated formaldehyde to raw surface areas (e.g., moist abrasions, desquamation, burned areas, opened pustules and blisters, and areas where tissue has been excised).

17. Align simple and compound fractures and if possible raise depressed fractures.

18. Apply massage cream to face and hands over intact tissues. Cream should not be applied to surfaces where wax, opaque cosmetics, or surface glue is to be used.

19. Apply compresses to swollen areas caused by trauma. Use compresses of phenol or concentrated formaldehyde to bleach bruised tissues. Place weighted compresses over the affected areas to help reduce swelling during arterial injection.

Guidelines for Restorative Treatments Made During Arterial Injection. During this time period, very few restorative and cosmetic treatments are performed. However, this phase of embalming is significant because this is when the embalming solution is introduced. For most restorative and cosmetic treatments, the surface tissues must be dry and firm. Well-preserved tissues are the key to successful restorative treatments.

Objectives. To establish good preservation so that the tissues will be firm and dry. In addition, adequate preservation will help to ensure that the facial features will be maintained in their posed positions. The contour of the facial areas can be altered by the injection of the arterial solution. Normal facial contours can be maintained by use of the proper arterial solution; swollen facial areas can be reduced, and emaciated and sunken facial areas can be restored by arterial solutions containing chemicals designed to restore tissue contour. Dyes in the arterial solution will add color to the skin surface and serve as an internal coloring.

Treatments Performed during This Time Period.

1. Establish good, even preservation to the tissues of the face and hands.

2. Surface compresses of concentrated formaldehyde (cavity fluid) or phenol compounds can be placed over areas where skin has been removed to help dry and firm these tissues.

3. Massage areas of the face and hands, which have been compressed to help to expand these tissues (e.g., if face was dependent or pushed against an object, or if hands were placed over one another).

4. Control swelling of facial tissues.

5. Reduce swollen facial tissues caused by edema by the use of mechanical embalming techniques and arterial chemicals.

6. Distend slightly emaciated facial areas by the use of additives to the arterial solution designed for this purpose.

7. Arterial solutions firm and set the facial tissues and features. Successful embalming will produce a dry skin surface.

8. Cosmetic dyes in the arterial solutions give a lifelike effect to the skin surface.

9. Clearing of intravascular blood discolorations (e.g., livor mortis).

10. Strong arterial solutions and supplemental fluids will bleach and lighten blood discolorations (e.g., hematoma, postmortem stain, ecchymosis, and purpura).

11. Facial tissues can be moisturized by supplemental fluids added to the arterial solution.

12. External application of massage cream moisturizes dry skin, prevents tissue dehydration, and cleanses the skin. Application by massage assists in relieving rigor mortis in the facial tissues, which will help promote distribution of the arterial solution.

Guidelines for Restorative Treatments Made after Arterial Injection (Postembalming). This time period occurs after arterial injection and cavity embalming have been completed. This phase usually begins with a **period of rest**, during which the tissues firm, the chemicals are given time to work, and it gives moist tissues an opportunity to dry. This is the time when the majority of restorative treatments are performed.

PERIOD OF REST. This time period can be very brief after arterial and cavity embalming, simply long enough to suture all embalming incisions, evaluate what areas need additional hypodermic and surface preservative treatments, and perform final washing and drying of the body. In the preparation of bodies with facial trauma, this may be a longer period of time, during which surface compresses will be placed over areas to bleach and reduce swollen tissues. With an extremely emaciated body, some embalmers attempt to distend the facial tissues using the arterial solution and a restorative chemical, then, allowing a long period of rest between arterial injection and cavity aspiration, the features of the face are able to thoroughly "set." Many funeral establishments will allow several hours of time between the completion of the embalming and the start of restorative and cosmetic treatments.

Objectives. The following are reasons for a period of rest:

1. To allow drying of areas where superficial tissues are missing (e.g., from desquamation and abrasions)
2. To allow tissues of the face and hands time to dry before the application of cosmetics
3. To allow time for the tissues of the face and hands to firm
4. To allow time for surface bleaching compresses to bleach discolorations (e.g., from ecchymosis, bruises, and purpura)
5. To allow time for hypodermically injected bleaches to lighten discolorations
6. To allow time for surface preservative compresses to penetrate and preserve underlying tissues
7. To allow time for hypodermically injected solutions to preserve injected tissues
8. To allow time for surface compresses placed over swollen tissues to reduce the distended area
9. To allow maximum drainage to occur and gases to escape
10. To observe if any additional treatments are necessary

Following a brief or extended period of rest, the majority of restorative and cosmetic treatments are performed. A careful examination of the body is necessary to check for evidence of gas formation, lack of preservation, and any previously unnoticed leakage.

Treatments.

1. Hypodermic injection of preservatives, bleaches, reducing agents, and so on
2. Hypodermic tissue building of face and hands
3. Suturing of disconnected tissues
4. Gluing of disconnected tissues
5. Gluing (sealing) of eyelids and lips
6. Application of surface glues over sutured areas and to replace skin
7. Application of surface waxes
8. Rebuilding of missing features or facial areas
9. General cosmetic treatments
10. Cosmetic treatments for discoloration
11. Facial expression changes made by tissue building and cosmetic shaping

12. Nail treatments
13. Hair grooming and restoration
14. Swelling reduction by use of heat, channeling, aspirating, gravitation, and excision
15. Excision of tumors and reconstruction of the affected area
16. Eye enucleation restoration
    a. Drying of the orbit
    b. Deep filling of the orbit with a moisture absorbent material such as mortuary mastic or incision seal powder
    c. Replacement of the missing eye with a material such as cotton, mortuary mastic, or wax
    d. Placement of an eyecap over the filler material
    e. Closure and sealing of the eyelids

It can be seen from these examples the majority of restorative treatments are performed during this postembalming period. It will be necessary to allow additional rest periods when certain treatments are performed to allow tissues to dry and chemicals to properly act on the tissues. It is necessary that the funeral director, when making arrangements, allow sufficient time for cosmetic and restorative treatments to be properly performed.

▶ SUMMARY

In 1965, G. Joseph Prager published in his *Manual of Restorative Art* the following summary that incorporates a general sequence of procedures for most restorative treatments:

1. Obtain permission for incisions or excisions necessary for restoration.
2. Cleanse the body thoroughly and remove all stains and foreign matter.
3. Straighten and replace fractures or missing bones.
4. Temporarily suture all disconnected tissues in visible areas.
5. Embalm the body.
6. Make incisions and excisions required for restoration; suture disconnected tissues.
7. Reduce swelling, bleach discolorations, and fill sunken areas as required.
8. Apply sealing compound to exposed subcutaneous tissues and fill cavities with a suitable foundation for wax surfacing.
9. When tissues are firm and dry, perform the wax restoration.

Time Period of Rest for Chemicals to React with the Tissues
10. Replace eyelashes.
11. Apply corrective cosmetics.

12. Replace eyebrows and cranial hair.
13. Reproduce skin pores in waxed areas.

▶ ESTABLISHMENT OF GOOD PRESERVATION

When facial conditions such as the following exist in the unautopsied body, the common carotid arteries should be used for arterial injection: trauma to the head (cranium) or the face; evidence of early or advanced decomposition; extensive pathological lesions; bruising, abraded, lacerated or burnt tissue; ecchymosis, hematoma, or lacerations of the eyelids; eye enucleation; facial or cranial tumor that must be excised; cranial or facial swelling from edema. This method of injection is called restricted cervical injection; it allows the best control over the amount and the strength of arterial solution entering the head and facial tissues.

Restricted cervical injection is performed by raising the right and the left common carotid arteries (some embalmers also prefer to raise both right and left internal jugular veins as sites for drainage from the head). (See Chapter 12) (Fig. 4).

Arterial solution for injection into the head and face for these restorative cases requires the use of a strong preservative solution. This is done to ensure firm and dry facial tissues. Swelling can be controlled with stronger

Figure 4. Restricted cervical injection.

arterial solutions because less volume of the solution is used to preserve the tissues. Concentrated arterial solutions also help to bleach blood discolorations, reduce facial swelling (edema), and dry moist tissues such as burns, desquamation, or abraded tissues. Dye may be added to the solution to assist in prevention of graying of the tissues and as a fluid tracer.

Instant tissue fixation is an embalming technique in which a minimal amount of concentrated arterial solution is injected by a series of pulses under high pressure. This technique achieves maximum preservation using

TABLE 1. CHEMICALS USED IN RESTORATIVE TREATMENTS

Chemical	Use	Application
Tissue builder	Raises sunken, emaciated tissues, rounds out wrinkled lips and fingers	Hypodermic injection
Tissue builder solvent	Cleans hypodermic syringe after any chemical is injected	Not injected into body tissues; use to flush out syringe
Hydrocarbon solvent dry hair washes (solvents)	Cleansing of skin; assists in removal of scaling skin; loosens scabs; dries skin surface; prepares skin for waxes, glues, and opaque cosmetics; removes surface stains, adhesive tape; can be mixed with a cream cosmetic to make an opaque undercoat; smoothes wax; cleans cosmetics from hair, eyebrows, and eyelashes	Applied on the skin surface with cotton, gauze or soft cotton, or brush
Cautery, bleaching, reducing agents (may contain phenol)	Bleaches tissue, bleaches blood discolorations, cauterizes broken tissue, preserves localized tissues; dries and firms tissues, reduces swollen tissues	Surface compress over affected area; chemical can also be injected by hypodermic syringe; may be painted or swabbed over the area
Formaldehyde (undiluted cavity fluid)	Used as a substitute for a phenol cautery preservative	Surface compress or hypodermic injection
Preservative gel	Preserves, bleaches, firms tissues	Surface compress or painted over area to be treated
Acetone	Fingernail polish remover; removes surface stains; loosens scabs, smoothes wax; cleans hair	Applied by cotton pad; gauze or cloth
Sodium hypochlorite	Used with water to clean blood from skin surface, hair, etc.	Gauze pad or soft cloth

TABLE 2. RESTORATION MATERIALS AND INSTRUMENTS AND THEIR USES

Material, Instrument Discussion, or Technique

Airbrush	A pressured atomizer used for the application of a liquid transparent or opaque cosmetic onto the skin surface.
Armature	A framework, commonly of metal or wood, used to provide support for a wax restoration. Examples would include pipe cleaners, lengths of wire, various small pieces of screen, or dowel rods of wood or metal. If a feature such as an ear were to be built on the body, the armature would be secured to the scalp or bony structures, and the modeled ear would then be built upon this framework.
Basket weave suture	A network of stitches that crosses the borders of a cavity or excision to anchor fillers and to sustain tissues in their proper position. A framework for attachment of wax or mortuary mastic where tissues or a feature is being rebuilt; also serves to hold the margins of the cavity or excision in a uniform position. The sutures are usually made into the subcutaneous areas of the skin.
Bridge suture	A temporary suture consisting of individually cut and tied stitches employed to sustain the proper position of tissues. Dental floss can be used for these temporary sutures. They are usually put into place during the preembalming time period.
Cotton	A highly absorbent natural white fibrous substance, it has numerous uses in restorative work; also available in a nonabsorbent form.
Cotton (webbed)	A nonwoven, lint-free absorbent fabric made from cotton. Can be used as a replacement for absorbent cotton.
Cyanoacrylate sealer (Superglue)	A strong and fast-acting bonding adhesive (viscosity can vary), used to seal lips and eyelids, lacerations and incisions, and bony fractures; primarily composed of alpha cyanoacrylate
Deep filler	A material used to fill cavities or excisions and to serve as a foundation for the superficial wax restoration. Examples include "wound filler," wax, mortuary mastic, plaster of Paris, cotton and sealer, cotton and plaster.
Electric spatula	An electrically heated blade used to dry moist tissues, reduce swollen tissues, and restore contour to natural form. Massage cream should be liberally applied to a skin surface before using the spatula. (This is not necessary when it is used to dry and/or cauterize deep tissues.)
Gauze	A light, open mesh variety of muslin or similar material; used over a mortuary mastic to prevent the mastic from separating from the edges of a cavity; used with a sealer to replace missing skin; by gently pressing onto a waxed area it imparts a porelike effect to the wax.
Hypodermic syringe	Used for the subcutaneous injection of liquid tissue builder, bleaches, and preservatives. A needle gauge of 17 works well for all of the liquids listed, but some embalmers prefer a higher gauge needle for lip treatments. Syringes and needles should be cleaned with tissue builder solvent after each use.
Intradermal suture	A suture used to close incisions such that the ligature remains entirely under the epidermis. It may be a double or single suture.
Inversion suture (worm or draw suture)	Parallel stitches are made in the surface edges of an incision and the skin from the stitch to the opening of the incision is inverted as the sutures are drawn tight. The suture is easily concealed with wax or surface glue; used to tighten loose skin.
Ligature	Thread, cord, or wire used for tying vessels, tissues, or bones. Cotton is the softest and weakest, linen is very strong, and for restorative work dental floss is often used.
Lip-eye cement	Fast setting liquid adhesive designed to bond the eyelids and lips.
Massage cream	A soft, white, oily preparation used as a protective coating for external tissues; a base for cream cosmetics and a wax softener; an emollient. It can also be used as a skin cleanser; to soften and loosen scabs; loosens and helps in the removal of loose scaling skin. Substitutes would include lanolin or baby oil. Massage cream should not be applied over an area where an opaque undercoat is going to be applied.
Mastic compound	A soft, puttylike substance; an absorbent sealing adhesive that can be injected under the skin or applied to surface tissues to establish skin contour. A substitute for incision powder. May be used as a deep cavity filler.
Needle injector	An instrument used to impel specially designed metal pins (with wires attached) into bone. Normal use would be as a method of mouth closure. It can also be used in trauma situations as a means of joining fractured bones.

TABLE 2. RESTORATION MATERIALS AND INSTRUMENTS AND THEIR USES (*Continued*)

Material, Instrument	Discussion, or Technique
Petroleum jelly	A semisolid, yellow mixture of hydrocarbons obtained from petroleum. It can be applied to the mucous membranes of the lips prior to embalming to hold the lips in a closed position. This technique also helps to remove horizontal wrinkles from the lips. Similar products to help affix free margins such as the eyelids and lips in a closed position are available through embalming suppliers.
Plaster of Paris	Calcium sulfate; a white powdery substance which forms a quick-setting paste when mixed with water. Drying time can be speeded by using warm water or slowed by mixing with cold water. Uses include repair of fractured bones, use with cotton as a deep filler, and as a means of attachment for the calvarium to the base of the skull in autopsied bodies.
Pneumatic collar	A plastic collar that surrounds the neck and is inflated with a rubber bulb pump; the collar places external pressure on the neck tissues and helps to reduce swelling.
Powder	Any solid substance in the state of fine, loose particles as produced by crushing or grinding. Talc or cornstarch is a common ingredient. Powder may be applied with an atomizer, puff, or brush. a. White drying—used for drying cream cosmetics; may be mixed with soft waxes to give more firmness to the wax; used for drying cream cosmetics placed over or within wax b. Tinted powders—contain a coloring agent; these will alter the color of complexion cosmetic when applied over the cosmetic. Do not apply this powder over a waxed area; apply a white drying powder first followed by a tinted powder. If used as a transparent cosmetic, a very light coating of massage cream should first be applied to the skin and then the powder applied.
Rubber cement	A viscous adhesive consisting of vulcanized rubber dispersed in an organic solvent; used for the attachment of hair patches to the scalp or face.
Sealer (collodion, liquid sealer, surface sealer)	A quick-drying liquid; available in a variety of viscosities; creates a firm, thin transparent coating through which moisture cannot pass. Used over sutured areas to prevent leakage; may be used as a replacement for epidermal skin. Surfaces must be dry for a sealer to adhere.
Spatula	A flat, blunt, knifelike instrument used for mixing cosmetics and modeling; a palette knife. The blade must be clean each time it touches the wax being modeled. The blade can be warmed by holding it between the thumb and index finger. The blade can be dipped in a solvent to make wax adjustments over delicate areas.
Undercoat	An opaque coloring applied to an area which, when dry, will be covered with wax or another cosmetic colorant. May be liquid or aerosol. Surface to which it is applied should first be cleaned with a solvent to remove any oils or grease. Surface to which it is applied should also be free of any moisture.
Wax	A restorative or surfacing material composed of beeswax, spermaceti, paraffin, starch, etc. and a coloring pigment that will soften at body temperature and will reflect light in a manner similar to normal skin. Most waxes need to be warmed prior to application. This can be done by mixing the wax with a spatula in the palm of the embalmer's hand. Cream cosmetic or colored powders can be added to neutral colored waxes to alter their color. Examples include: a. Lip wax—a soft restorative wax, usually tinted, used to surface the mucous membranes or to correct lip separations. b. Surface restorer (soft wax)—a surface filler wax used to fill shallow depressions; softer and more pliable than wound filler. c. Medium wax—a derma surgery or restorative wax. d. Firm wax (wound filler)—the most viscous type of wax; a puttylike material used to fill large cavities or model features.
Worm suture	See Inversion suture.

as little embalming solution as possible, keeping any swelling to a minimum. The left side of the face is injected first, then the right side. (See Chapter 12.)

Below are several **waterless** formulas for arterial solutions used to embalm the head and face when conditions such as extensive facial trauma or early decomposition exist.

1. 16 oz of a high index arterial fluid (25 index or higher)
   16 oz of coinjection chemical $\frac{1}{2}$ oz dye
2. 16 oz of a medium index arterial fluid (16 to 22 index)
   16 oz of a high index arterial fluid (30 to 35 index)
   16 oz of coinjection chemical
   $\frac{1}{2}$ oz fluid dye
3. Chemical companies make a special purpose high-index arterial fluid for difficult cases. Directions for use by the manufacturer should be followed.
4. Chemical companies have their own waterless formulas using their arterial fluids, coinjection, and water corrective products.

Some embalmers prefer not to use the solutions described above. They prefer to use a standard arterial solution and add several ounces of a high-index arterial fluid.

Arterial treatment may need to be supplemented by local hypodermic and surface embalming. A bleaching-cautery chemical or concentrated cavity fluid can be used to make surface compresses. The phenol-cautery solutions work much faster than the formaldehyde compresses, but the formaldehyde compresses penetrate deeper into the tissues. These surface compresses can be applied in all three restorative time periods. They should be covered with thin plastic to contain fumes and prevent the chemicals from dehydrating. Preservative or autopsy gels can be painted over affected areas to preserve and dry tissues. The gels should also be covered with plastic. When gels or chemical compresses are removed, the area needs to be cleaned using a hydrocarbon solvent. These chemical compresses or gels will bleach blood discolorations, preserve, dry and firm tissues, and act as a cautery to sear torn or excised tissues.

Hypodermic preservative treatment is usually done after the arterial injection. Injection into tissues should be done from hidden points of entry because chemicals such as formaldehyde or phenol compounds can leak. As a substitute, undiluted cavity chemical may be used as a bleaching, preservative, and reducing agent. Hypodermic injection of an arterial chemical should be avoided if it contains a tissue dye; in time, this dye can stain tissues and create a discoloration.

Broken skin areas need to be dried before wax or cosmetic treatments can be done. Examples include skin-slip, torn skin, moist abrasions, and second-degree burns. These areas can be dried by, chemical cautery agents, a heated spatula or hair dryer. If time permits, allowing air to pass over the raw tissues will dry these skin areas. Intact tissues can be protected with a coating of massage cream; this prevents stains from chemicals and dehydration.

Tables 1 and 2 list the chemicals, materials, and instruments used in restorative procedures.

RESTORATIVE ART—PART 2

▶ DEEP CAVITY RESTORATION

In this section, we will look at deep cavity restoration. It is an extensive and radical restoration and it outlines the basic order of steps that must be followed to achieve a natural-looking restored area that will not change over the period of time the body is viewed (Figs. 5, 6A–K, and 7A–E).

The following case presentation will assume there is a cancerous growth on the lower right lateral cheek of the deceased. It is not possible to remove the growth from inside the mouth. Therefore, the cancerous protrusion must be removed by excising the tumor directly from the surface of the face. The tumor should be re-moved **after** arterial embalming if it **is not** distorting another feature of the face. If it is distorting another feature of the face, it should be excised **prior to** arterial injection, and several bridge sutures can be made across the cavity to align the margins. The cavity can be filled with a compress of a preservative-cautery chemical during the arterial embalming of the body.

To better match the cosmetized skin colors of the undamaged tissues with the restored waxed area, it is recommended that the undamaged areas of the face be cosmetized first. A cream cosmetic can be mixed with the wax or applied over the wax to match complexion coloring.

Protocol	Discussion
1. Obtain permission from the persons in charge of disposition of the body.	Permission from the arranging party will assure the embalmer in writing that the tumor is to be removed and the resulting excised area restored. (Other options might include using a full-couch casket, turning the body and viewing the deceased from the left side; leaving the malignant growth on the face and covering it with a clean bandage.)
2. Sanitize and clean the affected area.	Cleansing the area with a surface disinfectant will destroy pathogenic surface bacteria and deodorize the tissues. If radiation treatments were given, marker stains such as gentian violet may be present on the intact skin surface. Cleaning with a solvent will remove these stains.
3. Protect undamaged skin areas.	Cover the undamaged skin areas surrounding the tumor with massage cream; this prevents chemicals from staining or drying the intact tissues.
4. Embalm the body.	If unautopsied, restricted cervical injection will insure good distribution of arterial solution to the tissues of the face. If autopsied, simply inject left and right sides of the face. Arterial solution should be strong enough to insure very firm and dry tissues.
5. Excise the tumor.	Cut around the tumor in a circular fashion holding the scalpel at an angle as if you were attempting to cut under the tumor. This is described as undercutting. The circular cut should be made in the undamaged tissue surrounding the growth. Excise as much of the tumor as possible. Dissect until undamaged tissues and bone are reached. Excise all diseased tissue. The excised material should be collected in a plastic container, treated with a preservative, and placed within the casket for burial or cremation with the deceased (see Fig. 6A–K). *(Text continues on page 533.)*

Protocol

6. Apply surface compresses to the surrounding subcutaneous walls; hypodermically inject the surrounding tissues from within the cavity.

7. Allow a period of rest.

8. Dry the subcutaneous surfaces.

9. Apply sealer to the cavity walls.

10. Fill the lower area of the cavity with a deep wound filler.

11. Apply a basket weave suture just beneath the top of the rim of the cavity.

12. Apply the surface restorer wax.

13. Apply the surface cosmetics over the waxed areas; complete with white drying powder.

14. Reinstate the pores.

15. Seal the cosmetics.

Discussion

Inspect the subcutaneous tissues to be certain the cavity is clean. If tissues appear moist, inject the surrounding tissues hypodermically with a preservative-cautery solution or undiluted cavity fluid. Pack the floor and walls of the cavity with cotton saturated with the same chemical. Cover the area with a thin layer of plastic.

If a phenol compound is applied to the raw tissues, it will work much faster than a compress of formaldehyde. The phenol should dry and firm the tissues very rapidly depending on the strength of the chemical. Formaldehyde may require 2 to 4 hours. It is very important that the tissues be dry and firm for this will prevent leakage and possible separation of the wax from the intact tissues.

Remove the compresses; some digital pressure can be applied to the surrounding intact tissues in an attempt to force out any leakage. The walls of the cavity can be swabbed with cotton or gauze saturated with cleaning solvent. If the walls seem moist, they can be force dried with a hair dryer or electric spatula. Time permitting, a fan blowing over the area can dry the tissue. Be certain the surrounding intact skin surface is protected with a coating of massage cream. Drying is important for it will prevent any leakage and wax separation.

A sealer can be applied to the base and walls of the cavity. Several coats of sealer will help to prevent the accumulation of moisture within the cavity. The glue may be force dried by using a hair dyer. This step can be omitted if the cavity is completely dry.

A variety of deep fillers may be used including mortuary mastic, deep-wound filler wax, cotton dipped in plaster of Paris, alternating strips of cotton or cotton webbing saturated with surface glue, and auto repair mastic.

Suture with dental floss or a linen thread using a sharp needle. Begin the suturing by tying the ligature in place; do not use a knot; leave about 3 inches of thread. When you are ready to end the suture, end at the same point as you began by tying two ends of suture thread together. Do not pull the basket weave sutures too tight or they will cause the marginal skin to "pucker." This lattice work of sutures helps to hold the margins of the cavity in alignment and holds the deep filler and surface wax in position.

A softer surface restorer wax can be placed over the deep filler and at the same time pushed into the threads of the basket weave suture. Mound the surface wax in the center of the excision, then feather it to the margins of the cavity, and extend it slightly over into the surrounding intact tissues. Smoothing of the wax can be done with a soft brush dipped in solvent or wax thinner. View the results from a variety of positions and adjust if necessary. Some cosmetic colorant may be added to the surface wax to obtain a good skin tone match. (See Fig. 7A–C.)

A cream cosmetic can be placed over a waxed surface. This step can be done if it is necessary to make a better match of the waxed area to the surrounding intact tissues. Never apply a tinted or colored powder directly to a wax surface.

Gently "dabbing" the waxed area with a soft powder brush will create the effect of skin pores. Other methods include gently pressing with moist lintless gauze or paper toweling, or lightly tapping a stippling brush over the area.

This can be done with a light spray of commercial hairspray.

Figure 5. Three-quarter profile of the face dissected. The orbicularis oculi muscle has been removed from the left side of the face exposing the tarsal plate of the upper eyelid. The skeleton of the nose has been exposed. The masseter muscle has been separated from its origin on the zygomatic bone and its insertion on the mandible, then retracted posteriorly. Key to the illustration: 1. frontalis muscle; 2. corrugator muscle; 3. superior tarsus; 4. procerus muscle; 5. orbicularis oculi muscle; 6. quadratus labii superior, angular head; 7. nasal branch of the angular artery; 8. cartilage of the nasal wing; 9. infraorbital nerve plexus; 10. orbicularis oris muscle; 11. superior mucous membrane; 12. inferior mucous membrane; 13. facial artery; 14. inferior labial artery; 15. quadratus labii inferior; 16. triangularis muscle; 17. temporalis muscle; 18. zygomatic arch; 19. zygomatic muscle; 20. zygomatic head of the quadratus labii superior muscle; 21. coronoid process of the mandible; 22. masseter muscle (reflected); 23. superior labial artery; 24. buccinator muscle; 25. sternocleidomastoid muscle; 26. submaxillary gland. (*Drawing courtesy of Jude Waples, Oakville, Ontario, Canada.*)

Figure 6. A. Tumor excised after embalming **B.** Massage cream protects intact tissues. **C, D.** Phenol treatments to dry the cavity. **E.** Basket weave suture applied. **F.** Sealer applied. **G.** Deep-filler (mortuary mastic) applied. (*Continued*)

Figure 6. (*Continued*) **H.** Gauze placed over filler and sealer applied. **I.** wax adjustments. **J.** Cosmetics applied. **K.** Completed restoration.

▶ RESTORATIVE TREATMENTS FOR DISCOLORATIONS

The majority of discolorations present on the visible body areas cannot be completely removed; most can be altered, and so, less cosmetic treatment will be needed. Those that can possibly be removed would include surface stains (discolorations) and antemortem and postmortem intravascular blood discolorations. Intravascular blood discolorations can be cleared through arterial solution injection and subsequent drainage.

Blood, some pathological, decomposition, and chemotherapeutic (drug) discolorations can be altered or lightened by (1) arterial injection and drainage, (2) surface bleaching compresses, and (3) hypodermic bleaches. Bleaching of a discoloration does not return the skin to its normal color, but the discoloration will be less intense. Use of these chemicals helps to ensure preservation of the area. Surface compresses provide a more uniform bleaching of the skin surface; hypodermic injection of a discolored area such as an eyelid does not always insure an even distribution of the chemical. Often both surface and hypodermic treatments are necessary, particularly when there is discoloration and swelling. Dehydrated and desiccated tissue or dried abraded tissues will not respond to bleaching.

For discussion in this text, discolorations are divided into three categories: (1) surface discolorations,

Figure 7. A. Entire orbit excised due to a cancer many years before death. Tissues are all dry. **B.** Orbit filled with mortuary mastic and an eyecap placed for convexity. **C.** Mastic covered with gauze and entire area coated with a surface sealer. **D.** Rebuilding of the lids (upper first) with surface wax. **E.** Completed.

(2) discolorations associated with nonbroken skin conditions, and (3) discolorations associated with broken skin conditions.

Surface Discolorations

Surface stains (discolorations) result from an external agent on the surface of the skin. Common examples include blood, dirt, nicotine stains, adhesive tape, betadine, and gentian violet. These discolorations need to be removed in the preembalming time period. Washing the discoloration with a soft washcloth using warm water and a liquid soap will loosen and remove a large number of discolorations. Adding sodium hypochlorite to the water will ease the cleaning of blood stains. A hydrocarbon solvent will remove most medicinal stains including adhesive tape. Whenever a solvent has been used to clean the face or hands, it should be followed by a light coating of massage cream to prevent dehydration. Fingernails should also be cleaned at this time. Acetone will assist in removing nail polishes and other paint products.

Nonbroken Skin Discolorations

Discolorations associated with nonbroken skin conditions can be local or general. Common local examples include blood discolorations such as ecchymosis, purpura, hematoma, first-degree burn, "black eye," vascular nevus or birthmark, small areas of dehydrated tissue, or postmortem stain. General discolorations would include jaundice, decomposition, or dehydration.

Blood decomposition discolorations will respond to mortuary bleaches. Many of these preservative-cautery-bleaching chemicals contain phenol (carbolic acid), a substitute can be undiluted cavity chemical. These chemicals can be applied in three ways: (1) as a compress on the surface of the body, (2) as a compress under the surface of the skin, for example, under eyelids, lips, mouth, or inside the nares, and (3) by hypodermic injection into or beneath the skin. Hypodermic injection makes it possible for cosmetic treatment to begin immediately. If the bleach is to be injected by hypodermic syringe, this is usually done in the postembalming time period. These bleaches should be injected into areas of the face and hands where any leakage of the chemical will not be noticed.

If preservative (bleaching) gels are used, they can be painted onto a surface. A surface compress or gel may be placed over the discoloration before, during, or after embalming the body. After the compress or gel is removed, the skin needs to be dried.

Dehydrated tissues do not respond to bleaching. Arterial injection of embalming solution does little to alter dehydrated tissues. Severely dehydrated areas will appear dark brown to black. If there is desiccation of the lips or eyelids, excision and rebuilding with wax may be necessary. Areas where the dehydration is less severe—perhaps the fingers or lips—can often be restored by hypodermic tissue building and the discoloration covered with opaque cosmetics.

Ecchymosis is frequently seen on the back of the hands. Treatment to lessen the discoloration is to inject (after embalming) a preservative-cautery-bleaching chemical (or undiluted cavity fluid) between the fingers into the discolored area. Inject sufficient chemical that a slight swelling of the discoloration is noted. Press on the raised areas to distribute the chemical throughout the discolored tissues. Leakage, from between the fingers, will stop in a short time. A semiopaque or opaque cosmetic should hide the now lighter discoloration.

Large discolorations such as jaundice, decomposition, or postmortem stain can be altered by the embalming technique. Special arterial fluids are available to assist in bleaching this type of discoloration. These treatments are followed by the application of opaque or semiopaque cosmetic treatments. In some situations, the embalmer may want to place a fluid compress over the entire face during and/or after the arterial injection (Fig. 8A–C).

Superficial Broken Skin Conditions and Discoloration

Superficial disconnected (broken) skin conditions include abrasions, razor abrasions, desquamation, torn epidermis (possibly associated with ecchymosis and purpura), second- and third-degree burns, blisters and pustules (which need to be opened and drained), and loose scabs. These conditions all involve the epidermis and possibly upper areas of the dermis (Fig. 9A–D).

Dehydration can be present over the broken skin areas. Dehydrated tissues can vary in color from light yellow to black. Wax, undercoat paints, and cosmetics can be applied over these dried tissues.

Depending upon the specific condition, the following treatments will be necessary to restore the face or hands where superficial broken skin conditions exist.

1. Disinfect and clean the area with solvent; protect unaffected tissues with massage cream, but do not apply massage cream over the affected tissues; establish a restoration plan.
2. Remove all loose tissues using a sharp scalpel or scissors.
3. Establish good preservation:
   a. Direct injection of a strong arterial solution into the affected region
   b. Application of surface compresses of a concentrated cautery chemical, undiluted cavity fluid, or preservative gels before, during, or after arterial injection

A

B

C

Figure 8. A. Ecchymosis of eye; early decomposition color changes. **B.** An opaque undercoat spray is applied. **C.** Cream cosmetics applied over the undercoat.

c. Postembalming subcutaneous hypodermic injection of a concentrated cautery chemical or undiluted cavity fluid beneath the affected areas and in the immediate surrounding area
4. Dry the tissues.
  a. Surface compresses preserve and dry tissues.
  b. Clean with a solvent.
  c. Use a hair dryer or electric spatula to dry the surface tissues.
5. Restore the area using wax, opaque paint, or surface glue.
  a. *Method 1:* Apply an opaque undercoat paint; after it dries, apply a cream cosmetic over it to match the surrounding cosmetized skin (Fig. 10A–C).

  b. *Method 2:* Apply a surface sealer to replace the missing skin; after the sealer dries, an opaque cosmetic can be applied over the sealer.
  c. *Method 3:* Apply an opaque undercoat paint; after it dries, apply a thin layer of surface restorer wax over the area.
    (1) Cream cosmetics may be mixed into the wax.
    (2) Cream cosmetics may be applied over the wax.
  d. *Method 4:* If the area is small (e.g., razor abrasion and fever blister), apply the cosmetic to the face including powder; make small adjustments with surface wax in which some of the cosmetic has been mixed.

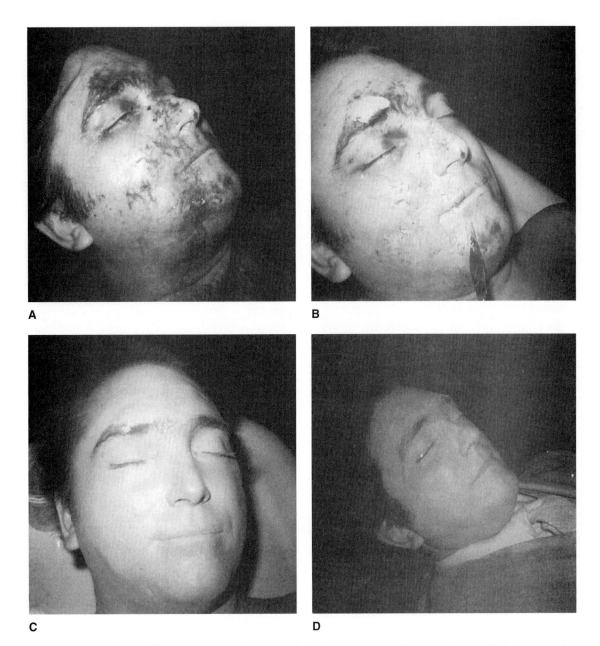

Figure 9. A. Multiple small lacerations and abrasions. **B.** Wax adjustments after embalming. **C.** Opaque undercoat sprayed over tissues. **D.** Cream cosmetics applied over the undercoat.

e. *Method 5:* Apply a surface sealer; when it has partially dried, apply a white powder with an atomizer or dropped from a brush. This will produce a skinlike color over the area where the sealer was applied.

▶ ESTABLISHING FORM—CORRECTING EMACIATED, DEPRESSED, AND COMPRESSED TISSUE

There are a variety of reasons why a body area such as the face or hands will require a reestablishment of form.

Examples include absence of teeth or dentures or a mild or extreme loss of weight. The emaciated body will exhibit unnatural depressions in various parts of the face and hands. Embalming itself can bring about dehydration to areas like the fingers and the lips making them appear slightly shrunken or wrinkled. For persons dying in a position in which the face, or a portion of the face or hands, is pushed against an immovable solid object, these contact areas will appear crushed. Trauma to the face or skull can cause a depressed fracture, resulting in a depression of the surface tissues.

There are natural depressions on the surface of the cranium and the face. These include the temple area

A

B

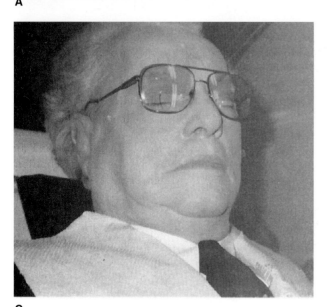

C

Figure 10. A. Desquamation (skin-slip); damaged skin removed and tissues dried. **B.** Dried skin surface painted with an undercoat paint, with cream cosmetics applied over it. **C.** Body dressed, glasses used.

and zygomatic arch depression in the cranium and the buccal depressions in the face. The deepest part of these depressions is located over the area of the teeth. These natural depressions have a tendency to deepen when there has been a loss of weight. Similarly, areas of the face containing fatty tissue may need to be rebuilt, areas including the cheeks, chin, and jawline (Fig. 11).

Correction of emaciated, depressed, or compressed tissue can be made using the following restorative treatments:

1. Embalming treatment—use of restorative coinjection fluids
2. Support inserted under sunken tissues
   a. Dentures
   b. Mouth formers; eyecaps
   c. Absorbent or nonabsorbent cotton, kapok, webbed cotton
   d. Mortuary mastics or feature posing mastic
3. Subcutaneous injection of hypodermic tissue builder
4. Subcutaneous injection of a mortuary mastic compound
5. Build upon the skin surface over the depressed area
   a. Lip wax or surface restorer wax
   b. Thick surface sealer (glue)
   c. Mortuary mastic + surface sealer + gauze + surface sealer
6. Excise damaged tissues and rebuild the area

Figure 11. A. Emaciation of the face. **B, C.** Hypodermic tissue building after embalming. **D.** Cosmetics applied.

Embalming Treatment

A restorative coinjection chemical can be added to the arterial preservative solution, usually during the last gallon of injection. When accompanied by restricted drainage, it is possible to distend sunken areas of the face, neck, and cranium. Directions of the individual chemical manufacturer should be followed. It is important to delay aspiration of unautopsied bodies for a period of several hours when using this treatment. It is not always possible to have complete control using this process; raising of the sunken areas is not always uniform. Some tissues will rapidly respond to this process and others will not respond at all. (See Selected Readings,

"Enhance Emaciated Features Arterially Using Split Injection and Restricted Drainage" by Sharon L. Gee.)

Mouth and Eyelid Support

Posing of the features is usually done in the preembalming time period. If dentures are absent, several types of supports or a combination of supports may be used. A mouth former of plastic or metal can be placed on the exposed portions of the mandible and maxillae within the mouth, or it can be placed over the few remaining teeth if the majority are missing. Absorbent or nonabsorbent cotton and kapok can be used to support the mouth when teeth and dentures are missing. For the eyelids, plastic eyecaps, cotton, or kapok can be used to keep the eyelids closed and elevated.

A feature-posing mortuary mastic compound can also be used as a support for missing teeth. The compound can be injected through the nozzle of a caulking gun. The compound alone can be used to fill out a sunken mouth or injected over the teeth (if present) or a mouth former. The mastic can also be used with eyecaps to elevate sunken eyelids. An advantage of the mastic compound is that the material does not dehydrate the tissues as cotton can.

Treatments for Sunken Eyes: Emaciated Borders of the Eye Socket

Raising sunken eyes with tissue builder is not always a successful process. Embalmers are divided on the entry point for the needle; some prefer the inner canthus of the eye and others prefer the outer corner of the eye. Once entered, direct the needle along the bony sidewall, being careful not to puncture the eyeball. Tissue builder is injected very slowly behind the eyeball. There is a tendency for the builder to flow into the upper eyelid and the supraorbital tissues giving the closed eye an unnatural appearance. Many find that using cotton as a method of eye closure is a more effective method of correcting sunken eyes. If cotton or a combination of cotton and eyecaps is used to raise the eyelids, the embalmer should also fill out the sharp bony inferior rim of the eye socket using tissue builder. Insert the needle through the nostril and direct it to the inferior rim of the eye socket. Slowly inject a small amount of tissue builder and with digital pressure distribute it along the inferior rim. This will help to remove the sharp margin of the lower eyelid.

Treatments for Underembalmed Eyelids

If the eyelids feel soft to the touch and appear underembalmed, use one of the following two methods:

1. Close the eyes using absorbent cotton saturated with several drops of undiluted cavity fluid and then seal the eyelids. The saturated cotton will act as an internal preservative compress. The glue will prevent separation of the lids. Cosmetics can be placed over the closed eyelids. It is recommended that cream cosmetics be used with this procedure.

2. A method that takes longer is to set and close the eyelids using caps or cotton and seal the eyelids with superglue. Place a preservative compress over the closed eyelids or coat the lids and surrounding area with preservative gel. Cover the compress or gel with a small sheet of thin plastic to prevent evaporation of the chemical and to help to control any fumes. Leave the preservative in place for several hours. Remove the chem-

ical, clean the eyelids with a solvent, and if necessary dry the tissues with a hair dryer. Proceed to cosmetize the eyelids. (See Selected Readings: Fountain's Method of Management Techniques for the Eyes.)

Treatments for Nasal Distortion and Tissue Erosion

If the anterior nares are depressed, cotton or mortuary mastic can be placed within the nares to hold them in correct position. These corrections should be made in the preembalming time period.

Plastic tubing (nasogastric tube) inserted through the nostrils and remaining in place for a long period of time may cause an erosion of the nasal tissue where the posterior, inferior portion of the wing of the nose attaches to the cheek. Often tissue is missing and the area appears brown and dehydrated. The tissues are generally dry. If they are moist, a preservative surface compress can be applied in the preembalming time period. When the tissues are completely dried, a surface restorer wax can be used to fill in the missing tissues.

Treatment for Earlobe Distortion

The earlobe may be depressed against the cranium and neck due to the body being wrapped in a sheet or improper placement on the headrest. The earlobes should be freed and properly positioned. A pledget of cotton coated with massage cream placed behind the lobe will hold it in position during the embalming process. This small correction is very important if earrings are to be worn by the deceased. A small amount of tissue builder injected into the lobe after embalming can also help to project the lobe (Fig. 12).

Treatment for Underembalmed Ear Tissue

If the tissues of the ear have received insufficient arterial solution, preservation is best accomplished by applying a preservative surface compress or coating the ear with a preservative gel. When sufficient time has been allowed for these chemicals to work, the tissues should be cleaned with a solvent and dried.

Treatment—Hypodermic Tissue Building

Hypodermic tissue building is done in the postembalming time period. A good rule to follow is to inject a minimum amount—more can be added later if necessary. Many embalmers still prefer to use hidden points of entry—inside nostrils and mouth or within the hairline or eyebrows. These points were used in past years to conceal possible leakage. Most quality tissue builders today leak only for a few moments following their injection. A 17-gauge needle works quite well (though some embalmers prefer a slightly smaller diameter). Tissue builder solvent should only be used for cleaning

Figure 12. Earlobe supported by cotton.

syringes. Syringes may be stored containing about 5 cubic centimeters (cc) of tissue builder solvent.

Treatment—Hypodermic Tissue Building of the Fingers

Tissue building of the fingers is often overlooked. It is especially necessary when the body is to be kept for any extended period of time, because it helps prevent dehydration of the fingertips. Tissue builder should also be injected into the area between the thumb and index finger; quite often, this area will dehydrate as a result of the embalming process. Tissue builder can be injected into the back of the hand between the tendons to compensate for weight loss and to help hide the discoloration produced by the lumbrical muscles (Fig. 13).

Treatment—Hypodermic Tissue Building of the Cheeks, Mouth, and Temple

Tissue builder injected into the anterior cheek and the angulus oris eminence (at the corners of the mouth) can help to produce a more pleasing expression. Some filling of the upper anterior cheek area may be required for almost every body because gravity has a tendency to cause the fleshy cheek areas to sag. The cheeks can be filled by inserting the needle through the respective nostril. The inferior lateral cheek area, especially over the teeth, may be depressed. This area can be filled out in the preembalming or postembalming period using cotton or mortuary mastic placed over the back teeth (see Fig. 11). If the temples are emaciated and sunken, they can be raised by tissue building. It may be also necessary to fill out the angle of the jaw and the inferior margin of the mandible. For extensive tissue building, a photograph is most helpful. DO NOT OVER FILL,

more tissue builder can be added. It is very difficult to reduce an area when excessive amount of tissue builder has been injected.

Treatment—Depressed Fractures of the Cranium, Forehead, and Cheek

Trauma, to the head, can create a depressed fracture of the cranium or areas of the face. If a cranial autopsy has been performed, this will provide easy access to the cranial cavity. If necessary, the floor of the cavity can be properly aligned and held in position by wooden splints, plaster of Paris, or strips of cotton dipped in plaster. The bone alignment should be done prior to arterial injection. After arterial injection, the cranium can be filled with packing, and the fractured bones of the calvarium placed in position over the packing. These bone fragments may be held in position by plaster of Paris or possibly superglue. (Some embalmers also prefer to drill and wire bone fragments.)

If a portion of the frontal bone has been depressed or crushed, the autopsy allows access to prop the bone in the correct position. If the body is NOT autopsied and the skin of the forehead and cranium is not torn, after embalming, an incision can be made in the scalp to gain access to elevate depressed areas of forehead and/or cranium. Cotton strips, mortuary mastic compound, and mortuary wax can be used to elevate the depressed areas (Fig. 14A–F).

Similarly if the cheekbone (maxilla) has been crushed and the surface skin is not broken, an incision can be made inside the mouth or inside the nostril to admit the nozzle of the mastic gun, the mastic compound can be injected into the area of crushed bone to raise the cheek to a normal position. The mastic compound treatments are done in the postembalming time period.

A

B

C

Figure 13. A. Wrinkled, dehydrated fingers. **B.** Tissue builder injected into each finger and area between thumb and index finger. **C.** Completed.

Treatment—Dehydrated Lips

Wrinkled mucous membranes of the lips are usually caused by dehydration. The lips can become dried (1) before death, (2) between death and embalming, (3) during embalming, and (4) between embalming and disposition of the body. Depending on the severity of the condition, correction can be made by cementing, tissue building, or waxing. Massage cream, lanolin spray, or a baby oil applied to the lips during the preparation of the body and during the interval between embalming and application of cosmetics will help to delay drying. During embalming, petroleum jelly or an adhesive emollient cream may help to gently "pull out" small wrinkles in the mucous membranes. The following are suggested postembalming treatments:

1. Part the lips, then using a spring forceps with cotton, dry the buccal cavity so that it is free of all liquids such as blood, arterial solution, or purge.
2. Make any adjustments within the buccal cavity by adding or removing cotton or mortuary mastic to achieve good curvature and projection of the mouth and lips; raise any depressed cheek areas.
3. If the tissues of the mucous membranes or the integumentary lips appear soft and underembalmed, place a thin layer of cotton over the teeth, dentures, or mouth former, and saturate it with undiluted clear cavity fluid. This will serve as an internal preservative compress, and it will remain in the buccal cavity. A surface preservative compress or preservative gel may also be used;

Figure 14. A. Self-inflicted gunshot into mouth; depressed frontal bone (no autopsy). **B.** Midline fracture of the mandible. **C.** Incision made in scalp after embalming. **D.** Depressed frontal bone raised with kapok. **E.** Small lacerations waxed, not sewn. **F.** Completed. Instant tissue fixation method of embalming treatment was used.

these will need to remain in place for several hours. When the compress or gel is removed, the tissues need to be cleaned with a solvent and dried.

4. Clean the lips with a solvent to remove any loose skin or scabs, massage cream, or emollient creams used to hold the lips together during embalming.
5. Observe any broken skin areas on the mucous membranes; these can be dried by placing a small compress of phenol or undiluted cavity fluid over the area for a period of time, or dry them with a hair dryer.
6. Tissue build the mucous membranes and/or integumentary lips.
7. Seal the lips using a small amount of superglue placed behind the weather line.
8. Apply wax if necessary.
9. Cosmetize the face and lips.

If tissue builder is used to restore dehydrated wrinkled lips, inject the **upper mucous membrane first** inserting the needle from right and left corners of the mouth. A finger placed firmly on the integumentary lip at its juncture with the mucous membrane will help to force the tissue builder into the mucous membrane portion of the lip. When injecting from the corners of the mouth, push the needle to the center of the mucous membrane, then carefully inject the filler as the needle is withdrawn. If the integumentary portions of the lips need filling, this can be done from the corners of the mouth.

Some wrinkled lips may be corrected by gluing the mouth closed. A superglue is recommended. The glue should be placed behind the weather line of the upper or lower mucous membrane. Be certain the mouth is free of any liquids prior to sealing. The mucous membranes must be cleaned with a solvent so that they are free of any moisture or oils before gluing.

Some embalmers prefer to correct wrinkled lips by waxing the lip. The upper lip should be waxed first. It may not be necessary to apply wax to both lips. A cosmetic may be mixed into the wax prior to application, either a "mortuary red" or a lipstick red. The color can also be applied by brush to the lips after they have been waxed. Wax can be smoothed and feathered into the margins of the mucous membranes using a solvent or acetone applied with a small brush. (See Mortuary Cosmetology section of this chapter.)

Treatment—Surface Restorations for Sunken, Crushed, or Eroded Tissues

With each of the conditions listed in the title of this section, it will be necessary to establish the form of the area. Sunken and crushed (or depressed) tissues need to be elevated, and eroded tissue needs to be replaced. In addition to establishing form, it may also be necessary to replace missing skin. Elevation of the tissue may come about during the arterial embalming of the face or hands. Firm massage of an area may help to bring about some swelling. There may be ruptured capillaries in the tissues, and leakage of fluid into the tissues could possibly swell the area.

Tissue elevation can also be done after embalming by tissue builder. If a large area has been crushed or depressed, the nozzle of a mortuary mastic gun can be placed deep into the tissues and the mastic injected to bring about the elevation. Some depressed areas can be corrected, after embalming, simply by application of surface wax.

Replacement of skin can be made with (1) wax, (2) a thick application (with a spatula) of a cream cosmetic, (3) surface glue (several applications), (4) alternate layers of surface glue and cotton, or (5) mortuary mastic painted with a surface glue over which a single layer of thin white gauze is placed, then the gauze is painted with surface glue.

Frequently, the angulus oris sulcus will be very long, and this can make the mouth look too long. Filling in the sulcus with a surface wax can conceal the depressed tissues. A cream cosmetic can be mixed with the wax or applied over the wax to blend with the surrounding skin cosmetic. Pronounced wrinkles in the lips can be concealed by placing a thin lip wax over the affected area. Tubes inserted into the mouth may leave deep erosion marks on the lateral corners of the mouth. During embalming, these areas can be firmly massaged to attempt making the tissues swell. If the tissues do not fill out, after embalming, seal the lips with glue, then rebuild the corners of the mouth with a surface restorer wax.

The deep mark of a rope or similar material on the neck following a trauma such as hanging can be treated by placing wax over the affected area. This treatment may need to be done after the body has been dressed and positioned in the casket. If the mark is low enough, the clothing may cover the injury to the neck. If it is not, a surface correction may need to be made. This can be done by (1) wax application; (2) cover the depressed tissues with several layers of a surface glue; and (3) apply a thin layer of mortuary mastic, coat the mastic with a surface glue, place a thin piece of gauze over the mastic and apply another layer of surface glue, when dried cosmetize the surface.

Treatment—Autopsied Neck Restoration and Tongue Excision

Several restorative problems are associated with the complete autopsy. If the neck organs have been removed, this area will need to be rebuilt. After embalming the autopsied body and prior to suturing, the neck can be filled out using cotton. Frequently the tissues of the neck will lack sufficient preservation. The cotton being used as a filler for the neck area may be saturated with undiluted cavity fluid or preservation gel and tightly packed into the neck area to replace the missing organs. This will serve not only to correct the depressed skin areas of the neck but will also provide an internal compress for preservation of the tissues.

If the tongue has been removed at autopsy, cotton saturated with undiluted cavity fluid, a cautery chemical, or autopsy gel can be inserted through the neck (if the neck organs have been removed) to reach the floor of the mouth, or it can be inserted through the mouth. Tightly pack the oral cavity before arterial injection. The internal compress assists in preservation and its pressure helps to reduce the loss of embalming solution from severed vessels. The cotton compress within the oral cavity does not have to be removed after embalming.

Treatment—Cranial Autopsy, Temple Area

Mastic compound is a good filler for the temple area when a cranial autopsy has been performed. It will remove the depression formed if the temporalis muscles have been severed or removed. With the calvarium in place, fill in the temple areas with the mastic (a soft surface restorer wax could be used as a substitute). Next, replace the scalp over the calvarium. The mastic is easily molded by pressure from moistened gloved fingers. This mastic compound (or incision seal powder) can also be placed along the scalp margins as the closure sutures are made. This will help to prevent any postembalming leakage from the cranial autopsy. The inversion suture is recommended for closure of the scalp incision, beginning on the right side of the head and ending on the left. The following protocol can be followed:

1. After arterial embalming, dry out the base of the cranial cavity.
2. Paint the inside of the cavity with a preservative gel.
3. Pack the foramen magnum and the base of the cavity with autopsy compound and cotton to absorb any leakage.
4. Attach the calvarium.
5. Fill the temple areas with mortuary mastic.
6. Paint the outside of the calvarium with an autopsy gel.
7. Place mortuary mastic or incision seal powder along the inside of the scalp as the suturing proceeds.
8. Suture closed using a worm (inversion) suture.

9. The inversion suture, properly done, leaves only a thin line on the scalp surface, which is easily waxed.

Treatment: Infant Cranial Autopsy

A problem with the infant cranial autopsy can be depressions in the cranial surface at the locations of the fontanels. Treat these depressions after embalming by tightly packing the cranial cavity with cotton or other filler material, then filling the fontanels with mortuary mastic compound. This compound can easily be smoothed by simply moistening the gloved fingers with water. The large cartilage segments forming the crown of the head can be held in position by bridge sutures made with dental floss after the cranial cavity is packed. If preservation of the scalp has been insufficient, the entire cranium can be painted with a preservative gel before the scalp is reflected back into position for suturing. A suggested protocol follows.

1. After arterial embalming, paint the floor of the cranial cavity with autopsy gel.
2. Place incision seal powder or autopsy compound in the base of the skull to absorb any moisture.
3. Tightly fill the cranial cavity with cotton or similar material.
4. Align the pieces of cartilage into their proper positions and if necessary suture them into position using dental floss.
5. At the fontanels place mortuary mastic over the cotton and blend over the cartilage (a soft surface restorative wax or several layers of thick surface glue may be used as substitute).
6. If the scalp needs additional preservative treatment, paint the inside of the scalp with autopsy gel and reflect the scalp into its normal position. If the scalp appears well preserved, a light layer of massage cream can be painted on the inside of the scalp to control dehydration.
7. Suture the scalp closed using thin suture cord or dental floss; an inversion suture is recommended, beginning on the right side of the head and ending on the left; as the suturing proceeds, place incision seal powder or mortuary mastic along the inside scalp margins to prevent leakage (Fig. 15).

Treatment—Eye Enucleation Restoration

This restoration is presented in the embalming portion of the text. Please refer to Chapter 18. Enucleation restoration is also found in the Selected Readings portion of this book, "Fountain's Method of Management Techniques for the Eyes," by Vernie Fountain.

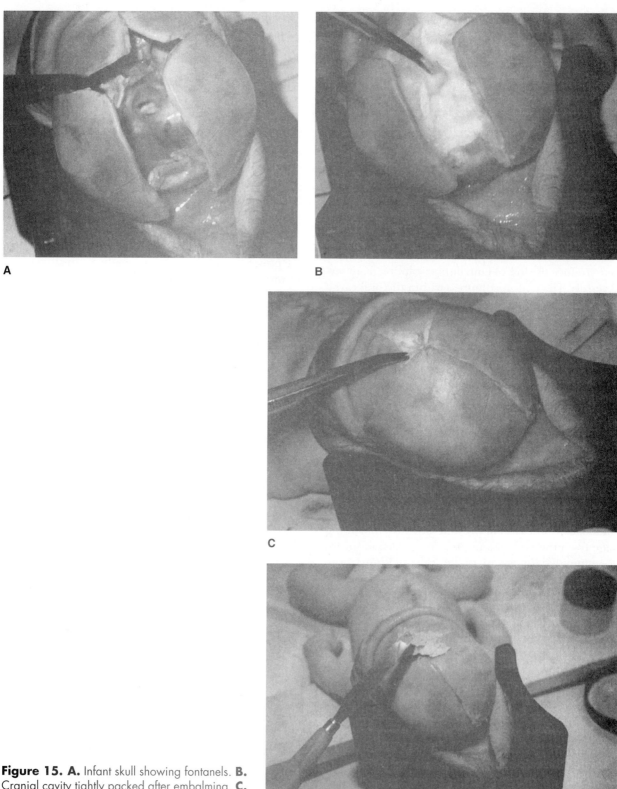

Figure 15. A. Infant skull showing fontanels. **B.** Cranial cavity tightly packed after embalming. **C.** Skull cartilage tied into position. **D.** Fontanels filled with mortuary mastic before suturing the scalp.

▶ ESTABLISHING FORM—REDUCTION OF SWOLLEN TISSUES

Swellings of the face may be general or localized. General swelling of the face may be the result of edema, gases, or extensive trauma to the facial tissues. General swelling can also be the result of the long-term use of corticosteroid drugs or an allergic reaction. Local swelling may be due to a tumor, disease such as exophthalmic goiter causing the eyes to protrude, or trauma. Distended and discolored eyes are frequently seen in cases of cranial trauma or surgery.

The following list summarizes these antemortem and postmortem causes of swelling.

1. Pathological—tumor, edema
2. Trauma—impact to head or face, surgery
3. Decomposition gases
4. Medical procedures—for example, tracheotomy, heart-lung procedures (allowing air to enter the tissues also called subcutaneous emphysema)
5. Embalming treatment—poor drainage from the face and neck; overly rapid injection of solution into facial tissues; glandular swelling in the face and neck; escape of embalming solution in areas with broken capillaries as a result of facial trauma

The actual types of distension created by the listed causes can be one or a combination of the following:

1. Liquid swellings—edema, blood, embalming solution
2. Gases—decomposition, subcutaneous emphysema, true tissue gas caused by *Clostridium perfringens*
3. Solid—neoplasm, goiter, swollen facial glands
4. Semisolid—pus

The embalmer must first determine the type of swelling before reducing the distended tissue. Restorative treatments for reducing swellings of the face and neck include the following methods. All of these treatments, with the exception of the embalming treatment, are done in the postembalming time period.

1. *Embalming treatment:* (1) Use of a strong embalming solution (hypertonic), (2) special purpose arterial fluids for edema, and (3) dehydrating coinjection fluids. These solutions and fluids are designed to dry moist tissues. Type of swelling reduced: liquids.
2. *Gravitation:* To move downward from an elevated position. Elevation of a body part (e.g., head or hands) to remove a liquid swelling. Type of swelling reduced: liquids.
3. *External pressure:* Weight applied to a surface; examples include compresses of fluid or water, pneumatic collar, water collar, small sandbags, elastic bandage, or digital pressure. Type of swelling reduced: liquids, gases, and semisolids.
4. *Channeling:* To make passages through tissues for the movement of gases or liquids. Depending on the body area, this can be done with a scalpel, trocar, or large hypodermic needle. May be combined with external pressure, gravitation, or aspiration. Type of swelling reduced: liquids and gases.
5. *Reducing chemicals:* Chemicals used to constrict or dry tissues, usually containing phenol or a phenol derivative. May be combined with other reducing techniques such as external pressure, channeling, incising, and aspiration. Type of swelling reduced: liquids and semisolids.
6. *Aspiration:* To draw out liquids or gases by means of suction. This may be done using a large hypodermic needle and syringe or infant trocar and hydroaspirator. It may be done along with channeling. Type of swelling reduced: gases, liquids, and semisolids.
7. *Incise:* To make a clean cut into tissue or skin. This would be done with a scalpel, bistoury knife, or hypodermic needle; after incising a localized swelling, pressure would be applied to express or drain the contents. Type of swelling reduced: liquids, gases, and semisolids.
8. *Excise:* To remove by cutting. This treatment would be used to reduce a localized area. Type of swelling reduced: solids.
9. *Heat:* To reduce a localized swollen area by increased temperature. This is done using an electric spatula. It may be applied to the skin surface to restore contour or natural form by drying moist tissues. The skin must be thoroughly coated with massage cream. It may also be applied directly to moist tissues under the skin. Type of swelling reduced: liquids and semisolids.
10. *Wicking:* The use of an absorbent material to draw moisture away from an area. The material (e.g., absorbent cotton) is inserted under the skin surface directly in contact with the moisture; the exposed end is outside the surface of the skin. Type of swelling reduced: liquids.

Restorative Treatments for Liquid Swellings

In recent years, generalized edema of the face has become a frequently encountered postmortem condition. This condition often accompanies extensive chemotherapeutic drug therapy, cardiac and vascular surgery, and organ transplantation. Diseases causing the axillary lymph nodes to swell or impairment to the vascular circulation of the arm can result in accumulation of edema in the arm and hand. There are several treatments for edema (liquid) swellings.

Embalming treatment—the area affected by the edema can be injected using a concentrated embalming solution. In addition to strong preservative solutions, coinjection chemicals designed to reduce edema can be added. Directions for these coinjections should be carefully followed. Epsom salts can also be used as an additive to the preservative solution to dry tissues where edema is present. When the face is swollen as a result of edema, and the body is not autopsied, restricted cervical injection and continuous drainage is recommended. If the facial edema is recent, for example, if it is a result of recent surgery, the edema will respond best to this treatment. When the face is swollen as a result of trauma, which may have occurred several weeks before death, these swellings do not respond as well to the chemical embalming treatment. Elevation of the head accompanied by external massage of the face and neck during and following arterial injection will assist in removal of the edema.

Elevation and Gravitation.
Elevation of the head and shoulders will help to gravitate edema from the facial tissues. Elevation of a distended hand after embalming can gravitate edema from the hand into the forearm. Removal of large quantities of edema from the face, hands, or a local area such as the eyelids may result in wrinkled tissues or broad flat areas. This can be seen particularly in the eyelids and hands. With the hands, it is prudent to limit the amount of edema removed so that the hand looks more presentable. After the edema is removed, tissue building may help restore a more natural appearance to the hands.

For treatment of extreme facial edema, some embalmers have taken the embalmed body, placed it on a removal cot, secured the body well with straps, then stood the cot in an upright position. Allowing the body to remain in this erect position for several hours promotes gravitation of the edema from the facial tissues.

Elevation and gravitation can be started in the preembalming time period and continued through the embalming and postembalming treatments. Thorough aspiration of the cavities is important, because this relieves internal pressure from the neck and face. Channeling the neck and the submandibular areas with a trocar by lowering the head and passing the trocar under the clavicles may help to provide passages for the facial fluids to drain into the thoracic cavity. External pressure applied by firm massage, working from the face to the neck, will help to promote drainage of the edema from the face or neck into the thorax. Time is necessary for gravitation to be effective, but when combined with aspiration, channeling, and external pressure, the time period may be shortened. In addition to the above methods after embalming, the embalmer may make a semilunar inci-

sion beginning above the center of the right clavicle and extending to a point above the center of the left clavicle. The flap formed can be lifted and the tissues of the neck and lower face channeled using an infant trocar. These channels will provide passage for the edema to the incised area. Cotton can be placed under the flap of tissue, which acts as a wick to draw the edema from the face and neck. Several hours time should be allowed for exit of the edema. When completed, the tissues under the flap can be filled with incision seal powder and the incision tightly sutured with a baseball suture or an inversion suture. The incision should be covered with surface glue.

> Wicking can be used to drain edema from a body area. A small puncture is made in the affected area and an absorbent material such as cotton or cotton webbing strips is inserted into the swollen area. The capillary attraction of the wick slowly draws the edema out of the body. If the punctures are small enough, they can be later closed with trocar buttons. This method is very effective but it does take time.

External Pressure.
Generalized facial edema can be treated to a limited degree by external pressure. This can be in the form of weighted compresses (e.g., cotton saturated with diluted cavity fluid) or by firm digital pressure (e.g., a rolling motion of the embalmer's fisted hand, rolling in a downward direction toward the neck). The pressure rolling may be done during injection of embalming solution and would be repeated many times in the postembalming time period. Methods discussed in the previous sections can be combined with external pressure and aspiration of the cavities.

A swollen neck will respond better than the face to external pressure. After arterial injection, several devices can be used to put pressure on the swollen neck tissues: water collar, pneumatic collar, or wrapping with an elastic bandage. These external pressure devices should be combined with aspiration of the cavities and channeling of the neck with the trocar passing under the clavicles. If these treatments are not successful, surgical excision may be necessary to treat a swollen neck.

Restorative Treatments for Solid and Semisolid Swelling

Excision (surgical reduction) is usually reserved for treatment of localized solid swellings such as a tumor or swollen glandular tissue and is sometimes also used to reduce swollen neck tissues. This section discusses the reduction of swellings caused by distended muscles and glands of the neck.

If there is general swelling of the neck and the glandular tissues (parotid, submandibular, and sublingual glands), an extensive excision of swollen tissues may be required. Two approaches can be used to accomplish this: method A uses two incisions and method B uses a single incision. These excision reductions are performed in the postembalming time period.

Method A.

1. Make a vertical incision on each side of the neck from a point behind and slightly below the ear, directed downward toward the superior border of the trapezius muscle.

2. Using a scalpel, dissect the skin away from the underlying structures in the area of the distension. Work over as far as the median line from the respective sides, upward and in front of the ear, removing the parotid gland if necessary.

3. Excise all structures necessary to return the neck to its normal size and shape. Grasp the tissues with lock forceps and dissect from the lower border of the mandible downward to the clavicle. Remove tissues in layers and avoid removing more than necessary. (Excised tissues should be retained in a plastic bag, preserved and buried or cremated with the body.)

4. Pack the cavity with cotton saturated with a phenol cautery solution or with undiluted cavity fluid. This will preserve and dry the remaining tissues (Fig. 16).

5. Allow at least 1 to 4 hours for chemical action (this will depend on the product used and its concentration), then remove the internal

A

B

C

Figure 16. A. Surgical neck reduction. Phenol applied after excision of swollen tissues. **B.** Worm (inversion) suture used to roll under excess skin. **C.** Completed reduction, glue applied over incision.

compresses and dry out the pocket with absorbent cotton.

6. Place mortuary mastic compound to help reshape the neck and to prevent leakage; if not available, place incision seal powder within the cavity.

7. Insert a long, straight needle on the left side through the subcutaneous tissues at a point posterior to the angle of the mandible. Direct the needle through the neck. Reinsert the needle in the subcutaneous tissue on the right side at the same position. Direct the needle back through the neck to the original point of entry. Tie the ends of the ligatures tight enough to give form to the angle of the jaw.

8. Suture the incision using an inversion suture. The amount of skin turned under should be proportionate to the amount of reduction that was necessary.

9. The incision is hidden in normal casket repose. To further minimize the possibility of leakage, paint the closure with a surface glue.

Method B. Method B involves the use of a single incision. A semilunar incision is carefully made beginning approximately 1 or 2 inches above the center of the right clavicle directed downward over the first or second ribs across the sternum and upward passing through the center of the left clavicle and continuing about 1 or 2 inches above the clavicle. This will create a large flap of skin. The skin is carefully dissected from the subcutaneous tissues. The flap is lifted and with a scalpel in an orderly fashion from superficial to deep the swollen muscles and glands are excised (Fig. 17). After sufficient tissue is excised, the cavity can be packed with cotton compresses saturated with phenol cautery solution or undiluted cavity fluid. These compresses can be left in place from 1 to 4 hours. When the tissues appear dry, remove the compresses. Insert mortuary mastic compound to reform the neck. This material will also help to prevent leakage. If the mastic is not available, incision seal powder can be liberally spread throughout the cavity. The incision can be aligned using one or two temporary bridge sutures. An inversion suture or a tight baseball suture can be used to close the incision. Coat the incision with surface glue and cover it with a piece of plastic to prevent leakage.

Treatment: Goiter Excision

With permission, after embalming, a goiter can be removed through a semilunar flap incision made from the center of the right clavicle to the center of the left clavicle. Lift the skin flap formed by the incision and dissect through the subcutaneous tissues until the enlarged lobes of the thyroid gland are reached. Using a scalpel or double-pointed scissors carefully excise the glandular

tissue. If reshaping of the neck is necessary, mortuary mastic compound can be injected into the region where the tissue was excised. The neck can be shaped by light pressure applied to the skin surface. Dry the subcutaneous marginal tissues and apply a liberal amount of incision seal powder or mortuary mastic compound along the margins of the incision. A tight baseball or inversion suture can be used to close the incision. Apply surface glue to the closed incision. If leakage is a concern, place a piece of plastic over the surface glue.

Treatment: Submandibular Swelling

Glandular swelling can be a problem when there is a long delay between death and embalming of the body. There may be a lengthy delay between death and embalming when there is an autopsy. During arterial injection of the head, there is frequently a tendency for the glandular tissues to swell (parotid, sublingual, and submandibular glands). Very firm external digital pressure applied immediately following injection will help to reduce the swollen glands. If this is unsuccessful, the head can be lowered, and entering through the neck (if the neck organs have been removed), the glandular tissues can be removed or incised using an infant trocar or bistoury knife, again followed by very firm external digital pressure applied to the swollen tissues. If the swelling remains, a scalpel or bistoury can be inserted up through the neck and the swollen glandular tissues excised. Care should be taken not to pierce the skin. Reshaping of the neck can be done with cotton saturated with cavity chemical.

Treatment: Solid/Semisolid Reduction by Incising

When the skin surface over a tumor or facial swelling is undamaged and the tumor is in such a position that it can be excised from inside the mouth, this approach should be given first consideration. If skin over a tumor or swelling is broken and discolored, it may be best to excise the swelling as well as the damaged skin.

The following protocol was used to reduce a very large growth on the left side of the face in the lateral cheek in front of the ear. The ear was unaffected. When pressed, the swelling did not appear to be solid tissue; it felt like liquid and semisolid material. The approach for incising, aspirating, and draining was from within the mouth (buccal cavity). Whenever possible, localized tumors of the face should be incised or excised from inside the buccal cavity. This approach leaves the surface skin intact, and any leakage occurs within the mouth and drains into the throat.

1. The body was disinfected, washed, and positioned.
2. The face was shaved and features set.
3. Arterial embalming of the body was performed.

A

B

C

D

Figure 17. A. Swollen neck, auto accident, no autopsy. **B.** Semilunar incision. **C.** Tissues removed; incision seal powder applied. **D.** Reduced neck.

4. The lips were parted and a scalpel inserted into the left cheek wall, puncturing the wall and entering the growth.

5. An infant trocar with the point removed attached to the hydroaspirator was inserted into the growth through the opening made by the scalpel.

6. The contents of the swelling were aspirated.

7. A long hypodermic needle was inserted through the opening made by the scalpel into the cavity of the collapsed swelling and 3 oz of undiluted cavity chemical was injected.

8. Thirty minutes were given for the chemicals to work, during which time the cavities were aspirated and injected. The trocar was inserted under the left clavicle from within the thoracic cavity, through the neck tissues, and into the collapsed area of the swelling to provide a drainage channel.

9. The temples and anterior cheek areas were filled with tissue builder.

10. Through the mouth, the cavity fluid was aspirated from the collapsed swelling with a blunt infant trocar, and cotton grasped by spring

forceps was inserted through the mouth to dry the treated area and the buccal cavity. This was repeated several times.

11. Cotton was placed over the teeth on the left side of the buccal cavity to absorb any accumulated cavity fluid.

12. The excess loose tissues over the collapsed swelling were rolled inward and secured with superglue, giving the appearance of a straight line. An inversion suture using a small circle needle and dental floss joined the two sides of the inverted tissue.

13. Surface glue was painted over the suture and allowed to dry.

14. Opaque paint was lightly sprayed over the entire area of discolored tissues and allowed to dry.

15. Cream cosmetics were applied to the face over the painted area; the face was dried using white talcum powder.

16. Hairspray was lightly sprayed over all areas of the cosmetized face.

Restorative Treatments for Facial Swelling from Gases

There are three causes for gases in the body tissues: (1) antemortem subcutaneous emphysema, (2) gas resulting from decomposition, and (3) gas from the growth of the bacterium *C. perfringens*, also known as tissue gas. Gas or air in the tissues tends to move in the postmortem period from the dependent tissues gradually into the more elevated areas of the body. Often these are the upper chest walls, neck, and facial tissues. Methods used to release gases include incising and channeling combined with external pressure and aspiration. The eyes and mouth should not be sealed with glue until every effort has been made to remove as much gas as possible.

Antemortem subcutaneous emphysema is the presence of air in the subcutaneous tissues, and it often remains in the deceased body. It is brought about by surgery or trauma when there has been a rupture of the pleural sac or an air passageway. It is frequently seen when CPR has been administered and a rib has fractured and pierced a lung or the pleural sac. Patients who die following surgery where a tracheotomy has been performed often exhibit gas or air in the tissues.

After death, these gases in the subcutaneous tissues have a tendency to move to the most elevated areas, often the face. Palpation of the affected tissue will move the gas and often a "crackling" sound can be heard as the gas moves. This is called **crepitation.** The condition can be quite severe, and the unsupported tissues of the face and upper chest can be greatly distended. There is (1) no odor, (2) desquamation, or (3) blebs on the skin surface with this condition. The distension does not intensify during the injection of arterial fluid; it is the movement

and relocation of the gas, which gives the impression that the amount of gas is increasing.

If the tissues of the face and the chest are affected, they can be treated with the following procedures.

1. *Prior to embalming:* Using the common carotid artery as an injection site creates an exit point for gases in the immediate vicinity. Some embalmers use a semilunar incision made from the center of the right clavicle to the center of the left clavicle. This provides a large opening for the exit of gases. Applying firm external pressure with the hands moves the gases toward the incision.

2. *Cavity embalming:* During aspiration of the cavities, the trocar can be directed over the ribs and into the tissues of the chest wall. This channeling will provide passages allowing gases to move into the abdominal cavity and then be aspirated. Channels can also be made into the tissues of the neck as passages for the gases to be drawn back into the thoracic cavity. Firm external pressure directing the gas from the face to the neck and chest will help to move the gas into the channels while aspirating the thoracic cavity.

3. *Postembalming:* The lips can be separated and a scalpel or bistoury knife inserted to incise the tissues and the buccal cavity. Channels can be made into the anterior and lateral cheek areas to release the gas. Passages for the gas can also be made within the hairline of the temples. From within the nostrils, a large hypodermic needle can be inserted to reach the lower eyelids and the inferior orbit. The eyelids can be gently everted and the tissues of the conjunctiva of the lids incised to release gas. Pressure is then exerted to move the gas from the lids to the openings. To prevent leakage, cotton can be used to close the eyelids; the cotton can be saturated with cavity fluid to ensure good preservation of the lids. If the embalmer wishes, the cotton compresses can be removed after several hours, and the eyes dried and closed with an eyecap and glued.

Gases from decomposition will also move to the high points of the body, especially the face. Thorough embalming is necessary to arrest the generation of the gas. Restricted cervical injection and use of a strong preservative solution are recommended to achieve the most complete preservation of the face and at the same time control facial swelling. It may be necessary to aspirate the cranial cavity if the body has not been autopsied. This can be done by passing a large hypodermic needle through a nostril and piercing through the ethmoid foramen located in the cribriform plate of the ethmoid bone. Undiluted cavity chemical should be injected after aspiration is completed. This treatment can help stop further generation of gases in the cranial cavity. Gases in the cranial cavity can move through the various cranial foramina to enter the facial tissues and create swelling, especially around the eye.

After thorough embalming, including multisite injection and the supplemental treatments of hypodermic injection and surface compresses, any gases present in the facial tissues can be removed by the methods previously discussed—incising and channeling combined with external pressure and aspiration. The embalmer may need to reaspirate and reinject the cavities several times prior to dressing and casketing the body.

True tissue gas is a rare condition—**but a very dramatic condition**—caused by the bacterium *C. perfringens*. The tissues rapidly fill with an immense amount of gas. In only a few hours, the face may become unrecognizable. There will be a very strong odor of decomposition, skin blebs will develop, and desquamation will occur. The origin of the gas may be in the dependent tissues, but as with the previous conditions, the gas rapidly moves into the elevated body areas, especially the tissues of the face.

The preparation of a body with true tissue gas necessitates the use of multisite injection, very strong preservative solutions, special purpose tissues gas fluids, and localized hypodermic injection. After thorough embalming, incising, channeling, and multiple aspiration of the body cavities may be necessary to remove the gases trapped in the tissues. Incisions should remain open for several hours to allow all gas to escape. All cutting instruments used on the body should be thoroughly sanitized because this bacterium can easily be passed from one body to another. Special care should be taken to disinfect the trocar used to aspirate and inject the cavities of these bodies. (See also Selected Readings, "Fountain's Method of Management Techniques for the Eyes," by Vernie Fountain.)

Restorative Treatments for Localized Swellings

Hematoma of the Eye—Chemical Bleaching and Reduction. A large blood discoloration is called an ecchymosis, and when the area is also swollen, it is called a hematoma. The discoloration and swelling is caused by an extravasation of blood into the tissues. The most common cause for this condition is trauma. The following treatments can be used to bleach the bluish-black discoloration and reduce the distension. Prior to any treatment of a "black eye," the unaffected tissues of the face should be coated with massage cream to protect them from the effects of the chemicals which will be used. No massage cream should be placed over the discolored tissues (Fig. 18A–D).

1. During arterial injection, a bleaching chemical or cavity fluid external compress may be placed over the swollen eyelids to retard further distension and begin the bleaching process.

2. After the arterial embalming, a hypodermic injection of a bleaching-cautery agent or undiluted cavity fluid may be made directly into the eyelids and affected surrounding tissues. Entry points can include the lateral corner of the line of closure, inner side of the eyelids, eyebrow, and the respective nostril. Insert the needle and in a "fanning" motion make a series of channels through as much tissue as possible. Each time the needle is withdrawn from its furthest point, slowly inject the chemical. There will be additional swelling as this is done.

3. About 2 cc of the concentrated chemical can be deposited behind the center of the eyeball. This can be done by inserting the needle at the medial or lateral canthus of the eye and slowly directing the needle along the bony margin of the respective wall until the back of the eyeball is reached. Care should be taken not to puncture the eyeball.

4. Using a cotton compress or webbed cotton pad apply firm pressure to the skin surface where the chemical has been injected and attempt to distribute the chemical under the skin.

5. Using cotton, pose the eyelids, saturating the cotton with the same bleaching chemical or cavity fluid. This places a bleaching-reducing chemical between the eyelids and the eyeball.

6. Allow 30 minutes to 1 hour for chemicals to work.

7. Remove the cotton from between the lids and the eyeball and replace it with dry cotton to help absorb any liquids.

8. Using cotton or a cloth begin to apply external pressure to the swollen upper lid and supraorbital tissues. Press the chemical and blood out through the points where the needle entered. Repeat this process for the lower lid and surrounding area.

9. If necessary, after as much liquid as possible has been expressed from the tissues, compresses of the bleaching solution or undiluted cavity chemical may again be placed on the lids, especially where they attach to the supraorbital and infraorbital areas, to help establish good form. These can remain in place for several hours.

10. Remove the compresses and clean the lids with a solvent and dry them with a hair dryer.

11. Pose the lids using cotton or eyecaps. The tissues should be quite firm at this point.

12. Seal the lids together with superglue.

Hematoma of the Eye—Heat Reduction and Chemical Bleaching. This treatment uses a heated electric spatula

Figure 18. A. Hematoma of the eyelids. **B.** Injection of a phenol cautery agent into the lids. **C.** Firm pressure applied as the phenol solution is pressed out of the tissues. **D.** Completed.

and a bleaching-cautery chemical for restoration of a "black eye."

1. Apply massage cream to the unaffected facial tissues.
2. Prior to arterial injection, place cotton under the swollen eyelids, saturated with a bleaching chemical or undiluted cavity chemical.
3. Apply a cotton compress saturated with the same bleaching chemical or undiluted cavity chemical to the surface of the swollen eyelids. This will help to preserve and bleach the tissues.
4. Embalm the body.

5. Remove the compresses over and under the distended eye.
6. Apply a thick coating of massage cream over the distended eye.
7. Preheat an electric spatula to its maximum setting.
8. Draw the heated blade across the swollen tissues of the lower and upper lids, moving from medial to lateral sides. After each pass, lift the spatula and wipe the blade clean with a dry cloth. The heat will dehydrate the tissues and reduce the swelling. Do not touch the heated spatula to the eyelashes.

9. Repeat the process reapplying massage cream to the swollen tissues each time.
10. Clean the eyelids with a solvent to remove all of the massage cream.
11. Pose the eyelids with cotton or eyecaps and glue eyes shut with superglue.
12. Apply an opaque cosmetic to match the normal complexion coloring.

A variation of this treatment is to apply the electric spatula to the underside of the eyelids to reduce the swelling.

Hematoma of the Eye—Reduction by Excision. A third treatment for swollen eyelids is surgical reduction. In the majority of cases, the eyeball proper is not protruding. The capillaries in the eyelids have ruptured and the result is both a distension and a discoloring of the eyelids. This treatment is well described in the Selected Readings section of this book, "Management Techniques for the Eyes," by Vernie Fountain.

Restorations for Separated Features
Separated lips and eyelids will be considered in this section. Conditions causing separation before and after embalming will be discussed.

Eyelid Separation—Prior to Embalming
Eye closure difficulties can be found in bodies with sunken eyes or the presence of a glass eye. Posing and closure of the eyes can be done prior to, during, or following arterial injection. Where a condition exists making closure difficult, it is best to attempt to close the eyelids prior to arterial injection. First the eyelids should be exercised. This can be done by inserting the rounded handle of an aneurysm needle or spring forceps under the eyelid. Move the instrument under the lids along the attached margins of the lids and gently raise and stretch each lid being careful not to tear the tissues. After exercising, attempt to close the eyelids using cotton or an eyecap to support the lids.

Sunken Eyes. If the body is extremely emaciated, the eyes will be sunken deep into the orbits. After the lids have been exercised, cotton can be used for eye closure. The cotton will help to raise the eyelids and keep them together. A combination of eyecaps and cotton can also be used, a cap over the eyeball, or a layer of cotton, and a cap on top of the cotton. Sealing (gluing) is usually not done until after the embalming of the body, but with sunken eyes, it may help to seal the eyelids prior to embalming.

Glass Eye. When a glass eye is present, there is frequently atrophy of the eyelids and closure may be diffi-

cult. The lids should be exercised and an attempt made to close the eyelids prior to arterial embalming. It may not be possible to raise the eye with a cap or cotton, so simply use the glass eye. To keep the lids closed, it may be necessary to glue the lids shut at this time. Using superglue, the lids can even be glued directly to the glass eye. In some cases, a better closure may be made by removing the glass eye and setting the lids with a cap and/or cotton. If closure is not possible at this time, set the eye after arterial embalming. After embalming, the lids can be exercised and if necessary the levator palpebrae superioris muscle and connecting tissues at the attached margin of the upper eyelid can be incised, and this will help to lower the upper lid.

Exophthalmic Goiter. This rare thyroid condition creates a protrusion of the eyes. It may be very difficult to insert any cotton or an eyecap under the lids. It may be necessary to simply seal the lids closed. This could be done prior to arterial injection. If superglue is being used, the sealing could be done prior to or following arterial injection.

Eyelid Separation—Postembalming
Eyelids that have separated slightly because of dehydration may be treated by exercising the lids and sealing the free margins with superglue. The superglues adhere better to the eyelids than the rubber-based glues, and they react faster and ensure a more secure closure.

Frequently in the case of an embalmed body shipped to a funeral home, the eyelids may show a marked degree of separation if they had not been glued prior to shipment. The lids can be stretched, and if absolutely necessary, the muscle (levator palpebrae superioris) high under the attached margin of the upper lid can be incised and the lid stretched to obtain closure. Closure can be maintained by an application of superglue to the free margins of the lids.

Prevention of eyelid separation can be accomplished by securing the lids with glue at the conclusion of embalming. Massage cream to retard dehydration can be placed under the lids by applying a light coating of the cream to an eyecap. A light coating of massage cream placed on the surface of the eyelids and later the use of cream cosmetics will retard dehydration. Well-embalmed tissue will not dehydrate as fast as underembalmed tissue. If the eyelids, at the conclusion of arterial embalming, appear to have insufficient arterial solution, cotton can be used for closure and the cotton slightly saturated with undiluted cavity chemical. The eyelids, after being set, should be sealed with superglue. In several hours, the lids and surrounding areas will feel firm and well preserved.

Lip Separation—Prior to Embalming

When teeth or dentures are present and the jaw is elevated to close the mouth, usually the lower lip rests on the inferior margin of the upper teeth. A difficult lip closure prior to embalming is usually caused by physical abnormalities of the jaw or teeth. Lip separation after embalming is more common, caused by dehydration of the mucous membranes or loosening of the wires used for mouth closure.

Disarticulated Mandible

A dislocated jaw can make mouth closure and lip contact almost impossible, caused when the condyle of the mandible has slipped out of the mandibular fossa of the temporal bone. When raising the mandible to close the mouth, the upper and lower teeth do not come into contact. The jaw will be thrust forward and instead of the teeth coming into contact, the lower teeth will be extended outward and actually above the upper teeth. The embalmer needs to take a firm grip on the mandible and attempt to push downward and backward to slip the condyle into the mandibular fossa. Several attempts may be necessary before this is accomplished. The jaw must be put into its proper place before the body is embalmed. When the jaw is in proper position, the upper and lower teeth should come into contact or the lower teeth should slip slightly behind the upper teeth. This same relationship should exist when dentures are used. The mouth can now be secured by needle injector or suture. Lip closure should be possible and the lips can be glued after the embalming of the body.

Dental Prognathism

Dental prognathism, or protrusion of the upper teeth, can make lip closure very difficult. A simple method of correction is to:

1. Close the mouth by needle injector or suture.
2. Stretch the lips as far as possible to attempt to bring the lips into contact.
3. Place a strip of cotton over the lower incisor teeth. This should nearly bring the lips into contact.
4. Coat the lips with an adhesive lip cream to hold the lips in contact. If the lips will not stay in contact, a rubber-based lip glue or superglue can be applied to hold them in position during embalming.
5. After embalming, the lips should be opened to ascertain if the buccal cavity is dry (free of purge material, embalming solution, or blood). Expression adjustments can be made with cotton or a posing mastic.
6. Reseal the lips with glue.

Postembalming—Slight Lip Separation After Mouth Closure

Some embalmers actually prefer to embalm the body with a slight separation of the lips (about the thickness of a nickel). This slight separation allows the lips to round out during the arterial injection. If this is not desired, first check if a needle injector was used to close the mouth. If it was, be certain the head of one or both needle injector barbs is not placed on the gum where the inner mucous membrane of the lip joins the gum. If so, the head of the barb may be pulling on the mucous membrane and not allowing the lips to come into contact. Using a hemostat pull the mucous membrane over the head of the barb. This will give more extension to the lip. An adhesive lip cream will assist in holding the lips together.

Lip Separation—Postembalming. A slight separation of the lips can be corrected by one of the following treatments:

1. The lips should be parted and using cotton attached to spring forceps thoroughly dry the buccal cavity. In addition to ensuring dryness of the cavity, the cotton passed over the inner tissues of the lips will help to exercise them. After the buccal cavity has been dried and the lips exercised, if the separation is small, an application of superglue just behind the weather line should firmly seal the lips together (Fig. 19A–D).
2. Inject tissue builder into the upper mucous membrane to expand the lip sufficiently to make contact with the lower lip. It may be necessary to tissue build both the upper and lower mucous membranes to bring the lips into contact.
3. A third treatment for closing small separations is to apply a thin layer of wax to the upper mucous membrane. If there is sufficient separation, both mucous membranes may need to be waxed.

Of the three methods described, securing the lips with superglue is generally the simplest and most satisfactory treatment. Some embalmers may want to combine two of these methods, for example, tissue building one or both mucous membranes followed by gluing of the membranes.

▶ RESTORATIONS FOR BROKEN TISSUES

In this section, treatments for deeply torn or disconnected tissues in visible areas of the head, face, neck, arms, and hands are discussed. Examples include trauma such as lacerations, compound fractures, and penetrating wounds; visible surgical incisions and tracheotomy; and postmortem treatments such as the autopsy scalp

Figure 19. A. Slight lip separation in a body shipped by air. **B.** Lips exercised with the handle of forceps. **C.** Glue applied. **D.** Completed.

incision and visible incisions related to embalming treatments. Small lacerations and surgical incisions of the eyebrow, eyelids, surrounding orbital tissues, and laceration of the lips are included in this section.

There are three objectives for performing these restorative treatments: (1) to realign and keep aligned the severed margins of the wound or incision; (2) to prevent any leakage from the wound or incision, because leakage could loosen and possibly free any cosmetic or wax treatment over the problem area; and (3) to hide the presence of the wound or incision by making the skin surface and contour appear natural (Fig. 20A–D).

The separations discussed in this section are cuts extending deeper than the skin level. Three treatments are used to close these separations: suturing, gluing, and waxing. These treatments are generally done in the postembalming time period. A suggested sequence of treatment is as follows:

1. Using a moist cloth or moist cotton carefully clean blood and debris from the cut and the surrounding tissues; use thick gloves if glass shards are present.
2. After cleaning the wound, evaluate the depth and extent of the separated tissues, apply

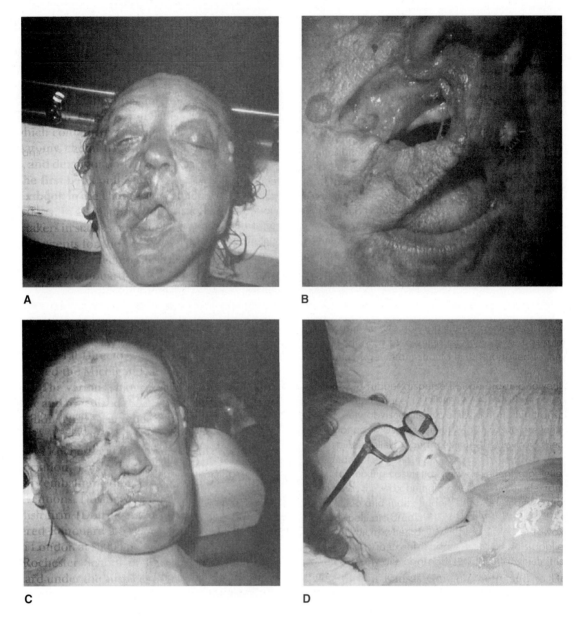

Figure 20. A. Deep laceration of cheek and hematoma of both eyelids. **B.** Deep laceration of cheek. **C.** Following embalming, laceration is sutured. **D.** Laceration waxed; eyes reduced by injection of phenol; discolorations undercoated before cream cosmetics were applied.

massage cream to the surrounding unaffected tissues, and excise dehydrated margins.

3. Align bony tissues if necessary.

4. Align deep tissues and suture into position using individual bridge sutures.

5. From within the wound hypodermically inject the walls using a cautery chemical or undiluted cavity fluid. A compress saturated with the same chemical can be placed between the separated tissues.

6. Align the surface margins using individual bridge sutures of dental floss.

7. Embalm the body.

8. Check for thorough preservation and dryness of the tissues and if inadequate renew compresses.

9. Remove the compresses and clean the wound with a solvent. A hair dryer or electric spatula can be used to dry the walls of the wound.

10. Place incision seal powder or a thin ribbon of mortuary mastic into the deep areas of the wound.

11. Close the wound:
    a. Using a single or double intradermal suture
    b. Using an inversion suture, if excess skin is present

c. Using a small baseball suture made with dental floss, which can be covered with wax or surface sealer

d. Using subcutaneous sutures placed about $\frac{1}{4}$ inch below the surface of the wound and superglue to close the skin surface

e. If the wound is not too deep seal edges with superglue

f. If the deep wound is small enough and suturing may cause the skin to "pucker" (e.g., small lacerations of the eyelid or lip) fill the separation with a surface restorer wax

12. Replace surface skin:

a. If the laceration or puncture has been waxed, simply blending the wax into the surrounding area will cover the problem area. Cream cosmetics can be mixed into the wax or applied over it to blend in with the surrounding intact tissues. Apply white drying powder and using the powder brush "stipple" lightly over the waxed areas to reproduce the pores of the skin.

b. If the laceration or puncture was closed with superglue or sutured

(1) and the area is discolored, spray or paint an opaque undercoat over the discolored area and the glued laceration or puncture. Once dry, make a wax adjustment along the laceration or puncture and blend the wax into the surrounding tissues. Cream cosmetics can be applied over the wax.

(2) and the area is not discolored, apply several thick layers of surface sealer over the laceration or puncture. Allow the sealer to dry and apply cream cosmetics over the sealer and the surrounding tissues.

(3) and the area is or is not discolored apply a transparent or opaque cosmetic and dry the cosmetic with a white drying powder. Apply a thin layer of matching surface restorer wax over the margins of the laceration or puncture and gently feather the wax into the surrounding areas. Powder can again be applied over the wax in a "stippling" fashion to give a porous effect to the wax (Fig. 21A–E).

Autopsy Scalp Incision

First, the base of the cranium needs to be dried and packed with an absorbent material. The calvarium may need to be anchored to the skull, and this can be done by suturing or with calvarium clamps. An inversion suture can be used to close this incision. Linen thread is stronger than cotton thread, and a seven-twist linen suture thread is strong enough that the thread does not have to be doubled. The suturing should begin on the right side of the head and end on the left side. If the incision is not uniform (e.g., a right angle second incision is present at some point along the autopsy incision), it will be necessary to align the margins using temporary bridge sutures before the primary autopsy incision is closed. A small baseball suture could substitute for an inversion suture. Tie the first stitch into position rather than relying on a knot to anchor the ligature.

Compound Fractures

Compound fractures should be realigned before arterial embalming. Rigor is often present in trauma cases, and this needs to be manually broken up before the fractured bone is placed back into its correct position. It may be necessary to temporarily hold the bones into position during arterial embalming. This can be done by placing a bandage of gauze or strips of cloth over the area to hold the bones in position until the tissues firm. To reset the bones, it may be necessary to use a flat-bladed instrument to force the bones into realignment. The blade is placed between the fractured ends of the bone and used to forcefully retract the ends of the bones into alignment. After the bone is reset and the body embalmed, the broken skin can be sutured. The 12-step protocol outlined above can be followed (Fig. 22).

Lacerations and Surgical Incisions

Conditions associated with trauma and surgical procedures are widely variable. The embalmer must see the existing conditions before a treatment plan can be made. It is important that the marginal tissues be realigned prior to embalming. For this reason, surgical staples and sutures should remain in place until arterial embalming is completed. The staples can be removed by grasping them, one at a time, in the center with a hemostat and with a right to left motion of the instrument they can be freed. Surgical sutures, if they are thin enough and there is no leakage from the incision, can be left in place and the incision covered with wax or with a surface sealer. Cosmetics can be applied over the wax or sealer. If there is any concern about leakage, after embalming, the surgical sutures can be removed, the incision cleaned, cautery chemicals applied, the incision dried and sealed with superglue or resuturing, and surface treatments performed as previously outlined.

Tracheotomy

Restorative treatments for the tracheotomy should be done after arterial and cavity embalming is completed. About 2 oz of a cautery chemical or undiluted cavity fluid can be gently poured or injected into the tracheotomy opening. This will help to disinfect and preserve any

Figure 21. A. Deep separation of chin; lower lip badly torn. **B.** Lower lip excised; deep filler of mortuary mastic. **C.** Lower lip rebuilt with surface wax. **D.** Chin waxed; lip color applied. **E.** Completed.

Figure 22. Compound fracture of the wrist.

materials in the air passageways. The passages can be filled with incision seal powder or mortuary mastic to help prevent any leakage. Finally, the tracheotomy can be tightly packed with cotton to almost the surface of the skin. A final layer of incision seal powder or mortuary mastic can be applied and the incision closed by suturing. The suture can be covered with surface sealer glue or wax to hide the sutures. If the tracheotomy has been present for a length of time, the edges will appear very firm and slightly swollen. Suturing will not be possible because the margins cannot be drawn together and the tissues easily tear. The aperture can be closed after the opening is packed as described above by (1) waxing over the opening with a surface restorer wax, (2) alternating strips of cotton or webbed cotton with surface sealer glue, or (3) applying several layers of a thick surface sealer glue.

Penetrating Wounds

These wounds are defined as deep wounds that penetrate an organ or cavity. Because these trauma wounds are so variable, it is necessary to view the body and the damage produced by the wound. A penetrating wound could be as small as the entry point for a small-caliber bullet or a thin bladed knife. With shooting victims, both entry and possibly exit wounds must be evaluated. Frequently the exit wound damages more tissues than the entry wound. The coroner or medical examiner may also enlarge these wounds if the tissue surrounding the wounds is excised for use as evidence. Most of these wounds would be cleaned and packed with a cautery chemical in the preembalming time period. After arterial and cavity embalming, the wound can be filled with incision seal powder or mortuary mastic to prevent leakage and closed by suture or superglue. If the margins of the wound cannot be drawn together, the wound can

be filled with (1) a surface restorer wax; (2) mortuary mastic then covered with surface sealer glue, gauze, and another coating of sealer; or (3) filled with alternate layers of sealer glue and cotton (Fig. 23A–E).

If the penetrating wound involves the cranium and if no autopsy was performed, it may be necessary to aspirate the cranial cavity to evacuate any blood or fluids, which may have accumulated there during the arterial injection. A small trocar can be inserted through the wound or the nostril. The injection of several ounces of undiluted cavity fluid or cautery chemical into the cranium will help to ensure good preservation of the contents of the cranial cavity. It is very important to seal the portion of the wound penetrating the bone. This may be done with a trocar button, cotton saturated with plaster of Paris, mortuary mastic, or packing with cotton. Hair replacement may be necessary with a penetrating cranial wound. Often hair can be taken from the back of the scalp and attached over the visible wound area using rubber cement or wax for attachment. A hair patch can also be cut from a matching wig. If this is done, cut the material to which the hair is sewn to a size that will cover the wound. Using superglue attach the piece of wig to the scalp. The attached hair can then be combed into the surrounding natural hair.

Small Laceration or Surgical Incision of the Lip or Eyelid

The suturing of a small laceration or surgical incision may cause a puckering of the skin. It may be best to let the small disconnected tissues dry and then wax over the separation with a surface restorative wax. These separations can be dried by heat or with chemicals. Air-drying and the use of a hair dryer may sufficiently dry the tissues that wax can easily be applied over the small wound.

Figure 23. A. Penetrating wound to the left temple area. **B.** Aspiration of the cranial cavity after embalming, through the wound entrance. **C.** Trocar button used to close wound to the cranium. **D.** Basket weave suture applied. **E.** Area waxed.

► HAIR TREATMENTS

The widespread use of chemotherapeutic and radiation treatments has greatly increased the number of bodies where cranial hair is absent. Today, very natural-looking wigs and toupees are available at relatively low prices. Often in life, the individual undergoing these treatments has already made use of these cosmetic hair replacements. These hairpieces can be styled by a hairdresser or barber and easily attached by the embalmer. The cranium should be thoroughly washed and sanitized during the embalming process. After embalming, the cranium can be wiped with a solvent to insure the removal of all oils. The wig or toupee can be placed on the head and if necessary held in position using drops of superglue on the cranium. If a wig or toupee is not available, a scarf or bandage could be used for women and a bandage or a hat for a man. For infants, a bonnet might be used.

If the left side of the cranium has been shaved, position the deceased straight—do not turn the head to the right, and comb some of the hair along the center of the cranium to the left to cover some of the nude scalp. A wig can also be cut and attached with superglue on the left side of the cranium, trimmed, and the wig and remaining hair blended together (Fig. 24A–G).

When hair replacement is necessary, it may be possible to use hair from the back of the deceased's head. The skin surface must be clean, so use a solvent such as a hydrocarbon solvent to remove all oils and debris. Short stubble need not be shaved; often it can aid in making a good attachment. A wig, toupee, or skein of artificial or real hair can be used as a hair source. Attachment can be made using rubber cement, hot wax, or surface restorer wax. Rubber cement makes the firmest attachment. Specific directions for replacing various hair styles, moustaches, eyelashes, and eyebrows by attaching hair can be found in textbooks dealing with postmortem restorative art and stage and theatrical makeup.

Eyebrows and eyelashes can often be corrected by lightly drawing them in using a brown eyebrow pencil. Moisten the point of the pencil and lightly sketch in the missing hair. Often this will give the illusion of the presence of hair. A moustache can also be thickened with the use of an eyebrow pencil.

► MEMORIAL MASK MAKING

A memorial mask (death mask) was once a very frequent request. Most older books on the subject of restorative art always carried a section on the preparation of the death mask, most often employing plaster of Paris. The American Board of Funeral Service Education no longer includes the teaching of this process. Some funeral establishments, particularly in the west coast area of the United States, still get requests for a death mask. David P. Carlson, a funeral director, embalmer, and special effects artist, along with Jon M. Snyder, embalmer from Upland, California, have prepared the following outline and suggestions for the making of a memorial mask. The process is done in two stages, first, a **negative mold** is formed, directly from the face (or hands) of the deceased, this is followed by creation of a **positive mold,** which is made from the negative mold. The positive mold is then painted and mounted for viewing.

Many families wish to preserve the memory of the departed by commissioning a memorial mask. The procedure involves taking a careful imprint of the face, and sometimes torso and so on, with a pliable, harmless substance. The mask is then created from this pliable "mold." What results is a realistic rendering of the face of the deceased.

The process is unique; it is, at once, both an old and new art form. Because the process is topical and entirely noninvasive, it has no effect on any postmortem study that may be performed, either immediately following mask creation or in the future. It is not necessary that the body be embalmed to get the proper results, either. After the mold "sets up," a high-grade gypsum compound is placed and leveled into the mold in stages, depending upon the size of the mold itself. Once the compound dries, an exact replica of the decedent's hands (and/or face) has been formed, right down to the smallest detail. After allowing ample time for the gypsum to dry, the cast is removed from the mold, then detailed and refined. The face is done in a similar manner, but a fiber foundation must also be built over the alginate to give the larger mold more rigidity and stability. The resulting impression can be mounted, tinted, or completed in any way that the family desires.

The following procedural steps give instructions for creating a memorial mask for the face. It is vital that all steps be carefully followed. Omitting any of the following steps may result in failure.

STEP 1—Preparation of the Negative Mold

- Clean face, making certain all substances (massage cream, etc.) have been completely removed.
- Set features, making certain eyes and mouth are securely closed.
- Insert cotton in nostrils and ear cavities to plug orifices.
- With a brush (massage cream brush) or gloved hand, apply very thin layer of massage cream or oil all over face, including moustache, beard,

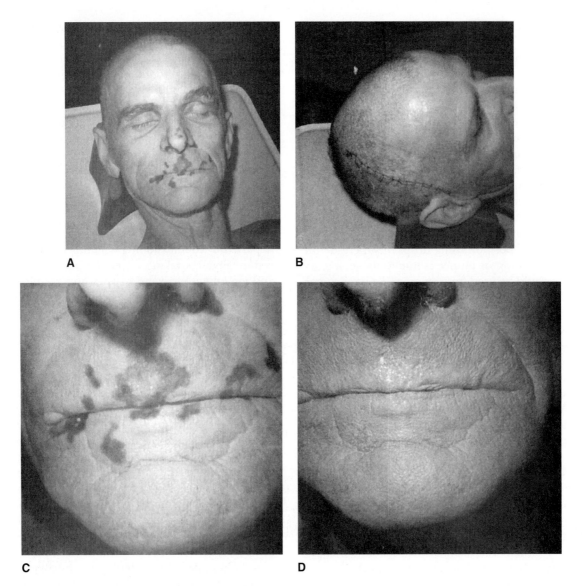

Figure 24. A. Craniotomy performed; vitamin B deficiency—note lesions around mouth. **B.** Craniotomy, right side. **C.** Mouth lesions. **D.** Lesions undercoated. (*Continued*)

eyebrows, eyelashes, and hairline; this will help prevent the mask material from sticking as much. Some sticking will still occur.

- Mix alginate (dental impression powder).
- Pour over subject's face and/or other chosen areas, making certain the area is covered to a depth of at least $\frac{1}{4}$ inch. Build up a small "barrier" around the edges of areas being covered to prevent material from moving onto other areas.
- Use Webril or other cotton while alginate is still wet. Cover areas thoroughly with Webril or cotton, working quickly; alginate must be wet while cotton is applied.
- Once cotton has been applied, casting material should be dampened, then applied to cotton. Casting bandages are applied in a crisscross or

herringbone pattern; for example, bandages may be applied down one side of the face, applying them at the same angle, then applied down the other side, creating the crisscross pattern.

- Allow to sit for 15 minutes; bandaging materials will become "hot" to the touch (this is an important chemical reaction, which helps alginate conform to face). Cut away any excess material.
- Slowly and gently "rock" material back and forth in preparation for removal from face. This will allow air pockets to form, which will facilitate removal. Continue to "rock" material until it is removed from face.
- Set mask aside to rest for about 10 minutes. During this time, the face of the deceased may be cleaned up.

Figure 24. (*Continued*) **E.** Sideburn rebuilt using rubber based glue for attachment. **F.** Cranial hair attached. **G.** Completed.

STEP 2—Preparation of the Positive Mold

- Look inside the mask. There will be flaking from the alginate, facial hairs, some excess run-off from alginate, and so on. Gently remove these with forceps and so on.
- If there is cutting or tearing of the mold, use superglue to repair these tears, cuts, and so on.
- For leftover oil, pat-dry the oil using cotton rather than attempting to rub it out or scrub.
- Mix gypsum (a form of cement) with water to "thin soup" consistency. Pour gypsum very slowly into mask, stopping frequently to rotate ("swirl") mask in order to distribute gypsum well. What you are doing is attempting to build up a thin layer of gypsum inside the mask. You will con-

tinue to do this until the inside of the mask is completely filled. Make certain to fill to edges. This can be done in stages, but should be completed while material is still wet and pliable.

- At this point, the mask is ready to sit and dry ("cure") for a minimum of about 15 to 20 days (longer if needed). Mask should be covered and protected, set aside and left alone.

STEP 3

- Move mask to work bench in preparation for next step.
- Peel off casting material first, then cotton, then alginate (which will still be wet to the touch), using your hands.

■ Allow mask to air-dry for at least a couple of days. There will be a powdery substance on mask, which will wipe off with a wet sponge. Remove this powder.

■ Where there are imperfections, some gypsum may be mixed with water and applied to mask with brush to smooth out areas. Use this gypsum to brush inside the nostril and eye cavity areas of the mask, to smooth area.

■ Allow to dry. Use "wet sandpaper" to slowly smooth out any areas on mask with excess materials and to smooth bottom of mask, to allow it to stand. A fine-textured file may also be used to help these areas.

■ Using a damp towel, wipe down mask.

RESTORATIVE ART—PART 3—MORTUARY COSMETOLOGY*

This section on mortuary cosmetology will study the procedures used to establish a receptive cosmetic surface foundation and the methods used in the application of postmortem cosmetics. When preparing the body for viewing, our main objective is to create an acceptable appearance or natural illusion of peaceful repose. This memory image is achieved through use of well-developed cosmetic skills.

The overapplication of cosmetics causing an artificially made-up appearance is a primary reason for the negative attitude toward viewing and embalming. The body placed in the funeral home refrigerator and later viewed unembalmed should receive the same considerations as the body to be arterially embalmed. Prerefrigeration treatments are as essential as preembalming treatments.

▶ BASICS OF MORTUARY COSMETOLOGY

Attaining perfection in mortuary cosmetology depends that a high degree of attention be given to disinfection, cleansing, and precosmetic surface treatments. Epidermal conditioning is the primary step in establishing a stable, receptive cosmetic surface foundation. Treating the face and hands with an emollient cream will have a positive effect to facilitate application of postmortem cosmetic media. Successful mortuary cosmetology depends on the following fundamental factors:

1. Effective employment of cosmetic coordination of arterial embalming, refrigeration, and use of surface cosmetics.
2. Familiarity with the tactical uses and blending characteristics of complexion colors.
3. Complete knowledge concerning the properties, uses, and limitations of various cosmetic types.

---

*C. Richard Sanders (The Dodge Company) contributed most of the material for this section.

4. Development of manual dexterity and artistic creativity, which are the driving forces behind all fine craftsmanship.

▶ VALUE OF PHOTOGRAPHS

A photograph of the deceased is an invaluable reference to have on hand when cosmetically treating the face and hands. Analysis of facial characteristics in the photograph will give the embalmer a better understanding of how to apply the toning cosmetics in accentuating the predominant facial lines and natural markings. If it becomes necessary to totally mask the entire epidermal surface of the face and hands, the photograph of the subject will become an essential aid in accurately duplicating the natural lines and markings on the opaque skin surface. Two or three recent photos of the deceased are considered the best reference for comparison between the facial features in life and the features seen after death. Avoid using older pictures. During the advancement in age, the contours of the facial features continually change. Avoid using a retouched "vanity photo" as a guide. Commercially produced portraits make the subject appear artificially more youthful and erase the age and character lines needed in establishing a true-to-life appearance. Recent pictures also give the hair stylist valuable information in grooming the hair for both men and women. Examination of the photos + under magnification often reveals character lines, wrinkle details, and natural markings invisible to the naked eye. Be certain photos are labeled. Place them in a clear plastic insert of the type used in photograph albums to protect them from damage (Fig. 1).

▶ PRECOSMETIC TREATMENTS

Epidermal Conditioning
After all disinfection and cleansing treatments have been completed, the epidermal surfaces of the face, neck, and

Facial Markings

Natural facial
markings

Acquired facial
markings

Figure 1. Classification of facial markings. (*Figure adopted from G. Joseph Prager, Manual of Restorative Art, 1965.*) (See the Glossary for detailed description of each marking). **Natural facial markings:** 1. oblique palpebral sulcus; 2. nasal sulcus; 3. nasolabial fold; 4. philtrum; 5. angulus oris eminence; 6. angulus oris sulcus; 7. labiomental sulcus; 8. submental sulcus; 9. dimple. **Acquired facial markings:** 10. transverse frontal sulci; 11. interciliary sulci; 12. superior palpebral sulcus; 13. optic facial sulci; 14. inferior palpebral sulcus; 15. nasolabial sulcus; 16. buccofacial sulcus; 17. labial sulci; 18. mandibular sulcus; 19. platysmal sulci; 20. cords of the neck.

hands should be treated with a skin conditioning cosmetic massage cream. Carefully apply the cosmetic massage cream, paying particular attention to the eyes, nose, lips, cheeks, and ears, and with your fingertips gently work the emollient cream into the epidermal surfaces. This breaks up rigor mortis, making feature posing easier. Before posing the features, all unnatural and downy hair growth should be removed from the face of infants

and females. After the shaving is completed, cleanse the lather from the face, and reapply a liberal coat of the massage cream. This procedure prevents any razor abrasions from turning brown. When a scaly skin condition must be treated, before shaving the body, massage a liberal amount of massage cream over the affected area. Leave the cream on the skin surface for approximately 10 minutes, then remove the cream with a gauze pad. It may be necessary to repeat the procedure two or three times to completely remove the roughened skin.

▶ POSING THE HANDS

The hands are often given only perfunctory attention when posing and cosmetizing the body. The hands are a powerful medium of expression both in life and in death and posing them should be given careful consideration.

After disinfecting treatments have been completed, the hands and fingers should be thoroughly cleansed with undiluted soap, making certain that the epidermal surfaces and fingernails are completely clean. Scrub the fingernails and cuticles with a stiff-bristled hand brush until every trace of soil above and below the nail is removed. Dried blood, grease, tobacco stains, and any stains caused by application of medicines should be removed **before embalming.** This is necessary because the protein-fixing action of the arterial solution will permanently bond the soil into the nail bed and cuticle, and so, it is imperative that the hands and nails be scrupulously clean before arterial injection.

Manual manipulation of the wrist and fingers is an important preembalming treatment in achieving correct hand alignment and natural contour. After manual manipulation is completed, apply cosmetic massage cream, working it into the tissues on the back of the hand, around the fingernails and fingertips. On female subjects also apply cream to the arms. The face, arms, hands, and legs of infants should be given thorough cosmetic cream massage before arterial injection. This helps to relieve rigor mortis and makes the delicate epidermal tissues of the infant more pliable and receptive to all cosmetic media. The contour of the relaxed hand during life is convex, with the fingers bent slightly inward toward the palm. This gives the hand a graceful semioval contour with the thumb and forefinger in natural parallel contact. The third, fourth, and fifth fingers of the hand should also appear in gentle contact with each other and parallel to the forefinger. To simulate the naturally curved contour of the reposed hand, place a pad of cotton or cloth saturated with humectant under the palm, molding the hand into a semioval contour over the pad. This will help sustain the natural contour of the hand. The three most commonly used poses when aligning the hands in a natural, relaxed manner are as follows:

1. Crossed hand position (right or left hand placed over the top of the opposite hand)—used primarily where religious tradition calls for this position
2. Left forearm and hand resting on the upper abdomen at the midline with the right forearm placed on the abdomen just below the left forearm parallel to it

3. Left forearm positioned at a right angle to the body with the center of the hand resting over the diaphragm at the midline. The right forearm is set with the elbow bent at an angle of about 60 degrees, and the hand resting at the midline on the lower abdomen.

Note: These three basic positions represent traditional customs for posing the hands and arms. However, reasonable variations may be made at the discretion of the embalmer/cosmetician or funeral director. The hands and arms should never be placed in a parallel position at the sides of the body. This produces a stilted effect, an attitude that detracts from the desired memory image. Moreover, in this position, the hands cannot be seen, obscuring their sensitive and expressive beauty in natural repose.

▶ COSMETIC APPLICATION

The art of color blending and the influence of textural values should be fully understood if we are to achieve perfection in embalming cosmetology. A natural appearance can only be achieved when the applied cosmetic medium approximates the true complexion color radiating from beneath the skin surface. The professional embalmer/cosmetician should have a good working knowledge of basic complexion tones and know how to make precosmetizing evaluations based on existing skin color. There are two factors to take into consideration when determining the composition of epidermal coloring: hemoglobin and melanin.

▶ HEMOGLOBIN

The most obvious characteristic of hemoglobin is its bright blood-red color appearing in the arteries as a rich scarlet and as a deep crimson in the veins. Skin coloring, therefore, is influenced by the amount of blood present in the superficial capillaries. These tiny vessels are so numerous and well distributed throughout the body that they are capable of holding enough blood near the epidermal surface to provide a radiating pink overtone under normal conditions. When more heavily charged with blood, these same capillaries will produce the ruddy, purplish-red complexion typical of an individual with high blood pressure. Under anemic conditions and instances where less than normal blood volume flows through the superficial capillaries, a pale complexion results. The pale, colorless skin coloring seen after death is caused by the absence of these radiant pink overtones present in healthy individuals. All living color includes microscopic amounts of red, blue, green, brown, yellow, and translucent flesh tones. For postmortem work, these colors must be present in embalming cosmetics before any true approximation of living skin coloring can be realized through surface cosmetizing.

▶ MELANIN

The amount of melanin present in the epidermis is an important element in determining complexion coloring, ranging from light tan through browns all the way to deep brown-blacks. It also determines the depth or intensity of complexion color at different ages and among various ethnic groups. Fair-complected individuals show only a faint trace of melanin, whereas darker-complected persons display an abundance of this skin coloring pigment. Exposure to the ultraviolet rays in sunlight stimulates production of melanin, producing a superficial suntan safeguarding underlying tissues against burn injury. An uneven distribution of melanin produces freckles on the skin, which appear more abundantly and deeper in color when exposed to sunlight. Duplication of freckles is an important aspect of embalming cosmetology, particularly when heavy opaque cosmetics are used. Failure to restore the individual characteristics produced by melanin pigmentation may cause inaccurate representation of the facial features and is frequently a source of frustration and anger for the family. In persons of advanced age, increased melanin production causes "liver spots" to appear on the face, neck, arms, and hands. Also, the skin color undergoes changes when moisture content changes in the underlying structures, primarily the blood vessels, and lymphatic system, and also when the melanin in the skin undergoes chemical changes. In selecting the proper cosmetic medium and color, consideration should be given to these factors: (1) complexion, (2) environment, (3) sex, (4) age, and (5) lighting.

Complexion
An important step in restoring the natural-looking appearance of the deceased is the determination of complexion coloring.

Environment
Environmental effects on complexion color should be considered when selecting the basic complexion color. The individual confined primarily to indoor activity does not, as a rule, have the sun-browned complexion of an outdoorsman, farmer, construction worker, or sportsman. For this reason, it is advisable that the embalmer/cosmetician know something about the vocation and activities of the deceased in order to achieve a faithful and natural-looking complexion color. True complexion values are often distorted by the pallor of death, but a few pointed inquiries concerning the employment and recreational activities of the deceased can help the

Figure 2. Heavy compound injector with attachments.

embalmer/cosmetician give each case the touch of realism needed to restore lifelike skin tones. During the arrangement interview, the funeral director should ask detailed questions about the facial characteristics, grooming habits, and general appearance of the deceased. This information is important to the embalmer/cosmetician in perfecting his or her work, will give the family confidence in the funeral home's professional staff, and assure the family that the deceased is being well cared for.

Sex
- ■ Ornamental cosmetics: For the female, it is desirable to accentuate her feminine characteristics by using cosmetic color distribution in accordance with current fashion trends and customs.
- ■ Natural cosmetics: For males and children, color distribution is more natural and should maintain traditional masculine values in appearance.

Age
The age of the individual is a significant element in determining complexion color. The process of aging modifies skin color, skin texture, and the configuration of facial tissues. Shadows fall differently with emaciation due to advanced age. Aging also changes feature contours, causes wrinkles, and accents the prominence of cheekbones, brows, and jawbones. In contrast, infants display a fresh, vibrant red-pink color. Changes in infant complexion occur at about the age of 2, when the skin takes on an aura of brown tones. Few further complexion changes other than those caused by sun exposure take place until the child is about 6 years old, when hereditary factors give the complexion its permanent identity.

Lighting
The same color and intensity of lighting to be used in the reposing room and chapel should also be used when applying cosmetics in the preparation room. Keep in mind

that cosmetics applied to appear natural under brilliant light in the preparation room will look pale and dull under the more subdued funeral home lighting. The importance of light equalization between working areas and viewing rooms cannot be too strongly stressed. Having the correct lighting is a dominant factor in cosmetic color control.

SUMMARY OF COSMETIC APPLICATION

1. Disinfect all tissues; thoroughly wash the face and hands; remove all facial hair
2. If necessary clean the face and hands with a solvent and thoroughly dry the skin
3. Apply surface or hypodermic treatments to discolorations, which can be bleached
4. For discolorations, apply an undercoat spray or liquid paint
5. Apply the base cosmetic
6. Adjust or alter the base cosmetic to achieve the correct foundation color
7. Reinstate the highlights and shadows of the face and hands
8. Apply the warm colors (reds) to the face and hands
9. Blend the cosmetic colors
10. Apply a drying powder to the cosmetics
11. Clean eyelashes, eyebrows, and hairline
12. Seal the cosmetic by a light application of hairspray

Figure 3. Distribution of warm color.

Color Blending

After the correct base complexion color is established, warm color distributed, and eye makeup and color correctly applied, these applications can be toned down with the brown toning cosmetics. Blending of the brown

Base Color

The fundamental function of the base color application is to replace the reds missing from the complexion due to blood drainage and bleaching action of embalming chemicals. Natural complexion color can be achieved only when the base cosmetic closely approximates the characteristic color values the individual possessed in life. The base complexion cosmetic is applied strictly as a background color.

Warm Color

The warm colors, namely, reds, pinks, and some deeper flesh tones, appear in specific areas of the face, namely, the chin, lips, nose, cheeks, ears, and forehead (Fig. 3). Distribution of warm color seldom extends beyond these limits. The most common exceptions are individuals with a lack of color in these areas and those with exceptionally ruddy complexions. The color of the cheeks in the elderly recedes below the tops of the cheekbones, while in younger subjects, the color glow rises higher, actually vanishing near the lower eyelids (Figs. 4 and 5).

Figure 4. Aged adult warm color on cheeks.

Figure 5. Youthful warm color on cheeks.

subdues the brilliance of the warm color just enough to allow a natural glow to emerge, reducing the reds to more lifelike values. The application of the toning medium should be made very lightly, so lightly in fact, that one should be unable to discern exactly where it has been applied. This will bring out the true complexion color, effectively simulating the radiant glow of the blood as it flows under the translucent sheath of skin. Working with the brown toning cosmetics goes a long way toward producing the perfect cosmetic finish. The complexion toning colors are light brown, dark brown, and black. The first consideration is to determine the color intensity category of the deceased: light, medium, or dark. Observe the amount of brown pigmentation in the skin, how deep the color appears in the face and hands. Choose the toning cosmetic from one of the three toning colors (light brown, dark brown, or black) to match the natural complexion of the individual. The correct matching shade should be applied over the basic and warm color application, using the classification of light, medium, or dark to select the correct toning color. All facial lines, wrinkles, freckles, and natural markings should be emphasized with one of the toning colors.

▶ GUIDE FOR COSMETIC APPLICATION

Brush Application

Transparent and opaque liquid cosmetics should be brush applied and dispensed directly from the container.

For brush application treatments, the liquid cosmetic medium is applied in short straight strokes confined to a small area. Immediately after application, the liquid cosmetic should be either blotted with a gauze pad or brushed out over the surface and blended such that there is no line of demarcation visible. This should be done quickly, because the vehicle in which the pigment is suspended evaporates almost immediately, limiting the time for distribution. The blotting and brush application procedures insure uniform distribution of color, preventing streaking and blotchy patches of uneven color.

Stipple Application

This method of applying color is done by tapping it off the end of the brush in a delicately controlled "pecking movement." The stipple application procedure is used in applying transparent, semiopaque, and opaque cream cosmetics. Opaque liquid cosmetics may also be stipple applied to achieve a more natural effect. The cream cosmetics are best applied from the palm of the hand where they are prewarmed and maintained at a good working consistency. Massage cream may be mixed with the cream cosmetic or applied directly to the skin surface. Begin stipple application with a small amount of cream held in the palm of the hand. Spread the cosmetic out in a fine film with the flat edge of a $2\frac{1}{4}$-inch spatula. Keep the thinly spread color restricted to the lower portion of the palm. Pick up a small amount of the cream with the brush. Apply with a light stippling movement. Continue with this method until the cosmetic has been stippled out into an even distribution over the desired area.

Finger Application

The finger application method is used in applying tinted emollient cream, semiopaque complexion cream, and opaque cream. Before applying the cosmetic medium, precondition the skin surface by massaging cosmetic massage cream into the tissues of the face and hands. Omit the use of massage cream when an opaque cosmetic is being used. Remove surplus massage cream with a lint-free gauze pad before applying the basic cosmetic medium. Place an ample amount of the cream cosmetic in the palm of the hand, allowing body heat to soften the material to an easy spreading consistency. Pick up a small amount of the cream with the tip of your index or middle finger. Position a dab of cream about the size of a penny on the middle of each cheek, in the center of the forehead, and on the high point of the chin. Wipe the finger clean, then using the tips of all three middle fingers, massage the cream gently into the tissues with a circular motion. Concentrate on producing a smooth, evenly distributed color. When properly massaged into the skin, the cosmetic finish takes on a uniform glow, free of a streaky or greasy looking surface. Treat the hands and fingers in the same manner as the face.

Spray Application

- Opaque undercoats (and some transparent tints) are available in aerosol spray containers. The spray nozzle should not be held closer to the working surface than 6 inches; however, when there is increased nozzle pressure, the container should be moved away up to 10 to 12 inches from the skin. The standard rule is the stronger the pressure, the greater the distance between the spray source and skin surface. Before commencing the basic spray application, position a protective cover carefully over the hair. Coat the hairline, eyebrows, and eyelashes with a light application of cosmetic massage cream. This will prevent discoloring and avoid troublesome, time-consuming cosmetic removal. The epidermal surface should be clean, dry, and free of all oily or heavy deposits of massage cream. Moisten a gauze pad with mortuary solvent and wipe the skin surface very gently until all massage cream is gone, creating a clean, dry surface foundation. Begin spray application just below the line of the mandible. Spray the basic cosmetic on the neck area, testing for proper color value, then proceed up the sides of the face, treating the chin, nose, eyes, ears, and forehead. Movement of the spray stream should be positive, swift, and smoothly executed so that no cosmetic buildup or runs appear. When excessive cosmetic buildup occurs, the most practical corrective treatment is to stipple out the surplus, distributing the excess cosmetic into the surrounding areas such that no line of demarcation is visible.
- The airbrush system of spray cosmetics—an early method of cosmetic application—has become popular in recent years. The cosmetic "paint" is propelled by a small air compressor. The cosmetic is available in a wide variety of complexion colorants. This system is recommended for cosmetizing the "normal" body as well as those that have large and small discolorations. The systems come with specific instructions for application.

Removal of Cosmetics

The following methods and materials are used in removing cosmetic media from the epidermal surface of the face and hands.

Gauze Pads. The use of 4-inch by 4-inch gauze pads is recommended for removal of cosmetic massage cream, as opposed to cotton or other material that may leave lint particles on the surface of the skin. It has an excellent surface with just enough texture in the weave to remove even heavy massage or stay creams from the face and hands. It is also used for blotting and smoothing out liquid surface cosmetics.

Massage Cream Removal of Cosmetics. Cosmetic massage cream removes all cosmetics from the skin surface with the exception of the resin base, adhesion-type opaque liquid, and opaque spray cosmetics, which require special solvents. Cosmetic removal is accomplished by applying a liberal coating of massage cream over the epidermal surface of the face and hands, rubbing the cream well into the hairline, eyebrows, and eyelashes. Allow the cream to remain on the skin surface for a few moments. To remove the lubricant film left by the massage cream, moisten a clean gauze pad with mortuary solvent and gently wipe the skin surface until all of the film is removed, establishing a receptive cosmetic foundation.

Solvent Removal of Cosmetics. Liquid opaque and opaque spray cosmetics often require special thinner solvent furnished only by the manufacturer of the cosmetic, but mortuary solvent will serve as a substitute. Apply the solvent with a brush, limiting the application to small areas, wiping away the cosmetic with gentle pressure on the gauze pad. Repeat this treatment until no trace of cosmetic color or greasy deposit appears on the skin surface. Apply cosmetic massage cream to reestablish the foundation for the new application of the basic complexion color. To prepare the skin for acceptance of transparent liquid tints or liquid opaques, make certain the tissue is totally free of greasy deposits by cleansing with mortuary solvent.

▶ BASIC COMPLEXION MATERIALS

Although there is an infinite variety of cosmetic materials, basic complexion materials may be classified as follows:

1. Transparent liquid tints
2. Liquid powder tint
3. Tinted emollient cream
4. Semiopaque emollient cream
5. Opaque cream
6. Liquid opaque
7. Spray cosmetics

Liquid Transparent Tint

The orange or red pigment in liquid transparents is suspended in a water-alcohol solution combining ultra-thin consistency with fast evaporation of the vehicle. It is generally used as a base color for the face and hands when no restorative or special treatments involving opaque cosmetics are required. They are compounded to simulate the basic natural coloring of the body. The major disadvantage of alcohol-based cosmetic solutions is their tendency to dehydrate the delicate surfaces around the eyelids and mucous lip surfaces due to their volatility and rapid evaporation.

Liquid Powder Tint

Liquid powder tints consist of a talc and clay base suspended in an aqueous-alcohol solution combined with a humectant, which helps the powder adhere to the cosmetized surface in a very thin, delicate, and barely visible matte film. When totally dry, they leave a smooth nonreflecting finish on the epidermal surface with the pores visible.

Tinted Emollient Cream

These cosmetics are compounded with an oil base similar to that used in cosmetic massage cream. Tinted emollient cream cosmetics become transparent when applied lightly over the skin surface, allowing the natural complexion to show through, imparting a delicate glow. These tinted creams are excellent basic complexion colors and retard dehydration of the skin.

Semiopaque Emollient Cream

The semiopaque emollient creams are virtually identical to the tinted emollient creams except that they are more opaque. Consequently, they allow less of the natural complexion to show through and reduce the conspicuousness of light-colored blemishes and mask the unsightly putty gray pallor of the face and hands, without creating a total blanket of artificial color. These semiopaque creams allow just enough of the natural undertones to show through to give the illusion of normal skin coloring.

Opaque Cream

The opaque cream cosmetic is a heavily pigmented oil-based cosmetic, used primarily to completely mask unsightly blemishes, discolorations, and restored surfaces on the face and hands. Although the objective is to conceal imperfections, it is equally important to avoid an artificial, overly made-up appearance. Opaque cream cosmetics work well over restored surfaces and are compatible with most all other cosmetic media. Light applications yield greater transparency. Opaque creams may also be used as a base cosmetic when applied very lightly.

Liquid Opaque

The liquid opaque medium is normally formulated with a resin base and used most commonly throughout the profession. Drying time is about 10 minutes. Once the liquid opaque is thoroughly dried, it will seal the epidermal surface and not rub off, and it also retards dehydration very effectively.

Spray Cosmetics

There are two types of aerosol spray cosmetics available for mortuary use: transparent cosmetic spray and opaque pigmented spray. The transparent aerosol sprays are used as a basic complexion colorant. The opaque pigmented aerosol is used for covering discolorations, restored surfaces, and total masking (undercoating) procedures on the face, arms, and hands.

Supplemental Complexion Color

The glowing undertones of color and textural control created by the **arterial injection** produces more true color radiance, skin translucence, and textural quality than can be created by even the most skillful cosmetizing. However, the use of harsh arterial chemicals reduces moisture in the skin and subcutaneous tissues. This brings about a darkening of the skin and creates a putty gray color as the chemical reacts with any hemoglobin present. Although the complexion coloring can be enhanced through the initial arterial injection, it is necessary to treat the warm areas, lines, wrinkles, and natural markings cosmetically to achieve a natural lifelike appearance.

Arterial Dyes

There are circumstances that require adding chromatic color to the arterial solution to prevent fading of the initial complexion color after the initial arterial injection has been completed. When it is necessary to increase the strength of the arterial chemical for thorough preservation, the increased volume of formaldehyde can cause fading in the epidermal tissues. Under these conditions, additional chromatic should be added to the arterial solution to compensate and stabilize the chromatic color in the tissues of the face and hands.

Warm Color Application

The illusion of natural repose is accomplished when the warm color application is blended into the correct background color of the complexion. Even though natural complexion color can be substantially enhanced by the use of advanced chemical formulas for the arterial injection, there is still no injectional chemical available that will color the warm areas of the face and hands. Surface cosmetics must still be used to supplement the underlying red skin tones in the warm areas of the face and hands. The need for surface cosmetizing becomes evident when we realize that in life the warm-toned areas of the face draw their color from the presence of strong reds in the blood (hemoglobin), reflected as a rosy glow through the translucence of the underlying epidermal layers. In analyzing warm color distribution, we see that nature does not normally vary the locations of warm color in the face. Areas of more intense color are uniformly distributed in nearly all individuals.

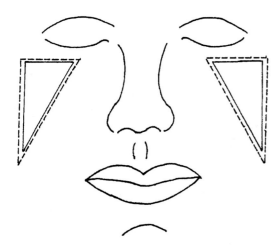

Figure 6. Widening the face.

Corrective shaping is usually only needed to create optical dimensional variations, most commonly when it is aesthetically advantageous to widen or narrow the face (Figs. 6 and 7). This is done by shifting the centers and scope of warm color cheek application to create the illusory effect. Women are usually given stronger color treatment of the warm areas—particularly in the cheeks. More cheek color has become a familiar personal trait through regular use of artificial cheek color throughout adult life. Questioning of family members will usually reveal the type and color intensity of the facial cosmetics favored by the deceased.

Other variations in color distribution include simulating the facial tones of naturally florid or ruddy complexions and duplicating the deeply sun-tanned skin tones of those with outdoor occupations or hobbies. The embalmer/cosmetician should always make a thorough evaluation of facial color characteristics in each individual before attempting treatment. The use of heavy-bodied opaque cosmetic media is frequently indicated

Figure 7. Narrowing the face.

for treating jaundice discolorations, diseased or abnormal skin conditions, and cosmetizing restored surfaces. Whenever opaque base complexion color is called for, it is advisable to choose *more vivid, more intense reds* for the warm facial areas because the brilliance of these colors will be considerably subdued as they are blended into the basic complexion colorant. Always blend the reds gradually into the surrounding tissues of each warm area so that no line of demarcation remains visible. When correctly blended, the warm color application will appear as a radiant glow emanating from an unseen subcutaneous source, more like a subtle radiance of pink undertone than a solid fleshlike color.

Method of Warm Color Application

The six dominant features of the face represent **nine warm color areas**; the chin, lips, and nose have only a single warm color area to be treated, whereas the cheeks, ears, and forehead require double area treatment. To define "warm (red) color" more specifically, it should be understood to mean those portions of the face and hands where high color accents appear normally in life.

■ *The Chin.* Red toning distributed over this prominent facial feature should be uniformly blended into a color value, which cannot be readily identified as red, but merely imparts a vibrant quality to the skin coloring. A small touch of warm color may be placed at the center of the chin and feathered out to remove every trace of a line of demarcation. Avoid excessive color on the chin.

■ *The Lips.* In evaluating lip color, careful comparison will show that it is identical to that of the cheeks, differing only in the intensity of the red common to both. For this reason, the lips should receive a heavier deposit of color and the cheeks a much thinner application of the same shade. Keep in mind the fact that the lips contain a large number of blood-filled capillaries that reflect strongly through a single layer of skin in the living body, whereas the cheeks, with far fewer capillaries, are seen through a triple-thick epidermal covering and therefore appear rosy rather than truly red.

When applying lip color, confine the color to the central and immediately adjacent areas of the mouth, following the normal lip outline carefully. Do not apply color to the extreme corners of the mouth unless you wish to create an illusion of increased width in this expressive facial feature. Stopping color about $\frac{1}{8}$ inch from each corner usually produces a more natural effect. If the mouth appears too wide in proportion to the other facial features, it may be necessary to block out color from the corners. The well-defined red area should be limited to the central parts of the lips and distributed gradually into the basic complexion color on both sides of the mouth. Lips that are too thin impart an undesirable expression to the face. To correct, extend the color above and below the lip outlines, but widen the color bands with care or even more objectionable distortion may result. Lips appearing too full and too short tend to give the face a pouting look.

- **The Nose.** Apply warm color to the wings, septum, sides, and bridge of the nose. All coloring applied to the sides, wings, and septum of the nose should be used sparingly and fully blended into the surrounding facial tissues so that only the slightest trace of color remains visible. The tip of the nose should always be kept free of strong color.

- **The Cheeks.** The cheeks represent two warm color areas that must be given carefully balanced symmetry in color and tonal values. The slightest variation in color intensity or an abnormal excess of color will produce noticeable facial distortion. Considerable variation in color location, distribution, and brilliance occurs in each specific age group. The following is a general guide in determining warm color distribution by age.

  - *Infant.* Unlike the warm color areas typical in the older individual, rosy color in the infant complexion is uniformly distributed over the entire facial expanse with the greatest red intensity centered on the cheeks. When treating infants, blend all red color (pink tones) into the basic complexion color until a uniform radiant glow spreads outward from a rosy red center at the highest contour of the cheek.

  - *Children.* Warm color distribution on children's cheeks should begin adjacent to the wings of the nose, making certain that equal color values are distributed on both sides. The color should be carried to the center of each cheek and then blended downward to the nasolabial fold. The red colorant must be very uniformly distributed and brought close to the nose without allowing it to extend beyond the uppermost terminus of the nasolabial fold.

  - *Juveniles and Adolescents.* Typical warm color distribution in this group begins high on the cheeks and disappears before it reaches the lower eyelid. Color is applied in a triangular pattern with the apex tangent to the upper margin of the cheekbone and extending toward the ears. It is important to note that the stronger red color values should be confined to the area above the middle of the cheek and not permitted to extend below that point. Reduced color, however, may be drawn downward in blending distribution and kept close to the

nose as it spreads to the area below the nasolabial fold.

  - *Young Adults.* In this group, warm color appears high on the cheekbones with the uppermost limits of tonality disappearing into the lower eyelid region. Heightened color should extend slightly beyond the outermost corners of the eyes. It may then be gradually spread downward in a triangular shape and made to vanish at the top limit of the nasolabial fold, establishing uniform tonal values on both sides of the face. Strong reds should be used very sparingly. It is far easier to add a touch of red where needed than to remove excess color.

  - *Middle-Aged Adults.* Warm color distribution in this age group appears well centered in the cheeks. Color deposit should be confined to below the edge of the cheekbone and then gradually extended to a point just beyond the middle of the cheek. Application of warm color is best made in the standard triangular pattern with the apex of the triangle terminating at the point where a horizontal line extending from the earlobe crosses the cheek. No warm color should appear below this imaginary line.

  - *Advanced Age.* Warm color application in cases of advanced age should be confined to a triangular area below the edges of the cheekbones and extending well into the hollow of each cheek. The tip of the color triangle should terminate at the upper margin of the jawbone. Blend the color so that the most vivid glow is located in the hollow of the cheek rather than high upon its prominence. This lowering of the cheek color is a normal characteristic of old age. This pattern of color should always be considered in treating males and those females who do not use rouge.

  - *Cheek Color in Females.* Because most women use rouge throughout adult life to heighten cheek color, more vivid facial cosmetizing becomes a routine complexion characteristic in the average female case. The position and extent of heightened color varies with personal preference. The most common position of cheek color in the adult woman is centered at mid-cheek (regardless of age) and distributed uniformly over the surface. Avoid excessive color accents. Powder lightly to reduce brilliance where necessary. A compressed dry rouge can be used *after* a drying powder has been applied.

  - *Cheek Color Summary.* Uniform rosy to pink coloring is a typical characteristic of the infant complexion. It is distributed over a broader area than in more mature individuals. At ages beyond the infant stage, children have cheek color centered and adjacent to the lower eyelid. Youthful cheek color is characterized by its elevated location on the cheekbones, fading into normal complexion color at the outer corners of the eyelids. At middle age and beyond, the warm color of the cheeks tends to recede, descending gradually to the hollow of the cheek where it remains during advanced age. Balanced color is a critical factor in treating all of the double-area features of the face. Both left and right surfaces must be given identical color intensity to achieve a natural look.

- *The Ears.* Warm color should be applied uniformly to both ears. Distribution of colorant should not extend beyond the tragus. Less color is used on the ears of elderly subjects, and more color on infants and youthful subjects. Color intensity should remain in the midrange of warm color, approximately the same color as the adjacent values at the sides of the face.

- *The Forehead.* Deposit above each eyebrow a half-inch-wide band of warm color about equal in length to the curved linear dimension of the eyebrow itself. Distribute warm color evenly across the forehead, blending the red colorant upward toward the hairline and outward over the temples, toward the ears. Impart equal color values on each side. In this procedure, the highest color values are placed immediately above the eyebrows with gradual reduction in intensity as the distribution approaches the hairline and sides of the head. Blend warm tones carefully into the basic complexion color so that no line of demarcation is visible. Create a subtle radiance or blushlike glow of color on this broad and prominent area rather than an identifiable red tone. Use *less* red on females than on males.

▶ APPLYING COSMETICS TO THE EYE

One of the most critical aspects in the art of mortuary cosmetology is the cosmetic treatment of the eyes, eyebrows, and eyelashes. In order to achieve a natural-looking result, we must consider the fact that the living individual is most commonly seen in an erect position. This posture, because of the protuberance of the eyebrows, creates a shadow effect that greatly influences the typical facial expression of the individual. In death, the individual is seen only in a reclining position with light falling directly on those facial areas that would normally remain shaded. This effect must be compensated for if

Figure 8. Shaded area under eyebrow, along upper eyelash line, and orbital pouch.

we are to achieve a natural, lifelike countenance for the deceased.

The eyelashes accent the margins of each eyelid with a line of short, closely set hairs curving outward and upward from the upper lid and outward and downward from the lower lid. When the eye is correctly closed, the upper lid and its lashes become the dominant feature of the upper half of the face, with the lower lid just barely visible. Most eyelashes are naturally dark in color. When cosmetizing the eye, it is important to pay special attention to the edges of the eyelids, where the lashes are rooted. There is a line of natural color (purple) where the upper lash enters the ridge of the eyelid.

Beneath the border of the lower lid is the orbital pouch, a puffy structure that follows the curvature of the orbit under the lower eyelid (Fig. 8). The surface of the pouch is slightly darker in color than the surrounding skin. In cases of advanced age or serious illness, the orbital pouch sags and becomes flabby and discolored. Overaccenting the orbital pouch will result in a major distortion of the facial expression. It must, however, be cosmetically treated when it is a familiar characteristic of the individual, particularly in aged individuals.

Method of Color Application

In applying the basic complexion coloring, the area surrounding the eyes should receive a light, evenly distributed application of base complexion color. When applying the eye shadow, it should be used very sparingly, so sparingly in fact, that it should never be apparent that any color has been applied. Stipple brush application is an effective procedure when simulating the eye shadow. To duplicate the shadow effect, apply a small amount of the correct shade above the upper eyelid (Fig. 9). Stipple this color out until it blends into the base color beneath the eyebrows and follow the natural curvature of the lid. Treat the lower eyelid, following the inner perimeter of the orbital ridge to conform to the natural curvature of the lower lid. The chromatic value of the eye shadow used is determined by the age and complexion coloring of the individual. There are four shades of eye shadow:

Figure 9. Eye shadow application.

(1) light brown, (2) dark brown, (3) purple, and (4) light blue. After applying the correct color, apply the purple colorant to the upper eyelid along the lash line and blend the purple into the lash where it enters the ridge of the eyelid (Fig. 10). The color is applied very sparingly, so much so that it should not be evident that it has been applied. The purple is smoothly blended along the lash line so that there is no line of demarcation. The purple shading produces a rounded contour of natural color. It is not necessary to treat the lower eyelid.

Shaping the Eyebrows

When the eyebrow is well formed, there is little shaping required. Usually all that is necessary is to lightly trim the eyebrow with barber shears, using a tapered barber comb as an aid. Corrective shaping is required when the line of the brow is unnatural. Such a condition could be caused from a long illness, old age, chemotherapy, or poor grooming. It is recommended that all corrective shaping be accomplished after the embalming treatments have been completed. Before trimming the eyebrow, rub massage cream well into the surface surrounding the eyebrow. Further shaping can be done with an eyebrow pencil. There will be times when you need to use an eyebrow pencil to create the appearance of hair where there is none. In such instances, inscribing short individual lines on the skin surface with the sharpened point of the eyebrow pencil, following the

normal growth pattern and curvature of the eyebrow, will establish a natural-looking result.

Eyebrow Pencil

Two factors affect the effectiveness of the eyebrow pencil. First is the need to restrain the tendency toward excessive use. The second consideration is the selection of the proper color. When using the pencil for its normal function (to darken hairs), be careful to darken only the hair—not the skin underneath. Use the correct color, rather than using the same shade for all cases. A black pencil should never be used unless necessary because it may be too conspicuous. The object is to darken the hair but not the skin underneath. Always apply the color very lightly, building it up to the desired degree. The pencil can also be used to effectively remove all traces of cosmetic powder by lightly stroking the hair with the pencil.

Lip Treatments

Mucous membrane surfaces. The professional embalmer/cosmetician must contend with three types of surfaces when applying color to the lips: the natural lip, the discolored lip, and the restored or waxed lip. When applying color to the mucous lip surface, certain procedures should be followed to ensure a natural appearance and to prevent troublesome buildup of lip cosmetics.

Widening the Mouth

Extend the topmost margin of the upper lip toward each corner of the mouth an equal distance on each side, retaining the existing thickness and contour at the middle portion (see Fig. 11). The bottom margin of the lower lip should be broadened gradually beginning at a point approximately $\frac{1}{8}$ inch from the corners of the mouth and terminating at its widest point at the center. The broadest band of color now appears at the middle of the lower lip giving the illusion of a larger mouth.

Shortening the Mouth

When it is necessary to shorten the width of the mouth, do not extend the color to the natural corners of the mouth; instead, terminate the color a bit short. Restraint

Figure 10. Purple colorant along lash line.

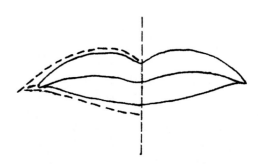

Figure 11. Widening the mouth.

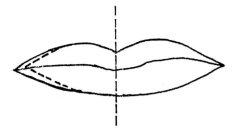

Figure 12. Shortening the mouth.

should be exercised or an unrealistic distortion will result. A small amount of surface restorer wax may be placed at the corners of the mouth to move the terminus of the lips inward on each side to create the illusion of a smaller mouth. When applying the lip color, retain the natural contour of the outer limits of the lips as faithfully as possible (Fig. 12).

Waxing the Mucous Lip Surface

The effects of age, disease, dehydration, emaciation, postmortem refrigeration, lip lesions caused by high fever prior to death, and traumatic injuries can damage the mucous lip surface and seriously detract from the illusion of natural repose. The condition must be corrected before a natural-looking effect can be achieved. Quality **lip wax** should work well on soft and slightly moist tissues and be effective in contouring the lips and simulating lip surface lines. If the lips are firm, after embalming, the use of a **surface or firm wax** may be employed.

Preparing the Mucous Lip Surface

Preparation of a clean, dry, and firm operational field is the first step. If the lip tissue is soft, flabby, or in any stage of putrefaction, it is important to correct this condition before proceeding. Fill a 10-cc hypodermic syringe with a solution of equal parts of cavity and humectant chemical and inject both the upper and lower lips. Insert a 1-inch hypodermic needle (22 gauge) just below the visible line of the lip (the point of entry is made in the center of the upper lip), directing needle thrust to the corner of the lip. Slowly withdraw the needle, injecting the solution at the same time. Keep the needle well within the rounded portion of the mucous lip surface. Repeat the same procedure for the lower lip, entering the needle just below the visible margin (weather line) in the center. This will preserve and firm the mucous tissues of the lips and establish the natural rounded contour at the same time. Allow a minimum of 30 minutes for firming. Note: this may also be done by inserting the needle at the innermost corners of the mouth. A tissue-builder containing a preservative may also be used for injection.

If time permits, a thin layer of cotton can be placed over the teeth and saturated with cavity fluid. The lips

can be glued and the saturated cotton will remain as an internal preservative pack. In several hours, the lips' mucous membranes and the integumentary lips will be firm.

To prepare the lip surfaces for waxing, using swabbed forceps saturated with mortuary solvent, remove all traces of soil, massage cream, and cosmetics. After cleansing operations are completed, the lips should be examined for the presence of scabs, fissures, dried, cracked or peeling skin, and traumatic injury. Loose edges of lacerated tissue should be trimmed away close to the lip surface. Fragmented tissue should be repositioned and sutured or cemented in correct alignment. Missing tissue areas should be trimmed to form a neat, well-defined perimeter. Moist lesions on the mucous membrane surface should be dried with a cauterant chemical and sealed with a surface sealant.

Application of Lip Wax

When resurfacing the mucous lip tissues, place a small amount of surface restorer wax in the palm of your hand where normal body heat will warm it to the right consistency for spatula application. Treat the upper lip first. The dip at the center of the upper lip gives fullness and accentuates the "cupid's bow" effect. Deposit more wax at the center of the lip to retain the effect of fullness and to create a naturally proportioned curvature.

Pick up a small amount of wax from the palm of your hand on the edge of the spatula blade (see Fig. 13). Start application at the lower margin of the upper lip. Pull the chin downward, separating the upper and lower lips. Place the deposit of wax slightly under the lower margin of the upper lip. Spread the wax upward using very light pressure to form the natural curve of the upper lip with the blade of the spatula.

In this illustration (Fig. 14), the wax has been applied to the lower lip. The procedure is the same as that used in forming the upper lip. Depress the chin,

Figure 13. First, apply wax to upper lip.

Figure 14. Wax applied to upper and lower lips.

Figure 16. Inscribing the vertical lines.

tapering the wax deposit to form smoothly underneath the upper lip in simulating the line of closure, making certain that the full, rounded contour is retained over the surface of the lower lip.

To establish the line of closure, apply an ample amount of massage cream to the bristles of a small brush, smooth the bristles into a sharp chisel edge (Fig. 15). (Form the chisel edge by running the bristles of the brush between your thumb and forefinger.) Using a horizontal stroke, pass the sharp edge of the brush from the left corner to the right corner of the mouth, along the line of closure. Repeat the procedure until you have established a natural contour of the line of closure.

Simulating the vertical lines of the lip in wax is a very important phase in lip waxing (Fig. 16). The procedure itself is a simple one when used with restraint and a light touch. When we study vertical lip lines, we observe the lines are spaced farther apart at the center of the lips and become closer together toward the corners of the mouth. To duplicate vertical lip lines and wrinkles, sharpen the end of a round-handled lip brush in a rotary pencil sharpener to a needle point. (The edge of a spat-

ula moistened with solvent could also be used.) Using very light vertical strokes, start at the center of the upper lip—inscribe the lines to the corners of the mouth. Treat the lower lip using the same procedure.

Observe the lip lines duplicated in the wax surface on the left side of the mouth. On the left side, the lines have been eliminated to illustrate the difference in natural appearance (Fig. 17).

Upon completion of scribing the vertical lines in the surface of the wax, it is necessary to reduce the "ridges" (caused by the scribing tool) into a smooth and natural contour (Fig. 18). To accomplish this, dip a small diameter brush into a mortuary solvent (remove the excess liquid from the brush by running the bristles between your thumb and forefinger). Using only the weight of the brush, smooth out the lines with vertical strokes of the brush.

Application of Cream Cosmetics over Waxed Lips

Before applying the lip cosmetics, allow the wax to dry and harden to its original consistency. Allotting the time for the wax to return to its original wax base will prevent

Figure 15. Line of closure established. Vertical lines begun.

Figure 17. No vertical lines on left side of lips.

Figure 18. Smoothing the attached margin on the lower lip.

Figure 20. Color applied to the lips.

the scribed vertical lines and line of closure from being altered when applying the lip cosmetics. Firming and resetting of the wax takes approximately 15 minutes at normal room temperature. Before applying the lip cosmetic, outline the upper and lower attached margins of the lips (Fig. 19). Mix the lip color to the desired shade. Using a fine-pointed brush outline the lips—follow the outside border in establishing their natural width and length.

Following the outlined shape of the upper and lower lip, apply the lip cosmetic over the surface of the wax (Fig. 20). Using the correct shade of lip color, place the cosmetic on the palm of your hand spreading the cream cosmetic in a downward direction with the blade of a spatula, forming a thin film of cream on the palm. Dilute the cream with mortuary solvent. Pick up a small amount of the cream with the brush from the palm of your hand. Apply the lip cream to the desired value—use two or three independent applications of the cream to establish the depth of color desired. The cosmetic can be applied using gentle vertical strokes.

Bring the basic (flesh colored) cosmetic downward to conform to the outer boarder of the upper of the upper lip; likewise bring the basic (flesh colored) cosmetic upward to meet the lower lip. Follow the configuration along the borders using a $\frac{1}{2}$-inch flat brush. Blend the basic (flesh colored) cosmetic outward into the epidermal surfaces surrounding the mouth (Figs. 21 through 23).

Stipple on of the toning creams (light brown or dark brown) over the basic (flesh colored) cosmetic applied along the outside border of the lips (see Fig. 22). This deposit of color should be applied (stippled) so lightly that it does not become apparent it has been applied. The brown toning medium will blend the lip color (red) into the basic (flesh) complexion cosmetic and remove any line of demarcation that is normally visible. This "hard line of demarcation" (where the red lip meets the flesh or complexion colored lip) is the major cause of artificial-looking lip contour. By stippling one of the brown toning creams lightly over the basic (flesh) complexion color, the "white line" surrounding the lips

Figure 19. Outlining lip margins.

Figure 21. Blending lip and skin colors.

Figure 22. Tone colors applied.

Figure 24. Natural look created by vertical lines on right side of these waxed lips.

becomes soft and natural looking (Fig. 23). A natural blended margin to the lips is desired for a natural look. A "sharp red lip" is used only for women when applying an ornamental lip color is desired. Ornamental cosmetic treatment of the lips uses an intense lip color (lipstick) and sharp edges are evident.

One of the most important procedures required to ensure the natural appearance of the deceased is a true simulation of contour and color of the lips. Lip color should be limited to the central areas of the lips and blended gradually into the basic complexion cosmetic. As seen in Figure 24, we observe the natural appearance of the lips with the lines duplicated in the wax (left side) and the natural lip color applied **compared to** where only the wax is applied and no further treatment made other than the application of lip cosmetics (right side).

▶ COSMETIC POWDER APPLICATION

The principal function of the powder application is to set and dry the various cosmetic media we have applied.

Figure 23. Stippling using a soft brush.

When powdering the skin where heavy opaque cosmetics have been applied, a very thin layer of white drying powder should first be evenly distributed. If the powder is applied heavily, it will cake on the surface. The general application procedure is to apply a light layer of powder, allow the powder to remain on the surface for a few minutes to set and dry the cosmetics, then remove the surplus. The normal skin texture exhibits a slight sheen on both the male and the female subjects. During the powder treatment, this natural sheen is eliminated, creating a dull matte finish. This dull finish would actually be characteristic of a person who wore makeup in life.

Matte Finish. A nonreflective finish will be the result any time powder is used over mortuary cosmetics. There is no type of powder that does not have the tendency to dull cosmetically treated epidermal surfaces. All other skin textures, with the exception of infants and children, require a sheen finish.

Sheen Finish. All normal adult male and female skin textures have a sheen finish. This is because all skin contains natural oils. Since males tend not to wear makeup, a slight sheen must be maintained for their complexion, particularly males with a dark complexion. To create the sheen finish after the powder has dried and set the cosmetics, all visible traces of powder should be removed using the powder brush. The skin is then patted with a gauze pad dampened with water. This treatment removes the dulling effect of the powder and reestablishes the natural sheen of the skin.

Hairspray. Aerosol hairspray can be used to lightly spray over the surface of cosmetic media after powder treatments have been completed. Lacquer hairspray is particularly effective for adult males with dark complexions in establishing a sheen finish. Non-lacquer spray dries with a matte finish. The use of either type of hairspray will help seal the skin surface and prevent cosmetics from rubbing off.

Method of Powder Application

Brush Application. A powder brush is the most common tool used in application procedures. Brush application consists of scooping up some of the powder on the bristles, holding the brush about 2 inches above the epidermal surface, and lightly tapping the handle with your index finger, to deposit a light layer of powder. When the brush load is too heavy, tap the brush over the palm of your hand to remove surplus powder before making the application. Allow the powdered surface to dry for approximately 5 minutes, then remove all excess powder with a clean brush.

Powder Blower Application. The powder blower gives the most control over the amount of powder being deposited. It is excellent for applying drying powder over restorative media. When using the powder blower, a fine layer of powder can be atomized, eliminating overuse of powder. Even when using the powder blower, it is necessary to remove some excess powder with the powder brush after application.

Powder Puff Application. This method of applying powder goes back many years in funeral service, to the time when dry rouge was the most commonly used mortuary cosmetic. The application is made by lightly blotting the powder puff over the epidermal surfaces. When using this method, care must be taken to avoid leaving excessive deposits of powder on the surface. After the application is completed, using a soft brush, lightly stipple and smooth out the powder over the epidermal surface.

Removal of Powder from Facial Hair

As a final treatment it is necessary to remove all powder from the facial hair. This surplus powder is easily removed with a small brush dipped in a mortuary solvent or simply clean water. Gently pass the brush through the eyelash or eyebrow. Another method of removing powder is the use of the eyebrow pencil. Sharpen the end of the pencil into a wedge shape. To treat the eyelash, place the blade of a spatula under the lash, so that the lash lies flat on the blade. Stroke the eyelash lightly with the flat edge of the pencil. This procedure removes the powder, darkens the lashes, and imparts a natural sheen to the hair of the lash. The eyebrows are treated by placing the flat edge of the pencil against the eyebrow, then stroking very lightly from the inner corner to the distal edge of the brow.

▶ COSMETIZING THE HANDS

Cosmetic procedures used in treating the hands and fingers call for the same degree of cosmetic skill as that used in treating the face.

Before applying the cosmetics to the hands, the final cleansing and manicuring should be done.

Dehydrated Fingertips

Troublesome problems concerning dehydration can easily be prevented by early recognition of warning signs that indicate incipient dehydration. One well-defined sign is the presence of abnormally soft tissue in the fingertips. It is an indication that these extremities have not received sufficient chemical preservation. Immediately upon detection, hypodermically inject the fingertips with a preservative-type feature builder or a 50/50 mixture of cavity solution and humectant chemical until they attain their normal contour and firmness. The natural contour of the fingertips is marked by a smooth roundness with no trace of wrinkling or flattening.

Dehydration of fingertips may also be the result of the arterial injection. When this condition exists, a postembalming injection of tissue builder into the finger tips will correct the problem.

Some embalmers tissue-build all fingertips as a routine procedure. This insures that dehydration of the fingertips will not occur.

▶ BASIC COLOR APPLICATION

The base cosmetic is applied to the hands and fingers as a background colorant, using the same method of application as that used for the face. For all normal applications, the following types of cosmetics are used for the basic color application: (1) transparent liquid tint, (2) liquid powder tint, and (3) tinted emollient cream. When it is necessary to use masking-type cosmetics to cope with discolorations and to cover restorative media, the covering qualities of the semiopaque emollient creams, opaque creams, and opaque liquid cosmetics are preferred. The opaque creams and opaque liquids may also be used to create transparent effects when applied sparingly.

Surface Preparation Procedure

When using transparent (alcohol-based) liquid tints, liquid powder tint, or opaque liquid cosmetics, the epidermal surface should be thoroughly clean and free of all massage cream and oily substances. To cleanse and degrease the skin, saturate a gauze pad with mortuary solvent and remove all traces of massage cream from the face and hands. On female subjects make sure that the lower arms (if a short-sleeved dress is to be used) are totally devoid of massage cream residue. A grease-free skin surface is essential for the successful application of all liquid cosmetics.

When applying emollient or cream cosmetics, degreasing is not required. All that is necessary is to wipe off all excess massage cream with a gauze pad until a clean, smooth foundation is established. This type of epidermal surface will respond very well to all cream cosmetic media.

Warm Color Application

Treating the warm-colored areas of the hands and fingers and reestablishing their natural lines and markings is a very important phase of mortuary cosmetology. The illustrations in Figures 25 to 28 show the specific areas of the hands and fingers subject to warm color cosmetic application and the captions explain the reasons why these warm color areas require special attention. The hands and fingers receive only minimal amounts of color through the arterial injection. The palms, fingertips, fingernails, cuticles, and inner surfaces of the thumbs are all areas of warm color in the living body. The skin around the thumb and forefinger and along the side of the hand usually appears unnaturally white in color with the waxy pallor indicative of embalmed tissue. A similar absence of natural color is also visible on dark-skinned Latinos and African-Americans after embalming. These missing warm color characteristics must be cosmetically restored if we wish to achieve a natural lifelike appearance in lifeless tissue.

Figure 26. This side and top view of the hand is seen with the little finger in the foreground, showing the distribution of warm color rising upward from the palm and extending around the contour of the hand, fingers, and fingertips and encircling the fingernails. A glow of warm color appears on the knuckles. Color is carried toward the wrist from the palmar surface of the hand. All warm color areas must be blended into the basic complexion colorant so that no distinct lines of demarcation are visible.

▶ DISCOLORATIONS

Postembalming Treatments of Discolorations

Broken Skin Surface. The arterial injection will normally cause swelling and leakage in broken skin. A cauterant chemical can be injected into the affected area before the arterial injection is made, which prevents swelling, dries, and seals the broken skin tissues, prevents leakage, and, most important, establishes a stable restorative foundation. (Some embalmers prefer to

Figure 25. This lateral view of the hand and fingers seen with the thumb in the foreground shows warm color locations indicated by the shaded areas. Note that warm color starts in the palm of the hand and spreads to the underside of the fingers and thumb and appears along the outer contour of the thumb and forefinger. Warm color also extends to the fingertips, encircles the fingernails (cuticles), and leaves a glow of warm color at each finger joint. Color is carried slightly beyond the thumb pad at the base of the palm and blended into the wrist.

Figure 27. Here the upturned palm is seen from above to indicate the characteristic natural distribution of warm color. Note that the warm color of the palm radiates into the lower surfaces and sides of the thumb, small finger, forefinger, all fingertips, and the palm itself. Although we normally do not apply warm color to the invisible palms of the hands, the illustration serves to show how the color radiates into the visible areas of the hands and fingers, where it contributes greatly to natural-looking cosmetic results.

Figure 28. This view of the back of the hand shows how warm color radiates from the palmar surface around the contours of the fingers and thumb. The illustration also shows how warm color accents begin at the fingertips and continue around the cuticles with a blush of color on the knuckles and tendons on the back of the hand. In some cases, the tendons on the back of the hand appear more prominently than in others. The warm color in this area would vary according to the prominence of this feature in each individual case. All red colorant should be blended to a full vanishing point for a realistic natural effect.

do all hypodermic treatments **after** arterial injection.) When it is not possible to treat the broken skin before the arterial injection and when delay is unavoidable, make sure that the subcutaneous injection of the cauterant is made at least one or preferably 2 hours before starting the restorative and cosmetic treatments. This will ensure a stable foundation.

Unbroken Skin Surface. Evaluate the preservative stability and extent of the discoloration before starting the cosmetic treatments. Small discolorations where the tissues have been well preserved by the arterial solution will require no further treatment beyond masking with opaque cosmetics. Large discolorations usually do not readily respond to preservation via the arterial injection and therefore should be given supplementary hypodermic treatment. Prepare a solution consisting of 50% cavity solution and 50% humectant (some embalmers use 100% cavity chemical or use of a cautery chemical). Inject it subcutaneously throughout the entire discolored area using a 22-gauge hypodermic needle. Distribute the solution in the tissues by manual manipulation until spread uniformly throughout. Always keep in mind that tissue breakdown in the dermal layer tends to retard the chemical circulation and these areas should be treated independently by subcutaneous hypodermic injection. Properly executed, this procedure will produce a smooth, natural skin texture and contour. The humectant in the hypodermic solution inhibits dehydration and wrinkling. The cavity chemical preserves the tissues and helps dispel the discoloration by its bleaching action. Ecchymosis is characterized by an intense,

purple-black discoloration of the skin, most commonly appearing on the back of the hand and it is frequently accompanied by swelling.

Discoloration on Back of Hand. Swelling may be associated with ecchymosis in the back of the hand caused by hypodermic needle punctures. This swelling may be reduced by injecting a cauterant chemical into the affected area before or after the arterial injection. Massage the tissues with your fingertips until the swelling is visibly reduced. The bleaching action of the cauterant chemical also dispels most of the discolorations. After the arterial injection is completed, apply an external pack by saturating absorbent cotton (premium grade) with the cauterant and placing it over the discolored area. Allow the compress to remain on the surface until a noticeable reduction of color intensity results.

Discolored and Swollen Eyelids. Swelling and discoloration of the eyelids (black eye) may be reduced by two methods: hypodermic injection and the electrical spatula. Because the arterial injection normally increases swelling in traumatized eyelids, it is imperative that the reduction be made before injection, while the tissues are still pliable and the blood is in its natural liquid state and not coagulated.* Hypodermically injecting a cauterant chemical into the eyelids will reduce the swelling and bleach out most of the purple-black discoloration. Both the upper and lower eyelids are injected subcutaneously, and excess serous liquid is pressed out through the needle-entry puncture. Use a 20-cc syringe fitted with a 22-gauge by 2-inch hypodermic needle. Starting with an empty syringe, insert the needle at the distal end of the eyebrow and channel underneath the eyelids by repeated back and forth movements. Upon completing the channeling, do not withdraw the hypodermic needle. Simply disengage the needle from the barrel of the syringe, fill the syringe with the cauterant chemical, and reattach it to the syringe. Inject both the upper and lower eyelids with the cauterant chemical. Inject the upper lid first and move the hypodermic needle back and forth so that the swollen tissue becomes completely saturated with the cauterant. Remove the syringe and needle.

Massage the eyelids and press downward with very firm pressure using your fingertips and thumb. Apply pressure in an outward direction toward the needle-entry point. Apply a heavy coat of cosmetic massage cream before rubbing the eyelids. Continue the massage until swelling is visibly reduced. Massaging should always immediately follow hypodermic injection. Any delay will allow the tissues to harden and become set, making it impossible to reduce the swelling.

---

*Some embalmers prefer to perform all invasive tissue corrections *after* arterial injection.

The electric spatula can be used effectively to reduce slight eyelid swelling or excessive wrinkling when the tissues are soft and pliable, even when no hypodermic reduction has preceded its use. However, maximum performance results when subcutaneous injection and heat reduction treatments are combined. (See also Selected Readings, "Management Techniques for the Eyes," by Vernie Fountain.)

Cosmetics Used in Treating Discolorations

In treating discolorations and restored skin surfaces, the combination of opaque liquid and opaque cream cosmetics is a very effective combination in establishing natural skin coloring. These cosmetics will mask virtually any type of discoloration or restored surface. Transparent and semiopaque cream cosmetics may be applied **over** dried opaque paints to adjust complexion coloring.

Liquid Opaque Cosmetic. This liquid opaque pigment is formulated to conceal difficult postmortem discolorations. They are available in liquid and aerosol media. The liquid opaques are fast drying and impart a natural-looking, noncaking translucent coloring with good stability to the skin surface and are used in all "undercoating" treatments.

Opaque Cream Pigments. The opaque cream pigments are widely used in cosmetic procedures involving the masking of skin discolorations, concealing minor blemishes and imparting natural color (basic complexion color) over surface restoration media.

Toning Creams. The toning cream cosmetic is very versatile and exceptionally well formulated for toning and color coordinating procedures when used over masked discolorations and restored skin surfaces. The following colors are used in toning treatments: light brown, dark brown, black, purple, blue, yellow, light rouge, and dark rouge.

Technical Procedure in Treating Discolorations

The following technical procedures are designed to treat discolored and restored skin surfaces, and these techniques are used for masking unbroken skin conditions such as yellow jaundice, petechial hemorrhage, ecchymosis, and contusions. The following steps list the order of application in masking epidermal surfaces and restorative media.

1. *Undercoat Application.* Brush apply liquid opaque cosmetic (or spray the aerosol media) directly over the discoloration. The color should match the natural (untreated) skin surface. Carefully apply the liquid opaque cosmetic evenly over the surface allowing it to extend about $\frac{1}{4}$ inch beyond the margin of the area being treated. Stipple out all lines of demarcation and allow to thoroughly dry.

2. *Basic Color Application.* Apply the correct shade of basic complexion colorant over the normal skin surfaces, extending it very lightly over the undercoat previously applied in step 1. Stipple and blend the basic colorant softly into the undercoating deposit. Smooth out the basic complexion cosmetic, stippling the opaque pigment very lightly over the treated surface, adjusting the application to attain a translucent effect.

3. *Toning Application.* Select the correct shade of toning cream to match the individual's natural complexion color as closely as possible. Using a light stippling movement with a camel hair stippling brush, apply the toning cream very lightly over the basic complexion colorant. This treatment replaces the melanin pigmentation naturally present in all complexions. Use light brown toning cream for all light to medium complexions; dark brown toning cream on dark complexions ranging in the brown to black category; and black toning cream is used on dark complexions ranging in the ebony to black range. The toning cream is applied very lightly, so lightly that it is barely visible. This light application tones the opaque cosmetic into a natural translucent skin coloring with an undertone of natural lifelike color.

4. *Drying and Finishing Powder Application.* Apply white drying and finishing powder over the cosmetized epidermal surfaces, using the powder blower for uniform distribution. Allow the powder to remain on the cosmetized surface for at least 5 minutes so that it will dry and set the cosmetics properly. Remove the surplus powder with a powder brush.

5. *Replacing Natural Facial Lines and Markings.* After removing all surplus powder, use light brown or dark brown toning cream to duplicate the characteristic coloring of facial lines, wrinkles, and natural markings. As the color is deposited, gently blend the cosmetic into a natural color intensity by lightly stippling over the skin with a clean and dry brush.

Individual Minor Discolorations

Opaque cosmetics (liquid spray or cream) applied over small discolorations will create a contrasting line on the skin surface. When treating small discolorations, liquid opaque cosmetic is applied as an undercoat to permanently obscure the discolored area. It is essential that this undercoat be a close approximation of the natural skin coloring. The basic complexion cosmetic should be lightly blended over the undercoat application. Upon completion of the basic complexion application, stipple a very light, thin coat of opaque cream cosmetic (matching the basic color application) over the discolored surface. With the basic complexion colorant properly blended over the undercoat application, the treated area is now perfected with the application of the correct shade of toning cream. The application of the toning cream removes all marginal lines of demarcation and brings out the true complexion coloring, achieving undetectable masking of the discoloration.

Warm Color Discolorations

When discolorations extend to the warm color areas of the face and hands, red colorant should be added to the liquid opaque undercoat. Brush apply the liquid opaque cosmetic and let it dry thoroughly. Blend the correct basic complexion color over the undercoat application, leaving a red undertone of color. Make the usual warm color application, blending the colorant out so that no line of demarcation is apparent. Apply toning cream and accent natural lines and markings as indicated.

Complete Surface Discoloration

In some situations, such as yellow jaundice, carbon monoxide poisoning, and petechial hemorrhage, it becomes necessary to totally mask the entire skin surface. Liquid opaque pigment is applied as an undercoat or an aerosol spray undercoat can be applied. The liquid opaque is brush applied in an overall application on the face and hands masking the discolored skin surface. This procedure will undercoat and seal the epidermal surface masking the discoloration. After the liquid opaque has thoroughly dried, match the complexion colorant with opaque cream cosmetic. Apply uniformly as lightly as possible, blending the cream over the undercoat. The opaque cream bonds with the undercoat and establishes a translucent background color of living tissue.

Apply the warm color (red) in a heavier deposit than normal because the soft texture of the opaque cream base will reduce and absorb the red colorant. A second application of red colorant may have to be applied over the warm color areas to produce a natural-looking effect. Blend the warm color into the basic complexion colorant until no line of demarcation can be seen.

Apply the correct shade of eye shadow to the upper eyelid and apply purple colorant along the lash line. The muted purple is applied where the lash enters the ridge of the eyelid, producing a rounded contour and natural color. When masking cosmetics have been used, it is necessary to apply white drying powder before cosmetically treating the facial lines and natural markings. Because of the absorbent quality of the opaque cream medium, it is nearly impossible to realistically duplicate the lines and markings. The skin surfaces must be completely dry and stable before these treatments can be accomplished. After the detailing treatments are completed, white drying powder is applied. Hairspray can be applied after excess powder is removed.

Cosmetically Treating Wax Surfaces

Epidermal surfaces restored with wax may be cosmetically treated by several different procedures to produce a natural texture and skin coloring. The three most commonly used methods are as follows:

1. *Surface Undercoating.* Liquid opaque cosmetic is brush applied as an undercoat over the restored surface or an aerosol spray undercoat may be used. After the opaque undercoat has completely dried, surface restorer wax is applied over the undercoated surface. This will mask the restoration and any discoloration associated with the traumatized tissue around the restoration. Opaque cosmetic medium (cream or liquid) is then lightly applied over the wax surface, matching the opaque application with the basic complexion colorant.

2. *Intermixing Wax Colors.* This procedure is based on matching the surface restorer wax by coordinating the color of the wax with the complexion or warm color tone. Various shades of wax are intermixed (usually two or three shades) until a basic or warm color equivalent is attained. The opaque cosmetic medium (cream or liquid) is then lightly blended over the wax surface, matching the natural complexion or warm colorant.

3. *Cosmetic Over Wax.* Restorations should be completed, including duplication of natural lines and wrinkles and simulation of pore texture, before applying the opaque cosmetic medium over the waxed surface. It is essential that the waxed restoration surface be allowed to firmly reset to its natural consistency before applying the opaque cosmetic medium. It usually takes about 20 minutes at room temperature for the wax to harden. After the wax has set, brush apply the opaque medium (cream or liquid) over the waxed surface. Very lightly stipple blend the opaque cosmetic over the wax surface. Avoid wax buildup on the bristles of the brush during this operation. Clean the brush frequently while working or the wax buildup on the bristles will damage and distort the restored surface.

► BIBLIOGRAPHY

Embalming Course Content Syllabus. American Board of Funeral Service Education; St. Joseph, MO, 2006.

Johnson EC. *Restorative Art.* Chicago: Worsham College of Mortuary Science, c. 1955.

Klicker RL. Restorative *Art and Science.* Thanos Institute, Buffalo, NY, 2003.

Mayer J. Sheridan. *Color and Cosmetics,* 3rd ed., Dallas Professional Training Schools, 1986.

Mayer J. Sheridan. *Restorative Art,* Dallas, Professional Training Schools, 2003.

More Thoughts on Postmortem Restorations, No. 434. Springfield, OH: Champion Expanding Encyclopedia, February, 1973.

Prager GJ. *Manual of Postmortem Restorative Art.* Cincinnati College of Embalming, Cincinnati, OH, 1965.

Principles of Restorative Art, No. 428–433. Springfield, OH: Champion Expanding Encyclopedia, June 1972–January, 1973.

Restorative Art Course Content Syllabus. American Board of Funeral Service Education, St. Joseph, MO, 2006.

Sanders C. Richard. Numerous articles 1960-2000. *Dodge Magazine.* The Dodge Company, Cambridge, MA, 1960–2000.

Strub CG. *The Principles of Restorative Art,* 2nd ed. *Embalmer's* Monthly, Westport, Conn., July 1933.

SECTION II
HISTORY OF MODERN RESTORATIVE ART

Edward C. Johnson, Gail R. Johnson, and Melissa J. Williams

The reader is advised to reread the section on Egyptian embalming procedures, entitled *Ancient Restorative Art*, found in the preceding section of this text.

Virtually all documented reports of embalming in the anatomical or middle period in Europe included the practice of enclosing the preserved body within a metal-lined, hermetically sealed coffin, which precluded viewing. To satisfy some medieval customs relating to funeral practices and chivalry, an imago or effigy of the decedent was created by preparing a death mask as the basis for the head. The features were painted to closely resemble the normal lifelike appearance, and effigies were often adorned with a wig. The completed head was attached to a torso, complete with arms and legs, proportional to the life size of the decedent. The effigy was dressed in the clothing or armor of the decedent and placed on the coffin containing the corpse, where it remained during the entire period preceding actual interment (Fig. 1).

A recent discovery suggests that in the early 1900s, there was a concern for the appearance of the deceased in Europe. Alfredo Salafia, a prolific embalmer from Palermo, Italy, describes his attention to former Italian Premier, Francesco Crispi, who died in Naples. Crispi was to be returned to Palermo and was unsuccessfully embalmed by another practitioner. Salafia reembalmed the body (possibly the first indication that this is a successful procedure) and replaced the eyes with glass eyeballs, reattached the hair and beard that had fallen out, and filled out the facial features with injections of paraffin to "regain the form and the lost volume."

During the U.S. Civil War, a few documents indicated that some effort was made to repair traumatic injuries. One such document in the Frank Hutton collection was a letter from the family of a Union Army soldier who was embalmed and sent home for burial. The family wrote in their letter to Hutton that the corpse "looked pretty good for being dragged by mules."

By and large, however, it can be stated without fear of contradiction that very little of what is referred to today as restorative art was practiced until the second decade of the twentieth century. There were exceptions occasionally, such as the treatment of the anarchist bomber's suicide in Chicago briefly described in the section on Felix Aloysius Sullivan (see the preceding section). Joseph H. Clarke briefly mentions the treatment of a tumor case in his book *Reminiscences of Early Embalming*.

What is termed restorative art today represents the greatest remaining challenge to the skill, the ability to improvise, and the courage of the practicing embalmer. It is the last frontier and poses problems to test those who choose to grapple with its manifest difficulties. Formerly known most commonly by several popular terms such as plastic surgery, demisurgery, and dermasurgery, it is today most commonly referred to as restorative art.

The term *restorative art*, not adopted until the early 1930s, is in reality a poorly contrived label for specialized postmortem treatment accorded those dying of trauma or debilitating disease, the practice of which is most often believed to have originated entirely in the United States in recent years. Such a premise is false inasmuch

Figure 1. Medieval funeral procession. Note effigy of deceased.

Figure 2. Arm of a mummy of the Egypt's twenty-first dynasty, showing the packing material.

as the practice of restorative art is dependent on and inseparable from the embalming procedure. Thus, one realizes that restorative art has been practiced from the origin of embalming in Egypt and so it was (Fig. 2).

The year 1912 marks the establishment of the modern era of what is today known as restorative art. The first articles appeared in the April 19, 1912, issue of *The Sunnyside. Demisurgery*, termed by its founder, was "the art of building or creating parts of the body which have been destroyed by accident, disease, decomposition or discoloration, and making the body perfectly natural and lifelike."

The science of restorative art as known today was founded by one man, Joel E. Crandall, then an embalmer in New York City. Although many others made important contributions to this science through the years, no other one person can claim the honor of stimulating the interest of fellow embalmers in this most difficult technical subject area.

An editorial in the April 19, 1912, issue of *The Sunnyside* stated that "the photographs of before and after appearance of a mutilated body show what can and should be done. The originator of the new art of demisurgery is Joel E. Crandall of New York City and his first article on the new technique appears in the pages of this issue of *The Sunnyside*" (Fig. 3).

Howard S. Eckels in a letter published in the May 14, 1914, issue of *The Sunnyside*, stating that the science of demisurgery was indeed founded by Joel E. Crandall, made an early acknowledgment of Crandall's primacy in the field.

A. Johnson Dodge, quoted in the June 1, 1917, issue of *The Casket*, states:

How to care for mutilated or postmortem cases, or bodies which from any cause have become unsightly and make them presentable, should constitute a part

of the education of the embalmer. Thorough instruction in this difficult part of the art should be given by the instructors in our schools. But this part of the work requires special experience and some study either to practice or teach it successfully. It was first taught as a specialty by Mr. Joel E. Crandall of New York City, and to him belongs the credit of introducing it. We think Mr. Crandall is the only person who has attained any great degree of success in the practice of this art, and would recommend the student who wishes to attain a high degree of proficiency in this part of his profession to apply to Mr. Crandall for instruction, as he appears to be the only known person really competent to teach it.

Joel E. Crandall (1878–1942) was born on September 16, 1878, in Whitesville, New York. Approximately at 20 years of age, he began working for a New York City undertaker. Deeply interested in embalming and becoming increasingly skillful, his services were much in demand and he was employed by both Frank E. Campbell and Stephen Merritt undertaking establishments as well as the National Casket Company.

Writing in 1912 about his efforts to repair mutilated cases, he stated that he had studied the problems over a period of 10 years. His early efforts to use conventional materials such as plaster of paris were abandoned for any use except as an interior deep filler in contact with bone. He formulated covering cosmetics and a waxlike putty to fill in missing or damaged areas.

His earliest experiments were on severely mutilated bodies that neither the family nor the undertaker believed could be restored to viewability. Little by little, over the years, by trial and error, he developed a successful system for treatment of mutilated cases that eventually embodied most present-day principles or techniques.

Among the requirements Crandall advocated were a recent photograph of the decedent as a reference for

Figure 3. Crandall's advertisement for his services.

the restoration, hardening of the soft tissues of the face as a prerequisite to demisurgery, and enough working time to carry out the entire treatment. Crandall also made the earliest mention of the use of "concealed stitches" to close lacerations and "corrective surgery" to remove remnants of features or tissue impossible to incorporate into the restoration. For his early research, he made use of plaster life-size heads that he mutilated and repaired: a procedure that was eventually adopted in one form or another by most embalming schools for laboratory practice and is generally used to this day.

Crandall began his career in demisurgery by offering his services anywhere within a 400-mile radius of New York City. Gradually, by demand, he was compelled to offer instruction in demisurgery. Each class was limited to 25 students for a 1-month period of instruction.

About the same time, he manufactured and sold the first demisurgical grip containing all required instruments, cosmetics, brushes, prefabricated mustaches and eyelashes, and preformed facial features of wax.

The use of prefabricated features as a base for individual modification of the decedent's facial topography enabled the unskilled or untrained embalmer to perform a reasonable restoration that is otherwise impossible. Crandall's brilliant concept was to be duplicated by others a number of times over the ensuing years.

Figure 4. Advertisement for Eckels molding masks.

A report of a restoration in 1924 mentions the use of prefabricated eyes and nose. The manufacturer of the parts, William Collier of New York City, advertised a kit containing prefabricated features in 1929 and patented the same in 1931. The Eckels Company of Philadelphia offered a similar kit in October of 1930 (Fig. 4), as did the Paasche Airbrush Company of Chicago in 1936. An interesting improvement on prefabricated features was developed by a dental plastic surgeon named C. J. Speas, who taught restorative art at Gupton-Jones College of Mortuary Science in Nashville, Tennessee, in the late 1940s. The basic concept was the "family resemblance theory," that is, members of the same family frequently resemble one another very closely. Thus, for example, when a nose is destroyed, a mold is made of the nose of a family member most closely resembling the decedent, cast in wax, and fitted into the decedent's face. Thus, a custom-made prefabrication is created.

Crandall purchased the Clerihew Undertaking Company located at 133 Broadway, Paterson, New Jersey, in 1913, and continued to maintain premises in New York City for his demisurgical supply company and school. Crandall must have written at some length on the subject of demisurgery, because *The Funeral Director's Encyclopedia*, a proposed three-volume work, each volume supposed to contain about 600 pages, was described in *The Sunnyside* in 1916 as having 100 pages on the art of demisurgery by Joel E. Crandall. No copies of this three-volume encyclopedia are known to exist, and it is suspected that it was never published. The 100 pages on demisurgery referred to were most likely the basic lectures by Crandall in the resident course of

DEMISURGERY
—OR—
THE NEW ART IN UNDERTAKING

WE WISH TO ANNOUNCE THE OPENING OF THE

DEMISURGICAL INSTITUTE
OF NEW YORK

On Feb. 18th, 1918, the Demisurgical Institute of New York will open its doors to the Profession with a complete course in the Art of Demisurgery.

The course will consist of Lectures, Experimental and Practical work and when completed every student will be able to restore nearly every mutilated case to its natural condition.

Each student will also receive a diploma, which will entitle him to the degree of "Demisurgeon," which name may be used in any way in connection with his business.

PROF. J. E. CRANDALL, Demisurgeon

The course will be given each month from Feb. 18th to June 18th, at which time the Institute will close to resume again on Sept. 18th.

As we have had many requests from prospective students, to be entered in the first class, we have decided that no applications will be considered until this announcement appears, and then each one accepted in turn, and as each class will be limited to 25 students, each applicant will be notified what month he may enter.

Write your application at once if you wish to enter one of the first classes and don't wait until your competitor forces you to do so.

ADDRESS ALL COMMUNICATIONS TO

DEMISURGICAL SUPPLY CO., 500 Fifth Avenue, New York City

Figure 5. Copy of the first ad for demisurgery in 1918.

instruction at the Demisurgical Institute of New York and the teaching text in his correspondence course in 1918 (Fig. 5).

The greatest impact of Crandall's influence on the embalmers of America resulted from his published photographs of mutilated cases taken before and after treatment, most of which were extremely difficult to restore even by today's standards. His work was exceptionally well done and was an inspiration to embalmers who desired to improve their skills, for he showed and proved that difficult cases could be restored to a viewable condition.

The effect of Crandall's announcement of the founding of the art of demisurgery on the embalming schools of the country varied. Some heads of schools such as Robbins of Boston, Charles O. Dhonau of Cincinnati, and Thorton Barnes of New York were rather vocal in their protest concerning Crandall's claim that he was the founder of the science (Fig. 6). All three claimed that their schools had taught the subject for years, although in truth, no mention of the matter in advertising nor listing of the subject matter in the school curricula is noted prior to April 1912. Barnes Schools began to advertise the teaching of DeMort-Ology, and the Cincinnati School added a course in demisurgery, whereas Robbins stated that his school taught artistic embalming, decoloration, and postmortem surgery. C. A. Renouard stated that he neither taught nor recommended the use of cos-

metics and, further, that much of demisurgery was unnecessary and unwelcome. Before his death, in 1953, Renouard was to reverse his opinion to the extent of even providing special short-term courses in restorative art.

Dhonau additionally accused Crandall of publishing retouched photographs of his restored cases. This so incensed Crandall that he secured affidavits from every one concerned—the undertaker, the photographer, lawyers, and family representatives, who attested to the authenticity of his work as represented by the case photographs.

The interest in the new art of demisurgery was immediate and has continued to the present day. The professional journals increasingly carried both photographs and case reports of successful treatment of mutilated cases, while advertisements multiplied for cosmetics, instruments, and demisurgical materials.

Among the cases Crandall treated was the famous Colonel Jacob Astor, who died at sea in 1912 as a passenger on the *Titanic*. His body, like hundreds of others, was taken from the sea near the site of the sinking and transported to Halifax, Nova Scotia, and from there returned to New York City for burial. Crandall was called by the New York undertaker in charge to treat Astor's badly discolored face. By means of Crandall's cosmetic skill, the casket was open for viewing of the body as it lay in state at the Astor estate near Rhinebeck, New York.

Figure 6. Carl L. Barnes (center) giving a demonstration in the Cook County Morgue, contiguous to the Barnes College building.

The February 1917 issue of *The Sunnyside* carried a notice that Crandall had taken motion pictures of a number of his demisurgical cases and that the films would be available for teaching purposes and presentations at conventions. Historically, this is the first known recording of any restorative procedures in motion pictures.

By 1918, the effect of World War I on the funeral profession was becoming evident and Crandall was interviewed by *The Sunnyside* for his views on the application of demisurgery to U.S. war casualties. He was most forthright in his conviction that all our war dead should be embalmed shortly after death and restored later at a convenient time and place.

From 1923 onward, however, Crandall faded in national mention, although he continued to operate his Paterson, New Jersey, funeral home until his death on July 19, 1942.

Joel E. Crandall demonstrated that any case, no matter how badly mutilated, could be restored to viewability. Furthermore, he devised not only the materials for his newly created science of demisurgery but also the technical instructions to accomplish this new skill.

All practicing embalmers owe a debt of gratitude to Joel E. Crandall, demisurgeon and founder of demisurgery, known today as restorative art.

The sudden and unforeseen arrival of Joel E. Crandall on the educational scene as the founder of the new art of demisurgery created the problem of partial loss of educational leadership for the American embalming schools. Recovering quickly from this threat, most schools began to teach the subject, although some, out of pride or vanity, refused to give the new art Crandall's title of demisurgery.

The immediate exception was Cincinnati College, which called the subject demisurgery but insisted that the subject had been taught there for years. Eckels College used the term "demisurgery" and acknowledged Crandall as the founder. Boston College called the course "postmortem surgery and the art of decoloration," and the Barnes School dubbed it Der-Mort-Ology *and* dermasurgery. An article describing Albert Worsham's demonstration of demisurgery calls it *plastic work*. The terms "dermasurgery" and "plastic surgery" also were noted as descriptive titles for the art, although one of the most original titles was used in 1917 by the New York School of Embalming (formerly Barnes School), which advertised derma sculpture taught by a sculptor and demisurgery taught by an embalmer. An advertisement for Dermatol Cosmetics in 1913 stated that it was not necessary to go to school to learn demisurgery or cosmetic application as everything one needed to know was in the pamphlet wrapped around each jar of cosmetics.

From 1912 onward, the pages of our professional journals disclose early contributions to the science of what today is termed restorative art. More and more advertisements are seen for cosmetics, demisurgery kits, and equipment (Fig. 7). Before-and-after case photos, pioneered by Crandall, appeared with some frequency in product advertisements as well as in articles. Demonstration of demisurgery at meetings and conventions became every bit as popular and as well attended as embalming demonstrations had been 30 years earlier.

Many prominent teachers and heads of embalming colleges wrote about the "new art." Some made first

Figure 7. This preparation, although not a preservative, is a valuable aid to the embalmer's art.

mention of standard basic procedures or techniques still employed today. Others advanced practices that were proven later to have little real value; for example, Robbins, in 1912, advocated the grafting of skin from another area of the body to replace damaged skin on the head. Such procedures were seldom very successful.

In 1912, Robbins, together with Lena Simmons, mentioned invisible or blind stitching (subcutaneous sutures), and C. O. Dhonau in the same year recommended baseball stitching with wax covering and concealing the sutured area, a rather unsatisfactory technique. Razorless shaving cream (a depilatory) made a brief but unsuccessful appearance in 1914, as it had a number of times since then.

Basic principles of demisurgery practice, such as using very concentrated fluid to produce firm tissue as ideal for final restoration and performing basic restoration to a near-normal anatomical relationship prior to arterial injection, were reiterated by C. O. Dhonau, Robbins, Worsham, Lena Simmons, and others. Some recommended removal of tumors and other surgical procedures prior to embalming, but Worsham and most modern authorities recommended that this be done after arterial injection. Most early authorities agreed that it was necessary to wait between completion of the arterial treatment and the final application of wax and cosmetics. Most recommended a minimum of 6 to 10 hours' time-lapse to ensure drying and halting of leakage from torn tissues.

In 1915, Worsham mentioned using cotton and collodion as a cavity filler to within one-sixteenth of an inch of the normal surface and then covering this surface with wax. He also used the cotton and collodion to form such basic features as lips, ears, nose, and eyelids.

Dhonau, writing at some length on demisurgery in 1915, called attention to the individuality of the human face, the differences in the lateral halves, as well as cosmetic skin variations. His suggestion, noted for the first time, to do the "work in the same light as that in which the body will rest until its final disposition," is still heeded today. In 1915, he demonstrated modeling of the facial features on a plaster skull, a technique that is today fairly standard throughout the schools for the teaching of restorative art.

One of the more dramatic demisurgical cases of the era was that treated by Worsham in Chicago in mid-1917. A lion tamer was attacked, mangled, and killed while performing in the lions' cage. A Chicago undertaker, Lafayette C. Ball, who was present at the place of attack, ran to his nearby funeral home, secured several bottles of formalin-based cavity fluid, returned to the circus cage, and poured the contents of the bottles over the dead lion tamer's torn body. This ingenious technique stopped the lions from further mangling the body and permitted the circus personnel to retrieve it. Worsham, called on to prepare the body, was confronted with the need to replace both ears, much of the face, and both arms and to close the torn open abdomen from which some viscera had been devoured. Before-and-after photos disclose a reasonable restoration.

Practicing embalmers were stimulated to try to repair difficult cases too. *The Sunnyside* issue of September 15, 1914, published a story and before-and-after photos of two cases, a murder and suicide by shotgun. In both cases, the skulls had been shattered by a 16-gauge shotgun. Mr. and Mrs. G. A. Rousevell of Lead, South Dakota, restored the bodies to a virtually normal appearance.

In 1917, C. O. Dhonau announced a new technique for treating swollen, blackened eyes. He incised the underside of the affected lid or lids, pressed out the accumulated blood and serum, and then applied 50% phenol solution to shrink and bleach the area.

At this time, the schools, which conducted courses of instruction of quite varying lengths averaging 3 months' duration at most, allotted some instruction time to demisurgery. Some schools scheduled regular periods in the laboratory for learning to form facial features in wax or clay on a plaster skull. Unique among these courses was that taught by Worsham, whose class in demisurgery was most often given at the end of the entire course of instruction. By the 1930s, it amounted to 25 to 40 total hours of laboratory work. The actual practice was carried out on mutilated human heads leftover from the anatomy dissection classes. The heads were stored in preservative fluid between class sessions and were, of course, rather wet, distorted, and chemically malodorous. The actual practice, however, was realistic, as all suturing, cavity filling, feature forming, and cosmetizing were practiced just as on an actual case.

In 1948, at the Postgraduate Institute of Restorative Art of Chicago, the laboratory teaching system was modified by the recreation of dozens of mutilated heads in plastic and rubber, which permitted suturing, waxing, and cosmetizing. The school was headed by Dean Edward C. Johnson.

Before-and-after photos of a case handled by the faculty and students of the Simmons School in 1921 indicate good results. In 1924, Cincinnati College featured its postmortem plastic surgery laboratory in an advertisement for the first time. In 1926, Dhonau criticized fluid manufacturers for issuing diplomas in demisurgery to those in attendance at their free clinics. This was a throwback to 35 years earlier when fluid manufacturers were criticized for issuing diplomas to those attending their embalming clinics.

Virtually every issue of *Casket and Sunnyside* during the 1920s carried at least one feature article about demisurgery, whether a case history, before-and-after photos, new products for the demisurgeon, or editorial praise and commendation for the procedure. In 1925, an advertisement appeared announcing that Clyde E. Richardson of Paterson, New Jersey, was available for dermasurgical cases. It is believed that he was trained by Joel E. Crandall. The April 1, 1925, issue of *Casket and Sunnyside* had a four-page insert by the Eckels Chemical Company of Philadelphia on dermasurgery. The copy was a combination of a sales pitch for the Eckels Company's cosmetics, instruments, and other materials and technical advice on case treatment.

Three notorious criminals—John Dillinger, Bonnie Parker, and Clyde Barrow—died at the hands of law enforcement agents in July 1934. Dillinger, dead from bullet wounds in a Chicago alley, was taken to the Cook County morgue, where a Worsham College of Mortuary Science instructor, Don Asheworth, was requested to make a death mask of Dillinger for the FBI. As he worth related to the writers that he was visited by the FBI at 2 AM and that he was persuaded to hand over the extra mask.

Bonnie and Clyde were slain near Arcadia, Louisiana, and taken to a mortuary there. Both were embalmed in Louisiana, but Clyde was taken to the Sparkman–Holly–Brand Mortuary in Dallas, whereas Bonnie was taken to McKamy–Campbell Funeral Home, also in Dallas. Clyde, his head shattered, received more than 100 bullet or shotgun pellet wounds; Bonnie received more than 50 bullet wounds. Both bodies were restored and viewed in their respective caskets by approximately 50,000 people.

In 1936, Bruno Hauptmann, the convicted kidnapper and murderer of Charles A. Lindbergh's baby, was executed by electrocution. Reports of his preparation state that restorative art procedures were required to repair burns on his face and head. Services were private, however, and followed by cremation.

In the December 1926 issue of *Casket and Sunnyside* appeared the first advertisement for the electric-heated spatula, manufactured by the Montez Manufacturing Company, Addison, Michigan (Fig. 8). This device, highly touted when first developed as an excellent spatula to smooth and model wax as well as to reduce swollen areas, was less effective than anticipated. The heat of the iron had a tendency to melt wax and leave an unnaturally shiny surface. When used to reduce swelling, the device produced only a very minor evident reduction after much effort. Perhaps its best use was to "iron" tissue.

In August 1927, during the Minnesota 37th State Convention at St. Paul, the term "restorative art" was first used. The Worsham College advertisement of December 1927 used the term "restorative art" but later reverted to the term "dermasurgery." In 1929, the McAllister School listed Robert C. Harper as professor of restorative art. In November 1928, William G. Collier, Collier School, New

Figure 8. Early heated spatula used to smooth wax and reduce swollen facial tissues, circa 1926.

York City, stated in an address, "Any man can be taught the principles of this restorative art." It was to take some years, however, before the term *restorative art* was adopted and uniformly applied to the subject area first termed demisurgery by Joel E. Crandall in 1912.

By the mid-1920s, articles by teachers and practitioners of embalming on restorative art appeared with frequency in most professional journals and house organs of chemical manufacturers and supply companies. One such writer and practitioner was William G. Collier, a trade embalmer of New York City, who became a prolific author of articles on restorative art. Collier, scion of a well-established funeral service family, first appeared in print in *Casket and Sunnyside* in 1925 with an article on jaundice treatment. From that moment, he was a more or less regular contributor of articles dealing with treatment of facial cancer, decapitation, general demisurgical procedures, and cosmetics.

Collier founded both a school of embalming instruction and a shipping service in New York City and was the holder of several patents for restorative wound fillers and preformed facial features. Collier is remembered as a patient teacher, excellent speaker, and excruciating writer.

The Champion Company in March 1929 introduced the subject area to the readers of its house organ, *Champion Expanding Encyclopedia of Mortuary Practice*, with an article entitled "The Art of Plastic Surgery." Such articles by the supervising chemist, A. O. Spriggs, on a variety of subjects (e.g., treatment of gunshot cases, subcutaneous suture, and hypodermic injection of tissue filler cream), were assembled into a textbook in 1934, which is still available today under the title *Champion Restorative Art*.

As early as 1927, C. F. Callaway was lecturing, demonstrating, and writing on the subject of restorative

Figure 9. Photograph of Clarence G. Strub.

art. Callaway became a special representative of the Undertaker's Supply Company of Chicago and wrote many articles on plastic surgery for its house organ as well as trade publications. Ten years later, he was joined in these activities by Ralph Hensen, who later taught mortuary science subjects at the College of Mortuary Science at St. Louis, and by Clarence G. Strub (Fig. 9), whose last years in a long and distinguished professional career in

funeral service were spent with the University of Iowa as curator of the Anatomy Department of the Iowa Medical College eye enucleation training program. Strub's early contribution to restorative art was his publication of a small textbook of 32 pages entitled *The Principles of Restorative Art As the Embalmer Should Know Them* in 1932 (Fig. 10). The little text was extremely well written in a simple and direct style with emphasis on the practical application of technique, although it did embody some elements of theory. Taken as a whole, the book can be recognized as the true prototype of the best contemporary restorative art textbook.

The Dodge Chemical Company, during this period, also had a team of talented writers, lecturers, and demonstrators in the persons of Frank Stallard, a voluminous writer whose articles appeared for years in trade publications and the Dodge Chemical Company house organ, and Ray Slocum, a most popular embalming and restorative art demonstrator on the Dodge "faculty." Both Stallard and Slocum produced pamphlets of instruction on the subject of embalming and restorative art, which were much sought after and highly prized by practicing embalmers.

In 1945, *Casket and Sunnyside* inaugurated a monthly feature, "Restoration Clinic," by E. C. Johnson. Each monthly article described treatment for a particular type of case and was illustrated by before-and-after photographs of each case. The series continued monthly for more than 14 years.

The spring of 1931 was marked by the untimely death of one of the early full-time embalming college teachers of restorative art, Ivan P. Bowsher. Bowsher,

---

The Principles of Restorative Art
As the Embalmer Should Know Them

By

CLARENCE G. STRUB

Professor of Embalming and Plastic Surgery,
Hohenschuh-Carpenter College of Embalming, St. Louis, Mo.

Figure 10. Title page of Clarence G. Strub's book.

dying at age 33, was a World War I veteran who had graduated from Cincinnati College in the class of 1921. While a student at the college, he was recognized as a gifted artist and was invited to join the faculty, on graduation, as a teacher of restorative art. For 10 brief years, he gave the students of Cincinnati College one of the best courses of instruction in restorative art available. On his death, the college instituted the Ivan P. Bowsher Medal for outstanding achievement in restorative art to be awarded to one member of each graduating class. Cincinnati College had another outstanding teacher of restorative art, G. Joseph Prager, who with Dean C. O. Dhonau wrote an excellent textbook entitled *Manual of Restorative Art*, published in 1934. Prager continued and expanded the restorative art curriculum inaugurated by Bowsher and in 1955 published another textbook entitled *Post Mortem Restorative Art*.

An excellent book that deals with a very limited area of the field of restorative art, written by Gladys P. Curry of Boston in 1947, is titled *A Textbook of Facial Reconstruction*. Gladys Curry was an internationally recognized authority on the identification of the dead, and her expertise was often requested in disasters such as the infamous Coconut Grove nightclub fire, which claimed more than 500 victims, and the recovery of decomposing bodies of the crew members of the submarine *Squalus* lost in U.S. waters in 1939.

The Curry text is devoted solely to instruction in reconstruction of the soft tissues of the head and neck with clay or wax and is devoid of any instruction on or concern with the ordinary restorative problems or embalming of such cases. This text is highly recommended as an invaluable addition to an embalmer's library for reference on modeling and identification techniques.

The contemporary standard textbook on restorative art was written by the late Sheridan Mayer (Fig. 11), published as a lengthy treatise in 1940 and as a fully hardbound textbook in 1943 entitled simply *Restorative Art*. This work has gone through many revisions and is now used in most mortuary science college programs. Mayer also wrote the treatises *Workbook on Color* published in 1947 and *Mortuary Cosmetology* published in 1948. In 1973, he published the textbook *Color and Cosmetics*, which is in use in mortuary science college programs.

It is noteworthy and to his great credit that Mayer overcame the handicap of not being a practicing embalmer and yet was able to impart instruction intelligently. Mayer is one of the very few, if not the only, truly successful teachers who had never been a practicing embalmer.

His introduction to the teaching of restorative art was at a clinic at the Eckels College of Mortuary Science in Philadelphia, September 6–8, 1939, where he appeared on the program with the famed Covermark

Figure 11. Photograph of J. Sheridan Mayer.

cosmetic formulator Lydia O'Leary. His dynamic and informative presentation was so well received by all in attendance that he was offered a position on the faculty, which he accepted and retained until 1947.

In 1947, he joined the faculty of the Pittsburgh Institute of Mortuary Science, where he met Otto S. Margolis and formed an admiration for him. In 1951, when Margolis assumed control of the American Academy of Mortuary Science in New York City, Mayer accompanied him there to strengthen the faculty. The American Academy merged with the McAllister Institute in 1964.

Mayer has written extensively on the subject of cosmetics and restorative art and has written articles for many professional journals. His greatest contribution to the subject of restorative art, however, has been his influence and steady guidance of mortuary colleges toward the development and acceptance of a uniform course of instruction, as well as the adoption of uniform standards of facilities for such instruction and relevant examination questions. He has been the chairman of the restorative art course content committee of mortuary science schools and colleges for many years, where he accomplished monumental tasks in curriculum studies and syllabus preparation and screening of a bank of examination questions on the subject of restorative art. Mayer taught until 1975. In December of 1993, he died in Cincinnati, Ohio, where he had retired.

The words of A. Johnson Dodge, as so well stated in 1917, are still valid today: "How to care for mutilated bodies and make them presentable should constitute a part of the education of the embalmer. Thorough instruction in this difficult art should be given by instructors in our schools. But this part of the work required *special experience* and some study either to practice or teach it successfully."

One area of instruction in restorative art that has been recognized increasingly as a valuable practical working asset is the study of physical anthropology. Physical anthropology has been defined as a science that deals with the physical likenesses and differences of the races and sexes as well as the changes wrought by age and disease of humans. Such study has been most helpful in the practice of restorative art. It has been particularly invaluable in identification and reconstruction of skeletal remains. Study of skeletal remains can reveal sex, race, age, general height range, as well as individual characteristics such as right- or left-handedness, old trauma, (e.g., healed fractures), and diseases. Perhaps, the most interesting use of such knowledge is the reconstruction of the face on a fleshless skull.

The technique used today by experts such as Betty Catliff, assistant to Clyde Snow, physical anthropologist, retired Chief of the Federal Aviation Authority, Physical Anthropology Unit, at Norman, Oklahoma, is virtually identical to the original system devised by Wilhelm His of Leipzig University in Germany.

In brief, in 1895, His was compelled to devise a method of identifying a skull as to whether or not it and its associated bones were the remains of the renowned composer Johann Sebastian Bach. The bones had been disinterred from the church cemetery during enlargement of the church of St. John and a new more elaborate grave and monument for the remains, if indeed they were his, were planned. Proof of the identity was imperative.

His began assembling measurements of the key points from the numerous undissected cadavers in his laboratory. He recorded each point thickness for each corpse and then averaged these measurements to secure a single working measurement for each such point. He had small metal markers constructed, which were labeled A, B, and so on, to correspond with the tissue thickness at that point.

He secured the services of a well-known sculptor who agreed to undertake the project of reconstruction of the skull using the His technique. The metal markers were put in position on the skull and embedded in clay. When they were all correctly placed, strips of clay were applied connecting the points, and these in turn were interconnected. Finally, the vacant spaces were filled in and the features formed. The reconstructed skull appearance obtained closely resembled contemporary portraits and sculptures of Bach, and the committee for construction of the new tomb and monument was satisfied.

This technique has been updated from time to time by creating new tables, as His did, of females and other races. The technique has produced good results even by those using the procedure for the first time.

Through the years, special schools were founded to teach cosmetic application and restorative art. An example of such a school, unaffiliated with an existing school of mortuary science, was the Embalmers Graduate College formed in Chicago in 1937 by L. Roy Davenport and Honora D. Mannix, which offered 30 hours of instruction and practice in both cosmetology and restorative art.

Edward C. Johnson (1914–2000) was recognized nationally and internationally as an educator, writer, and demonstrator in the field of embalming and restorative art. He was born in Chicago in 1914 and worked for 66 years in funeral service throughout the greater Chicago area. He graduated in 1936 from the Worsham College of Mortuary Science in Chicago. He worked at this time for Oscar G. Merager, a Chicago undertaker. He developed an interest in restorative art. This was during a time when bodies were still embalmed in the home without gloves, in front of the family of the deceased!

Johnson taught embalming, restorative art, and the history of embalming at the Worsham College and served at its associate dean. Years later, he taught in the mortuary program at Malcolm X Community College in Chicago. Over his teaching career, he taught more than 10,000 students. He authored more than 650 scholarly articles on the history of embalming and American funeral service. In 1950, he was a major contributor to the National Funeral Directors Association publications, *Funeral Customs the World Over* and *The History of American Funeral Directing*.

In 1948, Professor Johnson organized the Postgraduate Institute of Restorative in Chicago. The curriculum included a short 2-week course and the standard 7-month course that offered 25 hours per week of instruction. When the school was merged into Worsham College in 1955, the course had been taken by 16 mortuary college restorative art instructors or their assistants.

Following his death, more than 90 boxes of books and educational materials were given by his family to the Museum of Funeral Customs in Springfield, Illinois. Edward Johnson was truly an indefatigable educator and practitioner in the fields of embalming, embalming history, and restorative art.

Restorative Art—Educational and In-Use Materials. Education of embalmers at all levels of skill in restorative art has been enhanced by the production of photographic records of actual restorative procedures. Some of these productions were in black and white, some in full color, some in motion, and others in still pictures. Most are silent and very few have either sound or voice accompaniment.

The truly classic motion picture on restorative procedures was produced in color in the early 1930s by the late Earle K. Angstadt (Fig. 12) of the Auman Funeral Home of Reading, Pennsylvania, who also performed all the actual restorative art techniques displayed in the

Figure 12. Photograph of Earle K. Angstadt.

film. The silent film has subtitles and is expertly photographed. It depicts classic technique, flawlessly performed, during the restoration of a surgically removed mandible, reduction of facial swelling, hypodermic tissue filling of face and hand, and replacement of eyelids and eyelashes damaged beyond salvage by an infection. This film, still available from the National Funeral Directors Association headquarters, will never be improved on.

Another much longer film recording many more cases of severe trauma was produced in the late 1930s by the late R. Victor Landig, founder of the Landig College of Mortuary Science at Houston. The photography of the 10 or 12 cases recorded on the film varies widely from poor to good, with respect to color fidelity, focus, and technique, whereas restorative skill is uniformly good except for the handling of hair restorations.

The Los Angeles College of Mortuary Science produced a fine color motion picture complete with sound and voice in the late 1940s. The film depicts no actual cases but does show how to produce plaster practice masks and provides excellent modeling instruction for producing the individual facial features. The Champion Company of Ohio has a motion picture in color made in the 1940s by A. O. Spriggs, featuring his technique in treating a small group of actual restorative cases. E. C. Johnson has slides recording the treatment of several hundred cases, including virtually every conceivable problem requiring restorative art treatment.

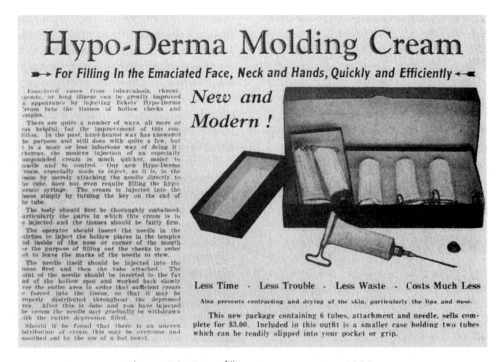

Figure 13. Tissue filler using cream, circa 1930.

Figure 14. Paasche Company's restorative art airbrush kit designed for embalmers' use.

Our profession desperately needs more visual aids such as the foregoing to provide wider exposure of our practitioners to successful techniques at conventions, meetings, seminars, and workshops.

In 1933, the Hydrol Chemical Company made a most significant announcement in the trade journals concerning the patenting of liquid tissue builder that coagulated or jelled on being hypodermically introduced into the body tissue. This, of course, was a vast improvement over ordinary liquids such as glycerin, then in use for this purpose, as such liquids, remaining liquid, tended to settle away from the high point in response to the pull of gravity. This failure of the hypodermically deposited material to maintain its position obviously ultimately destroyed the effect of such treatment.

Another equally vexatious problem resulting from the use of such permanent liquid-state tissue builders was the most disturbing occurrence of seepage from the point of insertion of the hypodermic needle. Both of these problems were corrected by the new jelling tissue builder as it would neither seep nor shift its position due to the change in its structure from liquid to semisolid to solid.

An alternative material such as hand cream or petroleum jelly had been used, but the technique for successful use required that both the filled syringe and the large-diameter needle be kept warm to permit a free flow of the semisolid material. Special hypodermic syringes with screw-threaded plungers were devised to make the ejection of thick creams easier, but they never did become very popular, and after introduction of coagulable liquid filler, they virtually disappeared from the market (Fig. 13).

In 1935, the Dodge Chemical Company introduced De-Ce-Co needle injector and needles as an improved means of securing mouth closure and in 1937 offered a complete set of eight specially designed restorative art instruments. In addition, the company, like many others, offered a complete range of cosmetics, waxes, and restorative art chemicals.

Methods of cosmetic application, but primarily application of highlight or accent cosmetics over waxed areas, had always required improvement. The difficulty in applying accent cosmetics evenly and naturally on waxed surfaces is a problem familiar to all experienced embalmers. The best solution is to apply the cosmetics

Figure 15. Master Nuance Aire-Tynt Unit.

with an airbrush or power sprayer. By these means, the cosmetics are literally floated into position, and disturbance of either the underlying base cosmetics or the wax surface is completely avoided.

As far back as 1911, spray applicators, powered by carbon dioxide cylinders, were available to the embalmer for cosmetic application, but it was not until the 1930s that the need and desire for sprayer-applied cosmetics became popular.

In 1934, the Undertaker's Supply Company announced the availability of the E-Z Way manually operated spray cosmetic applicator and a compatible cosmetic. The device was well received because it was most efficient and was generally conceded to be the best of the non-power-operated sprayers, many of which are still in use today.

In 1936, the Paasche Company of Chicago, a manufacturer of industrial and artistic airbrush equipment, offered a restorative art airbrush kit designed for embalmers' use (Fig. 14). The kit contained an electric-powered air compressor; an airbrush applicator of high quality; restorative art wax; cosmetic instruments; preformed features such as ears, nose, and lips; and an instruction pamphlet. The Nuance Aire-Tynt cosmetic applicator was advertised in 1937 by J. Horace Griggs of Amarillo, Texas (Fig. 15). The airbrush applicator could be adapted to apply cosmetics, whether powered by a manually operated pump, an electric-powered air compressor, or a carbonic gas cylinder.

Today many embalmers have been using, when the need arises, inexpensive easily available handheld model paint sprayers that are powered by small replaceable containers of Freon gas. These units, readily available in hobby shops, hardware stores, or paint stores, serve the purpose equally as well as the more expensive air compressor-powered sprayers (Fig. 16).

Restorative art was considered of sufficient importance in 1945 to have Richard G. Reichle, registrar of Worsham College, address the National Funeral Directors Association convention in Chicago on the continuing value and need for these procedures.

Now, as in the origin of the art, it is necessary for the individual embalmer, in charge of the case, to initiate the restoration of that case and to bring it to a successful conclusion. No amount of material, equipment, or training can substitute for the individual will and determination to overcome a most distressing case. The individual, now as always, is the key to success. The will to succeed and the ability to improvise are more often of value than any other asset.

It is therefore necessary that we in funeral service rededicate ourselves to the fulfillment, to the very best of our ability, of the American way—the funeral with the body present and viewable (Fig. 17).

Figure 16. Handheld model paint sprayer powered by small replaceable containers of Freon gas.

Figure 16. Robert G. Mayer (left) and Edward C. Johnson are instructors of embalming and restorative art. They are the primary authors of *Embalming: History, Theory, and Practice.*

▶ BIBLIOGRAPHY

Benkard E. *Undying Faces.* London: Hogurth Press, 1929. [A collection of death masks from the fifteenth century to the present]

Clarke CH. *Practical Embalming.* Cincinnati, OH: C. H. Clarke, 1917.

Crane EH. *Manual of Instruction to Undertakers,* 8th ed. Kalamazoo, MI: Kalamazoo, 1888.

Curry GP. *Facial Reconstruction.* Boston, MA, 1947.

Dhonau CO, Prager GJ. *Manual of Restorative Art.* Cincinnati, OH: Embalming Book Co., 1932.

Dodge AJ. *The Practical Embalmer.* Boston, MA: A. Johnson Dodge, 1908.

Dutra FR. Identification of person and determination of cause of death. *Archives of Pathology* 1944;38:339.

Eckles HS. *Derma Surgery.* Philadelphia, PA: H. S. Eckles, 1925.

Espy JB. *Espy's Embalmer.* Springfield, OH: Espy's Fluid Co., 1895.

Gerasimov MM. *The Face Finder.* Philadelphia, PA/New York, NY: Lippincott, 1971.

Gradwohl RBH. *Legal Medicine.* St. Louis, MO: C.V. Mosby, 1954.

His W. *Anatomische Forschungen über Johann Sebastian Bach's Gegeine und Antlitz Nebst Bermerkungen über dessin Bilder.* Leipzig: S. Hirzel, 1895.

Hooten EA. *Up from the Ape.* New York, NY: Macmillan, 1946.

Johnson EC. *Restorative Art.* Chicago, IL: Worsham College, 1948.

Krogman W. *A Guide to the Identification of Human Skeletal Material.* Washington, DC: FBI Law Enforcement Bulletin.

Krogman W. *The Human Skeleton in Forensic Medicine.* Springfield, IL: Charles C. Thomas, 1962.

Mayer JS. *Workbook on Color.* Philadelphia, PA: Westbrook Publishing Co., 1947.

Mayer JS. *Mortuary Cosmetology.* Philadelphia, PA: Westbrook Publishing Co., 1948.

Mayer JS. *Color and Cosmetics.* Bergenfield, NJ: Paul Publishing, 1973.

Mayer JS. *Restorative Art.* Dallas, TX: Professional Training Schools, 1993.

Michel G. *Scientific Embalmer.* Cleveland, OH, 1922.

Piombino-Mascali D, Williams MJ. Rosalia Lombardo and her master embalmer. *The Director,* July, 2009.

Quiring DP. "Skeletal identification." Address to Ohio State Coroners Association, May 23, 1951.

Reichle RG. "Practical problems in restorative art." Lecture National Funeral Directors Association 63rd Convention, Chicago, 1945.

Smith E, Dawson WR. *Egyptian Mummies.* New York, NY: Dial Press, 1924.

Spriggs AO. *Plastic Surgery,* 4th ed. Springfield, OH: Champion Chemical Co., 1946.

Stewart TD. *Essentials of Forensic Anthropology.* Springfield, IL: Charles C. Thomas, 1979.

Strub CG. The principles of restorative art. *Embalmer's Monthly,* 1932.

Wentworth B, Wilder HH. *Personal Identification.* Chicago, IL: T. G. Cooke Fingerprint, 1932.

PART

III

SELECTED READINGS AND
GLOSSARY

SECTION I
SELECTED READINGS

The following articles have been reprinted for extra research and information:

1. Summary of Guidelines Submitted to OSHA from the National Funeral Directors Association Committee on Infectious Disease (Summer, 1989)
2. Armed Services Specification for Mortuary Services (Care of Remains of Deceased Personnel and Regular and Port of Entry Requirements for Caskets and Shipping Cases). Appendix D Federal Acquisition Regulation AR 638-2.9, February 1996
3. Identification: An Essential Part of What We Do, by Michael Kubasak (2002)
4. *The Mathematics of Embalming Chemistry: Part I. A Critical Evaluation of "One Bottle" Embalming Claims,* by Jerome F. Frederick (1968)
5. The Measurement of Formaldehyde Retention In the Tissues of Embalmed Bodies, by John Kroshus, Joseph McConnell, Jay Bardole (1983)
6. The Two Year Fix: Long-Term Preservation for Delayed Viewing, by Kerry Don Peterson (1992)
7. Occupational Exposure to Formaldehyde in Mortuaries, by L. Lamont Moore and Eugene C. Ogrodnik (1986)
8. The Strange Case of Dr. Jekyll and Formaldehyde (Is It Good or Evil), by Maureen Robinson (2009)
9. The Preparation Room: Ventilation, by Jack Adams, CFSP (2004)
10. Risk of Infection and tracking of work-related infectious diseases in the funeral industry, by Susan Salter Davidson and William H. Benjamin, Jr. (2006)
11. Creutzfeldt-Jakob Disease, by Ruth Carrico, Christian Davis Furman, Curtis Rostad and Dorothy Cannan Hyde (2005)
12. Hepatitis From A to G, by Kim Collison (1999)
13. The Increase in MRSA and VRE, by Mike Cloud, Jr. (1999)
14. The Antimicrobial Activity of Embalming Chemicals and Topical Disinfectants on the Microbial Flora of Human Remains, by Peter A. Burke and A. L. Sheffner (1976)
15. The Microbiologic Evaluation and Enumeration of Postmortem Specimens from Human Remains, by Gordon W. Rose and Robert N. Hockett (1970)
16. Professional Hair Care for Human Remains, by Darla A. Tripoli (2010)
17. Management Techniques for the Eyes, by Vernie R. Fountain (2005)
18. Enhance Emaciated Features Arterially Using Split Injection and Restricted Drainage, by Sharon L. Gee (2005)
19. Embalming—United Kingdom and European, by Peter J. Ball (2005)
20. The Art of Embalming and Its Purpose, by Ron Hast (2006)

Summary of Guidelines Submitted to OSHA from the National Funeral Directors Association Committee on Infectious Disease (Summer, 1989)

PUBLIC HEALTH PRECAUTIONARY REQUIREMENTS AND STANDARDS

I. Background. Prevention of the transmission of recognized classical and/or opportunistic pathogens from human remains to the embalmer, from the embalmer to his or her family, and to the families and friends of the deceased is a reasonable public health expectation.

Many of the infectious agents associated with medical and paramedical environments are classified as "opportunistic" pathogens or microbial agents considered to be of lower or reduced virulence. The increasing association of "opportunistic" pathogens with symptomatic infectious diseases has all but eliminated the reference to the category "nonpathogen."

The implementation of minimum professional practice standards in embalming is necessary to provide a standard of quality control and quality assurance in the preservation and disinfection of human remains. It is important that when embalming is performed, a significant measure of uniformity of professional skills will be employed by all funeral service practitioners.

Following somatic or functional death, normally structurally intact epithelial, facial, and other tissue barriers undergo a loss of structural integrity and permit the bodywide translocation and distribution of systemic microflora and create alternate body fluid and body tissue reservoir sites of host contamination.

During life, the body fluids or body secretions most frequently associated with the transmission of potentially infectious doses or densities are quite definable. After death, this is no longer true. All body fluids and body tissues may become reservoirs of infectious agents within a relatively short postmortem interval.

Cellular death may not be complete for up to 12 hours after somatic or functional death. During this postmortem interval, the viability and potential infectivity of blood-borne viruses, for example, HIV and hepatitis B, may persist, and the exiting of the agents from any body opening, natural or artificial, may occur.

Funeral service practitioners normally have more than casual contact with parenteral (including open wound) and mucous membrane exposure to blood and body tissues. Such individuals occupationally exposed to blood, body fluid, or tissues can be protected from the recognized risks of blood-borne agents such as HIV and HBV (hepatitis B virus) by imposing barriers in the form of engineering controls, work practices, in-service training, and protective equipment and attire.

II. Recommendations. It is recommended that every funeral service firm/facility in the United States adopt the following policies and guidelines for implementation: (1) public health guidelines, (2) personnel health precautions for the prevention of blood-borne microbial agent(s) and infections, and (3) minimum standards for the embalming and disinfection of human remains. The recommendations and guidelines within each of the three categories described above are as follows.

1. PUBLIC HEALTH GUIDELINES

A. Care of the Human Remains. Thoroughly cleanse and disinfect the body surface and natural or artificial body orifices/body openings with a suitable EPA-registered, hospital, or health care facility acceptable agent, for example, tuberculocidal, germicidal detergent. The tuberculocidal germicidal detergent, for example, a phenylphenol or a third-generation quaternary ammonium compound complex, should be an EPA-registered product offering confirmatory evidence of all label claims, including the recommended use dilution. The disinfected body surfaces should be thoroughly rinsed following a minimum of a 10-minute exposure interval.

Injection and drainage procedures should include (1) multisite injection and drainage procedures, (2) intermittent or restricted drainage, (3) the use of a 3.0% v/v formaldehyde-base arterial injection solution or a 2.0% glutaraldehyde-base solution, and (4) the use of 1 pint of concentrated cavity chemical per major or primary body cavity, for example, abdominal, pelvic, and thoracic, or 1 pint of concentrated cavity chemical per 50 pounds of body weight.

B. The Embalmer (Universal Precautions). This category of barrier attire utilization and precautions has replaced the health care facility category of Blood and Body Fluid Precautions. The category requires the *minimum* barrier attire utilization of a whole body gown or apron and gloves. The wraparound, moisture-repellent, or moisture-proof gown or apron of rubber, plastic, or

impregnated fabric is considered to be disposable or a single-use barrier attire item. The same is true for the gloves. Double rubber or plastic gloves are recommended for funeral service personnel.

This minimum standard of barrier attire protection is to be employed in the preparation of *all* human remains, no matter what the indicated cause of death reported. The risk of blood and body fluid exposure is significantly high for all funeral service personnel, and frequently, the infectious disease status of the deceased is unknown. Therefore, it is recommended that all persons performing postmortem procedures consider the use of additional barrier attire items such as protective eyewear, oral–nasal masks, and shoe and head covers.

Hands should be thoroughly scrubbed, using an EPA-registered* medicated liquid soap, before and after gloving. If a glove is penetrated by a sharp or the uneven edge of a bone, the glove is to be removed and replaced as soon as possible.

All instruments employed during the embalming should be sterilized or disinfected prior to reuse. A high-level disinfecting liquid immersant may be employed in lieu of a steam sterilizer if the latter is not available. Chemical germicidal detergents registered with EPA as "cold chemical sterilants" can be used either for sterilization or for high-level disinfection, depending on the interval or contact.

C. Air Handling Within the Environment "at Risk." An efficient air supply and air exhaust system or an air purification system must be operative within the embalming environment. The air handling system should protect the embalmer from a hazardous airborne density of biologic particulates as well as from the accumulation of formaldehyde monomers exceeding 0.75 ppm, the permissible exposure limit or 8-hour time-weighted average (TWA) concentration. The TWA "action level" is 0.5 ppm of formaldehyde monomer concentration.

D. Terminal Disinfection and Decontamination. All instruments, horizontal surfaces such as floor, operating table, sink, and countertop, waste receptacles, and any other surface in direct or indirect contact with the preparation site must be cleansed and disinfected upon removal of the human remains from the preparation environment.

All instruments, including trocars and venous drainage tubes, must either be steam sterilized or immersed in a suitable cold chemical sterilant. *Note:* The use of a hypochlorite, 1000 to 5000 ppm, may be used for the "spot" disinfection of body fluid spills on hard, nonporous surfaces. However, immediate rinsing is necessary to prevent the formation of BCME (bischloromethyl

---

*For example, *para*-Chloro-*meta*-xylenol (PCMX) or chlorhexidene gluconate (CHG) biocidal additive.

ether), a confirmed carcinogen, in the presence of formaldehyde monomers.

E. Solid Waste Management. Potentially infective, contaminated solid wastes associated with the preparation of human remains should be placed in "alert" colored plastic bags, for example, red, the bag twist-closed and securely tied prior to ultimate disposition. Local codes permitting bulk blood and suctioned/aspirated fluids may be carefully drained into the sanitary sewer system, and vacuum breakers must be installed on all involved water lines to prevent the back-siphoning of contaminated liquids into potable water supply lines.

F. Hearse/First Call Vehicles. Cleanse and disinfect all mortuary cots or trays following exposure to the unembalmed human remains. Employ cleansed and disinfected cot or tray covers for each transfer of unembalmed human remains from the home or from the health care facility to the preparation room. Cleanse and sanitize the internal horizontal surfaces of the hearse/first call vehicle following the transfer of the remains to the preparation room.

G. Funeral Service Personnel Health Recommendations.

1. Annual physical examination
2. Annual TB skin testing
3. Immunizations—annual influenza, single-dose/single-series Pneumovax, hepatitis B, Rubella vaccine—are recommended for all women of pregnancy age if not protected and for all male employees because they can transmit to the female employee.

2. PERSONNEL HEALTH PRECAUTIONS FOR PREVENTION OF BLOOD-BORNE AGENT(S) AND INFECTIONS

A. Removal/Transfer of Human Remains.

1. Removal personnel (licensees, resident trainees, nonlicensees, and nonresident trainees)—disposable whole-body barrier attire and plastic or rubber gloves.
2. Avoid contact with covering of remains at sites of body fluid or exudative contamination. Place the remains in an impervious plastic whole-body pouch and effect zipper closure.
3. Sanitize the transfer vehicle following the transfer of remains to the preparation room.

B. Transfer of the Remains to the Preparation Room, Using a Team of Two Employees. Transfer the pouched remains to the preparation room table, open pouch, and loosen body coverings. Allow the body coverings to fall into the pouch. Carefully position the remains from side to side for the careful removal of the pouch and contents. Dispose of the pouch and contents as contaminated solid wastes.

C. Terminal Disinfection

1. Disinfect all horizontal inanimate surfaces in direct or indirect contact with preparation site.
2. Sterilize or disinfect all instruments by cold chemical sterilizer immersion or by steam sterilization.
3. Remove all barrier attire items, place in plastic bag, and treat as contaminated solid wastes in terms of final disposition.
4. Scrub ungloved hands and wrists with a medicated liquid soap preparation, preferably one that is recommended as a health care personnel hand wash.
5. Complete whole-body bathing or showering and shampooing prior to return to home or office.

3. MINIMUM STANDARDS FOR THE EMBALMING AND DISINFECTION OF HUMAN REMAINS.

The following professional profile of standards for embalming practices and procedures is based on laboratory evaluations and post-embalming observations.

A. Multiple-Site Injection and Drainage. Multiple-site (two or more) injection and drainage procedures assure a more consistent distribution and ultimate diffusion of the disinfection and preservation chemicals to all receptive tissue sites, deep and superficial. This will more consistently provide public health protection as expected from the thorough preparation of human remains for ultimate disposition.

B. Rate of Flow of Arterial Injection Chemicals. A moderate rate of flow, 12 to 15 minutes per gallon of arterial injection solution, accompanied by a sufficient arterial injection pressure to maintain the desired rate of flow, 2 to 10 psi, are recommended for the assurance of distribution and diffusion of the arterial injection chemicals.

C. Intermittent or Restricted Drainage. This method of venous drainage should produce maximum preservation and disinfection. It is considered to be one of the most effective procedures for the assurance of adequate distribution of arterial injection solution(s). It is especially recommended following the removal of surface discolorations.

D. Total Volume of Arterial Injection Solution Employed. Consideration should be given to the use of a minimum of 3 to 4 gallons of arterial injection solution in adult remains weighing 125 to 175 pounds. Injection and drainage procedures may involve the removal of 4 to 6 quarts of body fluids. To properly restore the loss of body fluids and overcome the loss, through drainage, of arterial injection chemicals, it becomes necessary to employ the recommended volume of arterial injection solution, for example, 1 gallon per 50 pounds of body weight, exclusive of the primary injection solution(s) volume.

E. Use of Supplemental Injection Chemicals. The enhancement of the arterial distribution of the arterial injection solution may often require the use of supplemental additives, for example, modifying and surface tension-reducing additives and water softeners. The use of such additives may increase the efficacy of injection solution distribution as well as the efficacy of venous drainage.

F. Concentration (%) of Preservative/Disinfecting Chemicals in the Arterial Injection Solution. Laboratory investigative data indicate that the percent of formaldehyde v/v in the formaldehyde-base arterial injection solution should not be less than 2.0. Formaldehyde concentrations ranging from 2.3 to 3.0% v/v will inactivate resident bacterial densities 95% or more. Formaldehyde concentrations less than 2.0%, for example, 1.0% v/v, may produce expected tissue fixation, but may not produce the desired level of microbial inactivation. Significant reduction in the endogenous microbial populations should always exceed 70% if public health expectations are to be fulfilled on a consistent basis.

Formaldehyde is categorized as an "intermediate" to a "high-level" chemical disinfectant when employed in concentrations ranging from 3.0 to 8.0% v/v. The recommended use of a minimum 2.0% v/v concentration of formaldehyde is based on this categorization as well as investigative data.

G. Cavity Chemical Utilization. Following the thorough treatment of the thoracic, abdominal, and pelvic cavities, including the aspiration of liquids and semisolids from nonautopsied remains, the injection of 1 pint (16 oz) of undiluted cavity chemical into each of the three trocar-prepared cavities is recommended. In remains weighing in excess of 150 to 200 pounds, it is recommended that the embalmer use 1 pint of concentrated cavity chemical per 50 pounds of body weight. The weight of the body viscera may approximate 15% of the total body weight. The chemically targeted hollow and solid organ tissues require maximal chemical contact following the trocar penetration and separation to ensure the prevention of the microbial generation of putrefactive activity, including body opening purge.

III. Administration. The funeral home owner/manager/employer should establish formal policies and procedures to ensure that all job-related tasks that involve an inherent potential for mucous membrane or skin contact with blood, body fluids, or tissues, or a potential for spills or splashes of blood or body fluids, will require appropriate preventive/protective measures. These preventive measures would be applicable to licensed, nonlicensed, resident trainee, and nonresident trainee personnel. Engineering controls, work practices, and protective barrier attire are critical to minimize exposure to HBV, HIV, and other blood- and body fluid–

transmitted microbial agents and to prevent infection(s). It is essential that the funeral home employee be fully aware of the reasons for the required preventive measures. Therefore, employee education programs must be implemented to assure familiarity with applicable work practices.

The employer should establish the following formal policies:

1. Develop and provide in-service training programs for all employees whose responsibilities include the direct or indirect exposure(s) to blood, body fluids, or tissues.
2. Document the attendance of employees at all scheduled and announced in-service training programs. The in-service training course content should include the approved Standard Operating Procedures (SOPs) for embalming practices and the required items of protective equipment and personnel barrier attire items.
3. Assure the convenient availability of all items of protective equipment and barrier attire items.
4. Surveillance of the workplace to ensure that the required work practices are being observed and that the protective barrier attire items and equipment are conveniently available and properly used.
5. Investigation of known or suspected parenteral exposures to body fluids or tissues to establish the conditions associated with the exposure and to improve training, work practices, or preventive equipment to prevent a recurrence.

IV. Training and Education. As recommended under the heading "Administration," the employer must establish an initial and periodic training program for all employees who may sustain direct or indirect exposure to blood, body fluids, or tissues. The employee must understand the following as a result of adequate in-service training:

1. Modes of transmission of HBV, HIV, and other blood- and body fluid–transmitted microbial agents.
2. The basis for the employment of the types of protective equipment and items of barrier attire.
3. The location of protective equipment and items of barrier attire, the procedures for the proper use of same and for the removal, decontamination, and disposition of contaminated barrier attire items or equipment.
4. The corrective actions necessary to disinfect blood and body fluid spills or splashes.
5. Concurrent and terminal disinfection and decontamination procedures. Disposable, puncture-resistant containers are to be employed for used needles, blades, and so on.

V. Work Practices.

1. Work practices should be developed on the assumption that all body fluids and tissues are infectious.
2. Provision must be made for the safe removal, handling, decontamination, and disposition of protective clothing items, equipment, soiled linens, and so on.
3. Work practices and SOPs should provide guidance on procedures to follow in the event of spills or personal exposure to fluids or tissues.

VI. Personal Protective Equipment. A required minimum of choice of barrier attire items or protective equipment should be specified by the firm's SOPs. As more departments of public health require the reporting of infectious disease causes of death by category of precautions implemented by the health care facility, it becomes increasingly important for the funeral service firm to be aware of the infectious diseases included in a given category or patient isolation precautions. The following is a recommended listing of barrier attire items that should be employed for a reported category of health care patient isolation precautions:

Category-Specific Health Care Facility Precautions	Recommended Funeral Service Personnel Barrier Precautions Attire
1. Strict precautions	Masks (face covers), gowns, gloves (double plastic or rubber gloves are recommended), head covers, shoe covers, eye protectors
2. Contact precautions	Gowns, gloves, shoe covers
3. Respiratory precautions	Masks, gowns, gloves, head covers, shoe covers
4. Enteric precautions	Gowns, gloves, shoe covers
5. Blood and body fluid or **universal precautions**	Gowns, gloves, masks, head covers, shoe covers, eye protectors

VII. Medical. The employer should make available, at no cost to the employee, the voluntary HBV immunization for all employees whose responsibilities involve the direct or indirect exposure to blood, body fluids, or tissues. The employer should also provide for the monitoring, at the request of the employee, for HBV or HIV antibodies following known or suspected parenteral exposure to blood, body fluids, or tissues.

VIII. Record Keeping. The employer should require the completion of a case report for the preparation of all re-

mains. Each case report should include (1) health care facility reporting of category of patient isolation precautions implemented, if applicable; (2) sites of injection and drainage employed; (3) volumes and concentrations of arterial injection and cavity treatment chemicals; (4) protective equipment and barrier attire items employed; (5) preembalming appearance and condition of the remains; and (6) any other observations or procedure relating to the public health status of the remains.

Armed Services Specification for Mortuary Services (Care of Remains of Deceased Personnel and Regular and Port of Entry Requirements for Caskets and Shipping Cases). Appendix D, Federal Acquisition Regulation AR 638-2.9, February 1996.

D-1. (1) Scope. (1.1.) This specification (in two parts) establishes minimum standards for the care and handling of deceased personnel. It encompasses professional services and requirements, caskets and shipping cases, transportation, and hygienic practices. This specification is applicable to regular and port of entry requirements.

SECTION I REMAINS

D-2. (2) Classification. a. (2.1) Remains defined. Autopsied (partial or complete) or unautopsied remains are defined as one of the following types.

b. (2.1.1) Nonviewable. Any remains where there exists extreme mutilation, advanced stages of decomposition, or severe burn wounds or charring and restoration of viewable exposed tissue surfaces to the known antemortem appearance of the deceased by restorative art is not possible, for example, floater, homicidal, suicidal, and major trauma cases.

c. (2.1.2) Viewable. Any remains (1) undamaged by trauma or disease or (2) remains damaged by trauma or disease, but the viewable tissue surfaces are restored to the known antemortem appearance of the deceased by restorative art work.

d. (2.1.3) Casket. The standard and oversize 18-gauge metal, sealer, cut-top casket shall be used for viewable and nonviewable adult remains.

D-3. (3) Applicable Documents. (3.1) There are no applicable documents to this part of this specification.

D-4. (4) Services. a. (4.1) General. The contractor shall be responsible for providing professional services of the highest quality to assure viewing of the remains under optimal conditions. The contractor shall practice hygienic measures that will assure complete and satisfactory disinfection and sanitation of the funeral establishment.

b. (4.2) Processing or reprocessing remains. See the following paragraphs.

c. (4.2.1) Processing of remains. The complete preservation (embalming) and disinfection, application of restorative art techniques and/or cosmetics, dressing and/or wrapping, casketing, and transportation of remains as directed by the contracting officer or his designee.

d. (4.2.2) Reprocessing of remains. The inspection and correction of all discrepancies noted in preservation (embalming). Application of restorative art techniques and cosmetics, dressing and wrapping, casketing, and transportation of remains as directed by the contracting officer or his designee.

e. (4.2.3) Unidentified remains. If identification of the remains is not officially established, the remains shall be placed under refrigeration at 38 to 40°F (3.3–4.4°C). If mechanical refrigeration is not available within a reasonable distance, ice chests or ice packs shall be used in lieu of the mechanical refrigeration. Processing (embalming) shall not be accomplished until the remains are released by a responsible official as identified.

f. (4.2.4) Restorative art. Major restorative art is an integral part of the processing and/or reprocessing of remains. It shall include, but not be limited to, rebuilding a large wound; rebuilding of facial features such as ear, nose, eye, mouth, chin, and so forth; removal of damaged tissue followed by restoration; restoration of scalp hair; and the application of cosmetics to render restored surfaces undetectable. Restorative art shall be accomplished in accordance with the highest professional standards.

g. (4.2.5) Chemical preservative preparations. Under this armed services specification, arterial, cavity, and other embalming chemicals used in the treatment of all remains shall effect the maximum preservation and disinfection of all body tissue, including that associated with body cavities (organs).

h. (4.2.6) Standards and techniques. The contractor shall provide high-quality service and a sufficient number of licensed embalmers to process (embalm) or reprocess any remains under this armed services specification on a timely basis. Interns (apprentices) may be used to assist the licensed embalmer in accordance with applicable state regulations. All supplies and technical procedures shall conform to standards and professional techniques acceptable to the funeral service industry. Embalmers shall utilize any and all optional techniques

available to assure complete and adequate treatment of remains.

D-5. (5) Treatment of Remains. a. (5.1) General. Frequently, final disposition of processed or reprocessed remains may not be effected for a period of 10 days or more; remains may be transported over long distances or subjected to hot, humid conditions. At all times, the remains must be free of putrefaction and infectious agents. This requires the thorough disinfection and uniform preservation of all body tissues. Employment of continuous injection and intermittent drainage will enhance chemical distribution and penetration. Use of humectants (moisture retention chemicals) in the arterial injection solution will help to achieve greater tissue penetration and to restore normal body moisture content.

b. (5.1.1) Preembalming procedures. The following basic steps shall be accomplished in the course of processing or reprocessing of all viewable remains and, to the extent possible, nonviewable remains.

c. (5.1.2) Washing and grooming. When possible, remains shall be bathed; male facial and scalp hair shall be washed and groomed to conform to military standards (suitable hair preparations shall be accomplished on females). Fingernails shall be cleaned and trimmed. The mouth shall be securely closed to form a natural expression and proper attention given to the eyes to prevent wrinkling of the eyelids and sunken appearance of the eyes. Cosmetics shall be applied only in the amount necessary to produce natural color and texture.

d. (5.1.3) Wounds and stains. All lacerations, abrasions, incisions, excisions, and burn wounds shall be sutured or sealed to prevent leakage. Swollen or distorted features shall be reduced to the normal contours enjoyed during life. Postmortem stains shall be chemically bleached by applying packs and/or needle injection. On viewable areas, further treatment shall consist of the use of masking cosmetics to render stains nondetectable.

e. (5.1.4) Body orifices and injured tissue. All body orifices shall be treated with a disinfectant nonastringent chemical (generic categories such as phenylphenols and iodophors) and then packed with cotton. Bedsores and ulcerated, burned, and necrotic tissue shall be treated either by hypodermic injection or by pack application of a deodorizing and preserving chemical.

f. (5.1.5) Insecticide treatment. Maggots and other insect larvae shall be destroyed and their breeding sites in or on the remains thoroughly treated with an insecticide chemical.

g. (5.1.6) Contractor's performance. The contractor's performance shall be such that all remains are effectively disinfected and uniformly preserved and that all offensive odors are eliminated before the remains are casketed.

D-6. (6) Preparation of Remains. *a. (6.1) General.* The military services require that all remains be processed or reprocessed in a manner reflecting the highest standards of the funeral service profession. Each remains, viewable and nonviewable, requires variation in the embalming treatment to accomplish the optimum results. A recommended procedure to achieve these goals is the injection of the solution at a moderate rate. The addition of a humectant to the solutions is also helpful in reducing overdehydration effects.

b. (6.1.1) Processing nonviewable remains. In all instances, multisite injection and drainage technique shall be attempted. When arterial injection is possible, each gallon of arterial fluid shall have a minimum concentration of 5% by volume aldehyde or aldehyde derivative preservative agents. The total volume of arterial solution injected shall be not less than 1 gallon per 50 pounds of body weight. All body areas shall be further treated by means of a trocar using undiluted cavity chemicals having a 30-index (percent) or greater. In addition, packs, special gel, and dry sanitizers shall be used, as required, to assure preservation, prevent leakage, and eliminate all offensive odor. Cranial, thoracic, and abdominal cavities, when present, shall be relieved of gases and distention. The cavities shall then be treated by injecting a minimum of 32 oz of a concentrated cavity chemical, having a 30-index (percent) or greater. When arterial injection or cavity treatment is impossible, all articulated and disarticulated anatomical portions shall be thoroughly disinfected and preserved via accessory chemical embalming techniques. Noninjectable intact remains and disarticulated anatomical portions shall be immersed or hypo injected with trocar or syringe and needle, using full strength cavity chemicals of 30-index (percent) or greater. Surface application of liquid, gel, or dry sanitizers and preservatives is also required to supplement primary needle or hypo injection techniques.

c. (6.1.2) Processing viewable remains. A thorough pre-embalming case analysis shall be made in order to determine the best embalming techniques to be used to obtain optimum results. The technique of arterial injection and venous drainage is of utmost importance as well as the need for adding humectants (moisture retention chemicals) to the arterial solution injected. Whenever possible, a six-point arterial injection with multisite drainage shall be accomplished. The arterial chemical injection solution shall contain a 2 to 3% concentration, by volume, of aldehyde or aldehyde derivative preservative agents, with equal parts of a humectant chemical also being added to the injection solution. The thoracic, abdominal, and pelvic cavities shall be thoroughly aspirated and injected with full strength cavity chemicals having a 30-index (percent) or greater, using a minimum of 16 oz for each cavity. In addition, needle injections, packs, or other special treatment shall be accomplished, as required, to assure the preservation and disinfection of all body tissues including those associated with body cavities (organs). A lanolin-base (or comparable) massage cream shall be applied on the face and the hands.

d. (6.1.3) Autopsied remains. If a partial or complete autopsy has been performed, a six-point injection with multisite drainage shall be accomplished, using arterial chemical injection solutions as specified for processing viewable remains. Thoracic and abdominal walls shall be hypoinjected using the same strength solution as injected arterially. On thoracic and abdominal autopsies, the viscera shall be removed and immersed in concentrated cavity chemical having a 30-index (percent) or greater. When a cranial autopsy has been performed, the calvarium shall be replaced and securely stabilized. The scalp shall be replaced over the calvarium and neatly sutured to avoid an unnatural appearance and the hair shall be washed. The inner surfaces of the body cavities shall be given a liberal application of gel preservative, the organs replaced within the cavities in normal anatomical location, and liberally covered with hardening compound.

e. (6.1.4) Treatment of scalp (viewable remains). When the scalp has been shaved because of medical treatment or surgery, processing or reprocessing shall be accomplished as specified for viewable remains, after which the head shall then be wrapped with gauze or equivalent in a neat and professional manner.

f. (6.1.5) Mutilated hands (viewable remains). When the hands are mutilated so that restoration is not possible, the hands shall be treated in a manner that shall render all tissue firm, dry, and thoroughly preserved. The hands will then be covered either by wrapping with gauze or equivalent in a neat and professional manner or by placing surgical gloves on the hands followed by white (military) gloves.

g. (6.1.6) Dressing remains, including intact nonviewable. Remains shall be dressed in the clothing provided by the contracting officer. Nonviewable remains that cannot be dressed shall be wrapped in the rubber or polyethylene sheeting and blanket furnished by the contracting officer. Wrapping shall be accomplished as follows: A blanket, furnished by the contracting officer, shall be spread on the dressing table with opposing corners at the head and the foot ends of the table. The blanket is then covered with a white cotton sheet followed by a sheet of polyethylene. Two strips of cotton are laid down the center of the plastic sheet and liberally sprinkled with hardening compound. The remains are then laid on the cotton strips, coated with hardening compound, and covered with additional cotton strips. The polyethylene sheet is then wrapped around the remains. The white cotton sheet is then wrapped around the plastic sheathed remains followed by the blanket that shall have as few creases as possible and be secured with large safety pins placed no more than 8 inches apart.

h. (6.1.7) Embalmer Evaluation. The embalmer (contractor's agent) processing or reprocessing the remains shall critically evaluate the completed treatment to ensure that any remains cared for under this contract are effectively disinfected, uniformly preserved, and shall arrive at destination in a satisfactory condition. The contracting officer or designate will authorize delivery or shipment of remains when he is assured that the services and supplies furnished by the contractor meet this specification. The contractor shall state on a certificate (Preparation Room History) furnished by the contracting officer that the services and supplies meet this specification in its entirety.

i. (6.1.8) Placement in casket. Remains shall be placed in the casket in a manner that will create an appearance of rest and composure and to ensure maintenance of position during transit. When remains are to be shipped, pads will be placed around the remains to prevent shifting. The pillow shall be turned over and a clean piece of cloth placed over the face. The casket shall be of sufficient size to prevent the appearance of crowding and cramping the remains.

j. (6.1.9) Quality assurance evaluation. Failure to pass inspector's evaluation after placement of remains in a casket and before delivery will require the contractor to remove remains from the casket and perform one or more of the following services as directed by the contracting officer or his designate: (1) additional disinfective or preservative treatment; (2) redressing; (3) change or add decorations or insignia; and (4) place remains in new casket. When services mentioned in this paragraph are performed, services as set forth in paragraphs 6.1.6, 6.1.8, and 6.1.10 shall again be performed by the contractor.

k. (6.1.10) Encasing casket. The casket shall be carefully and professionally placed in the protective *outer* container, as directed by the contracting officer. All shipping documents will be affixed or enclosed.

l. (6.1.11) Loading remains. The remains shall be carefully and professionally placed in the type of vehicle designated by the contracting officer for the delivery of remains.

D-7. Transportation of Remains. *a. (7.1) Removal of remains.* Transport remains in a suitable funeral coach, ambulance, or service car to the place where processing or reprocessing is performed. This transportation shall include calling at the place where death occurs or remains are located when such place is on the activity(ies) or any place designated by the contracting officer or his designate.

b. (7.2) Escorted delivery. Delivery of remains, including escort in:

(1) (*a*) Contractor's funeral coach to a place of religious service and then to a common carrier, another funeral home, or to a government or nongovernment cemetery.

(2) (*b*) Contractor's funeral coach shall arrive at any location at the time specified by the contracting officer.

c. (7.3) Rail or air delivery. Remains being shipped by common carrier shall be delivered to airport or rail terminal not later than 2 hours before scheduled departure of aircraft or train.

d. (7.4) Escort attire. Personnel used in transportation of the remains or escort, off the installation, shall be dressed in a seasonal suit with shirt and tie. Other vehicle operators may wear clean cotton twill matching shirt and trousers in dark or neutral colors.

D-8. Cremation. *a. (8.1) Cremation.* This paragraph explains services, supplies, and transportation for local cremation when called for by the contracting officer or designated representative. Remains shall be prepared, dressed, and cosmetized as prescribed in these specifications. The casket provided shall meet or exceed the armed services hardwood casket specification. Transportation of the remains (including escort and escort's return) shall be provided to the crematory engaged under contract by the government and return of cremated remains to the government facility. The contracting officer or designated representative shall specify whether a bronze or hardwood urn is to be provided. The contractor shall provide an urn that meets or exceeds the applicable urn specification. The urn shall be engraved (the urn itself shall be engraved if a bronze urn or if a hardwood urn, the specified engraving plate shall be engraved) with the name, rank, date of birth, and date of death of the deceased. The contractor will place all the cremated remains received from the crematory in the urn.

Note. Cremation charges will be paid by the government directly to the crematory engaged by the government.

b. (8.2) Processing procedure. Following the preparation, dressing, and cosmetizing of the remains according to these specifications, the contractor shall attach to the right ankle of the deceased or to the top of the blanket, when remains are wrapped, and to the casket handle at the head end of the casket a tag exhibiting the decedent's name, rank, social security number, and date of death. The contractor shall deliver the casketed remains to the crematory in sufficient time to ensure cremation is accomplished and completed on the same day as delivery to the crematory. The contractor shall return the cremated remains to the funeral service establishment or port mortuary facility not later than the day following cremation for inurnment in the designated urn. The cremated remains shall be inurned promptly upon return to the contractor's facility or port mortuary facility.

D-9. Hygienic Practices. *a. Concurrent and terminal disinfection and decontamination.* The contractor shall employ protective, precautionary hygienic measures and techniques designated to accomplish concurrent and terminal disinfection and decontamination of the entire funeral service establishment or port of entry mortuary preparation room and shipping area environment. The application of appropriate in-use concentrations of chemical disinfectants (generic categories such as phenyphenols or iodophors) to body surfaces and orifices, instruments, preparation room, floor, walls, and equipment surfaces and general sanitation of public visitation areas (as applicable) will help prevent the transmission of actual and potential pathogens to personnel.

b. Inhalation protection. Also recommended is the wearing of a protective surgical-type oral-nasal mask designed to prevent the inhalation of infectious particles originating from the surface, orifices, and cavities of human remains.

D-10. Additional Requirement—Port of Entry (POE) Mortuary. *a. (10.1) Processed remains (embalmed).* The contractor (responsible licensed embalmer) shall remove remains from the transfer case or casket and with the contracting officer or designate determine:

(1) (*a*) Whether remains are viewable or nonviewable.

(2) (*b*) Effectiveness of disinfection, uniformity of preservation, and any additional disinfective and preservative treatment and restorative art work and cosmetic work required.

(3) (*c*) Size casket to be used.

b. (10.2) Unembalmed remains. The contractor (responsible licensed embalmer) shall remove the remains from the transfer case or casket and with the contracting officer or designate determine:

(1) (*a*) Whether the remains are viewable or nonviewable.

(2) (*b*) The treatment to effectively disinfect and uniformly preserve the remains and also eliminate all offensive odors emanating from the remains.

(3) (*c*) Restorative art and cosmetic work required.

(4) (*d*) Size casket to be used.

c. (10.3) Reprocessing viewable remains. Tissue areas requiring further or special attention shall be treated to assure that the remains are effectively disinfected and uniformly preserved. The treatment shall be accomplished by one or more of the following: trocar or hypodermic injection and external pack application using full strength cavity chemicals having a 30-index (percent) or greater. Thoracic, abdominal, and pelvic cavities shall be relieved of gases and distension and reinjected with a minimum

of 32 oz of concentrated cavity chemical having a 30-index (percent) or greater.

d. (10.4) Reprocessing nonviewable remains. Those tissues requiring further or special attention shall be treated to assure the remains are effectively disinfected and uniformly preserved. This treatment shall be accomplished by means of one or more of the following: trocar or hypodermic injection and external pack application using full strength cavity chemicals having a 30-index (percent) or greater. Thoracic and abdominal cavities, when present, shall be relieved of gases and distension and reinjected with a minimum of 32 oz of concentrated cavity chemicals having a 30-index (percent) or greater.

e. (10.5) Processing unembalmed adult remains. The contractor shall perform those requirements enunciated in paragraph 6 of this armed services specification for preparation of remains.

f. (10.6) Infant and child remains. Treatment of infant and child remains—neonatal, infant, and child remains (birth through 60 months)—follows.

g. (10.6.1) Viewable and injectable remains.

h. (10.6.2) Nonviewable and noninjectable remains. Nonviewable and noninjectable remains shall be disinfected and preserved by means of accessory embalming techniques. Superficial and deep tissues shall be injected by infant trocar or syringe and needle. The arterial injection solution shall have a minimum concentration of 3% by volume aldehyde or aldehyde derivative preservative agents. The supplemental use of liquid (packs), gel, or dry sanitizers for the confirmed disinfection and preservation of superficial tissue shall also be accomplished. The cranial, thoracic, abdominal, and pelvic cavities shall be thoroughly aspirated. The cavities shall then be injected by means of trocar and sufficient amount of cavity fluid (having a 30-index or greater) to thoroughly saturate the organs and contents.

i. (10.6.3) Autopsied remains. If a partial or complete autopsy has been performed, a six-point arterial injection with multisite drainage shall be accomplished. The arterial chemical injection concentration solution requirements indicated in paragraph 10.6.1, as applicable, shall also apply. Following the arterial injection, the thoracic and abdominal walls shall be hypo injected by means of a trocar or syringe with an arterial solution of the same strength as injected arterially. Treatment for organs or portions of organs that have become separated during autopsy investigation shall be removed from the cavities and immersed in concentrated cavity chemical having a 30-index (percent) or greater. Inner surfaces of body cavities shall be treated with a liberal application of a gel preservative, then the organs or portions of organs are returned to the cavities in their normal anatomical location and covered with hardening compound. The calvarium shall be replaced, scalp sutured, and hair treated as indicated for adult autopsied remains.

j. (10.6.4) Treatment of scalp (viewable). When scalp has been shaved, procedures indicated in paragraph 6.1.4 shall apply.

k. (10.6.5) Mutilated hands (viewable). Procedures indicated in paragraph 6.1.5 shall apply.

l. (10.6.6) Dressing remains. Procedures indicated in paragraph 6.1.6 shall apply.

m. (10.6.7) Embalmer evaluation. Procedures indicated in paragraph 6.1.7 shall apply.

n. (10.6.8) Placement in casket. Procedures indicated in paragraph 6.1.8 shall apply.

o. (10.6.9) Quality assurance. Procedures indicated in paragraph 6.1.9 shall apply.

p. (10.6.10) Encasing casket. Procedures indicated in paragraph 6.1.10 shall apply.

q. (10.6.11) Loading remains. Procedures indicated in paragraph 6.1.11 shall apply.

Identification: An Essential Part of What We Do*

Michael Kubasak

Requests for both cremation and burial without formal ritual are becoming common in funeral homes throughout the country. As requests for these and other abbreviated services increase, so does the decision not to view the body. This poses several challenges for the funeral director:

- Regardless of what services are requested, we must perform certain legal functions. Everything we do in caring for a decedent and in serving a family has legal implications and carries liability.
- We cannot treat even minimal service requests casually.
- No matter how simple or complex the service, we must perform all duties in an ethical, professional manner.
- Abbreviated services of any type carry a higher risk of misidentification than traditional (full) services.

Viewing is rarely an easy matter for newly bereaved families. As funeral directors, we can identify with a family's reluctance to view. At the same time, to fulfill our professional and legal responsibilities, we must involve the next of kin or their designated representative in verifying the identity of the body in our custody. We are like

*Reprinted from *Mortuary Management*, Vol. 89, No. 9, Monterey, CA: Abbott and Hast Publications, Inc.; 2002, with permission.

the physician who knows that in order to accomplish a beneficial outcome and give peace of mind to the patient or confirm a diagnosis, the patient may have to endure some discomfort.

Funeral directors offer a wide spectrum of services. *Identification is central to all of them.* Identification is imperative before performing a cremation or any type of abbreviated service without formal viewing, including burial, entombment, or shipping of the body. This makes sense from a risk-management point of view. We are responsible for preventing misidentification *even if the error was made before the body came into our custody.* If the wrong body is cremated, buried, or shipped, there is serious liability for the funeral home and for everyone who participated in the chain of custody.

The need for positive identification is not something new or unique in funeral service. The best funeral directors have always required it. Even in those states where it is not required by law, we have a clear responsibility to ensure the positive identification of every deceased person we serve, just as a surgeon must be sure of the patient's identity and the procedure planned before beginning. It is a standard of care. The only exception to requiring verification of the deceased *might* occur when the deceased dies at home in the presence of family or legal representative, and the funeral home transfers the deceased from the residence *directly* to the funeral home.

Identification makes sense professionally, practically and legally for several reasons:

1. Identification certifies that this is the right person beyond any doubt.
2. Identification underscores the professional responsibilities we assume in providing disposition.
3. Identification stresses the irreversibility of the cremation process.
4. Identification facilitates the process of grieving. The majority of memories are visual. Seeing the person dead is a powerful confrontation that undercuts the normal tendency to deny that a death has occurred. If at least one person in the family certifies personally to the death, it becomes easier for others to accept the finality of death and to proceed with their mourning. The "Missing person" phenomenon teaches us that the absence of positive identification can complicate bereavement.
5. Identification serves as a preventive mental health measure for the bereaved by establishing a basis for certifying the death has occurred and for setting in motion the supportive and therapeutic benefits of whatever ethnic, social, and spiritual services follow the death.

Some funeral directors take exception to having a firm policy on identification before disposition or treat it with indifference. However, today's litigious climate and the tendency of courts and juries to award enormous settlements make a profound statement. *Verifying the identity of the deceased prior to any disposition, especially when cremation is selected, is the foundation of all risk reduction methods.*

A recent legal case provides an example. A hospital released the wrong decedent to a funeral home. The funeral home cremated the body that was transferred into their custody. When it became known that the wrong body was cremated, the funeral home was sued. During a trial that received front-page newspaper coverage, the funeral home claimed it did not start the problem. The court agreed but determined that the funeral home "acted below the Standard of Care by not verifying the identity of the deceased," before performing cremation. The court further stated that they were the last ones that could have remedied the error, but failed to do so. In the *chain of custody*, the funeral director occupies a vital position that carries liabilities even for misidentification that may have occurred previously.

Practicing risk management, including identification, is not done merely for the funeral director but also for the survivors. Today, funeral service deals with a skeptical consumer. Any attempt to distance the family or their designated representative from the reality of our services, no matter how well intentioned, especially when cremation is chosen, or to save them from the need to verify the identity can come back to haunt us. For the family, a lack of understanding can contribute to doubts and mistaken assumptions.

For the funeral director, making funeral arrangements today is substantially different from what it was 30 years ago. Then we were making adjustments to comply with FTC regulations. Today, funeral service is scrutinized by Wall Street, the media, consumer watchdogs, and the legal community. As society becomes less trusting, families question what they once took for granted. We can no longer assume that people understand what we say or do. Most people are inexperienced in planning a cremation, burial service, or shipment of the body. They are well aware of reports of alleged wrongdoing by some in funeral service. To be more consumer-focused means more disclosure, more explanation and information about what we do, where it is done, and how it is accomplished. By explaining, we build trust. **A policy requiring verification of the identity of the deceased builds trust. It is the foundation of all risk reduction methods and the best way to ensure that the wrong person will never be cremated, buried, or shipped.**

Every funeral director has heard people raise doubt about whether the person really died. In the absence of viewing, it is easy for people to question the identity of the person buried or cremated. Many of us have experienced misidentification of remains from a medical center, nursing home, coroner's office, or other institution. We cannot put our reputation and business in someone else's hands. Trusting the name that is imprinted on a toe tag or wristband without question is no longer safe practice. Positive identification means having the next of kin or their legal representative *verify* that the identity is correct. I can recall two legal cases as examples. At a medical center, two males died on the same day. One occupied a room on the second floor, the other on the fifth floor. Unrelated to one another, they shared the same common last name. Hospital personnel were unaware of this unique situation, but correct wristbands and toe tags were attached after the death. As you might guess, at the time of transfer from the hospital, the morgue attendant and the funeral home representative only looked for comparison using the last name. This serious error was discovered at the funeral home the next day when a grandson wanted to place a handwritten letter with his grandpa. In the other case, two people died at a nursing facility, one male, the other female, only a few rooms apart. While preparing both for transfer, the nurse was sidetracked by an emergency. In her haste, she gave another nurse the body tags. The second nurse attached the wrong identification tags to each decedent. One body was mistakenly cremated. Three days later, out-of-town relatives arrived at the other funeral home to claim the body for transport and burial in a native American cemetery and discovered the mistake. Knowing nightmares like these can occur, how can you prevent them in your practice?

You can develop a policy of identification at your funeral home. Here are some guidelines to consider for each decedent that comes into your custody:

1. Identification should be performed by the next of kin or their *designated-in-writing* representative (relative, clergy, best friend) and presented as policy, NOT an option.
2. If identification is done by photograph, the funeral home should take the photograph after obtaining written permission to do so. If the family brings their own photograph, it must be recent enough for valid comparison and must be retained in the decedent's file. The person making the identification should sign the back of the photograph, noting the date and time the identification occurred.
3. Identification should take place at the funeral home in an appropriate room, such as a small chapel or slumber room. Viewing should *never* be done in a garage, flower room, storage room, preparation room, or carport area.
4. During the arrangement conference, families should be informed that identification viewing is not the same as formal viewing but is a very

time-limited act, usually taking from several seconds to several minutes. Frank discussion reduces the possibility of misunderstanding about its purpose.

5. Whenever possible, identification should take place with the deceased in the casket or container to be used for the cremation, burial, entombment, or shipment.

6. Prepare the person who will be making the identification before it occurs. Inform them where it will take place, what they will see, and how the deceased is covered. Disclose that the body may not be embalmed, dressed in normal attire, or clean-shaven. If there was a postmortem examination or there are manifestations of trauma or disfigurement, mention this as well as any other relevant details.

7. Prepare a form on your letterhead stating the name of the deceased, date of death, and the name and relationship of the person with the right of disposition. If the next of kin designates another person to make the identification, *it should be done in writing*, noting the relationship of the person designated by the next of kin. Once the identification is complete, have the person making the identification sign the form and indicate the date and time it occurred.

8. If at all possible, after the identification has been performed, invite the person who made the identification to sit in your office and answer any questions they may have.

9. Some funeral homes present a flower or other small token to the person making the identification.

Some funeral homes provide attention to the body prior to identification. Your state may have laws or statutes governing what may or may not be done to a body for this purpose. The circumstances as well as the condition of the body can vary and the attention rendered may involve some or all of the following:

1. Unwrap or undress the remains and inspect the physical condition, noting the condition on the embalming case report.

2. Be certain the *funeral home identification tag* is securely attached to the body and that all forms of identification *are the same.*

3. Inventory and record valuables, personal belongings, or other items on the deceased.

4. Document the presence of any medical or mechanical devices or equipment on the body. Inform the family of devices that must be removed, such as pacemakers, when cremation is chosen.

5. Position the deceased with arms and legs straight, when possible.

6. Comb and brush the hair.

7. Clean the face, close the eyelids, and deodorize the body with a topical disinfectant spray.

8. Cover the deceased with undergarments or an apron and wrap the deceased in a clean sheet.

9. Refrigerate the body. If the body is placed in a pouch, ensure that another identification tag is securely attached to the exterior of the pouch.

We must also consider what to do when the body is decomposed or the death was due to violence. Both of these conditions can create a problem for the funeral director regarding identification. In both instances, people who do not understand our liability in disposing of a body, especially by cremation, can accuse us of adding to a family's emotional stress or being insensitive. Yet, for our peace of mind and that of the family, we must be assured of the identity of the body before proceeding. When conventional viewing is impossible, identification can also be accomplished by alternative methods that can include photographs, scars or tattoos, physical deformities, or dental records. Advanced decomposition and violent deaths can render identification almost impossible. Often, the coroner or another agency is involved in these instances, and they generally establish the identity of the remains before releasing them to the family or funeral home. *Make it a practice to ask the coroner for written acknowledgment of the identity of the remains.* On your letterhead, have the next of kin sign a statement acknowledging that identity was established by the coroner or other agency, that the remains are in such a condition that renders them not viewable, and that the funeral home is held harmless from any claims relating to the failure or inability to identify the remains at the funeral home.

When the next of kin or legal representative declines to verify the identity, some funeral homes have them sign a waiver. To the funeral home, a waiver may provide a sense of ease in reducing liability and a way of helping the family by not having them visually identify the body. However, it can also provide the funeral home with a false sense of security. A waiver can be useless unless *all of the next of kin* sign it or if your funeral home operates in a state whose laws permit fewer than all of the next of kin to waive each person's rights. Using a waiver raises numerous questions and is not the "cure all" that some funeral directors want it to be. No matter how assuring such a form may appear on paper, even when properly executed by all of the next of kin, legally *it will not protect your funeral home from the other family whose loved one has been mistakenly cremated, buried, or shipped.* All courts may not recognize waivers. It is suggested that you seek counsel from an attorney before using any type of waiver.

Today, we deal with a skeptical and demanding consumer. With cremation, you only get one chance to do it right. As we know and as the courts have stated, cremation is final and irreversible. The funeral home is normally the last in a line of those who can ensure the identity of the deceased person. This responsibility does not end with the identification at the funeral home. Identification is not just an event but is a *continuous process throughout the entire sequence of disposition*. Our obligation to the family and the resultant liability extends to outside contractors and agents as well. Funeral directors will be held accountable for everything their employees and organizations did or failed to do while serving a bereaved family. Our practices, procedures, and policies are now held to higher standards than ever before. Just because we never employed certain professional practices in the past is no excuse. Standards of care change and we must adapt to change. Verifying the identity of decedents in our care prior to any form of disposition is a standard of care. Funeral service can no longer give excuses. Risk management and risk reduction must be a part of our professional practice in 2005 and beyond. *It makes good sense for all concerned and is an essential part of what we do.*

About the author: Michael Kubasak has a life-long career in funeral service and formerly owned his own funeral home for 30 years. He is a licensed funeral director, embalmer, and certified crematory operator and is the author of the book *Cremation and the Funeral Director: Successfully Meeting the Challenge.* In addition to providing frequent presentations and workshops throughout the United States on leadership, management, customer service, operational topic, and consultation to funeral-cremation providers, Mr. Kubasak serves as an expert witness in litigation cases. Known as "the funeral director's coach," he is President of Kubasak Associates and can be reached at 702.345.3212 or *mike@kubasak.com.*

The Mathematics of Embalming Chemistry*: Part I. A Critical Evaluation of "One-Bottle" Embalming Chemical Claims

Jerome F. Frederick, Ph.D
Director of Chemical Research, Dodge Chemical Company.

Few concepts can be more misleading and destructive to the professional future of the modern embalmer than

the belief that "one-bottle embalming" is technically possible or even ethically admissible. The faulty reasoning behind this kind of wishful thinking is predicated on the premise that one single 16-oz bottle of embalming chemical can be made to contain *all* of the essential chemical components required for the complete embalming of the "average" case, regardless of the condition variables present in such a case.

Certain unscrupulous "fluid merchants," who are actually not bona fide embalming chemical manufacturers at all, have good reason to foster this misleading and unrealistic view. They do so with an obvious ulterior motive in mind. To put it plainly, they hope to win favor in the profession on the strength of a sensational economy appeal by claiming that embalming can be accomplished far more inexpensively with just one bottle of their super-duper elixir. Nothing could be further from the truth. To those who really understand the science of tissue preservation, such a claim smacks strongly of the chicanery and flim-flam of the old-time "medicine men" who in earlier days ranged the frontiers in their flashy horse-drawn vans and sold cure-alls "good for man or beast" to the trusting pioneer folk in the far-flung outposts of expanding America. Times have changed, but credulity, it seems, remains a dominant factor of human nature even in this enlightened day and age. Although stemming more from trustfulness than ignorance, unquestioning belief in the impossible and impractical still threatens the success of the misguided individual, but even more important, tends to undermine the very foundation of funeral service itself.

Misleading, illogical, and technically faulty, the "one-bottle" concept must be explored in depth before its pitfalls can be made clear to all ethical embalming practitioners, for if allowed to gain momentum unopposed, such a trend can only give the critics and detractors of funeral service valid evidence to win public support for their destructive efforts.

In order to guide our readers toward a true and realistic evaluation of the hazards inherent in the "one-bottle" concept, we will divide discussion of the subject into two parts. In the first portion, we will center our analysis upon a hypothetically "perfect case"—one in which no type of chemotherapy had been administered prior to death and where no problems other than those met within the normal course of tissue preservation face the embalmer. We must realize, of course, that no such case actually exists. But it gives us the unbiased starting point needed to expose the fallacies of the "one-bottle" embalming chemical concept and so reveal its hidden threat to the profession.

In cases where modern chemotherapy has been brought into play prior to death—and this encompasses some 90% of the cases treated by embalmers nowadays—the calculations for the analysis and critical evaluation must be revised. For here, the hazards of "one-bottle embalming" take a sharp upward turn—and its inadequacy becomes greatly intensified.

We know, for instance, that cases in which the new antibiotic *kanamycin* has been used for some time prior to death require a much greater concentration of the arterial chemical than that indicated for cases that have not been treated with this drug. Expressed in its simplest terms, this requirement stems from the fact that the antibiotic causes changes in the kidneys. In consequence, the kidney tissues accumulate large concentrations of nitrogenous and ammoniacal wastes. And, as every embalmer knows, there is no more effective way to neutralize formaldehyde than reacting it with ammonia.

We shall take this part of our discussion, however, later and for the present confine ourselves to an analysis of the "perfect case," keeping in mind that it is purely hypothetical—for nowhere in our present chemotherapeutic era will the professional embalmer ever encounter such a case! Remember also that in any discussion concerning a topic such as this one, it is necessary to establish and accept certain basic scientific assumptions. While these may not apply directly to 100% of our cases in actual practice—"perfect" or otherwise—they do take into consideration the most common variables and so hypothesize a truly realistic and typical "specimen" case. For example, an *average* adult cadaver weighing 65.3 kg (or 65,300 g) has been shown to contain a *total protein* content of 10.7 kg (or 10,700 g of protein), by Brozek et al. (*Annals of the New York Academy of Sciences* 1963;110:123).

When formaldehyde reacts with protein, and *only* protein—and here again, we simplify the discussion by deliberately overlooking the fact that formaldehyde will also react with *other* components of the human body besides protein—it requires about 4.0 to 4.8 g (or 4.4 g average) of formaldehyde to totally react with and fix exactly *100 g of a soluble protein*. Nonsoluble proteins require even more preservative.

Now, as pointed out by J. F. Walker in his treatise (*Formaldehyde*, 2nd ed. New York: Reinhold, 1953, 315), the 4.4 g of formaldehyde is required to totally fix and preserve, for "all times," the 100 g of soluble protein.

The average cadaver has about 10,700 g of protein. To totally and "forever" preserve *all* the protein present in this average cadaver, we would need

$$10,700/100 \times 4.4 = 470.8 \text{ g of formaldehyde}$$

Let us consider, then, an average 16-oz bottle of arterial fluid. If it contains only 30% formaldehyde (most modern arterials contain other preservatives in addition to formaldehyde), it would be technically defined as a "firming" or "high-index" fluid. Its formaldehyde content is computed as follows:

$$1 \text{ U.S. fl oz} = 29.6 \text{ mL}$$

$$16 \text{ fl oz} = 473.6 \text{ mL of fluid, of which 30\% is formaldehyde,}$$

$$\text{hence } 0.30 \times 473.6 = 142.08 \text{ g of formaldehyde.}$$

If we require 470.8 g of formaldehyde to totally preserve all the protein in an average body, then that amount of this chemical in a 30% fluid will contain only enough formaldehyde to preserve

$$142.08/470.8 = 0.3 \text{ or 30\% of all the protein in that average cadaver.}$$

These calculations, as we pointed out earlier in this article, are necessarily predicated upon assumptions that must be accepted to establish a basis for computation. But even allowing the most liberal margin of error, it can be readily seen that *no single 16-oz bottle of fluid* could possibly deliver the minimal acceptable degree of preservation—even in a "high-index" formulation! And this, remember, is calculated on the conditions of an *average* case!

Yet, as theoretical figures, these must not be construed as applicable to every like instance. There are many truly capable and excellent embalmers whose professional standards demand the most critical technical perfection who can point to instances where they have achieved adequate preservation with as little as $1\frac{1}{2}$ or 2 bottles of arterial fluid.

But none among them would rightfully claim that he uses *only one* bottle of arterial per case as *standard operating procedure*, for to do so would reflect unfavorably upon his professional judgment. Even the most ingenious and careful practitioners must admit that they are compelled to vary the concentrations of arterial chemical to meet the exigencies and special conditions present in each specific case. Most conscientious embalmers, in fact, use the full complement of "adjunct" chemical when the need for them is indicated—restorative humectants when there is evidence of emaciation or dehydration, water conditioners to neutralize chemical conflict in their solutions, modifiers, preinjections, coinjections, and vascular conditioning expedients. It is their familiarity with these "tools of the trade" that sets them apart as an elite professional class, where attitude and course of action are closely patterned on that of the medical man who employs every pharmaceutical and surgical expedient available to him as the need becomes apparent and modifies his treatment according to the conditional factors present in the case at hand.

Imagine, if you can, a doctor who would be content to use the *same drug* in the *same concentration* on every case he treats! The analogy is very close to "one-bottle embalming."

But even if it were possible to produce a reasonably acceptable, if not perfect, embalming result with the "one-bottle" tactic, the embalmer who chose to place such paltry economy above the true objectives of his profession would indeed be asking for trouble. For the value of his reputation can scarcely be counted in fluid ounces of arterial chemical. Sensibly enough, few are ready to risk so much for so little in return—and the profession can well spare those who fall by the wayside with "one-bottle embalming."

Now, back to the hard facts of embalming chemistry. Even if it were technically possible to increase the amount of formaldehyde in a 16-oz bottle of arterial chemical to an absolute 100%, we would have barely enough to "fix" the total protein present in the "average perfect case." This, of course, is not feasible because of the intrinsic chemical–physical nature of formaldehyde. But mere "fixation" or stabilization of the body proteins does not constitute total embalming. The result of using such an arterial would be a rock-hard, ghastly gray cadaver—a far cry indeed from the lofty standards of modern embalming! And where would we put our diffusion stimulating constituents in a 100% formaldehyde fluid?—or our cosmetic modifiers, blood solvents, and vascular conditioning components? Without these, could this super-duper 100% formaldehyde arterial do the job we want it to do? Could it penetrate and preserve *all* the proteins in our hypothetical "average" case? Could it get past the "average" number of circulatory obstacles we would be almost certain to encounter in such a case? Lacking its normal complement of supporting constituents, it is hardly likely that this 100% formaldehyde fluid would win any applause from experienced professionals.

It should be plainly apparent at this point in our discussion that the "one-bottle" technique offers more danger to embalming results and professional reputation than the earnest, ethical embalmer is willing to risk. But our analysis and evaluation would not be quite complete if we did not take a moment to quiet the suspicion that "one-bottle" embalming might become valid through technical advances in injection equipment. We refer specifically to the use of high-pressure embalming. Although embalming under such pressures may *appear* to use only one bottle of arterial chemical to achieve preservation, the technique merits the most critical scientific scrutiny. There is now evidence that high-pressure embalming actually causes the preservation to be "blown" to the superficial areas of the body. The result is a "taut skin" appearance that gives the *impression* of true preservative firming, but actually fails to embalm the deep underlying tissues, creating a condition that can obviously cause the embalmer a great deal of trouble.

In any event—no matter which technique is employed—we must face the incontrovertible mathematical truths of embalming. Knowing the way proteins react with preservatives leaves no illusions that one-bottle embalming will ever become a practical reality. Claims to the contrary should be viewed with cautious skepticism, for there is every indication that they will prove wholly false and unworthy of acceptance by the ethical professional.

The Measurement of Formaldehyde Retention In the Tissues of Embalmed Bodies*

John Kroshus ● *Joseph McConnell* ● *Jay Bardole*
Editor's Note: John Kroshus is Chairman of the Funeral Service Education Program and Jay Bardole is Chairman of the Chemistry Department at Vincennes University. Joseph McConnell is an Evansville (Indiana) Funeral Director.

INTRODUCTION

As a result of tests conducted jointly by the Funeral Service Education Program and Chemistry Department at Vincennes (Indiana) University, a procedure has been developed by which the amount of formaldehyde retained in the tissues of a dead human body can be measured. It appears as though this project, which can provide a quantitative analysis of formaldehyde retention, might be used to evaluate the efficiency of new embalming techniques or products and thereby create the possibility of reducing the material expenditures in embalming.

In addition, improved techniques may also upgrade the quality of embalming results. Reducing material expenditures means that costs can be reduced, and if this can be accomplished without sacrificing results, it will constitute a significant advance for funeral service.

Embalmers have long suspected that a substantial amount of chemicals injected into a body during arterial embalming simply pass through the blood vascular system and are lost with the other fluids that drain from the body. Other tests have indicated that this was perhaps true. Now it is possible to measure quite accurately

---

*Reprinted from the Director, Vol. 54, No. 3, Milwaukee, WI: National Funeral Directors Association, NFDA Publications Inc., 1983, with permission.

just how much chemical is lost and how much remains in the body.

The research project has indicated that approximately 50 to 55% of the arterial fluid injected into a body is lost along with the venous drainage. It seems evident that funeral service needs to examine ways by which embalming can be made more efficient and thereby reduce the waste of arterial fluid. Again, this procedure can be used to evaluate the efficiency with which embalmers are operating.

The procedure for measuring formaldehyde retention in the tissue of embalmed bodies has been adopted from a quantitative analysis experiment used to determine the amount of formaldehyde in pesticides.[1] Basically, the formaldehyde retention experiment involves reacting a sample of the venous drainage with sodium hydroxide and hydrogen peroxide.

The ratio of sodium hydroxide to formaldehyde is one to one in the reaction. This means that for every mole of formaldehyde present, one mole of sodium hydroxide will be used up in the reaction. Thus, by determining how much sodium hydroxide is used, the amount of formaldehyde present in the venous drainage can be calculated. That amount is then subtracted from the amount of formaldehyde originally injected into the body, and the amount of formaldehyde retained in the body is known.

The hydrogen peroxide is reduced during the reaction and provides hydroxide ions to the formaldehyde, which oxidizes to formic acid. The formic acid reacts with the sodium hydroxide to produce a sodium salt and water.

That solution is then titrated with sulfuric acid, and the data gathered are used to calculate how much sodium hydroxide reacted with the formaldehyde in the venous drainage sample.

METHODOLOGY OF THE STUDY

Standardization of Chemicals. The sodium hydroxide and sulfuric acid used in the experiment must be standardized before being used. The procedure for the standardization of these chemicals is similar to that used in most elementary chemistry courses, and in this instance, the object is to make solutions that have a normality of one. What this means basically is that the acid and the base will react in such a way that they will neutralize one another if mixed in equal amounts.

Practice Titration. Once the chemicals have been standardized, it is also necessary to test them in laboratory conditions. For this reason, the solutions of sodium hydroxide and sulfuric acid were tested against a solution where the amount of formaldehyde was known. This allowed for a comparison of the calculations based on data gathered by titrations with predictable results.

PROCEDURE. Embalming chemicals were mixed with water to produce 150 mL of 1% formaldehyde solution. This was possible because of the standard "index" of arterial fluids, which states that index is the amount of formaldehyde present in 100 mL of solution. By using the formula, volume one times concentration one is equal to volume two times concentration two, the formaldehyde solution was mixed to contain 1% formaldehyde. Since the experiment used a 30-index fluid, 5 mL of the arterial fluid was mixed with 145 mL of water to produce the solution.

Using a volumetric flask, the 150 mL of formaldehyde solution was divided into three 50-mL portions, each of which was poured into separate 500-mL flasks.

Fifty milliliters of the sodium hydroxide was then added to each of the flasks.

Fifty milliliters of hydrogen peroxide was then added to each of the flasks.

Heat was then added to each of the 500-mL flasks to stimulate the reaction. The heat was continued until the bubbles of the reaction stopped and then for about 10 minutes longer.

When the reaction was completed, the flasks were cooled.

Next, a 50-mL burette was thoroughly cleaned and rinsed and filled with sulfuric acid. The amount was recorded on a data sheet.

Indicator was then added to the now cool "basic" solution, and the titration was begun. This procedure was repeated for each of the 50-mL portions of the formaldehyde solution with the initial and final burette readings recorded on the data sheet.

OBSERVATION. The titration is a back titration. The amount of acid delivered to reach the point of equilibrium was inversely proportional to the amount of formaldehyde that was present in the original solution. Therefore, the greater the amount of sulfuric acid delivered, the less the amount of formaldehyde present.

At the end point of the titration, the equivalents of the base and the equivalents of the acid should be equal. The difference between the equivalents in the calculations indicates that a certain amount of the sodium hydroxide was used up as formaldehyde was oxidized. As previously mentioned, the formaldehyde and the sodium hydroxide react on a one-to-one basis. The amount of sodium hydroxide absent from the original 50 mL is therefore directly proportional to the amount of formaldehyde that is in the drainage taken from a body, or in this case, to the amount of formaldehyde mixed to create the 1% solution.

TITRATION DATA. The burette readings indicate the amount of acid delivered in the titrations. The amounts are averaged, and the average is used to calculate the amount of base that reacted with formaldehyde.

CALCULATIONS. The difference of the equivalents of acid and base will determine the amount of base equivalents that react with formaldehyde. That figure is then multiplied by the formula weight of formaldehyde (which equals one equivalent of formaldehyde) that has as its product the grams of formaldehyde that reacted with the sodium hydroxide.

The Embalming Procedure. The embalming procedure in the experiment was done using the legs of a dead human body as subjects in obtaining samples. This was done for two main reasons. One, to insure that there were no adverse effects from the embalming that would distort the normally exposed portions of the body, namely, the face, neck, and hands. Two, it allowed the experimenter to strike a comparison on tissue that was very similar in nature.

The researcher made every effort to keep the procedures identical for the injection of each limb. It should also be pointed out there is no deviation from normal embalming procedure.

Femoral arteries and veins were raised and ligated on both the left and right legs of the deceased.

Two gallons of preinjection was then mixed in 1-gallon quantities. Six ounces to the gallon of a formaldehyde-free preinjection chemical was added to each gallon. The embalming machines were then filled and set for pressure and rate of flow.

One machine was set to a pressure gauge reading of 6 pounds per square inch, with a rate of flow of 1 gallon per 5 minutes. The other machine was set to a pressure gauge reading of 60 pounds per square inch, with pulsation, and a rate of flow of 1 gallon per 5 minutes.

Arterial injection tubes and venous drain tubes were then inserted into the arteries and veins, respectively.

The embalming machines were then started and the legs were injected simultaneously.

During the preinjection, the drainage was not saved. The object of the preinjection was to "flush" out the vascular system and replace the blood and tissue fluids with the preinjection solution. This is a very important point because the preinjection solution was composed of known elements, while the embalmer could not be sure what was in the blood and tissue fluids of the body.

Once the preinjection was completed, hoses were placed on the venous drain tubes, and collection containers were installed to collect the drainage from the preservative injection.

The preservative solution was mixed in a 1-gallon container with a dilution of 6 oz of arterial fluid per gallon. The arterial fluid used was 30 index. The solution was then divided into 1.5-gallon portions, and each machine was filled with 0.5 gallon of the arterial solution.

Again the limbs were injected simultaneously, and this time the drainage was saved from the beginning to the end of the injection of the 0.5-gallon portions. By saving the drainage throughout the injection, it was felt that the samples saved constituted a representative sample of the drainage total.

It should be pointed out that the independent variable in this experiment was a variation in pressure gauge readings on the embalming machines being used. As mentioned previously, the independent variable could be changed to include a new technique, new product, or new solution mixture. Whatever the independent variable being tested happens to be, the remainder of the experiment stays the same.

Titration of Drainage Samples. The drainage samples saved from the embalming were kept in separate containers. Care was taken throughout the titration to make sure the samples were not mixed.

A 150-mL portion of the "low-pressure" sample was divided into three 50-mL portions and placed into three 500-mL flasks.

To each flask, 50 mL of sodium hydroxide was added.

To each flask, 50 mL of hydrogen peroxide was added.

The flasks were then placed over heat. The heat served to speed up the reaction and was maintained until the tiny bubbles of the reaction ceased. As the reaction was in full progress during heating, the mixture in the flasks tended to foam over. Toward the end of the reaction, the foam would gradually disappear.

The same procedure was then followed for a 150-mL portion of the "high-pressure" sample.

All flasks were carefully labeled and observed during the course of the reaction. It should be pointed out that heat has no adverse effect on the final results. The solutions cannot be overheated.

When all reactions were complete, the flasks were placed in an ice bath until they were cool.

The contents of a flask were then placed into a clean 250-mL beaker. A magnetic stirring rod was placed in the beaker, and the beaker was placed on an automatic magnetic stirring device.

An electrode was then placed into the beaker, and the pH of the solution was registered on a pH meter connected to the electrode. The pH reading was recorded on a graph sheet. The graph sheet was contained in a grapher that was connected to the pH meter. The grapher would make a graph of the pH changes during the titration.

To begin the titration, an Automatic Constant Rate Burette and the grapher were turned on simultaneously. The Automatic Burette would deliver sulfuric acid into the 250-mL beaker of drainage sample. The automatic stirring device would mix the solution as the titration progressed.

The researcher was able to monitor the titration through the end point and until it could be determined that the basic solution present at the outset of the titration had become an acid solution.

The final pH reading was recorded on the end of the graph, and the amount of sulfuric acid delivered by the Automatic Burette was also recorded on the end of the graph. The initial and final pH and burette readings were used to calculate the amount of sulfuric acid needed to reach equilibrium in the solution.

That amount would help determine the amount of sodium hydroxide, which had reacted with formaldehyde in the solution. That figure, in turn, was used to determine the amount of formaldehyde in the drainage sample. The difference of the amount of formaldehyde in the drainage sample and the amount of formaldehyde injected was the amount of formaldehyde retained in the tissues.

This entire experiment was repeated over 10 times during the course of about 2 and 1.5 years. The object was to find a pattern that would indicate proof of the superiority of either "high" or "low" pressure in embalming. At no time was any direct comparison made between bodies. Direct comparisons were made between legs of the same body until an overall pattern was established. In this case, the experiment showed that there was very little difference in formaldehyde retention in bodies embalmed with "high" pressure as compared to bodies embalmed with "low" pressure. It has already been pointed out that an independent variable of pressure could be switched for any number of variables that would warrant testing.

The procedure is precise and accurate. It would seem to open countless possibilities for improvement of presently accepted arterial embalming techniques as well as for the testing of newly developed techniques. It may also provide definitive answers to questions about the value of the multitude of preinjects, coinjects, water correctives, and supplemental chemicals that are on the market today.

REFERENCE

1. Welcher FJ, ed. *Standard Methods of Chemical Analysis*, 6th ed., Volume Two—Industrial and Natural Products and Non-instrumental Methods. Part B. Princeton, NJ: D. Van Nostrand Company, Inc., 1963:1878–1879.

The Two-Year Fix: Long-Term Preservation for Delayed Viewing*

by Kerry Don Peterson

This article is taken from excerpts of a workshop presented at NFDA's 1991 annual convention by Kerry Don Peterson, Director of the Body Donor Program—University of Utah School of Medicine.

Operating a body donor program is in many ways an enlightening experience, and I have found a number of similarities exist between funeral service and anatomic science. Just one of these similarities is the practice of embalming.

The history of funeral service and anatomic science merged for a brief period at the close of the Civil War as a result of the work of Anatomist Thomas Holmes who developed a method to preserve dead human bodies to elongate and enhance the dissection process. Holmes capitalized on the idea after the war by offering his embalming services to Washington, D.C., funeral homes and from this embalming evolved into what it is today.

Anatomic embalming is unique when compared to mortuary embalming as we in the anatomic sciences have the opportunity to view our embalming successes or failures over a period of 2 years. As a result, we must learn the necessary techniques for long-term preservation or suffer the consequences.

One of the last cases I embalmed while a full-time employee of a funeral home 8 years ago was the body of a 39-year-old woman who had been stabbed 109 times. The family desired a traditional funeral with embalming followed by cremation. Being a homicide, the body was autopsied and could not be cremated until the county attorney cleared the case because cremation would have destroyed potential unfound evidence. It was going to be 6 to 9 months until the cremation could be performed; yet, the family indicated a desire to see the body just prior to cremation for a final goodbye. So here I was, presented with an autopsied body carrying 109 stab wounds on every part of the body, including the face. It was the beginning of summer and the family wanted a final viewing in 6 to 9 months.

I embalmed the woman as thoroughly as I knew possible by using a higher volume of more concentrated arterial fluid, hypoed the autopsy flaps, quadruple bagged the viscera and treated it with three bottles of cavity

*Reprinted from the Director, Vol. 63, No. 4, Milwaukee, WI: National Funeral Directors Association, NFDA Publication Inc., 1992, with permission.

chemical, packed pledgets of cotton soaked in insecticide and cavity chemical in the body's orifices, and used an inordinate amount of drying compound in the abdominal and thoracic cavities. At the time of the funeral, the body looked great. Afterward, it was stored in the coolest room in the funeral home, which usually stayed between 60 and 70 degrees Fahrenheit. Stone oil and lanolin cream were applied to the face and hands throughout this time. Over the storage period of 7 months, the body manifested increasing signs of dehydration and tissue shrinkage, some graying and darkening of the tissues, and development of a slight odor.

All in all, I did not feel too bad about the results given the circumstances. With deodorant powder in the casket and some opaque makeup and wax, the body looked okay. The family did not sing praises at the final viewing, but they seemed happy. Again, this all took place about 8 years ago, and since then, I found I could have done a much better job.

Over the last 5 years, I have experimented with normal mortuary supplies and chemicals on 135 cadavers (these cadavers exhibited a full compliment of physical and pathologic conditions including edema, ascites, jaundice, chemotherapy, obesity, skin slip, and so on; there were even a few "normal" cases) and through trial and error have devised what I consider to be the best method to preserve and store a body for extended periods of time. Each of these 135 cadavers was held and observed for 2 years. The majority of them exhibited minute dehydration, no discoloration, no blebs, no odor, and no mold. Using this method, I have also reinjected cases that were embalmed a week prior and it has not affected the end result, provided cavity work was not performed. I would like to mention the method was derived on the prep room table, not on a computer or through chemical equations on paper.

I have arbitrarily broken the long-term preservation process into three steps: (1) preinjection details, (2) application of chemicals, and (3) method of storage. Most of the steps covered are no doubt part and parcel of your normal routine, but it is the sum of all these steps that leads to long-term embalming success. Negligence in one or two of the procedures can lead to partial or total embalming failure.

PREINJECTION

To achieve long-term preservation, the embalmer must employ all known and accepted techniques of thorough embalming; shortcuts will cause future headaches. The body should be thoroughly disinfected using a reputable disinfectant and warm water, and the body's orifices should be sprayed or swabbed. *Rigor mortis* should be broken up. Elevate the body above the preparation table with positioning devices under the buttocks, shoul-

ders, and ankle bones. This will take the weight off of most tissues on the back of the body, allowing for better fluid distribution to the area. Prior to the use of positioning devices, I had some bodies exhibit fluid distribution failure on only the weight-bearing posterior portions of the body. Once positioned, the face can be shaved and the facial and body features posed. In setting the facial features, I suggest you restore as much natural contour to the cheeks and eyelids as possible because the arterial fluid recommended will set the facial features firmer than you may be used to. Hypoing of tissue builder will still be an option after the injection of the arterial chemical but, once again, the tissues will be more rigid and less susceptible to tissue builder distension.

An embalmed body is like a petri dish for mold to grow on when stored for long periods of time. Since cotton and absorbent paper products (tissues and paper towels) are likely to harbor mold spores, they should be treated with a sporicide, such as phenol, prior to contact with the body during all three steps of the process.

APPLICATION OF CHEMICALS

To begin step two, select the vessel to be raised. I have had success with both the femoral artery and the carotid arteries, although I personally prefer the latter because it allows for better draining of the internal jugular vein. Most important is that you use the vessel you are most familiar working with. Be advised that venous drainage is of the utmost importance for cosmetic effect but is of no consequence for preservation; in fact, many medical schools do not drain a drop of blood when injecting their cadavers.

After you have raised the selected vessel, make a "T" incision in the artery with the base of the "T" pointing the direction of cannula insertion. This should be part of your normal embalming routine. When a cannula is inserted in the "T" incision, it is less likely that the tunica intima or tunica media will separate from the tunica adventitia. Ligature compression will also do less damage to the arterial layers when the "T" incision is used, which is very important in those cases you reinject. I generally insert a closing drain tube in the vein as it seems a superior way to regulate venous drainage and resistance, when it works! About 60% of the time I replace the drain tube with drainage forceps at some point during the injection process.

Chemical selection and storage techniques are the crux of long-term preservation. In mixing your chemicals, you want a sufficient amount of preservatives, antidehydrants, mold retardants, and accessory chemicals to break up clots, lubricate the vessels, and reduce surface tension. Water has none of these qualities. If you only have arterial and cavity chemicals on your shelves, your success will be no better than what I had with the stab victim. Every reputable manufacturer of embalming chemicals has an array of chemicals that preserve, break up clots, lubricate vessels, reduce surface tension, act as an antidehydrant, and contain phenol or specific retardants. The truth of the matter is you *do not* need most of these chemicals to inject the average case, but you *do* need all of them to inject a case you are going to keep around the funeral home for a couple of years unless you want to deal with dehydration, blebs, mold, odor, discoloration, and so on.

The minimum amount of chemical I have injected with 100% satisfactory results is two tanks of the following:

First Injection. Formaldehyde: Sixty-four ounces (four 16-oz bottles) with an index range of 21–27%. I have tried using less, but some of those cases failed.

Water corrective: Use 64 oz, even if your morgue has soft water. Water corrective has an array of qualities that enhance the injection process, some of which include: (1) it inactivates the minerals in body fluids just as it inactivates minerals in the water supply, (2) it extracts inert gases from the water supply and the body, (3) it defibrinates the blood, (4) it maintains a proper acid–base relationship between chemicals and the body, (5) it intensifies permeability of arterial solutions, and (6) it maintains the potency of formaldehyde and coinjectants against the body's natural chemical barriers.

Vascular lubricant/clot dispenser: Sixty-four ounces, which not only aids in drainage but also protects the capillaries from searing when using harsher chemicals and makes the tissues more receptive.

Mold retardant: Thirty-two ounces of mold retardant or 8 oz of phenol-containing cauterant *or* 16 oz of phenol-containing cavity fluid. *Note:* To avoid jelling, this chemical is usually best when premixed with your vascular lubricant or clot disperser before adding it to the embalming machine tank. When mixing new chemicals, it is a good idea to test mix a small batch.

Dye: More or less than normally added, but the amount of time you hold a body will be the main factor in determining how much dye to use if you choose to dye at all.

Water: Add enough water to make a solution totaling no more than 16 oz over 2 gallons.

Second Injection. The second injection is the same as the first *unless* you are using an arterial formaldehyde that does not contain a humectant or if one of the accessory chemicals does not contain a glycol (such as ethylene or propylene glycol), which acts as a humectant. If you have not injected a humectant in the first injection, add humectant to the second injection by reducing the water corrective and vascular lubricant by 16 oz each (a total of 32 oz) and replacing it with 32 oz of humectant.

If you do not keep a humectant in stock, add 32 oz of Downy fabric softener instead.

Usually two injections of this chemical mixture will suffice, but at times, I have had to mix and inject subsequent batches. Do not be tempted to shortcut chemicals on subsequent batches and remember that other rules of embalming apply, so do what you always do when you successfully embalm a case. Sometimes you will need to inject multiple points, and sometimes you will need to hypo an area to get adequate fluid to the tissues. Contrary to what I was told in mortuary science school, I have found hypoing to be a very effective treatment for any tissues not receptive to arterial injection. Hypoing the flaps of an autopsy with the same chemical is a must. Also on autopsy, a liberal application of external preservation cream on the underside of the scalp is warranted.

I do not recommend a preinjection before the injection of this arterial formula. Preinjection was part of my normal routine in the funeral home, and I tried to incorporate it into the anatomical routine, but my results were less than satisfactory. Tissues only have the capacity to absorb limited amounts of fluid, and when embalming for long-term preservation, you want the more stringent fluid absorbed by the tissues.

Particular items to be aware of during the injection procedure include:

- *Manifestations of the chemical:* While embalming, you may note the skin manifesting what I call an orange peel demarcation. The skin sometimes takes on the color and texture of a dehydrated orange peel. This demarcation is normal and passes in 24 to 48 hours. When using phenol, you might also note 1/8th- to 1/4th-inch white patches; this is also normal and goes away shortly after embalming.
- *Drainage:* When phenol is used, your drainage may become gritty. But regardless of whether or not phenol is used, the more stringent chemicals inherently lead to poor drainage late in the embalming process. It is also a good practice to tie off the vein while injecting the last quart or two of chemicals.
- *Swelling considerations:* Weigh the variables. If you see swelling of facial features occurring and the body is well perfused except the feet, stop injecting and hypo the feet. If the face starts swelling and the body is a long way from being embalmed, lower the pressure or flow, raise and clamp both carotids, and open the jugulars. Be aware that when the body is in storage, swelling diminishes to near normal contours naturally within a month's period of time.
- *Purge:* The more stringent fluids often lead to copious purge. This purge is often the same color as the fluid you are injecting and seems to run

out as fast as it is injected, but most of the time, fluid distribution is unaffected.

■ *Pressure and flow considerations:* I find the pressure versus flow debate to be one of the most confusing issues of embalming science. With the flow closed on my machine, I set the pressure gauge at 25 pounds and open the flow until the pressure drops to 18–20 pounds; on my machine, this is an unencumbered rate of flow of 22 oz per minute. I do adjust the pressure down when injecting those bodies that appear prone to swell and often increase the rate of flow later in the embalming process when the body is taking fluid well and not swelling. If your normal pressure and flow settings give you good results, I advise you to continue using these settings. **Always use the pulse—** studies prove the slight pause in fluid movement increases the amount of fluid absorbed into the tissues. If your machine does not have a pulse feature, turn the machine off for 5 minutes at each quarter tank interval; also wait 10 minutes between the first and the second injection as the rest periods give the tissues a chance to absorb the fluid and offer you a chance to evaluate your progress.

■ *Bright dye effect:* The accessory chemicals you mix in this arterial formula not only make the tissues more receptive to formaldehyde but also make the tissues more receptive to dyes. The catch here, however, is that over a period of 2 months the dye starts to bleach or wash out. When embalming, if you know how long you will have to hold the body, add dye accordingly. What appears bright red at the conclusion of embalming will be very light red in a year. Take this into consideration.

■ *Monitor body features for displacement during embalming.*

■ *Chemistry:* Provided you have injected two tanks of formula and feel you have adequately preserved the body, you have actually injected twice as much formaldehyde as embalming chemistry tells us it is necessary to react with and preserve the soluble proteins of a 160-pound person. Considering you lose arterial formula during drainage and that there are other factors to consider when embalming besides soluble proteins, it should become apparent that this dilution of fluid is in line with the accepted chemical principles of embalming.

When the body has received enough fluid, ligate the arteries and veins, treat the internal incision, suture, and apply incision sealer to the outside of the incision.

Using a 30-cc syringe and your longest hypo needle, inject the brain. Direct the needle through the medial canthus of the eye (pretty much straight back, but you may have to feel around a bit to locate the superior orbital fissure), through the superior orbital fissure, and into the cranial cavity. Inject 30 cc of formaldehyde slowly through each eye socket into the cranial cavity, drawing the needle outward. Avoid swelling the eye sockets by injecting the bulk of fluid well within the cranial cavity.

At this point, I suggest you do any hypo tissue building or restorative work necessary. Then apply a liberal amount of cream to the face, neck, hands, and wrists.

If the body does not warrant immediate cavity treatment, delay cavity work for 12 to 24 hours and then perform the work in the usual manner followed by an injection of 16 to 32 oz of cavity chemical.

METHOD OF STORAGE

In storage you want to create an environment for the body that (1) maintains an osmotic balance of moisture between the body and its environment to prevent dehydration, (2) protects the body from mold growth, and (3) provides a preservative buffer between the body and its external environment. The storage technique is easily accomplished and requires 5 minutes a week, at most, to maintain. The required supplies include:

1. A thick, plastic sheet large enough to loosely wrap the body with excess to tuck beneath.
2. A hospital gown or cloth shroud.
3. A spray bottle.
4. A chemical wetting agent consisting of two-thirds of a gallon of humectant (glycol or antifreeze), 4 oz of mold retardant (thymol or phenol), and 1 gallon of water.
5. A body rest or wooden two-by-fours or four-by-fours.

PROCEDURE

1. Lay the large plastic sheet on a table surface.
2. Place the body rest or cut wood on the plastic sheet (body rests should be high enough to keep all parts of the body off of the table surface).
3. Semisaturate the hospital gown or shroud with the wetting agent. Dress or wrap the body in the gown or shroud but do not cover the face or feet. Put the rest of the wetting agent in a spray bottle.
4. Place the draped body on the body rests and wrap the plastic sheet loosely around the body. Tuck the free ends of the plastic snugly under the body, trapping a moderate amount of air in with the body (do not wrap the body tightly in the plastic sheet).
5. Place the body in a cool spot. Refrigeration is not necessary but it does help.

Check the body every 3 or 4 days for the first couple of weeks. Aspirate or sponge out free liquids in the bag (it is quite normal for some bodies to precipitate 2 gallons of fluid), keep the cloth shroud moist with the spray bottle, and apply cream to the face and the hands as necessary. The plastic wrapping normally creates a rain garden environment.

After the first 2 weeks have passed, weekly maintenance consisting of spraying the shroud with wetting agent, draining pooled liquids, and reapplying cream to the face and hands is more than sufficient to maintain the body in its environment. Mix more wetting agent when necessary. If a part of the body seems to be going soft (which I have never had happen), hypo treatment is still an option.

Before final viewing, remove the body from the wraps, wash thoroughly with an ample amount of soap, and proceed with the normal cosmetic routines.

I do not suggest this method of preparation for every case as the method is costly and time consuming. As embalmers, we know it is not our charge to preserve artifacts for future centuries, but to disinfect and prepare bodies of the dead for therapeutic funeralization of the presently living. I do, however, suggest this method for long-term preservation or when a firm base is required for reconstruction or restoration.

Occupational Exposure to Formaldehyde in Mortuaries*

L. Lamont Moore, CIH CSP
Safety Sciences Department, Indiana University of Pennsylvania, Indiana, Pennsylvania

Eugene C. Ogrodnik, MS
Dean, Pittsburgh Institute of Mortuary Science, Pittsburgh, Pennsylvania

---

A short-term project was conducted to evaluate occupational exposure to formaldehyde in mortuaries. The study group consisted of 23 mortuaries located in Allegheny County, Pennsylvania. These establishments had business volumes ranging from 35 to 500 embalmings per year. On-site surveys were conducted at each location to examine ventilation systems and review work practices. Breathing zone and room air samples were subsequently collected during actual embalming procedures in a number of the smaller facilities with less well-designed ventilation systems. One of the primary objectives of the project was to educate par-

*Reprinted from the *Journal of Environmental Health* 1986;49(1), with permission.

ticipating mortuary directors about the potential health hazards associated with occupational exposure to formaldehyde. An extensive literature review was completed to summarize related epidemiological and environmental studies for participants. Additionally, the monitoring data were compared to previous observations and exposure estimates. Results of this study did not reveal employee exposures that approached existing limits established by the Occupational Safety and Health Administration (OSHA).

Formaldehyde is a colorless, pungent, irritant gas that is water soluble and most frequently marketed as 37 to 56% aqueous solutions, commonly known as formalin. Formaldehyde vapor is very irritating to the respiratory tract, eyes, and exposed surfaces of the skin. Inhalation of high concentrations can cause laryngitis, bronchitis, and bronchopneumonia. Liquid formaldehyde solutions may cause severe burns on contact with the eye. Formaldehyde will act as a primary skin irritant, causing an erythematous or eczematous dermatitis reaction.

Formaldehyde solutions do not have a high degree of systemic toxicity, and acute and chronic exposures generally result in varying degrees of irritation, which are usually localized. Symptoms commonly experienced by the general population are nonspecific, transient, exposure dependent, and usually mild. In some cases, however, formaldehyde may act as an allergic (immunologically mediated) skin sensitizer, and it may also exacerbate respiratory distress in individuals with preexisting or formaldehyde-induced bronchial hyperactivity. It may not be feasible for sensitized persons to work in an area where there is any possibility of exposure, even at very low levels.

Formaldehyde has an odor threshold far below 1 part per million (ppm). Stern[1] reported the lower limit for odor detection to be 0.05 ppm with throat irritation first occurring at 0.5 ppm. Bourne and Seferman[2] established the threshold for eye irritation at 0.13 to 0.45 ppm. The experience of numerous investigators has been that rapid inurement to such concentrations develops and there is a general absence of complaints from most workers exposed below 2 or 3 ppm.[3] According to existing OSHA regulations, the permissible limit for 8-hour time-weighted average exposure to formaldehyde is 3 ppm. The acceptable ceiling concentration is 5 ppm and the acceptable maximum peak is 10 ppm for 30 minutes. This standard was adopted in the mid-70s based on the irritant properties of formaldehyde.

The American Conference of Governmental Industrial Hygienists[3] has listed formaldehyde as a substance suspect of carcinogenic potential for man. In 1983, they proposed an 8-hour time-weighted average exposure limit of 1 ppm with a short-term exposure limit of 2 ppm for a maximum of 15 minutes. They point out that these concentrations may not be sufficient to prevent sensitized persons from suffering irritation but should be adequate to avoid development of persistent adverse effects.

In 1976, the National Institute for Occupational Safety and Health[4] recommended to OSHA that occupational exposure to formaldehyde be limited so that no employee is exposed at concentrations that exceed 1 ppm during any 30-minute period. This recommendation presumably was designed to protect the health of employees over their working lifetime, but may not be adequate to protect sensitized or hypersensitive individuals.

Plunkett and Barbela[5] completed a mail survey of 57 embalmers in 20 California funeral homes during 1976. Nine had symptoms compatible with acute bronchitis, and 17 were considered to have chronic bronchitis. No data on formaldehyde exposure levels, work practices, ventilation, or frequency of exposure were gathered. Nevertheless, there was enough evidence to suggest that more in-depth studies of this profession should be considered.

Levine et al.[6] studied nearly 100 West Virginia morticians who were attending an educational program during 1978. Standardized respiratory disease questionnaires and pulmonary function tests were administered to the group. The pulmonary function of morticians compared favorably with that of residential populations in Oregon and Michigan. Among the study group, those who had presumably embalmed the largest number of bodies did not demonstrate a higher than expected incidence of chronic bronchitis or pulmonary function deficits. The authors concluded that long-term intermittent exposure to low levels of formaldehyde had exerted no meaningful chronic effect on respiratory health. No actual data on formaldehyde exposures, ventilation, or work practices were gathered as part of this study.

Williams et al.[7] recently published the results of exposure studies conducted in seven West Virginia funeral homes. Area and personal samples were used to evaluate the embalmers' exposure to formaldehyde, phenol, and 23 organic solvents and particulates. Twenty-five personal samples revealed time-weighted average formaldehyde concentrations that ranged from 0.1 to 0.4 ppm during the embalming of intact bodies, and ranging between 0.5 and 1.2 ppm during preparation of autopsied cases. The overall average exposures were 0.3 ppm and 0.9 ppm, respectively. Concentrations of other airborne chemicals and of particulates were negligible. Time-weighted averages were calculated over the length of time actually required for the embalming. Embalming technique and condition of the body appeared to be the major determinants of formaldehyde exposure in preparing autopsied bodies. The importance of room air exchange rate could not be determined from this study. Overall, exhaust ventilation appeared to reduce formaldehyde concentrations in general room

air but had little effect on the embalmer's personal exposure.

Kerfoot and Mooney[8] completed an extensive study of six funeral homes in the Detroit area, collecting 187 air samples under various conditions. The vapor concentrations encompassed a range between 0.09 and 5.26 ppm. The average formaldehyde concentrations ranged between 0.25 and 1.30 ppm under normal working conditions with an overall average of 0.74 ppm.

It was not clear whether personal or area samples were obtained. Ventilation systems were evaluated in terms of air changes per hour and compared with average concentrations of formaldehyde found in each facility. The largest number of air changes did not always correspond to the lowest concentration of vapors. The authors concluded that the location of the fan and size of the room were also significant factors. They also pointed out that all six establishments were above average facilities and inferred that formaldehyde concentrations in smaller, less well-designed funeral homes might be markedly higher.

In 1979, NIOSH[9] conducted a health hazard evaluation of the embalming laboratory at the Cincinnati College of Mortuary Science. The request had been prompted by the early disability retirement of an embalming instructor who had developed asthmatic bronchitis after 5 years of laboratory exposure. Air samples were collected via general area and personal breathing zone sampling during actual work conditions and simulated accidents involving spillage of embalming fluids. Formaldehyde concentrations exceeded the proposed ACGIH threshold limit value of 1 ppm in 7 of 13 samples collected. All of the excessive concentrations were detected during simulated (worst case) situations, or during one afternoon when the ventilation system was inoperable.

A study of mortality among undertakers licensed in Ontario, Canada, was completed by R. J. Levine[10] in late 1982. He selected a cohort of 1477 embalmers licensed between 1928 and 1957 and examined the cause of death in 337 men who had died before 1978. The ratio of observed to expected deaths from each cause was expressed as a percentage or standard mortality ratio. No significant increase in mortality was detected for any form of cancer. Deaths from cancers at sites of potential contact with formaldehyde—skin, nose, oropharynx, larynx, and esophagus—were less than expected, as were deaths from cancer of the lung.

Walrath and Fraumeni[11] of the National Cancer Institute published a study in 1983, which investigated whether embalmers in New York State, compared with the general population, had a greater proportion of cancer deaths that might be associated with exposure to formaldehyde. The study group consisted of approximately 1132 deceased embalmers who had been licensed to practice in New York State between 1902 and 1979. The difference between observed and expected numbers of deaths from malignant neoplasms was elevated, but not significantly. Skin cancer mortality was significantly elevated, primarily among those licensed for more than 35 years. Mortality was slightly elevated for kidney cancer, leukemia, and brain cancer. No excess mortality was observed for cancers of the respiratory tract and no deaths ascribed to nasal cancer.

Walrath and Fraumeni[12] published the results of a similar study of California embalmers in 1984. The authors examined the death certificates of 1007 embalmers and calculated proportionate mortality ratios for the major causes of death. Mortality was significantly elevated for total cancer, arteriosclerotic heart disease, leukemia, as well as cancers of the colon, brain, and prostate. There were no deaths from nasal cancer, and the pattern of lung cancer mortality was unremarkable. One of the inherent weaknesses of both the California and the New York studies is that sample sizes were of insufficient size to detect rare conditions such as nasal cancer. Although the respiratory tract would presumably be the prime target site for formaldehyde carcinogenicity, the authors conclude that available epidemiological evidence suggests attention should be given to possible cancer risks at other sites, including the brain, bone marrow, and colon. It may be of significance to note that the Ontario study[10] did not indicate an elevated risk of cancer based on a study of 300+ death certificates. However, larger studies performed in New York[11] and California[12] both showed excess deaths from leukemia and brain cancer.

Patty's text[13] suggests that aldehydes cannot be regarded as potent carcinogens. The irritant properties of the compounds preclude substantial worker exposure under normal conditions. The extreme reactivity of formaldehyde, acrolein, and chloroacetaldehyde, for example, produces reactions at epithelial surfaces that tend to limit their absorption into the body. The rapid metabolic conversion to innocuous materials also may limit those critical reactions necessary to initiate systemic tumorigenesis. However, formaldehyde-induced tissue irritation may promote tumor formation initiated by another compound. Therefore, caution is warranted, and certainly, further epidemiologic studies must be performed to define any hazard that may exist.

Since 1979, there have been several research reports linking formaldehyde exposure to cancer. These studies were based on exposure of rats and mice to concentrations of 2, 6, and 15 ppm for 30 hours per week over a period exceeding 2 years.[14] On the basis of these findings, NIOSH recommended in 1981 that as a prudent measure, occupational exposure be reduced to the lowest feasible limit.

MATERIALS AND METHODS

On-site surveys were conducted at each facility to interview the funeral director about work procedures, evaluate the overall floor plan, calculate room volume, and record air flow measurements where appropriate. Subsequently, air sampling was conducted in a number of the funeral homes with poorly designed ventilation systems. Where feasible, samples were collected from the breathing zone of the embalmer during the entire period required for the embalming, usually 45 to 75 minutes.

Air was drawn through a liquid sampling medium using MSA Model G pumps set at a flow rate of 500 cc per minute. Calibration was accomplished prior to the surveys using a primary standard (soap-bubble meter) as suggested by the manufacturer. Pumps were adjusted as necessary to maintain the desired flow rate throughout the sampling period. A midget impinger with fitted glass bubbler containing 15 mL of a 10% aqueous methanol solution was used to collect air samples to be analyzed for formaldehyde. At the conclusion of the sampling period, samples were transferred to polyethylene bottles, sealed, labeled, and shipped to an approved industrial hygiene laboratory.

At the laboratory, samples are reacted with hydrazine reagent to form a hydrazone derivative, then analyzed by differential pulses polarography. This sampling and analytical technique (ID-102) was developed at OSHA's Analytical Laboratory in Salt Lake City, Utah. The coefficient of variation (CY_T) for the total sampling and analytical technique is 0.08. This value corresponds to a standard deviation of 1 mg/m^3 at the OSHA permissible exposure limit of 3 ppm.

RESULTS AND DISCUSSION

The embalming rooms examined as part of this study varied significantly in terms of their size, layout, and the effectiveness of the ventilation system. Preparation rooms were equipped with ventilation systems that produced from 0 to 20 air changes per hour with a mean of 7.6 air changes per hour. Three facilities had exhaust systems that produced no measurable air movement at all. Only 17% of these rooms had an exhaust grate or fan that was positioned to prevent fumes from being drawn through the breathing zone of the employee.

The size of embalming rooms ranged from 735 to 5000 ft^3 with a mean of 1950 ft^3. Less than 10% of the establishments had any provisions for the introduction of makeup air into the work area. The only source of makeup air would have been leakage around doors or windows throughout the structure.

Eight personal samples were collected from the breathing zone of funeral directors during separate

TABLE 1. SUMMARY OF FORMALDEHYDE EXPOSURE MEASUREMENTS BASED ON PERSONAL SAMPLING

	Low (ppm)	High (ppm)	Average (ppm)
Time-weighted average exposure during the period required for the embalming procedure	0.03	3.15	1.1
Exposure estimate for the full workshift, an 8-hour time-weighted average	0.01	0.49	0.16

Note: Calculation of 8-hour time-weighted averages was completed making the assumption that exposure would have been zero during the unsampled portion of the workshift.

embalming procedures in six different funeral homes. None of these establishments had ventilation systems that would be considered above the norm described above. Exposure concentrations summarized in Table 1 show a range of 0.03 to 3.15 ppm with an overall average of 1.1 ppm during the period required for the embalming. Embalming procedures typically last 45 to 75 minutes depending on the condition of the subject. When we assumed zero exposure during the unsampled portion of the shift, 8-hour time-weighted average exposures ranged from 0.01 to 0.49 ppm, with an overall mean of 0.16 ppm.

The data summarized in Table 2 provide a comparison of our limited data with that of more extensive studies by Kerfoot and Mooney[8] and Williams et al.[7] Allegheny County exposure estimates reflect slightly higher formaldehyde concentrations that may be associated with the smaller, poorly designed preparation rooms where sampling was conducted. Plans for a longer-term study were abandoned when our initial monitoring revealed 8-hour time-weighted average exposures to be well below the OSHA permissible exposure limit of 3 ppm.

TABLE 2. COMPARISON OF ALLEGHENY COUNTY EXPOSURE DATA WITH PREVIOUS STUDIES

	Estimated Formaldehyde Exposure During Embalming (in ppm)		
	Low (ppm)	High (ppm)	Average (ppm)
Kerfoot/Mooney (1975)[8]	0.25	1.39	0.74
Williams/Levine/ Blunden (1984)[7]			
Intact cases	0.10	0.40	0.30
Autopsied cases	0.50	1.20	0.90
Allegheny County (1984)	0.03	3.15	1.10

TABLE 3. COMPARISON OF FORMALDEHYDE CONCENTRATIONS DETECTED IN WORKROOM AIR DURING EMBALMING PROCEDURES—AREA VERSUS PERSONAL SAMPLING

	Low (ppm)	High (ppm)	Average (ppm)
Area samples taken in proximity to preparation tables	N.D.[a]	0.84	0.45
Personal samples collected from the breathing zone of embalmers	0.03	3.15	1.1

[a]N.D. signifies "not detected."

Six area samples were also collected from general workroom air in proximity to preparation tables, usually in conjunction with personal sampling. Results summarized in Table 3 suggest that area sampling is not representative of the embalmers' actual exposure. Where concurrent sampling was carried out, concentrations found in the employee's breathing zone were up to twice as high as measurements taken from general workroom air several feet away.

There are a number of conclusions to be drawn from this study, despite its limited scope. First, the authors found many funeral directors to be largely unaware or poorly informed about the continuing controversy over the carcinogenic potential of long-term exposure to formaldehyde. Second, it was clear that most funeral homes in this study had ventilation systems or floor plans that were largely ineffective in controlling exposure during embalming procedures. The position of the exhaust grate commonly draws contaminants through the embalmer's breathing zone. Third, the authors' data suggest that personal breathing zone samples are likely to provide the most accurate indicator of employee exposure in the embalming room.

Occupational exposure to formaldehyde in funeral homes should rarely exceed permissible exposure limits established by OSHA. These limits were adopted in the early 1970s to protect employees against the irritant properties of formaldehyde and may not be sufficiently stringent in view of the chemical's suspected carcinogenic potential. It is reasonable to assume, however, that there are regular occasions where embalmers' exposures exceed the short-term exposure limits of 2 ppm during any 15-minute period recommended by ACGIH in 1983 and the NIOSH recommendation of 1981, which suggests exposure be kept at the lowest feasible limit.

More extensive epidemiological and laboratory studies will be carried out before the issue of formaldehyde carcinogenicity is resolved. Funeral directors or embalmers represent a profession that should be of continuing interest to epidemiological researchers studying the long-term exposure to formaldehyde. Should more definitive evidence be developed with regard to the carcinogenic effects of formaldehyde, large-scale education efforts and installation of improved engineering controls will become priority within the funeral home industry.

REFERENCES

1. Stern AC. *Air Pollution.* New York: Academic Press, 1968; Vol. 1, p. 484.

2. Bourne HG, Seferman S. Wrinkle proofed clothing may liberate toxic quantities of formaldehyde. *Industrial Medicine & Surgery* 1959;28:232.

3. American Conference of Governmental Industrial Hygienists. *Documentation of the Threshold Limit Values.* Cincinnati, OH: ACGIH, 1983:197.1.

4. National Institute of Occupational Safety and Health. *Criteria for a Recommended Standard. ... Occupational Exposure to Formaldehyde.* Baltimore, MD: NIOSH, 1976:P.B. 76-273805.

5. Plunkett ER, Barbela T. Are embalmers at risk? *American Industrial Hygiene Association Journal* 1977;38:61–62.

6. Levine RJ, DalCorso RD, Blunder PB, Battigelli MC. The effects of occupational exposure on the respiratory health of West Virginia morticians. *Journal of Occupational Medicine* 1984;26:91–98.

7. Williams TM, Levine RJ, Blunden RB. Exposure of embalmers to formaldehyde and other chemicals. *American Industrial Hygiene Association Journal* 1984; 45:172–176.

8. Kerfoot EJ, Mooney TF. Formaldehyde and paraformaldehyde study in funeral homes. *American Industrial Hygiene Association Journal* 1975;36:533–537.

9. National Institute of Occupational Safety and Health. *Health Hazard Evaluation.* Cincinnati: College of Mortuary Science Embalming Laboratory; 1980:HHE 79-146-670, NTIS Pub. PB80-192099.

10. Levine RJ. Mortality of Ontario undertakers. In: *C.I.I.T. Activities.* Research Triangle Park, NC: Chemical Industry Institute of Toxicology, 1982.

11. Walrath J, Fraumeni JF. Mortality patterns among New York embalmers. *International Journal of Cancer* 1983;31:407–411.

12. Walrath J, Fraumeni JF. Cancer and other causes of death among California embalmers. *Cancer Research* 1984;44:4638–4641.

13. Clayton GD, Clayton FE, eds. *Patty's Industrial Hygiene and Toxicology*, 3rd ed. New York: John Wiley & Sons, 1981:Vol 2A.

14. National Institute of Occupational Safety and Health. *Intelligence Bulletin 34: Formaldehyde: Evidence of Carcinogenicity*, Baltimore, MD: NIOSH, 1981.

The Strange Case of Dr. Jekyll and Formaldehyde (Is It Good or Is It Evil?)

by Maureen Robinson

FORMALDEHYDE'S SPLIT PERSONALITY

Formaldehyde, is it good or is it evil? It is a carcinogen, it is not a carcinogen, it is a probably carcinogen, it is not.... I think you get the picture. There is a lot of uncertainty in the data. Where there is no uncertainty is in the benefits formaldehyde provides an as an embalming agent. Where there has been some misguided information, is in the reporting to the public that there is enough formaldehyde put in the ground each year in the United States to fill eight Olympic size swimming pools, and that the dead human body poses no health risks to those that come in direct contact with the body. Individuals making these claims are not scientists. Information is being taken out of context from extremely reputable sources and being inaccurately presented to the public.

There is a social movement, which seems to imply that, as a group, funeral service professionals are not concerned about the environment. Are funeral directors that are using formaldehyde saying that there is no need for us as an industry to look at being more "green" and more responsible with our environment? I would hope that this is absolutely not a true statement. Funeral service professionals should be looking at ways to make changes that can benefit our planet earth. How that is presented and marketed to the public should be done in a responsible way. The use of formaldehyde is not a major environmental issue. Its misuse can, however, potentially create very serious health issues. It is true that going out in the sun unprotected could cause skin cancer. There are, however, billions of people outside enjoying that sun each day. The informed individual will reduce their risk of skin cancer by wearing protective sunscreen. The responsible embalmer will use personal protective equipment and ventilation to minimize formaldehyde exposure.

In an effort to help the environment, each funeral home and funeral service professional should identify things they can do differently at their place of business and in their homes that would help sustain our planet for our children, our children's children, and so on. The current track we are on, in which the burning of fossil fuels is our primary energy source, is not sustainable. Projections indicate that if we continue burning fossil fuels at this current rate, we will deplete this natural resource in the next 5 to 100 years. Fossil fuel prices cannot remain artificially low, nor can government continue to subsidize their producers.

In the United States, we are approximately 95% dependent on these nonrenewable resources. We need to see a paradigm shift from the use of conventional oil, coal, and natural gas to alternative fuel sources that do not contribute to global warming. Solar energy, wind energy, and geothermal energy need to take the forefront. This shift will not occur without our pressure on local, state, and national politicians.

Our world population cannot continue to grow at its current rate. How about the issue of trying to sustain 8.9 billion people on this planet by 2050: If as a country or a world we do not start addressing some of these bigger environmental and social issues, soon the debate on a choice of an arterial fluid will be laughable at best. As funeral service professionals and responsible stewards of our planet earth, we can work together in developing a lifestyle that is more environmentally sustainable. There will be "an environmental corner" in this publication each quarter to aid in communicating our strategies within our profession and our daily lives. We can learn from one another and show that in solving large-scale environmental problems, individuals do matter.

This is not to imply that we should disregard any potential health effects or safety issues. It is just to state that the use of formaldehyde in funeral service cannot even begin to make its way onto the list of top environmental global issues. If current scientific studies reveal that formaldehyde is a known carcinogen and poses a threat of nasopharyngeal cancer in embalmers, then appropriate measures should be taken to better protect embalmers from this threat. The National Funeral Directors Association (NFDA) has already started to address this issue. In the face of renewed worldwide focus on formaldehyde and its risks, they have issued formaldehyde-specific best management practices (BMPs).

BEST MANAGEMENT PRACTICES

NFDA formed a panel to draft the BMPs that then underwent a peer review by funeral directors, educators, and leading chemical suppliers to make sure that the BMPs were protective, workable, and sensible. The Funeral Service Environmental Working Group also reviewed the BMPs, which were then approved by the NJDA Executive Board in January 2009. Brining in the Environmental Working Group for part of the peer-review process is another positive indication that funeral service professionals are concerned about the environment. The BMPs have been designed as a dynamic tool that can change to reflect any new evaluations of formaldehyde by domestic and international organizations, including

the current study released by the National Cancer Institute (NCI).

The first BMP addresses preparation room ventilation. Preparation room ventilation is the single most important factor in reducing health risks associated with formaldehyde exposure. The BMPs state that there should be no fewer than 10 to 15 air changes per hour supplied to the preparation room for each active embalming table. Jack Adams, in his November 2004 *Dodge Magazine* article, "The Preparation Room: Ventilation," recommends 20 air changes per hour. A properly functioning HVAC system aids in reducing the risk of formaldehyde exposure in the workplace. This seems to indicate that it would be prudent to shoot for a range of 10 to 20 air changes per hour. To ensure use of the ventilation system, wire the ventilation system's activation to the preparation room's light switch. Monitor the effectiveness of the preparation room HVAC system no less than annually. Jack also emphasizes the importance of having the preparation room under negative pressure. That is, more air is exhausted than is taken into the room. This keeps the other parts of the building from being contaminated with air from the preparation room.

The second BMP states that in addition to a properly ventilated preparation room, a thorough case analysis of the condition of the remains should be made before embalming. When performing the embalming, only use the amount of formaldehyde necessary to achieve a quality result. I think this is supportive of the overall environmental strategy of "reduce, reuse, and recycle," as well as an excellent strategy to reduce potential formaldehyde exposure to the embalmer.

Which actually moves us to the third BMP, which indicates the importance of taking precautions in the preparation room to limit formaldehyde exposure and emissions during routine embalming. A simple strategy to greatly reduce the embalmer's exposure to formaldehyde would be to always add the arterial fluid to the water in the embalming machine. A sign should be posted near each embalming machine as a constant reminder to employees of this simple procedure. At Worsham College of Mortuary Science, where I teach microbiology, chemistry, and anatomy, my students have assured me that this procedure is taught in their embalming labs. Hopefully, they will continue this work practice long after leaving Worsham College.

Formaldehyde exposure to the embalmer will be greatest when a formaldehyde spill occurs. Sit down as a staff and brainstorm a list of your specific work practices that could help to minimize the potential for formaldehyde spills. Post the list and institute the work practices. Conduct short training sessions with new employees and refresher training sessions for current employees. If you are the boss, lead by example. If you teach embalming laboratories, this would be an excellent team exercise to conduct in your laboratories. Feel free to e-mail your results, and I will be sure to share them with others.

Even with these work practices in place, formaldehyde spills will occasionally occur in the workplace. Formaldehyde spills should be cleaned up immediately. There are spill kits available; however, an ammonia solution can be used as an inexpensive and effective formaldehyde neutralizer: When formaldehyde and ammonia react, a compound called urotropin is formed. Urotropin is an organic nitrogen compound. The formation of urotropin demonstrates the affinity of formaldehyde for nitrogen. Any source of nitrogen can bring about a similar neutralization reaction. Many decomposition products are derivatives of ammonia (NH_3) and would therefore neutralize the effects of formaldehyde. Therefore, embalming the body as soon after death as is possible can limit the concentration of formaldehyde necessary for a successful embalming, which in turn is an effective way to limit the formaldehyde exposure to the embalmer.

There are many other simple ways to limit formaldehyde exposure. Always keep the lid on the embalming machine, always use a sink cover to limit splashing and exposure, and use all appropriate personal protective equipment to avoid skin and eye contact with formaldehyde. Another good recommendation is to switch from latex gloves to nitrile gloves. The BMPs point out that nitrile has high chemical resistance against formaldehyde without the failure rate of latex. These recommendations, and others, are all easy and inexpensive to incorporate into your work practices. Posting friendly reminders for personnel will help to minimize bad habits from creeping into daily work routines.

One of the most effective strategies in limiting formaldehyde exposure to the embalmer would be to capture the formaldehyde emissions before those emissions enter the breathing zone of the embalmer. This can be accomplished by utilizing a local exhaust ventilation (LEV) system. Employees may choose to wear a properly fitted respirator. The key here is wearing a *properly fitted* respirator. Respirators should not be interchanged between employees. Each employee must be properly fitted, and they should then store their respirator where they store their other personal belongings, so that others do not inadvertently grab their personal protective gear. An improperly fitted respirator is not effective. Respirators should be worn when cleaning up a formaldehyde spill.

The fourth BMP reminds us that special cases such as embalming organ procurement cases and autopsied remains can increase the embalmer's formaldehyde exposure risk. It becomes even more imperative that embalmers follow the above-mentioned strategies when dealing with these types of cases.

The fifth BMP requires embalmers to be familiar with and follow federal, state, and local environmental, OSHA and health requirements that apply when an embalming is performed. Unfortunately, the longer we are at a job, the less familiar we become with these requirements. To keep formaldehyde in a good light, we need to change this strategy. I think it is also a natural progression that the longer we work at a job, the more shortcuts we tend to take, and the more complacent we can become in regard to personal safety and protection. I caution embalmers to keep this thought in the back of their minds.

Here is a true story. I was performing a test in an organic testing laboratory, a test I had performed safely and without incident thousands of times. One of the safety precautions was to bring down the glass sash on the ventilated hood in which I was performing my tests. During the test, the glassware that I was using exploded. The material in the glassware at the time was boiling. An additional safety precaution that took me less than 10 seconds most likely saved me from serious injury or a potentially fatal accident. After the accident, we reevaluated the entire laboratory procedure and found an additional step that could be added to hopefully avoid this incident from happening again in the future. This type of strategy could be incorporated when an accident occurs in the preparation room as well.

FORMALDEHYDE COUNCIL IS HOLDING CONSTANT VIGIL

The Formaldehyde Council is a nonprofit organization that represents the leading producers and users of formaldehyde in the United States. The National Funeral Directors Association is one of its many members. The Formaldehyde Council is dedicated to promoting the responsible use and benefits of formaldehyde and ensuring its scientific evaluation. Their organization is focused on the relationship between formaldehyde and the public health and assuring that the utilization of formaldehyde and the public policies governing its use are based on sound science. Sound science is science that has undergone the rigors of a scientific community peer review. Junk science has not undergone the rigors of a scientific peer review. Social movements often present junk science as sound science and in the process often do more damage to the case they are trying to make. Some of the current articles and advertisements that are being published about formaldehyde and funeral service professionals are perfect examples of why environmental science and other forms of sound science should be driving regulatory change, and not emotionalism, social movements, marketing schemes, or media hype based on junk science.

WHAT IS FORMALDEHYDE?

Let us take a closer look at the chemical that has drawn so much attention at the national and international level and has provided a full-time job for both those defending its use and those proposing a ban of its use. Here is an age-old question: what is formaldehyde? Formaldehyde is a simple molecule made of hydrogen, oxygen, and carbon and is a natural part of our world and the product of many natural processes. Lots of organisms use formaldehyde for the carbon it contains. It is made by our bodies and occurs naturally in the air that we breathe. In fact, metabolic processes break it down to simple carbon dioxide and water. Plants and animals also produce formaldehyde. If organisms that live in soil and water do not break down the formaldehyde, sunlight breaks it down through a process known as photo degradation. It is even emitted as a by-product of certain vegetables such as brussel sprouts and cabbage when they are cooked. Beware, there may be a proposal banning farmers' markets!

Formaldehyde is soluble in water, so it does not accumulate in the fatty tissues of terrestrial or aquatic organisms. Processes like bioaccumulation and biomagnifications are not a primary concern. Certain pesticides, for example, may bioaccumulate in organisms and then biomagnify in the environment. DDT is an example of a persistent organic chemical, which, due to its fat solubility, will accumulate in the fatty tissues of aquatic and terrestrial organisms. This sets up the potential for biomagnifications through simple food chains and complex food webs. Chemicals such as DDT can be found as a pollutant in water in the parts per trillion level be consumed by plankton, small fish, large fish, and by the time a bird consumes that large fish, be present in the parts per million level. This was the primary drive behind the ban of the use of this pesticide in the United States. Rachel Carson feared that without a ban on DDT, we would one day have a "Silent Spring" without the voices of birds in spring. Unlike DDT, formaldehyde is water-soluble and will not bioaccumulate in the fatty tissues.

THE CHEMISTRY OF FORMALDEHYDE AND ITS ACTION IN FIRMING PROTEINS

The molecular formula for formaldehyde is HCHO of CH_2O. Formaldehyde is a colorless gas. It is very soluble in water. Formaldehyde is generally available as formalin, an aqueous solution containing 37% formaldehyde gas by weight of 40% by volume. This expresses the limits of the solubility of formaldehyde in water. To increase the solubility above this level, ethanol can be added to the solution.

Formaldehyde can polymerize to form paraformaldehyde. The more CH_2O units that add into the structure, the heavier the molecule becomes, until it precipitates out of solution in the form of waxy-like flakes. If the arterial solution on your shelf has exceeded its shelf life, you may observe these flakes in the bottom of the bottle. This precipitation also occurs in acidic solutions. Methanol is generally added to arterial fluids as an antipolymerizing agent for formaldehyde. Remember if the formaldehyde in your arterial has formed paraformaldehyde, the available formaldehyde for an embalming has been reduced.

In a very alkaline solution, formaldehyde is unstable. Formaldehyde has a very limited pH range. If the surrounding medium becomes too acidic, it polymerizes; if it becomes too alkaline, it breaks down. Again, if the formaldehyde breaks down, there will be less formaldehyde available for an embalming. The breakdown of proteins as the body decomposes will form organic nitrogen compounds, such as amino acids, which further break down to produce amines and ammonia. Each of these products contributes to producing an alkaline environment and may contribute to the formation of foul odors. Therefore, the more advanced the decomposition, the more nitrogen is available to neutralize the formaldehyde, hence a greater formaldehyde demand on the need for a higher index solution to adequately embalm and firm the tissues of the body. Uremic poisoning can also increase formaldehyde demand. When someone has died as a result of kidney failure, the potential of urea (an organic nitrogen compound) in the blood is greatly increased. Hence, the importance of completely flushing this contaminated blood from the system. Again, increased nitrogen content would call for increased formaldehyde demand, thus increasing the risk of formaldehyde exposure to the embalmer.

The chemistry between formaldehyde and the proteins of the body is very fascinating. When formaldehyde reacts with water, it forms methylene glycol. There is very little free formaldehyde in a formalin solution. The methylene glycol forms methylene bridges between the nitrogen atoms of adjacent proteins. In the process of this reaction, water is lost. Cross-linking of protein removes one molecule of water for every cross-link that is formed. As water is lost, the proteins become more viscous or firm. In other words, the main chemical action of formaldehyde in embalming is the coagulation of protein. The protein's resistance to digestive enzymes is also increased. The proteins also become less susceptible to hydrolysis. An abundance of water could reverse the embalming results. Hence, cases of edema would increase the formaldehyde demand. Any process that can reduce the amount of excess tissue fluid prior to embalming would again decrease the need for a higher index fluid and would protect the embalmer from increased formaldehyde exposure.

BESIDES AS AN EMBALMING AGENT, HOW IS FORMALDEHYDE USED?

According to the Formaldehyde Council, formaldehyde is used in thousands of products. Chemistry has allowed the responsible use of formaldehyde in personal hygiene products, vaccines, film used in x-rays, soaps, detergents, cosmetics, plastics, carpeting, clothing, resins, glues, and medicines, to name a few. Table 1 lists many products that depend on formaldehyde in their manufacture.

Did you know that funeral service only accounts for approximately 1% of the total usage of formaldehyde in the United States? Imagine the number of jobs that would be eliminated with a ban on formaldehyde if funeral service only accounts for 1% of the usage of formaldehyde in the United States. With these types of economic ramifications, decisions on formaldehyde must be based on sound science, not junk science, media-hype, or the "flim-flam" of marketers. Our economy is already fragile, unemployment rates are very high, and government spending must be wise and prudent.

Interestingly enough, formaldehyde is instrumental in the manufacture of many products, but often little or no formaldehyde is present in the final product. Also, glues and adhesives that are made with formaldehyde are exceptional bonding agents. Formaldehyde-based products are key to the manufacture of automobiles, including the paint, as well as the production of dollar bills, the ink used in books, magazines, and newspapers, wood products, and agricultural products including fertilizers. In textiles, formaldehyde-based material helps bind dyes to fabrics and improves a fabric's resistance to wrinkles.

In many instances, because of formaldehyde's unique physical and chemical properties, few compounds can replace it as a raw material without reducing performance and making the final product more expensive. Whether it is plywood for home construction, fuel system components for automobiles, or components of heart valves and pacemakers, using formaldehyde translates into enormous health and safety benefits, more affordable housing and automobiles, and many products with a consistent quality.

EVERYDAY MEDICAL APPLICATIONS

The microbiologist and anatomist in me found the following applications very fascinating. Urinary tract infections can be treated using a derivative of formaldehyde. Using formaldehyde-based drugs to treat UTIs eliminates the creation of bacterial resistance to antibiotics. We are seeing the emergence of many drug-resistant

TABLE 1. FORMALDEHYDE'S MANY USES

Home Construction Applications	Home Interiors	Aerospace Applications	Automotive Applications
Asphalt shingles, sheathing, cladding, and roofs	Electrical boxes and outlets	Brake pads, landing gear, lubricants,	*Fuel System Components*
Walls, wall panels, and floors	Furniture, countertops, cabinets, and cabinet doors	Tire cord adhesives	Pump housings and filters
	Bedding, seating, and carpet underlay	Seats, seatbelt buckles	Impellers, reservoirs, senders, and gas caps
	Appliances: Washers, dryers, and dishwashers	Insulation of doors and windows, and interior walls and floors	*Under the Hood*
	Plumbing: Faucets, showerheads, and valve mechanisms		Molded components and engine and metallic parts, automatic transmission parts, and carburetor floats
	Paints and varnishes		*Exterior*
			Exterior primer, clear coat, and trim
			Tire cord adhesive, bumper
			Interior
			Seats, steering wheel, and interior trim
			Brake pads, dashboard, and fascias
			Instrument knobs, hooks, fasteners, and clips, locks, speaker grilles
			Trunk release levers
			Door handles, door panels, and window cranks
			Seatbelt buckles
			Windshield wiper parts
			Cup holders and head rests

strains of bacteria, caused by the use, misuse, and overuse of antibiotics and other antimicrobials. Bacteria are incapable of developing resistance to formaldehyde. Formaldehyde is used to create the hard capsules of many time-released drugs. The formaldehyde-based pill coatings allow the capsule to dissolve slowly and promote maximum absorption of the medicine. In both of these instances, the body's metabolic processes would naturally break down any small residual amounts of formaldehyde. Formaldehyde is used to make plastics used in artificial heart valves, pacemakers, and artificial limbs. More than 10 types of vaccines are made each year that use formaldehyde as the delivery system.

THE LIFE SCIENCES

Formaldehyde provides many benefits to the life sciences. Formaldehyde is used in research laboratories throughout the world as tissue preservative. It has been used for more than 100 years in embalming for its preservative and disinfecting qualities. Being able to adequately preserve tissue samples allows researchers to identify proteins, DNA, and RNA. The ability to preserve tissues has benefited those in the field of medicine, the pharmaceutical industry, the field of forensics, funeral service, and those involved in the training of these esteemed professionals.

CONSUMER AND OCCUPATIONAL SAFETY

The fact has been established that formaldehyde and formaldehyde-based products are used to manufacture thousands of products that are purchased daily in the United States. It should make American consumers more comfortable about purchasing these products, knowing that three agencies, the United States Environmental Protection Agency (US EPA), the Consumer Product Safety Commission (CPSC), and the United States Department of Housing and Urban Development (HUD), have addressed indoor air exposure to formaldehyde. With the combination of governmental regulation and voluntary product emission standards, indoor formaldehyde emissions have declined significantly. Formaldehyde is an extensively regulated material. Mandatory government regulations set standards to protect health and the environment. These requirements allow for the safe production, storage, handling, and use of formaldehyde.

Governmental regulations that help to protect consumers and the environment, the United States Department of Labor's Occupational Safety and Health Administration (OSHA) sets standards for workplace exposures to formaldehyde. These comprehensive health standards include limits on permissible exposures, requirements for monitoring employee exposures in the workplace, protective measures including engineering controls, medical surveillance, and communication and training about hazards. OSHA provides comprehensive health standards for formaldehyde exposure by embalmers in their Formaldehyde Standard. The permissible exposure limit (PEL) is 0.75 ppm (parts of formaldehyde per million parts air) measured as a time-weighted average (TWA). A TWA is the level of formaldehyde gas present in the air, averaged over a 9-hour time period. The short-term exposure limit (STEL) is a high formaldehyde gas limit to which employees may be safely exposed for a short time; the limit is 2 ppm for a time not to exceed 15 minutes; the employee may not be exposed to this higher limit for this limited amount of time more than 4 times per 8-hour work day. The STEL was included in the standard mainly to allow for autopsy procedures.

FORMALDEHYDE UNDER FIRE IS NOTHING NEW

Formaldehyde has been under continuous fire for close to 40 years. In March of 1972, Dr. Jerome F. Fredrick published the first in a new series, "Ecological Factors in Embalming." Here were some of his comments as they applied to the public's growing concern over embalming and air pollution:

1. Even if the embalmer were to inject the body with chemically required quantities that would insure the thorough conversion of all protein, the fumes emanating from such a cadaver would be nonexistent.
2. The embalmer should also be mindful of pathogenic organism release, which is much more important insofar as the public health goes.
   a. Limit the manipulations of a cadaver.
   b. Thorough disinfection of the skin surfaces prior to arterial embalming.
   c. Another very important source of bacterial air pollution is via the forced expiration of entrapped air in the lungs of a cadaver. Airborne diseases such as tuberculosis and some of the fungal lung diseases can be guarded against if the embalmer, during the course of his embalming procedures, is on his/her guard to avoid pressures on the thoracic cavity of the case he/she is working on. In support of Dr. Fredrick, I would point to the documented case in *Mortuary Management*, 2000, where an embalmer acquired tuberculosis from the deceased that he had embalmed. The John Hopkins School of Medicine verified this with DNA analysis. Yet, we still hear that the "dead human body poses no health threat to the public or the embalmer."

d. The thorough disinfection of the cadaver is the most important way in which the professional embalmer can contribute to the public health, and to the ecology, at the same time. I would say Dr. Fredrick was ahead of his time.

In November, 1982, Margaret S. Boothe, then the Director of the Dodge Cambridge Research Laboratories, published a three-part article "Formaldehyde: Friend of Foe?" Ms. Boothe, also an analytical chemist, reported on many interesting findings on formaldehyde:

1. She described a cancer study that was conducted by the Chemical Industry Institute of Technology (CIIT) in 1979, in which laboratory rats exposed to formaldehyde vapor developed nasal cancer. Here is a summary of the study:
   a. It indicated that for exposures of 15 ppm for 6 hours/day, 5 days/week, for 16 months, formaldehyde is carcinogenic. At this level after 16 months, 3 rats out of 120 animals had developed nasal cancer.
   b. Up to 18 months, no cancer had developed in rats exposed to 2 and 6 ppm.
   c. Also, mice that were exposed at 2, 6, and 15 ppm formaldehyde over the same time period of time showed no occurrences of cancer.
   d. At 15 ppm, a human being would run screaming from the room the instant of first exposure. A man would be blind from tearing and unable to stand the pain of breathing at 15 ppm.
2. Formaldehyde manufacturers, EPA, TSCA, NIOSH, Formaldehyde Institute (now called the Formaldehyde Council), and other research facilities are constantly collecting, reviewing, and publishing data on the effect of formaldehyde on laboratory animals and upon people who are in contact with it in the workplace. The information coming out of these studies so far has been the foundation for the decision by the EPA not to include formaldehyde in its list of carcinogens at this time. I would add that since the time of Ms. Boothe's work, the EPA has classified formaldehyde as a probable carcinogen, but has not succumbed to pressures by the Sierra Club, or others, to upgrade this classification, or pose a ban on formaldehyde. It is my hope that the EPA would not make such a ruling without a thorough review of all the scientific and historical data currently available on formaldehyde by the National Academy of Sciences, as per the recommendation of the Formaldehyde Council.
3. Again it is well to warn that, as with all chemicals, care and good management practices should be

the watch words of the day. Despite the date this article was written by Ms. Boothe, this is still excellent advice. Please refer again to the best management practices (BMPs) developed by the NFDA.

In 1991, Dr. Fredrick, published an article "Formaldehyde-Phobia: Friend or Foe?" Dr. Fredrick begins his article, "Probably no chemical has ever had the publicity and reputation that formaldehyde has acquired over the last 20 years." Some of his findings can be summarized as follows:

1. It has been publicized as the basic chemical responsible for all life in the universe.
2. It has been found by spectroscopic analysis in the huge clouds that occupy interstellar space.
3. It is probably the first step in synthesis of sugars during the process of photosynthesis in green plants.
4. This primeval chemical is one of the building blocks of all life on the earth.
5. Formaldehyde is a carcinogen; formaldehyde is not a carcinogen. Formaldehyde is an irritant; it is not an irritant. The upshot was to make the public really formaldehyde phobic!
6. The nonscientific sector of the public became wary of whether formaldehyde would leak out of the embalmed bodies. All of the formaldehyde is reacted with the excess proteins in the body. And hence, there is none left over to leak out. In other words, what Dr. Fredrick would say today is that there are not eight Olympic-sized swimming pools full of formaldehyde in the ground. There are not even eight Olympic-sized bathing suits full of formaldehyde in the ground as a result of the embalming process.
7. Even if the modern embalmer were to use enough formaldehyde to "over embalm" and the excess leaked out, it would immediately react with the nitrogenous components contained in all soils to form innocuous urotropin. Any small amount of the chemical that theoretically could "leak" into the atmosphere would be rapidly broken down to water and carbon dioxide by ultraviolet light or by heat from the sun. Remember back to my earlier discussion on the neutralization of formaldehyde by nitrogen compounds. This is the primary reason OSHA does recommend the use of ammonia (NH_3) in a formaldehyde spill. It will neutralize the formaldehyde. Likewise, with an advance case of decomposition, there will be more organic nitrogen compounds and a greater demand for formaldehyde.
8. At the time of Dr. Fredrick's article, the State of New Jersey's Department of Environmental Protection, Division of Hazardous Waste considered

formaldehyde that has been used to embalm a body no longer a "generically hazardous waste" under the state's listing of chemical hazards. In other words, the formaldehyde is not present as such (in leakages from embalmed bodies), but rather as the spent reaction products (which are not hazardous wastes). Leakage of formaldehyde from embalmed cadavers in our cemeteries does not constitute any possible threat to soils and/or potable waters in the area. Any research that I conducted in this area also supports Dr. Fredrick's findings.

SCIENTIFIC STUDIES ON HEALTH EFFECTS

Since we have established that formaldehyde does not bioaccumulate in the environment, let us discuss its health effect from a purely scientific standpoint. There has been much work done in this area both past and present. There have been irritation studies, exposures studies, and cancer studies. Epidemiologists, oncologists, and toxicologists have devoted careers to studying formaldehyde. Scientific endeavors with no promise of fame and fortune. Pure science. No gimmicks, no marketing schemes. Just sound science on which environmental regulation can be based. The following is a summary of some of the findings from these studies.

Irritation Studies

Formaldehyde can be irritating to the eyes, nose, and throat, but for most people, the irritation appears to be highly subjective. An expert panel review of over 150 published studies found that eye irritation does not become significant until around 1 ppm (par per million), and moderate to severe eye, nose, and throat irritation occurs at 2 to 3 ppm. The expert panels found that a level of 1 ppm would not cause eye irritation in 75 to 95% of all people exposed. In any case, normal environmental exposures and embalming occupational exposures are less than these levels.

Cancer Studies

In the area of evaluating the cancer risk associated with formaldehyde, the Formaldehyde Council brought in experts in the field to evaluate the many studies that have been conducted. One such expert, Dr. Gary Marsh, since 1978 has conducted more than 25 occupational epidemiology studies of health effects from various workplace exposures. A major focus of his research has been the evaluation of human health effects from formaldehyde exposure.

Dr. Marsh reports that most of the epidemiology evidence for assessing human cancer risk from formaldehyde exposure comes from three large cohort studies of industrial workers: one in Britain and two in the United States by the National Institute of Occupational Safety and Health (NIOSH) and the National Cancer Institute (NCI). In 2004, the International Agency for Research on Cancer or IARC reclassified formaldehyde as carcinogenic in humans based largely on evidence from the NCI study that formaldehyde causes nasopharyngeal cancer. The NCI finding was based on only eight nasopharyngeal deaths among exposed workers, an increase of only two nasopharyngeal deaths from IARC's 1995 classification of formaldehyde as a probable carcinogen. Only one nasopharyngeal cancer death was observed in the other two cohort studies combined. The evidence that formaldehyde causes other cancers, such as leukemia, was deemed nonsufficient by IARC.

Recent literature reviews and reanalysis of the NCI cohort data conducted by Dr. Marsh's research group have cast considerable doubt on the validity of NCI's findings and IARC's reclassification. For example, his research group showed that NCI's findings for nasopharyngeal cancer were driven entirely by an anomalous finding in 1 of 10 study plants, termed Plant 1. Six of the eight nasopharyngeal cancer deaths occurred among exposed workers in this single plant, resulting in a statistically significant 10-fold excess in nasopharyngeal cancer with a 35% deficit in nasopharyngeal cancer deaths among exposed workers in the remaining 9 plants.

Dr. Marsh's group also conducted an independent and expanded cohort study of Plant 1. They concluded in their latest published report that the anomalous finding of the nasopharyngeal cancer in Plant 1 may be related to previous work in the extensive local metal industry. These jobs entailed possible exposures to several risk factors for nasopharyngeal cancer, including sulfuric acid mists, mineral acid, metal dust, and heat.

In summary, Dr. Marsh's group concluded that their analysis of the NCI cohort data did not support NCI's suggestion of a causal association with formaldehyde and nasopharyngeal cancer. They believe that the 2004 decision by IARC to reclassify formaldehyde as a Group 1 substance was premature, considering the small number of nasopharyngeal cancer deaths, the missing evidence from the British and NIOSH cohort studies, the anomalous finding for nasopharyngeal cancer in Plant 1, and their new evidence that the nasopharyngeal cancer risk in the influential Plant 1 may be related to previous work in the metal industry.

On November 27, 2005, the Formaldehyde Council was encouraged that the US Environmental Protection Agency intended to wait until it had the benefit of enhanced scientific data from the National Cancer Institute (NCI) before updating its carcinogenic classification for formaldehyde under its Integrated Risk

Information System (IRIS) program. EPA currently classifies formaldehyde as "probably carcinogenic to humans" under the IRIS program. As was stated earlier in this article, there still seems to be a lot of uncertainty in the data, again warranting an extensive study by the National Academy of Sciences.

In August 2008, the EPA denied a Sierra Club petition to promulgate national formaldehyde regulations similar to those adopted in California by the California Air Resource Board (BCARB). The EPA ruled that there was insufficient data to assess the risk proposed by formaldehyde or to identify the least burdensome means of protecting against such a risk. Instead, the EPA said it would initiate a proceeding to investigate whether and what type of regulatory or other action might be appropriate. The Formaldehyde Council brought in experts that support the current stance taken by the EPA. Here is a summary of Dr. F. J. Murray of San Jose, California, in regard to the CARB proposal to lower formaldehyde emissions:

"The health benefits of CARB's proposal to lower formaldehyde emissions have been over-estimated by a cancer risk assessment that does not use the most current peer-reviewed scientific information. Importantly, more recent and sophisticated risk assessments of formaldehyde by other respected regulatory agencies, including US EPA, Health Canada, and the World Health Organization (WHO), predict the cancer risk is as much as 36,000 times lower than the estimate relied upon by the CARB study. These assessments indicate that the proposed reductions in formaldehyde emissions will not produce any meaningful reduction in cancer cases in California.

CARB should carefully evaluate the proposal to reduce exposure to formaldehyde, particularly the extremely low limits proposed in Phase 2, in light of the tenuous public health benefits represented by the estimated reduction in cancer cases in California. If reducing exposure to formaldehyde will not result in any meaningful reduction in cancer risk in California, the proposed action must be questioned. Given the fact that over 100,000 Californians are expected to die annually from cancer, it is especially important to focus the state's resources on actions that will result in cancer and improvement in public health."

On May 12, 2009, the Formaldehyde Council was kept busy responding to the latest article on formaldehyde that was published in the *Journal of the National Cancer Institute*. The NCI article was entitled, "Mortality From Lymphohematopoietic Malignancies Among Workers in Formaldehyde Industries: The National cancer Institute Cohort." This study was a continuation of a study that followed through December 31, 1979, and updated through December 31, 1994, in which formaldehyde exposure was associated with an increased risk of leukemia.

NCI extended the follow-up through December 31, 2004. Evaluation of risks over time suggests a possible link between formaldehyde exposure and leukemia. The NCI reported that observed patterns could be due to chance or could be consistent with a causal association within the relatively short induction-incubation period, characteristic of leukemogenesis. The NCI conclusion was that further epidemiological study and exploration of potential molecular mechanisms are warranted.

The Formaldehyde Council believes that the significant disparity between the author's conclusions and the actual data underscores the need for reevaluation of this latest report in conjunction with the broader body of existing formaldehyde research. The Formaldehyde Council supports the commission of a scientific peer review of formaldehyde by the prestigious National Academy of Sciences (NAS). This intensive scientific peer review would consider all existing research data on formaldehyde. The Formaldehyde Council is hopeful that NAS will produce a scientifically sound interpretation of all current research on formaldehyde and that our government will use the NAS analysis as the basis for developing appropriate formaldehyde policies and regulations to enhance public health. This recommendation of the use of sound science to make policy decisions with large-scale ramifications makes good environmental and economic sense and is a very responsible and ethical approach.

SUMMARY

Since the 1990s, the National Cancer Institute studies have shown that effective ventilation is the single most important factor in protecting embalmers exposed to formaldehyde from harm. NFDA is considering conducting a study that will investigate strategies for keeping the air in the prep room formaldehyde free. The study would ultimately lead to the design of a cost-effective prep room ventilation system.

As always, consumers need to be careful that some products may be presented as better for the environment and truly are not. Sometimes the only thing green about the product you are buying is the container it comes in or the cash ending up in the marketer's pocket. The good news is we already know that, based on current information available, formaldehyde use in funeral service is not a serious environmental issue. So let us work together to follow BMPs in funeral service that could help protect the health and safety of funeral service professionals. As professionals, we can band together to promote the strict implementation of the BMPs in our funeral homes and businesses. In doing so, we can cast a shadow over the evil personality of formaldehyde and let the good personality shine brightly.

WORKS CITED

Bastionon D, Matos BS, Aquino WF, Pacheo A, Mendes JMB. Geophysical surveying to Investigate Groundwater Contamination by a Cemetery. Proceedings of the Symposium on the Application of Geophysics to Engineering and Environmental Problems: The Annual Meeting of the Environmental and Engineering Geophysical Society: February 20–24, 2000:709–718.

Bean LE, Blair A, Leubin JH, Stewart PA, Hayes RB, Hoover RN, Hauptmann M. Mortality from lymphohematopoietic malignancies among workers in formaldehyde industries: The National Cancer Institute Cohort. *Journal of the National Cancer Institute* 2009;101:751–761.

Boothe MS. Formaldehyde: friend or foe? Parts I-III *The Dodge Magazine*, November 1982:4+

Chan GS, Scafe M, Emami S. *Cemeteries and Groundwater: An Examination of the Potential Contamination of Groundwater Preservatives Containing Formaldehyde.* Queen's Printer for Ontario, 1992.

Corley C. Burials and cemeteries go green. *NPR*, April 26, 2009.

Dempsey PA. The future of formaldehyde. *The Forum*, January 2009:22–28.

Dent BB. Cemetery Decay Product Profiles: Two Cases in Australia, Unconsolidated, Sandy Aquifers. Searching for Sustainable Future: 15th Australian Geological Convention, July 3–7, 2000; Sydney:130.

Dorn JM. *Thanatochemistry*, 2nd ed. Upper Saddle River, NJ: Prentice Hall, 1998.

"FCI Fact Sheet on JNCI Study on Occupational Exposure to Formaldehyde." May 12, 2009. May 18, 2009.

"FCI JNCI Talking Points." Formaldehyde Council, 12 May 2009. 18 May 2009 http://www.formaldehyde. org. Formaldehyde Council. "Formaldehyde Industry Disputes Findings of JNCI Report." Press release. Formaldehyde Council. 12 May 2009. Formaldehyde Council. 18 May 2009 http://www.formaldehyde.org.

"Formaldehyde: Hazard Recognition." January 27, 2009.

"Formaldehyde." January 27, 2009.

Fredrick JF. Ecological factors in embalming: Parts I-IV. *The Dodge Magazine*, March 1972: 20+.

Fredrick JF. "Formaldehyde-phobia: Friend or foe. *The Dodge Magazine,* June 1991: 11+.

Gary M. Reevaluation of mortality risks from leukemia in the formaldehyde Cohort Study of the National Cancer Institute. *Regulatory Toxicology and Pharmacology* 2004;40:113–124.

Green CL, Fitch JH. Death Knell for Formaldehyde. *The Director,* May 2009: 48–51.

Hayes R. Mortality of U.S. embalmers and funeral directors. *American Journal of Industrial Medicine* 1990;18: 641–652.

Hopkins DW, Wiltshire PEJ, Turner BD. Microbial characteristics of soils from graves: An investigation at the interface of soil microbiology and forensic science. *Applied Soil Ecology* 2000;14:238–288.

Levine R. The mortality of Ontario undertakers and a review of formaldehyde-related mortality studies. *Journal of Occupational Medicine* 1984;26:740–746.

Loh, MM, Levy JI, Spengler JD, Houseman EA, Bennett DH. Ranking cancer risks of organic hazardous air pollutants in the United States. *Environmental Health Perspectives* 2007;115:1160–1168.

Mayer RG. *Embalming: History, Theory, and Practice*, 4th ed. New York: McGraw-Hill, 2006.

Miller GT. *Environmental Science*, 11th ed. Belmont, CA: Thomson, 2006.

National Funeral Directors Association. Formaldehyde best management practices. *The Director,* May 2009: 52–56.

National Funeral Directors Association. NFDA green funeral service Q&A. The Director, February 2009: 32–36.

Q&A on JNCI. *Formaldehyde Council.* May 12, 2009. May 18, 2009.

United Nations Environment Publications. OECD SIDS. Formaldehyde. Paris, France, 2002.

Untitled. The Australian Institute of Embalming (December 2008).

Walrath J. Mortality patterns among embalmers. *International Journal of Cancer* 1983;31:407–411.

Walrath J, Fraumeni JF, Jr. Cancer and other causes of death among embalmers. *Cancer Research* 1984; 44:4638–4641.

What Will Be Formaldehyde's Fate? Funeral Service Insider 24 Nov. 2008. World Health Organization. Concise International Chemical Assessment Document 40: Formaldehyde. Geneva, 2002.

World Health Organization. *Environmental Health Criteria for Formaldehyde.* Geneva, 1989.

The Preparation Room: Ventilation*

Jack Adams, CFSP

Care and custody for the dead human body is and will always be the most important activity a funeral home does. The work done in the preparation room is the foundation for the funeral home. The preparation room itself

*Reprinted by permission from The Dodge Magazine, Nov.–Dec., Vol. 96, No. 5, 2004. Copyright: The Dodge Company.

needs to provide a comfortable and safe work environment. A room of adequate size, with proper ventilation and lighting, and furnished with the necessary working equipment will often result in higher-quality work results.

With OSHA and public health concerns, there is greater interest in preparation room safety and design. In addition to having properly sized doors, sanitary flooring and walls, and lighting and environmental controls, the room needs to reflect comfort and safety measures that do not interfere with but rather enhance the work routines of the embalmer.

The size and location of the prep room is important when building a new funeral home or remodeling. If possible, the room should be large enough to accommodate three remains and have private access, with doors of sufficient size, opening into hallways that lead to casket storage rooms, chapels, and garage reception areas. As call volume goes over 150 per year, the preparation room needs to be larger to accommodate the greater volume.

An enclosed garage for delivering remains and loading vehicles should be near or adjacent to the prep room. The garage entry and exit into the preparation room needs to be private and away from any public visibility.

The ventilation system is a safety as well as a comfort factor for employees using the preparation room. New and remodeled preparation rooms need to comply with local building codes and OSHA standards. Ideally, the room should have its own independent heating, cooling, and ventilation system. Unfortunately, this type of independent system is rare, especially in older funeral homes. Air from the prep room should not be recirculated to other parts of the building. Once the size and space of a room has been determined, a proper ventilation system can be designed.

Embalmers know the effects, such as watery eyes and coughing spells, brought about by inadequate ventilation in the preparation area. In addition to formaldehyde, even common cleaning chemicals such as ammonia, household bleach and many of the disinfectants employed will have irritating side effects.

Proper ventilation is the most important factor in any prep room. Too many prep rooms are designed without input from an embalmer. Eight-inch-diameter kitchen exhaust fans seemed to be the normal ventilation for preparation rooms in older funeral homes. Of course, this fan does not come close to supplying proper ventilation for the prep room. A properly ventilated embalming room must be able to handle any aerosol pathogen or chemical concerns, including a chemical spill, as well as the odors associated with decomposition.

Certain infections are circulated by the airborne route including varicella, measles, and tuberculosis. The usual mode of contaminating the air is breathing, coughing, and sneezing. When death occurs, these functions stop, so why the concern? During removals and embalming, tasks like transferring bodies to cots and tables, washing and embalming remains, and aspirating are common ways to create aerosols. Even unwrapping or undressing remains can cause potentially dangerous breath-like aerosol action in a preparation room. Gentle unwrapping or removing remains from a transfer pouch can reduce aerosols dramatically.

These potential aerosol exposures and exposures to blood and body fluids are the reasons that embalmers are required to use universal precautions and personal protection equipment. Physicians are aware of airflow patterns to limit transmission of airborne pathogens. The duration of time that airborne viruses remain in a room depend on the rate of air exchanges. The CDC recommends that patients requiring isolation for infectious diseases such as TB be placed in rooms having negative airflow. These rooms should have frequent air changes. The air should be exhausted directly outside without recirculation.

The American Society of Heating, Refrigeration and Air Conditioning Engineers (ASHRAE) design airflow systems for health control within hospitals and industries using chemicals in their everyday operation.

The Centers for Disease Control and Prevention (CDC), the National Institute for Occupational Safety (NIOSH), and the American National Standard Institute (ANSI) are all active in recommending guidelines for proper ventilation for health facilities and the workplace. Because of that, we have used them for part of our sources for this article. The two most common reasons for controlling ventilation would be for infection control and control of chemical contaminants.

The armed forces are presented with unique situations because of their exposure to medical isolation, pathology, and chemical exposure. The Navy for instance has ventilation requirements for their ships that give us a good source for recommended air changes per hour. For instance, acid store rooms aboard ship are required to have 15 air changes per hour. Chlorine gas cylinder rooms are required to have 30 air changes per hour. Paint lockers on ships are required to have 15 air changes per hour.

The Air Force requirements on Heating, Ventilation, and Air Conditioning (HVAC) systems are geared to infection control. Contaminated areas, such as infectious isolations areas and autopsy rooms, should maintain a negative air pressure relative to adjoining rooms and corridors. Air from these rooms should not be recirculated through a cold air return back through the central air system. The negative air pressure ensures that other rooms in the building will not be contaminated from the isolation or autopsy room. This principle should be the same for our prep rooms.

Some of the Air Force requirements for ventilation in medical facility rooms by air changes per hour (ACH) are as follows:

Location	Outdoor Air (ACH)	Total Air (ACH)	Exhaust Air to Outside
Trauma room	5	12	Optional
Nursery suite	5	12	Optional
Infectious isolation	2	12	Yes
Autopsy rooms	2	12	Yes

You can see that the infectious disease rooms and the autopsy rooms are considered to be high risk and require air to be exhausted outside without any recirculation. Preparation rooms certainly should be considered high risk, and they are rooms where potential chemical exposure is possible. So now that we realize that we work in areas that are potentially hazardous to us, how many air changes per hour would be adequate for our preparation room?

While researching this topic and contacting NIOSH, AIA, ASHRAE, ANSI, and various other sources for ventilation information, it was made obvious that preparation room ventilation was not covered under any existing guidelines or standards. As long as an embalming room passes a Formaldehyde Monitor test, it is considered safe. Because it is relatively easy to stay within the acceptable limits for formaldehyde, too many prep rooms still have the older ventilation systems, and this might consist of only a 14-inch exhaust fan.

Just because a preparation room can pass a monitoring test, it does not mean that it is a comfortable place to work. It could be a room that is recirculating pathogens and chemical fumes into other parts of the building. Autopsy rooms are considered high risk and are recommended to have 12 air changes per hour, and two of those changes should consist of outside air.

So, once again we are in a position to use our own common sense for the safety of our own workers. Because a preparation room presents a greater degree of chemical exposure than an autopsy room, this embalmer would like to work in a room with 20 air changes per hour. I have personally recommended 20 air changes per hour (ACH) to funeral homes, and those that have complied are the best ventilated and most comfortable preparation rooms that I have ever worked in. The room should be under negative pressure. That is, more air is exhausted than is taken into the room. This keeps the other parts of the building from being contaminated

with air from the preparation room. If the funeral home does not have an independent heating and ventilation system for the prep room, a one-pass system can be utilized when remodeling. This means that any air going into the preparation room will not be allowed to reenter or recirculate into any part of the funeral home.

FIGURING AIRFLOW IN AIR CHANGES PER HOUR

Fans are usually rated in CFMs (cubic feet per minute). In order to relate these "per minute" ratings to our ACHs (air changes per hour), we must divide ACH by 60 (the number of minutes in an hour). So the formula for determining the CFMs of the fan to purchase is:

Divide the number of air changes per hour you desire by 60 and then multiply that figure by room size in cubic feet

Calculate the volume of the preparation room by multiplying length, width, and height of the room in feet, or

length in feet × width in feet × height in feet = volume in cubic feet

(feet × feet × feet = cubic feet)

For example, a room 20 ft. × 10 ft. and 10 ft. high will have a volume of 2000 CF (cubic feet). If one wants 20 air changes per hour, then they will have to simply calculate the volume in cubic feet, divide by 20/60, and you will have the minimum required CFM rating of an exhaust, which could achieve the 20 air changes per hour (667 CFM, in this case). Once the funeral director knows the volume of the preparation room area and calculates the exhaust requirement, then the equipment supplier or installer can easily help.

To achieve a desired 20 air changes per hour, you could use the following chart to help choose the proper size of exhaust fan.

(Cubic Ft. Per Minutes)

Room Size	Volume – Divided by 3 = CFM
(a) 10 × 15 and 10 ft. high:	10 × 15 × 10 = 1500 cubic ft./3 500 CFM
(b) 10 × 20 and 10 ft. high:	10 × 20 × 10 = 2000 cubic ft./3 = 667 CFM
(c) 20 × 20 and 10 ft. high:	20 × 20 × 10 = 4000 cubic ft./3 = 1333 CFM

Risk of Infection and Tracking of Work-related Infectious Diseases in the Funeral Industry

Susan Salter Davidson, MS.MT (ASCP) and William H. Benjamin, Jr. PhD
Birmingham Alabama

The routine tasks carried out by funeral service professionals (FSPs) would seem to put them at significant risk of exposure to several infectious agents. Exposure by way of splashes to the mucus membranes, inhalation of aerosolized body fluids, and direct inoculation can result in infectious diseases caused by multiple species of bacteria, viruses, and prions. The purpose of this review is to determine what is known of the risk of exposure to infectious agents that FSPs experience in the workplace, identify prevention and postexposure strategies utilized in the funeral business, and determine occupationally acquired infection rates among this group.

METHODS

A literature search was carried out using the PubMed service of the National Library of Medicine (April, 2006). Abstracts were reviewed, and applicable articles were obtained. Internet sources included the web sites of the Centers for Disease Control and Prevention (CDC), the United States Department of Labor, the US Census Bureau, the National Funeral Directors Association (NFDA), and the American Board of Funeral Service Education.

RESULTS

Risk of Exposure

The risk of exposure to infectious agents in the health care setting is well documented; however, one occupational group that appears to be underrepresented in the infectious disease literature is FSPs. A recent literature review sponsored by the British Institute of Embalmers found that the risk of exposure is well documented but that there is a need for additional studies focusing on the suggested link between reported infections and the embalming procedure.[1] That review, as well as this one, also found a lack of studies in the literature focusing on the implementation of effectiveness of infection control practices in the funeral business.[1]

There were 2,448,288 reported deaths in the United States during 2003, the majority of which was followed by embalming according to the NFDA.[2,3] An infectious disease was the reported cause in 99,232 of these individuals and is recognized as a frequent contributor to mortality, even when not documented as the primary cause of death.[2] The infectious nature of cadavers, regardless of their cause of death, has been documented.[1,4-8] The routine transport and embalming of cadavers place the FSP in a position to be exposed to multiple infectious agents that are transmissible by mucocutaneous contamination, aerosolization, and direct inoculation.[1,8-15]

Two common bacterial pathogens that may be contracted through mucocutaneous contamination are methicillin-resistant *Staphylococcus aureus* (MRSA) and *Streptococcus pyogenes*. Long recognized as a nosocomial pathogen, MRSA is establishing itself as a community-acquired infectious agent with increasing frequency.[10,16,17] Because of the prevalence of MRSA in the population both as a commensal and as a pathogen, the FSP has a potential exposure risk from the remains of individuals who expired in health care facilities and those who died in other settings.[18,19] Group A streptococcus has been shown to survive on the cadavers of victims of invasive disease, presenting a serious infectious risk to the FSP because it may be transmitted by direct contact and as a result of direct inoculation following even minor nicks to the skin during autopsy.[8,12,17,20-22]

FSPs may be exposed to gastrointestinal organisms through direct contact with leaking fecal material when manipulating corpses, which can lead to transmission via the fecal-oral route.[8] The two microorganisms of greatest concern for transmission are non-typhi Salmonella and hepatitis A, whereas *Salmonella typhi*, Shigella species, Cryptosporidia, Helicobacter pylori, and other microorganisms are less of a risk in the developed world.[12,23-25] Another group of Enterobacteriaceae that have the potential to present a risk to FSPs are the extended-spectrum B-lactamase producers (ESBLs) because of their growing prevalence and refractoriness to treatment, resulting in higher mortality rates when responsible for bacteremia.[26,28]

Infectious agents transmitted primarily by the airborne route that should be of concern for the FSP include *Mycobacterium tuberculosis* and the virus responsible for severe acute respiratory syndrome (SARS).[1,8,13,29,30] Tuberculosis is a leading cause of disease and death, with more than one-third of the global population being infected. Attempts to control the infections are complicated by the high prevalence of multiple drug-resistant strains, which are common in some populations.[31] The risk of exposure to *M. tuberculosis* experienced by FSPs is documented for airborne transmission and through direct inoculation.[1,6-8,10,32,34]

SARS is a newly recognized infection disease, and there are no published reports of transmission from cadavers to FSPs. Moore et al. analyzed the data available on SARS and published guidelines for infection control in the health care setting, which were tested in Toronto.[30] Others have also published reviews of the infection control literature concerning SARS, and the World Health Organization (WHO) has released guidelines addressing management of known or suspected cases.[29,30,35,36] Because of the virulent and contagious nature of the SARS virus, it is of special concern to both the health care worker (HCW) and the FSP.[29]

The three most common blood-borne pathogenic viruses FSPs are at risk of exposure to are the hepatitis B virus (HBV), the hepatitis C virus (HCV), and the human immunodeficiency virus (HIV).[1,8,9,11,12,15,37-42] The risk of exposure to blood and other body fluids for this occupational group has been the subject of a limited number of studies.[9,11,37,42,43] Studies focusing on the occurrence of HBV among FSPs show that members of this occupational group have a higher rate of infection than control groups.[1,6,9,12,37] However, widespread implementation of vaccination programs has dramatically lowered the infection rate among HCWs and FSPs.[39,41,44] HCV is the most prevalent blood-borne pathogen in health care settings, with many chronically infected individuals being asymptomatic. Currently, there is no HCV vaccine available.[12,45-48] The long-term viability of HIV in cadaver tissue is recognized, and the literature reports a documented case of seroconversion in a pathologist following necropsy, along with two possible and one documented seroconversions in FSPs.[12,38,49-54] Thus, the importance of the prevention of transmission of HCV and HIV during the embalming procedure is clear, especially in light of these documented cases of transmission of HIV.

The Marburg and Ebola hemorrhagic fever viruses are not endemic in the United States, but the continuing sporadic outbreaks on the African continent, the previous occurrence of infection in European countries, the ease and speed of international travel, and their classification as category A bioterrorism agents warrant their inclusion in a discussion of potential exposure risks for FSPs.[7,55-57] Secondary transmission of these two viruses is known to occur following unprotected exposure to patients and cadavers through mucocutaneous contact and blood and body fluid exposure.[7,58,59] Aerosolization cannot be definitively excluded as a mode of transmission.[58,60] Guidelines have been published for the management of suspected or confirmed cases of these viral infections and include postmortem instructions.[7,56-58,61]

Another important group of infectious diseases of concern to FSPs is the transmissible spongiform encephalopathies (TSEs) or Creutzfeldt–Jakob disease (CJD) in humans, including kuru, iatrogenic, and new variant CJD (vCJD).[62-64] The mode of transmission of prions is not completely understood, with 85% of patients showing no recognizable pattern of transmission, but it is known that iatrogenic CJD has been passed from cadavers to recipients of human growth hormone, dura mater, and corneal grafts as well as between living patients following use of contaminated neurosurgical equipment.[62-64] Blood-borne transmission has been implicated in two cases of secondary vCJD infections in the United Kingdom, prompting concern that the blood supply could be contaminated with the responsible prion because of asymptomatic donor contributions.[63-68] Because prions are not destroyed by formaldehyde or embalming is not recommended for autopsied or traumatized bodies, but, if the procedure is necessary, the CDC suggests following the WHO guidelines.[62,69]

Although most cases of TSE have been located in countries other than the United States, the government is vigilant in monitoring CJD and vCJD cases and has taken steps to prevent an outbreak.[64] Transmission of TSE between patients, to HCW, and to FSP is a major concern because supportive treatment is all that can be done for victims because these diseases are invariably fatal.[63,64]

The potential for transmission of multiple infections agents while engaging in the routine tasks of FSPs has been demonstrated. The nation's primary source of occupational information is the Occupational Information Network (O*NET) sponsored by the US Department of Labor Employment and Training Administration, and their Summary Report for Embalmers and Funeral Directors provides a detailed description of the tasks performed by FSPs that place them at risk.[70] There have been a limited number of published studies documenting actually exposure events.[1,9,11,42,55] The use of sharp implements during the embalming procedure places the FSP at risk of blood-borne pathogen exposure via needlestick, cuts, and splashes. The routine aspiration of blood and other body fluids carries the risk of aerosolization of droplet nuclei. The collection of fluid in the chest cavity of the deceased because of putrefaction of tissue can lead to frothing and gurgling through the nose and mouth of the corpse.[1,9,11]

Exposure Prevention and Management Strategies

Evaluation of exposure prevention and postexposure strategies utilized in the funeral business is difficult. There are few published references focusing on infection control in this setting.[1,9-11,37,42] Funeral homes fall under the mandates of the Occupational Safety Hazard Association's Bloodborne Pathogens Standard (number 1910.13100), which requires that employers have a written exposure control plan and meet the methods of compliance.[71] These methods include the practice of universal precautions, the implementation of engineering and work practice controls, and the provision of personal protective equipment. There does not appear to be a monitoring system in place to determine the effectiveness of adherence to the standard by tabulating exposure events or infection rates among FSPs.[71] The CDC maintains the National Surveillance System for Health Care Workers, which is a voluntary program that monitors exposure events among hospital-based HCWs to HIV, HBV, HCV, and *M. tuberculosis* to assess trends, prevention strategies, and postexposure prophylaxis, but funeral homes are not part of this surveillance program.[72]

A further reason evaluation is difficult is the absence of infection control activities in funeral homes analogous to those found in most health care facilities. These activities are implemented to analyze policies and procedures to control infectious disease transmission. Although compliance among FSPs has not been studied to the degree that it has for HCWs, much of the data from the HCWs can be applied to the funeral business. It is known that compliance is greater if employees feel that their organization is interested in safety, if they have current and correct knowledge of the availability of personal protective equipment, and if they perceive that compliance is mandatory.[30] There has been speculation concerning the usefulness of disclosing to FSPs the specific infectious nature of particular cadavers, but it has been shown that this knowledge does not affect compliance in a significant percentage of employees.[10] The autonomous nature of the work performed by FSPs might be a factor contributing to noncompliance issues. Postexposure actions followed by the FSP might be less than those of the HCW because of the expectation and relative ease of reporting exposure events and receiving postexposure care in most health care settings.

The role continuing education plays in compliance among FSPs is another area that appears not to have been evaluated fully. The American Board of Funeral Service Education, the accrediting agency for schools offering degrees in funeral service, requires students to complete successfully the basic science courses, including microbiology and pathophysiology, and the examinations for licensure administered by each state include sections covering these subjects.[73,74] More than 30 states require annual continuing education credits for licensed funeral directors and embalmers, but there are no specific requirements for infection control subject matter.[73,74] Studies have suggested a need for continuing education to ensure adherence to infection control policies.[29,30,75]

Occupationally Acquired Infection Rates

It is difficult to determine the occupationally acquired infection rate among FSPs. One possible explanation for the apparent underrepresentation of FSP in the infection control literature could be that embalmers and funeral directors are placed under the Personal Care and Service Occupations group rather than being included in the Healthcare Practitioners and Technical Occupations or Healthcare Support Occupations groups in the Bureau of Labor Standard Occupational Classification (SOC) system.[76] This SOC system is consistent with the Census 2000 Alphabetical Indexes of Industries and Occupations used in coding information gathered by governmental and private agencies for statistical reporting programs.[76,77] Another contributing factor is the lack of standardized coding on death certificates for the occupation of the decedent, although multiple governmental agencies are working together to make improvements in the coding system to standardize this data.[78] Underreporting of exposure events by individual employees along with the lack of infection control oversight programs in the funeral business could also be factors making this determination difficult.

An additional topic that is worthy of mention is the exposure risk experienced in countries other than the United States and Canada, which are the only two countries that routinely embalm the deceased. Other countries have various types of funeral services available, but embalming is reserved for cases requiring a prolonged viewing period or for shipment of the corpse. In most areas, family members wash the dead and prepare them for internment, and only rudimentary steps are taken to prevent the spread of communicable disease if it is known to be present.[79] According to the WHO mortality records, worldwide, there were 10,903,977 deaths attributed to infectious and parasitic diseases in 2002, and the majority of these deaths occurred in areas other than the United States and Canada.[80] Thus, as with many issues related to infectious diseases, the developing world could benefit from better surveillance as well as implementation of controls to prevent transmission related to handling of the dead.

DISCUSSION

This review of published literature demonstrates that FSPs have a risk of exposure to bacterial and viral pathogens as well as to prion-mediated diseases. It reveals a lack of published studies focusing on the implementation and effectiveness of infection control policies for this occupational group as well as the difficulty involved in determining actual infection rates related to workplace exposure events. Questions that should be the focus of future studies include determining the level of employee compliance with existing infection control policies, accessing factors that influence compliance, and evaluating the effectiveness of existing policies in preventing exposure events and actual infections as well as implementing better systems to determine the infection rates of the various agents in this occupational group.

REFERENCES

1. Creely KS. Infection risks and embalming. Institute of Occupational Medicine. 2004. Available at http://www.iom-World.org/pubs/IOMTMO401.pdf (accessed April 1, 2005).

2. National Center for Health Statistics. Death: final data for 2003. National Vital Statistics Reports 2006. Available at http://www.cec.gov/nchs/data/hestat/finaldeaths03_tables.pdf#2 (accessed January 38, 2006).

3. National Funeral Directors Association. National Funeral Directors Association fact sheet 2005. Available at http:www.nfda.org/nfdafactsheets/php (accessed July 27, 2005).

4. Rose GW, Hockett RN. The microbiologic evaluation and enumeration of postmortem species from human remains. Health Laboratory Science 1971;8:75–78.

5. Hinson MR. Final report on literature search on the infectious nature of dead bodies for the Embalming Chemical Manufactures Association. Embalming Chemical Manufacturers Association 1968. In: Mayer RG, ed. *Embalming History, Theory, and Practice*, 3rd ed. New York: McGraw-Hill, 2000:649–652.

6. Rendon LR. Dangers of infection. In: Mayer RG, ed. *Embalming History, Theory, and Practice*, 3rd ed. New York: McGraw-Hill, 2000:652–654.

7. Nolte KB, Taylor DG, Richmond JY. Biosafety considerations for autopsy. *The American Journal of Forensic Medicine and Pathology* 2002;23:107–122.

8. Healting TD, Hoffman PN, Young SE. The infection hazards of human cadavers. Communicable Disease Report. *CDR Review* 1995;5:R61–R68.

9. Gershon RR, Vlahov D, Farzadegan H, Alter MJ. Occupational risk of human immunodeficiency virus. Hepatitis B virus, and hepatitis C virus infections among funeral service practitioners in Maryland. *Infection Control and Hospital Epidemiology* 1995;16:194–197.

10. Gershon RR, Vlahov D, Edsamilla-Cejudo JA, Badawi M, McDiarmid M, Karkashian C, Grimes M, Comstock GW. Tuberculosis risk in funeral home employees. *Journal of Occupational and Environmental Medicine* 1998;40:497–503.

11. Nwanyanwu OC, Tabasuri TH, Harris GR. Exposure to and precautions for blood and body fluids among workers in the funeral home franchises of Fort Worth, Texas. *American Journal of Infection Control* 1989;17:208–212.

12. Burton JL. Health and safety at necropsy. *Journal of Clinical Pathology* 2003;56:254–260.

13. Morgan O. Infectious disease risks from dead bodies following natural disasters. Revista Panamericana de Salud Publica 2004;15:307–312.

14. Hanzlick R. Embalming, body preparation, burial, and disinterment: An overview for forensic pathologists. *American Journal of Forensic Medicine and Pathology* 1994;15:122–131.

15. Claydon SM. The high-risk autopsy: Recognition and protection. *American Journal of Forensic Medicine and Pathology* 1993;14:253–256.

16. Fridkin SK, Hagerman JC, Morrison M, Sanza LT, Como-Sabetti K, Jernigan JA, Harriman K, Harrison LH, Lynfield R, Farley MM, Active Bacterial Core Surveillance Program if the Emerging Infections Program Network. Methicillin-resistant *Staphylococcus aureus* disease in three communities. *The New England Journal of Medicine* 2005;352:1436–1444.

17. O'Brien KL, Beall B, Barrett NL, Cieslak PR, Reingold A, Farley MM, Danila R, Zell ER, Facklam R, Schwartz B, Schuchat A. Epidemiology of invasive group A streptococcus disease in the United States, 1995-1999. *Clinical Infectious Disease* 2002;35:268–276.

18. Kuehnert MJ, Hill HA, Kupronis BA, Tokars JI, Solomon SL, Jernigan DB. Methicillin-resistant-*Staphylococcus aureus* hospitalizations, United States. *Emerging Infectious Diseases* 2005;11:868–872.

19. Lowy FD. Staphylococcus aureus infections. *The New England Journal of Medicine* 1998;339:520–532.

20. Greene CM, Van Beneden CA, Javadi M, Skoff TH, Beall B, Facklam R, Abercrombie DR, Kramer SL, Arnold KE. Cluster of deaths from group A streptococcus in a long-term care facility-Georgia, 2001. *American Journal of Infection Control* 2005;33:108–113.

21. Centers for Disease Control and Prevention. Active Bacterial Core Surveillance (ABCs) Report Emerging Infections Program Network: Group A streptococcus. 2004-provisional. 2005. Available at http://www.cec.gov/ncidod/dbmd/abcs/survreports/gas04prelim.pdf (accessed January 28, 2006).

22. Hawkey PM, Pedler SJ, Southall PJ. *Streptococcus pyogenes*: A forgotten occupational hazard in the mortuary. *British Medical Journal* 1980;281:1058.

23. Sepkowitz KA. Occupationally acquired infections in health care workers. Part II. *Annals of Internal Medicine* 1996;125:917–928.

24. Swaminathan B, Barrett TJ, Fields P. Surveillance for human Salmonella infections in the United States. *Journal of AOAC International* 2006;89:553–559.

25. Niyogi SK. Shigellosis. *Journal of Microbiology* 2005; 43:133–143.

26. Schwaber MJ, Navon-Venezia S, Kaye KS, Ben-Ami R, Schwartz D, Carmeli Y. Clinical and economic impact of bacteremia with extended spectrum-β-lactamase-producing Enterobacteriaceae. *Antimicrobial Agents and Chemotherapy* 2006;50:1257–1262.

27. Tumbarello M, Spanu T, Sanguinetti M, Citton R, Montuori E, Leone F, Fadda G, Cauda R. Bloodstream infections caused by extended-spectrum-β-lactamase-producing Klebsiella pneumonia. Risk factors, molecular epidemiology, and clinical outcome. *Antimicrobial Agents and Chemotherapy* 2006;50:498–504.

28. Moolman GJ, Jankowits CE, Bezuidenhout S, Pitout JD. Beta-lactamases in Enterobacteriaceae-an ever-present threat. *South African Medical Journal* 2006; 96:331–334.

29. Gamage B, Moore D, Copes R, Yassi A, Bryce E. Protecting health care workers from SARS and other respiratory pathogens: A review of the infection control literature. *American Journal of Infection Control* 2005;33:114–121.

30. Moore D, Gamage B, Bryce E, Copes R, Yassi A. Protecting health care workers from SARS and other respiratory pathogens: Organizational and individual factors that affect adherence to infection control guidelines. *American Journal of Infection Control* 2005;33:88–96.

31. Centers for Disease Control and Prevention. Tuberculosis in the United States. 2004. Available at http://www.cec.gov?nchstp/tb/surv/surv2004/default.htm (accessed October 1, 2005).

32. Lauzardo M, Lee P, Duncan H, Hale Y. Transmission of *Mycobacterium tuberculosis* to a funeral director during routine embalming. *Chest* 2001;119:640–642.

33. Sterling TR, Pope DS, Bishai WR, Harrington S, Gershon RR, Chaisson RE. *Transmission of Mycobacterium tuberculosis* from a cadaver to an embalmer. *The New England Journal of Medicine* 2000; 342:246–248.

34. Demiryurek D, Bayramoglu A, Ustacelebi S. Infective agents in fixed human cadavers: A brief review and suggested guidelines. *Anatomical Record* 2002;269:194–197.

35. World Health Organization. Hospital infection control guidance for severe acute respiratory syndrome (SARS). 2003. Available at http://www.who.int/csr/sara/infectioncontrol/en/ (accessed October 1, 2005).

36. World Health Organization. Consensus document on the epidemiology of severe acute respiratory syndrome (SARS). 2003. Available at http://www.who.int/csr/sars/en/WHOconsensus.pdf (accessed October 1, 2005).

37. Turner SB, Kunches LM, Gordon KF, Travers PH, Mueller NE. Occupational exposure to human immunodeficiency virus (HIV) and hepatitis B virus (HBV) among embalmers: A pilot seroprevalence study. *American Journal of Public Health* 1989; 79:1425–1426.

38. Douceron H, Deforges L, Gherardi R, Sobel A, Chariot P. Long-lasting postmortem viability of human immunodeficiency virus: A potential risk in forensic medicine practice. *Forensic Science International* 1993;60:61–66.

39. Beltrami EM, Williams IT, Shapiro CN, Chamberland ME. Risk and management of blood-borne infections in health care workers. *Clinical Microbiology Reviews* 2000;13:385–407.

40. Riddell LA, Sherrard J. Blood-borne virus infection: The occupational risks. *International Journal of STD & AIDS* 2000;11:632–639.

41. Twitchell KT. Bloodborne pathogens: What you need to know. Part II. *AAOHN Journal* 2003;51:89–97.

42. Beck-Sague CM, Jarvis WR, Fruehling JA, Ott CE, Higgins MT, Bates FL. Universal precautions and mortuary practitioners influence on practices and risk of occupationally acquired infection. *Journal of Occupational Medicine* 1991;33:874–878.

43. McDonald L. Blood exposure and protection in funeral homes. *American Journal of Infection Control* 1989;17:193–195.

44. Mahoney FJ, Stewart K, Hu H, Coleman P, Alter MJ. Progress toward the elimination of hepatitis B virus transmission among health care workers in the United States. *Archives of Internal Medicine* 1997;157:2601–2605.

45. Memon MI, Memon MA. Hepatitis C: An epidemiological review. *Journal of Viral Hepatitis* 2002;9:84–100.

46. Williams I. Epidemiology of hepatitis C in the United States. *The American Journal of Medicine* 1999;107:52–59.

47. Alter MJ, Kruszon-Moran D, Nainan OV, McQuillian GM, Gao F, Moyer LA, Kaslow RA, Margolis HS. The prevalence of hepatitis C virus infection in the United States. 1988 through 1994. *The New England Journal of Medicine* 1999;341:556–562.

48. Lanphear BP. Transmission and control of blood-borne viral hepatitis in health care workers. *Occupational Medicine* 1997;12:717–730.

49. Henry K, Dexter D, Sannerud K, Jackson B, Balfour H, Jr. Recovery of HIV at autopsy. *The New England Journal of Medicine* 1989;321:1833–1834.

50. deCraemer D. Postmortem viability of human immunodeficiency virus-implications for teaching

of anatomy. *The New England Journal of Medicine* 1994;331:1315.

51. Johnson MD, Schaffner W, Atkinson J, Pierce MA. Autopsy risk and acquisition of human immunodeficiency virus infection: A case report and reappraisal. *Archives of Pathology & Laboratory Medicine* 1997;121:64–66.

52. Bankowski MJ, Landa AL, States B, Shuburg R, Krizler M, Hajakian V, Kessler H. Postmortem recovery of human immunodeficiency virus type I from plasma and mononuclear cells: Implications for occupational exposure. *Archives of Pathology & Laboratory Medicine* 1992;116:1124–1127.

53. Nyberg M, Suni J, Haltia M. Isolation of human immunodeficiency virus (HIV) at autopsy one to six days postmortem. *American Journal of Clinical Pathology* 1990;94:422–425.

54. Do AN, Ciesielski CA, Metler RP, Hammett TA, Li J, Fleming PL. Occupationally acquired human immunodeficiency virus (HIV) infection: National case surveillance data during 20 years of the HIV epidemic in the United States. *Infection Control and Hospital Epidemiology* 2003;24:86–96.

55. Centers for Disease Control and Prevention. Brief report: Outbreak of Marburg virus hemorrhagic fever–Angola. October 1, 2004-March 29, 2005. *MMWR* 2005;54:308–309.

56. Centers for Disease Control and Prevention. A guidebook for surveillance medical examiners, coroners, and biologic terrorism and case management. *MMWR* 2004;53:RR08.

57. Ligon BL. Outbreak of Marburg hemorrhagic fever in Angola: A review of the history of the disease and its biological aspects. *Seminars in Pediatric Infectious Diseases* 2005;16:219–224.

58. Borio L, Inglesby T, Peters CJ, Schmaljohn AL, Hughes JM, Jahrling PB, et al. Hemorrhagic fever viruses as biological weapons: Medical and public health managements. *Journal of American Medical Association* 2002;287:2391–2405.

59. Peters CJ. Marburg and Ebola-arming ourselves against the deadly filoviruses. *The New England Journal of Medicine* 2005;352:2571–2573.

60. Leffel EK, Reed DS. Marburg and Ebola viruses as aerosol threats. *Biosecurity and Bioterrorism* 2004; 2:186–191.

61. Centers for Disease Control and Prevention. Management of patients with suspected viral hemorrhagic fever. *MMWR* 1988;37:1–16.

62. Centers for Disease Control and Prevention. CEC. Questions and answers: Creutzfeldt-Jakob disease infection control practices. 2005. Available at http://wwwcec.gov/ncidod/dvrd/cjc/infection_control_cjd.htm (accessed October 1, 2005).

63. Chesebro B. Introduction to the transmissible spongiform encephalopathies or prion diseases. *British Medical Bulletin* 2003;66:1–20.

64. Belay ED, Schonberger LB. The public health impact on prion diseases. *Annual Review of Public Health* 2005;26:191–212.

65. Brown P, Will RG, Bradley R, Ashes DM, Detwiler L. Bovine spongiform encephalopathy and variant Creutzfeldt-Jakob disease: Background, evolution, and current concerns. *Emerging Infectious Diseases* 2001;7:6–16.

66. Llewelyn CA, Hewitt PE, Knight RS, Amar K, Couses S, Mackenzie J, Will RG. Possible transmission of variant Creutzfeldt-Jakob disease by blood transfusion. *Lancet* 2004;363:417–421.

67. Peden AH, Head MW, Ritchie DL, Bell JE, Ironside JW. Preclinical vCJD after blood transfusion in a PRNP codon 129 heterozygous patient. *Lancet* 2004;364:527–529.

68. Brown P. Pathogenesis and transfusion risk of transmissible spongiform encephalopathies. *Developmental Biology (Basel)* 2005;120:27–33.

69. World health Organization. WHO infection control guidelines for transmissible spongiform encephalopathies: Report of a WHO consultation. Geneva, Switzerland, 23–26 March 1999. Available at http://www.who.int/csr/resources/publications/bse/WHO_CDS_CSR_APH_2000_3/en/ (accessed October 1, 2005).

70. Occupational Information Network. Summary report for: 11-9061.00 Funeral Directors. 2004. Available at http://online.onetcenter.org/link/summary/11.9061.00 (accessed October 1, 2005).

71. Occupational exposure to bloodborne pathogens-OSHA. *Final rule. Rred Regist* 1991:56-64004-182.

72. Centers for Disease Control and Prevention. Surveillance system for hospital health care workers. 2005. Available at http://www.cec.gov/niosh/docs/chartbook/ (accessed October 1, 2005).

73. National Funeral Directors Association. Careers in funeral service. 2005. Available at http://www.nfda.org/careers.php (accessed April 6, 2005).

74. Bureau of Labor Statistic. US Department of Labor Occupational outlook handbook. 2004-05 edition. Available at http:/www.bls.govioco/acos011.htm (accessed May 21, 2005).

75. Berhe M, Edmond MB, Bearman GM. Practices and an assessment of health care workers' perceptions of compliance with infection control knowledge of nosocomial infections. *American Journal of Infection Control* 2005;33:55–57.

76. US Department of Labor Standard Occupational Classification System. Available at http://www.bls.gov/soc/home.htm (accessed May 21, 2005).

77. US Census Bureau. Housing and Household Economics Statistics Division. 2004. Available at gov/hhes/www/ioindex.overview.html (accessed May 13, 2005).

78. Department of Health and Human Services. Mortality by occupation, industry, and cause of death: 24 reporting states (1984-1988). 1997. Available at http://www.cdc.gov/niosh/bk97114.html (accessed March 25, 2005).

79. Habenstein RW, Lamers WM. Funeral customs the world over, 4th ed. Milwaukee, WI: Bulfin Printers, Inc, 1994.

80. WHO. Burden of disease estimates by region in 2002. World Health Report: 2004.

Creutzfeldt-Jakob Disease: A Comprehensive Guide for Healthcare Personnel Section 3—Information for Embalmers*

Curtis D. Rostad, CFSP.

FOREWORD

CJD is a baffling disease. Not only because there is so much we do not know, but even what we do know has been misunderstood, exaggerated or understated, misrepresented, and miscommunicated.

On the one hand, CJD is a fatal disease; yet, we know little of its transmission. Its threat to our health is often minimized to the public to avoid undue panic; yet, health care workers are given specific cautions to protect themselves.

In our attempts to avoid unnecessary fear of the disease, we sometimes fail to separate the differences in exposure that exist between living with a person with CJD, caring for a patient in the hospital setting, handling lab and pathology samples, and caring for the body after death—especially when an autopsy has been performed.

This section includes what the funeral director and the embalmer need to know about CJD. While the exposure to CJD is limited when the person is alive, mortuary care increases that exposure. Even then, we can say little about what risk that exposure presents other than that it appears to be small.

Still, we must present the facts (as we know them today), issue our cautions, and offer our suggestions as to how to care for the remains in a safe, yet professional manner.

Admittedly, the extent of care the funeral director feels is prudent to offer is a matter of professional evaluation and personal decision.

We hope we have presented in this section the information they need to make those decisions and the tools to complete their tasks in as safe a manner as possible.

Curtis Rostad, CFSP.

INTRODUCTION

Throughout the 130 plus years of modern embalming, funeral service has faced many infectious and potentially fatal diseases and has still found ways to serve families and protect the public health.

We have survived the emergence of TB, polio, hepatitis, and HIV/AIDS because we have formaldehyde and other embalming chemicals that effectively kill the bacteria and viruses that cause these diseases and we have learned to protect ourselves from infection during the embalming process.

As long as we never encounter an organism that is resistant to formaldehyde and other embalming chemicals, and as long as we have the means to protect ourselves, we will always be able to serve the public with our skills.

But *what if*, in the future, an organism comes along that we cannot destroy through embalming? What then?

Well, the future is now. *Such a disease exists.*

- There is no diagnostic test for it.
- You can have it for up to 25 years and not know it.
- There is no vaccine.
- There is no cure.
- There is no treatment.
- It is infectious.
- It is always fatal.
- Formaldehyde does not touch it.
- There are no embalming chemicals that will kill it.
- Common methods of disinfection and sterilization will not kill it.

It is called *Creutzfeldt–Jakob disease.*

WHAT IS CREUTZFELDT-JAKOB DISEASE?

Creutzfeldt–Jakob disease, or CJD, is a one of a family of diseases known as transmissible spongiform encephalopathies (TSEs). It was first identified and described by both Creutzfeldt and Jakob in the 1920s.

It is a fatal neurological disease for which there is no treatment and no cure.

There is no vaccine available.

*Ruth Carrico, PhD, RN, CIC, Christian Davis Furman, MD,MSPH, Curtis D. Rostad, CFSP, Dorothy Cannan Hyde, MSW, Med. Chicago Spectrum Press, Louisville, KY., 2005. *Reprinted with permission of the author.*

Other TSEs include kuru (a disease associated with cannibalism in New Guinea) and Gerstmann–Straussler–Scheinker syndrome.[1]

There are also similar diseases among animals. In sheep and goats, it is called scrapie. In deer and elk, it is known as chronic wasting disease. In cows, it is called bovine spongiform encephalopathy (BSE) or "mad cow disease." An outbreak of this disease in Great Britain in 1995 caused worldwide concern over whether or not this disease could be transferred from animal to human through the eating of contaminated meat or other animal products.[2] As a result, shipment of cattle or meat products into the United States was halted.

The first case of BSE in the United States was discovered in a single cow in Washington state in December of 2003. The cow reportedly came from Canada where mad cow disease had been found earlier.

A new variant of CJD called nvCJD has been identified in Britain and has been proven to be associated with BSE. Humans apparently contract the disease from eating beef from cows with BSE. The new variant kills younger people (average age 28), and unlike classic CJD, the incubation period appears to be months (7–24) rather than years in length. As of this writing, no cases of nvCJD have been diagnosed in the United States.[3,4]

WHO GETS CJD?

Creutzfeldt–Jakob disease affects both men and women worldwide usually between the ages of 50 and 75.

WHAT CAUSES IT?

CJD results when abnormal protein accumulates in the brain cells. Scientists do not know what triggers the conversion of protein from the normal to the abnormal form, although a genetic defect has been identified that might provide a clue.[5,6] Some believe the conversion is caused by a spontaneous mutation of the normal protein itself, whereas other scientists believe a virus or virus-like entity may be involved.[7]

This abnormal protein, believed to be the causative agent of CJD, is known as a *prion* (pronounced "pry-on"),[8] a protein-based molecule with no RNA or DNA that is smaller than a virus.[9]

Actually, because the prion disease we see today differs in many respects from the original description of CJD, some scientists question whether or not the disease we see today is indeed the same disease described by Creutzfeldt and Jakob some 70 years ago.[10]

WHAT ARE THE SYMPTOMS OF CJD?

The initial symptoms are subtle and can include insomnia, depression, confusion, personality/behavioral changes, strange physical sensations, balance and coordination disorders, loss of memory, and visual problems.

Rapidly the patient deteriorates with progressive dementia and usually myoclonus (involuntary irregular jerking motions) as the disease progresses. Language, sight, muscular weakness, and coordination problems worsen.

The patient finally loses all mental and physical functions. Coma follows and death is usually due to pneumonia precipitated by the bedridden, unconscious state.

The duration of CJD from the onset of symptoms to death is usually 1 year or less, most commonly 2 to 6 months.[11]

HOW COMMON IS IT?

The official mortality rate is approximately 1 death per million population worldwide per year.[12] CJD is still classified as a rare disease (although the National Center for Infectious Diseases considers it an "emerging infectious disease").[13] This figure appears to be understated because CJD is often misdiagnosed. Because of the dementia it causes, it is often confused with Alzheimer.

One study done by Yale University showed that 13% of patients with Alzheimer were found upon autopsy to actually have CJD.[14]

[1] Ricketts, Maura, et al, *Emerging Infectious Diseases*, Volume 3, Number 2, 1997. National Center for Infectious Diseases, CDC.

[2] Division of Viral and Rickettsial Diseases, National Center for Infectious Diseases, CDC.

[3] Ibid.

[4] Brown, P. The human spongiform encephalopathies: Kuru, Creutzfeldt-Jakob Disease, and the Gerstmann-Straussler-Scheinker Syndrome. *Current Topics in Microbiology and Immunology*, vol. 172. New York, 1991.

[5] The gene is known as the scrapie amyloid precursor gene and is located on chromosome 20.

[6] Brown, Paul, M.D. National Institute of Neurological Disorders and Strokes.

[7] Manuelidis L. The dimensions of Creutzfeldt-Jakob disease. *Transfusion* 1994;34:915–928.

[8] Sanders et al. *Dorland's Medical Dictionary*, 28th edition, 1998.

[9] Ozel M. Small virus-like structure in fractions from scrapie hamster brain. *Lancet* 1994;343:894–895.

[10] Adams, R. D. et al. *Principles of Neurology*, 6th ed., 1998:771–773.

[11] De Silva R. Human spongiform encephalopathy: clinical presentations and diagnostic tests. In: *Methods in Molecular Medicine: Prion Diseases*; 1996:15–33.

[12] Masters CL et al; Creutzfeldt-Jakob disease: patterns of worldwide occurrence and the significance of familiar and sporadic clustering. *Annals of Neurology* 1979;5:177–188.

[13] Holman R. Creutzfeldt-Jakob Disease in the United States, 1979–1994: *Emerging Infectious Diseases*, Vol 2, Number 4, 1996.

[14] Campbell, D. et al. CJD Fact Sheet, *CJD Voice*.

Approximately 80% of deaths were among persons aged 60 or older. Among this age group, the death rate from CJD is 4.5 per million persons.[15]

HOW IS IT DIAGNOSED?

There is no definitive diagnostic test for CJD. The disease is suspected when a patient develops a rapid dementia and myoclonus. A 14-3-3 spinal test is 95% effective in supporting a clinical diagnosis of CJD. Unfortunately, the only 100% effective diagnostic tool available is an autopsy with appropriate tests.[16]

The postmortem finding of a coarse spongy-like surface of the brain (and the underlying microscopic cellular changes) is characteristic of CJD, thus the term, spongiform.

HOW LONG DOES IT TAKE FOR SYMPTOMS TO DEVELOP?

A person can become infected with CJD and have no symptoms for typically 12–25 years, although the disease can run its course and result in death in less than 3 years from the time of infection.

HOW DO YOU GET IT?

Three epidemiologic forms of CJD are well recognized. The familiar (genetic) form (5 to 10% of cases) results from a genetic mutation.

Approximately 1% of cases are iatrogenic (resulting from a medical procedure) including neurological procedures using contaminated instruments, corneal transplant, from electroencephalographic electrodes, cadaveric dura mater grafts, and pituitary hormone administration.[17]

Sporadic CJD accounts for 80 to 85% of all cases. These cases result from the mutation of the protein by some unknown cause.[18]

SO IT IS INFECTIOUS?

Yes. Although CJD was first described in the 1920s, it was not considered a transmissible disease until 1966.[19]

In 1974, a case of CJD transmission as the result of a corneal transplant was reported.[20]

In 1977, CJD transmission caused by silver electroencephalograph electrodes previously used in the brain of a person with CJD was reported. The transmission occurred despite decontamination of the electrodes between patients.[21]

In 1985, there were a series of case reports showing that cadaver-extracted pituitary human growth hormone could transmit CJD.[22] Shortly thereafter, it was shown that human gonadotropin administered by injection could also transmit CJD from person to person.[23]

CJD was first reported in a recipient of a dura mater transplant in 1987.[24]

IS CJD A DANGER TO HEALTH CARE AND MORTUARY STAFF?

As of today, over two dozen cases of CJD exist among health care workers including physicians, neurologists, pathologists, and laboratory technicians exposed to CJD. There are as yet no documented cases of transfer of the disease from a deceased patient to mortuary staff.

However, the cause of 80 to 85% of the cases of CJD is unknown and because it can take up to 25 years for symptoms of CJD to develop, it could be decades before we find out the true number of infections of CJD in health care workers exposed to patients with the disease.

WHAT BODY FLUIDS AND ORGANS ARE INFECTIOUS?

Since this is a neurological disease, the cerebrospinal fluid is highly infectious. The transmissible agent has also been shown to be present in the brain, spleen, liver, lymph nodes, lungs, spinal cord, kidneys, cornea and lens, bone, and to a much lesser degree, blood.

It is not found in tears, nasal mucous, saliva, urine, or feces. Therefore, there is little risk involved in becoming infected by casual contact or by living with a person with CJD.[25]

[15]Ibid.

[16]Gibbs CJ. National Institutes of Health.

[17]Collinge J. et al. Genetic predisposition to iatrogenic Creutzfeldt-Jakob disease. *Lancet* 1991;337:1441–1442.

[18]Lasmezas CI. et al. Transmission of the BSE agent in mice in the absence of abnormal prion protein. *Science* 1997;275:402–405.

[19]Will RG. et al. A new variant of Creutzfeldt-Jakob disease in the UK. *Lancet* 1996;347:921–925.

[20]Gibbs CJ. et al. Creutzfeldt-Jakob disease: transmission to the chimpanzee. *Science* 1968;161:388–391.

[21]Brown, P. Environmental causes of human spongiform encephalopathy. Methods in molecular medicine: prion diseases. Humana Press; 1996:139–154.

[22]Esmonde T. et al. Creutzfeldt-Jakob disease and lyophilised dura mater grafts. *Journal of Neurology, Neuosurgery, and Psychiatry* 1994;56:999–1000.

[23]Centers for Disease Control. *Morb Moral Wkly Rep.* 1985;34:359–60, 365–366.

[24]Nevin S. et al. Subacute spongiform encephalopathy: A subacute form attributable to vascular dysfunction. *Brain* 1960;83:519–564.

[25]National Institutes of Health, Biomedical Laboratory Safety, Section VII, Viral Agents.

It is important to understand this when dealing with the family of the deceased. During life, they were able to have normal contact with their family member with no adverse health consequences or risk of infection.

Now that the person is dead, they may not be able to understand why you hesitate to care for the person they loved.

This is simply because during life, the points of contact with a CJD patient are not infectious. It is after death, when invasive procedures are done, when contact with the prion is possible.

CAN YOU GET CJD FROM BLOOD?

That is the question being debated and researched at the present time. Although there have been no documented cases of CJD resulting from blood or blood transfusion, consider the following.

The Red Cross will not accept blood from a person with CJD symptoms or family history of CJD. A history of CJD disqualifies a patient from being an organ donor.

Human CJD has been reported to have been transmitted to mice by the injection of infected blood from human patients into mouse brain.[26]

Studies of experimental CJD in guinea pigs and mice have shown that the infectious agent is present in the blood before clinical disease develops.[27]

Sufficient evidence of animal transmission suggests that the disease has the potential to be transmitted through blood. Human epidemiological evidence only indicates that if blood transmission occurs, it is likely rare.[28]

Cases of CJD have been found among persons who have received blood transfusions, but the link between the disease and the transfusion has not been proven. Four Australians have been reported with CJD following transfusion. However, the source of the blood transfusions was undocumented.[29] There is a recent report in the western United States of three patients contracting CJD and dying after receiving a transfusion from a person who had CJD. This has not been confirmed.

Several cases of CJD following a blood component (albumin) transfusion have been reported. Two cases have been confirmed to have come from a person who died of CJD.[30]

The members of the Special Emphasis Panel on Creutzfeldt–Jakob disease, National Heart, Lung, and Blood Institute, have agreed that "an unqualified and irreducible risk of exposure to CJD through blood and blood products does exist...."[31]

Since there is no definitive direct evidence of infection from blood *transfusions*, there obviously can be no answer to whether or not CJD can be contracted by other blood *contact*. However, the absence of evidence is not evidence of the absence of transmission of CJD through blood.[32]

So there is as yet no definitive answer to the question, but the evidence would suggest that extreme caution in exposure to blood is warranted.

IS IT AIRBORNE? CAN YOU GET CJD BY BREATHING IT?

The risk of infection from aerosols, droplets, and exposure to intact skin, gastric, and mucous membranes is not known.

Nevertheless, the National Institutes of Health strongly cautions laboratory workers to avoid the generation of aerosols and droplets during the manipulation of tissues or fluids known or suspected to be contaminated with CJD.[33]

AND CJD IS HARD TO KILL?

Yes, the organism is not destroyed by formaldehyde, phenol, glutaraldehyde, alcohol, dry heat, boiling, hydrogen peroxide, ultraviolet radiation, or standard gravity sterilization.

The only effective sterilization technique is steam pressure sterilization (a process not commonly available to most funeral homes). However, even this method is not foolproof. In 2001, a major hospital in Denver reported the exposure of CJD to six patients who had undergone neurosurgery, as a result of the use of CJD contaminated surgical instruments *after* autoclaving. As a result, they have changed their procedure to include disposal of all surgical instruments used on a known or suspected CJD patient. Other medical centers are known to double autoclave these surgical instruments.

[26]Manuelidis EE. et al. Transmission to animals of Creutzfeldt-Jakob disease from human blood. *Lancet* 1985;2:896–897.

[27]Lavelle GC. et al. Isolation from mouse spleen of cell populations with high specific infectivity from scrapie virus. *Infection and Immunity* 1972;5:319–323.

[28]Heye N. et al. Creutzfeldt-Jakob disease and blood transfusion. *Lancet* 1994;343:298–299.

[29]Creange A. et al. Creutzfeldt-Jakob disease after liver transplantation. *Annals of Neurology* 1995;38:269–272.

[30]Patry, D. Neurology, 1998, June. Dept. of Medicine, University of Calgary.

[31]Minutes of the Special Emphasis panel on Creutzfeldt-Jakob Disease and Blood Transfusion. Sept 24–25,1997.

[32]Ricketts Maura, et al, *Emerging Infectious Diseases*, Volume 3, Number 2, 1997. National Center for Infectious Diseases, CDC.

[33]National Institutes of Health, Biomedical Laboratory Safety, Section VII, Viral Agents.

Incineration is also effective but obviously destroys equipment along with the organism.

The use of sodium hypochlorite (household bleach) is often mentioned as a potential disinfectant, but its results are inconsistent. It is highly corrosive to metal instruments, gives off irritating fumes, and cannot be used as an embalming agent.[34] For maximum effectiveness, soaking for 2 hours is recommended. Wiping floors or countertops with bleach therefore would not produce this level of disinfection.

Sodium hydroxide (lye) is also mentioned as a disinfectant but has also shown inconsistent results and is also corrosive. In addition, it is a hazardous substance itself, which must be neutralized prior to disposal, thus raising OSHA and EPA concerns for handling and disposal. Finally, it deteriorates with age, so it loses whatever effectiveness it may have while in storage.[35]

Finally, it has been shown that the disease organism has long-term survivability. It is still viable and can be transmitted after an inactive period of a year or more.[36,37]

EMBALMING CONSIDERATIONS

First of all, a basic review of some embalming fundamentals. Embalming is defined by the following three terms:

1. Disinfection
2. Preservation
3. Restoration

A person who dies from CJD will not present any particular challenges to preservation. The selection of embalming fluid, fluid strength, and fluid volume will be the same as a similar body deceased from any other cause.

Similarly, the appearance of the body will be no different than that of a similar body deceased from any other cause. No special restorative techniques will be necessary.

However, CJD is resistant to formaldehyde and every other embalming fluid component or disinfecting chemical including glutaraldehyde, phenol, and alcohol. Nothing you can do with the body will render it disinfected.

Therefore, *by definition*, you cannot technically embalm a person who is deceased from CJD.[38]

You can produce tissue firmness and preservation. You can produce a pleasant cosmetic effect. But you have not really embalmed the body.

When you have completed the arterial injection, the disease organism is just as much alive as it was when you began.

PERSONAL PROTECTION MEASURES

While there are no industry-specific standards of protection for mortuary staff when discussing CJD, we can emulate what is done in the medical field.

Most pathology departments have additional guidelines for handling patients deceased from CJD.

Typically, this includes wearing two or three pairs of disposable gloves (rubber or latex, never vinyl), protective eye covering and face shield, mask, cap, jumpsuit, waterproof apron, and shoe coverings. (Hospital guidelines go beyond what is normally considered "standard" universal precautions when dealing with CJD.)

Avoid causing aerosol distribution of contaminants. Avoid contact with all tissues and body fluids.

All solid waste should be placed in a leakproof container and disposed of by incineration.

Instruments should be disinfected by autoclave or incinerated. They can also be containerized and disposed of as medical waste.

All surfaces should be wiped with sodium hypochlorite. Despite its shortcomings, the use of ordinary household bleach is recommended for general disinfective use in the embalming room and especially when dealing with CJD. Surfaces that may be contaminated should be wiped with a .5% solution (1:10 dilution) of bleach.[39,40]

Since the organism has also been isolated in several internal organs, aspiration of the body should not be attempted.[41] Minute pieces of the internal organs can be aspirated into the trocar, exposing the embalmer to the organism, and the trocar will remain contaminated after the process is completed.

Like other diseases, we are going to be exposed to CJD unknowingly. But when we know or suspect the presence of CJD, we can take steps to protect ourselves. We

---

[34]Brown, P. Guidelines for High Risk Autopsy Cases: Special Precautions for Creutzfeldt-Jakob Disease. College of American Pathologists, Autopsy Performance and Reporting, 1990.

[35]Ibid.

[36]Adams, R.D. et al. *Principles of Neurology*, 6th ed, 771–773.

[37]Bernoulli C. et al; Danger of accidental person to person transmission of Creutzfeldt-Jakob disease by surgery. *Lancet* 1977;1.

[38]Strub CG, Frederick LG. *The Principles and Practice of Embalming*. LG Frederick, Dallas Texas, 1967.

[39]Guidelines for Control of Infections in Hospital Pathology, University of Washington Medical Center, 1998.

[40]Dilution of bleach should be done at the time of use. Bleach diluted with water loses its effectiveness within hours of being diluted. Maximum effectiveness of bleach takes at least 10–30 minutes of contact. In the case of CJD, 2 hours of soaking is recommended.

[41]National Institutes of Health, Biomedical Laboratory Safety, Section VII, Viral Agents.

cannot totally eliminate the risk of exposure to any disease, but when we know it is present, special care is warranted.

Finally, you would be well advised to consult with local public health authorities before attempting preparation to see if special handling of the case is required. Most states and counties have regulations concerning the handling of infectious disease cases. Whether or not it is specifically named in the regulations, CJD is an infectious disease. There may be restrictions on shipping, public viewing, or other exposure to the general public.

ADDITIONAL CONCERNS FOLLOWING AUTOPSY

The CJD organism is concentrated in the brain and the spinal column. While we might assume that exposure to the CJD organism is rather limited when handling the "normal" case, the embalmer is fully exposed to the organism when an autopsy has been performed, when death follows neurosurgery, or when death is due to head trauma.

The embalmer is well advised to request that the body be placed in a body pouch following autopsy to minimize contamination of the cot and removal vehicle or exposure of the removal personnel.

If restoration of the remains is attempted, all instruments, the embalming table, embalming room, and embalming room personnel are exposed to the organism, and there are no procedures available that will guarantee rendering the organism harmless. The organism can remain viable for over a year.

Limit the number of people who are exposed to the body by limiting admission to the preparation room during the preparation process. Exposure to others after the body has been repaired should also be limited. This would include other embalmers, hairdressers, cosmetologists, and so on.

WHAT SHOULD BE THE FINAL DISPOSITION?

There have been no specific tests done to determine if the prion is destroyed during the cremation process. This has led some to speculate that the prion is some type of superbug that cannot be destroyed. Incineration has been shown to destroy the prion at 1000 degrees Fahrenheit. Therefore, it is reasonable to assume that cremation, which is also essentially incineration, also destroys the prion. Also, since the prion is normally destroyed during autoclaving, which is steam under pressure at 130+ degrees Celsius, we can safely assume that the 1660+ degree Fahrenheit crematory will also destroy it.

Likewise, there have been no specific tests as to what happens to the prion when it is buried. Since we know that the prion can live for a year under normal condi-

tions, there is no reason to believe that it can survive any longer than that underground. Assuming that the body remains intact inside the casket or casket and vault for at least a year, the interred body should pose no threat to the environment or underground water sources.

SHOULD PREPARATION BE ATTEMPTED?

Knowing what we know about CJD (and probably more importantly, what we *do not* know), the question as following must be asked:

Should an embalmer attempt to embalm a body with CJD?

Some funeral directors who have been called on to serve a family where CJD is the cause of death have had this question answered for them. The family physician has already told the family that they cannot expect to have the body embalmed, have a public viewing, or a funeral. Some families have been told that the body should be cremated immediately upon death.

There is no reason for a family to feel obligated to choose cremation. By use of a body pouch and/or a sealing-type casket, there is no reason why an unprepared body with CJD cannot have a public funeral and an earth burial.

While we may not agree with the conclusion reached by the physician, we should at least note the seriousness he attaches to this disease.

We must also note, however, that misinformation within the medical community has also led some physicians to tell families that the disease cannot be easily transmitted and there should be no concerns on the part of the funeral home. Even the medical community has a long way to go in educating its members about CJD.

Whether or not an embalmer agrees to prepare the body is a personal decision that should be weighed carefully.

It is quite different from the questions we faced years ago when AIDS was first identified. Even though we did not know much about AIDS initially, we had an effective embalming technique and the chemicals available to render it harmless if we were careful in our procedures.

While the Americans With Disabilities Act (The ADA) has made AIDS a disability and requires embalmers to embalm AIDS cases or risk civil liability, the refusal to attempt to do what is impossible is an entirely different matter.

Since neither the Department of Justice nor the courts have ruled on the issue of handling CJD, a funeral home refusing to attempt preparation may indeed have to defend their decision if an ADA enforcement action is brought against it.

The case will hinge on whether this risk of CJD can be eliminated by "reasonable modifications" to the embalming process.[42]

Since no embalming fluid exists that will render the prion harmless, it would be argued that there is no "reasonable modification" to be made.

The threat of defending oneself from an ADA complaint must be weighed against the personal health risks involved.

The other difference that we can note between the history of AIDS and the history of CJD is that within months of its discovery, we knew a lot about AIDS, what it was, how it was transmitted, and so on. CJD was identified over 70 years ago and still we know very little about it.

With CJD, the question of preparation can only be answered after carefully considering the facts and weighing the consequences.

- We are being confronted with a 100% fatal disease.
- There is no cure; there is no treatment.
- There is no vaccine.
- The mode of transmission of this disease in humans is largely unknown.[43]
- There is no effective embalming treatment.
- There is no effective disinfecting technique for instruments, equipment, or the preparation room itself.
- The organism can survive and remain viable for over a year, possibly infecting others during that time.
- You may become infected with this disease and not know it for decades.

It would appear that CJD is not a vicious, rampant, killer organism intent on wiping the human race from the face of the planet. The numbers indicate something far less than a worldwide epidemic, to say the least. There is no need for panic or hysteria. We are not facing Black plague or Ebola.

However, it is a fatal illness and we cannot take that lightly. And it is not a disease we can do much with, either by way of protective measures or by embalming technique.

Universal precautions coupled with cautious, deliberate work practices, and a dose of plain common sense will do much to reduce the exposure risk.

But the risk cannot be eliminated and the full extent of that risk is unknown. Is it worth it?

How much risk are you willing to take?

If you determine that the risk of infection is minimal in the "normal" case and attempt preparation, do you still refuse to attempt preparation of the autopsied case where the highly infectious brain, spinal column, and cerebrospinal fluid are exposed?

Should you refuse to attempt preparation when there is no concrete evidence that you can be infected with CJD in the preparation process? What happens if it is proven that there is no risk of CJD infection from a dead human body? What happens if it is proven that infection *is* possible?

If you refuse to prepare the body, will the family choose another funeral home? What effect could this refusal have on your reputation of service within the community? What liability might a funeral home face if they refuse to attempt preparation?

What liability might your funeral home face if it is shown that an employee contracted CJD from a body that they prepared in your funeral home?

What moral obligation do you have to protect your employees versus your moral obligation to serve the public?

Although not specifically addressed by OSHA, the "General Duty Clause" of the Bloodborne Pathogen Standard would require the employer to protect employees from a known hazard. Since CJD is certainly a known hazard, employers would be required to protect their employees from this hazard.

It would appear that CJD would require steps beyond that of "universal precautions" and indeed the question is—can the employer adequately protect their employees from CJD if preparation is attempted?

Some surgeons have refused to operate on a person known to be infected with CJD. Some pathologists have refused to perform an autopsy on a deceased patient who is known or suspected to harbor the CJD organism. Can you base your own decision on theirs?

Indeed knowledgeable authorities within the medical community flatly advise against embalming, including the National CJD Surveillance Unit in the United Kingdom.[44]

Can you justify embalming a CJD case for what you charge knowing that equipment may have to be destroyed after use and additional precautions must be taken? (Which might illustrate the fact that embalming *any* case is worth a lot more than what you might presently charge?)

These are questions that funeral home staff members should discuss before accepting a person deceased from CJD or suspected CJD.

The embalmer deserves to be fully informed about CJD before they make that decision. That decision

---

[42]Gilligan, T. Scott, ADA vs CJD, The Director, 2000.

[43]National Center for Infectious Diseases, Hospital Infections Program. Creutzfeldt-Jakob Disease:Epidemiology, Risk Factors and De-contamination.

[44]Will, R.G. Professor, National CJD Surveillance Unit, West General Hospital, Edinburgh. 2000.

should be respected and there should be no thought that there is a shirking of "professional responsibility" by electing not to attempt preparation.

CONCLUSIONS

Ideally, there would be definitive answers. Unfortunately, science has not yet provided them.

Ideally, we would have all of the answers. Unfortunately, such is not the case. We simply do not have definitive answers to many of our questions.

Even knowledgeable people within funeral service have honest points of disagreement. Some see little risk, at least in the nonautopsied case. Some flatly refuse to touch a CJD case, autopsied or not.

Add to that the complications of OSHA obligations to protect employees and ADA requirements to provide services as a "public accommodation" and we can see that the situation becomes even more complicated.

Too many in funeral service know nothing at all about CJD. Too many have never even heard of it.

Some will attempt embalming only because that is what embalmers do. Anything less might appear cowardly, especially when the foe is unseen.

That means that too many are going to be exposed to CJD without ever having considered the long-term effects of their decision to handle or not handle a CJD case.

While we may not have definitive answers, what we do have are cautions.

What we do have are warnings.

Someday we should have more.

Someday this report will be outdated.

Until then . . .

PROCEDURAL GUIDELINES FOR MORTUARY CARE OF CRUETZFELDT-JAKOB DISEASE

. . . And that is where the original manuscript ended in 1998.

Since that time, we really have not learned that much more about CJD, but as more and more embalmers become aware of it and the potential danger it presents, it becomes obvious that we as a profession need some guidelines or protocols on the handling of a known or suspected case of CJD.

What follows then is what we hope is a reasonable set of procedural guidelines for the embalmer based on what we know today.

Before using them, read the entire article on CJD so that you better understand the disease and its risks to you and other employees. You also need to know the legal and business risks of not preparing the body. We recommend that you read the other material available listed in Appendix A to make a fully informed decision.

NOTICE AND DISCLAIMER

These CJD preparation guidelines are based on the knowledge available to the industry at the date of writing. These procedures may become outdated based on more current information. The embalmer must keep apprised of the latest information available.

The procedures outlined are, in the professional opinion of the author, a reasonable response to the potential risks posed by CJD. The individual funeral home owner and embalmer must make their own independent decisions based on the risks presented by preparing or not preparing a person with known or suspected CJD and be responsible for them.

The decision then to proceed or not to proceed is purely the decision of the funeral home and/or the individual embalmer. The author cannot be held responsible for the consequences or results of either decision.

The **"exposure level"** rating of 1 (low) to 5 (high) indicates the level of potential exposure to the prion. Basically, no exposure to blood or cerebrospinal fluid creates a negligible or very low potential exposure level. Exposure to blood or certain other body fluids produces a medium potential exposure level, since the causative agent for CJD is found in the blood, although in small amounts. Exposure to the brain and/or cerebrospinal fluid produces a high potential exposure level because these (and to a lesser degree, other internal organs) are the primary reservoirs for the prion.

It does not in any way imply a risk of developing CJD, because the chances of contracting the disease from exposure to blood, body fluids, brain, and spinal fluid, and so on are not known, but are admittedly low.

It simply makes sense, however, that the lower the exposure to the prion, the lower the chances of contracting CJD. But even maximum exposure to the prion is no indicator that a person will eventually contract CJD.

The term **"intact"** as used here is defined as a body that has not been autopsied, has no brain or spinal column injury, and does not display any excessive blood or body fluid leakage.

Since we maintain that a person deceased with CJD cannot technically be "embalmed" (since the body cannot be disinfected, which defines embalming) we will use the words "prepare" or "inject" to refer to the procedures that on any other body would be considered "embalming."

"Universal Precautions" refers to an approach to infection control that considers all deceased human bodies to be infectious and must be handled as such. OSHA regulations require that universal precautions be practiced. This requires the proper use of **personal protective clothing and equipment (PPE).** In the case of a CJD case, universal precautions must also take into consideration the possibility that the deceased could have other diseases of concern to the embalmer. Therefore, recommendations concerning universal precautions will be based on other diseases also and indeed should be utilized on every case regardless of any assumed cause of death. For instance, we recommend the use of face masks not because CJD is an airborne disease (there is no evidence to suggest that) but because TB is an airborne disease and the principle of universal precautions says we assume the person may have this and other diseases also and we must protect ourselves accordingly.

CJD GUIDELINES

TASK:
Removal of remains

BODY CONDITION:
Intact

EXPOSURE LEVEL:
0–1 (Negligible/very low)

RECOMMENDATION:
The body can be removed and transported with little if any risk to mortuary personnel.

**UNIVERSAL PRECAUTIONS/
PRE-RECOMMENDED:**
Minimum: Gloves
　　　　Face mask or barrier cloth over face of
　　　　the deceased.
　　　　Additional protective clothing and
　　　　equipment as indicated.

PROCEDURE:
Follow basic sanitary procedures that should be utilized on any removal.
　　Cover the cot surface with a protective plastic such as a casket cover.
　　Transfer remains to cot. Wrap body completely in protective plastic to eliminate contact with the cot.
　　Place used gloves and other PPE in sealed plastic bag for later disposal.
　　Wash hands with disinfectant soap.
　　Transport.
　　If the body exhibits any bleeding, open wounds, or other leakage, a body pouch is recommended.
　　Leave body wrapped until disposition is determined.
　　Disinfect cot with Clorox.

CJD GUIDELINES

TASK:
Removal of remains

BODY CONDITION:
Nonintact (autopsied)

EXPOSURE LEVEL:
2 (low) if body is pouched to 4 (high) if mortuary personnel must directly handle remains.

RECOMMENDATION:
The body can be removed and transported, but extra precautions are warranted.

**UNIVERSAL PRECAUTIONS/
PRE-RECOMMENDED:**
Minimum: Gloves
　　　　Face mask or barrier cloth over face of
　　　　the deceased.
　　　　Additional protective clothing and
　　　　equipment as indicated.

PROCEDURE:
The hospital or autopsy facility should be asked to place the remains in a body pouch taking care not to contaminate the outside of the pouch. The removal personnel should monitor this task to observe any contamination of the outside of the pouch.
　　Hospital or autopsy facility should retain all organs removed, especially the brain.
　　This pouch should then be placed in an outer pouch to further insure no contamination of the cot.
　　Place used gloves and other PPE in sealed plastic bag for later disposal.
　　Wash hands with disinfectant soap.
　　Transport.
　　Leave body pouched until disposition is determined.
　　Disinfect cot with Clorox.

CJD GUIDELINES

TASK:
Preparation (injection) of remains

BODY CONDITION:
Intact

EXPOSURE LEVEL:
3 (Medium)

RECOMMENDATION:
We recommend the body not be prepared by arterial injection.

UNIVERSAL PRECAUTIONS/PRE-RECOMMENDED:
Minimum: Gloves, gown, face mask/eye shield, head, and shoe covers.

PROCEDURE: (If injection is attempted)
Restrict embalming room access to necessary personnel only.

Follow preparation procedures as indicated by body condition.

Fluid strength, quantity, and dilution will be determined by overall condition of the body, because this will have no effect on the CJD prion.

Use drain hose to sewer system to minimize exposure to blood.

Minimize the number of instruments used.

Do not aspirate body.

Containerize and dispose of all instruments, tubes, hoses, needles, and so on.

Place all gloves and other PPE in sealed plastic bag for disposal.

Clean table and other embalming room surfaces with Clorox.

Wash hands with disinfectant soap.

NOTE: There are no practical procedures available to ensure destruction of the prion once it has contaminated the preparation room.

CJD GUIDELINES

TASK:
Preparation (injection) of remains using "no drainage" method*

BODY CONDITION:
Intact

EXPOSURE LEVEL:
2 (Low)

RECOMMENDATION:
We recommend the body not be prepared by arterial injection. This method reduces the level of exposure if injection is attempted.

UNIVERSAL PRECAUTIONS/PRERECOMMENDED:
Minimum: Gloves, gown, face mask/eye shield, and shoe covers.

PROCEDURE: (If injection is attempted)
Restrict embalming room access to essential personnel only.

Inject body with no drainage.*

Do not aspirate body.

Minimize the number of instruments used.

Containerize and dispose of all instruments, tubes, needles, and so on.

---

*See Appendix B for "no-drainage" injection method.

Clean table and other embalming room surfaces with Clorox.

Place all gloves and other PPE in sealed plastic bag for disposal.

NOTE: There are no practical procedures available to ensure destruction of the prion once it has contaminated the preparation room.

CJD GUIDELINES

TASK:
Preparation of remains

BODY CONDITION:
Nonintact (autopsied)

EXPOSURE LEVEL:
5 (Full exposure to the causative agent)

RECOMMENDATION:
Preparation and/or restoration of the body should not be attempted and is strongly discouraged.

UNIVERSAL PRECAUTIONS/PRERECOMMENDED:
Minimum: Gloves, gown, face mask/eye shield, and shoe covers.

PROCEDURE: (If injection is attempted)
Restrict embalming room access to essential personnel only.

Minimize the number of instruments used.

Follow preparation procedures as indicated by body condition.

Fluid strength, quantity, and dilution will be determined by overall condition of the body, because this will have no effect on the CJD prion.

Use extreme care in not contaminating embalming room with blood.

Containerize and dispose of all instruments, tubes, needles, and so on.

Clean table and other embalming room surfaces with Clorox.

Place all gloves and other PPE in sealed plastic bag for disposal. Wash hands with disinfectant soap.

NOTE: There are no practical procedures available to ensure destruction of the prion once it has contaminated the preparation room.

CJD GUIDELINES

DISPOSITION AND OTHER HANDLING:

Refrigeration—Body should remain wrapped in plastic or body pouch while under refrigeration.

Viewing—Viewing the unembalmed intact remains does not present a particular hazard beyond that of any other disease.

Utilizing universal precautions, body can be sanitized (body surfaces) and features can be set.

To avoid unnecessary manipulation of the body and exposure to body fluids, body should remain wrapped in plastic and clothing should be draped over remains after casketing or placement on viewing table.

This may be an acceptable alternative for the family that desires a viewing.

If viewing is requested after cranial restoration, exposure to the prion is present, especially in the hair. A hairdresser would be exposed, if the hair is to be done before viewing as would those who touch the body during viewing. Since the risks here are unknown, we strongly caution the funeral home against restoration or viewing of autopsied remains.

Cremation—Body should already be wrapped in plastic or placed in a body pouch. Body should also be in a rigid alternative cremation container or casket. With no direct contact with the body, no special precautions are required by crematory personnel.

While there have been no specific studies to definitively determine that the CJD prion is destroyed during the cremation process, it is normally destroyed by routine autoclave procedures (>130° Celsius for 15 minutes), which is done at a much lower temperature. Indeed the preheating of the retort alone is likely to be sufficient to destroy the prion.

Incineration at a temperature of 1000° Fahrenheit is considered effective against the CJD prion.

Therefore, we can safely assume that the prion is destroyed during the cremation process (1600+ degrees Fahrenheit) and the handling of the cremated remains (ashes) poses no threat to crematory personnel.

Entombment—Body should already be placed in a body pouch. Using appropriate universal precautions, body should be treated with external embalming powder to minimize odors. Body should be placed in an inner sealer case or sealer-type casket. (Note: Mausoleum regulations may require embalming or have regulations concerning communicable diseases. Check mausoleum requirements before assuring family that entombment will be allowed.)

Since the CJD prion can survive under normal conditions for up to a year, we assume that it will also survive for that long within the mausoleum. Assuming that the casket remains intact for at least a year, it should present no further health hazard if later re-moved. Even then, the casket should not be opened for any reason.

Burial—Body should already be wrapped in plastic or be in a body pouch before casketing. Body should be placed in an inner sealer case or sealer type casket.

Since the CJD prion can survive under normal conditions for up to a year, we assume that it will also survive for that long underground. To assure that the casket remains intact for at least a year, a vault or graveline should also be used.

Disinterment—Since the CJD prion can survive under normal conditions for up to a year, we assume that it will also survive for that long underground or in a mausoleum. We recommend that no disinterment be made for at least the first year following interment. Even prior to that time, if the casket is intact and sealed, the body should not present any appreciable risk. Even then, the casket and/or vault should not be reopened during the disinterment and reinterment.

Disposal of liquid waste (drainage)—If injection with drainage is attempted, it presents the additional problem of what to do with the drainage. Since formaldehyde has no effect on the prion, normal disposal into the sewer system means introducing an unknown quantity of the prion into the sewer system.

As an alternative, some have proposed treating the drainage with a chemical known to have some effectiveness against the prion, such as sodium hydroxide (lye) or sodium hypochlorite (bleach).

This presents further complications however.

Formaldehyde, which would also be in the drainage, should never be mixed with bleach.

Lye mixed with water produces heat and presents its own handling and disposal hazards.

Any attempts at treating the drainage further expose the embalmer to the prion as well as additional chemical hazards.

Therefore, although it may not seem to be an adequate solution, the most logical answer is to dispose of the drainage directly into the sewer system with a minimum of exposure to the embalmer.

This situation alone should be further justification for not attempting arterial injection of the body.

Disposal of solid waste (PPE, etc.)—All solid waste including gloves, gowns, sheets, and so on that have been used or that may have come into contact with the CJD case should be sealed in plastic and disposed of as hazardous waste.

Treatment of instruments—Disposable instruments should be used and also disposed of as hazardous waste or sharps. Nondisposable instruments should likewise be disposed of and not reused. Since the CJD prion has been shown to survive autoclaving if not done at proper temperature (and since most funeral homes do not have access to an autoclave), attempts at sterilization are not recommended.

Appendix A

ADDITIONAL RECOMMENDED READING

"A CJD Primer"
   James F. Burnside, CFSP
   Curtis D. Rostad, CFSP
   Kurt Soffe, CFSP
   The Director, July 2000

"ADA vs. CJD"
   T. Scott Gilligan, Esq.
   The Director, August 2000

"CJD and OSHA"
   Edward M. Ranier, Esq.
   The Director, September 2000

"CJD and the Environment"
   Carol Green, Esq.
   The Director, April 2001

"Should Funeral Homes Embalm CJD Cases"
   James F. Burnside, CFSP
   The Director, May 2001

Appendix B

"NO DRAINAGE" INJECTION METHOD

While injection of a known or suspected CJD case is not recommended, the exposure level can be greatly reduced if injection of the intact body is done with no drainage.

With this method, exposure is limited to incidental leakage at the injection site.

Restrict embalming room access to essential personnel only.

Minimize the number of instruments used.

Use universal precautions as with all embalming procedures, that is, gloves, gown, face mask and eye shield, and head and shoe covers.

Prepare remains for injection like any other case, that is, position body, wash remains, set features, and so on.

Cover table with disposable plastic sheet or place small disposal emesis basin under incision site to catch incidental leakage and avoid contamination of table.

Soak up any incidental leakage and dispose of towel or cotton in sealed plastic bag.

INJECTION POINT: Single injection point of the embalmer's preference. Carotid injection is recommended to eliminate need to reverse tube to inject lower leg and ease in controlling incidental leakage.

FLUID: Standard arterial fluid chosen based on overall condition of body.

CONCENTRATED FLUID: Same as would be used if this were a normal injection based on overall body condition.

DILUTED FLUID SOLUTION: No more than 2 gallons total. A "normal" body can easily retain this amount of fluid in the arterial/venous system without swelling. For a small or emaciated case, this amount may be reduced to 1 to 1.5 gallons. Mix total amount of concentrated fluid to be used to make this amount of solution.

That is, if you would normally use 16 oz of arterial to 2 gallons of fluid to embalm this body and then use another 16 oz in a final 2-gallon injection—in this case, you would mix the entire 32 oz of fluid into 2 gallons (or less) of diluted solution.

PRESSURE: Use same injection pressure as if this were a normal injection based on overall body condition.

RATE OF FLOW: Use minimum rate of flow. This is the secret to success. Monitor body closely for signs of swelling. If distention or swelling occurs, it is because of too high a rate of flow, not too much pressure or too much fluid.

Note that some older machines are incapable of operating at a rate of flow low enough to prevent distention or swelling.

Do not aspirate body. If abdominal gases must be relieved, use a large bore needle into the intestinal spaces taking care not to produce leakage or puncture of internal organs that may house the prion.

Containerize and dispose of all instruments, tubes, needles, and so on.

Clean table and other embalming room surfaces with Clorox.

Place all gloves and other PPE in sealed plastic bag for disposal.

Wash hands with disinfectant soap.

ABOUT THE AUTHOR

Curtis D. Rostad, CFSP, is a licensed funeral director and embalmer with over 30 years experience as an employee, manager, funeral home owner, and consultant.

He also serves as executive director of the Wyoming Funeral Directors Association, a position he has held since 1987, and served as the executive director of the Colorado Funeral Directors Association from 1988 to

1992. He is a member of the American Society of Association Executives (ASAE), the Colorado Society of Association Executives (CSAE), and the Council of Funeral Association Executives.

He has an extensive background in forensics and death investigation with 7 years of serving as a county coroner. He is a member of the American College of Forensic Examiners and is a Board Certified Forensic Examiner with a specialty in death investigation through the American Board of Forensic Examiners.

Curtis D. Rostad, CFSP
6138 Trailhead Rd.
Highlands Ranch, CO 80130
1 (303) 471-6072
e-mail crostad@aol.com

Hepatitis from A to G*

Kim Collison

Viral hepatitis is a worldwide health problem. It is estimated that 300 million people throughout the world carry the hepatitis B virus, whereas over 4 million Americans have hepatitis C. Considering the frequency of contact with blood and body fluids when working in funeral service, it is important to understand how the hepatitis viruses are transmitted and what precautions you need to follow to protect yourself.

Hepatitis is defined as an inflammation of the liver that can damage this organ and even cause death. While there are several etiologic agents that may be responsible for liver inflammation, the term "hepatitis" is most commonly associated with several distinct viruses. Hepatitis has been documented for centuries including accounts of human hepatitis appearing in Babylonian texts and Hippocrates' works. However, it has only been in the last 40 years that the hepatitis viruses have been discovered and identified. The signs and symptoms of all types of hepatitis are similar, so blood tests are necessary to determine which of the nine known viruses is causing the disease.

Viral hepatitis can be separated into two basic groups based on their mode of transmission. Hepatitis A and E are transmitted via the fecal-oral route, while hepatitis B, C, D, G, and GBV are blood-borne. The blood-borne viruses are spread whenever there is the possibility of the exchange of blood or body fluids.

Reprinted with permission from The Dodge Magazine, Jan.–Feb., Vol. 91, No. 1, 1999. Copyright: The Dodge Company.

HEPATITIS A

Hepatitis A, formerly called infectious hepatitis, is caused by the enterically transmitted hepatitis A virus. The Centers for Disease Control and Prevention (CDC) estimate that over 140,000 cases of acute hepatitis A occur in the United States each year, accounting for approximately 80 deaths. Worldwide, the incidence of hepatitis A (HAV) infection exceeds 1.5 million cases. HAV is especially common in parts of Asia, Africa, South America, and Mexico. HAV enters the body through the digestive system, when one eats food or drinks water that has been contaminated with fecal material. Hepatitis A can also be spread via fresh fruits, salads, or vegetables washed in contaminated water.

The virus can be transmitted between family members, within institutions, by food handlers, and through sexual contact. An HAV positive person can spread the disease even if he or she has no symptoms. Hepatitis A generally produces a mild infection that lasts 6 to 10 weeks. Children and young adults account for 50% to 60% of the reported cases of HAV. Once you have the infection, you develop a natural immunity, so you never become infected again. Being vaccinated or just following good hand washing practices will protect you from acquiring hepatitis A in the prep room.

HEPATITIS E

In 1990, the virus that is responsible for enterically transmitted non-A, non-B hepatitis was discovered. Hepatitis E (HEV) is prevalent in Asia, Africa, and the Middle East and has caused epidemics in Mexico. Like hepatitis A, hepatitis E is transmitted in water contaminated with infectious human waste. HEV generally produces a mild infection with an overall fatality rate of 1 to 3%. However, this disease does pose a serious risk to pregnant women, causing a fatality rate of 15 to 25%. There is not a blood test available for diagnosing hepatitis E, and researchers are currently testing a possible vaccine. Because there is the potential for contamination with fecal material in the prep room, strict adherence to universal precautions should protect you from both hepatitis A and E.

HEPATITIS D

Hepatitis D, or delta hepatitis, is a blood-borne virus that only exists in combination with the hepatitis B virus. The prevalence of hepatitis D in the United States is low, except in IV drug users and multiple transfused individuals. The coinfection of hepatitis B and D results in a severe disease state and often results in severe chronic liver disease. There is no vaccine available for hepatitis D. However, because it can only exist with hepatitis B, the hepatitis vaccine will therefore offer protection against hepatitis D.

HEPATITIS G

Hepatitis G virus (HGV) is spread in the same manner as other conventional blood-borne viruses. The risk factors for HGV are similar to those of hepatits B and C—namely, IV drug use, multiple blood transfusions, and accidental sharps injuries. Chronic infection develops in 90 to 100% of individuals infected with HGV.

HEPATITIS GBV

In June 1995, hepatitis GBV was discovered. It also appears to be transmissible through contaminated blood and body fluids. Extensive hepatitis research is still necessary, since approximately 20% of cases of acute and chronic hepatitis cannot be attributed to any of the known viruses.

HEPATITIS C

Most hepatitis cases that were once referred to as blood-borne non-A, non-B are now known to be due to the hepatitis C virus (HCV). The recent identification of HCV and the development of screening tests for it have brought to light the enormity of the worldwide health problem. According to the American Liver Foundation, over 4 million people in the United States have chronic hepatitis C. In addition, each year an estimated 150,000 people are infected with HCV, and about 10,000 die of hepatitis C. The CDC now predicts that over the next 10 years, the hepatitis C death toll will triple. Hepatitis C has been responsible for most cases of transfusion-related hepatitis. However, since 1989, blood products have been screened for hepatitis C, and no longer pose a risk. Today, one of the leading causes for liver transplantation is the presence of cirrhosis and/or liver cancer due to hepatitis C.

Hepatitis C is transmitted in many of the same ways as hepatitis B, and therefore, they share many of the same risk factors. Essentially any activity that results in the transfer of contaminated blood or body fluids can result in the transmission of HCV. Common risk factors are IV drug use, chronic hemodialysis, accidental sharps injuries, tattooing, body piercing, being the offspring of HCV-positive mothers, and intranasal cocaine use. Studies show that the incidence of household (nonsexual) transmission of HCV range from 0 to 11%. They also estimate that the risk of hepatitis C transmission from a single needlestick involving HCV-positive blood is 3 to 10%.

An average of 6- to 7-week incubation period follows infection with the hepatitis C virus. The early stage of HCV infection is termed acute hepatitis, and it may be mild or severe. Unlike the illness that occurs following infection with hepatitis A or B, many people with HCV will initially suffer flu-like symptoms, while the virus quietly damages the liver. According to recent studies, up to 80% of people with acute hepatitis will develop chronic hepatitis—that is, hepatitis that continues beyond a 6-month period—and they may remain infected for several years or life. Up to 25% of these patients will progress to hepatic cirrhosis. Also, hepatitis C is a known predisposing factor in the development of liver cancer.

In 1992, the FDA approved the use of interferon-alpha 2b for treating selected cases of chronic hepatitis C. Although studies have shown that this treatment can lead to significant improvement in liver function tests, it has some major drawbacks. First of all, it is expensive and has numerous side effects. Also, fewer than half of HCV-infected individuals respond to treatment, and most trials report at least a 50% relapse rate within 6 months of completing therapy. In October 1997, the FDA approved the use of Infergen, a biologically engineered version of interferon. Unfortunately, Infergen is about as effective as interferon against the hepatitis C virus.

Any accidental sharps injury or mucous membrane exposure to blood or body fluids in the prep room should be immediately documented and reported. Because postexposure testing of the source will be difficult, you should assume the source is positive for HCV. You should have a blood test to check for anti-HCV immediately following the exposure and you should be tested again for anti-HCV and for the liver enzyme ALT. There is no established postexposure prophylaxis for hepatitis C.

HEPATITIS B

It is estimated that 300 million people throughout the world carry the hepatitis B virus (HBV). In China, Southeast Asia, and Africa, up to 12% of the population carries the hepatitis B virus. In this country, approximately 200,000 to 300,000 people become infected with HBV each year. On the basis of estimates from the CDC, there are approximately 1.25 million chronic carriers, or people with ongoing hepatitis B infection, in the United States alone. Of these people, nearly 5000 die from cirrhosis or liver cancer each year. The CDC reports that almost 12,000 health care workers become infected with HBV each year, with about 200 dying from the disease.

The hepatitis B virus can be found in blood, saliva, semen, vaginal secretions, cerebrospinal fluid, peritoneal fluid, pericardial fluid, and basically any other body fluid contaminated with blood. Blood is the single most important source of hepatitis B and other blood-borne pathogens in the occupational setting. Often overshadowed by the fear of AIDS, hepatitis B is a greater threat in terms of infection, sickness, and death—mainly because it is a much hardier virus.

The hepatitis B virus is passed either directly from an infected individual by contact with his or her body fluid or indirectly, by contact with dried blood or body fluids on clothing or other surfaces. HBV is acquired through the skin by way of cuts, scrapes, hangnails, or needle sharing. Other means are by tattooing, by ear or body piercing, or by sharing razors, pierced earrings, toothbrushes, or nail clippers. It is also acquired through the mucous membranes such as the eyes, nose, or mouth by exposure to infected blood or body fluids, through sexual contact, and through contact between an infected mother and her newborn child. Also, hemophiliacs are a high-risk group due to their need for numerous blood products, many of which were not screened for HBV before 1975.

Needlesticks continue to be the main source of occupational exposure. More than 800,000 needlesticks and sharps injuries are reported each year, although the number of actual injuries is believed to be much higher. Because there can be 500 million hepatitis B viral particles in 1 cc of carrier's blood, the risk of acquiring HBV from a needlestick ranges from 6 to 30%. After an exposure and an incubation period of 60 to 180 days, symptoms such as fatigue, enlarged liver, and jaundice will appear. The short-term consequences of an HBV infection include an average 8 to 12 weeks off work and risk of permanent liver damage. Long-term effects include chronic active hepatitis, cirrhosis, liver cancer, and death.

The best methods for protection against HBV are strict adherence to universal precautions and the hepatitis B vaccine. The first hepatitis B vaccine was derived from human plasma and became available in 1982. In 1986, a genetically engineered vaccine was licensed by the FCA. When given in the deltoid muscle, the hepatitis B vaccine produces protective antibody in more than 90% of healthy individuals. A blood test to check for the development of protective antibodies can be done 1 to 6 months after completing the three-injection vaccine series. Currently, there are different theories regarding the need for booster doses and how to treat those individuals who fail to produce protective antibodies following the vaccination series.

Should an exposure occur in the prep room, testing and treatment should be initiated within 72 hours. The exposure source should be assumed to be positive. You will require blood tests and should also receive one dose of hepatitis B immune globulin and one dose of the hepatitis B vaccine. Follow-up testing is generally done 6 months postexposure.

Hepatitis is a worldwide health problem and a major occupational hazard in funeral service. It is important that you understand how these different viruses are transmitted, because you are most likely embalming undiagnosed hepatitis positive remains. Your best protection against hepatitis B is the hepatitis B vaccine. Your best protection against all forms of hepatitis is following universal precautions.

BIBLIOGRAPHY

Department of Labor, Occupational Safety and Health Administration, 29CFR Part 1920.1030, Occupational exposure to bloodborne pathogens, final rule. *Federal Register.* 1991;56:64004–64182.

Hepatitis C: Improved Options Available for Diagnosis and Treatment. *Mayo Clinic Update* 1993;9:7–8.

Kuhns MC. Viral hepatitis. *Laboratory Medicine* 1995;26: 650–659.

Larsen JT, Larsen HS. Viral hepatitis: An overview. *Clinical Laboratory Science* 1995;8:169–173.

Mordechai E, Belmont M. The pivotal role of serum hepatitis C viral load in disease progression. *Advance for Medical Laboratory Professionals* 1998;10:17–19.

Pallatroni L. Needlesticks: Who pays the price when the costs are cut on safety? *Medical Laboratory Observer* 1998;30–36, 88–91.

Protection Against Viral Hepatitis: Recommendations of the Immunization Practices Advisory Committee. *MMWR* 1990;39:1–23.

Shute N. Hepatitis C: A silent killer. *U.S. New and World Report,* June 22, 1998;60–66.

Witthaus D. New federal guidelines for HCV lookback. *Medical Laboratory Observer.* September 1998;22–26.

Zuckerman AJ. The new GB hepatitis virus. *Lancet* 1995;345:1453–1454.

The Increase in MRSA and VRE*

Mike Cloud, Jr.

Let us take a few moments to explain the pathogens of MRSA, VRE, and VRSA. Then, I will make some recommendations as to the disinfection and preparation of a deceased body with these conditions.

---

*Reprinted with permission from *The Dodge Magazine,* September–October 1999, Volume 91, No. 4. Copyright: The Dodge Company.

Staphylococcus aureus (also referred to as Staph aureus and abbreviated *S. aureus*) is one of the most common causes of nosocomial (hospital-acquired) and community-acquired infections worldwide. In 1992, the 19,000 deaths directly caused by nosocomial infections made them the 11th leading cause of death in the US population.[1] In 1998, Dr. William Jarvis of the CDC stated, "We estimate that today two million patients develop a hospital-acquired infection in the United States each year. Of that number, 90,000 die as a result of those infections."[2]

These Staph pathogens are mutating so as to become resistant to a series of drugs including penicillin and methicillin. Until recently, doctors were treating *S. aureus* with methicillin. Some of these Staph organisms have become resistant to methicillin (and so are called methicillin-resistant *Staphylococcus aureus* or MRSA). The antibiotic vancomycin is effective against MRSA pathogens, but is considered a last ditch defense. As time passes, these pathogens may become resistant not only to a single type of antibiotic but even perhaps to two or more antibiotics in combination. The initials MRSA can also be an acronym for a similar but different set of words: multiple-resistant Staph aureus.

Of course, each of you can see that these Staph aureus pathogens that are methicillin resistant could become VRSA (vancomycin-resistant Staph aureus). Sad to say, that has happened. At the beginning of 1999, the third reported case of VRSA killed a middle-aged Hong Kong woman. Many people naturally carry the Staph aureus organism as part of their normal flora with no sign of illness. These people are said to be colonized with the bacteria.

The growth of VRE, MRSA, and VRSA may be attributed to more invasive procedures, using breathing tubes and intravenous catheters, for example. *The Surgical Infection Society Position of Vancomycin-Resistant Enterococcus* (October, 1996), a publication of the American Medical Association, stated, "Presumably much of this spread occurs as a result of carriage of enterococci on the hands of health care workers and through interhospital transfers of patients colonized with these enterococci." Later in their report, they note, "This problem is growing rapidly; the incidence of VRE infections has increased 20-fold in the United States between 1989 and 1993, and 34-fold in intensive care units."[3]

Even at the removal site, one should use universal precautions. We should not guess whether the deceased has VRE, MRSA, or even HIV. Remember, if we are to err, let us err on the side of caution. All bodies should be treated as if they are contagious. Rectal swabs were taken from 30 patients known to be harboring VRE. All were tested, but only 14 showed positive for the disease. Even our best tests are imperfect. Of secondary but real concern should be the professional image we convey to the family and others who see us in the performance of our work. Certainly we cannot allow ourselves to become passive carriers who might infect others because of our lack of appropriate procedures.

After the body has been transferred to the cot, hand washing and disinfection are imperative. The paper by the AMA that I have been quoting stated, "The CDC has since published guidelines establishing hand washing as the most important procedure for preventing nosocomial infections." The publication further states, "The institution of universal precautions to protect health care workers from human immunodeficiency virus and other virus, by promoting the use of gloves, may have given workers a false sense of security, with neglect of hand washing."[3]

Upon returning to the preparation room, we should spray a topical disinfectant such as Dis-Spray over the entire sheet covering the deceased before transferring the body from the cot to the embalming table or before removing the sheet. Fold the sheet back from the face while liberally spraying the face with topical disinfectant. Remember that Staph aureus is part of the normal flora of the nasal tract and even the mouth. Therefore, I recommend the use of a swab saturated with Dis-Spray along the walls and the opening of the oral and nasal cavities. Continue to topically disinfect the surface of the body before positioning on the table.

Once the body is on the embalming table, spray the remaining linen on the cot before placing it in the linen disposal. Next, liberally spray the cot and pillow. I have noticed that many times we fail to completely disinfect the cot. One must be mindful to allow the disinfectant to remain on the area long enough to do its job.

Continue with the arterial embalming procedure as usual. During aspiration and cavity fluid injection, I suggest that specific attention be given to the digestive tract. Also use a cavity fluid that has additional disinfectant properties such as Metafix. At the end of the embalming process and prior to final disinfection of the preparation room, it is advisable to pack the vagina, rectum, and any other areas that have folds with a cotton pack saturated with formaldehyde-based chemical.

It is vital for embalmers to remember that organisms that have become resistant to antibiotics inside the living human body do not become in any way more resistant to the disinfecting chemicals such as formaldehyde, which we use in our embalming procedures. If we achieve thorough distribution, we will achieve disinfection, and families viewing the body will not be at any greater risk than from nonresistant (equally disinfected) bacteria. Moreover, if we follow universal precautions properly, embalmers should not become infected while performing their work (before the chemicals have had a chance to disinfect).

REFERENCE

1. Reuters-May 14, 1998
2. Reuters-Mike Cooper-March 11, 1998
3. AMA, *Surgical Infection Society Position on Vancomycin-Resistant Entero,* October 1996.

ABOUT THE AUTHOR

Mike Cloud is a licensed embalmer and funeral director from Newnan, GA. He has been an OSHA coordinator for 4 years. Mike graduated with honors from Gupton-Jones, and is a member of the Academy of Graduate Embalmers of Georgia.

The Antimicrobial Activity of Embalming Chemicals and Topical Disinfectants on the Microbial Flora of Human Remains*

Peter A. Burke and A. L. Sheffner
Department of Microbiology, Foster D. Snell, Inc., Florham Park, New Jersey

The antimicrobial activity of embalming chemicals and topical disinfectants was evaluated to determine the degree of disinfection achieved during the embalming of human remains. The administration of arterial and cavity embalming chemicals resulted in a 99% reduction of the postmortem microbial population after 2 hours of contact. This level of disinfection was maintained for the 24-hour test period. Topical disinfection of the body orifices was also observed. Therefore, it is probable that present embalming practices reduce the hazard from transmission of potentially infectious microbial agents within the immediate environment of embalmed human remains.

INTRODUCTION

For many years, embalming chemicals have been utilized to preserve and disinfect biological tissues for anatomical studies, environmental storage, and hygienic safety. The majority of these embalming chemicals are formaldehyde-based products, whose disinfectant properties have been described by Walker,[1] Lawrence and Block,[2] and Spaulding.[3] It has been reported that pathogenic organisms, such as *K. pneumoniae, H. influenzae, M. tuberculosis,* and *H. capsulatum,* are recoverable

*Reprinted from *Health Lab Sci* 1976;13(2):267–270, with permission from the American Public Health Association.

from embalmed human remains.[4-6] Thus, conceivably, infection could occur from contact with post-embalming microbial fluids and swabs of areas around orifices from cadavers to determine if commercially available embalming chemicals produce a significant reduction in the microbial flora.

MATERIALS AND METHODS

Samples of biological fluids and swabs of the area around orifices were taken from eight cadavers to determine the antimicrobial activity of embalming fluids in vivo as a function of time. Four of the bodies were embalmed, whereas the other four cadavers were not and served as controls. The primary cause of death of the subjects was diagnosed to be other than an infectious disease (i.e., coronary thrombosis, cerebrovascular accident, and arteriosclerosis).

Embalming Procedure. The bodies were embalmed by a professional licensed mortician using the following procedure. The body was washed with an antiseptic soap containing 0.75% hexachlorophene and thoroughly rinsed. The cadaver was sprayed with a topical embalming disinfectant and the orifices swabbed with the same disinfectant. This disinfectant was a solution of 1.0% (w/v) formaldehyde and 0.5% (w/v) quaternary ammonium compounds in a base of isopropanol and ethylene dichloride.

Prior to dilution of the arterial embalming chemical, the tap water was treated with a water conditioning mixture formulated specifically for embalming use. This conditioner is a complexing agent that removes chemical constituents found in municipal water supplies, which could interfere with the preservative and disinfecting properties of the arterial solutions. This conditioner is basically a mixture of trisodium ethylenediaminetetraacetate and polyvinylpyrrolidone in a base of various glycols.

The arterial embalming chemical consisted of 29.8% (w/v) formaldehyde, 3.8% (w/v) anionic detergents, 4.0% (w/v) borate and germicides, 9.6% (w/v) alcohol, and various inert ingredients in a water base. The arterial embalming chemical was then diluted 6 oz to $\frac{1}{2}$ gallon of water. An equal amount of coinjection chemical for the purpose of stimulating drainage and inducing penetration was added to the solution. This chemical consisted of 8.9% (w/v) chelating agents, 0.1% (w/v) reducing agents, 0.7% (w/v) preservatives, 2.0% (w/v) plasticizers, 9.9% (w/v) humectants, and various inert ingredients in a water base.

The total amount of solution injected into the body was approximately 2 to $3\frac{1}{2}$ gallons, depending on the body size and weight. Two pints of cavity embalming chemical (24–28% [w/v] formaldehyde) were

TABLE 4. ANTIMICROBIAL ACTIVITY OF EMBALMING CHEMICALS AND TOPICAL DISINFECTANTS ON MICROFLORA OF HUMAN REMAINS

Treatment	Anotomical Site	Preembalming	Treatment Period (hours)				% Reduction After 24 Hours
			2	4	8	24	
			Mean Microbial Populations[a]				
Embalmed	Heart	8.0×10^5	1.8×10^2	1.6×10^2	2.0×10^2	70	>99
Embalmed	Lung	2.5×10^1	<10	<10	<10	<10	>99
Embalmed	Colon	7.4×10^1	80	<10	<10	<10	>99
Embalmed	Bladder	1.3×10^5	3.8×10^2	<10	<10	<10	>99
Embalmed	Oral cavity	$++^b$	0	0	0	0	—
Embalmed	Nasal cavity	+	0	0	+	0	—
Embalmed	Anus	+++	0	+	0	0	—
Unembalmed	Heart	2.8×10^5	7.2×10^5	7.8×10^5	7.5×10^5	9.0×10^5	—
Unembalmed	Lung	2.5×10^5	3.2×10^5	3.0×10^5	2.4×10^5	3.8×10^5	—
Unembalmed	Colon	1.5×10^6	1.6×10^6	1.7×10^6	1.5×10^6	2.2×10^6	—
Unembalmed	Bladder	2.9×10^6	2.3×10^6	2.3×10^6	2.4×10^6	2.5×10^6	—
Unembalmed	Oral cavity	+	+	+	+	+	—
Unembalmed	Nasal cavity	+	+	+	+	+	—
Unembalmed	Anus	+++	+++	++	++	+++	—

[a]Organisms (mL) (mean of four subjects per group).
[b]Scale of growth from swab cultures: 0 = none, + = slight, ++ = moderate, +++ = heavy.

injected into each subject, one into the thoracic cavity and the other into the abdominal cavity. All products used in the study were commercially available embalming chemicals.

Sample Collection. Samples were drawn from superior and inferior anatomical sites, with sterile 18-gauge needles and 30-mL syringes. Needle puncture sites were topically disinfected with 95% ethanol. Swab samples were taken with sterile polyester swabs, which just before swabbing were immersed in sterile phosphate-buffered saline.* Biological fluids and swab cultures were taken from the following areas.

FLUID SAMPLES

- **Lung:** The needle was inserted 3 inches to the right of the midline, through the fifth intercostal space. Pulmonary fluids or aspirates were extracted from the middle lobe of the right lung.
- **Heart blood:** The needle was inserted 1 inch to the left of the midline, through the fifth intercostal space.
- **Descending colon:** A longitudinal incision 3 inches long was made midway between the tip to the 12th rib and the anterior iliac spine; the descending colon was identified and the fecal extracted from the lumen of the colon.

*Phosphate-buffered saline prepared by diluting 0.25M phosphate buffer 1/1000 in physiological saline (0.9% NaCl).

- **Urinary bladder:** The needle was inserted through the external urethral orifice and the urine extracted from the lumen of the bladder.

Dehydrated or coagulated sample sites were injected with sterile phosphate-buffered saline.

Swabs of Orifices

- **Oral cavity:** Samples were taken from the buccal furrow between the mucous membrane of the upper lip and the gingiva.
- **Nasal cavity:** Swabs were made from the vestibule of the left half of the nasal cavity.
- **Anus:** Swabs were taken from the terminal inch of the anal canal.

Immediately after taking samples, the swabs were placed in Stuart's transport medium.

Samples were taken before embalming and then 2, 4, 8, and 24 hours after embalming. The bodies were covered with plastic sheeting while sampling procedure was not in process. All samples were packed in dry ice during transportation to the laboratories of Foster D. Snell, Inc., where they were immediately plated.

Quantitative Measurement of Microbiological Flora. Immediately following receipt in the laboratory, the biological fluids were serially diluted in thiotone peptone water blanks and subsequently plated on MacConkey and Heart Infusion Agar with 5% defibrinated sheep blood. Into both agar preparations, 0.5% Tween-80 and 0.1% lecithin were incorporated to neutralize residual

TABLE 5. ISOLATION AND DISTRIBUTION OF MICROFLORA ASSOCIATED WITH HUMAN REMAINS: ANATOMICAL SITES

Heart	Lung	Colon	Bladder
Proteus mirabilis	Escherichia coli	Escherichia coli	Escherichia coli
Pseudomonas sp.	Pseudomonas aeruginosa	Micrococcus sp.	Klebsiella aerogenes
Staphylococcus aureus	Staphylococcus aureus	Proteus mirabilis	Proteus vulgaris
Staphylococcus epidermidis	Staphylococcus epidermidis	Proteus vulgaris	Proteus morganii
Streptococcus	Streptococcus sp.	Pseudomonas aeruginosa	Pseudomonas aeruginosa
Bacillus sp.	Alcaligenes faecalis	Staphylococcus aureus	Staphylococcus aureus
Escherichia coli		Staphylococcus epidermidis	Staphylococcus epidermidis
		Streptococcus sp.	Bacillus sp.
		Bacillus sp.	
		Klebsiella aerogenes	

microbial activity from the embalming fluids. The plates were incubated at 35–37°C for 48 hours following which a colony count was performed.

Microbial Identification. Isolates were identified using standard morphological and biochemical tests with the general outline utilized for identification as defined in *Bergey's Manual of Determinative Bacteriology,* eighth edition,[7] and Skerman's *Identification of the Genera of Bacteria,* second edition.[8]

RESULTS AND DISCUSSION

In vitro, germicidal activity of formaldehyde has been established and documented for many years.[2] However, the amount of microbiological data concerning the in vivo efficacy of embalming chemicals on human remains is scant. In the present study, formaldehyde-based embalming fluids were found to be highly active in reducing the microbial flora in human remains. The microbial population was reduced greater than 99% at every site 2 hours after embalming; with control bodies, as anticipated, a continuous microbial growth pattern was observed (Table 4). The antimicrobial action of formaldehyde-based embalming chemicals was apparently not limited or adversely affected by the proteinaceous material or other macromolecules present in the biological fluids and tissues.

Following topical disinfection of the areas around the orifices, no growth or limited growth could be detected after 24 hours of exposure. Disinfection of the orifices occurred within 2 hours of contact. Random positive results after disinfection, however, were seen because the bodies were not protected from the environment with the exception of a nonsterile plastic cloth.

Differential monitoring of the microbial population revealed that microorganisms translocate across anatomical barriers, which during life prevent penetration and translocation. These body defenses are as follows: epithelial and mucous membrane coverings, reticuloendothelial system, blood drainer barrier.

The organisms that were isolated from the human remains are listed in Table 5.

Comparison of the microbial flora before and after embalming produced no pattern or general trend. Specific microbial resistance to the antimicrobial action of formaldehyde-based embalming chemicals was not observed. No pathogenic bacteria were found following embalming.

In conclusion, it was found that the use of formaldehyde-based embalming chemicals is a satisfactory disinfectant when applied as a public health measure to reduce microbial hazards when human remains are handled.

ACKNOWLEDGMENTS

We thank J. B. Christensen of the George Washington School of Medicine, Department of Anatomy, Washington, D.C., and R. Swaminathan, Foster D. Snell, Inc., for their professional assistance. This study was supported by the Embalming Chemical Manufacturers Association.

REFERENCES

1. Walker JF. *Formaldehyde.* American Chemical Society Monograph Series, 3rd ed. New York: Reinhold, 1964.
2. Lawrence CA, Block SS. *Disinfection, Sterilization, and Preservation.* Philadelphia: Lea & Febiger, 1968.
3. Spaulding EH. Role of chemical disinfection in the prevention of nosocomial infection. In: *Proceedings of the International Conference on Nosocomial Infections.* Atlanta: Centers for Disease Control and Prevention; 1970.
4. Meade GM, Steenken W. Viability of tubercle bacilli in embalmed human lung tissue. *American Review of Tuberculosis* 1949;59:429.
5. Weed LA, Baggerstoss AH. The isolation of pathogens from tissues of embalmed human bodies. *American Journal of Clinical Pathology* 1951;21:1114.

6. Weed LA, Baggerstoss AH. The isolation of pathogens from embalmed tissues. *Proceedings of the Staff Meetings. Mayo Clinic* 1952;27:124.
7. Buchanan RE, Gibbons NE, eds. *Bergey's Manual of Determinative Bacteriology*, 7th ed. 1957.
8. Skerman VK. *Identification of the Genera of Bacteria*, 2nd ed. 1967.

The Microbiologic Evaluation and Enumeration of Postmortem Specimens from Human Remains*

Gordon W. Rose, Ph.D.
Associate Director, Department of Mortuary Science, Wayne State University, Detroit, Michigan

Robert N. Hockett, M.S.
Research Associate, School of Dentistry, University of Michigan, Ann Arbor, Michigan

Several recognized and potential pathogens, both bacterial and mycotic, were recovered consistently from body fluids and/or aspirates withdrawn from human cases certified to have died from causes other than an infectious disease. Samples were taken from five anatomic sites of varying postmortem time intervals. Filter membrane culture techniques were used for primary isolation and enumeration. Some isolates seemed to imitate classical growth curve indications of exponential increase at the 6-hour to 8-hour postmortem interval. Densities reached a level of 3.0 to 3.5 million organisms per milliliter or gram of sample at the 12- to 14-hour interval, the time period of maximal microbiologic translocation and proliferation. These studies indicate that unembalmed human remains are capable of contributing a multitude of infectious doses of microbial agents to a body handler, the body storage area, or to the environment adjacent to the body storage area.

INTRODUCTION

Research in postmortem microbiology is not new; Achard and Phulpin presented data on the recovery of microorganisms from human remains in 1895.[1] Sampling has generally followed the opening of body cavities.[2-4] One improvement in technique was the use of animal model systems[5] as an investigational tool. The amount of scientific data originating from this area of microbiologic investigation remains scant. The bibliography of the Embalming Chemical Manufacturers Association[6] is to be recommended for background.

The study utilized the application of the relatively new technique of membrane filtration (MF) to the qualitative and quantitative microbiological evaluation of body fluids and/or aspirates. Winn et al. reported the use of this technique in postmortem studies in 1966.[7] They described two advantages of the MF technique: (1) the MF method provides a three-dimensional approach to the cultivation of microorganisms and (2) it yields more accurate and reproducible quantitative results.

METHOD

Death certifications on all human remains sampled indicated the primary cause of death to be other than an infectious disease (e.g., coronary thrombosis, cerebrovascular accident, and arteriosclerotic disease). Samples were secured from refrigerated cases over a postmortem period of 72 hours for temporal profile purposes. Samples were withdrawn from upper or superior to lower or inferior anatomic sites, with 18-gauge needles and 25-mL Luer syringes. Dehydration or coagulation of some samplings required aspirates of injected sterile phosphate-buffered saline (PBS). Topical disinfection of needle puncture sites was effected with an iodophore (Hi-Sine (R), Huntington Laboratories, Huntington, IN). The sampling needle was directed into the cisterna magna (cisterna cerebellomedullaris) at the base of the cerebellum via the foramen magnum for the withdrawal of cerebrospinal fluid. Heart blood samples were taken from the left ventricle by directing the needle to the upper border of the fifth rib just to the left of the sternum. Pulmonary fluids and/or aspirates were taken from the lungs for the third sampling. The needle was directed into the transverse colon at the level of the umbilicus to sample the lumen contents. Finally, urinary bladder needle taps were made from a site marking the intersection of the median line and the pubic bone.

All samples were initially diluted 1:3 or 1:4 in PBS, and 0.1 mL of each diluted sample impinged on 0.45-em MF, and then washed with 10.0 mL of PBS. The MFs with impinged organisms were rolled onto primary isolation agar plates of MacConkey, phenylethyl alcohol/blood, and chocolate blood. Aerobic incubation at 35 to 37°C for 24 to 48 hours and preliminary picking of isolates were routinely practiced. Isolates were characterized by pertinent methods.[8,9]

RESULTS AND DISCUSSION

Table 6 lists the bacterial isolates from the five anatomical areas sampled.

*Reprinted from *Health Lab Sci* 971; 8(2), with permission from the American Public Health Association. Presented before the laboratory section at the Ninety-Eighth Annual Meeting of the American Public Health Association, Houston, TX, Oct. 29, 1970.

TABLE 6. BACTERIAL ISOLATES FROM FIVE ANATOMICAL SITES

Organism	Cerebrospinal Fluid	Lung	Heart Blood	Transverse Colon	Bladder Urine
Alcaligenes faecalis	×	×		×	×
Bacillus sp.			×	×	
Corynebacterium diphtheriae[a]	×	×		×	
Escherichia coli	×	×	×	×	×
E. coli (A–D)					×
Klebsiella aerogenes	×	×	×	×	×
Micrococcus sp.	×	×	×	×	×
Proteus mirabilis			×	×	×
Proteus vulgaris				×	
Providencia				×	
Pseudomonas aeruginosa	×	×	×	×	×
Shigella flexneri		×		×	
Staphylococcus aureus	×	×	×	×	×
Staphylococcus epidermidis	×	×	×	×	×
Streptococcus (Group D)	×	×	×	×	×
Streptococcus pneumoniae		×		×	×

[a]Not a typical isolate.

The selection of sampling sites was based on anatomic considerations of the normal microbial flora associated with specific anatomic areas during life. The epithelial and mucous membrane coverings and linings are normally during life intact anatomic barriers to bacterial penetration and translocation. The reticuloendothelial system is a second nonselective barrier that helps to deter translocation during life. The blood–brain barrier is probably the last line of anatomic defense against many potential microbial invaders. The cerebrospinal fluid, a filtrate of circulating blood, maintains its biologic integrity in a closed system of circulation.

All of the selected sampling sites were easily accessible and, with the exception of the colon, yielded essentially liquid specimens. The colon contents occasionally required a presampling injection of sterile PBS. Needle penetration of the selected sites involved minimal manipulation of the body areas and permitted the rapid procurement of specimens in a state best suited for MF processing.

Thorough washing of each impinged MF reduced or removed the possible effects of specific and nonspecific inhibitors that might have been associated with the specimens. Each MF was quickly transferred to the basic group of primary isolation agars. The direct rolling of the MFs onto the agar surfaces facilitated contact between the matrix- and surface-oriented microorganisms and growth substrates.

The MF allowed the impingement of a standardized volume (0.1 mL) of diluted specimen that gave total plate colony counts that were mathematically referable to densities per milliliter or per gram of original sample. Gridded MFs improved the accuracy of colony counting; plate counts in excess of 200 per plate were not recorded. Processed MFs were sterilized with ethylene oxide and stored for possible future serotaxonomic or other studies.

Bacteria *normally* associated with the transverse colon during life, with the exception of clinically opportunistic conditions, do not translocate. They are, by description of the US Public Health Service Ad Hoc Committee on the Safe Shipment and Handling of Etiological Agents,[10] "Agents of no... [to] ordinary potential hazard." This general statement assumes a knowledge of infectious disease and immunology. There might well be logical disagreement originating from those who have attempted the treatment of infections from enteric "commensals."

The colon was chosen as the translocation reference baseline for indicator organisms isolated from other sampling sites. The brain, lung, and heart samples frequently yielded recognized pathogens in addition to the indicator commensals and opportunists. Many of the same indicator organisms were isolated from all five sampling sites. This is indicative of the extent to which bacteria, both pathogenic and nonpathogenic, can be translocated within a period of 6 to 8 hours after death.

The quantitative results (Fig. 1) of the study indicate that a postmortem multiplication of the isolates begins approximately 4 hours after death and assumes a logarithmic-like increase between 6 and 8 hours after death. The bacterial cell densities reach a peak of approximately 3 to $3\frac{1}{2}$ million organisms/mL or gram of fluid or tissue within 24 to 30 hour after death.

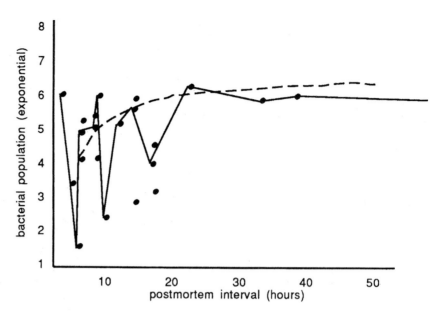

Figure 1. Bacterial population versus postmortem interval.

Within a postmortem interval of 4 to 6 hours, there is a body-wide redistribution of endogenous flora. Postmortem chemical changes in and manual manipulation of human remains may cause these organisms to exit from any of the body orifices and contribute contamination to adjacent environments. This places the body handlers and other personnel in or near the body storage area at higher risk.

ACKNOWLEDGMENT

Support for this study was received from the National Funeral Directors Association.

REFERENCES

1. Achard C, Phulpin E. Contribution a l'etude de l'envahissement des organes par les microbes pendant l'agonie et apres le mort. *Archives of Medical Expert Anatomical Pathology* 1895;7:25–47.
2. Burn CG. Experimental studies of postmortem bacterial invasion in animals. *The Journal of Infectious Diseases* 1934;54:388–394.
3. Carpenter HM, Wilkins RM. Autopsy bacteriology: Review of 2,033 cases. *Archives of Pathology* 1964; 77:73–81.
4. De Jongh D, Lottis JW, Green GS, Shinely JA, Minckler TM. Postmortem bacteriology. *American Journal of Clinical Pathology* 1968;49:424–428.
5. Burn CG. Postmortem bacteriology. *Journal of Infectious Diseases* 1934;54:395–403.
6. Hinson MR. Final report on literature search on the infectious nature of dead bodies for the Embalming Chemical Manufacturers Association. Mimeo, 1968.
7. Winn WR, White ML, Carter WT, Miller AB, Finegold SM. Rapid diagnosis of bacteremia with quantitative differential membrane filtration culture. *Journal of American Medical Association* 1966;197:539–548.
8. Cowan ST, Steel KJ. *Manual for the Identification of Medical Bacteria.* London: Cambridge University Press, 1966.
9. Harris AH, Coleman MB. *Diagnostic Procedures and Reagents.* Washington, DC: American Public Health Association, 1963.
10. Anonymous. *Classification of Etiologic Agents on the Basis of Hazard.* Atlanta: Centers for Disease Control (US DHEW, USPHS), 1970.

Professional Hair Care for Human Remains

Darla A. Tripoli, CO, LFD, CFSP

When the words restoration or restorative art are mentioned in the funeral profession, one usually thinks of a trauma case where extensive restoration skills are needed to repair damaged head and facial features. However, embalmers practice the art of restoration on each and every case in the embalming room. Sometimes, dramatic restoration is needed, but most often, it is the smaller details of care of human remains, which demonstrate our skills in restoration and professionalism in body preparation.

Attention to detail when caring for the hair of human remains is essential for authenticity of the decedent's appearance and a pleasing visual experience for the family members and the public.

The task of grooming the hair and the application of tastefully chosen cosmetics can have a dramatic impact on the final appearance of the deceased. Perhaps, the smaller details of restoration, like professional hair care, are considered secondary because they are not perceived to be true "restoration." This is an incorrect assumption. When it comes to hair care, sometimes trained professionals are hired by the funeral home to care for the deceased's hair. From a business perspective, this can become quite costly to the funeral home. With basic knowledge of hair, techniques, and products, a funeral professional can begin to take responsibility for more of the hair care and grooming themselves. Not only can this raise the level of professionalism of the worker, but it can also prevent valuable service dollars being lost at the funeral home by hiring an outside source. In some cases, it is wise to hire a professional, but oftentimes with the right knowledge and the right skills, a funeral professional can achieve quality and professional hair care results.

HAIR BASICS

Hair strands are primarily made up of a protein called keratin. Keratin is a tough, water insoluble type of protein that is also found in skin, fingernails, and toenails. Individual hair strands are made up of three layers. The outer layer, called the cuticle, is microscopically demonstrated as clear cells that appear flat and tight to the hair strand giving them the appearance of "shingles." The inner layer is called the cortex. The medulla is found inside the cortex.

With undamaged hair, the outer layer, the cuticle, which has the appearance of scales or shingles, appears flat, tight, and imbricate on this strand of hair. This gives us many clues to the condition of the hair. This hair is, most likely, virgin hair. Virgin hair has never been chemically altered by perms or colors and will visually demonstrate a shiny, healthy appearance. This type of hair is easy to identify because virgin hair will be easy to comb, easy to style, and have superior shine. This is not the type of hair we often see in the preparation room.

With damaged hair, the cuticle of this hair strand is not smooth. The cuticle is damaged, rough, broken, and does not imbricate. This indicates that the hair has been damaged in some way, by either by hair color, bleach, permanent waves, or the misuse of heating devices used on the hair. This hair will be difficult to comb or brush, is usually very dry, tangles very easily, and is visually dull and flat with little or no luster. This is often the type of hair observed in the preparation room.

HAIR CLEANSING

There are many types of hair care products available on the market. Purchasing professional shampoos and conditioners in a beauty supply store will ensure the best products at reasonable prices. Oftentimes, employees are trained licensed cosmetologists who can answer any questions about which products to purchase. A 32-oz bottle with a pump for one-handed efficiency in the preparation room is ideal.

Step one is properly cleansing the hair. There are three basic types of shampoo that are recommended in the preparation room. They are described in the following paragraphs.

Stripping Shampoo—These shampoos have a high alkaline content. They range from 7.5 to 8.5 on the pH scale. These shampoos are considered a deep cleansing type. This shampoo will rid hair of grease, dirt, blood, medication, and styling product buildup (gels and hairsprays) on hair strands. Depending on the cleansing needs, one application of this type of shampoo is generally effective in cleansing the hair.

Medicated—May be used to rid hair of obvious dandruff flakes on the hair/scalp.

Acid Balanced—These shampoos are used for color-treated or permanently waved hair. Typically, these types of shampoo have a pH of 4.5 to 5.5. This type of shampoo is considered nonstripping and will not dull, strip, or harm hair color. It will remove dirt effectively without harming the hair or dulling hair that has been artificially colored. It is also recommended to have a pediculicide available to treat pediculosis capitis (commonly known as head lice). Pediculosis capitis is a communicable disorder and can be contagious to the embalmer. Proper use of PPE (personal protective equipment) at all times, which includes a head covering, will help keep the embalmer protected. If infestations on the scalp of the human remains are found, it is wise to check the eyebrows, eyelashes, and any facial hair for infestation as well, and treat accordingly. Sometimes, cases seen with a severe infestation of pediculosis capitis must be treated more than one time.

Hair Cleansing Procedures

Wet the hair with water. While the hair is wet, pump a small amount of the selected shampoo into a gloved hand, rub your hands together, and then evenly apply the shampoo, beginning at the scalp and then throughout the hair to the ends. Lather, rinse well, and repeat if necessary. Rinse the hair thoroughly.

If a buildup of styling products is observed in the hair, do not comb or brush the hair first. This can break the hair or tear it from the root. Saturate the hair with water and then shampoo as indicated above.

HAIR CONDITIONING/INSTANT DRAMATIC RESTORATION

Hair that is damaged is matte, nonreflective, dry, drab, dull, and difficult to comb or brush. Application of a hair conditioner can dramatically change the appearance of the hair, adding shine, luster, and manageability. Hair conditioner can help to correct any physical or chemical damage observed in the hair.

The main ingredients in hair conditioners are moisturizers, surfactants, glossers, fatty oils, polymers, lubricants, detanglers, and thermal protectors. Conditioners are frequently acidic with a low pH. Hair conditioners work on the outside of the hair strand, (where the cuticle is found) to help close or "fill in" the damaged spaces on the cuticle. This will smooth the hair strand and change the appearance of the hair. By utilizing this product, the hair will better reflect light, be easier to comb, and it will give the hair a healthy, sleek, and shiny appearance.

Conditioning Procedures

After the hair is cleansed and rinsed properly, pump a small amount of conditioner into the palm of a gloved hand and work the conditioner from the scalp to the ends of the hair strands. Follow by using a wide-tooth hair pick to evenly distribute the conditioner throughout the hair. Start from the scalp and comb the conditioner to the ends of the hair strands. Leave the conditioner on the hair strands for a few minutes and then rinse thoroughly. Typically, only one application of hair conditioner is necessary. Sometimes if the hair is badly damaged, the conditioner can be left on for a longer period of time and then rinsed thoroughly. This product dramatically restores shine and luster and positively changes the appearance of the hair. Visually this is an important restorative step that must not be omitted.

CRANIAL INCISIONS

If the body has been autopsied and the decedent has long, thick, and/or extremely tangled hair, care is essential as to not to pull or tear the hair from the scalp when embalming/suturing the cranium. Hair conditioner and a wide-tooth hair pick can help alleviate frustration for the embalmer in this situation. This also will prevent damage to the hair caused by pulling or tearing hair from the scalp.

Procedure

With your hands, apply a small amount of hair conditioner to the hair, working from the scalp to the ends of the hair strands. Using a wide-tooth hair pick, comb through the hair until the hair is tangle-free. Part the hair along the cranial incision. Gather half the hair on the top of the head and secure it with a clamp. Keep the bottom half of the hair secure with a clamp at the nape of the neck. After embalming, shave or cut the hair to the scalp 1/8' above and below the incision. This will help prevent the hair from becoming tangled when suturing. Suture the incision, take the hair out of the clamp(s), shampoo the hair properly again, and then condition the hair again, if needed.

SCALP DISORDERS

The most common scalp disorders observed in the preparation room are pityriasis steatoides and pityriasis capitis simplex. Pityriasis capitis simplex is dry, scaly dandruff. Pityriasis steatoides disorder is often seen as a greasy, waxy, thick scaly type of dandruff commonly seen in the elderly. This is often caused by an excess of sebum production that causes flaking skin to stick together and form scales over the scalp. It is common to see scratch marks or gouge marks on the scalp as this disorder can itch and can be quite uncomfortable during life. These types of scales can be difficult to remove without causing the appearance of brown marks visible on the skin, called demarcation marks. However, they can be unsightly if left untreated and present on the scalp. It is wise to attempt to gently remove these thick scales before the embalming process begins.

Procedure

For the disorder pityriasis capitis simplex, a medicated shampoo can be used to cleanse the hair and the scalp. For the disorder pityriasis steatoides, another method can be utilized. Treat pityriasis steatoides observed on the scalp before the embalming process. Pump a generous amount of creamy hair conditioner into a gloved hand and, using fingertips, work the conditioner directly onto the scalp **only**. Allow the conditioner to penetrate the scales until the scales start to loosen and dissolve. Then, carefully comb through the hair until all the scales are removed from the scalp. Using a proper shampoo, shampoo the hair thoroughly until the scales are removed from the hair strands and the hair appears clean. Rinse and repeat until all the scales are removed. Use hair conditioner again this time working a small amount through the hair strands to help close the cuticle and to restore health and shine. Rinse thoroughly.

CURLY HAIR

Curly hair tends to have a coarser texture than straight hair and has greater tensile strength than fine hair. It is typically drier and more brittle and has a tendency to frizz.

Shampoos/conditioners that have a cream base work best with curly hair. Before drying or styling, apply a small amount of serum, a thick honey-like substance that is used to combat frizz. It is best to let curly hair dry naturally. By letting hair air-dry, the curls will be more natural and there will be less chance of frizz.

If time is of the essence, it is possible to speed up drying time. Blot excess moisture from curly hair with paper towels. Do not rub curly hair vigorously with a towel to remove moisture. A diffuser can be used to dry curly hair quickly. Diffusers can be purchased at a beauty supply store or drugstore and are relatively inexpensive. A diffuser diffuses air onto the hair through the hair dryer to remove moisture but retains the curl. Attach a diffuser on the end of a standard hair dryer. While drying curly hair with a diffuser, use a low-temperature setting and a low air flow setting and try not to touch the hair with your hands or fingers as this will cause the hair to frizz. When drying curly hair with a diffuser, begin at the root level and work in circular motions until the hair is dry.

BLOW DRYING

It is always best to let hair air-dry, especially if the hair is damaged or fragile. Fragile hair has less tensile strength and has a tendency to break easily. Great care and caution must be taken when caring for this type of hair.

If the hair is in a good condition, and time is a factor, utilizing a blow-dryer will help remove moisture from the hair quickly. It is wise to have a variety of brushes to dry/style hair. A round brush, a vent brush, and a natural bristle brush will work on most hair types. A round brush is used for styling and volume, a vent brush for hairstyles that lay flat against the head, and a natural bristle brush for ethnic hair or straight hair.

Be sure to keep the blow-dryer moving at all times and on a medium- to low-temperature setting. Begin at the nape of the neck and move forward, drying the roots first and then the ends of the hair strand. Be sure to thoroughly dry the nape of the neck, as this is a common place for mold growth.

PROFESSIONALLY FINISHED HAIR

Embalmers can enhance any final hairstyle with professional finishing products. One product that works well on most hair types is a glosser or finishing spray. These coat the hair with silicone polymers that reflect light and give the hair a shiny, finished appearance. A spray that lists, among its ingredients, mica, is a superb choice. This mica spray is highly reflective and gives a professional looking shine to any hairstyle. It can be used on any hair type, including male facial hair, creating extraordinary shine and the appearance of healthy hair. This type of spray is nonsticky and is the finishing touch to a professional appearance. It can be applied without buildup on the hair. It especially works very well with overhead lighting seen in viewing rooms. This product is reflective, eye catching, and positively enhances any finished hairstyle.

ETHNIC HAIR

African-American hair is much more fragile than Caucasian hair. It tends to be extremely dry and breakage is quite common. Damaging the hair can be done if you are not careful or experienced with this type of hair. When cleansing the hair, a hydrating shampoo is a must with African-American hair. A moisturizing conditioner must be used as well. African-American hair should be oiled using a small amount of shea butter, jojoba oil, olive oil, or sunflower oil. When caring for African-American hair, it is essential to use a wide-toothed hair pick, not a standard comb or brush. A standard comb or brush can be very harsh on ethnic hair and can tangle very easily and/or pull the hair from the scalp. When using a brush on ethnic hair, use a natural bristle brush, and brush hair gently to prevent breakage.

Many African-American women use hair extensions or weaves to accent their hair in an ornamental manner. It is always wise to consult a professional hairdresser if you are not familiar with the proper care and arrangements or extensions or weaves.

TRIMMING HAIR BASICS

Many times, especially in the final stages of an illness, personal grooming is not a priority. It is important to communicate with the family the possibility of hair cutting or trimming. If the remains need a bit of hair trimming or grooming, here are a few tips to achieve professional results.

Begin by securing the proper tools. It is wise to have hair-trimming shears. These can be purchased in a beauty supply store. Shears are balanced, sharp, and specific for hair cutting. A balance comb is a wise purchase. These inexpensive plastic combs have units of measure on the comb, which makes it easier to have accurate measurements when cutting hair. A few hair clips or butterfly clamps will help keep the hair manageable while trimming.

Basic Hair-Trimming Procedure

Before beginning, ensure that the hair is clean, conditioned, and tangle-free. Trim hair when the hair is wet (unless it is a hair replacement, then trim when dry). When hair is wet, it appears longer than it will when it is dry. Hair will appear shorter when dry. This is called the "drying factor." Take into consideration the "drying factor," especially when trimming or cutting curly hair and/or bangs.

Part the hair in small sections at a time, securing the hair with a hair clamp. Make parts approximately a half-inch wide and less than a quarter of an inch thick. Ensure the parts are very straight. When trimming, use the index finger and the middle finger to hold the section of hair securely between them and cut the hair straight across. Use fingers as a guide to cut along the fingers in a straight line. While cutting or trimming hair, only move the thumb up and down while trimming for maximum control. Hair has elasticity and can easily stretch when wet and pulled. Do not pull or tug on the hair when holding the hair to trim. When possible, lay hair flat on the skin when trimming. Use the nose, ears, and/or the mandible as measurement guides to keep both sides even. When trimming or cutting, start conservatively. It is possible to go back and trim more hair if necessary.

BALD SCALP

For a finished, professional appearance for bald scalps, it is essential to follow a few simple steps. First, exfoliate any dry skin flakes seen on the scalp. For mild flakes, use generous amounts of massage cream before, during, and after embalming. Before cosmetics are applied, remove the massage cream with a lint-free gauze pad to gently remove all visible dry skin flakes from the scalp. The preferred method of applying cosmetics to a bald scalp is by airbrushing the cosmetics onto the skin. Airbrush cosmetics are highly pigmented and water-based. These cosmetics dry to a matte finish and are rub-resistant. Airbrushing cosmetics on the scalp will minimize the chance of soiling the pillow or the interior of the casket with cosmetic.

WIG CARE/SECURING TO SCALP

Sometimes, a family will bring in a wig that their loved one wore in life to be attached to the scalp for an authentic look of the deceased. With a little knowledge about wigs and wig care, we can be confident that the appearance will be pleasing to the family.

There are two types of hair used when making wigs: human hair and synthetic hair. Both need to be treated with care.

Before securing the wig to the scalp, a little preparation is needed. If the natural hair is long, secure the hair tightly to the head with bobby pins. Then identify which is the front of the wig and which is the back. The label is always in the back of the wig. There are usually two tabs (one on either side) that should line up with the ears. Before putting the wig on the decedent, give the wig a shake to fluff the style. Stand at the end of the embalming table where the head is. Grab the wig by each tab (on the side) and slip the wig over the head with the label toward the back. Line up the front of the wig with the hairline. Lift the head from the neck block and gently pull the wig down toward the nape of the neck. In some wigs, there are Velcro tabs to adjust the tightness of the wig to the scalp. Once the wig is placed properly, lined up with the hairline and secure at the nape, then adjust tightness using the Velcro tabs. Style the wig with fingers or comb.

Soiled Wigs

Dirty or soiled wigs should be properly cleansed before placing on the decent. First, gently brush through the wig with a wide-tooth comb or brush. Fill a sink with cold water and add a capful of gentle shampoo (baby shampoo works well). Immerse the wig in the cold water for a few minutes and agitate gently. Rinse the wig in cold water until the shampoo is completely removed. Allow the wig to air-dry naturally. Do not brush the wig when wet, as this will damage or remove the wig fibers. Heat will damage the wig and so do not use a blow-dryer or heated appliances on the wig hair. Blot any excess moisture with a towel. Allow the wig to air-dry on an empty plastic bottle covered by a towel. A Styrofoam head should be avoided as they can possibly stretch the wig.

FACIAL HAIR

When trimming or shaping facial hair on the deceased, clear, concise communication with the families is essential. Examining close-up photos of the facial hair and asking good questions regarding shape and styling will ensure the family is satisfied with the end result.

Begin by shampooing and conditioning facial hair. Dry gently with a towel and comb the hairs into place so that the hairs are all in the same direction.

Beards

Secure the proper tools before beginning. Choose a wider-toothed comb for trimming beards. Either scissors or clippers can be used to trim the hair. This is generally the personal preference of the embalmer. Begin by an ear and then clip the upper edges of the beard, cheeks, the jaw line (work top to bottom), and then lastly, the neckline. Reduce facial hair length slowly and conservatively as to not remove too much, working one side and then the other, and check for balance and symmetry on both sides.

Rechargeable cordless clippers work best in the prep room. These offer more control and precision. When determining length, choose the proper attachments and place on the end of the clippers. Double-check that the attachment is securely and firmly attached to the clippers before beginning. While choosing to trim without attachments, use a balance comb for length and control. Comb through the beard hairs and run the clippers along the length of the comb.

Scissors can also be used to trim beards. The scissor over comb technique takes practice and skill to get the beard uniform in length and shape. The tools chosen to trim beards are a personal preference.

Moustaches

For trimming moustaches, a small mustache comb and scissors or clippers are needed. Begin by combing the moustache hairs straight down toward the upper lip.

Start trimming in the middle and trim toward one side of the mouth and then the other. Use a fluff brush to remove hair clippings from the skin. Finish with a small amount of pomade or petroleum jelly to hold the hair in place. Set the facial hair with hair spray and finishing spray with mica for luster and shine.

CONCLUSION

Learning new skills and techniques, and incorporating them in body preparation, will lead to a higher level of professional care of human remains. Understanding basic fundamentals of hair care will allow embalmers to take a more active role in hair care of the deceased. This will prevent valuable service dollars being lost, while still providing exceptional care to the deceased, resulting in a positive lasting memory image for family members.

Fountain's Method of Management Techniques for the Eyes*

Practical Techniques

Vernie R. Fountain, Embalmer, Founder[†]

Vernie Fountain has been associated with funeral service since 1965 and became licensed as a funeral director in 1972 and as an embalmer in 1977. For 18 years, until December 1995, he owned and operated Fountain Mortuary Service in Columbia, Missouri, which responded to over 1000 deaths annually. He currently owns and operates Fountain National Academy of Professional Embalming Skills, Fountain Embalming Services, Forensic Investigative Resources of the Midwest (F.I.R.M.), a private detective agency, specializing in death investigations, surveillance, employee theft, background checks, and locating individuals that skip out on paying their bills. All of Fountain's businesses are headquartered in Springfield, Missouri.

Fountain National Academy, founded in May 1990, is a full-time venture for Fountain who is the Academy's founder and primary instructor. In addition to conducting spring and fall Embalming Seminars at FNA's training facility in Springfield, Missouri, he travels the United States and abroad teaching postgraduate education to embalmers, including specialized embalming techniques and postmortem reconstructive surgery. As a long-time supporter of Organ and Tissue Donation, he has consulted with numerous Organ and Tissue Agencies and presented seminars for them across the country. He is well known for his very strong advocacy of open casket viewing, the body being present, and the values associated with it for the family, friends, and the future of funeral service.

VALUES ASSOCIATED WITH EMBALMING AND RECONSTRUCTIVE SURGERY

As professional embalmers, we must always remember that the dead human body is the main taproot for all we do in funeral service. It should always be our main focus. Embalming and reconstructive surgery management should be performed with the desire to transform the appearance of the body in such a way that will enable the family to have open casket viewing if desired. The professional embalmer will be called upon by families to serve as the "Expert" regarding the proper embalming and reconstruction of their loved one to create an acceptable appearance. Your community expects you to be the "Expert" and it expects nothing but the best.

1. The psychological value to the family and friends
   a. It is well known that seeing is believing and that viewing the body will bring forth the true reality of the death. It will dramatically help the family and friends with closure and minimize the potential mind-set of denial.
   b. Viewing normally provides an extra degree of comfort to the family and friends.
   c. Having the body present with viewing is THE MOST PERSONALIZED service we can provide to the family during the ceremonial process.
2. Embalming and postmortem reconstructive surgery
   a. *As* a professional embalmer, you should be reminded that you are considered by your community to be the "Expert" regarding your expertise.
   b. No other professional can perform your expertise.
   c. Embalming and reconstructive surgery should translate to revenues gained for the embalmer and funeral establishment. Your expertise is worth a fair and reasonable professional fee for your time and effort.
3. Embalmer's mission
   a. The first objective is to preserve and sanitize the body. With some *preparations*, it may be necessary to sacrifice normal skin color and flexibility to achieve quality preservation and sanitation.
   b. When authorized, restore or perform postmortem reconstructive surgery to achieve a more acceptable and identifiable appearance

---

*Reprinted by permission of the author, January 2005.
[†]Founder, Fountain National Academy of Professional Skills, 2211 West Norton Road, Springfield, Missouri.

Embalming & Post Mortem Reconstructive Surgery

should transform the body from

UNACCEPTABLE to ACCEPTABLE and more

APPEARANCE for viewing

Before Fountain's Techniques

After Fountain's Techniques

of the facial features. This is particularly important when the victim has suffered disfiguring injuries. The objective or mission of postmortem reconstructive surgery is to transform the body **from an UNACCEPTABLE to an *ACCEPTABLE* and more *IDENTIFIABLE* appearance. It should not be confused with perfection of the appearance.** (See Exhibit 1 before and after.)

SPECIALIZED EMBALMING MANAGEMENT OF EYES

All case management strategies begin with a thorough preembalming analysis. One should identify all aspects of the case and then identify techniques to manage each aspect.

PROCEDURES FOR NORMAL EYES WITH NO TRAUMA OR ABNORMALITIES

Recommendations:

1. Use caution when cleaning debris from the eyelashes and lids. Briefly soak the eyelids with a humectant. This will help with removal and will not dehydrate the edges of the eyelids.
2. Use caution if you spray the eyelids with a topical disinfectant. Some disinfectants may produce excessive dehydration of the edges of the eyelids.
3. Position eyelids in the lower one-third of the orbit prior to arterial embalming. I do not recommend overlapping the eyelids as it creates a very unnatural appearance.
4. Use eye caps, not cotton. Cotton has a dehydrating effect.
5. Use a rounded type eye cap. I do not recommend the long shallow oval type because they tend to give the curvature of the eye an abnormal appearance.

6. Use a smaller eye cap rather than a larger one. Eye caps that are too large will tend to cause puffiness in the orbital area during arterial injection.
7. Eye caps should be covered with Vaseline or massage cream before placement over the globe of the eye.

PROCEDURE FOR ENUCLEATED EYES WHEN THE ENTIRE GLOBE HAS BEEN REMOVED AND THERE ARE NO ABNORMALITIES TO THE EYE LIDS

(Note: Hospitals and organ procurement organizations should be instructed **NOT** to place ice packs on the eyes. **Ice packs do not reduce** the threat of swelling in the eyelids, but rather they greatly **INCREASE** the chance of swelling during arterial injection.)

Recommendations: (**Prior** to arterial injection)

1. Remove all cotton or prosthetic devices from the orbital sockets.
2. Perform arterial embalming as appropriate for the condition of the body. Use a slightly stronger injection solution.
3. Following the completion of arterial injection and final bathing of the body, perform the restoration of the eyes.

Recommendation for restoration: (**After** arterial injection)

1. Place a light coating of massage cream surrounding the eyes on the tissues of the cheek and temple to protect these tissues.
2. Carefully swab the inside of the orbits with a cauterant chemical and then dry the socket of any excess chemical.
3. Place a small amount of "nonswelling" or "minimal-swelling" dry incision powder into the back of the sockets. Some dry incision powders will swell significantly when they absorb moisture. This may produce undesirable swelling in

the eyes. The powder should be moved around with a small instrument to lightly coat the entire raw tissue surface of the orbit.

4. Use modeling clay to make a prosthetic eyeball or use the one provided by the eye procurement agency. Use caution if you elect to use a soft material to make the prosthetic device because the pressure caused by touching the area during the family viewing can easily alter the contour of the finished eye. Cover the chosen device with an eye cap and coat it with Vaseline or massage cream and insert it into the socket.

5. With an instrument manually stretch the eyelids and close them in the lower one-third of the orbit.

6. Analyze the facial features from a profile view and make a judgment for appropriate projection of the eye outward. Some people will have protruding eyes while others are more retracted into the facial features. A useful technique is to place a straight edge on an imaginary vertical line from the midline of the eyebrow to the midline of the cheek to check for protrusion of the eye. Most individuals will look normal if the eyelid is protruding to a point where it barely touches the straight edge. Often, eyes appear abnormal because the prosthetic device was made too small. If you are not satisfied with the appearance, you may need to consider enlarging the prosthetic device.

7. Glue the edge of the eyelids together.

PROCEDURES FOR EYE DONATION WITH CORNEA REMOVAL ONLY

Recommendations: (**Prior** to arterial injection)

1. Remove any eye cap or prosthetic device placed in the eye.
2. Arterial inject the body.
3. Restore eyes after arterial injection is completed.

Recommendations: (**After** arterial injection)

1. Remove the vitreous humor by swabbing out the inside of the globe with cotton.
2. Swab inside of the globe with a cauterant.
3. Fill the eyeball with cotton soaked in a humectant or use a mortuary putty material.
4. Coat an eye cap with Vaseline or massage cream and insert under eyelids.
5. Close eyelids in lower one-third of the orbit.
6. Manually stretch eyelids and glue the edges together.

PROCEDURES FOR ANY FORM OF ENUCLEATED EYES WITH ASSOCIATED TRAUMA SUCH AS DISCOLORATION AND SWELLING

Recommendations: (**Prior** to arterial injection)

1. Remove all cotton or prosthetic devices from the orbital sockets.
2. Bleach all blood discolorations as outlined in Figures 1–1 through 1–3 (see next section).
3. Begin the arterial injection with the head. I recommend that the head of all head trauma cases be injected, by way of the carotids, with the "Waterless" method (see **Exhibit 1**). This method will minimize additional swelling and you would expect it to significantly reduce any edematous swelling present in the facial features. Following injection of the head, perform arterial embalming to the trunk.
4. Following the completion of arterial injection and final bathing of the body, perform reconstructive surgery on the eyes.

Exhibit 1: Waterless Method of Injection

Mix equal parts of the chemicals listed and **do not add water.** You can expect to use a total volume of 48 to 96 oz to inject the head. I recommend beginning with one 16-oz bottle of each to create 48-oz total solution. A volume of 48 oz will usually be adequate for the entire head. If necessary, mix additional amounts in equal proportions.

　　Chemicals:
　　Water Corrective Chemical
　　Coinjection Chemical
　　Arterial Chemical (use a nonhumectant type)

PROCEDURES FOR BLEACHING BLOOD DISCOLORATIONS OF THE EYES

Step 1. As an option, you may want to coat the side of the face with Vaseline or massage cream to protect the skin surface from the draining of excess bleaching chemical. Without the coating, you will likely experience streaking on the side of the face. Inject a bleaching chemical just under the surface of the eyelids PRIOR to injecting the head using the "Waterless" method (see Figs. 1–1 and 1–2).

　　Step 2. Supersaturate the area with the bleaching chemical. Even though you produce additional swelling in the eye, it is necessary to be successful with this technique. An adequate amount of bleaching/cauterant chemical must come in contact with all the entire discolored area (see Fig. 1–3).

Figure 1–1.

Step 3. Inject the head via the carotids with the "waterless" method.

Step 4. Inject the trunk of the body using an adequate strength and volume of injection solution.

Step 5. Immediately after final bathing or within a few hours, perform reconstructive surgery on the eyes to reduce the swelling (see Figs. 2–1 through 2–6).

PROCEDURES FOR POSTMORTEM RECONSTRUCTIVE SURGERY ON THE EYES

Recommendations: (All surgery procedures should be performed after arterial injection)

Step 1. Use a 20-gauge or larger hypodermic needle and syringe. Insert the needle into the sclera (white of the eyeball). Pass the needle tip to the center of the eyeball and withdraw as much of the vitreous humor as possible. Dispose of the vitreous humor. This step de-

Figure 1–3.

flates the eyeball and allows better access to perform surgical removal of the swollen tissue under the eyelids and within the orbital area (see Fig. 2–1).

Step 2. Use double-pointed sharp scissors, a hemostat or forceps, and aneurysm hook. Lift the upper eyelid and insert the point of the scissors under the eyelid. Then begin to excise the swollen tissue. The hemostat or forceps will allow you to grab tissue to pull it slightly outward where it can be excised (see Figs. 2–2 and 2–3).

Step 3. During excising of the swollen tissue, evaluate the eye frequently. Following removal of an adequate amount of swollen tissue make aggressive channels underneath the eyelids with the scissors (see Fig. 2–4).

Step 4. Apply a liberal amount of Vaseline or massage cream to the eyelids and apply very aggressive digital pressure. Press the eyelids until they are almost back to normal thickness (see Fig. 2–5).

Step 5. Evaluate and position eyelid to check for appropriate reduction of swelling (see Fig. 2–6). If you

Figure 1–2.

Figure 2–1.

Figure 2–2.

are comfortable that enough reduction has occurred, move to step 6.

Step 6. Inflate the eyeball using tissue builder.

Step 7. Insert and position an eye cap.

Step 8. Position the eyelids and evaluate for wrinkles. Analyze general facial characteristics and age of deceased to determine if too many wrinkles are present. Wrinkles usually can be reduced using a tissue dryer (heat spatula) (see Fig. 2–7).

Recommendations for using a tissue dryer (Heat Spatula):

1. Remember a tissue dryer must be hot to be effective. Let it heat up for several minutes to reach its maximum temperature.
2. Apply a liberal coat of Vaseline or massage cream to the area.

Figure 2–4.

3. Do not drag the spatula tip across the eyelid, as this tends to cause undesirable burning and leatherizing of the tissue. Rather quickly press it down onto the skin and quickly raise it off. Touch quickly and remove quickly. Work in small areas until you heat that area up enough to shrink the tissue.
4. Evaluate the area frequently by wiping off the cream to check if wrinkles have been removed. When wrinkles are removed to your satisfaction, then move to another small area.
5. Upon completion, remove the heavy coating of cream.

Step 9. Position the eyelids in the lower one-third of the orbit. Remember to recreate the natural contour of the eye. As with any reconstructive surgical process, remember the three-dimensional aspect of facial features.

Figure 2–3.

Figure 2–5.

Figure 2–6.

To achieve normal curvature of the eye, you can use your thumb finger and index finger to press the inner canthus and outer corner closer together.

Step 10. Glue the edges of the eyelids together. In order to achieve a more natural curvature of the eyelids, it may be necessary to glue the underside of the eyelid down. This can be accomplished using a 20-gauge needle and syringe to inject superglue through the skin into the superorbital area and pressing it into the desired position. Hold it there until the superglue cures.

PROCEDURES FOR EYES THAT POSSESS EITHER SUBCUTANEOUS EMPHYSEMA (AIR WITHIN THE TISSUE) OR TISSUE GAS

Before you can develop a management strategy, you must establish whether the swelling is caused by subcutaneous emphysema or tissue gas. Since it is impossible to determine this by visual inspection or palpation of the

Figure 2–7.

After Fountain's techniques

area, it is important to carefully analyze and consider all factors surrounding the history and circumstances of the death. For example, persons who die a traumatic death may have a puncture or laceration of the lung(s) from things such as fractured ribs, blunt force trauma impact injury, or an invasion of the lung by a projectile type of object. If the person took a few breaths for a while following the event, or if life-support measures were administered, it is possible for air or oxygen to escape from the lung(s) and move into the subcutaneous tissues. Another condition to consider is chronic obstructive pulmonary disease (COPD). With this condition, it is not uncommon for life-saving measures such as, but not limited to, CPR to rupture the lung(s). This can allow oxygen to escape into the tissues and **mimic** tissue gas. Remember that subcutaneous emphysema has no odor, whereas tissue gas possesses an odor and tends to spread rapidly.

To determine if tissue gas is present, you must consider numerous factors such as cause of death, environment where death occurred, how the death occurred, length of time from death to embalming, length of time of any refrigeration, visual signs of external decomposition, or any indication through the chain of events of the case history of possible internal decomposition. A good understanding of all the facts about the case will be paramount to making the determination. If you determine it is tissue gas, the management strategy will need to be different than that of subcutaneous emphysema. As a safeguard, I recommend the policy of **when in doubt, treat it as tissue gas.**

Recommendations: (Prior to Arterial Injection)

Note: If the eyelids are grossly swollen, I do not recommend attempting to place an eye cap over the globe. Instead leave the swollen eyes alone because you can reconstruct after arterial injection.

Step 1. Assuming the swelling is only slight to moderate, I would recommend placing an eye cap over the globe and proceeding as though it was a normal embalming case. If discoloration is present, follow the steps of bleaching techniques.

Step 2. Inject the arterial system. If it is subcutaneous emphysema, a slightly stronger-than-normal injection solution can be used. If it is tissue gas, use a waterless injection solution on the head accompanied by a tissue gas chemical. The entire body should then be injected with a very strong arterial solution accompanied by a tissue gas chemical.

Recommendations: (After arterial injection)

Step 1. Follow the reconstructive surgery steps previously outlined, in most cases of subcutaneous emphysema or tissue gas, it will not be necessary to excise tissue. Aggressive channeling and digital pressure will likely solve the problem.

Step 2. On tissue gas cases, make sure the tissue gas chemical has thoroughly saturated the eyelids. If you are not comfortable that the area is saturated, I would recommend direct hypodermic injection of nondiluted tissue gas chemical into that area before you reconstruct or perform any surgery on the eye

---

Enhance Emaciated Features Arterially Using Split Injection and Restricted Drainage*

By Sharon L. Gee

If you poll the ranks of embalmers, the majority place feature "building" after embalming just prior to cosmetic application, dressing, and casketing. Therefore, academically, feature enhancement is a post-embalming treatment, separate, and distinct from arterial injection. The instrument of choice for this application is the needle and syringe. Consider the challenges of uniformly addressing the entire facial terrain in this manner while maintaining the integrity of natural and acquired facial markings. Consider eliminating this post-embalming treatment in favor of enhancing features DURING the arterial embalming.

Split injection, one-point injection, and restricted cervical injection are all injection methods that utilize the blood vascular system to deliver preservative chemicals. The split injection method (using the femoral artery as an injection site) affords the embalmer the

*Sharon L. Gee, is Assistant Professor-Clinical, Embalming, at Wayne State University, Detroit. She is manager of the Pixley Funeral Home Godhardt-Tomlinson Chapel in Keego Harbor and President of the Michigan Embalmers Society. By permission of the author, 2005.

most control in yielding uniform fluid distribution and symmetry in the facial tissues. The result can parallel a natural weight gain and present a healthy appearance. Feature enhancement through arterial injection can allow the embalmer to improve rather than change the decedent's appearance.

Split injection requires two vessel sites, one for injection and the other for drainage. It is understood that embalming fluid is more readily assimilated in the tissues nearest the site of injection and in the highest concentrations. Distance matters. To achieve symmetry of facial enhancement, the femoral (or common Iliac) vessel is raised for injection. A large volume of well-coordinated solution is injected toward the face without fear of over-embalming these viewable features. The femoral vessel should be injected first distally to observe for fluid distribution, diffusion, and cosmetic coloring in the leg and to allow for adjustments of pressure and rate of flow before injecting superiorly. The benefit of distance from the femoral injection site to the head affords higher pressure and rate of flow settings to overcome vascular obstructions or resistances.

The most copious drainage is taken from the center of venous drainage in the dead human body, the heart. The site of drainage is the right atrium of the heart via a drainage instrument inserted into the right internal jugular vein. Blood, body fluids, and coagula are evacuated directly from the heart to reduce the opportunity for unwanted facial swelling. In facially emaciated decedents, the technique of restricting drainage (intermittent or alternate drainage) creates intravascular pressure so that large volumes of solution enter and remain in the facial tissues. Drainage restriction gives the embalmer the most control over fluid retention in the face and in combination with distance injection, which is the secret to enhancing contour uniformly.

While injecting, note the expansion of the intact right common carotid artery. Engorgement of this vessel is evidence of arterial preservative traveling to the head and of the intravascular pressure necessary to perfuse the preservative into the deep tissues. Pressure filtration is the passive transport mechanism chiefly responsible for preservative distribution and is created by the centrifugal embalming machine. The success of pressure filtration relies directly on the embalmer's ability to set the controls on the machine accordingly to overcome vascular resistances. Two other mechanisms, osmosis and dialysis, work concurrently with the force of the embalming machine to deliver and perfuse the tissues with preservative.

The embalmer optimizes the performance of the arterial chemical with the addition of coinjection and specialty chemicals. These additive chemicals boost the ability of the arterial preservative to distribute within the vascular system, to diffuse the deeper tissues to bind ultimately, with the protein molecules, and to create a necessary moisture balance within the tissues. Because large volumes of solution are injected toward the delicate facial tissues, the arterial formulation must not be too harsh. Hypertonic solutions may sear the capillary beds, hindering further distribution. Coinjections temper the harshness of formaldehyde, adjust pH, soften coagula, and condition the vascular system to readily accept the preservative. Coinjections act as a substitute for water. Water has no benefit to the embalmer save its function to dilute the chemicals. Lanolin-based specialty chemicals promote moisture retention to yield natural skin contour and pliability for the best and most natural presentation of the decedent. Humectant fluids also hydrate the tissues to prevent shrinking, wrinkling, and discoloration and reduce the surface evaporation that will occur over the course of the visitation and funeral. A word of caution as too much humectant will actually yield a reverse effect and draw moisture from the tissues, thus accelerating dehydration!

It is important that during injection of the last portion of the arterial solution, attempt to fully restrict drainage so that a very positive pressure is built within the vascular system. Once the embalmer is satisfied that a sufficient volume of solution has reached all tissues of the body and there has been a noted improvement of the sunken facial features, injection can be stopped. Carefully remove instruments and immediately tie off the vessels so that a positive pressure is maintained in the vascular system. Delay aspiration as long as possible giving tissues a time to fully firm and react to the arterial chemicals.

The embalmer of today faces new challenges brought forth by medical science advancements that extend the life span. Terminal patients are actively dying over longer intervals of time. Extended agonal periods create numerous embalming complications. One-point injections are a luxury and not the standard. Embalmers no longer believe multiple incisions symbolize defeat, rather the use of multiple sites for injection and drainage yields obvious value.

Embalming—United Kingdom and European

Peter J. Ball, FBIE
Secretary, The European Association of Embalmers

The subject of this discussion is embalming or, as it is often called in Europe—thanatopraxy. The European name of thanatopraxy was created to distinguish between the perception that embalming was in some way similar to mummification as practiced by the ancient Egyptians (among others): it is likely that the word embalming does not translate readily into non-English languages without attracting this inference. This is further underlined in some countries where embalming is forbidden by law, whereas thanatopraxy is a legitimate practice.

There is often a distinction between what is perceived as embalming by the medical profession and that practiced by the funeral business in the United Kingdom and other countries of similar funeral customs. It is as much a question of custom and purpose that serves to define the difference between the two types; for the sake of clarity, I intend to use the term "thanatopraxy" to differentiate between "funeral" embalming and "medical" embalming. Medical embalming is concerned only with preservation; thanatopraxy is concerned with preservation and presentation because of the practice of viewing the body by relations and friends of the bereaved. Thanatologists will argue the psychological benefits of this practice, but I do not propose to dwell on this subject that in itself provokes lengthy discussion. It has been part of funeral customs for many years within the United Kingdom and other countries to view the deceased, before the final disposal of the body; I am aware that this is not the case with many other countries where different cultures and therefore differing customs prevail. However, there does seem to be a common psychological need for some form of ceremony surrounding the disposal of the dead human body, and in many countries, a need to view the body is part of that ceremonial.

Medical embalming of the nonautopsied subject is achieved by the injection of a preservative mixture containing formaldehyde as the basic chemical—usually into the common carotid artery. This is supplemented by the injection of strong preservative into the thoracic and abdominal cavities. Drainage of blood is not often attempted, and the final appearance of the deceased is not an important consideration, preservation is the objective. High volumes of chemical are injected, which causes swelling of tissues in the face and limbs, and these tissues also tend to turn a gray color because of the reaction to formaldehyde. If the body has been the subject of an autopsy, medical embalming techniques vary. Some procedures involve the injection of preservative into the common carotid, subclavian, and femoral arteries supplemented by hypodermic injection into trunk tissues; others may simply inject straight into the tissues without use of the blood vessels. These techniques are not designed to accommodate viewing of the body and were never intended for this purpose. Modern usage outside of medical school subjects is more concerned with the safe and hygienic transport of deceased persons over long distances for the benefit of the transporting agent and the hygiene laws of any country or state who authorize entry of the body.

Thanatopraxy is concerned with the preservation, hygiene, and appearance of the dead human body, and in that sense shares two of the same objectives achieved by medical embalming, that is, those of preservation and hygiene. However, the crucial difference of rendering the remains fit for viewing demands a different approach. The chemicals used for injection into the arterial system are made from carefully compiled formulae with the end of achieving a natural appearance. Of necessity, these are stable compounds designed to overcome or, at worst, neutralize the effects of morbid conditions within the body to be treated, it is not surprising therefore that there are specialized formulations for some of the more common conditions such as jaundice, edema, and tissue gas.

In its simplest form, thanatopraxy is the injection of preservative chemical under pressure into the arterial system, which is then forced out into the capillaries to reach the tissue cell. Protein is coagulated by reaction with the embalming chemical, and blood is forced back toward the heart. In the nonautopsied subject, it is a matter of the introduction of a canula into a major artery, the injection of preservative chemical under pressure, and the removal of the blood via a vein drainage tube inserted into the internal jugular vein to reach the right atrium of the heart. The major arteries in normal use for adults are the common carotid, axillary, or femoral artery; the veins normally used are the internal jugular or the axillary vein. The technique is to inject through the artery until sufficient pressure is present in the vascular system, which is then relieved by opening a tap on the vein drainage tube; the blood flows through the tube and connects into a collecting jar for ultimate disposal. The vein tube is then closed, and injection is continued to build up pressure before opening the vein tube again to drain more blood, this alternation continues until the operator is satisfied that preservative has been distributed to all parts of the body. If for any reason drainage through a vein is not possible, the introduction of a trocar into the right atrium of the heart is an effective means of blood drainage, the blood being drawn through the trocar into a closed container under a vacuum. On completion of injection, the trocar and aspiration apparatus is employed for removal of body fluids within the trunk cavities. As well as achieving preservation and disinfection, the effect of the injection is to restore normal color to the tissues and remove postmortem discoloration.

If the body has been the subject of an autopsy, a different technique is necessary and is dependent very much on the extent of the examination. Where there has been the complete removal of the organs in the trunk cavities during autopsy, these are again removed by the operator and treated, allowing access to the major arteries. Where they are intact, it is normal to inject distally into the common carotid, subclavian, and common iliac arteries; where there is damage to these, injection commences from the point distally beyond the damage. The blood drainage flows back into the cavities and is subsequently removed by aspiration. It is normally with the arteries of the head that the majority of difficulties occur, often as a result of careless removal of the tongue. I am fortunate in the area where I work to have a skilled postmortem technician who is able to remove the tongue, trachea, and esophagus without excising the common carotid arteries. In many instances, the damage is severe, and injection may only be possible via the external carotid, internal carotid, and external maxillary or facial arteries, and even these are often sufficiently damaged as to be of no practical use. The face is the most important area for viewing with the hands next in order of visual importance and it seems at times that some of the persons engaged in autopsy work are not aware of the consequences of their actions. For example and again in my area, some forensic pathologists are removing the facial tissues from the bones of the face, to leave the face held in place only by the tissues around the nose and eyes. This almost eliminates the possibility of arterial injection and removal of discoloration's caused by blood remaining in the blood vessels and significantly reduces the chance of viewing without signs of putrefaction. Further difficulties can be caused by the nature of the incision used for opening the trunk and head. The "V" incision causes the most damage to the neck and facial tissues, this consists of an incision from the pubes to the sternal notch and from that point across the neck on each side behind the ears and across the skull; the line of the incision is continuous. The incision causing the least damage extends from the sternal notch to the pubes, and the incision for cranial examination extends from behind one ear across the back part of the skull to a point behind the other ear.

These, briefly, are the methods employed by the qualified practitioner; there are many other complications and variations to the basic injection techniques described today. On completion of the injection, all tissues should be restored to a natural color with discoloration removed. The operator then washes and disinfects the body, cleaning all orifices and placing the features in an attitude of repose. Dressing of the body may be by the use of the deceased's own clothes or of funeral clothing as supplied by the funeral director. Injuries are treated and covered with cosmetics; the use of these varies according to the customs and beliefs of the deceased. The end result is that the deceased is presented with a more acceptable appearance than that of a person with the more obvious signs of death, so providing a more pleasant memory of the last time that it is possible to see them.

This then defines the major objective of thanatopraxy—to render the experience of viewing the deceased less of an ordeal to those who are taking their final leave. Clearly, the appearance can only remain acceptable if preservation is achieved, equally disinfection is a vital feature because of the need for some mourners to touch and even kiss their loved one.

Thanatopraxy does not set out to achieve permanent preservation; there are many additional factors that influence this as I feel sure this assembly is already aware, and additional or even different techniques would be employed to achieve that objective. It is concerned only with the delay of putrefactive changes until after final disposal of the body.

There have always been difficulties with the transport of people who die many miles away from their home; the numbers of these have increased dramatically with the advent of ease of travel. On an international scale, a significant number of people die abroad and repatriation is required. In most of these cases, embalming or thantopraxy is a requirement by the transporting agency or the receiving country itself. In those countries where viewing is part of the funeral customs, it is often the case that this is impossible because of either poor quality treatment or the deceased has become unrecognizable. The latter instance arises from medical embalming because embalming by anybody other than members of the medical profession is forbidden in the country where the death has occurred. Unless the individual concerned has undergone training in modern embalming techniques, at best, it is unlikely that anything more than preservation will be achieved. This causes genuine distress to the bereaved, and if they insist upon viewing will leave only an unpleasant memory. I make no comment on the many examples of poor quality embalming received in some international transports, as professionals yourselves you would not condone incompetence. The worst examples of incompetent treatment seem to occur where the remains have been hermetically sealed and the coffin reopened for viewing on arrival at its destination. It may be that opening the coffin again was not considered to be a possibility; however, embalming has been paid for and should be carried out efficiently.

In conclusion, I would like to refer to the modern operator who may not be a qualified doctor. In Europe, it is only in France that a state qualification is required to practice thanatopraxy although other European countries are starting to legislate at local government level. In some cantons in Switzerland, it is now permissible for qualified operators to treat bodies for international transport, where until recently only doctors were permitted to do this. This is welcomed because there is a need for a qualified operator, properly trained for the care of the dead as a service to the bereaved person at a difficult time. In general, the interest of the medical profession is not concerned with the disposal of the deceased after life has become extinct. In some European countries, there is no prohibition against the use of unqualified persons. Suffice it to say that knowledge of disease, hygiene, anatomy and physiology, and other disciplines are an essential background to an efficient performance of the work in the modern scenario, and these form the basis of study for the modern embalmer or thanatopractitioner.

The Art of Embalming and its Purpose

Ron Hast

Mortuary Management, October 2006

Whenever I am asked to explain embalming, my response has been " Embalming is the best known method of presenting a deceased person in a state that will last well through the memorial event." If more information is requested, I say, "Blood is replaced with preservative chemicals, similar to a transfusion."

It is the privilege of any funeral director to decide whether an unembalmed body will be publically viewed, but to say the reason for requiring embalming is "to protect the public health" is not substantiated by any known scientific study. It is fair to expect anyone making such a claim would also enforce strict universal precautions from the instant mortuary personnel touch an unembalmed decedent, which is often not practiced, nor is it practiced in most health care institutions. If any health issues exist, they relate to those who handle, transport, and embalm bodies. Occupational hazards are not family or public risks. Handling an unembalmed body from initial care, refrigeration, casketing, and final cosmetic details can be more difficult than handling an embalmed body. But public presentation without embalming has been successfully and safely accomplished.

We know of the formal traditions and practices in Japan, England, and Jewish and Muslim communities, where refrigeration and frozen gel packs are routinely used throughout their services for stabilization and presentation, including those for large public audiences. For generations, these procedures have been practiced.

There are some who go so far as to claim that I am "anti-funeral" and opposed to the principles of proper funeral services. This is not true. I recognize the art of embalming, but also recognize the fact that bodies are often effectively and cosmetically presented throughout the world, including the United States, without embalming and health issues. I have observed this technique and results on numerous occasions. There are certainly instances and circumstances where embalming may be the best choice for temporary preservation and cosmetic enhancement. But it is not mandatory; it is a choice. If laws requiring embalming in certain states exit "for public health reasons," it is possible they are unfounded or politically based.

It is sad to note that certain death care "professionals" openly admit that if a family insists on viewing an unembalmed body, they make little attempt to enhance its appearance. If a client complains, their ready answer is that permission to embalm was denied and therefore appearance may be unsatisfactory.

With this topic coming to the forefront, several credentialed individuals were interviewed and contributed statements.

Dr. Lakshmanan Sathyavagiswaran, M.D., pathologist and chief medical examiner for the Los Angeles County for the past 15 years – well respected, appreciated, and honored by the medical profession and funeral service – says, "there is no reason that an unembalmed dead human body should be infectious to anyone attending visitation or public services. Persons transporting and handling bodies or cutting into them may be vulnerable in rare instances, with little or no risk if proper precautions are taken. To refuse to present a body unembalmed because of public health risk is unfounded. On rare occasions of certain deaths resulting from contagious disease, our office may encourage placing a face mask on the decedent before and during transportation and containment, and disposing without embalming or viewing. In the event, however, it becomes necessary to hold a body for an extended period of time before public services can be held, arterial embalming is recommended. Riding on an airplane or a bus may be a public health risk; the presence of an unembalmed body is not."

"The fact that dead bodies are a potential cause of epidemics after a disaster is almost always broadcast after major disasters. This 'fact' is a myth, and depriving survivors of appropriate burial ceremonies for their relatives may administer yet another blow to already injured or weakened persons. The only situation in which handling corpses is a risk is during epidemics of infectious diseases such as cholera. Even in these situations, no reason exists to totally deprive families from honoring their dead if they follow certain precautions. We have not at any point prescribed embalming as a method of protecting public health," says Bernadette Burden, Centers for Disease Control and Prevention (CDC), Atlanta, Georgia.

The question posed to the Dodge Company is whether they believe that a dead human body is a potential health risk. Their answer is "yes," because disease organisms do not die when a body dies. Rather, the lack of an immune system allows many of these organisms to reproduce very quickly. "We are not saying that a body, properly handled, is a health risk in every sit-

uation; rather, that it should be treated with care and that the person handling the body should use universal precautions as required by OSHA."

Should embalming be required in every situation if there is to be a viewing? Their answer is "no, we do not feel that embalming should be required as a condition to view unless the individual died from an infectious disease. We are of threat opinion only if the viewing family or individual is made aware of the natural process of decomposition, of how the body may look and of the time constraints placed on planning and holding a service when there is no embalming. Everyone has a different level of expectation and what one family or individual may find acceptable, another may find totally unacceptable. In today's litigious society (even with signed legal agreement indicating awareness of potential health risks and other potential problems) these issues need to play an important role in whether or not a business owner requires embalming if there is to be a public viewing," according to Debbie Dodge, The Dodge Chemical Company, Cambridge, Massachusetts.

"Representing that something, such as embalming, is legally required when that isn't the case is a violation of the FTC Funeral Rule and may give rise to liability under state laws as well," says Douglas O. Meyer, attorney and death care specialist, Woodland Hills, California.

"The art of embalming raises far above the clinical descriptions and opinions of direct handling of a human dead body. We must acknowledge that in many cultures, families take hold of a deceased person and intimately relate to the body from the moment of death to final disposition. It is unprofessional to primarily claim embalming is to protect public health. Our talents and artistry have proven to comfort survivors, giving them the best opportunity to embrace their dead without offensive natural occurrences. We do our work with pride, confidence and our contribution to the dignity of life through the death experience. It is the highest level of care through the death experience. It is the highest level of care and support to those who appreciate its values," notes Robert G. Mayer, author of *Embalming: History, Theory and Practice* (four editions), Pittsburgh, Pennsylvania.

Two long-term professors of accredited colleges of mortuary science were asked the following questions and gave the following answers (indicated as A1 and A2).

Q: Do the Schools teach methods and techniques of care for unembalmed bodies to be viewed?
A1: Yes, for identification purposes.
A2: Yes, briefly mentioned, but more on the subject is in order.

Q: Are students taught that embalming protects public health:
A1: Yes.
A2: Yes, and we test on that.

Q: Do students who graduate from your program understand that embalming protects public health?
A1: Yes.
A2: Yes.

Q: If a friend died and the spouse requested the unembalmed body to be present and viewed for a large public service, would you refuse to accommodate?
A1: No.
A2: No.

Q: Would you warn the family of public health exposure risks:
A1: No.
A2: No.

The content of what they are teaching is inconsistent with the facts. One admitted, "Your information is indefensible. Changes need to be made to the curriculum." Their candid comments and open discussion on the subject were impressive, and one instructor expressed willingness to change what he teaches in light of professional opinions and scientific conclusions.

The American Board of Funeral Service Education defines embalming as "The process of chemically treating the dead human body to reduce the presence and growth of microorganisms – to temporarily inhibit organic decomposition and to restore an acceptable physical appearance."

If a reason for embalming is to slow decomposition (and provide a base for cosmetic enhancement), refrigeration must also be acknowledged as a method of temporary preservation that yields similar stabilizing results. Is there some reason that many funeral directors do not have refrigeration facilities?

I emphasize that this information is not an attempt to promote death care without embalming. The values of embalming are well known. But firsthand knowledge of many who believe and claim to their clientele (when asking permission to embalm) if viewing is planned, embalming is required to protect the public health is misleading. To say embalming is a requirement of your firm to present the body for visitation and funeral services may be closer to the truth.

All said, here is a thoughtful way to request permission to embalm: "Trusting us to provide care and services includes certain choices and authorizations. If you intend to have formal viewing and public services, embalming is proper to control natural changes that may occur. May we have your authorizations to proceed?" If further information is requested about embalming, it may be said that "Natural discoloration, gasses, fluids and odors may occur. Embalming controls these and other concerns."

SECTION II
GLOSSARY

Embalming, Restorative Art and Mortuary Cosmetology Terms*

*Portions prepared by the Embalming (2008) and Restorative Art (2006) Syllabus committees of the
American Board of Funeral Service Education.

Abdominal anatomical regions. (1) Nine regions of the abdomen as demarcated by four imaginary planes, two of which are horizontal (indicated by lines drawn across the right and left tenth ribs and across the right and left anterior superior iliac spines) and two sagittal (indicated by lines drawn from the midpoint of inguinal ligament to the nipples on the chest and right and left sides). Upper row: right hypochondriac, epigastric, left hypochondriac. Middle row: right lateral, umbilical, left lateral. Lower row: right inguinal, pubic, left inguinal. (2) Four regions of the abdomen as demarcated by two imaginary planes, one horizontal and the other midsagittal: upper right quadrant, upper left quadrant, lower right quadrant, and lower left quadrant.

Abrasion. Antemortem injuries resulting from friction of the skin against a firm object and causing removal of the epidermis.

Abscess. Localized accumulation of pus.

Abut. To touch or contact, as with the tarsal plates of the closed eyelids.

Accessory chemicals. Chemicals used in addition to vascular (arterial) and cavity embalming fluids. Include but are not limited to hardening compounds, preservative powders, sealing agents, mold-preventive agents, and compress application agents.

Acetone. Dimethylketone; a colorless liquid used to soften and remove scabs; a solvent for restorative wax; a stain remover.

Acquired facial markings. Facial markings that develop during one's lifetime, primarily as a result of repetitious use of certain muscles.

Acquired immunodeficiency syndrome (AIDS). Specific group of diseases or conditions that are indicative of severe immunosuppression related to infection with the human immunodeficiency virus (HIV). Persons who died with AIDS may exhibit conditions such as wasting syndrome, extrapulmonary tuberculosis, and Kaposi sarcoma.

Action level (AL). Exposure limit usually one half of the Occupational Safety and Health Administration (OSHA) legal limit for a regulated substance. This level is established to ensure adequate protection of employees at exposures below the OSHA limits, but to minimize the compliance burdens for employers whose employees have exposures below the 8-hour permissible exposure limit (PEL). The AL for formaldehyde is 0.5 ppm.

Actual pressure. See Pressure.

Adipocere/Grave wax. Soft, grayish-white to brown, waxlike material composed of oleic, palmitic, and steric (fatty) acids. Formed by the postmortem hydrolysis and hydrogenation of body fats. Most prominent in the subcutaneous tissue but can occur wherever fat is present. Recent research indicates bacterial enzymes may be primarily responsible by converting unsaturated liquid fats (oleic acid) to saturated liquid fats.

Aerobic. In the presence of free oxygen.

Aerosol. Colloidal solution dispensed as a mist.

Aerosolization. Dispersal as an aerosol. Minute particles of blood and water become atomized and suspended in air when water under pressure meets the blood drainage or when flushing an uncovered flush sink.

Agglutination. Intravascular: increase in viscosity of blood brought about by the clumping of particulate formed elements in the blood vessels.

Agonal algor. Decrease in body temperature immediately before death.

Agonal coagulation. In reference to blood, a change from fluid to thickened mass.

Agonal dehydration. Loss of moisture from the living body during the agonal state.

Agonal edema. Escape of blood serum from an intravascular to an extravascular location immediately before death.

Agonal fever. Increase in body temperature immediately before death.

Agonal period. Period immediately before somatic death.

Agonal translocation. See Translocation.

Airbrush. Pressured atomizer used for spraying liquid paint or cosmetic on a surface.

Algor mortis. Postmortem cooling of the body to the surrounding temperature.

Alopecia. Absence or loss of hair.

Alternate drainage. Method of injection-drainage in which embalming solution is injected and then injection is stopped while drainage is open.

Alveolar process. Bony ridge found on the inferior surface of the maxilla and the superior surface of the mandible that contains the sockets for the teeth.

American Congress of Governmental Industrial Hygienists (ACGIH). An organization of professional personnel in government agencies or educational institutions who are employed in occupational safety and health programs.

Amino acids. Building blocks of which proteins are constructed and the end products of protein digestion or hydrolysis. The basic formula is NH_2–CHR–COOH–amino group, an alpha carbon, any aliphatic or aromatic radical, and a carboxyl group.

Anaerobic. In the absence of free oxygen.

Anasarca. Severe generalized edema.

Anatomical guides. Descriptive references for locating arteries and veins by means of the anatomical structures that are known.

Anatomical limits. Points of origin and points of termination in relation to adjacent structures. Used to designate the boundaries of arteries.

Anatomical position. The body is erect, feet together, palms facing forward, and thumbs pointed away from body.

Anchor. Material or technique employed to secure tissues or restorative materials in a fixed position; an armature.

Aneurysm. Localized abnormal dilation or outpocketing of a blood vessel resulting from a congenital defect or a weakness of the vessel wall.

Aneurysm hook. An embalming instrument that is used for blunt dissection and in raising vessels.

Aneurysm needle. An embalming instrument used for blunt dissection and in raising vessels that have an eye in the hook portion of the instrument for placing ligatures around the vessels.

Angle of the mandible. Body angle formed by the junction of the posterior edge of the ramus of the mandible and the inferior surface of the body of the mandible.

Angular spring forceps. Multipurpose instrument (size can vary) used in the embalming process (e.g., as a drainage instrument).

Angulus oris eminence. Small, convex prominence found lateral to the end of the line of closure of the mouth; a natural facial marking.

Angulus oris sulcus. Groove found at each end of the line of closure of the mouth; a natural facial marking.

Anomaly. Deviation from the normal.

Antecubital. In front of the elbow/in the bend of the elbow.

Antemortem. Before death.

Antemortem subcutaneous emphysema. A distension of the body tissues by the presence of gas or air beneath the skin; an antemortem condition brought about by a surgical procedure, trauma, or by a puncture or tear in the pleural sac or the lung tissue.

Anterior. Before or in front of; an anatomical term of position and direction, which denotes the front or forward part.

Anterior nares. External nostril openings.

Anterior superior iliac spine. A bony protuberance that can be palpated topographically, found on the ilium, the superior broad portion of the hip bone; the origin of the inguinal ligament and the sartorius muscle.

Anticoagulant fluid. Ingredient of embalming fluids that retards the natural postmortem tendency of blood to become more viscous or prevents adverse reactions between blood and other embalming chemicals.

Apparent death. Condition in which the manifestations of life are feebly maintained.

Aqueous. Watery; prepared with water as a solvent.

Aqueous humor. Clear, thin, alkaline fluid that fills the anterior chamber of the eyeball.

Armature. Framework; a material, commonly of pliable metal or wood, employed to provide support for a wax restoration.

Arterial (solution) delivery. Movement of the vascular solution from its source (e.g., embalming machine tank) through the machine apparatus, connective tubing and arterial tube into an artery.

Arterial (vascular) fluid. Concentrated, preservative, embalming chemical that is diluted with water to form the arterial solution for injection into the arterial system during vascular embalming. Its purpose is to inactivate saprophytic bacteria and render the body tissues less susceptible to decomposition.

Arterial solution. Mixture of arterial (vascular) fluid and water used for the arterial injection. May include supplemental fluids.

Arterial tube. Tube used to inject embalming solution into the blood vascular system.

Arteriosclerosis. Term applied to a number of pathological conditions causing a thickening, hardening, and loss of elasticity of the walls of the arteries.

Articulation. Place of union between two or more bones.

Ascites. Accumulation of serous fluids in the peritoneal cavity.

Asepsis. Freedom from infection and from any form of life. Sterility.

Asphyxia. Insufficient intake of oxygen. Numerous causes.

Aspiration. Withdrawal of gas, fluids, and semisolids from body cavities and hollow viscera by means of suction with an aspirator and a trocar.

Asymmetry. Lack of symmetry, balance, or proportion.

Atheroma. Fatty degeneration or thickening of the walls of the larger arteries occurring in atherosclerosis.

Autoclave. Apparatus used for sterilization by steam pressure, usually at 250°F (121°C) for a specific time.

Autolysis. Self-destruction of cells. Decomposition of all tissues by enzymes that form without microbial assistance.

Autolytic enzyme. The body's own digestive enzymes that are capable of destroying body cells (autolytic decomposition).

Autopsy. Postmortem examination of the organs and tissues of a body to determine cause of death or pathological condition. Necropsy.

Bactericidal agent. Agent that destroys bacteria.

Bacteriostatic agent. Agent that has the ability to inhibit or retard bacterial growth. No destruction of viability is implied.

Balsamic substance. Resin combined with oil. A fragrant, resinous, oily exudate from various trees and plants.

Base. (1) In cosmetology, the vehicle in a cosmetic (oil base); the initial application of cream or cosmetics. (2) The lower part of anything, the supporting part.

Base of the axillary space. Armpit.

- **Anterior boundary.** Established by drawing a line along the fold of skin that envelops the lateral border of the pectoralis major muscle.
- **Lateral boundary.** Established by drawing a line that connects the two points where the pectoralis major and latissimus dorsi muscles blend into the arm.
- **Medial boundary.** Established by drawing a line that connects the two points where the pectoralis major and latissimus dorsi muscles blend into the chest wall.

- **Posterior boundary.** Established by drawing a line along the fold of skin that envelops the lateral border of the latissimus dorsi muscle.

Basket weave suture. (Cross-stitch) Network of stitches that cross the borders of a cavity or excision to anchor fillers and sustain tissues in their proper position.

Bilateral. Having two sides.

Bilateral differences. Dissimilarities existing in the two sides or halves of an object.

Bilateral silhouette. The bilateral view; an inferior or superior viewpoint that permits the comparison of the two sides or halves of an object or facial feature.

Biohazard. Biological agent or condition that constitutes a hazard to humans.

Biological death. Irreversible somatic death.

Bischloromethyl ether (BCME). A carcinogen potentially produced when formaldehyde and sodium hypochlorite come into contact with each other. Normally occurs only in a controlled laboratory setting and requires a catalyst.

Bleach. Chemical that lightens or blanches skin discoloration.

Bleaching. Act of lightening a discoloration by hypodermic means or by surface compress.

Bleaching agent. A chemical that lightens a skin discoloration.

Blister. Thin vesicle on the skin containing liquid matter.

Blood. Cell-containing fluid that circulates through the blood vascular system and is composed of approximately 22% solids and 78% water.

Bloodborne pathogens. See Bloodborne Pathogen Rule.

Bloodborne Pathogen Rule. Occupational Safety and Health Administration (OSHA) regulation concerning exposure of employees to blood and other body fluids. The following are OSHA definitions.

- **Blood.** Human blood, human blood components, and products made from human blood.
- **Bloodborne pathogens.** Pathogenic microorganisms that are present in human blood and can cause disease in humans. These pathogens include, but are not limited to, hepatitis B virus (HBV) and human immunodeficiency virus (HIV).
- **Contaminated.** Marked by the presence or reasonably anticipated presence of blood or other

potentially infectious materials on an item or surface.

■ **Contaminated laundry.** Laundry that has been soiled with blood or other potentially infectious materials or may contain sharps.

■ **Contaminated sharps.** Any contaminated object that can penetrate the skin including, but not limited to, needles, scalpels, broken glass, and exposed ends of wires.

■ **Engineering controls.** Those mechanical systems and devices engineered into the architecture of a building, for example, exhaust systems and sanitary plumbing.

■ **Exposure incident.** Specific eye, mouth, other mucous membrane, nonintact skin, or parenteral contact with blood or other potentially infectious materials that results from the performance of an employee's duties.

■ **Occupational exposure.** Reasonably anticipated skin, eye, mucous membrane, or parenteral contact with blood or other potentially infectious materials that may result from the performance of an employee's duties.

■ **Parenteral.** Introduced into the body by way of piercing the mucous membranes or the skin barrier, for example, by needlesticks, human bites, cuts, and abrasions.

■ **Personal protective equipment (PPE).** Specialized clothing or equipment worn by an employee for protection against a hazard.

■ **Universal Precautions.** An approach to infection control in which all human blood and certain human body fluids are treated as if they are contaminated with HIV, hepatitis B virus (HBV), and other bloodborne pathogens.

■ **Work practice controls.** Controls that reduce the likelihood of exposure by altering the manner in which a task is performed (e.g., prohibiting recapping of needles, not allowing blood splatter or aerosolization of blood while draining during the embalming process).

Blood discoloration. Discoloration resulting from changes in blood composition, content, or location, either intravascularly or extravascularly.

Blood pressure. Pressure exerted by the blood on the arterial wall in the living body and measured in millimeters of mercury.

Blood vascular system. Circulatory network composed of the heart, arteries, arterioles, capillaries, venules, and veins.

Blunt dissection. Separation and pushing aside of the superficial fascia leading to blood vessels and then the deep fascia surrounding blood vessels, using manual techniques or round-ended instruments that separate rather than cut the protective tissues.

Body of the mandible. Horizontal portion of the lower jaw.

Boil. Acute, deep-seated inflammation in the skin. Usually begins as a subcutaneous swelling in a hair follicle.

Bridge. Raised support; the arched portion of the nose, which is supported by the nasal bones; a structure or span connecting two parts of a mutilated bone.

Bridge suture. (Interrupted suture) A temporary suture consisting of individually cut and tied stitches employed to sustain the proper position of tissues.

Bruise. (Ecchymosis) An injury caused by a blow without laceration; a contusion.

Buccal cavity. The space between the lips and the gums and teeth; the vestibule of the oral cavity.

Buccal depressions. Natural, shallow concavities of the cheeks that extend obliquely downward from the medial or lateral margins of the cheekbones.

Buccinator. Principle muscle of the cheek that compresses the cheeks and forms the lateral wall of the mouth.

Bucco-facial sulcus. Vertical furrow of the cheek; an acquired facial marking.

Buffer. Embalming chemical that effects the stabilization of acid–base balance within embalming solutions and in embalmed tissues.

Bulb syringe. Self-contained, soft rubber manual pump designed to create pressure to deliver fluid as it passes through one-way valves located within the bulb. It is used only to deliver fluids; it cannot be used for aspiration.

Burn. To oxidize or to cause to be oxidized by fire or equivalent means; a tissue reaction or injury resulting from the application of heat, extreme cold, caustic material, radiation, friction, or electricity.

Cadaver. Dead human body used for medical purposes, including transplantation, anatomical dissection, and study.

Cadaveric lividity. Postmortem intravascular red–blue discoloration resulting from hypostasis of blood (livor mortis).

Cadaveric spasm. Prolongation of the last violent contraction of the muscles into the rigidity of death.

Calvarium. Domelike superior portion of the cranium. That portion removed during cranial autopsy.

Calvarium clamp. Device used to fasten the calvarium to the cranium after a cranial autopsy.

Canalization. Formation of new channels in a tissue.

Cancer. Any malignant neoplasm marked by uncontrolled growth and spread of abnormal cells.

Capillaries. Minute blood vessels, the walls of which comprise a single layer of endothelial cells. Capillaries connect the smallest arteries (arteriole) with the smallest veins (venule) and are where pressure filtration occurs.

Capillary permeability. Ability of substances to diffuse through capillary walls into the tissue spaces.

Capri garment. Plastic protective garment designed to cover the legs, buttocks, and abdomen. A combination of pants and stockings.

Carbohydrate. Compound containing hydrogen, carbon, and oxygen. Sugars, starches, and glycogen are carbohydrates.

Carbuncle. Circumscribed inflammation of the skin and deeper tissues that ends in suppuration and is accompanied by systemic symptoms such as fever and leukocytosis.

Carcinogen. Cancer-causing chemical or material.

Carmine. (Crimson) Purple-red in coloration.

Carotene. The yellow pigment of the skin.

Cartilage. A specialized type of dense connective tissue; attached to the ends of bones and forming parts of structures, such as the nasal septum and the framework of the ear.

Cast. Casting; any object that has been made from a mold; the positive reproduction obtained from a negative impression.

Cauterizing agent. A chemical capable of drying tissues by searing; caustic.

Cavitation. Formation of cavities in an organ or tissue. Frequently seen in some forms of tuberculosis.

Cavity embalming. See Embalming.

Cavity fluid. Embalming chemical that is injected into a body cavity following aspiration in cavity embalming. Cavity fluid can also be used as the chemical in hypodermic and surface embalming.

Cellular death. Death of the individual cells of the body.

Cement. Substance used to promote the adhesion of two separated surfaces such as the lips, eyelids, or margins of an incision.

Center of fluid distribution. Ascending aorta and/or arch of the aorta.

Center of venous drainage. Right atrium of the heart.

Centers for Disease Control and Prevention (CDCP, CDC). Major agency of the Department of Health and Human Services, with headquarters in Atlanta, Georgia, concerned with all phases of control of communicable, vectorborne, and occupational diseases.

Centrifugal force machine. Embalming machine that uses motorized force; pulsating and nonpulsating types.

Channeling. Restorative treatment usually accompanied by aspiration, gravitation, or external pressure to remove gases or excess liquids from tissues; passages are made through the tissues with a scalpel, hypodermic needle, or trocar.

Charred. Reduced to carbon; the state of tissues destroyed by burning.

Chelate. Substances that bind metallic ions. Ethylenediaminetetraacetic acid (EDTA) is used as an anticoagulant in embalming solutions.

Chemical postmortem change. Change in the body's chemical composition that occurs after death, for example, release of heme leading to postmortem staining.

Chemotherapy. Application of chemical reagents in the treatment of disease in humans. May cause an elevated preservation demand.

Chin. The prominence overlying the mental eminence; located at the medial-inferior part of the face; mentum.

Chin rest. One of several methods used for mouth closure (antiquated).

Cilia. Eyelashes.

Clinical death. Phase of somatic death lasting from 5 to 6 minutes during which life may be restored.

Closed drainage technique. A drainage procedure that limits the exposure of the embalmer to the drainage. Tubing is attached to a drain tube allowing drainage to flow directly from a vein into a sanitary disposal system; tubing may also be attached to a trocar and aspirator allowing drainage to be taken from the right atrium of the heart to the sanitary disposal system.

Clostridium perfringens. Anaerobic, saprophytic, spore-forming bacterium, responsible for tissue gas. Referred to as a gas bacillus.

Coagulating agents. Chemical and physical agents that bring about coagulation.

Coagulation. Process of converting soluble protein into insoluble protein by heating or contact with a chemical such as an alcohol or an aldehyde. Solidification of a sol into a gelatinous mass. Agglutination is a specific form of coagulation.

Co-injection fluid. Supplemental fluid used primarily to enhance the action of vascular (arterial) solutions.

Collodion. Clear syruplike liquid that evaporates, leaving a contractile, white film; a liquid sealer.

Columna nasi. Fleshy termination of the nasal septum at the base of the nose; located between the nostrils; the most inferior part of the mass of the nose.

Coma. Irreversible cessation of brain activity and loss of consciousness. Death beginning at the brain.

Communicable disease. Disease that may be transmitted either directly or indirectly between individuals by an infectious agent.

Complexion. Color and texture of the skin, especially that of the face.

Compound fracture. A broken bone piercing the skin.

Compress. Gauze or absorbent cotton saturated with water or an appropriate chemical and placed under or upon tissues to preserve, bleach, dry, constrict, or reduce swelling.

Concave. Exhibiting a depressed or hollow surface; a concavity.

Concha. Concave shell of the ear; the deepest depression of the ear.

Concurrent disinfection. Disinfection practices carried out during the embalming process.

Concurrent drainage. Method of drainage in which drainage occurs continuously during vascular (arterial) injection.

Condyle. Rounded articular process on a bone.

Congealing. See Coagulation and Agglutination.

Conjunctiva. Mucous membrane that lines the eyelid and covers the white portion of the eye.

Constrict. To contract or compress.

Contagious disease. Disease that may be transmitted between individuals, with reference to the organism that causes a disease.

Contaminated. See Bloodborne Pathogen Rule.

Contour. Outline or surface form.

Contusion. Bruise.

Cords of the neck. Vertical prominences of the neck; an acquired facial marking.

Cornea. Transparent part of the tunic of the eyeball that covers the iris and pupil and admits light into the interior.

Corneal sclera button. That portion of the cornea recovered for transplantation in situ.

Coroner. Official of a local community who holds inquests concerning sudden, violent, and unexplained deaths.

Coronoid process. The anterior, nonarticulating process of the ramus of the mandible, which serves as the insertion for the temporalis muscle.

Corpulence. Obesity.

Corrective shaping with cosmetics. (Corrective shaping) Cosmetic technique consisting of highlighting those parts of the face or individual features to enlarge or bring them forward or shadowing them to reduce the appearance of size or deepen a depression.

Corrugator. Pyramid-shaped muscle of facial expression that draws the eyebrows inferiorly and medially.

Cosmetic. Preparation for beautifying the complexion and skin.

Cosmetic base. Initial application of a cream or paste cosmetic to skin tissues.

Cosmetic fluid. Embalming fluid that contains active dyes and coloring agents intended to restore a more natural skin tone through the embalming process.

Counterstaining compound. Dye that helps to cover internal discolorations such as jaundice or postmortem stain.

Coverall. Plastic garment designed to cover the body from the chest down to the upper thigh.

Cranial embalming. Method used to embalm the contents of the cranial cavity through aspiration and injection of the cranial chamber by passage of a trocar through the cribriform plate.

Cranium. That part of the human skull that encloses the brain.

Cremated remains. Those elements remaining after cremation of a dead human body.

Crepitation. Crackling sensation produced when gases trapped in tissues are palpated, as in subcutaneous emphysema or tissue gas.

Creutzfeldt–Jakob disease (CJD). Disease of the central nervous system with unknown etiology, assumed to be caused by a prion.

Cribriform plate. Thin, medial portion of the ethmoid bone of the skull.

Crimson. Deep purplish-red in coloration.

Cross-linkage of proteins. In embalming, the chemical joining of proteins brought about by the chemical reaction of aldehydes with different forms of nitrogen. Cross-linkage results in firmness of embalmed tissue.

Crown. (Vertex) Topmost part of the head.

Cuticle remover. Commercially prepared solvent used to remove dead cuticle from the nails and obstinate scabs.

Cyst. Closed sac, with a definite wall, that contains fluid, semifluid, or solid material.

Death. Irreversible cessation of all vital functions—nonlegal definition.

Death rattle. Noise made by a moribund person caused by air passing through a residue of mucus in the trachea and posterior oral cavity.

Death struggle. Semiconvulsive twitches that often occur before death.

Decapitation. Separation of the head from the body; to decapitate is the act of such separation.

Decay. Decomposition of proteins by enzymes of aerobic bacteria.

Decomposition. Separation of compounds into simpler substances by the action of microbial and/or autolytic enzymes.

Deep filler. Material used to fill cavities or excisions and to serve as a foundation for the superficial wax restoration.

Defibrillator. An automatic implanted cardioverter defibrillator is surgically implanted into the body. It sends an electronic impulse to the heart to maintain the rhythm of the heat. It must be removed, from the deceased, if the body is to be cremated.

Dehydration. Loss of moisture from body tissue that may occur antemortem or postmortem (antemortem: febrile disease, diarrhea, or emesis; postmortem: injection of embalming solution or through absorption by the air).

Denatured protein. Protein whose structure has been changed by physical or chemical agents.

Dental prognathism. (Buck teeth) Oblique insertion of the teeth.

Dental tie. Ligature around the superior and inferior teeth employed to hold the mandible in a fixed position; antiquated method of mouth closure.

Dentures. Artificial teeth.

Depression. Hollow or concave region; the lowering of a part.

Depressor anguli oris. Facial expression muscle that depresses the angle of the mouth.

Depressor labii inferioris. Facial expression muscle that draws the lower lip inferiorly and slightly lateral.

Derma. (Dermis, skin) Corium, or true skin.

Desiccation. Process of drying out.

Desquamation (skin-slip). Sloughing off of the epidermis, wherein there is a separation of the epidermis from the underlying dermis.

Dialysis. Separation of substances in solution by the difference in their rates of diffusion through a semipermeable membrane.

Differential pressure. See Pressure.

Diffusion. Movement of molecules or other particles in solution from an area of greater concentration to an area of lesser concentration until a uniform concentration is reached.

Diffusion (arterial solution). Passage of some components of the injected embalming solution from an intravascular to an extravascular location. Movement of the embalming solutions from the capillaries into the interstitial fluids.

Digastricus. Double-bellied muscle that draws the hyoid bone superiorly.

Digits. Fingers and toes. The thumb is the number one digit for each hand and the large toe is the number one digit for each foot.

Dimples. Shallow depressions located on the cheek or chin in a rounded or vertical form; natural facial markings.

Disarticulate. Disjoining of bones.

Discoloration. Any abnormal color in or on the human body.

Disease. Any deviation from or interruption of the normal structure or function of a body part, organ, or system.

Disinfectant. An agent, usually chemical, applied to inanimate objects/surfaces to destroy disease-causing microbial agents, but usually not bacterial spores.

Disinfection. Destruction and/or inhibition of most pathogenic organisms and their products in or on the body.

Dissection. Act of cutting apart.

Distend. To expand or swell.

Distortion. State of being twisted or pushed out of natural shape or position.

Distribution (fluid). Movement of embalming solutions from the point of injection throughout the arterial system and into the capillaries.

Dorsum. Top; the anterior protruding ridge of the nose from the root to the tip of the lobe.

Dowel. Wooden or metal rod used as an armature.

Drain tube. Embalming instrument, inserted into a vein, used to aid the drainage of venous blood from the body.

Drainage. Discharge or withdrawal of blood, blood clots, interstitial and lymphatic fluid, and embalming solution from the body during vascular embalming, usually through a vein.

Drench shower. Occupational Safety and Health Administration–required safety device for release of a copious amount of water in a short time.

Dry ice. Carbon dioxide cooled to the point at which it becomes solid; this occurs at −110 degrees fahrenheit.

Dry gangrene. See Gangrene.

Dryness. Freedom from wetness; a condition of tissues necessary for the adhesion of cement, sealer, deep filler, or wax.

Dye. (Coloring agent) Substances that, on being dissolved, impart a definite color to the embalming solution. Dyes are classified as to their capacity to permanently impart color to the tissue of the body into which they are injected.

Ecchymosis. (Bruise) Discoloration of the skin caused by the escape of blood within the tissues; generally accompanied by swelling.

Edema. Abnormal accumulation of fluids in tissues or body cavities.

Electric aspirator. Device that uses a motor to create a suction for the purpose of aspiration.

Electric spatula. Electrically heated blade that may be used to dry moist tissue, reduce swollen tissue, and restore contour.

Electrocardiogram (ECG, EKG). Record of the electrical activity of the heart.

Electroencephalogram (EEG). Record of the electrical activity of the brain.

Emaciated. (Emaciation) Excessive leanness; a wasted condition resulting in sunken surfaces of the face.

Embalming. Process of chemically treating the dead human body to reduce the presence and growth of microorganisms, to temporarily inhibit organic decomposition, and to restore an acceptable physical appearance.

- **Cavity embalming.** Direct treatment other than vascular (arterial) embalming of the contents of the body cavities and the lumina of the hollow viscera. Usually accomplished by aspiration and then injection of chemicals using a trocar.
- **Hypodermic embalming.** Injection of embalming chemicals directly into the tissues through the use of a syringe and needle or a trocar.
- **Surface embalming.** Direct contact of body tissues with embalming chemicals.
- **Vascular (arterial) embalming.** Use of the blood vascular system of the body for temporary preservation, disinfection, and restoration. Usually accomplished through injection of embalming solutions into the arteries and drainage from the veins.

Embalming analysis. (Case analysis) That consideration given to the dead body before, during, and after the embalming procedure is completed. Documentation is recommended.

Embalming Care Report. (Case report) Detailed listing of body conditions and treatments performed by funeral personnel for all bodies received into a facility for preparation, sheltering, shipping to another facility, or shipped in from another funeral facility.

Eminence. Prominence or projection of a bone.

Engineering controls. See Bloodborne Pathogen Rule.

Enucleation. Removal of an entire mass or part, especially a tumor, or the eyeball, without rupture.

Environment. Surroundings, conditions, or influences that affect an organism or the cells within an organism.

Environmental Protection Agency (EPA). Governmental agency with environmental protection regulatory and enforcement authority.

Enzyme. Organic catalyst produced by living cells and capable of autolytic decomposition.

Epidermis. Outermost layer of skin; cuticle or scarf skin.

Erythema. A reddening of the skin, caused by a dilation of the superficial blood vessels in the skin. Erythematous rash. Antemortem pathological discoloration.

Ether. Clear, volatile liquid used as a wax solvent or to remove grease, oil, and adhesive tape stains.

Excise. To remove as by cutting out.

Excision. Area from which tissue has been removed.

Expert test of death. Any procedure used to prove a sign of death, usually performed by medical personnel.

Exposure incident. See Bloodborne Pathogen Rule.

External auditory meatus. Opening or passageway of the ear.

External pressure. Weight applied to a surface.

Extravascular. Outside the blood vascular system.

Extravascular blood discoloration. Discoloration of the body outside the blood vascular system, for example, ecchymosis, petechia, hematoma, and postmortem stain.

Extrinsic. From outside the body.

Eye enucleation. Removal of the eye for tissue transplantation, research, and education.

Eye enucleation discoloration. Extravasation of blood as a result of eye enucleation.

Eye socket. (Orbit) Bony region containing the eyeball; the orbital cavity.

Eyebrows. (Supercilium) Also the superficial hairs covering the superciliary arches.

Eyecap. Thin, domelike shell made of hardened cloth, metal, or plastic placed beneath the eyelids to restore natural curvature and to maintain the position of the closed eye.

Eyelids. (Palpebrae) Two movable flaps of skin that cover and uncover each eyeball.

Eyelid overlap. Method of eye closure in which the upper lid is placed on top of the lower lid.

Eyewash station. Occupational Safety and Health Administration–required emergency safety device providing a steady stream of water for flushing the eye.

Face. Anatomically, the region from the eyes to the base of the chin; physiognomically, the region from the normal hairline to the base of the chin.

Facial markings. Character lines of the face and neck; wrinkles, grooves, cords, and dimples.

Facial profiles. Silhouettes of the face from the side view.

Fat. Organic compound containing carbon, hydrogen, and oxygen. Chemically, fat is a triglyceride ester composed of glycerol and fatty acids.

Fatty acids. Product of decomposition of fats.

Febrile. Characterized by high fever, causing dehydration of the body.

Federal Trade Commission (FTC). The agency of federal government created in 1914 to promote free and fair competition by prevention of trade restraints, price fixing, false advertising, and other unfair methods of competition.

Fermentation. Bacterial decomposition of carbohydrates.

Fever blisters. Lesions of the mucous membrane of the lip or mouth caused by herpes simplex type I or II virus or by dehydration of the mucous membrane in a febrile disease.

Filler. Material used to fill a large cavity (e.g., plaster of Paris and cotton; liquid sealer and cotton).

Firming. Rigidity of tissue due to chemical reaction.

Firm wax. (Wound filler) The most viscous type of wax; a puttylike material used to fill large cavities or to model features.

First-degree burn. (Hyperemia) Injury caused by heat that produces redness of the skin.

Fixation. Act of making tissue rigid. Solidification of a compound.

Fixative. Agent employed in the preparation of tissues, for the purpose of maintaining the existing form and structure. A large number of agents are used, the most important one being formalin.

Floater. A dead human body, in a body of water, which has generated sufficient decomposition gasses to float to the surface of the water (face down).

Florid. Flushed with red, when describing a complexion; not as vivid as ruddy.

Fluorescent light. Illumination produced by a tubular electric discharge lamp; the fluorescence of phosphors coating the inside of a tube.

Flush (flushing). Intravascular blood discoloration that occurs when arterial solution enters an area (such as the face), but due to blockage, blood and embalming solution are unable to drain from the area.

Fold. Elongated prominence adjoining a surface.

Foramen magnum. Opening in the occipital bone through which the spinal cord passes from the brain.

Forehead. That part of the face above the eyes.

Formaldehyde (HCHO). Colorless, strong-smelling gas that when used in solution is a powerful preservative and disinfectant. Potential occupational carcinogen.

Formaldehyde gray. Gray discoloration of the body caused by the reaction of formaldehyde from the embalming process with hemoglobin to form methylhemoglobin.

Formaldehyde rule. Occupational Safety and Health Administration regulation limiting the amount of occupational exposure to formaldehyde gas.

Fossa. Depression; concavity.

Fourth-degree burn. Total evacuation (absence) of tissue.

Fracture. Broken bone.

Frenulum. Vertical restraining fold of mucous membrane on the midline of the inside of each lip connecting the lip with the gum.

Frontal. Anterior; anterior view of the face or features.

Frontal bone. Anterior third of the cranium, forming the forehead and the anterior portion of the roof of the skull.

Frontal eminences. Paired, rounded, unmargined prominences of the frontal bone found approximately 1 inch beneath the normal hairline.

Frontal process of the maxilla. Ascending part of the upper jaw that gradually protrudes as it rises beside the nasal bone to meet the frontal bone; the ascending process of the upper jaw.

Furrow. (Wrinkle) Crevice in the skin accompanied by adjacent elevations.

Furuncle. See Boil.

Gangrene. Necrosis, death, of tissues of part of the body usually due to deficient or absent blood supply.

■ **Dry gangrene.** (Ischemic necrosis) Condition that results when the body part that dies had little blood and remains aseptic. The arteries but not the veins are obstructed.

■ **Gas gangrene.** Necrosis in a wound infected by an anaerobic gas-forming bacillus, the most common etiologic agent being *Clostridium perfringens*.

■ **Moist (wet) gangrene.** Necrotic tissue that is wet as a result of inadequate venous drainage. May be accompanied by bacterial infection.

Germicide. Agent, usually chemical, applied either to inanimate objects/surfaces or to living tissues to destroy disease-causing microbial agents, but usually not bacterial spores.

Glabella. Single bony prominence of the frontal bone located between the superciliary arches in the inferior part of the frontal bone above the root of the nose.

Glycerin. Syrupy, colorless liquid obtained from fats or oils as a by-product of the manufacturing of soaps and fatty acids; used as a vehicle for some cosmetics.

Gooseneck. Rubber stopper containing two tubes, one to create vacuum or pressure and the other to deliver fluid or achieve aspiration. Possibly used in conjunction with a hand pump.

Grave wax. See Adipocere.

Gravity filtration. The settling of fluids by gravitational force to the dependent areas of the body.

Gravity injector. Apparatus used to inject arterial fluid during the vascular (arterial) phase of the embalming process. Relies on gravity to create the pressure required to deliver the fluid (0.43 pounds of pressure per 1 foot of elevation.).

Green (natural) burial. Bodies not embalmed or temporarily preserved using a non-formaldehyde biodegradable temporary preservative. All preparation of the body including the clothing worn and the casket (if used) must be biodegradable. Green cemeteries do not use traditional grave markers.

Groove. Elongated depression in a relatively level plane or surface.

Groove director. Instrument used to guide vein tubes into vessels.

Hairline. Outline of hair growth on the head or face; the lowest centrally located part of the hair of the cranium.

Hand pump. Historical instrument resembling a large hypodermic syringe attached to a bottle apparatus. Used to create either pressure for injection or vacuum for aspiration.

Hard palate. Anterior portion of the roof of the mouth.

Hard water. Water containing large amounts of mineral salts. These mineral salts must be removed from or sequestered in water (vehicle) to be used in mixing vascular embalming solutions.

Hardening compound. Chemical in powder form that has the ability to absorb and to disinfect. Often used in cavity treatment of autopsied cases.

Hazard Communication Standard (Rule). Occupational Safety and Health Administration regulation that deals with limiting exposure to occupational hazards.

Hazardous material. Agent or material exposing one to risk.

Headrest. Piece of equipment used to maintain the head in the proper position during the embalming process.

Helix. Outer rim of the ear.

Hematemesis. Blood present in vomitus. Vomiting of blood.

Hematoma. A swelling or mass of clotted blood caused by a ruptured blood vessel and confined to an organ or space.

Heme. Nonprotein portion of hemoglobin. Red pigment.

Hemoglobin. Red respiratory portion of the red blood cells. Iron-containing pigment of red blood cells functioning to carry oxygen to the cells.

Hemolysis. Destruction of red blood cells that liberates hemoglobin.

Hepatitis. Inflammation of the liver that may be caused by various agents, including viral infections, bacterial invasion, and physical or chemical agents. It is usually accompanied by fever, jaundice, and an enlarged liver.

Hepatitis A (HAV). Formerly called infectious hepatitis. It is caused by the enterically transmitted (oral-fecal route) hepatitis A virus.

Hepatitis B virus (HBV). Severe infectious bloodborne virus.

Hepatitis C virus (HCV). Spread by contaminated blood or body fluids.

Hepatitis D virus (HDV). A bloodborne virus, it can only exist in combination with the hepatitis B virus. HBV vaccine will offer protection against HDV.

Hepatitis E virus (HEV). Transmitted by contaminated water and human waste.

Hepatitis G virus (HGV). A bloodborne virus.

Herpes. Inflammatory skin disease marked by small vesicles in clusters, usually restricted to diseases caused by herpes virus.

High-index fluids. Special vascular (arterial) fluid with a formaldehyde content of 25 to 36%.

Holding room. An area of a funeral home, crematory or embalming facility exclusively used for preparation of deceased human bodies by means other than embalming.

Horseshoe curve. Roughly U-shaped, with the front being narrower than the sweep of the curve.

Household bleach. Five percent sodium hypochlorite solution. Mixing 12 ounces of household bleach with 116 ounces of water yields 1 gallon of a 10% household bleach solution (5000 ppm sodium hypochlorite).

Human immunodeficiency virus (HIV). Retrovirus that causes acquired immunodeficiency syndrome (AIDS).

Human remains. Body of a deceased person, including cremated remains.

Humectant. Chemical that increases the ability of embalmed tissue to retain moisture.

Humor. Any liquid or semiliquid of the body, as the aqueous or vitreous humor of the eyeball.

Hunting bow. Shaped as a bent wood weapon with a central belly; resembling a cupid's bow. Shape of the attached margin of the upper red lip; shape of the lip line of closure.

Hydroaspirator. Apparatus that is connected to the water supply. When the water is turned on, suction is developed and is used to aspirate the contents of the body's cavities.

Hydrocele. Abnormal accumulation of fluids in a saclike structure, especially the scrotal sac.

Hydrocephalus. Abnormal accumulation of cerebrospinal fluids in the ventricles of the brain.

Hydrolysis. Reaction in which water is one of the reactants and compounds are often broken down. In the hydrolysis of proteins, the addition of water accompanied by the action of enzymes results in the breakdown of protein into amino acids.

Hydropericardium. Abnormal accumulation of fluid within the pericardial sac.

Hydrothorax. Abnormal accumulation of fluid in the thoracic cavity.

Hygroscopic. Absorbing moisture readily.

Hypertonic solution. Solution having a greater concentration of dissolved solute than the solution with which it is compared.

Hypodermic embalming. See Embalming.

Hypodermic tissue building. Injection of special creams or liquids into the tissues through the use of a syringe and needle to restore natural contour.

Hypostasis. Settling of blood and/or other fluids to dependent portions of the body.

Hypotonic solution. Solution having a lesser concentration of dissolved solute than the solution with which it is compared.

Hypovalve trocar. A long thin trocar used for supplemental hypodermic embalming.

Imbibition. Absorption of the fluid portion of blood by the tissues after death, resulting in postmortem edema. Postmortem swelling and softening of tissues and organs as a result of absorbing moisture from adjacent sources.

Incision. A clean cut made with a sharp instrument. In embalming, a cut made with a scalpel to raise arteries and veins.

Incisive fossa. Depression between the mental eminence and the inferior incisor teeth.

Incisor teeth. Four teeth located anteriorly from the midline on each jaw, used for cutting.

Index. Strength of an embalming fluid, indicated by the number of grams of pure formaldehyde gas dissolved in 100 mL of water. Index usually refers to a percentage; an embalming fluid with an index of 25 usually contains 25% formaldehyde gas.

Infant. Child less than 1 year of age.

Infant trocar. A short hollow tubular instrument with a sharp point. Used for aspiration and injection of an infant's thoracic and abdominal cavities.

Infectious disease. Disease caused by the growth of a pathogenic microorganism in the body.

Infectious waste. See Biohazard.

Inferior. Beneath; lower in plane or position; the undersurface of an organ or indicating a structure below another structure; toward the feet.

Inferior nasal conchae. Lowermost scroll-shaped bones on the sidewalls of the nasal cavity.

Inferior palpebral sulcus. Furrow of the lower attached border of the inferior palpebra; acquired facial marking.

Inflammation. Reaction of tissues to injurious agents, usually characterized by heat, redness, swelling, and pain.

Inguinal ligament. Anatomical structure forming the base of the femoral triangle; extends from the anterior superior iliac spine to the pubic tubercle.

Injection. Act or instance of forcing a fluid into the vascular system or directly into tissues.

Injection pressure. See Pressure.

Inner canthus. Eminence at the inner corner of the closed eyelids.

Instant tissue fixation. Embalming technique that uses a very strong arterial solution (often waterless). The solution is injected under high pressure in spurts into a body area. Very little solution is injected; the technique attempts to limit swelling; for example, in bodies with facial trauma or early decomposition.

Instantaneous rigor mortis. Instantaneous stiffening of the muscles of a dead human body.

Integumentary lips. Superiorly, the skin portion of the upper lip from the attached margin of the upper mucous membrane to the base of the nose, and inferiorly, the skin portion of the lower lip from the attached margin of the lower mucous membrane to the labiomental sulcus.

Intercellular. Between the cells of a structure.

Intercellular fluid. Fluid outside or between the cells of the body.

Interciliary sulci. Vertical or transverse furrows between the eyebrows; acquired facial markings.

Intercostal space. Space between the ribs.

Intermittent drainage (restricted drainage). Method of drainage in which the drainage is stopped at intervals while the injection continues.

Interstitial fluid. Fluid in the supporting connective tissues surrounding body cells (about one-fifth the body weight).

Intracellular fluid. Fluids within the cell.

Intradermal suture. (Hidden suture) Type of suture used to close incisions in such a manner that the ligature remains entirely under the epidermis.

Intravascular. Within the blood vascular system.

Intravascular blood discoloration. Discoloration of the body within the blood vascular system, for example, hypostasis, carbon monoxide, and capillary congestion.

Intravascular fluid. Fluid contained within vascular channels (about one-twentieth of the body weight).

Intravascular pressure. See Pressure.

Intrinsic. From within the body.

Inversion. Tissues turned in an opposite direction or folded inward.

Inversion suture. See Worm suture.

Ischemic necrosis. See Gangrene.

Isotonic solution. A solution having a concentration of dissolved solute equal to that of a standard of reference.

Jaundice. Conditions characterized by an excessive concentration of bilirubin in the skin and tissues and deposition of excessive bile pigment in the skin, cornea, body fluids, and mucous membranes with the resulting yellow appearance of the patient.

Jaundice fluid. Arterial fluid with special bleaching and coloring qualities for use on bodies with jaundice. Usually, formaldehyde content is low.

Jawline. Inferior border of the mandible.

Jugular drain tube. Tubular instrument of varying diameter and shape, preferably with a plunger, which is inserted into the jugular vein to aid in drainage.

Juxtaposition. (Simultaneous contrast) Any two hues seen together that modify each other in the direction of their complements.

Labial sulci. (Furrows of age) Vertical furrows of each lip extending from within the mucous membranes into the integumentary lips; acquired facial markings.

Labiomental sulcus. Junction of the lower integumentary lip and the superior border of the chin, which may appear as a furrow; a natural facial marking.

Laceration. Wound characterized by irregular tearing of tissue.

Lanolin. Oil from sheep wool.

Lanugo. (Peach fuzz) Downy hair of a fetus, child, or woman.

Larvicide. Substance used to kill insect larvae.

Lateral. Away from the midline.

Legionnaires disease. Severe, often fatal bacterial disease characterized by pneumonia, dry cough, and sometimes gastrointestinal symptoms (*Legionella pneumophila*).

Lesion. Any change in structure produced during the course of a disease or injury.

Levator anguli oris. Muscle of facial expression that elevates the angle of the mouth.

Levator labii superioris. Muscle of facial expression that elevates and extends the upper lip.

Levator labii superioris alaeque nasi. Muscle of facial expression that elevates the upper lip and dilates the nostril opening; the common elevator.

Levator palpebrae superioris. Muscle of facial expression that raises the upper eyelid.

Ligate. To tie off, as in ligating an artery and vein on completion of embalming or ligating the colon in autopsied bodies.

Ligature. Thread, cord, or wire used for tying vessels, tissues, or bones.

Linear guide. Line drawn or visualized on the surface of the skin to represent the approximate location of some deeper lying structure.

Line of closure. Line that forms between two structures such as the lips or the eyelids when in a closed position, which marks their place of contact with each other.

Linear sulci. Eyelid furrows that are short and broken, extending horizontally on the palpebrae themselves and that may fan from both the medial and lateral corners of the eyes.

Lipolysis. Decomposition of fats.

Lip wax. Soft restorative wax, usually tinted, used to surface the mucous membranes or to correct lip separations.

Livor mortis. See Cadaveric lividity.

Loop stitch. Single, nooselike suture, not pulled taut before knotting, that stands away from the skin and anchors restorative materials.

Lumen. Cavity of a vein, artery, or intestine.

Lysin. Specific antibody acting destructively on cells and tissues.

Lysosome. Organelle that exists within a cell, but separate from the cell. Contains hydrolytic enzymes that break down proteins and certain carbohydrates.

Maggot. Larva of an insect, especially a flying insect.

Major restoration. Those restorations that require a long period of time, are extensive, require advanced technical skill, and require expressed written consent to perform.

Mandible. Horseshoe-shaped bone forming the inferior jaw.

Mandibular fossa. Glenoid fossa; the small oval depression on the zygomatic process of the temporal bone into which the condyle of the mandible articulates, just anterior to the external auditory meatus. Forms the temporal mandibular joint (TMJ).

Mandibular sulcus. Furrow beneath the jawline that rises vertically on the cheek; an acquired facial marking.

Mandibular suture. Stitch used to hold the mouth closed; placed behind the lips, one part is passed through the inferior jaw at the median plane, whereas the other part extends through the nasal septum or the superior frenulum.

Manual aid. Those treatments or procedures that are applied by the use of hands. Scrubbing with soap and water to remove a surface discoloration; flexing, bending, rotating, and massage of the limbs to stimulate the circulation of arterial solution and movement of blood and body fluids.

Marbling. A greenish-black coloration along the vessels (veins) produced by hemolysis of the blood in the vessels. Hemoglobin mixes with hydrogen sulfide to produce the discoloration observed on the skin surface when decomposition is present.

Masking agent. See Perfuming agents.

Massage. Manipulation of tissue in the course of preparation of the body.

Massage cream. Soft, white, oily preparation used as a protective coating for external tissues; a base for cream cosmetics and a wax softener; an emollient.

Masseter muscles. Muscles of mastication that close the mandible.

Mastic compound. Puttylike substance; an absorbent sealing adhesive that can be injected under the skin or applied to surface tissues to establish skin contour.

Mastoid process. The rounded projection on the inferior portion of the temporal bones just posterior to the lobe of the ear.

Material Safety Data Sheet (MSDS). Form that must accompany a hazardous product. Requirement of the Department of Labor and Occupational Safety and Health Administration under the Hazard Communication Standard.

Matte. Having a dull finish; as afforded by the application of loose powder, lack of sheen.

Maxilla. Paired bone with several processes that form the skeletal base of most of the superior face, roof of the mouth, sides of the nasal cavity, and floor of the orbit.

Mechanical aid. The application of treatments or procedures that utilize machines or instruments. Adjustments of pressure and rate of flow on the embalming machine; utilization of properly sized arterial tubes and/or drainage instruments. Opening and closing of drainage instruments.

Medial. Toward the midline.

Medical examiner. Official elected or appointed to investigate suspicious or unnatural deaths.

Medium wax. Dermasurgery or restorative wax.

Melanin. The brown to black-brown pigment in the epidermis and hair.

Meningitis. Inflammation of the meninges.

Mental eminence. Bony triangular projection on the inferior portion of the anterior mandible.

Mentalis muscle. Elevates and protrudes the inferior lip, wrinkles the skin over the chin.

Methicillin-resistant *Staphylococcus aureus* **(MRSA).** Pathogenic bacterial *Staphylococcus aureus*, resistant to most drugs. A causative agent of bedsores, surgical wound infections, skin and nose infections, and pneumonia.

Microbe (microorganism). Minute one-celled form of life that cannot be distinguished as being of either vegetable or animal nature.

Microbial enzyme. The enzymes of microorganisms; a source of the enzymes that contribute to decomposition.

Midaxillary line. Vertical line drawn from the center of the medial border of the base of the axillary space.

Millicurie (mCi). That amount of radioactive material in which 37 million atoms disintegrate each second.

Minor restoration. Those restorations requiring a minimum effort, skill, or time to complete.

Mixture. Composition of two or more substances that are not chemically bound to each other.

Modifying agents. Chemical components of vascular fluids that control the rate and degree of tissue firmness by the fluid utilized (e.g., humectants and buffers); chemicals for which there may be greatly varying demands predicated on the type of embalming, the environment, and the embalming fluid used.

Mold-preventive agents. Agents that prohibit the growth of mold.

Mortuary mastic compound. See Mastic compound.

Mottle. To diversify with spots or blotches of different color (or shade).

Moribund. In a dying state. In the agonal period.

Mouth former. Device used in the mouth to shape the contour of the lips.

Mucous membranes. The visible red surfaces of the lips; the lining membrane of body cavities that communicate with the exterior.

Multi-point injection (multisite). Vascular injection that utilizes two or more injection sites.

Musculature suture. Method of mouth closure in which a suture is passed through the septum of the nose and through the mentalis muscle of the chin.

Nasal bones. Directly inferior to the glabella and forming a dome over the superior portion of the nasal cavity.

Nasal cavity. Space between the roof of the mouth and the floor of the cranial cavity.

Nasal spine of the maxilla. Sharp, bony projection located medially at the inferior margin of the nasal cavity.

Nasal sulcus. Angular area between the posterior margin of the wing of the nose and the nasolabial fold; a natural facial marking.

Nasal tube aspirator. Embalming instrument used to aspirate the throat by means of the nostrils.

Nasolabial fold. The eminence of the cheek and adjacent to the mouth; extending from the superior part of the posterior margin of the wing of the nose to the side of the mouth; a natural facial marking.

Nasolabial sulcus. Furrow originating at the superior border of the wing of the nose and extending to the side of the mouth; acquired facial marking.

Naso-orbital fossa. Depression superior to the medial portion of the superior palpebrae.

Natural facial markings. Those that are present at birth; hereditary facial markings.

Necrobiosis. Antemortem, physiological death of the cells of the body followed by their replacement.

Necropsy. See Autopsy.

Necrosis. Pathological death of a tissue still a part of the living organism.

Needle injector. Mechanical device used to impel specially designed metal pins into bone.

Neoplasm. New and abnormal formation of tissue, as a tumor or growth.

Nephritis. Inflammation of the kidneys.

Nevus. Birthmark; congenital skin blemish; any congenital anomaly, including various types of birthmarks and all types of moles.

Nitrogenous waste. Metabolic by-products that contain nitrogen, such as urea and uric acid. These compounds have a high affinity for formaldehyde and tend to neutralize embalming chemicals.

Noncosmetic fluid. Type of arterial fluid that contains inactive dyes that will not impart a color change on the body tissues of the deceased.

Nonformaldehyde fluids. Fluids that are designed to be nontoxic and environmentally friendly. They provide a limited sanitization and preservation of the deceased body.

Norm. The most common characteristics of each feature; typical, common, average.

Obese. Having an unhealthy accumulation of fat on the body. Corpulent.

Oblique palpebral sulcus. Shallow, curving groove below the medial corner of the eyelids; natural facial marking.

Occipital bone. Lowest part of the back and base of the cranium, forming a cradle for the brain.

Occipital protuberance. The prominence at the center of the external surface of the occipital bone.

Occipitofrontalis muscle. Epicranius; draws the scalp posteriorly and anteriorly and raises the eyebrows.

Occupational exposure. See Bloodborne Pathogen Rule.

Occupational Safety and Health Administration (OSHA). A governmental agency with the responsibility for regulation and enforcement of safety and health matters for most U.S. employees. An individual state OSHA agency may supersede the U.S. Department of Labor OSHA regulations.

One-point injection. Injection and drainage from one location.

Opaque. Not transparent or translucent; not allowing light to pass through a concealing cosmetic.

Opaque cosmetic. A cosmetic medium able to cover or hide skin discolorations.

Operative corrections. Invasive treatments or procedures to correct a problem area. Examples include channeling, incisions, and excisions.

Ophthalmoscope. Optical instrument with an accompanying light that makes it possible to examine the retina and to explore for blood circulation.

Optic facial sulci. (Crow's feet) Furrows radiating from the lateral corner of the eye; acquired facial markings.

Optimum. Most favorable condition for functioning.

Oral cavity. Mouth and vestibule, or the opening to the throat.

Orbicularis oculi muscle. Closes the eyelids; compresses the lacrimal sacs.

Orbicularis oris muscle. Closes the lips.

Orbital cavity (orbit). Eye socket.

Orbital pouch. Bags under the eyes; the fullness between the inferior palpebrae and the oblique palpebral sulcus.

Orifice. Entrance or outlet of any body cavity; an opening.

Ornamental. Adornment or embellishment; a cosmetic material manufactured for street wear; the technique of cosmetic application to beautify the face.

Osmosis. Passage of solvent from a solution of lesser to one of greater solute concentration when the two solutions are separated by a semipermeable membrane.

Pacemaker. A device that can trigger mechanical contractions of the heart by emitting an electrical discharge. These devices can be surgically implanted. These devices must be removed if a body is to be cremated.

Packing forceps. Embalming instrument used in closing the external orifices of the body.

Palatine bone. One of the bones forming the posterior part of the hard palate and lateral nasal wall between the interior pterygoid plate of the sphenoid bone and the maxilla.

Palpate. To examine by touch.

Palpebrae. Eyelids both superior and inferior; singular palpebra.

Parallel incision. Incision on the surface of the skin to raise the common carotid arteries. It is made along the posterior border of the inferior one-third of the sternocleidomastoid muscle.

Parenteral. See Bloodborne Pathogen Rule.

Parietal bones. Two bones that form the roof and part of the sides of the skull.

Parietal eminence. Rounded peak of the external convexity of the parietal bones; determines the widest part of the cranium.

Parts per million (ppm). In contaminated air, the parts of vapor or gas (formaldehyde) per million parts of air by volume. In solution, the parts of chemical per million parts of solution.

Passive transport system. Method by which solutes and/or solvents cross through a membrane with no energy provided by the cells of the membrane. In embalming, examples include pressure filtration, dialysis, diffusion, and osmosis.

Pathological condition. Diseased; due to a disease.

Pathological discoloration. Antemortem discoloration that occurs during the course of certain diseases such as gangrene and jaundice.

Pediculicide. Substance able to destroy lice.

Penetrating wounds. Wounds entering the interior of an organ or cavity.

Percutaneous. Effected through unbroken skin.

Perfuming agents. (Masking agents) Chemicals found in embalming arterial formulations having the capability of displacing an unpleasant odor or of altering an unpleasant odor so that it is converted to a more pleasant one.

Perfusion. To force a fluid through (an organ or tissue), especially by way of the blood vessels. Injection during vascular (arterial) embalming.

Peritonitis. Inflammation of the peritoneum, the membranous coat lining the abdominal cavity and covering the viscera.

Permissible exposure limit (PEL). Maximum legal limit established by the Occupational Safety and Health Administration for a regulated substance. These are based on employee exposure and are time-weighted over an 8-hour work shift. When these limits are exceeded, employers must take proper steps to reduce employee exposure. For formaldehyde, the PEL is 0.75 ppm.

Perpendicular plate of the ethmoid bone. Superior portion of the bony nasal septum.

Personal protective equipment (PPE). See Bloodborne Pathogen Rule.

Petechia. Antemortem, pinpoint, extravascular blood discoloration visible as purplish hemorrhages of the skin.

Petroleum jelly. Semisolid, yellow mixture of hydrocarbons obtained from petroleum.

Pharmaceutical. Drug or medicine.

Phenol. (Carbolic acid) Antiseptic/disinfectant employed to dry moist tissues and to bleach discolored tissues.

Philtrum. Vertical groove located medially on the superior lip; a natural facial marking.

Physiognomy. Study of the structures and surface markings of the face and features.

Pitting edema. Condition in which interstitial spaces contain such excessive amounts of fluid that the skin remains depressed after palpation.

Plaster of Paris. Calcium sulfate; a white powdery substance that forms a quick-setting paste when mixed with water.

Platysma muscle. Thin layer of muscle covering anterior aspect of neck.

Platysmal sulci. Transverse, dipping furrow of the neck; acquired facial marking.

Pneumonia. Acute infection or inflammation of the alveoli. The alveolar sacs fill up with fluid and dead white blood cells. Causes include bacteria, fungi, and viruses.

Positioning devices. Preparation room equipment for properly positioning bodies before, during, and after vascular embalming.

Postembalming. That time period after the arterial injection.

Posterior. Toward the back.

Postmortem. Period that begins after somatic death.

Postmortem caloricity. Rise in body temperature after death due to continued cellular metabolism.

Postmortem chemical changes. Change in the body's chemical composition that occurs after death (e.g., decomposition, change in body pH, rigor mortis, postmortem stain, and postmortem caloricity).

Postmortem examination. See Autopsy.

Postmortem physical change. Change in the form or state of matter without any change in chemical composition, for example, algor mortis, hypostasis, dehydration, livor mortis, increase in blood viscosity, and translocation of microbes.

Postmortem stain. Extravascular color change that occurs when heme, released by hemolysis of red blood cells, seeps through the vessel walls and into the body tissues.

Potential of hydrogen (pH). Degree of acidity or alkalinity. The scale ranges from 0 to 14 with 0 being completely acid, 14 completely basic, and 7 neutral. Blood has a pH of 7.35 to 7.45.

Potential pressure. See Pressure.

Precipitant. Substance bringing about precipitation. The oxalates formerly used in water conditioning chemicals are now illegal because of their poisonous nature.

Preembalming. That period of time before the arterial injection.

Pre-injection fluid. Fluid injected primarily to prepare the vascular system and body tissues for the injection of the preservative vascular (arterial) solution. This solution is injected before the preservative vascular solution is injected.

Preparation room. That area or facility wherein embalming, dressing, cosmetizing, or other body preparation is effected.

Preservation. See Temporary preservation.

Preservative. Chemicals that inactivate saprophytic bacteria, render unsuitable for nutrition the media upon which such bacteria thrive, and will arrest decomposition by altering enzymes and lysins of the body as well as converting the decomposable tissue to a form less susceptible to decomposition.

Preservative demand. Amount of preservative (formaldehyde) required to effectively preserve and disinfect remains. This amount depends on the condition of the tissues as determined in the embalming analysis.

Preservative powder. Chemical in powder form, typically used for surface embalming of the remains.

Pressure. Action of a force against an opposing force (a force applied or acting against resistance).

- **Actual pressure.** That pressure indicated by the injector gauge needle when the arterial tube is open and the arterial solution is flowing into the body.
- **Blood pressure.** Pressure exerted by the blood on the vessel walls, measured in millimeters of mercury.
- **Differential pressure.** Difference between potential and actual pressures.
- **Injection pressure.** Amount of pressure produced by an injection device to overcome initial resistance within (intravascular) or on (extravascular) the vascular system (arterial or venous).
- **Intravascular pressure.** Pressure developed as the flow of embalming solution is established and the elastic arterial walls expand and then contract,

resulting in filling of the capillary beds and development of pressure filtration.

■ **Potential pressure.** Pressure indicated by the injector gauge needle when the injector motor is running and the arterial tubing is clamped off.

Pressure filtration. Passage of embalming solution through the capillary wall to diffuse with the interstitial fluids by application of positive intravascular pressure. Embalming solution passes from an intravascular to an extravascular position.

Primary dilution. Dilution attained as the embalming solution is mixed in the embalming machine.

Primary disinfection. Disinfection carried out before the embalming process.

Prion. A protein particle that lacks nucleic acid (smaller than a virus); implicated as the cause of various neurodegenerative diseases, for example, CJD.

Procerus muscle. Draws the skin of the forehead inferiorly.

Procurement. Recovery of organs or tissues from a cadaver for transplantation.

Professional portrait. Photograph or painting in which the subject has been posed and lighted flatteringly by a professional photographer or artist.

Profile. Side view of the human head.

Prognathism. Projection of the jaw or jaws that may cause problems with mouth closure and alignment of the teeth.

Protein. Organic compound found in plants and animals that can be broken down into amino acids.

Proteolysis. Decomposition of proteins.

Ptomaine. Any one of a group of nitrogenous organic compounds formed by the action of putrefactive bacteria on proteins, for example, indole, skatole, cadaverine, and putrescine.

Pubic symphysis. Fibrocartilage that joins the two pubic bones in the median plane.

Purge. Postmortem evacuation of any substance from an external orifice of the body as a result of pressure.

Purpura. An antemortem, extravascular blood discoloration. Caused by blood cells leaking into the skin or mucous membranes. Frequently seen with persons using blood thinners. Purpura lesions are larger than pin-point petechia: large purpural lesions are called ecchymosis.

Pursestring suture. Suture made around the circumference of a circular opening or puncture to close it or to hold the margins in position.

Pus. Liquid product of inflammation containing various proteins and leukocytes.

Pustular lesion. Characteristic pus-filled wound of a disease such as smallpox, syphilis, and acne.

Pustule. Small elevation of the skin with an inflamed base, containing pus.

Putrefaction. Decomposition of proteins by the action of enzymes from anaerobic bacteria.

Pyramid. Apparently solid structure having a square base and four triangular sides that meet at a central point.

Radiate. To spread out from a common point.

Radiation protection officer. Supervisor, in an institution licensed to use radionuclides, who has the responsibility to establish procedures and make recommendations in the use of all radioactive matter.

Radionuclide. Chemical element that is similar in chemical properties to another element, but differs in atomic weight and electric charge and emits radiation. An atom that disintegrates by emission of electromagnetic radiation.

Ramus. Vertical portion of the mandible.

Rate of flow. Speed at which fluid is injected, measured in ounces per minute.

Razor burn (razor abrasion). Mark of desiccation. A darkened, air-dried area on the skin resulting from removal of the epidermis while shaving the remains.

Reaspiration. Repeated aspiration of a cavity.

Reducing agent. Substance that easily loses electrons and thereby causes other substances to be reduced. Formaldehyde is a strong reducing agent.

Repose. To lay at rest.

Resinous substance. Amorphous, nonvolatile solid or soft side substance, a natural exudation from plants. Any of a class of solid or soft organic compounds of natural or synthetic origin.

Restoration. Treatment of the deceased in the attempt to recreate natural form and color.

Restorative art. Care of the deceased to recreate natural form and color.

Restorative fluid (humectant). Supplemental fluid, used with the regular arterial solution, whose purpose is to retain body moisture and retard dehydration.

Restricted cervical injection. Method of injection wherein both common carotid arteries are raised.

Restricted drainage. See Intermittent drainage and Alternate drainage.

Right atrium. Chamber on the right side of the heart seen as the center of drainage. Used as a site of drainage via instruments from the right internal jugular vein and direct via the trocar or through the thoracic wall.

Rigor mortis. Postmortem stiffening of the body muscles by natural body processes.

Risorius muscle. (Laughing muscle) Narrow superficial band of muscle that pulls the angle of the mouth laterally.

Ruddy. Red complexion; having a healthy reddish color, said of the complexion, more vivid than florid.

Saccharolysis. Decomposition of sugars.

Sallow. Yellowish, sickly color of the complexion.

Sanitation. Process to promote and establish conditions that minimize or eliminate biohazards.

Saturation. Visual aspect indicating the vividness of the hue in the degree of difference from gray of the same lightness.

Saponification. Process of soap formation. As related to decomposition, the conversion of fatty tissues of the body into a soapy waxy substance called adipocere or grave wax.

Saprophytic bacteria. Bacteria that derive their nutrition from dead organic matter.

Scab. Crust over a healing sore or wound.

Scalpel. Two-piece embalming instrument consisting of a handle and a blade used to make incisions and excisions.

Sealer. Quick-drying liquid that leaves a hard, thin transparent coat or layer through which moisture cannot pass.

Sealing agents. Agents that provide a barrier or seal against any leakage of fluid or blood.

Sear(ing). To cauterize tissues by heat or chemical to provide a dry foundation.

Second-degree burn. Those resulting in acute inflammation of the skin and blisters.

Secondary dilution. Dilution of the embalming fluid by the fluids in the body, both vascular and interstitial.

Sectional hypodermic embalming. Embalming of a large body area (e.g., hand or side of face) by the injection of embalming chemicals directly into the tissues through the use of a syringe and needle or a trocar.

Sectional vascular embalming. Embalming of a body area or region (e.g., arm or side of face) by the injection of an embalming solution into an artery that in life supplied blood to that particular body region.

Semilunar incision. Crescent shaped or flaplike incision.

Sepsis. Pathologic state resulting from the presence of microorganisms or their products in the blood or other tissues.

Septicemia. Condition characterized by the multiplication of bacteria in blood.

Septum. Vertical cartilage dividing nasal cavity into two chambers, responsible for asymmetry of the nose.

Sequestering agent. Chemical agent that can "fence off" or "tie up" metal ions so that they cannot react with other chemicals.

Serrated. Notched on the edge like a saw, as seen with forceps.

Sharps. Hypodermic needles, suture needles, injector needles, scalpel blades, razor blades, pins, and other items sharp enough to cause percutaneous injury, penetration of unbroken skin. May include other items normally not disposed of following use such as scissors, teeth, fingernails, and ribs.

Sharps container. Occupational Safety and Health Administration–required receptacle for proper disposal of sharps.

Sheen. Shine; as of the reflection of natural oils of the skin.

Short-term exposure limit (STEL). Legal limits established by the Occupational Health and Safety Administration to which workers can be exposed continuously for a short period without damage or injury. Exposures at the STEL should not be longer than 15 minutes and not repeated more than four times per workday.

Sign of death. Manifestation of death in the body.

Simple fracture. Fractured bone that does not pierce the skin.

Six-point injection. A multipoint injection in the autopsied or unautopsied body in which six areas of the body are separately injected: right and left common carotid, axillary, and femoral arteries are six arteries frequently used for a six-point injection.

Skeletal edema. Edema in the body appendages, trunk, and/or head as contrasted with edema of the body cavities.

Sodium hypochlorite. Unstable salt usually produced in an aqueous solution and used as a bleaching and disinfecting agent. See Household bleach.

Solute. Substance that is dissolved in a solution.

Solution. Liquid containing dissolved substance.

Solvent. Liquid holding another substance in solution.

Somatic death. Death of the organism as a whole.

Spatula. Flat, blunt, knifelike instrument used for mixing cosmetics and modeling; a palette knife.

Split injection. Injection from one site and drainage from a separate site.

Sponge. Elastic, porous mass of interlacing horny fibers that are permanently attached; remarkable for its power of absorbing water and becoming soft when wet without losing its toughness.

Squama. Vertical surface of the temporal bone.

Stabilization. A treatment of the dead human body to temporarily slow or inhibit decomposition physically by the use of refrigeration, wet or dry ice, or chemically by the use of non-fromaldehyde or phenol fluids.

Stain removers. Any substances or agents that will cause an external discoloration to be removed or lessened.

Sterilization. Process that renders a substance free of all microorganisms.

Sterilizers. Oven or appliance for sterilizing. An autoclave that sterilizes by steam under pressure at temperatures above 100°C.

Sternocleidomastoideus muscle. Muscle of the neck that is attached to the mastoid process of the temporal bone and superior nuchal line and by separate heads to the sternum and clavicle. They function together to flex the head and form the lateral boundaries of the cervical triangle and the widest part of the neck.

Stethoscope. Delicate instrument used to detect almost inaudible sounds produced in the body.

Stillborn. Dead at birth. A product of conception either expelled or extracted dead.

Subcutaneous. Situated or occurring beneath the skin.

Subcutaneous emphysema. Distension of the tissues beneath the skin by gas or air. An antemortem condition brought about by a surgical procedure or trauma.

Submandibular. Describing those portions that lie immediately inferior to the mandible.

Submental sulcus. Junction of the base of the chin and the submandibular area, which may appear as a furrow; a natural facial marking.

Superciliary arches. Inferior part of the forehead just superior to the median ends of the eyebrows.

Supercilium. Eyebrows.

Superficial. Toward the surface.

Superior. Anatomically toward the head.

Superior palpebral sulcus. Furrow of the superior border of the upper eyelid; acquired facial marking.

Supplemental fluid. A fluid the embalmer injects prior to the preservative solution (e.g., preinjection fluid) or adds to the preservative solution to enhance certain qualities of the preservative fluid (e.g., coinjection, dye, humectant, and water conditioner).

Supraorbital area. Region between the supercilium and the superior palpebrae.

Supraorbital margins. Superior rim of the eye sockets.

Surface compress (pack). An absorbent material saturated with an embalming chemical and placed in direct contact with the tissue.

Surface discoloration. Discoloration due to the deposit of matter on the skin surface. Surface discolorations may occur antemortem or during or after embalming of the body. Examples are adhesive tape, ink, iodine, paint, and tobacco stains.

Surface embalming. See Embalming.

Surfactant (surface tension reducer; wetting, penetrating, or surface-active agent). Chemical that reduces the molecular cohesion of a liquid so that it can flow through smaller apertures.

Surgical reduction. Restoration to a normal position or level through surgical excision.

Sustain. To provide support for; to hold in a fixed position.

Suture. Act of sewing; also the completed stitch.

Swab. Bit of cotton or cloth used for removing moisture or discharges from mucous membranes as well as for applying bleaches or liquid disinfectants.

Swarthy. Dark-colored complexion, as a face made swarthy by the tropical sun.

Tache noire. A brown to black band of discolored sclera of the eye. Created by the postmortem drying of the sclera by the air.

Tardieu spots. Minute petechial hemorrhages caused by the rupture of minute vessels as blood settles into the dependent areas of organs and tissues; it is accompanied by livor mortis. Postmortem, extravascular blood discoloration. Most common in asphyxial or slow deaths.

Temporal bones. Inferior portion of the sides and base of the cranium, inferior to the parietal bones and anterior to the occipital bone.

Temporal cavity. Concave surface of the head overlying the temporal bones.

Temporalis muscles. Muscle of mastication that helps to close the mandible (the strongest chewing muscles).

Temporary preservation. Science of treating the body chemically so as to temporarily inhibit decomposition.

Terminal disinfection. Institution of disinfection and decontamination measures after preparation of the remains.

Test of death. Any procedure used to prove a sign of death.

Thanatology. Study of death.

Thanatopraxy. Embalming as practiced in European countries, it involves preservation and presentation of the body so that the body may be viewed by friends and family. This distinguishes the preparation from that of medical embalming where only preservation is a concern.

Third-degree burns. Burns that result in destruction of cutaneous and subcutaneous tissues (seared, charred, or roasted tissue).

Three-quarter view. In reference to a photograph, a view revealing the fullness of the cheeks.

Time-weighted average (TWA). Exposure that is time-weighted over an established period. It allows the exposure levels to be averaged generally over an 8-hour period.

Tissue builder. Substance used to elevate sunken (emaciated) tissues to normal level by hypodermic injection.

Tissue coagulation. See Coagulation.

Tissue gas. Postmortem accumulation of gas in tissues or cavities brought about by an anaerobic gas-forming bacillus, *Clostridium perfringens*.

Tobacco tar. Yellowish-brown discoloration of the fingernails and fingers from excessive use of cigarettes.

Topical disinfection. Disinfection of the surface of the body or an object.

Tragus. Elevation protecting the ear passage (external auditory meatus).

Translocation. Agonal or postmortem redistribution of host microflora on a hostwide basis.

Transplantation. Grafting of living tissue from its normal position to another site or of an organ or tissue from one person to another.

Transverse. Lying at right angles to the long axis of the body.

Transverse frontal sulci. Furrows that cross the forehead; acquired facial markings.

Trauma. Physical injury or wound caused by external force or violence.

Trocar. Sharply pointed surgical instrument used in cavity embalming to aspirate the cavities and inject cavity fluid. The trocar may also be used for supplemental hypodermic embalming.

Trocar button. Plastic, threaded screwlike device for sealing punctures and small round trocar openings.

Trocar guide. Line drawn or visualized on the surface of the body or a prominent anatomic structure used to locate internal structures during cavity embalming, from a point of reference 2 inches to the left of and 2 inches superior to the umbilicus.

Tumor. Spontaneous new growth of tissue forming an abnormal mass.

Undercoat. Coloring (opaque) applied to an area, which, when dry, will be covered with wax or another colorant.

Undercut. Angled cut of the borders of an excision, made so that the skin surface will overhang the deeper tissues.

Unionall. Plastic garment designed to cover the entire body from the neck down to and including the feet.

Universal precautions. See Bloodborne Pathogen Rule.

Vacuum breaker. Apparatus that prevents the backsiphoning of contaminated liquids into potable water supply lines or plumbing cross-connections within the preparation room.

Vascular (arterial) embalming. See Embalming.

Vehicle. Liquid that serves as a solvent for the numerous ingredients incorporated into embalming fluids.

Vertex. Top of the head.

Vertical. Perpendicular to the plane of the horizon, balanced.

Viral hepatitis. Inflammation of the liver caused by a virus (possibly as many as seven in number) capable of causing acute or chronic hepatitis illness. The transmission can be oral-fecal, parenteral, or sexual.

Viscera. Internal organs enclosed within a cavity.

Viscosity. Resistance to the flow of a liquid. Thickness of a liquid.

Vitreous humor. Semifluid, transparent substance that lies between the retina and lens of the eyeball.

Vomer bone. Bone of the nasal cavity situated between the nasal passages on the median plane; forms the inferior and posterior portion of the septum of the nose.

Vancomycin-resistant enterococci (VRE). A drug-resistant bacterium found in feces and open wounds. It can also be found associated with nasogastric tubes often in patients who have had long hospitalization.

Vancomycin-resistant *Staphylococcus aureus* (VRSA). *Staphylococcus aureus* pathogens that have become resistant to the drugs methicillin and vancomycin.

Warm color areas. Areas of the skin surface that, during life, are naturally reddened; places where cosmetics will be applied to restore the warmth that red will give.

Water conditioner. Complexing agent used to remove chemical constituents that could interfere with arterial formulations from municipal water supplies.

Water hardness. Quality of water containing certain substances, especially soluble salts of calcium and magnesium.

Waterless embalming. Arterial injection of an embalming solution composed of arterial fluid, humectant, and coinjection fluid. No water is added to the solution.

Waterlogged. Condition resulting from the use of an embalming solution containing an insufficient amount of preservative to meet the preservative demand of the tissues. The interstitial spaces are overly filled, engorged with water.

Wax. Restorative modeling or surfacing material composed of beeswax, spermaceti, paraffin, starch, and so on and a coloring pigment that will soften at body temperature and will reflect light in a manner similar to normal skin.

Weather line. Line of color change at the junction of the wet and dry portions of each mucous membrane.

Wet gangrene. See Gangrene.

Wet ice. A solid form of water; this occurs at 32 degrees fahrenheit.

Wetting agent. See Surfactant.

Wicking. Operative or mechanical aid where an absorbent material, such as webbed cotton, is inserted into a body area where moisture is present, the absorbent material draws the moisture to the outside of the body.

Width. Dimension of an object measured across from side to side.

Work practice controls. See Bloodborne Pathogen Rule.

Worm suture. (Inversion, draw stitch) Method of sewing an incision along the edges without entering the opening whereby the suture becomes invisible and the line of suture becomes depressed, which lends it ease of concealment by waxing.

Zygomatic arch. Processes on the temporal and zygomatic bones; determines the widest part of the face.

Zygomatic arch depression. One of the lesser concavities of the face located on the lateral portion of the cheek inferior to the zygomatic arch.

Zygomatic bones. Small bones of the cheeks; widest part of the cheek.

Zygomaticofrontal process. Lateral rim of the eye socket formed by a process of the frontal bone and a process of the zygomatic bone.

Zygomaticus major muscles. Muscles of the face that draw the superior lip posteriorly, superiorly, and anteriorly.

Zygomaticus minor muscles. Muscles of the face that draw the superior lip superiorly and anteriorly.

▶ ACRONYMS

ACGIH	American Congress of Governmental Industrial Hygienists
AIDS	Acquired immunodeficiency syndrome
AL	Action level
ANSI	American National Standard Institute
BCME	Bischloromethyl ether
CDCP	Centers for Disease Control and Prevention
ECG	Electrocardiogram (also EKG)
EEG	Electroencephalogram

EPA	Environmental Protection Agency
FCI	The Formaldehyde Council, Inc.
FTC	Federal Trade Commission
HBV	Hepatitis B virus
HIV	Human immunodeficiency virus
IVP	Intravascular pressure
mCi	Millicurie
MRSA	Methicillin-resistant *Staphylococcus aureus*
MSDS	Material Safety Data Sheet
NCI	U.S. National Cancer Institute
NIOSH	National Institute for Occupational Safety and Health
OPIM	Other potentially infectious material
OSHA	Occupational Safety and Health Administration
PEL	Permissible exposure limit
pH	Potential of hydrogen
PPE	Personal protective equipment
ppm	Parts per million
STEL	Short-term exposure limit
TLV	Threshold limit value
TWA	Time-weighted average
VRE	Vancomycin-resistant enterococci
VRSA	Vancomycin-resistant *Staphylococcus aureus*

▶ REFERENCES

Benenson AS. *Control of Communicable Diseases in Man*, 15th ed. Baltimore: Victor Graphics, 1990.

DiMaio VJ, DiMaio D. *Forensic Pathology*, 2nd ed. Boca Raton, FL: CRC Press, 2001.

Embalming Course Content Syllabus. American Board of Funeral Service Education, 2008.

Frederick LG, Strub CG. *The Principles and Practices of Embalming*, 5th ed. Dallas, TX: Professional Training Schools, 1989.

Mayer JS. *Color and Cosmetics*. Dallas, TX: Professional Training Schools, 1991.

Mayer JS. *Restorative Art*, 13th ed., Dallas, TX: Professional Training Schools, 1993.

Mayer RG. *Embalming: History, Theory and Practice*, 3rd ed. New York: McGraw-Hill, 2006.

Merriam Webster's Collegiate Dictionary, 10th ed. Springfield, MA: Merriam-Webster, 1993.

Restorative Art Course Content Syllabus. American Board of Funeral Service Education, 2006.

Spitz WU. *Medicolegal Investigation of Death*, 3rd ed. Springfield, IL: Charles C. Thomas, 1993.

Thomas CL. *Taber's Cyclopedic Medical Dictionary*, 19th ed. Philadelphia: F.A. Davis, 2001

Page numbers followed by f indicate figures; page numbers followed by t indicate tables.

715